Surgical Oncology

Quyen D. Chu • John F. Gibbs
Gazi B. Zibari
Editors

Surgical Oncology

A Practical and Comprehensive Approach

Springer

Editors
Quyen D. Chu, MD, MBA, FACS
Department of Surgery
LSU Health Sciences Center-Shreveport
Shreveport, LA, USA

Gazi B. Zibari, MD, FACS
John C. McDonald Regional Transplant Center
Willis Knighton Health System
Shreveport, LA, USA

John F. Gibbs, MD, FACS
Department of Surgery
Jersey Shore University Medical Center/Meridian Health
Neptune, NJ, USA

ISBN 978-1-4939-1422-7 ISBN 978-1-4939-1423-4 (eBook)
DOI 10.1007/978-1-4939-1423-4
Springer New York Heidelberg Dordrecht London

Library of Congress Control Number: 2014950229

Printed on acid-free paper

Springer is part of Springer Science+Business Media (www.springer.com)

To our wives, Trina Chu, Theresa Gibbs, Maysoon Zibari, and our children, Thuy-Tien Chu, Yen Chu, Matthew Gibbs, Zachary Gibbs, Brianna Gibbs, Susan Seepan Zibari, Renas Zibari, Rona Connie Zibari, and Lehat Zibari.

To our parents, Trinh V. Chu and Nhan T. Chu, (the late) William L. Gibbs, Sr, and Betty G. Gibbs, and (the late) Baderkhan Zibari and Khanzad Zibari.

Foreword

This is a unique surgical oncology text. It is written in a very user friendly format that is somewhat unusual for a standard text. Each chapter starts out with Learning Objectives, followed by an Abstract of the chapter. The chapter itself then follows, each chapter being comprehensive and complete, but brief. This is followed by a list of Salient Points, and a section on Questions concerning the chapter, with Answers. This is followed by a comprehensive list of references. I believe this format will be particularly effective for individuals in terms of learning and retention. This book should be appropriate for medical students, residents, fellows, faculty, and surgeons out in private practice. Each chapter is written by experts in their field. The editors, Drs. Chu, Gibbs, and Zibari, have all contributed to the text, and have done an excellent job in editing those chapters contributed by outside experts. Many surgical oncology texts are so large and cumbersome, that they are difficult to handle. They are also written in a format that does not encourage retention. I would predict that this text will be a great success, following the format of other textbooks and concentrate on being brief, but comprehensive. I believe this text will attract a large audience.

The Johns Hopkins Medical Institutions
Baltimore, MD, USA

John L. Cameron, MD

Preface

Learning the correct approach for managing solid tumors represents a large part of medical/surgical residency training. The demand for an oncology textbook that is tailored to the needs of both learners and teachers is high. One might expect to see a plethora of surgical oncology textbooks readily available to accommodate such a demand; unfortunately, this is not the case. Despite a handful of excellent surgical oncology textbooks out there, most either lack sufficient depth and/or contain information that may not be practical or germane to the learners.

This textbook, *Surgical Oncology: A Practical and Comprehensive Approach*, provides a comprehensive perspective on surgical oncologic diseases that are relevant to those who have an interest in surgical oncology. Its purpose is to distill a voluminous amount of information into one book so that readers can readily access relevant information and knowledge according to their particular needs. Medical students and residents will find this textbook useful in preparing for surgical case presentations and written/oral tests. For the surgical oncology fellows, the book not only provides the already mentioned advantages, but also serves as a guide and a beginning point to help them further explore specific topics more in-depth. For the busy general surgeons who care for cancer patients, this book serves an invaluable source to help them better manage their patients while staying abreast with the latest advances in the field. Finally, for the educators (staff members, academicians, etc.), this book can serve as a valuable teaching tool to save them from spending countless hours searching for relevant teaching materials.

Each chapter is written by experts and their colleagues in their respective field of expertise. The chapters provide concise and in-depth information on the topic at hand. Seminal articles are highlighted throughout the book to reinforce the principle that optimal management depends not only on good clinical judgment, but also on evidence-based medicine. Plenty of illustrations, diagrams, tables, and photographs are included to assist the visual learners. The unique outline of the book is that each chapter begins with key points to focus the readers on the materials covered and concludes with an appendix that summarizes the chapter with salient points. This unique set-up can be used as a tool to quickly review the topic at hand. *Surgical Oncology: A Practical and Comprehensive Approach* also includes a set of short questions and answers at the end of each chapter to reinforce key learning points.

One of the problems with currently published surgical textbooks is that the information contained therein may become outdated and obsolete by the time they are published. However, by publishing a textbook with (eBook) capability, we can achieve our objectives – mainly to publish a practical oncology text that is geared towards the needs of the practicing surgeon, surgical oncology fellow, surgical residents, and medical students while at the same time have the flexibility to readily update the information to match current practices.

Surgical Oncology: A Practical and Comprehensive Approach is a book that includes topics that are germane to a broad range of audiences who have an interest in surgical oncology. Those interested in surgical oncology will gain an in-depth knowledge on traditional topics such as breast cancer, thyroid cancer, melanoma, gastric cancer, colorectal cancer, esophageal cancer, hepatobiliary cancers, sarcomas, and gastrointestinal stromal. In addition, topics such as local treatment of early rectal cancer, breast cancer in pregnancy, and management of colorectal metastases to the liver are examples of other topics that will be emphasized.

Although topics such as urologic cancers, neurosurgical cancers, and childhood cancers are important, they are not necessarily an important part of general surgical training in many healthcare centers in the USA. Therefore, these topics are excluded from *Surgical Oncology: A Practical and Comprehensive Approach*.

We believe that *Surgical Oncology: A Practical and Comprehensive Approach* will be an invaluable resource for any serious learners of surgical oncology and will become a must-have textbook for training programs.

Shreveport, LA, USA — Quyen D. Chu, MD, MBA, FACS
Neptune, NJ, USA — John F. Gibbs, MD, FACS
Shreveport, LA, USA — Gazi B. Zibari, MD, FACS

Acknowledgement

We would like to thank our illustrators, Thuy-Tien Chu, Yen Chu, Lory Tubbs, Paul Tomljanovich, M.D., F.A.C.S., Karen Howard, and Kimberly Wooten, M.D., as well as Beverly Wright, Yvette Sanchez, Monica Laurents, RN, and J. Karen Miller for their administrative assistance.

Contents

Editors and Contributors

Editors

Quyen D. Chu, M.D., M.B.A., F.A.C.S. Department of Surgery, LSU Health Sciences Center-Shreveport, Shreveport, LA, USA

John F. Gibbs, M.D., F.A.C.S. Department of Surgery, Jersey Shore University Medical Center/Meridian Health, Neptune, NJ, USA

Gazi B. Zibari, M.D., F.A.C.S. John C. McDonald Regional Transplant Center, Willis Knighton Health System, Shreveport, LA, USA

Contributors

Ernest Kwame Adjepong-Tandoh, M.Bch.B. Department of Surgery, University of Ghana Medical School, Accra, Ghana

Mazin F. Al-Kasspooles, M.D. Department of General Surgery, University of Kansas Medical Center, Kansas City, KS, USA

Salim Amrani, M.D. Department of Surgery, Carlsbad Medical Center, Carlsbad, NM, USA

Tania K. Arora, M.D. Department of Surgery, Geisinger Health System, Danville, PA, USA

Rachel D. Aufforth, M.D. Division of Surgical Oncology and Endocrine Surgery, University of North Carolina, Chapel Hill, NC, USA

Justin John Baker, M.D. Department of Surgery, Maine Medical Center/Tufts University School of Medicine, Portland, ME, USA

Joaquina C. Baranda, M.D. Internal Medicine, University of Kansas Medical Center, Westwood, KS, USA

Harry D. Bear, M.D., Ph.D. Department of Surgery, Virginia Commonwealth University, Richmond, VA, USA

Richard J. Bold, M.D. Division of Surgical Oncology, UC Davis Cancer Center, Sacramento, CA, USA

Jeffrey J. Brewer, M.D. Department of Surgery, University at Buffalo, Buffalo, NY, USA

Jocelyn F. Burke, M.D. Department of General Surgery, University of Wisconsin Hospital and Clinics, Madison, WI, USA

Michael R. Cassidy, M.D. Department of Surgery, Boston University School of Medicine, Boston Medical Center, Boston, MA, USA

Herbert Chen, M.D. Department of General Surgery, University of Wisconsin Hospital and Clinics, Madison, WI, USA

Edward Eun Cho, M.D., Sc.M. Department of Surgery, Kaleida Health/ Buffalo General Med Center, State University of New York at Buffalo, Buffalo, NY, USA

Quyen D. Chu, M.D., M.B.A., F.A.C.S. Department of Surgery, Louisiana State University Health Sciences Center – Shreveport, Shreveport, LA, USA

Linus T. Chuang, M.D., M.P.H., F.A.C.O.G. Division of Gynecologic Oncology, Department of Obstetrics, Gynecology and Reproductive Science, Icahn School of Medicine at Mount Sinai, New York, NY, USA

Mark S. Cohen, M.D. Department of General Surgery, University of Michigan Hospital and Health Systems, Ann Arbor, MI, USA

Phillip A. Cole, M.D., M.H.C.M., F.A.C.S., F.A.S.C.R.S. Department of Surgery, LSUHSC/University Health-Shreveport, Shreveport, LA, USA

Rouzbeh Daylami, M.D. Department of Surgery, Kaiser Permanente, Sacramento, CA, USA

Liane Deligdisch, M.D. Department of Pathology, Obstetrics-Gynecology and Reproductive Science, Ichan School of Medicine at Mount Sinai, New York, NY, USA

Peter J. DiPasco, M.D. Department of General Surgery, University of Kansas Medical Center, Kansas City, KS, USA

Lesly A. Dossett, M.D., M.P.H. Department of Surgery, Naval Hospital Jacksonville, Jacksonville, FL, USA

Rosemary Bernadette Duda, M.D., M.P.H. Department of Surgery, Beth Israel Deaconess Medical Center, Howard Medical School, Boston, MA, USA

John F. Gibbs, M.D. Department of Surgery, Jersey Shore University Medical Center/Meridian Health, Neptune, NJ, USA

David Gleason, M.D. Department of Surgery, Kaleida Health/Buffalo General Medical Center, State University of New York at Buffalo, Buffalo, NY, USA

Stephen R. Grobmyer, M.D. Section of Surgical Oncology, Cleveland Clinic, Cleveland, OH, USA

William R. Jarnagin, M.D. Hepatopancreatobiliary Service, Memorial Sloan-Kettering Cancer Center, New York, NY, USA

Martin S. Karpeh, Jr., M.D. Department of Surgery, Mount Sinai Beth Israel Medical Center, New York, NY, USA

Elizabeth P. Ketner, M.D. Department of Surgery, Mount Sinai Beth Israel Medical Center, New York, NY, USA

Nikhil I. Khushalani, M.D. Department of Medicine, Roswell Park Cancer Institute, Buffalo, NY, USA

Hong Jin Kim, M.D. Division of Surgical Oncology and Endocrine Surgery, University of North Carolina at Chapel Hill, Lineberger Comprehensive Cancer Center, Chapel Hill, NC, USA

Roger H. Kim, M.D. Department of Surgery, Louisiana State University Health Sciences Center – Shreveport and the Feist-Weiller Cancer Center, Shreveport, LA, USA

Bas Groot Koerkamp, M.D., Ph.D. Hepatopancreatobiliary Service, Memorial Sloan-Kettering Cancer Center, New York, NY, USA

David A. Kooby, M.D. Division of Surgical Oncology, Winship Cancer Institute, Emory University, Atlanta, GA, USA

Moshim Kukar, M.D. Surgical Oncology, Roswell Park Cancer Institute, Buffalo, NY, USA

Mahmoud N. Kulaylat, M.D. Department of Surgery, Buffalo General Medical Center, University at Buffalo-State University of New York, Buffalo, NY, USA

Edward A. Levine, M.D. Department of Surgery, Wake Forest School of Medicine, Salem, NC, USA

Parham Mafi, M.D. Department of Surgery, SUNY Buffalo, Buffalo, NY, USA

Jane E. Méndez, M.D., F.A.C.S. Department of Surgery, Surgical Oncology, Boston Medical Center/Boston University School of Medicine, Boston, MA, USA

Nipun B. Merchant, M.D., F.A.C.S. Department of Surgical Oncology and Endocrine Surgery, Vanderbilt University Medical Center, Nashville, TN, USA

Kimberly E. Miller-Hammond, M.D. Department of Surgery, Kaleida Health/Buffalo General Medical Center, State University of New York at Buffalo, Buffalo, NY, USA

Jacqueline Oxenberg, D.O. Surgical Oncology, Roswell Park Cancer Institute, Buffalo, NY, USA

John H. Park, M.D. Radiation Oncology, University of Kansas Medical Center, Kansas City, KS, USA

Elena Pereira, M.D. Department of Obstetrics, Gynecology and Reproductive Science, Mount Sinai Hospital, New York, NY, USA

Michael Polcino, M.D. Department of Surgery, Memorial Sloan Kettering Cancer Center, New York, NY, USA

Reese W. Randle, M.D. Department of Surgery, Wake Forest School of Medicine, Salem, NC, USA

Luz Maria Rodriguez, M.D. Department of Surgery, Walter Reed National Military Medical Center/National Cancer Institute, Bethesda, MD, USA

Miguel Rodriguez-Bigas, M.D. Department of Surgical Oncology, UT MD Anderson Cancer Center, Houston, TX, USA

Matthew Sanders, B.A., M.D. Department of Surgery, LSUHSC-Shreveport, Shreveport, LA, USA

Guillermo Pablo Sangster, M.D. Department of Radiology, Louisiana State University Health Sciences Center – Shreveport, Shreveport, LA, USA

Christopher N. Scipio, M.D. Department of General Surgery, University of Michigan Hospital and Health Systems, Ann Arbor, MI, USA

Dhruvil Shah, M.D. Department of Surgery, UC Davis, Sacramento, CA, USA

Christiana Shaw, M.D. M.S., F.A.C.S. Surgery, University of Florida, Gainesville, FL, USA

Perry Shen, M.D. Department of Surgery, Wake Forest School of Medicine, Salem, NC, USA

Junichi Shindoh, M.D., Ph.D. Department of Surgical Oncology, Anderson Cancer Center, Houston, TX, USA

Hosein Shokouh-Amiri, M.D. John C. McDonald Regional Transplant Center, Willis Knighton Health System, Shreveport, LA, USA

Joseph Skitzki, M.D. Surgical Oncology, Roswell Park Cancer Institute, Buffalo, NY, USA

Jillian K. Smith, M.D., M.P.H. Department of Surgery, University of Massachusetts Medical School, Worcester, MA, USA

Richard R. Smith, M.D. Department of Surgery, Tripler Army Medical Center, Honolulu, HI, USA

Malcolm H. Squires III, M.D. Division of Surgical Oncology, Winship Cancer Institute, Emory University, Atlanta, GA, USA

John H. Stewart IV, M.D., M.B.A. Department of General Surgery, Wake Forest Baptist Health, Salem, NC, USA

Jennifer F. Tseng, M.D., M.P.H. Department of Surgery, Beth Israel Deaconess Medical Center and Harvard Medical School, Boston, MA, USA

Benjamin W. Vabi, M.D. Department of General Surgery, University at Buffalo School of Medicine, Buffalo, NY, USA

Jean-Nicolas Vauthey, M.D. Department of Surgical Oncology, Anderson Cancer Center, Houston, TX, USA

Konstantinos I. Votanopoulos, M.D., Ph.D. Department of Surgery, Wake Forest School of Medicine, Salem, NC, USA

Nathalie C. Zeitouni, M.D.C.M. Dermatology, University of Arizona, Tucson, AZ, USA

Gazi B. Zibari, M.D. John C. McDonald Regional Transplant Center, Willis Knighton Health System, Shreveport, LA, USA

Giuseppe Zimmitti, M.D. Department of Surgical Oncology, Anderson Cancer Center, Houston, TX, USA

Part I

Skin

Melanoma

1

Christiana Shaw and Stephen R. Grobmyer

Learning Objectives

After reading this chapter, you should be able to:

- Recognize risk factors for melanoma.
- Understand how to evaluate and stage patients with melanoma.
- Appreciate how prospective randomized controlled trials have impacted the treatment of patients with melanoma, and apply these trials to treatment paradigms.
- Be familiar with novel target-specific therapy for advanced melanomas.
- Select options for local, regional, and systemic control of the disease.

C. Shaw, M.D., M.S., F.A.C.S.
Surgery, University of Florida, 1600 Southwest Archer Road, Box 100109, Gainesville, FL 32610, USA
e-mail: christiana.shaw@surgery.ufl.edu

S.R. Grobmyer, M.D. (✉)
Section of Surgical Oncology, Cleveland Clinic, 9500 Euclid Avenue A81, Cleveland, OH 44195, USA
e-mail: Grobmys@ccf.org; Stephen.grobmyer@gmail.com

Background and Historical Perspective

Melanoma is an important health problem. In the United States, it is estimated that 76,690 people (45,060 men and 31,630 women) will be diagnosed with melanoma in 2013 [1], and lifetime risk for development of melanoma is currently estimated at 2 % [1]. An increase in episodic exposure to intense sun of fair-skinned individuals has led to a 600 % rise in melanoma incidence from 1950 to 2000 [2]. Despite an increased incidence, survival rates improved over the same time period, although melanoma is responsible for 80 % of skin cancer deaths. Education and early diagnosis, resulting from better skin cancer screening, have resulted in this improvement in survival. One of its most important public health features is that melanoma often affects younger patients, with a median age at diagnosis of 61 and median age at death of 69. Thus, an average of 18.6 years of potential life are lost for each melanoma death, one of the highest rates for an adult onset cancer [3].

Risk Factors

When taking a history of a patient with a skin lesion, certain risk factors for melanoma are important to understand. Relative risk is one way of understanding a risk factor for development of

Q.D. Chu et al. (eds.), *Surgical Oncology: A Practical and Comprehensive Approach*,
DOI 10.1007/978-1-4939-1423-4_1, © Springer Science+Business Media New York 2015

a disease. Relative risk is the chance of developing a disease, when comparing an exposed group of individuals to a nonexposed group. A history of severe, episodic sunburns in early life is the most widely recognized risk factor for the development of melanoma, although with a relative risk of 2.5, a history of blistering sunburn is often not the strongest risk factor for its development. Perhaps the most important risk factor is a family history of melanoma. A weak family history accounts for a threefold increase in risk, whereas a strong family history (≥3 first degree relatives) carries a relative risk of 35–70. Heritable mutations have been identified, and a genetic modification in *CDKN2A* or *CDK4* confers a 60–90 % lifetime risk of melanoma [4]. Having multiple benign or atypical nevi confers a relative risk of 11, whereas a personal history of melanoma is responsible for an 8.5 times higher risk. Additional risks include dysplastic nevus syndrome (RR=2.3–12) [5], xeroderma pigmentosum (1,000-fold increased risk for developing skin cancer, including cutaneous melanoma) [6, 7], a personal history of previous nonmelanoma skin cancer (RR=2.9), immunosuppression (RR=1.5–3), and markers of sun sensitivity such as type I skin, freckling, blue eyes, or red hair (RR=1.6–2.5) [3].

Diagnosis

Melanoma can be recognized using the ABCDE features (Table 1.1, Fig. 1.1). Often patients may complain of a mole that has changed in characteristics and is associated with itching, bleeding, or ulceration. When thinking of any cancer patient, the first step in management is to obtain an accurate diagnosis. Biopsy of suspicious cutaneous lesions is of critical importance in making an early diagnosis of melanoma or other skin cancers. Excisional biopsies are the most accurate but are best suited for small lesions. Other types of biopsies that can be performed include punch biopsies and shave biopsies [8, 9]. Each biopsy type has benefits and drawbacks. Punch biopsies while easy to perform may misrepresent the depth of a lesion. Shave biopsies are quick and easy to perform but have been criticized traditionally for not providing accurate depth of a lesion, although a large recent study suggests that shave biopsies provide reliable information in planning surgical treatment and staging [10]. When performing a wide local excision of a melanoma on the extremity, the incision should be placed longitudinally along the long axis of the extremity (Fig. 1.2).

Useful immunohistochemical stainings include S100, HMB-45, MART-1/Melan-A, tyrosinase, and MITF [11].

Table 1.1 The ABCDEs of melanoma

A: **A**symmetry
B: **B**order (irregular)
C: **C**olor changes
D: **D**iameter > 6 mm (size of a pencil eraser)
E: **E**volving (any change in characteristics such as size, shape, color, elevation, new symptoms such as bleeding, itching, or ulcerating)

Staging and Prognosis

The next step in management of a cancer patient is to accurately stage the disease. This allows appropriate treatment decisions to be made through risk-benefit analysis, often based on prognosis. Two scales are used to determine the depth of invasion: (1) Breslow's thickness and (2) Clark's levels (Fig. 1.3).

Melanomas are staged according to the American Joint Committee on Cancer (AJCC) TNM system, where tumor depth (Breslow's thickness), ulceration, nodal status, and metastases form the basis of prognosis (Table 1.2). Tumor depth is the strongest prognostic factor, whereas ulceration is the second most important prognostic indicator (Tables 1.3 and 1.4). Tumors with a Breslow's thickness of less than 1 mm (1 mm ≈ width of a dime) are known as "thin" melanomas, whereas those between 1 and 4 mm are "intermediate thickness" and those greater than 4 mm (4 mm ≈ width of two nickels) are "thick." Tumor depth forms the basis of the margin needed for excision and is also predictive of node positivity. For tumors ≤ 1 mm, 4 % have positive regional lymph nodes; 1.01–2.00 mm,

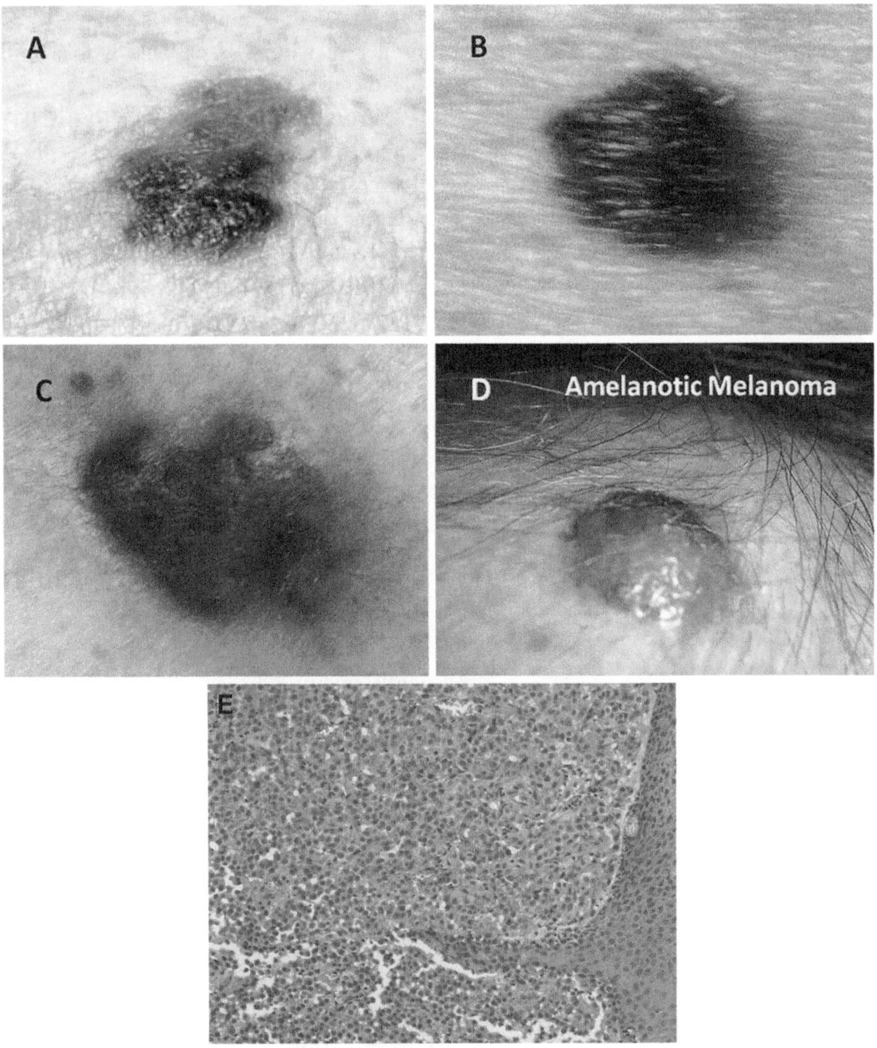

Fig. 1.1 (**a**–**c**) Melanoma and (**d**) amelanotic melanoma. (**e**) Photomicrograph showing sheets of neoplastic melanocytes deep to the epidermis with amphophilic cytoplasm, large ovoid nuclei and prominent nucleoli. Pigment deposition is relatively sparse in this example (hematoxylin and eosin X 200) (**a**–**d**: With kind permission from Ilene Rothman, M.D., Roswell Park Cancer Institute; **e**: Courtesy of Barry DeYoung, MD, Wake Forest School of Medicine)

12 %; 2.01–4.00 mm, 28 %; and >4.00 mm, 44 % [12]. The relationship between depth and the risk of lymph node metastasis forms the basis for recommendations regarding surgical nodal staging.

The incidence of ulceration is also greater with thicker tumor depth and is present in 6–12.5 % of thin melanomas versus 63–72.5 % in thick (>4 mm) melanomas. Ulceration decreases survival in all tumor thickness categories and is the only primary tumor factor that impacts prognosis of patients who have node-positive disease [13].

Other prognostic factors include age, gender, and anatomic location [13–15]. In a recent analysis , female gender was prognostically favorable, as 10-year survival rate for women was 86 % compared to 68 % for men [14]. Locations that were associated with higher risk of death included the **b**ack, back of upper **a**rms, **n**eck, and **s**calp (BANS).

Mitotic rate, which is measured as the number of mitoses per square millimeter, has also been shown to be an important independent prognostic factor [16–18]. For patients with stage I melanoma, the adjusted odds ratio of survival for patients with a mitotic rate of 0 was 12 times higher than that of patients with a mitotic rate of $>6/\text{mm}^2$ [17].

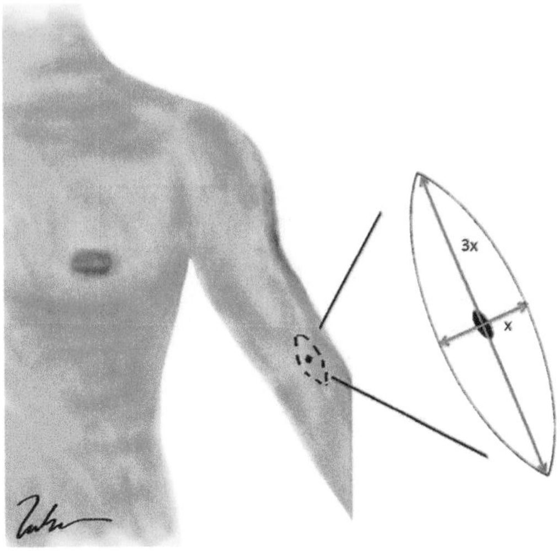

Fig. 1.2 *Wide local excision of a melanoma*. Note that the incision should be placed longitudinally along the long axis of the extremity. The length of the incision is generally 3× the width (Courtesy of Thuy-Tien Chu and Quyen D. Chu, MD, MBA, FACS)

Serum lactate dehydrogenase (LDH) level is one of the patient factors most predictive of decreased survival. LDH remains predictive even after accounting for site and number of metastatic lesions. In stage IV melanoma, LDH level has a 79 % sensitivity and 92 % specificity in detecting disease progression [15]. LDH has been recommended by certain practice guidelines as part of surveillance for patients with melanoma.

Clinical nodal staging is an important part of the physical examination of patients with a diagnosis of melanoma. Whereas microscopic disease is clinically occult and only found on microscopic examination of excised lymph nodes, macroscopic disease is clinically or radiographically apparent. Survival rates between microscopically positive disease and macroscopically positive disease differ significantly. Balch et al. (2001) demonstrated a survival difference of 63 % for a single microscopic positive node versus 47 % for a single macroscopic positive node ($p<0.001$) [15].

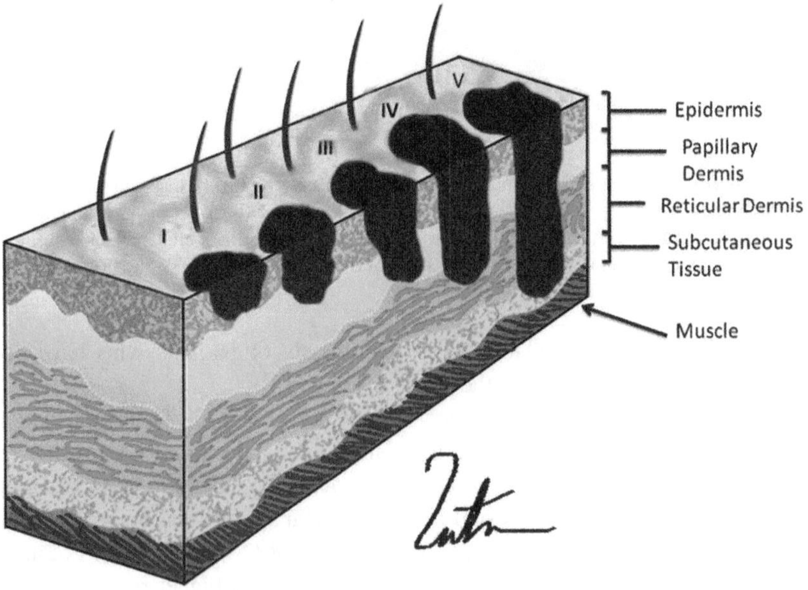

Fig. 1.3 *Clark's level*: level 1, tumor confined to the epidermis; level II, tumor invades papillary dermis; level III, tumor fills the papillary dermis, but does not extend into the reticular dermis; level IV, tumor invades the reticular dermis; level V, tumor invades the deep subcutaneous tissue (Courtesy of Thuy-Tien Chu and Quyen D. Chu, MD, MBA, FACS)

Table 1.2 American Joint Committee on Cancer (AJCC) TNM staging for cutaneous melanoma (7th edition)

Primary tumor (T)	
TX	Primary tumor cannot be assessed (e.g., curettage or severely regressed melanoma
T0	No evidence of primary tumor
Tis	Melanoma in situ
T1	Melanomas ≤ 1.0 mm
T2	Melanomas 1.01–2.0 mm
T3	Melanomas 2.01–4.0 mm
T4	Melanomas > 4.0 mm

Note: a and b subcategories of T are assigned based on ulceration and number of mitoses per mm², as shown below

T classification	Thickness (mm)	Ulceration status/ Mitoses
T1	≤1.0	a: w/o ulceration and mitosis <1/mm²
		b: with ulceration or mitoses ≥1/mm²
T2	1.01–2.0	a: w/o ulceration
		b: with ulceration
T3	2.01–4.0	a: w/o ulceration
		b: with ulceration
T4	>4.0	a: w/o ulceration
		b: with ulceration

Regional lymph nodes (N)	
NX	Patients in whom the regional nodes cannot be assessed (e.g., previously removed for another reason)
N0	No regional metastases detected
N1-3	Regional metastases based upon the # metastatic nodes and presence or absence of intralymphatic metastases (in-transit or satellite metastases)

Note: N1–3 and a–c subcategories assigned as shown below

N classification	# of metastatic nodes	Nodal metastatic mass
N1	1 node	a: micrometastasis[1]
		b: macrometastasis[2]
N2	2–3 nodes	a: micrometastasis[1]
		b: macrometastasis[2]
		c: in-transit met(s)/ satellite(s) *without* metastatic nodes
N3	4 or more metastatic nodes, or matted nodes or in transit met(s)/satellite(s)	

(continued)

Table 1.2 (continued)

Distant metastasis (M)	
M0	No detectable evidence of distant metastases
M1a	Metastases to skin, subcutaneous, or distant lymph nodes
M1b	Metastases to lung
M1c	Metastases to all other visceral sites or distant metastases to any site combined site combined with an elevated serum LDH

Note: Serum LDH is incorporated into the M category as shown below

M classification		
	Site	Serum LDH
M1a	Distant skin, subcutaneous, or nodal mets	Normal
M1b	Lung metastases	Normal
M1c	All other visceral metastases, Any Distant metastasis	Normal elevated

Clinical staging[3]				Pathologic staging[4]			
Stage	Tis	N0	M0	0	Tis	N0	M0
Stage 1A	T1b	N0	M0	I A	T1a	N0	M0
Stage 1B	T1b	N0	M0	I B	T1b	N0	M0
	T2a	N0	M0		T2a	N0	M0
Stage IIA	T2b	N0	M0	II A	T2b	N0	M0
	T3a	N0	M0		T3a	N0	M0
Stage IIB	T3b	N0	M0	II B	T3b	N0	M0
	T4a	N0	M0		T4a	N0	M0
Stage IIC	T4b	N0	M0	II C	T4b	N0	M0
Stage III	Any T	≥N1	M0	III A	T 1–4a	N1a	M0
					T 1–4a	N2a	M0
				III B	T 1–4b	N1a	M0
					T 1–4b	N2a	M0
					T 1–4a	N1b	M0
					T 1–4a	N2b	M0
					T 1–4a	N2c	M0
				III C	T 1–4b	N1b	M0
					T 1–4b	N2b	M0
					T 1–4b	N2c	M0
					Any T	N3	M0
Stage IV	Any T	Any N	M1	IV	Any T	Any N	M1

[1]Micrometastases are diagnosed after sentinel lymph node biopsy and completion lymphadenectomy (if performed)

(continued)

Table 1.2 (continued)

[2]Macrometastases are defined as clinically detectable nodal metastases confirmed by therapeutic lymphadenectomy or when nodal metastasis exhibits gross extracapsular extension

[3]Clinical staging includes microstaging of the primary melanoma and clinical/radiologic evaluation for metastases. By convention, it should be used after complete excision of the primary melanoma with clinical assessment for regional and distant metastases

[4]Pathologic staging includes microstaging of the primary melanoma and pathologic information about the regional lymph nodes after partial or complete lymphadenectomy. Pathologic stage 0 or stage IA patients are the exception; they do not require pathologic evaluation of their lymph nodes

Adapted from Ref. [78]. With permission from Springer Verlag

Table 1.3 Impact of tumor thickness and ulceration on survival in melanoma

Tumor thickness (mm)	5 years survival: no ulcer (%)	5 years survival: ulcer (%)
≤1	95	91
1.01–2.00	89	77
2.01–4.00	79	63
>4	67	45

Table 1.4 Prognostic factors for cutaneous melanoma

Breslow's thickness
Ulceration
Age
Gender
Anatomic location
Lactate dehydrogenase
Mitotic index
Radial versus vertical phase of tumor growth
Lymphovascular invasion
Microsatellites
Regression
Tumor-infiltrating lymphocytes

Clinical suspicion and understanding of prognosis may also dictate a metastatic workup be performed prior to surgical resection and sentinel lymph node biopsy. The National Comprehensive Cancer Center (NCCN) guidelines state that fine-needle aspiration biopsy of any clinically positive nodal disease, in-transit disease, or metastatic disease be performed prior to resection of the primary lesion. Furthermore, a metastatic workup can be considered if clinical suspicion is present in stage IB or stage II disease or without clinical suspicion in clinical stages III or IV disease [19]. Many forms of metastatic workup exist, and there is disagreement as to which is preferred. Chest x-ray, CT of chest, abdomen, and pelvis, and PET/CT with or without brain MRI are all used for metastatic workup and surveillance. The authors favor PET/CT with brain MRI for all deep (>4 mm) lesions, for patients with constitutional symptoms, and for those who are a high surgical risk due to comorbid conditions, although there is no one practice considered standard.

Treatment Principles

Surgery remains the mainstay of treatment for patients with locoregional melanoma, and survival for those with localized disease is greater than 98 % [1]. Locoregional control is achieved through a combination of wide local excision, sentinel node biopsy, completion lymphadenectomy, and adjuvant radiation. Immunotherapy and targeted therapy are reserved for high-risk, metastatic, or recurrent disease. There is no role for chemotherapy in the adjuvant treatment of melanoma. The most appropriate treatments for melanoma have been demonstrated through prospective randomized controlled clinical trials, many of them multi-institutional.

Treatment Specifics

Margins

Thin Melanoma

The appropriate margin needed for local control in melanomas of varying depths was long a source of debate, and historically margins were treated with massive local excisions, typically 4 cm or greater. In 1991, the World Health Organization (WHO) Melanoma Program Study

Table 1.5 Recommended margins and indications for sentinel lymph node biopsy based on melanoma thickness

Tumor thickness	Recommended clinical margins (cm)	Sentinel lymph node biopsy?
In situ	0.5	No
≤1 mm	1	±[a]
1.01–2 mm	1–2	Yes
2.01–4 mm	2	Yes
>4 mm	2	Controversial[b]

Courtesy of Quyen D. Chu, MD, MBA, FACS
[a]May be considered for those with high-risk factors such as ulceration or mitotic rate ≥ 1/mm^2, especially for those with melanomas with Breslow's thickness 0.75–0.99 mm [29]
[b]May be considered for staging purposes or to facilitate regional disease control [29]

completed a prospective randomized controlled trial of patients who had primary melanomas <2 mm in thickness to excision with margins of either 1 cm or ≥3 cm. There was neither disease-free nor overall survival rate difference between the two groups at a mean follow-up of 90 months, although some recurrences were noted in those >1 mm in depth with a 1 cm margin. The authors concluded that thin melanomas (≤1 mm thick) were adequately treated with a 1 cm margin, and this became the gold standard resection margin for treatment of thin melanomas [20, 21] (Table 1.5).

Intermediate-Thickness Melanoma

Similarly, the US Intergroup Melanoma Surgical Trial prospectively randomized patients with 1–4 mm thick melanomas to be treated with either 2 or 4 cm excision margins. Overall recurrence rates were not significantly different: 2/244 (0.8 %) in the 2 cm group compared to 4/242 (1.7 %) in the 4 cm group. There was no significant difference in overall 5-year survival (80 % vs. 84 %). Those patients who had a 4 cm resection margin had significantly greater treatment morbidity. A 2 cm margin became the standard for intermediate-thickness melanomas as it was found to be equivalent to a larger margin but decreased the need for skin grafting and decreased hospital length of stay [22].

As a follow-up, Thomas et al. in 2004 randomized 900 British patients with truncal or extremity melanomas ≥2 mm to either surgery with 1 cm or 3 cm excision margins. Median follow-up was 5 years. Locoregional recurrence was 26 % higher in the group with a 1 cm margin, and the difference in disease-free survival approached statistical significance ($p=0.06$). The authors concluded that in a small number of patients, the melanoma cells that remain after excision with 1 cm margin will prove fatal. The use of 1 cm margins is thus avoided in patients with melanomas ≥ 2 mm, and the 2 cm margin remains standard of care except when not technically feasible [23] (Table 1.5).

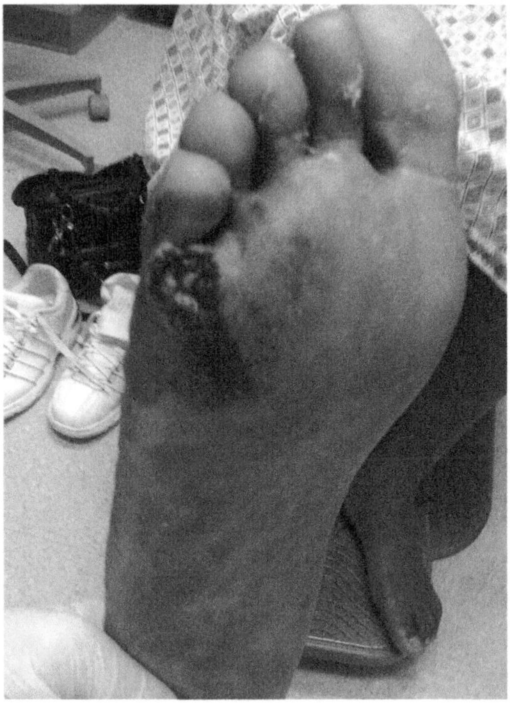

Fig. 1.4 Advanced melanoma (Courtesy of Quyen D. Chu, MD, MBA, FACS)

Thick Melanoma

In 1998, Heaton et al. retrospectively reviewed 278 patients in an attempt to determine an adequate margin in patients with thick melanomas (Figs. 1.4 and 1.5). They found that nodal status, thickness, and ulceration were significantly associated with overall survival in patients with melanomas greater than 4 mm in thickness.

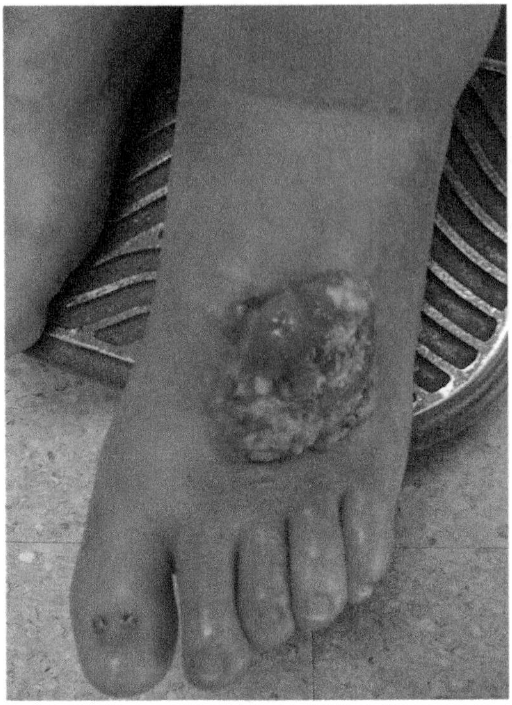

Fig. 1.5 Advanced melanoma (Courtesy of Quyen D. Chu, MD, MBA, FACS)

However, when compared using multivariate analysis, neither local recurrence nor excisional margin (<2 cm vs. >2 cm) significantly affected disease-free or overall survival. It was concluded that a 2 cm margin was adequate for intermediate and thick melanomas [24].

A 1 cm margin for melanomas less than or equal to 1 mm and 2 cm for those greater than 1 mm remains the standard of care today (Table 1.5).

Regional Lymph Nodes

Sentinel Node Biopsy

Historically, melanoma was treated by performing a wide local excision and regional lymphadenectomy. Lymphadenectomy carries significant morbidity, namely, lymphedema in approximately 20–30 % of patients. Sentinel node biopsy was developed as a potential technique that would provide prognostic information and minimize the morbidity associated with traditional lymphadenectomy (Figs. 1.6 and 1.7). It was also postulated to improve the accuracy of nodal staging, by identifying the most likely (sentinel) node to which disease would spread.

In 1994, Dr. Morton and colleagues challenged the standard of immediate lymphadenectomy by applying the technique of sentinel lymphadenectomy to patients with melanoma. The Multicenter Selective Lymphadenectomy Trial (MSLT-1) [25] randomized 1269 patients with an intermediate-thickness primary melanoma to wide excision of melanoma and either observation of regional lymph nodes with lymphadenectomy if nodal relapse occurred or sentinel node biopsy with immediate completion lymphadenectomy if metastases were found in the sentinel node (Fig. 1.8). Among patients with a positive sentinel node, 5-year survival rates were higher among those who underwent immediate completion lymphadenectomy than among those in whom lymphadenectomy was delayed (72.3 ± 4.6 % vs. 52.4 ± 5.9 %; hazard ratio for death of 0.51; $p = 0.004$). It must be noted that although there was a survival difference within the subgroups of patients with nodal involvement, there was no significant difference in overall survival for the entire population. This was thought to be due to the dilution effect [26]. What this means is that because the rate of sentinel node metastasis was 16 %, the number of patients who could derive benefit from early lymph node dissection was diluted by the larger number of patients who had tumor-free nodes [26].

Due to its staging and prognostic value, this landmark trial established sentinel node biopsy as standard of care for patients with intermediate-thickness melanomas (Breslow's thickness, 1–4 mm). The technique was later established to be prognostically useful in patients with high-risk thin melanomas (Breslow's thickness < 1 mm) where the node positivity rate is approximately 10 % [27] but remains controversial as to its utility in thick melanomas [28, 29]. High-risk thin melanomas are those that have evidence of ulceration or mitotic rate $\geq 1/\text{mm}^2$, especially in those with Breslow's thickness 0.75–0.99 mm [29] (Table 1.5).

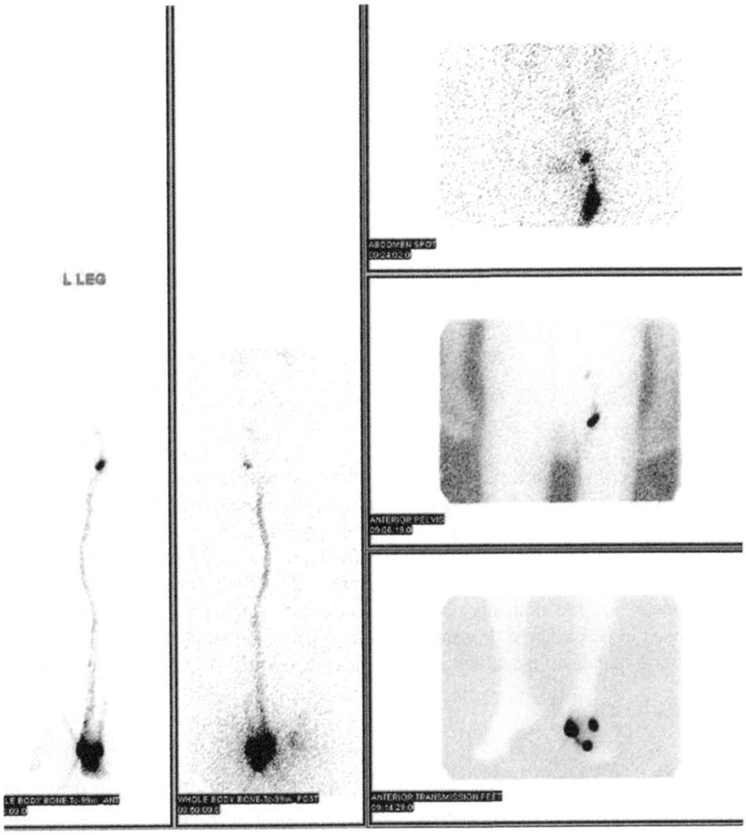

Fig. 1.6 *Sentinel lymph node mapping of a melanoma of the left foot using lymphoscintigraphy*. Radiotracer used was Tc-99 m sulfur colloid (Courtesy of Quyen D. Chu, MD, MBA, FACS)

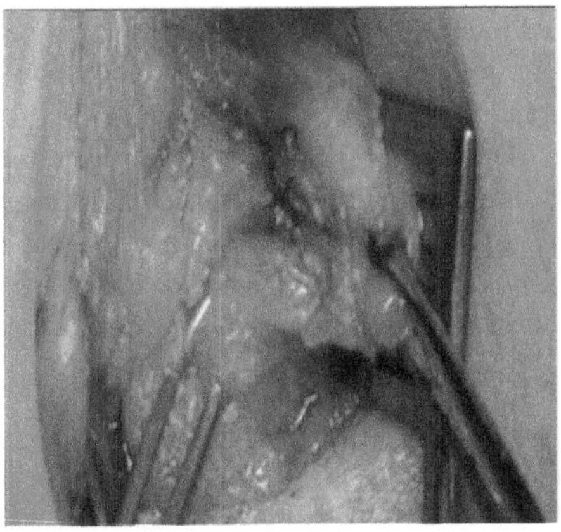

Fig. 1.7 Blue sentinel lymph node (Courtesy of Quyen D. Chu, MD, MBA, FACS)

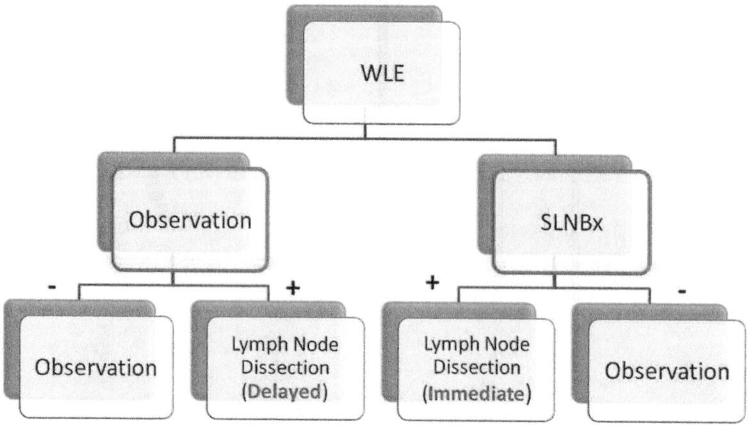

Fig. 1.8 *Multicenter Selective Lymphadenectomy Trial (MSLT) design*: Patients with intermediate-thickness melanoma underwent wide local excision and then randomized to either (1) observation or (2) sentinel lymph node biopsy. For those in the observation arm, a delayed node dissection is performed when the node(s) become clinically relevant; otherwise, patients continued to be observed. For those in the sentinel lymph node arm, a negative sentinel lymph node biopsy is observed, while a positive is subjected to a completion lymph node dissection. For those with nodal disease, immediate nodal dissection had better outcome (melanoma-specific survival) than those who had delayed nodal dissection. However, when comparing the two groups as a whole (red outlines), there was no overall survival benefit. This was thought to be due to the "dilution effect" (see text) (Courtesy of Quyen D. Chu, MD, MBA, FACS)

Completion Lymph Node Dissection

When a sentinel node biopsy demonstrates a lymph node metastasis, completion lymph node dissection is recommended. This remains the standard of care in the United States today [19], although it has become a controversial topic. Both sides of the debate agree that completion lymph node dissection has additional staging benefit, but randomized trials have not shown a survival benefit attributable to the procedure [30–33]. Furthermore, multiple trials have shown that only 18 % of patients will have disease within the remaining lymph nodes [25, 28]. An ongoing multicenter trial, the MSLT-II, aims to answer the question of completion lymph node dissection in patients with positive sentinel lymph node(s). Patients with positive sentinel node(s) will be randomized to either a completion lymph node dissection or observation with serial ultrasound of the nodal basin. Results are anxiously awaited, and until the clinical trial has been completed, patients should be recommended to have a completion lymph node dissection for positive sentinel node biopsy (Fig. 1.9).

Initial Lymphadenectomy

As mentioned above, clinically positive regional nodes portend a poor prognosis. The estimated 5-year overall survival (OS) rates range from 20 % to 40 % [34–36]. The NCCN guidelines recommend fine-needle aspiration biopsy to confirm the presence of metastases followed by immediate lymph node dissection at the time of initial operation [19]. Patients who are clinically node positive should be carefully staged to evaluate for systemic

Fig. 1.9 (continued) sartorius muscle, which can be detached at its origin and transferred medially as a flap without disrupting the neurovascular supply, which is located laterally. The muscle flap can be sutured to the inguinal ligament and/or adjacent tissue with 3–0 or 4–0 absorbable sutures (**a**: Courtesy of Thuy-Tien Chu and Quyen D. Chu, MD, MBA, FACS; **b**–**d**: Reprinted from Ref. [76]. With permission from Elsevier)

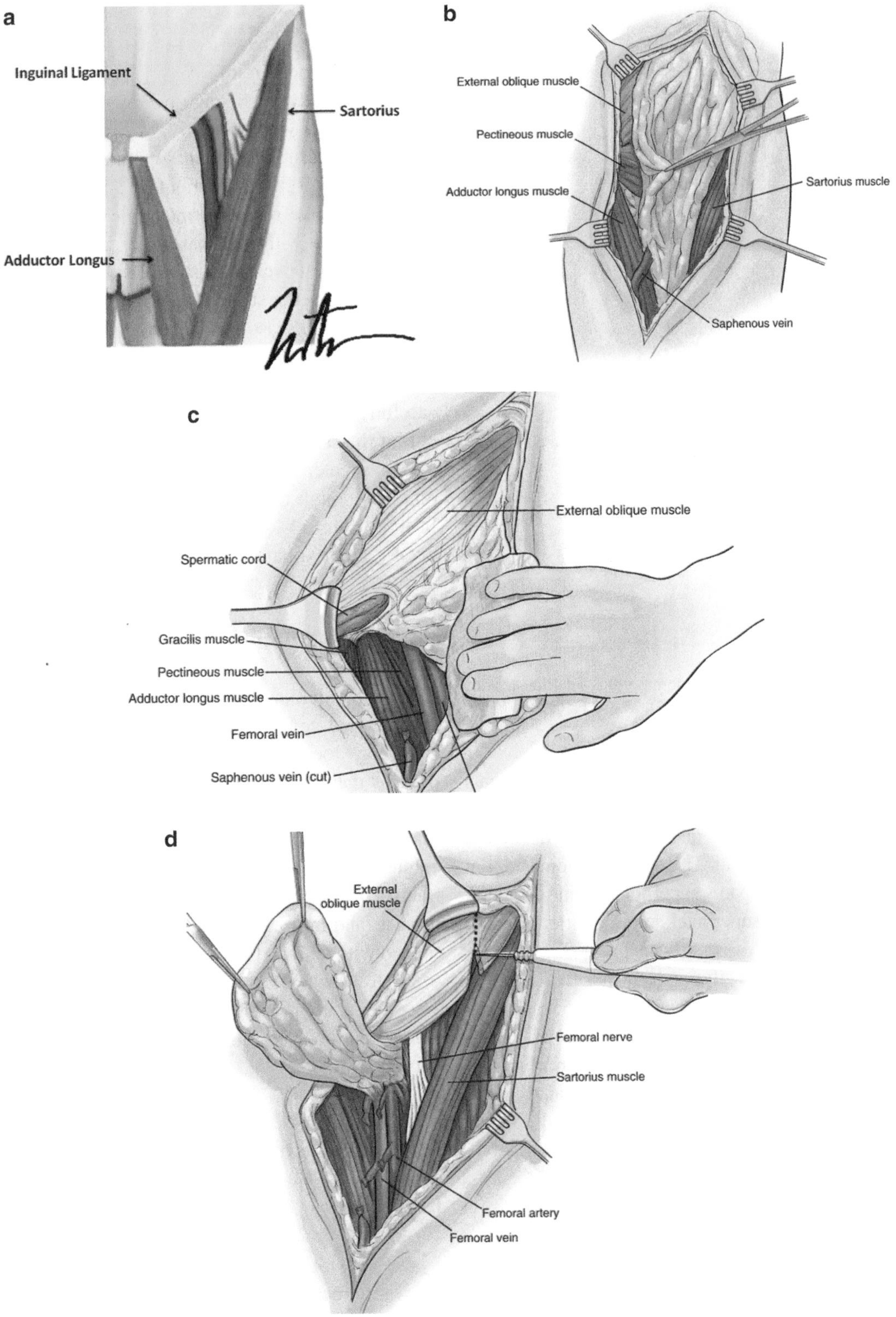

Fig. 1.9 *Groin lymph node dissection*. The lymph node-bearing area is located within the femoral triangle, which is bounded by the inguinal ligament superiorly, the Sartorius muscle laterally, and the adductor longus muscle medially. The floor of the triangle is formed by the fascia over the adductor longus, iliopsoas, and pectineus muscles, while the roof is formed by the fascia lata. Exposed vessels are generally covered with the

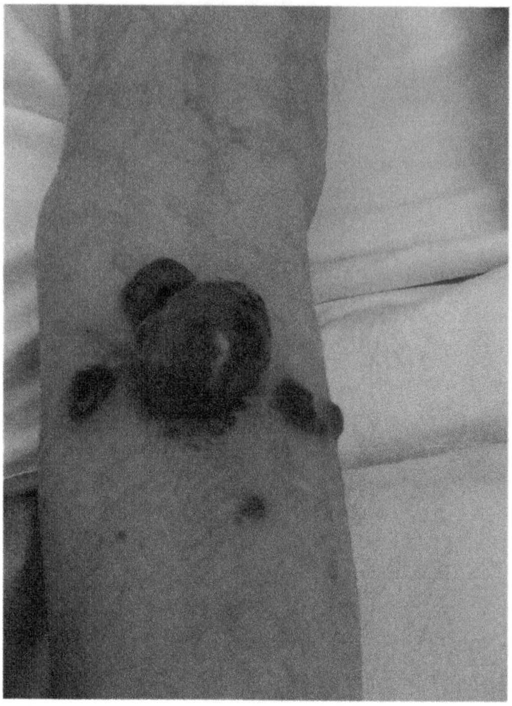

Fig. 1.10 Advanced melanoma with satellite lesions (Courtesy of Quyen D. Chu, MD, MBA, FACS)

disease prior to surgical therapy. Whether patients should undergo a superficial groin dissection or a combined superficial and deep groin dissection remains controversial. There is no randomized trial that directly compares superficial groin dissection with combined superficial and deep groin dissection. In general, a superficial groin dissection is recommended for those with positive sentinel lymph node, while a combined superficial and deep groin dissection is reserved for those who have clinically gross involvement of the groin, clinically detectable deep lymph nodes, histologically positive Cloquet's node (node medial to the femoral vein at the level of the inguinal ligament), or pelvic lymphadenopathy as seen on CT scans [35].

Surgery for Oligometastatic Stage IV Disease

Historically, patients with advanced melanoma (Figs. 1.10 and 1.11) have been offered surgery for palliation only, and the lack of efficacy of this approach has been reinforced by a stable rate of survival for advanced stage melanoma over the past 30 years. Median survival of patients with stage IV disease is less than 8 months in numerous studies. A subset of patients exists, however, where palliative resection may prove beneficial [37]. Patients with a disease-free interval of 3 years prior to developing stage IV disease have significantly better survival ($p<0.001$) than those with shorter disease-free intervals [38]. When isolated and a few number of lesions, surgical excision can be safe and effective if patients are carefully selected. Excision should be performed before disease is bulky and symptomatic, and a margin greater than 1 cm minimizes local recurrence, although repeat excision is often needed. In these carefully selected patients, median survival is approximately 2 years [39].

Adjuvant Radiation Therapy

Adjuvant radiation may also provide improved locoregional control in patients who are at high risk for locoregional recurrence. High-risk patients include those with recurrence after prior surgery, more than three positive lymph nodes, nodes greater than 3 cm in size, extracapsular extension, incomplete regional node dissection, microscopically positive margins, gross residual disease, and in-transit metastases [19, 40]. When treated with adjuvant radiation, locoregional control rates range from 74 % to 94 % [41–44]. Despite an improvement in local control, adjuvant radiation has not been shown to improve survival [45].

Adjuvant Systemic Therapy

Interferon

Systemic cytotoxic chemotherapy is the standard adjuvant treatment for many types of cancer; however, its efficacy in melanoma (not in combination with other therapy) is low. In the late 1990s, immunotherapy began to show signs of promise for patients with melanoma. Interferon-alpha

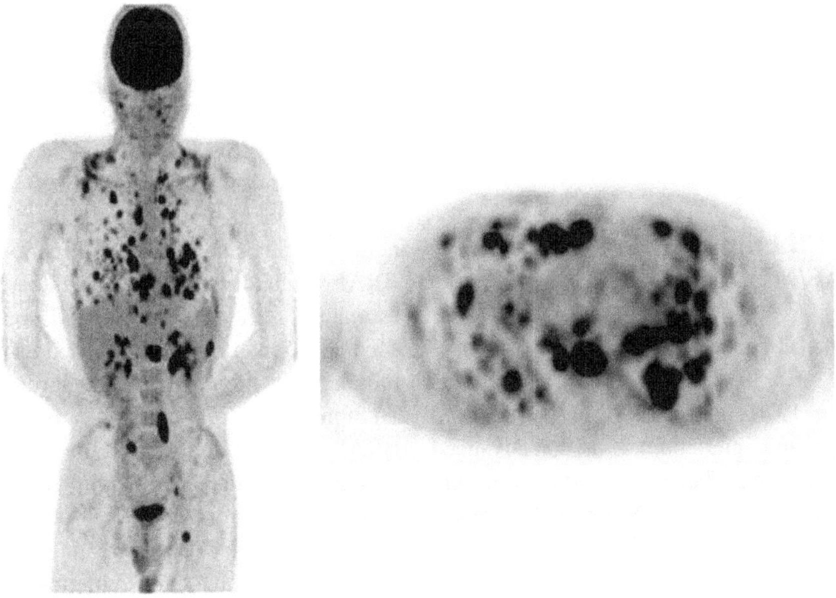

Fig. 1.11 PET scan of a patient with widely metastatic melanoma (Courtesy of Quyen D. Chu, MD, MBA, FACS)

(IFN-α) was one of the first therapies to demonstrate activity in patients with melanoma. The Eastern Cooperative Oncology Group (ECOG) evaluated the use of interferon in a series of randomized controlled clinical trials, the first being E1684. E1684 compared high-risk patients receiving IFN-α to placebo. Following publication of an initial overall survival benefit [46], IFN-α was FDA approved. Further analysis with longer follow-up demonstrated the survival benefit to no longer be significant [47], although IFN-α is still FDA approved for adjuvant treatment of patients with high-risk melanoma.

After E1684 and subsequent trials evaluated IFN-α, several reviews and meta-analyses further explored the IFN-α question. Lens et al. (2002) performed a review of US and European randomized controlled trials using IFN-α in melanoma. No trial demonstrated significant overall survival benefit [48]. Kirkwood et al. (2004) then performed a pooled analysis of ECOG and intergroup trials of adjuvant high-dose IFN-α. They reviewed updated data on nearly 2,000 patients from four clinical trials: E1684, E1690, E1694 (intergroup), and E2696. In comparison to observation, high-dose IFN-α was superior with respect to disease-free survival ($p<0.006$) but showed no benefit with regard to overall survival ($p=0.42$) [47]. The EORTC 18952 trial published in 2005 was a randomized controlled trial comparing different doses of IFN-α versus observation. IFN-α used in the regimen studied did not improve outcome for patients with either thick melanomas or positive nodes, and the authors concluded that IFN-α cannot be recommended. Equally important, the authors noted that a substantial number of patients (18 %) treated with intermediate dose IFN-α treatment had side effects that resulted in discontinuing therapy and 10 % had severe toxicities. Of those treated with high-dose IFN-α, 75 % had severe toxicity. Among subgroup analyses, duration of treatment seemed more important than dose [49].

Because of the toxicity associated with IFN-α, adjuvant pegylated interferon alfa-2b was then tested in clinical trials. The EORTC 18991 trial demonstrated that pegylated interferon alfa-2b for stage III melanoma has a significant effect on disease-free survival (46 % vs. 39 % at 4 years), but not on overall survival. Despite its improved risk profile over IFN-α, treatment was still discontinued due to toxicity in 31 % [50]. Although IFN-α is still FDA approved for melanoma, newer agents have begun to show promise with less toxicity.

Targeted Therapy: CTLA-4 Inhibitor and BRAF/MEK Inhibitors

Ipilimumab (Yervoy®)

In the late 1970s and 1990s, FDA approved dacarbazine and interleukin-2 in the advanced melanoma setting. Their response rates are approximately 10–20 %, although neither medication showed an overall survival benefit [51, 52]. More recently, an overall survival benefit in patients with metastatic melanoma was demonstrated in 2010 using ipilimumab, a monoclonal antibody that blocks cytotoxic T-lymphocyte-associated antigen 4 (CTLA-4) receptor. These lymphocytes then target cancer cells including melanoma. The use of ipilimumab in patients with melanoma was first tested against a tumor vaccine (gp100), and either ipilimumab alone or in combination with gp100 showed an improved median survival by 4 months over the vaccine alone (10 months vs. 6 months) [53] (Table 1.6). Ipilimumab is FDA approved for use in the unresectable and metastatic setting. A second trial published a few months later showed a survival benefit of 2 months when given in combination with dacarbazine [54].

BRAF and MEK Inhibition

Targeted therapies for melanoma have also shown a significant improvement in survival. Investigations began into the mitogen-activated protein (MAP) kinase pathway (Fig. 1.12), demonstrating that about half of melanomas have a mutation in the gene encoding the serine-threonine protein kinase BRAF. Ninety percent of BRAF mutations in melanoma affect a single residue (V600E) of the BRAF gene ($BRAF^{V600E}$), and 10–20 % affects the V600K residue. Knowledge of $BRAF^{V600E}$ mutation led to the development of vemurafenib (Zelboraf®). A prospective, randomized trial was published in 2010, demonstrating the first substantial improvement in progression-free survival (PFS) and overall survival (OS) in patients with metastatic melanoma. Eighty-one percent of patients with a BRAF mutation responded to therapy, with an estimated PFS of more than 7 months [55]. Median OS had not been reached at the time of initial publication but was later reported to be 16 months [56]. Dabrafenib (Tafinlar®), another $BRAF^{V600E}$ inhibitor, has also been demonstrated to improve median PFS, but not OS [57].

BRAF inhibitors were soon followed by MEK inhibitors, which is downstream of BRAF in the MAP kinase pathway, and trametinib (Mekinist®) was developed and later FDA approved when it demonstrated improved median PFS (4.8 months vs. 1.5 months; $p < 0.001$) and 6-month OS (81 % vs. 67 %; $P = 0.01$) over dacarbazine [58].

Despite these advances, durability of response is short-lived. Approximately 50 % of patients who are treated with BRAF or MEK inhibitors exhibit disease progression within 6–7 months of treatment [56, 59]. Recent data suggest that compared to monotherapy, combination of BRAF and MEK inhibitors (dabrafenib and trametinib) may be better. The median progression-free survival was 9.4 months in the combination group versus 5.8 months in the monotherapy group ($P < 0.001$) [60]. Pyrexia was increased in the combination therapy group, whereas the rate of proliferative skin lesion (i.e., cutaneous squamous cell carcinoma) was nonsignificantly reduced [60].

Since 2011, ipilimumab, vemurafenib, dabrafenib, and trametinib have all been FDA approved for the treatment of melanoma (Table 1.6). With four exciting new treatments on the market, the most recent challenge has been to understand which adjuvant systemic treatments are best. Several clinical trials are now underway or have recently been published comparing different immunotherapies, targeted therapies, combinations, and sequences of these drugs.

Table 1.6 Selected clinical trials of FDA-approved targeted therapy against advanced melanoma

Drugs	Mechanism of action	Patient population	*N*	Study groups	Outcomes	Highlights of study
Ipilimumab [53] (Yervoy®)	Monoclonal antibody against cytotoxic T-lymphocytes-associated antigen 4 (CTLA-4)	Unresectable or metastatic	676	gp100 (vaccine) Ipilimumab Ipilimumab + gp100	**Median OS (mos)**: Ipilimumab + gp100: 10.0 Ipilimumab: 10.1 gp100: 6.4 ($P<0.001$) **2-year OS**: Ipilimumab + gp100: 21.6 % Ipilimumab : 23.5 % gp100 : 13.7 %	Significant improvement in OS with ipilimumab ± gp100 vaccine over gp100 alone
Vemurafenib [56] (Zelboraf®)	BRAF inhibitor, targets mutated V600E ($BRAF^{V600E}$)	Unresectable or metastatic	675	Vemurafenib Dacarbazine	**OS**: Vemurafenib: 84 % Dacarbazine: 64 % ($P<0.001$) RRR: 63 %[a] **Median PFS (mos)**: Vemurafenib: 5.3 Dacarbazine: 1.6 ($P<0.001$) RRR: 74 %[a]	Significant improvement in OS and PFS with vemurafenib over dacarbazine
Dabrafenib [57] (Tafinlar®)	BRAF inhibitor, targets mutated V600E ($BRAF^{V600E}$)	Unresectable or metastatic	733	Dabrafenib Dacarbazine	**Median PFS (mos)**: Dabrafenib: 5.1 Dacarbazine: 2.7 ($P<0.0001$)	Significant improvement in PFS with dabrafenib
Trametinib [58] (Mekinist®)	MEK inhibitor, targets mutated V600E ($BRAF^{V600E}$) or V600K ($BRAF^{V600K}$)	Unresectable or metastatic	322	Trametinib Dacarbazine	**6 month OS**: Trametinib: 81 % Dacarbazine: 67 % ($P=0.01$) **Median PFS (mos)**: Trametinib: 4.8 Dacarbazine: 1.5 ($P<0.001$)	Significant improvement in OS and PFS with trametinib

Courtesy of Quyen D. Chu, MD, MBA, FACS
RRR relative risk reduction, *PFS* progression-free survival, *OS* overall survival; *mos* months
[a]In favor of novel drugs

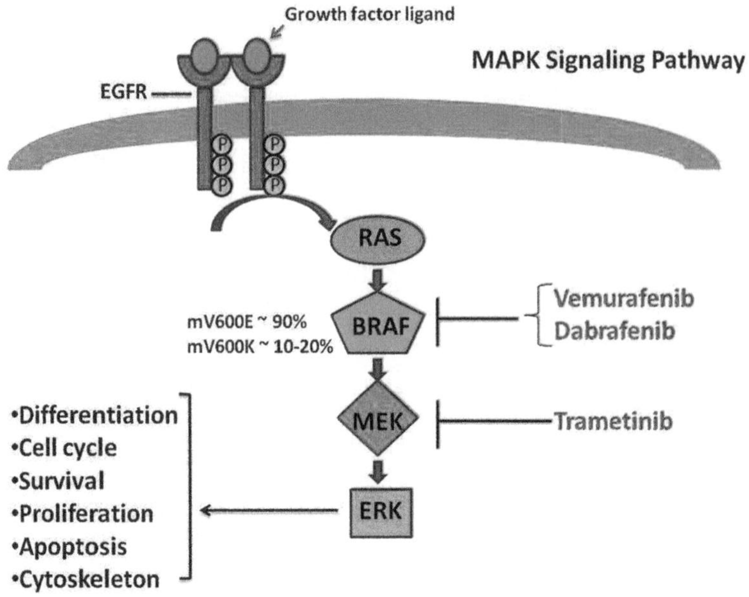

Fig. 1.12 *Mitogen-activated protein kinase (MAPK) pathway*: 50 % of melanomas have BRAF mutation, of which 90 % occurs at a single residue (V600E), while 10–20 % occurs at the V600K residue. Novel drugs that target BRAF are vemurafenib and dabrafenib. Trametinib targets MEK, which is downstream of BRAF (Courtesy of Quyen D. Chu, MD, MBA, FACS)

Other Therapeutic Strategies for Advanced Disease

Historically, in-transit metastases were differentiated from satellite lesions based on the distance of the lesions from the primary melanoma; satellite lesions are those that are within 2 cm of the primary melanoma, whereas in-transit metastases are those that are located greater than 2 cm from the primary melanoma and between the primary extremity site and the primary nodal basin (Fig. 1.13). However, given their overall poor prognosis [61], both are considered by the AJCC as stage III disease.

In-transit, satellite lesions, or locally recurrent melanoma can be a very challenging and difficult to manage clinical problem in a small subset of patients with extremity melanoma. In-transit metastases have been reported to develop in 6–19 % of patients with stage II melanoma at presentation [62]. The presence of in-transit, satellite lesions, or locally recurrent disease is associated with a poor overall survival as most patients ultimately fail systemically. A workup to exclude systemic disease should be considered. Local control for symptom palliation is a major priority in these patients.

Regional Chemotherapy

In order to limit systemic toxicity and increase the dose of delivered drug to the site of in-transit disease, isolated limb perfusion (ILP) was developed by Creech and Krementz in 1956 [63] (Fig. 1.14). Melphalan or melphalan in combination with other cytotoxic drugs has been most commonly used for regional chemotherapy [64]. ILP has been demonstrated to have high overall response rates in the range of 90 % and to improve local control in patients with in-transit melanoma; however, it has not been shown to have an impact on overall survival [64]. The combination of hyperthermia with isolated limb perfusion has been demonstrated in some studies to be associated with improved response rates [64]. Limitations of ILP are the need for surgical

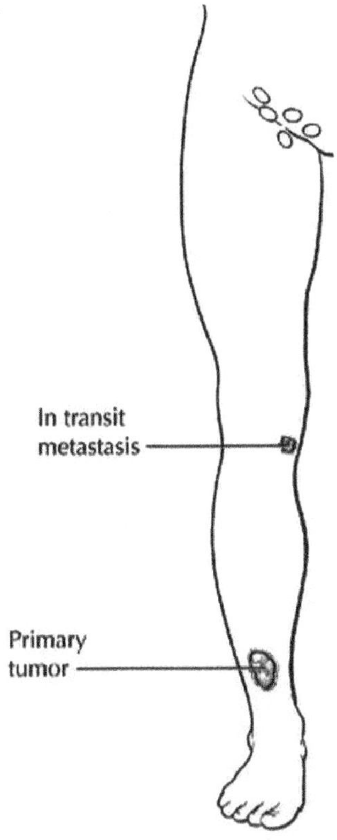

Fig. 1.13 *In-transit metastasis from melanoma (N2)*: Defined as a tumor distinct from the primary lesion and located either (1) between the primary lesion and the draining regional lymph nodes or (2) distal to the primary lesion (Reprinted from Ref. [77]. With permission from Springer Verlag)

access to the arterial and venous vessels of an involved extremity, prolonged recovery, difficulty in repeating the procedures, and a high incidence of mild to moderate regional and systemic toxicity [64].

A catheter-based minimally invasive approach to regional chemotherapy, isolated limb infusion, in patients with advanced melanoma of the extremity was developed by Thompson and colleagues at the Sydney Melanoma Unit in 1992 [65]. This catheter-based technique has gained popularity as it has been associated with similar response rates and less side effects and faster patient recovery [66].

Other Local Therapies for Recurrent Disease

Palliative measures that have been employed to achieve local control in patients with local or in-transit recurrent melanoma include surgical excision, laser ablation, and cryotherapy (reviewed in Squires et al [67]). Intralesional injection (e.g., IL-2 and bacilli Calmette-Guerin), topical therapies, and electrochemotherapy have also been studied and associated with improved local control in some cases of locally or regionally recurrent melanoma [67].

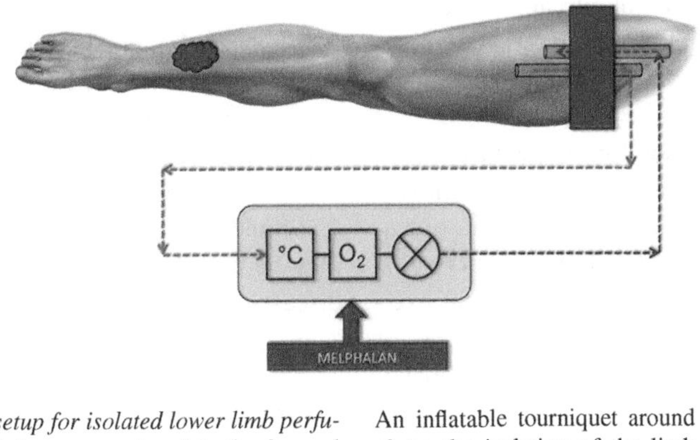

Fig. 1.14 *Schematic setup for isolated lower limb perfusion for melanoma*: Catheters are placed in the femoral artery and vein and then connected to the perfusion circuit consisting of a heater, an oxygenator, and a roller pump. An inflatable tourniquet around the thigh further completes the isolation of the limb (With kind permission from Roger Olofsson, M.D., In: Isolated Regional Perfusion for Metastases of Malignant Melanoma)

Non-cutaneous Melanomas

While the vast majority of melanomas arise in the skin, a small percentage (<2 %) occurs in the mucosal area such as the head and neck, vulvar, and anorectum. Mucosal melanoma (MM) portends a poor prognosis and is believed to be biological distinct from the skin melanomas. Because of its rarity, a standardized approach is not well defined. Surgery plays a central role, but the extent of surgical resection remains controversial. Management of anorectal and vulvar melanomas will briefly be discussed.

Anal Melanoma

Anal melanoma is the third most common location for malignant melanoma following cutaneous melanoma and ocular melanoma [68]. The biology for anal melanoma is poorly understood, but unlike cutaneous melanoma, it is not related to ultraviolet (UV) exposure and there is no evidence of BRAF mutation in anal melanoma [69]. Approximately 60 % of patients present with lymphatic spread, while 25 % have either distant disease or inoperable locoregional diseases [70].

Optimal treatment for this rare entity is not known. For patients with clinically negative lymphadenopathy, sentinel lymph node biopsy might be a viable option to allow early completion lymphadenectomy. In selected cases, radiotherapy might play a role in providing locoregional disease control.

Often, a major operation is required (i.e., abdominoperineal resection or APR) to achieve a complete R0 resection, although such an operation can be highly morbid and overall survival is not significantly different from wide local excision (WLE) [71]; the 5-year OS was 17 % for APR and 19 % for WLE [71]. The primary goal of surgery should be to resect the tumor to negative margins without having to resort to a highly morbid operation, if possible. Margin has an impact on outcome. The 5-year OS was 19 % for an R0 resection versus 6 % for an R+resection [72].

Survival is predicated on extent of disease. Using the Surveillance, Epidemiology, and End Results (SEER) database from 1973 to 2003, Iddings et al reported the median survivals for localized, regional, and distant disease to be 24 months, 17 months, and 8 months, respectively, and the 5-year OS to be 26.7 %, 9.8 %, and 0 %, respectively ($P<0.001$) [71].

Vulvar Melanoma

Vulvar melanoma is rare but represents the second most common vulvar malignancy, accounting for 8–10 % of all vulvar malignancies [73]. It generally afflicts the elderlies in their 70s, and outcome is poor with a 5-year survival rate ranging from 27 % to 54 % [73]. The most common location of primary vulvar melanoma is the labia majora followed by the labia minora [74]. The most common symptoms include pruritus, lumps, tumor mass, swelling, or abscess.

Similar to anal melanoma, management is controversial. Management is mainly based on a review of sporadic case reports/series [74]. Preoperative staging to rule out distant disease should be performed. Extent of surgical resection is predicated by the extent of disease. For those that are localized, a wide local excision with a 1 cm margin for melanoma<1 mm thick and 2 cm margin for intermediate thickness (1–4 mm) is recommended [73]. For lesions that extend beyond the labia (i.e., urethra or rectum), more extensive surgery may be required. The role of prophylactic lymphadenectomy is controversial. A sentinel lymph node biopsy might serve useful for those with a primary lesion>1 mm and clinically negative node. The 5-year OS for node-negative and node-positive vulvar melanomas is 65 % and 27 %, respectively [75]. Radiotherapy may be useful in select cases of advanced stage disease to control symptoms.

Conclusions

Melanoma is a challenging malignancy with a wide spectrum of disease. Proper diagnosis and staging are crucial to determine prognosis. Surgery remains the mainstay of treatment, including wide local excision, sentinel node biopsy, and lymph node dissection. Adjuvant treatment was transformed in 2010 with systemic biologic agents showing an overall survival benefit for patients with advanced disease. Advancement in the treatment of melanoma has been highlighted by randomized, prospective clinical trials.

Salient Points

- Important risk factors for developing melanoma are family history of melanoma, personal history of melanoma, dysplastic nevus syndrome, xeroderma pigmentosum, having multiple benign or atypical nevi, and having light skin, freckles, blue eyes, or red hair.
- Melanomas can be recognized using the "ABCDE" features (see Table 1.1).
- IHC stains for melanomas include S100, HBM-45, tyrosinase, MART-1/Melan-A, and MITF.
- Tumor depth and ulceration are two strongest prognostic factors. Others include mitotic index, LDH, location, microsatellites, and TIL (see Table 1.4).
- Locations that are associated with poor prognosis are "BANS" (back, back of upper arm, neck, scalp).
- Surgical treatment requires knowledge of tumor thickness, which assists in determining the width of excision and the need for sentinel lymph node biopsy (See Table 1.5).
  - Lesions that are between 1.01 mm and 4 mm thick should undergo a 2 cm wide local excision and a sentinel lymph node biopsy.
  - MLST-1 Results
    - Improved survival for those who undergo immediate node dissection versus delayed in those with nodal disease
    - No overall survival difference between observation group and sentinel lymph node biopsy group (maybe due to dilution effect)
  - MLST-2 Trial
    - Randomizes SLNBx(+) to either observation or lymphadenectomy (i.e., is a completion node dissection for positive sentinel lymph node(s) necessary?).
    - Final results not yet available.
  - SLNBx should not be performed in patients with palpable lymphadenopathy.
- Palpable lymph node(s) should undergo FNA for confirmation of metastases before subjecting a patient to a full lymph node dissection.
- A completion lymph node dissection is required when the SLNbx is positive.
- Deep lymph node dissection can be considered in the following situations:
  - Clinically detectable deep lymph nodes
  - Positive Cloquet's nod
  - Pelvic adenopathy as seen on CT scans
- The following treatments do not improve overall survival:
  - Interferon-alpha
  - Dacarbazine
  - Interleukin 2
- Ipilimumab (monoclonal antibody against CTLA-4R; FDA approved) improves median OS over vaccine by 4 months (10 months vs. 6 months).
- BRAF is involved in the MAP kinase pathway and is mutated in melanoma.
  - Ninety percent BRAF mutation occurs at the V600E residue, while 10–20 % occurs at the V600K residue.
  - Vemurafenib (BRAF inhibitor) improves progression-free survival and *overall survival* in patients with metastatic melanoma.
  - Other BRAF inhibitors are dabrafenib and trametinib (MEK inhibitor).
- In-transit metastases and satellite lesions are considered stage III disease; they carry poor prognosis.
  - Isolated limb perfusion using melphalan is an option to treat in-transit metastases.
- Anal melanomas and vulvar melanomas are rare but highly aggressive. The role of prophylactic lymphadenectomy is controversial.

Questions

1. A 37-year-old man presents to your clinic with a history of a pigmented skin lesion on his back. His dermatologist performed a biopsy demonstrating a 1.4 mm thick melanoma. He has no palpable axillary or inguinal adenopathy. The next step in management is:
   A. Staging PET/CT scan
   B. Wide local excision with 1 cm margin
   C. Wide local excision with 1 cm margin and sentinel node biopsy

   D. Wide local excision with 2 cm margin and sentinel node biopsy
   E. Wide local excision with 2 cm margin and axillary dissection
2. A 45-year-old woman presents with a new diagnosis of a 3.5 mm thick melanoma of the foot. On examination, she has palpable inguinal adenopathy. What is the next step in management?
   A. Fine-needle aspiration biopsy of the palpable inguinal node
   B. Wide local excision with 2 cm margin and sentinel node biopsy
   C. Wide local excision with 2 cm margin and inguinal node dissection
   D. Systemic immunotherapy alone
   E. Systemic immunotherapy with radiation to the inguinal nodes
3. A history of blistering sunburns is the most significant risk factor for developing melanoma.
   A. True
   B. False
4. Sentinel node biopsy should be considered on all melanoma patients with:
   A. Primary melanoma > 0.5 mm thick
   B. Primary melanoma 0.75–1 mm thick with high-risk features
   C. Lymphedema
   D. Palpable adenopathy
   E. Metastatic disease
5. Completion lymph node dissection:
   A. Has a 5 % risk for lymphedema
   B. Will demonstrate additional nodal disease in 50 % of patients
   C. Confers a survival benefit in patients with node-positive disease
   D. Should be recommended after a positive sentinel node biopsy
   E. Should be performed on all patients with melanoma > 4 mm deep
6. Overall survival in metastatic melanoma is NOT improved with treatment with which medication?
   A. Interferon-alpha
   B. Ipilimumab
   C. Vemurafenib
   D. Dabrafenib
   E. Trametinib

Answers

1. D
2. A
3. B
4. B
5. D
6. A

References

1. Howlader N. SEER cancer statistics review, 1975–2010. Available at: www.seer.cancer.gov(2013).
2. Miller AJ, Mihm Jr MC. Melanoma. N Engl J Med. 2006;355(1):51–65.
3. Thompson JF, Scolyer RA, Kefford RF. Cutaneous melanoma. Lancet. 2005;365(9460):687–701.
4. Bishop DT, Demenais F, Goldstein AM, et al. Geographical variation in the penetrance of CDKN2A mutations for melanoma. J Natl Cancer Inst. 2002; 94(12):894–903.
5. Elder DE. Precursors to melanoma and their mimics: nevi of special sites. Mod Pathol. 2006;19 Suppl 2:S4–20.
6. Paszkowska-Szczur K, Scott RJ, Serrano-Fernandez P, et al. Xeroderma pigmentosum genes and melanoma risk. Int J Cancer. 2013;133(5):1094–100.
7. Kraemer KH, Lee MM, Andrews AD, Lambert WC. The role of sunlight and DNA repair in melanoma and nonmelanoma skin cancer. The xeroderma pigmentosum paradigm. Arch Dermatol. 1994;130(8): 1018–21.
8. Riker AI, Glass F, Perez I, Cruse CW, Messina J, Sondak VK. Cutaneous melanoma: methods of biopsy and definitive surgical excision. Dermatol Ther. 2005;18(5):387–93.
9. Roses DF, Ackerman AB, Harris MN, Weinhouse GR, Gumport SL. Assessment of biopsy techniques and histopathologic interpretations of primary cutaneous malignant melanoma. Ann Surg. 1979;189(3): 294–7.
10. Zager JS, Hochwald SN, Marzban SS, et al. Shave biopsy is a safe and accurate method for the initial evaluation of melanoma. J Am Coll Surg. 2011;212(4):454–60; discussion 460–452.
11. Ohsie SJ, Sarantopoulos GP, Cochran AJ, Binder SW. Immunohistochemical characteristics of melanoma. J Cutan Pathol. 2008;35(5):433–44.
12. Rousseau Jr DL, Ross MI, Johnson MM, et al. Revised American Joint Committee on Cancer staging criteria accurately predict sentinel lymph node positivity in clinically node-negative melanoma patients. Ann Surg Oncol. 2003;10(5):569–74.
13. Balch CM, Buzaid AC, Soong SJ, et al. Final version of the American Joint Committee on Cancer staging system for cutaneous melanoma. J Clin Oncol. 2001;19(16): 3635–48.

14. Schuchter L, Schultz DJ, Synnestvedt M, et al. A prognostic model for predicting 10-year survival in patients with primary melanoma. The Pigmented Lesion Group. Ann Intern Med. 1996;125(5):369–75.
15. Balch CM, Soong SJ, Gershenwald JE, et al. Prognostic factors analysis of 17,600 melanoma patients: validation of the American Joint Committee on Cancer melanoma staging system. J Clin Oncol. 2001;19(16):3622–34.
16. Spatz A, Shaw HM, Crotty KA, Thompson JF, McCarthy SW. Analysis of histopathological factors associated with prolonged survival of 10 years or more for patients with thick melanomas (>5 mm). Histopathology. 1998;33(5):406–13.
17. Clark WH, Elder DE, Guerry D, et al. Model predicting survival in stage I melanoma based on tumor progression. J Natl Cancer Inst. 1989;81(24):1893–904.
18. Nagore E, Oliver V, Botella-Estrada R, Moreno-Picot S, Insa A, Fortea JM. Prognostic factors in localized invasive cutaneous melanoma: high value of mitotic rate, vascular invasion and microscopic satellitosis. Melanoma Res. 2005;15(3):169–77.
19. Coit DG, Andtbacka R, Anker CJ, et al. Melanoma, version 2.2013: featured updates to the NCCN guidelines. J Natl Compr Canc Netw. 2013;11(4):395–407.
20. Veronesi U, Cascinelli N. Narrow excision (1-cm margin). A safe procedure for thin cutaneous melanoma. Arch Surg. 1991;126(4):438–41.
21. Veronesi U, Cascinelli N, Adamus J, et al. Thin stage I primary cutaneous malignant melanoma. Comparison of excision with margins of 1 or 3 cm. N Engl J Med. 1988;318(18):1159–62.
22. Balch CM, Urist MM, Karakousis CP, et al. Efficacy of 2-cm surgical margins for intermediate-thickness melanomas (1 to 4 mm). Results of a multi-institutional randomized surgical trial. Ann Surg. 1993;218(3):262–7; discussion 267–269.
23. Thomas JM, Newton-Bishop J, A'Hern R, et al. Excision margins in high-risk malignant melanoma. N Engl J Med. 2004;350(8):757–66.
24. Heaton KM, Sussman JJ, Gershenwald JE, et al. Surgical margins and prognostic factors in patients with thick (>4 mm) primary melanoma. Ann Surg Oncol. 1998;5(4):322–8.
25. Morton DL, Thompson JF, Cochran AJ, et al. Sentinel-node biopsy or nodal observation in melanoma. N Engl J Med. 2006;355(13):1307–17.
26. Morton DL, Cochran AJ, Thompson JF. Authors' response to a letter to the editor re: sentinel node biopsy for early-stage melanoma. Ann Surg. 2007; 245(5):828–9.
27. Puleo CA, Messina JL, Riker AI, et al. Sentinel node biopsy for thin melanomas: which patients should be considered? Cancer Control. 2005;12(4):230–5.
28. Jacobs IA, Chang CK, Salti GI. Role of sentinel lymph node biopsy in patients with thick (>4 mm) primary melanoma. Am Surg. 2004;70(1):59–62.
29. Wong SL, Balch CM, Hurley P, et al. Sentinel lymph node biopsy for melanoma: American Society of Clinical Oncology and Society of Surgical Oncology joint clinical practice guideline. J Clin Oncol. 2012; 30(23):2912–8.
30. Veronesi U. Regional lymph node dissection in melanoma of the limbs. Stage I. A cooperative international trial (WHO collaborating centers for diagnosis and treatment of melanoma). Recent Results Cancer Res. 1977;62:8.
31. Balch CM, Soong S, Ross MI, et al. Long-term results of a multi-institutional randomized trial comparing prognostic factors and surgical results for intermediate thickness melanomas (1.0 to 4.0 mm). Intergroup Melanoma Surgical Trial. Ann Surg Oncol. 2000;7(2):87–97.
32. Sim FH, Taylor WF, Pritchard DJ, Soule EH. Lymphadenectomy in the management of stage I malignant melanoma: a prospective randomized study. Mayo Clin Proc. 1986;61(9):697–705.
33. Cascinelli N, Morabito A, Santinami M, MacKie RM, Belli F. Immediate or delayed dissection of regional nodes in patients with melanoma of the trunk: a randomised trial. WHO Melanoma Programme. Lancet. 1998;351(9105):793–6.
34. Mann GB, Coit DG. Does the extent of operation influence the prognosis in patients with melanoma metastatic to inguinal nodes? Ann Surg Oncol. 1999; 6(3):263–71.
35. Hughes TM, A'Hern RP, Thomas JM. Prognosis and surgical management of patients with palpable inguinal lymph node metastases from melanoma. Br J Surg. 2000;87(7):892–901.
36. Meyer T, Merkel S, Göhl J, Hohenberger W. Lymph node dissection for clinically evident lymph node metastases of malignant melanoma. Eur J Surg Oncol. 2002;28(4):424–30.
37. Young SE, Martinez SR, Faries MB, Essner R, Wanek LA, Morton DL. Can surgical therapy alone achieve long-term cure of melanoma metastatic to regional nodes? Cancer J. 2006;12(3):207–11.
38. Essner R, Scheri R, Kavanagh M, Torisu-Itakura H, Wanek LA, Morton DL. Surgical management of the groin lymph nodes in melanoma in the era of sentinel lymph node dissection. Arch Surg. 2006;141(9):877–82; discussion 882–874.
39. Ollila DW. Complete metastasectomy in patients with stage IV metastatic melanoma. Lancet Oncol. 2006; 7(11):919–24.
40. Mendenhall WM, Amdur RJ, Grobmyer SR, et al. Adjuvant radiotherapy for cutaneous melanoma. Cancer. 2008;112(6):1189–96.
41. Ballo MT, Garden AS, Myers JN, et al. Melanoma metastatic to cervical lymph nodes: can radiotherapy replace formal dissection after local excision of nodal disease? Head Neck. 2005;27(8):718–21.
42. Ballo MT, Strom EA, Zagars GK, et al. Adjuvant irradiation for axillary metastases from malignant melanoma. Int J Radiat Oncol Biol Phys. 2002;52(4): 964–72.
43. Ballo MT, Zagars GK, Gershenwald JE, et al. A critical assessment of adjuvant radiotherapy for inguinal lymph node metastases from melanoma. Ann Surg Oncol. 2004;11(12):1079–84.

44. Mendenhall WM, Shaw C, Amdur RJ, Kirwan J, Morris CG, Werning JW. Surgery and adjuvant radiotherapy for cutaneous melanoma considered high-risk for local-regional recurrence. Am J Otolaryngol. 2013;34(4):320–2.
45. Burmeister BH, Henderson MA, Ainslie J, et al. Adjuvant radiotherapy versus observation alone for patients at risk of lymph-node field relapse after therapeutic lymphadenectomy for melanoma: a randomised trial. Lancet Oncol. 2012;13(6):589–97.
46. Kirkwood JM, Strawderman MH, Ernstoff MS, Smith TJ, Borden EC, Blum RH. Interferon alfa-2b adjuvant therapy of high-risk resected cutaneous melanoma: the Eastern Cooperative Oncology Group Trial EST 1684. J Clin Oncol. 1996;14(1):7–17.
47. Kirkwood JM, Manola J, Ibrahim J, Sondak V, Ernstoff MS, Rao U. A pooled analysis of eastern cooperative oncology group and intergroup trials of adjuvant high-dose interferon for melanoma. Clin Cancer Res. 2004;10(5):1670–7.
48. Lens MB, Dawes M. Interferon alfa therapy for malignant melanoma: a systematic review of randomized controlled trials. J Clin Oncol. 2002;20(7):1818–25.
49. Eggermont AM, Suciu S, MacKie R, et al. Post-surgery adjuvant therapy with intermediate doses of interferon alfa 2b versus observation in patients with stage IIb/III melanoma (EORTC 18952): randomised controlled trial. Lancet. 2005;366(9492):1189–96.
50. Eggermont AM, Suciu S, Santinami M, et al. Adjuvant therapy with pegylated interferon alfa-2b versus observation alone in resected stage III melanoma: final results of EORTC 18991, a randomised phase III trial. Lancet. 2008;372(9633):117–26.
51. Carbone PP, Costello W. Eastern Cooperative Oncology Group studies with DTIC (NSC-45388). Cancer Treat Rep. 1976;60(2):193–8.
52. Atkins MB, Lotze MT, Dutcher JP, et al. High-dose recombinant interleukin 2 therapy for patients with metastatic melanoma: analysis of 270 patients treated between 1985 and 1993. J Clin Oncol. 1999;17(7):2105–16.
53. Hodi FS, O'Day SJ, McDermott DF, et al. Improved survival with ipilimumab in patients with metastatic melanoma. N Engl J Med. 2010;363(8):711–23.
54. Robert C, Thomas L, Bondarenko I, et al. Ipilimumab plus dacarbazine for previously untreated metastatic melanoma. N Engl J Med. 2011;364(26):2517–26.
55. Flaherty KT, Puzanov I, Kim KB, et al. Inhibition of mutated, activated BRAF in metastatic melanoma. N Engl J Med. 2010;363(9):809–19.
56. Chapman PB, Hauschild A, Robert C, et al. Improved survival with vemurafenib in melanoma with BRAF V600E mutation. N Engl J Med. 2011;364(26):2507–16.
57. Hauschild A, Grob JJ, Demidov LV, et al. Dabrafenib in BRAF-mutated metastatic melanoma: a multicentre, open-label, phase 3 randomised controlled trial. Lancet. 2012;380(9839):358–65.
58. Flaherty KT, Robert C, Hersey P, et al. Improved survival with MEK inhibition in BRAF-mutated melanoma. N Engl J Med. 2012;367(2):107–14.
59. Sosman JA, Kim KB, Schuchter L, et al. Survival in BRAF V600-mutant advanced melanoma treated with vemurafenib. N Engl J Med. 2012;366(8):707–14.
60. Flaherty KT, Infante JR, Daud A, et al. Combined BRAF and MEK inhibition in melanoma with BRAF V600 mutations. N Engl J Med. 2012;367(18):1694–703.
61. Singletary SE, Tucker SL, Boddie AW. Multivariate analysis of prognostic factors in regional cutaneous metastases of extremity melanoma. Cancer. 1988;61(7):1437–40.
62. Kam PC, Thompson JF. Isolated limb infusion with melphalan and actinomycin D in melanoma patients: factors predictive of acute regional toxicity. Expert Opin Drug Metab Toxicol. 2010;6(9):1039–45.
63. Creech O, Krementz ET, Ryan RF, Winblad JN. Chemotherapy of cancer: regional perfusion utilizing an extracorporeal circuit. Ann Surg. 1958;148(4):616–32.
64. Moreno-Ramirez D, de la Cruz-Merino L, Ferrandiz L, Villegas-Portero R, Nieto-Garcia A. Isolated limb perfusion for malignant melanoma: systematic review on effectiveness and safety. Oncologist. 2010;15(4):416–27.
65. Thompson JF, Kam PC. Isolated limb infusion for melanoma: a simple but effective alternative to isolated limb perfusion. J Surg Oncol. 2004;88(1):1–3.
66. Beasley GM, Caudle A, Petersen RP, et al. A multi-institutional experience of isolated limb infusion: defining response and toxicity in the US. J Am Coll Surg. 2009;208(5):706–15; discussion 715–707.
67. Squires MH, Delman KA. Current treatment of locoregional recurrence of melanoma. Curr Oncol Rep. 2013;15(5):465–72.
68. Carcoforo P, Raiji MT, Palini GM, et al. Primary anorectal melanoma: an update. J Cancer Educ. 2012;3:449–53.
69. Edwards RH, Ward MR, Wu H, et al. Absence of BRAF mutations in UV-protected mucosal melanomas. J Med Genet. 2004;41(4):270–2.
70. Chang AE, Karnell LH, Menck HR. The National Cancer Data Base report on cutaneous and noncutaneous melanoma: a summary of 84,836 cases from the past decade. The American College of Surgeons Commission on Cancer and the American Cancer Society. Cancer. 1998;83(8):1664–78.
71. Iddings DM, Fleisig AJ, Chen SL, Faries MB, Morton DL. Practice patterns and outcomes for anorectal melanoma in the USA, reviewing three decades of treatment: is more extensive surgical resection beneficial in all patients? Ann Surg Oncol. 2010;17(1):40–4.
72. Nilsson PJ, Ragnarsson-Olding BK. Importance of clear resection margins in anorectal malignant melanoma. Br J Surg. 2010;97(1):98–103.
73. Irvin WP, Legallo RL, Stoler MH, Rice LW, Taylor PT, Andersen WA. Vulvar melanoma: a retrospective analysis and literature review. Gynecol Oncol. 2001;83(3):457–65.

74. Suwandinata FS, Bohle RM, Omwandho CA, Tinneberg HR, Gruessner SE. Management of vulvar melanoma and review of the literature. Eur J Gynaecol Oncol. 2007;28(3):220–4.
75. Ragnarsson-Olding BK, Nilsson BR, Kanter-Lewensohn LR, Lagerlöf B, Ringborg UK. Malignant melanoma of the vulva in a nationwide, 25-year study of 219 Swedish females: predictors of survival. Cancer. 1999;86(7):1285–93.
76. Hockstra HJJ, Wobbes T. Radical superficial and deep groin dissection. In: Khatri V, editor. Atlas of advanced operative surgery. Philadelphia: Elsevier; 2012. p. 474–81.
77. Compton C, Byrd DR, Garcia-Aguilar J, et al. Merkel cell carcinoma. In: Compton C, Byrd D, Garcia-Aguilar J, editors. AJCC cancer staging atlas. 2nd ed. New York: Springer; 2012. p. 371–83.
78. Compton C, Byrd D, Garcia-Aguilar J, et al. Melanoma of the skin. In: Compton C, Byrd D, Garcia-Aguilar J, Kurtzman S, Olawaiye A, Washington M, editors. AJCC cancer staging atlas. 2nd ed. New York: Springer; 2012. p. 385–416.

Nonmelanoma Skin Cancers

2

Moshim Kukar, Jacqueline Oxenberg,
Edward Eun Cho, Nathalie C. Zeitouni,
and Joseph Skitzki

Abbreviations

5-FU	5-fluorouracil
AJCC	American Joint Committee on Cancer
AK	Actinic keratosis
AS	Angiosarcoma
BCC	Basal cell carcinoma
CCI	Crude cumulative incidence
CK-20	Cytokeratin 20
CLL	Chronic lymphocytic leukemia
DFSP	Dermatofibrosarcoma protuberans
ED&C	Electrodesiccation and curettage
EMPD	Extramammary Paget's disease
EPC	Eccrine porocarcinoma
MCC	Merkel cell carcinoma
MCV	Merkel cell polyomavirus
MPD	Mammary Paget's disease
NCCN	National Comprehensive Cancer Network
NMSC	Nonmelanoma skin cancer
PDT	Photodynamic therapy
PTCH1	Patched 1 gene
RT	Radiation therapy
SCC	Squamous cell carcinoma
SEER	Surveillance epidemiology and end results
SLNB	Sentinel lymph node biopsy
TTF-1	Thyroid transcription factor 1
UV	Ultraviolet light

M. Kukar, M.D. • J. Oxenberg, D.O.
J. Skitzki, M.D. (✉)
Surgical Oncology, Roswell Park Cancer Institute,
Elm and Carlton Street, Buffalo, NY 14263, USA
e-mail: moshim.kukar@roswellpark.org;
Jackieofrg@yahoo.com; joseph.skitzki@roswellpark.org

E.E. Cho, M.D., Sc.M.
Department of Surgery, Kaleida Health/Buffalo
General Med Center, State University of New York
at Buffalo, 100 High St. Buffalo, 14203 NY, USA
e-mail: eecho@buffalo.edu

N.C. Zeitouni, M.D.C.M.
Dermatology, University of Arizona,
1515 N Campbell Avenue #1907, PO Box 245024,
Tucson, AZ 85724, USA
e-mail: nathaliezeitouni@email.arizona.edu

Learning Objectives

After reading this chapter, you should be able to:

- Describe the most common nonmelanoma skin cancers (NMSC) in terms of epidemiology and etiology
- Identify how NMSC types are diagnosed and select the proper biopsy method
- Define the surgical management options and considerations for NMSC
- Identify the variety of other nonsurgical treatment options and their indications including radiation therapy and topical therapies
- Understand the pattern of metastases for the range of NMSC
- Describe the surveillance for treated NMSC

Q.D. Chu et al. (eds.), *Surgical Oncology: A Practical and Comprehensive Approach*,
DOI 10.1007/978-1-4939-1423-4_2, © Springer Science+Business Media New York 2015

Basal Cell Carcinoma

Basal cell carcinomas (BCC) are the most common type of skin cancer and arise from the basal layer of the epidermis and its appendages. These tumors were referred to as "epitheliomas" because of their low metastatic potential. It is extremely rare for BCC to metastasize to lymph nodes or distant organs. However, the term carcinoma is appropriate, since they are locally invasive and aggressive. The incidence of BCC is rapidly rising [1].

Ultraviolet (UV) light is the greatest risk factor for developing BCC with sun exposure being the most common mechanism. Populations at risk include people with fair skin, light-colored eyes, red hair, northern European ancestry, older age, farming occupations, and family history of BCC [2]. There is also an association between chronic arsenic exposure, ionizing radiation, and chronic immunosuppression [3].

The sonic hedgehog signaling pathway has emerged as having a pivotal role in the pathogenesis of BCC. Mutations in the patched 1 gene (PTCH1) on chromosome 9q, which codes for the sonic hedgehog receptor, are the underlying cause of nevoid basal cell carcinoma syndrome and are frequently seen in sporadic BCC. Specific UV-induced mutations in the tumor suppressor gene p53 also appear to be a common event in developing a malignant phenotype [4].

Approximately 70 % of BCCs occur on the face, consistent with the etiologic role of solar radiation. Fifteen percent present on the trunk, and only rarely is BCC diagnosed on penial, vulvar, or perianal skin. BCC can be divided into several groups, and the three most common ones, based on histopathology, are nodular, superficial, and infiltrative/morpheaform. Nodular BCC is most frequently seen and presents as a pearly or translucent-appearing papule or nodule. Approximately 30 % of BCCs are superficial and most commonly occur on the trunk as a scaly plaque that is erythematous in color. Infiltrative/morpheaform BCCs account for about 5 % of BCCs and are characterized by their ill-defined borders, plaque-like appearance, and high risk of recurrence [5, 6]. A typical, superficial BCC is contrasted to a locally advanced infiltrative BCC as depicted in Fig. 2.1a, b. The current American Joint Committee on Cancer (AJCC) TNM staging classification for BCC overlaps with squamous cell carcinoma of the skin and is listed in Table 2.1 [7].

Surgical Considerations

A detailed clinical examination is paramount, and most BCC can be diagnosed by their appearance. A skin biopsy is usually performed to provide histologic confirmation of the diagnosis. Shave biopsies, punch biopsies, and excisional biopsies can be used for the diagnosis of BCC.

Surgical options for BCCs at low risk for recurrence include conventional surgical excision, Mohs surgery, and electrodesiccation and curettage (ED&C). Typically, surgical excision of the BCC is the preferred option and can often be performed under local anesthesia. Generally, surgical excision of the trunk, extremity, or small facial BCCs of the head or neck with anywhere from 1 to 10 mm margins has been associated with 5-year cure rates exceeding 95 %; therefore, 3–5 mm surgical margins are commonly used for the excision of these lesions [8]. Infiltrative/morpheaform lesions may require wider (5–10 mm) margins due to their indistinct borders. Mohs surgery is usually reserved for lesions that exhibit features associated with an increased risk for recurrence and for locations in which tissue sparing is of great value due to cosmetic or functional concerns. When standard surgical excision is performed, all extremity lesions should be removed in a longitudinal fashion. While a longitudinal incision of the extremity may not be the most cosmetic, it allows for an easier re-excision if the lesion recurs and also disrupts less lymphatic tissue so that lymphedema is minimized (See Chap. 1, Fig. 2.2). The concept of longitudinal excisions of the extremities is critical for all NMSCs and should be considered the standard. Cryosurgery may be used for small superficial lesions, but for larger nodules, its use is infrequent. With proper lesion selection and operator skill/experience, ED&C is capable of achieving a high cure rate.

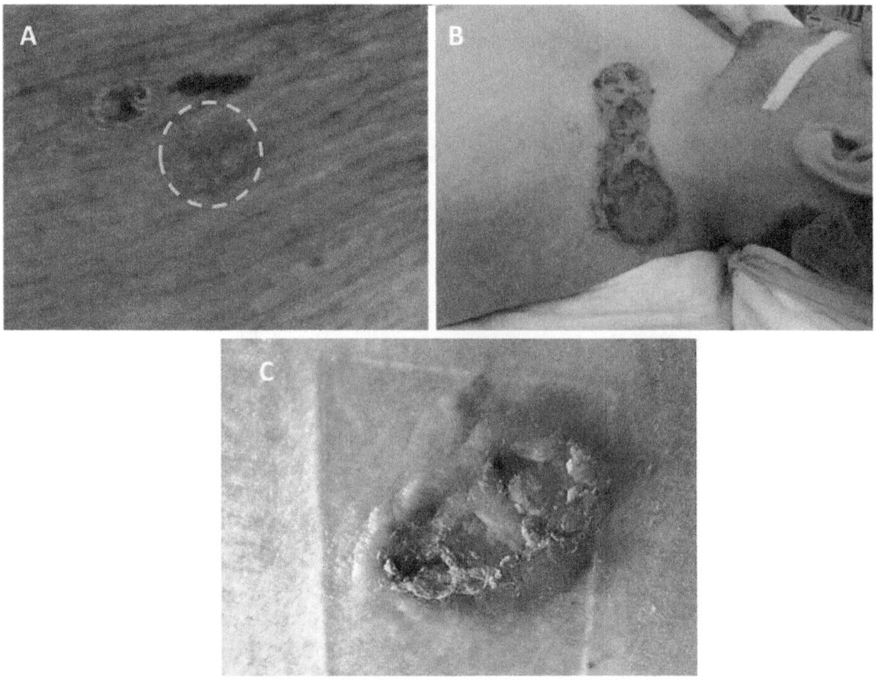

Fig. 2.1 A superficial basal cell carcinoma (BCC) with a characteristic raised, "pearly" appearance is depicted (**a**, *yellow circle*, **c**). A locally advanced infiltrative BCC is shown on the left shoulder/neck area (**b**). While this advanced lesion has low metastatic potential, it was infiltrative into the underlying muscle and along the spinal accessory nerve

Other Treatments

Photodynamic therapy (PDT) is a nonsurgical treatment option for superficial BCCs. The three components of PDT are a light source; exogenous photosensitizer, such as aminolevulinic acid or methyl-aminolevulinic acid; and oxygen. Excellent response rates have been reported for this modality in selected BCC.

The superficial nature of early BCCs allows for effective topical treatments of these lesions. Options for topical therapy include 5-fluorouracil (5-FU) and imiquimod. 5-FU is a pyrimidine analogue that induces cell cycle arrest and apoptosis. Extensive experience with topical 5-FU indicates that this treatment should be restricted to superficial BCCs in non-critical locations. Imiquimod 5 % cream is an immune response modifier that is approved by the US Food and Drug Administration for the treatment of superficial BCCs in low-risk sites. Topical agents require active patient participation and close practitioner surveillance to prevent BCC progression and/or recurrence. All nonresponding lesions should be biopsied for persistent or recurrent disease. Radiation therapy (RT) is utilized as a primary modality in patients who are poor surgical candidates. As an adjuvant therapy, radiation therapy can achieve good results with excellent cosmetic results if applied appropriately especially in patients with high risk of recurrence. A randomized study in 347 patients receiving either surgery or RT as primary treatment of BCC found RT to result in higher recurrence rates than surgery alone (7.5 % vs 0.7 %) [9]. For multiple recurrent BCC that have failed to be cleared by surgical excisions, RT is often a useful option, particularly for microscopically involved margins.

Advances in the understanding of the molecular mechanisms that lead to BCC formation has led to the FDA recently approving a novel agent Vismodegib, a first-in-class Hedgehog pathway inhibitor. This agent can be used for refractory

Table 2.1 American Joint Committee on Cancer (AJCC) TNM staging for cutaneous squamous cell carcinoma and other cutaneous carcinomas (7th edition)

Primary tumor (T)*	
TX	Primary tumor cannot be assessed
T0	No evidence of primary tumor
Tis	Carcinoma in situ
T1	Tumor ≤ 2 cm in greatest dimension with less than two high-risk features**
T2	Tumor > 2 cm in greatest dimension or tumor any size with two or more high-risk features**
T3	Tumor with invasion of maxilla, mandible, orbit, or temporal bone
T4	Tumor with invasion of skeleton (axial or appendicular) or perineural invasion of skull base

* Excludes cSCC of the eyelid

* High-risk features for the primary tumor (T) staging

Depth/invasion	>2 mm thickness
	Clark level ≥ IV
	Perineural invasion
Anatomic location	Primary site ear
	Primary site hair-bearing lip
Differentiation	Poorly differentiated or undifferentiated

Regional lymph nodes (N)	
NX	Regional lymph nodes cannot be assessed
N0	No regional lymph nodes metastases
N1	Metastasis in a single ipsilateral lymph node, ≤3 cm in greatest dimension
N2	Metastasis in a single ipsilateral lymph node, >3 cm ≤ 6 cm in greatest dimension; or in multiple ipsilateral lymph nodes, none > 6 cm in greatest dimension; or in bilateral or contralateral lymph nodes, none > 6 cm in greatest diameter
N2a	Metastasis in a single ipsilateral lymph node, >3 cm but not more than 6 cm in greatest dimension
N2b	Metastasis in multiple ipsilateral lymph nodes, none > 6 cm in greatest dimension
N2c	Metastasis in bilateral or contralateral lymph nodes, none > 6 cm in greatest dimension
N3	Metastasis in a lymph node, >6 cm in greatest dimension

Distant metastasis (M)	
M0	No distant metastasis
M1	Distant metastasis

(continued)

Table 2.1 (continued)

Anatomic stage/prognostic groups			
Group	T	N	M
Stage 0	Tis	N0	M0
Stage I	T1	N0	M0
Stage II	T2	N0	M0
Stage III	T3	N0	M0
	T1-T3	N1	M0
Stage IV	T1-T3	N2	M0
	Any T	N3	M0
	T4	Any N	M0
	Any T	Any N	M1

Reprinted Ref. [46]. With permission from Springer Verlag

locally advanced BCCs that have failed all other options or for the rare metastatic BCC patient. While this treatment is currently quite expensive, the results can be significant in clearing the tumors. Multiple side effects have been reported with this agent which may limit its use in certain patients.

Close follow-up is required following treatment to diagnose both local recurrences and new skin cancers and to assess posttreatment outcomes. Most dermatologists recommend reevaluation every 3–6 months for the first year following treatment and then every 6–12 months thereafter. About 30–50 % of patients may develop another NMSC within 5 years. Therefore, close skin surveillance is mandatory.

Squamous Cell Carcinoma

Squamous cell carcinoma (SCC) is the second most common type of NMSC, accounting for approximately 20 % of all NMSC cases. SCCs can arise de novo, but unlike BCCs, SCCs often arise from precursor lesions that show partial-thickness epidermal dysplasia, such as actinic keratosis (AK). AK presents as slightly scaly papules with ill-defined borders, on sun-exposed skin. Seborrheic keratosis is tan to dark brown stuck-on appearing benign, warty growths located anywhere on the body. The rate of malignant transformation from AK to SCC is estimated to range from 0.025 % to 16 % per year for an individual lesion [10]. Intraepithelial SCC or

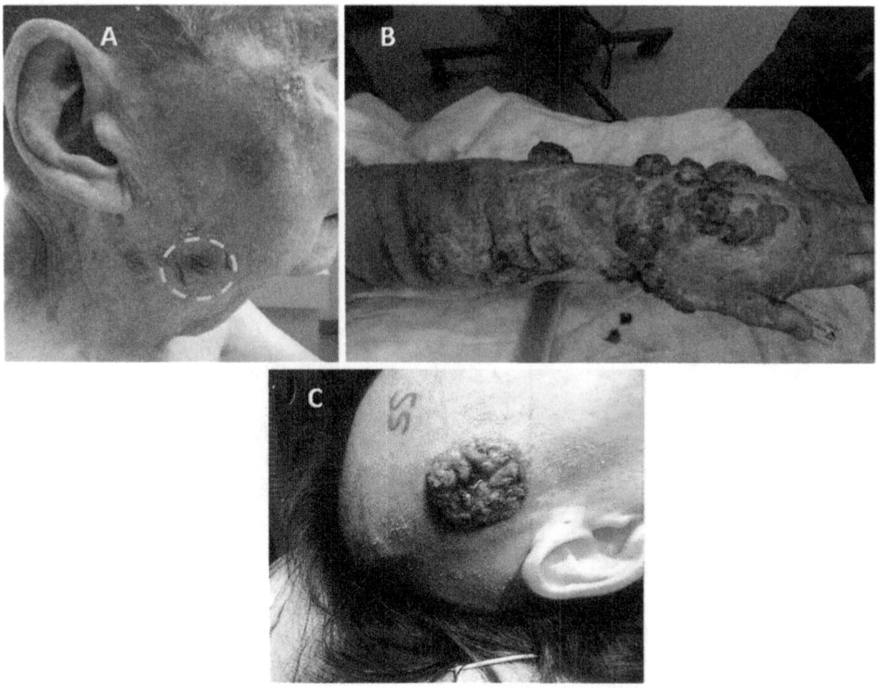

Fig. 2.2 A superficial squamous cell carcinoma (SCC) is noted with a typical raised, scaly/crusty appearance (**a**, *yellow circle*) in the background of multiple actinic keratosis (scaly, *red* patches) or possibly SCC in situ. An advanced SCC of the left hand/forearm demonstrated rapid growth and nodal and visceral metastases (**b**). This local disease was not responsive to systemic treatment, and despite the presence of metastatic disease, surgery was required in the form of an amputation for palliation of pain, bleeding, and infection. (**c**) A neglected SCC of the right scalp was completely excised with clear margins (**c**: Courtesy of Quyen D. Chu, MD, MBA, FACS)

carcinoma in situ is believed to be the next step in the progression to invasive SCC. Risk factors for developing SCC include sun exposure, radiation, chronic inflammation, immunosuppression, and virally induced.

SCC typically develops on areas that are commonly exposed to the sun, including the head and neck, scalp, face, dorsum of hand, shoulder, and chest. The majority of these lesions occur on the head and neck areas. SCCs appear as ill-defined keratotic papules and nodules which may be ulcerated. They can be reddish brown, erythematous, or flesh colored. Occasionally, cutaneous horns from hyperkeratosis may be seen, and bleeding can occur with SCC. A typical SCC in the background of extensive AK is compared to a locally advanced SCC as depicted in Fig. 2.2a, b. Histologically, they show nests of atypical keratinocytes with dermal invasion. In situ lesions, also known as Bowen's disease, are characterized by full-thickness atypical epidermal involvement. Histologic grading is divided into well, moderately, or poorly differentiated. Poorly differentiated lesions have a higher recurrence (28.6 % versus 13.6 %) and metastatic rate (32.8 % versus 9.2 %) compared to well-differentiated lesions [11].

Clinical workup includes a complete history and physical examination, with emphasis on full skin and regional lymph node examinations. Patients may have concurrent cancer located in various sites, and individuals with SCC may be at increased risk of developing BCC and/or melanoma.

A skin biopsy is performed, making sure to obtain full-thickness sample down to the deep reticular dermis. Punch biopsies are simple to perform in the clinic under local anesthesia and yield

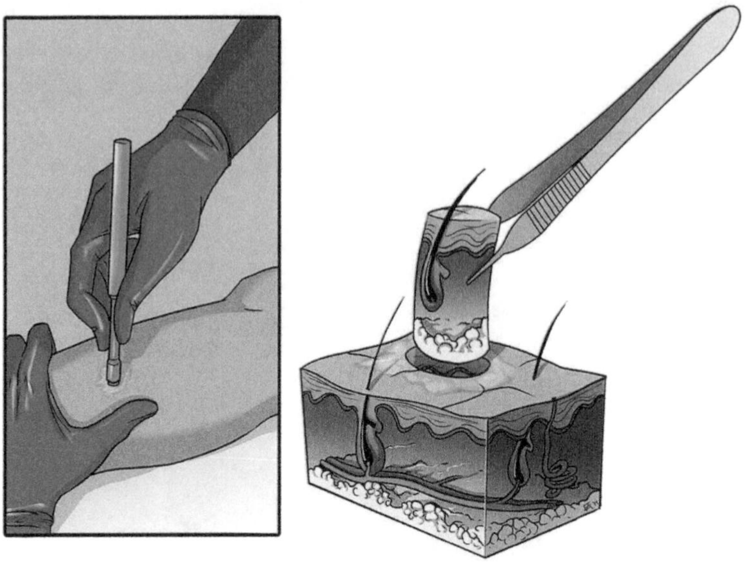

Fig. 2.3 A standard punch biopsy is depicted. The skin lesion is prepped with alcohol, anesthetized with 1 % lidocaine, and a punch biopsy is performed to obtain a full-thickness specimen for further pathologic analysis. An absorbable suture or steri-strip can be placed for re-approximation of the skin (Illustrator-Karen Howard; Courtesy of Quyen D. Chu, MD, MBA, FACS)

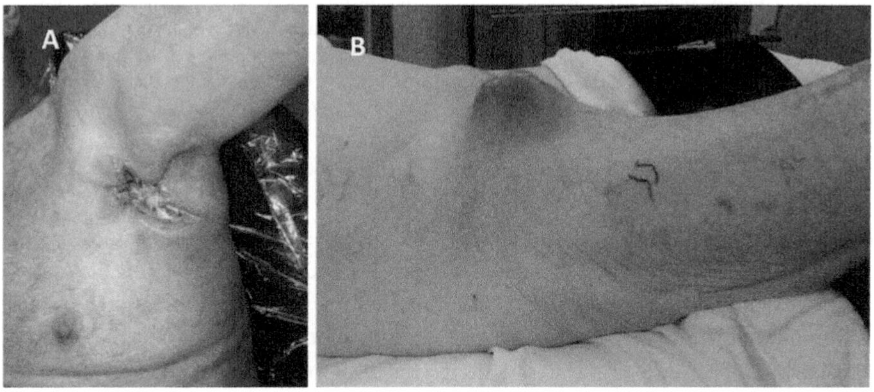

Fig. 2.4 Advanced metastatic lymph nodes to the axillary (**a**) and groin (**b**) lymph node basins. As depicted, these lesions are locally destructive and are prone to necrosis, infection, and significant disability. Extensive surgical resection is required often with the need for soft tissue coverage for closure and adjuvant radiation therapy to improve regional control (**a**: Courtesy of Quyen D. Chu, MD, MBA, FACS)

good full-thickness samples for pathologic evaluation (Fig. 2.3). Imaging studies are rarely necessary and typically reserved only for locally advanced or clinically detected metastatic lesions.

The presence of palpable lymph nodes identified by clinical examination or imaging studies should prompt a fine-needle aspiration for diagnosis. Regional nodal involvement significantly increases the risk of recurrence and mortality and is often associated with other histologic findings including lymphovascular invasion, poor differentiation, and perineural invasion (Fig. 2.4a, b). A fine-needle aspiration or core biopsy is generally sufficient for pathologic diagnosis, and excisional biopsies are discouraged as they may confound future definitive surgical interventions.

Fortunately, the rate of lymph node metastasis from cutaneous SCC is estimated to only be 0.1 % for early lesions, but increases with more advanced lesions.

The American Joint Committee on Cancer (AJCC) TNM staging classification for cutaneous squamous cell carcinoma is listed in Table 2.1 [7].

Surgical Considerations

Surgical excision with at least 4–6 mm margins is the standard of care for small, low-risk squamous cell cancers and is the current recommendation in the NCCN guidelines. Zitelli and colleagues reported that for SCC less than 2 cm in diameter, a 4 mm clinical margin of surgical specimen yielded a complete removal with negative margins with a 95 % confidence interval [12]. Postoperative margin assessment should be performed, and re-excision is indicated for positive margins.

Mohs surgery is an excellent surgical technique for high-risk SCC and those in cosmetically sensitive areas. A meta-analysis reported a 5-year disease-free survival rate after Mohs surgery of 97 % for SCC [11]. Another surgical option is excision with compete circumferential peripheral and deep margin assessment using intraoperative frozen sections or delayed closure/skin grafting with a detailed postoperative margin assessment.

Curettage and electrodesiccation is a process of scraping away tumor tissue then denaturing the area. Up to three cycles can be performed in one session. Overall 5-year cure rate reported for low-risk SCC is 96 % [13]. Three caveats are underscored in the NCCN guidelines: (1) this technique should not be used to treat areas with hair growth due to tumor extending down the follicular structures; (2) if the subcutaneous layer is reached during the course of curettage, surgical excision should be used instead; and (3) biopsy samples should be taken at the time of curettage to analyze for high-risk pathologic features.

The current NCCN recommendations for low-risk SCC are surgical excision with 4–6 mm margins with primary closure, skin graft, or healing by secondary intention, curettage with electrodessication, or radiotherapy for nonsurgical candidates. For high-risk SCC, or those in cosmetically sensitive areas, Mohs surgery or resection with intraoperative frozen sections or radiotherapy is indicated. Sentinel lymph node biopsy (SLNB) for the evaluation of occult nodal metastatic disease can be performed and may allow for more accurate staging in high-risk feature patients. Criteria to perform an SLNB for SCC are not standardized but often include high-risk features of the primary tumor (size >2 cm, poorly differentiated, evidence of perineural or lymphatic invasion) [14]. Positive sentinel lymph node biopsies should be followed by imaging for complete staging and then completion lymphadenectomy in the absence of distant metastatic disease.

If suspicious lymph nodes are seen clinically or by imaging, FNA or core biopsy is indicated. If the lymph nodes return positive for SCC, regional lymph node dissection is recommended. Those with multiple nodes involved should be considered for adjuvant radiotherapy as multiple studies have shown decreased locoregional recurrence and improved 5-year disease-free survival with this modality [15] . Surgical interventions for widely metastatic SCC are limited to palliative procedures to control bleeding, infection, and/or pain when systemic therapy and/or radiation therapy fails. Although exceedingly uncommon, amputation for uncontrolled tumor is a potential option in advanced SCC arising in the extremities.

Other Treatments

Photodynamic therapy (PDT) is a nonsurgical treatment option for actinic keratosis and superficial SCC. Although superficial BCC is most responsive to PDT, there has been some success with SCC. In a retrospective study of 35 superficial SCC defined as carcinoma confined to the papillary dermis, complete response rate was reported to be 54 %. However, projected disease-free rate at 36 months after treatment was only 8 % [16]. A few case reports and series report a high recurrence rate, up to 52 %, for SCC in situ and even higher, 82 %, for invasive SCC lesions [17]. Therefore, PDT is not a recommended treatment modality for invasive SCC tumors.

Topical 5-FU applied twice daily or once daily under occlusion for 1.5–2 months has been reported to have a 54–85 % cure rate for intraepithelial SCC. Less intense regimen reduces the clearance rate to only 27–56 % [18]. Imiquimod stimulates the innate immune response by activating cytokines that ultimately induces interferon-gamma release by T cells. Use of imiquimod for SCC is limited. A randomized, double-blind placebo-controlled trial showed 73 % of SCC in situ lesions that achieved clearance after 16 weeks of imiquimod therapy [19]. Current evidence supports the use of topical imiquimod in poor surgical low-risk candidates with SCC in situ lesions.

Diclofenac is a nonsteroidal anti-inflammatory drug (NSAID) that inhibits cyclooxygenase 2 (COX 2) and thereby reduces the production of prostaglandins. COX 2 enzymes are believed to be upregulated in NMSC lesions. Thus far, topical diclofenac 3 % gel has been approved only for the treatment of actinic keratosis.

Epidermal growth factor receptor (EGFR) is an extracellular signaling receptor in the tyrosine kinase receptor family. Activation of this receptor by various ligands stimulates keratinocyte proliferation. It has been shown that advanced SCC lesions contain EGFR mutation causing overexpression in 43–73 % of cases [20]. Cetuximab is a chimeric monoclonal antibody directed against EGFR. It is currently approved for treatment of recurrent or metastatic SCC of the head and neck. A study comparing radiotherapy alone versus cetuximab combined with radiotherapy showed improved locoregional control and overall survival rate in those that received cetuximab [21]. Erlotinib and gefitinib, which disrupt the intracellular signaling cascade after EGFR is activated, are being investigated for use in cutaneous SCC.

External beam radiation therapy can function both as a primary treatment, especially for advanced head and neck SCC in poor surgical candidates or as adjuvant therapy after surgical excision. A meta-analysis reported a 5-year recurrence rate of 10 % after radiotherapy on patients with high-risk primary SCC [11].

Merkel Cell Carcinoma

Merkel cell carcinoma (MCC) is an aggressive neuroendocrine malignancy that arises in the dermoepidermal junction. It commonly affects elderly Caucasians and was originally described by Toker in 1972 as trabecular carcinoma of the skin. Other names include Toker tumor, primary small cell carcinoma of the skin, primary cutaneous neuroendocrine tumor, and malignant trichodiscoma. Although rare, MCC incidence rates are increasing rapidly. The tumor often appears as an asymptomatic erythematous nodule and may resemble a basal cell carcinoma, a common misdiagnosis both clinically and histologically (Fig. 2.5). The pathogenesis of MCC is controversial. One thought is it arises from Merkel cells, which are part of the amine precursor uptake and decarboxylation system located in the basal layer of the epidermis and hair follicles. Another hypothesis is that MCCs originate from immature stem cells that acquire neuroendocrine features during malignant transformation.

MCCs can be characterized by **AEIOU** features: **A**symptomatic/lack of tenderness, **E**xpanding rapidly, **I**mmune suppression, **O**lder than 50 years, and **U**ltraviolet-exposed site on a person with fair skin [22]. In a SEER data review of 1,034 patients, MCC was more common in males and patients geographically located in sun-exposed climates; 94 % were Caucasian, 76 % were older than 65 years (median 75), and 48 % occurred on the head [23]. MCC has been shown to be more common in immunosuppressed populations such as solid organ transplant recipients and HIV patients. Accordingly, MCC can be aggressive and should be considered to have a high lethal potential with an estimated 1 in 3 patients succumbing to the disease. Of the patients for which MCC is the cause of mortality, half of the patients will die within 4 years of the initial diagnosis.

In 2008, Merkel cell polyomavirus (MCV) was discovered and found to be integrated into the host genome of over 80 % of patients with MCC, and this association has been validated by multiple other studies [24]. An increased incidence of MCCs was found in patients with chronic lymphocytic leukemia (CLL) who are

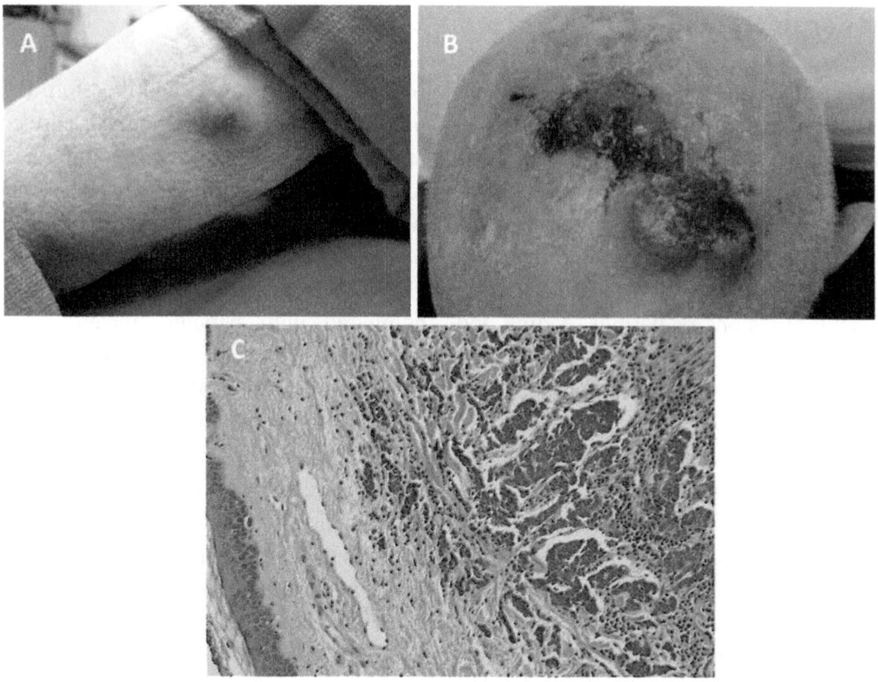

Fig. 2.5 A typical Merkel cell carcinoma (MCC) is shown on the extremity as an erythematous nodule that exhibited a rapid growth phase (**a**). MCC can be locally aggressive and has a high potential for recurrence and metastasis (**b**). Adjuvant radiation therapy following the wide excision of MCC has proven benefit in reducing the local recurrence rate for advanced lesions. (**c**) Photomicrograph depicting clusters of neoplastic cells within the dermis having the finely granular chromatin pattern characteristic of Merkel cell carcinoma (hematoxylin and eosin X 200) (**c**: Courtesy of Barry DeYoung, MD, Wake Forest School of Medicine)

relatively immunosuppressed and have a high rate of MCV detected in their MCC tumors [22].

When MCC is suspected, a punch biopsy or full-thickness biopsy should be performed. There are three main histologic patterns: (1) solid type-most common type, composed of irregular groups of tumor cells interconnected by strands of connective tissue; (2) trabecular type- well-defined cords of cells that form invading columns or cords; and (3) diffuse type- exhibits poor cohesion and a lymphoma-like diffuse type of growth. The pathologic diagnosis is difficult due to its similarity to small round blue cell tumors (small cell carcinoma of the lung, cutaneous large cell lymphoma, neuroblastoma, metastatic carcinoid, amelanotic melanoma, sweat gland carcinoma, Langerhans cell histiocytosis, and Ewing sarcoma). Hematoxylin and eosin (H&E) staining should be confirmed by immunohistochemistry (IHC). CK-20 is both sensitive and specific for MCC with a positivity in 89–100 % cases, and thyroid transcription factor 1 (TTF-1) is consistently negative in MCC [25].

Histologic features that may have prognostic significance include: tumor thickness, presence of lymphovascular invasion, and tumor growth pattern. The AJCC lists site-specific prognostic factors: measured thickness (depth), tumor base transection status, profound immune suppression, tumor infiltrating lymphocytes in the primary tumor, growth pattern of primary tumor, size of tumor nests in regional lymph nodes, clinical status of regional lymph nodes, regional lymph nodes pathologic extracapsular extension, isolated tumor cells in regional lymph node(s) [7]. The majority of patients die from distant metastases involving liver, bone, lung, brain, or distant lymph nodes. Tumors greater than 2 cm in diameter at the time of diagnosis have been shown to have a negative influence on survival.

Surgical Considerations

MCC has a propensity for local recurrence and regional lymph node metastases. Diagnosis is typically made with a skin biopsy after a complete skin and lymph node examination. In 2010, the AJCC published the new staging system for MCC, which is based on primary tumor size and nodal status. The primary lesion should be examined for satellite lesions or dermal seeding and the extent of disease assessed. If lymph nodes are clinically involved, fine-needle aspiration or core biopsy should be performed with consideration of open biopsy if negative. Diagnostic imaging such as CT, MRI, and/or PET/CT should be performed to evaluate disease extent and rule out distant visceral metastases particularly when signs or symptoms of metastatic disease warrant further investigation.

Surgical management continues to be the primary treatment for clinically localized MCCs. Wide local excision with 1–2 cm margins to investing fascia and SLNB are the current recommendations for early stage cancers. In one study, an average margin width of 1.1 cm had a low (8 %) recurrence rate if negative, and a decreased local recurrence rate was not associated with a margin of more than 1 cm [26]. In areas of difficult margins, Mohs micrographic surgery may be an additional option. Primary radiation therapy has also been used successfully in selected patients.

SLNB, although not clearly proven to impact survival, is recommended. The techniques performed are similar to melanoma. Sentinel lymph nodes should be assessed using IHC for more effective metastatic identification, including CK-20 staining. A low rate of lymph node metastases from primary tumors <1 cm has been observed, but the low risk has not been clearly reproducible, and omitting the SLNB procedure for smaller tumors does not appear to be widely accepted. If lymph nodes are clinically positive, FNA or core biopsy should be performed for confirmation followed by either complete lymphadenectomy and/or radiation therapy (RT) for regional control.

Other Treatments

MCC is radiosensitive, and therefore RT is often used adjunctly for locoregional disease control. In an extensive review of the literature, a decreased local recurrence of 10.5 % with RT versus 52.6 % without was found [27]. SEER data review of patients stage I–III had an increased overall survival when treated with surgery plus radiation compared with patients treated with surgery alone. Adjuvant radiation was a component of therapy in 40 % of the surgical cases, and the median survival for those patients receiving adjuvant RT was 63 months compared with 45 months for those treated without. The use of RT was associated with an improved survival for patients with all sizes of tumors, but the improvement was particularly prominent for primary lesions larger than 2 cm [28]. However, not all studies have found an increased survival benefit. NCCN guidelines recommend a total radiation dose of 50–56 Gy in patients with clinically negative margins who are considered to be at significant risk for residual subclinical disease at the resection site.

Data on chemotherapy for MCC is scarce. It is used more often for stage IV and node-positive disease. The Trans-Tasman Radiation Oncology Group (TROG 96:07) performed a phase II trial using carboplatin and etoposide that did not demonstrate an improvement in survival, although the study was thought to be underpowered. When evaluating chemoradiation, TROG 96:07 had 87 % patients complete all 4 cycles of chemotherapy, with a locoregional control rate of 77 % in patients treated in an adjuvant manner and 71 % for those treated therapeutically [29]. The small numbers of patients diagnosed annually with MCC have limited the ability to conduct meaningful clinical trials regarding optimal chemotherapy regimens.

Follow-Up

Close follow-up is recommended for nearly all stages and includes a physical examination of the skin and regional lymph nodes. Current recommendations include exams performed every 3–6 months for the first 2 years and then every 6–12 months.

Dermatofibrosarcoma Protuberans

Dermatofibrosarcoma protuberans (DFSP) is a relatively unusual, locally aggressive cutaneous tumor, characterized by high rates of local recurrence, but low risk of metastasis. DFSP is a rare tumor that constitutes 0.1 % of all malignancies and 1 % of all soft tissue sarcomas. Nevertheless, DFSP is the most common sarcoma of cutaneous origin [30]. The age spectrum varies from congenital cases to patients>90 years old and is equally represented in both sexes. DFSP is an asymptomatic tumor with a slow growth. DFSP is preferentially located on the trunk with 40–50 % of cases found to occur in this area. In 30–40 % of cases, the tumor is located in the proximal portion of the limbs (more often on the arms than the legs), and in 10–15 % of cases, DFSP affects the head and neck areas [30].

Over 90 % of DFSPs are characterized by a unique chromosomal translocation t(17;22)(q22;q13). This translocation results in the gene for platelet-derived growth factor beta polypeptide (PDGFB) being fused with the highly expressed collagen type 1A1 (COL1A1) gene. The resulting PDGFB/COL1A1 fusion protein is processed to produce fully functional PDGFB, which results in continuous autocrine activation of the PDGF receptor b, a tyrosine kinase. This molecular alteration, which has been demonstrated in over 90% of DFSPs, is thought to be fundamental to the development of the tumor [31].

Histologically, DFSP appears as a poorly circumscribed tumor that infiltrates the whole dermis down to fat and muscle and spreads in a tentacle-like fashion into the cellular subcutaneous tissue. The tumor is composed predominantly of a dense, uniform array of cells with spindle-shaped nuclei embedded in varying amounts of collagen. DFSP should be suspected in any patient with a history of a firm, slow-growing cutaneous nodule, and definitive diagnosis requires an incisional or deep punch biopsy representative of the lesion (Fig. 2.6).

Surgical Considerations

The primary treatment of DFSP is surgical removal to obtain clear margins. A wide excision of 2 cm margins including the investing fascia is often definitive; however, larger margins (3–4 cm) can be taken for recurrent or extensive tumors. Deep undermining or raising large flaps should be avoided. Alternatively, Mohs micrographic surgery has been shown to be associated with high cure rates and very low recurrences. Recent reviews have suggested that either wide local excision with appropriate margins or Mohs surgery may have similar outcomes, but that Mohs surgery may be preferable for head and neck tumors or tumors located in areas where tissue sparing is of importance. Irrespective of the approach, the status of the surgical margins is the most important prognostic factor in patients with DFSP. The prognostic importance of resection margins was shown in a series of 159 patients (134 DFSP, 25 DFSP with sarcomatous transformation). At a median follow-up of 57 months, there were 34 recurrences, 29 of which developed in patients with positive or close margins [32].

Other Treatments

Given DFSPs' characteristic chromosomal translocation, t(17;22), orally active small molecule tyrosine kinase inhibitors (TKIs) have been utilized for the rare unresectable or metastatic tumor. The most commonly used agent is imatinib followed by sunitinib and sorafenib often with mixed and transient responses [33].

Although DFSP is a radiosensitive tumor, radiation is rarely used a primary treatment. Despite the absence of randomized clinical trials proving benefit, adjuvant RT may be recommended in conjunction with wide local resection of large tumors or when the surgical margins are

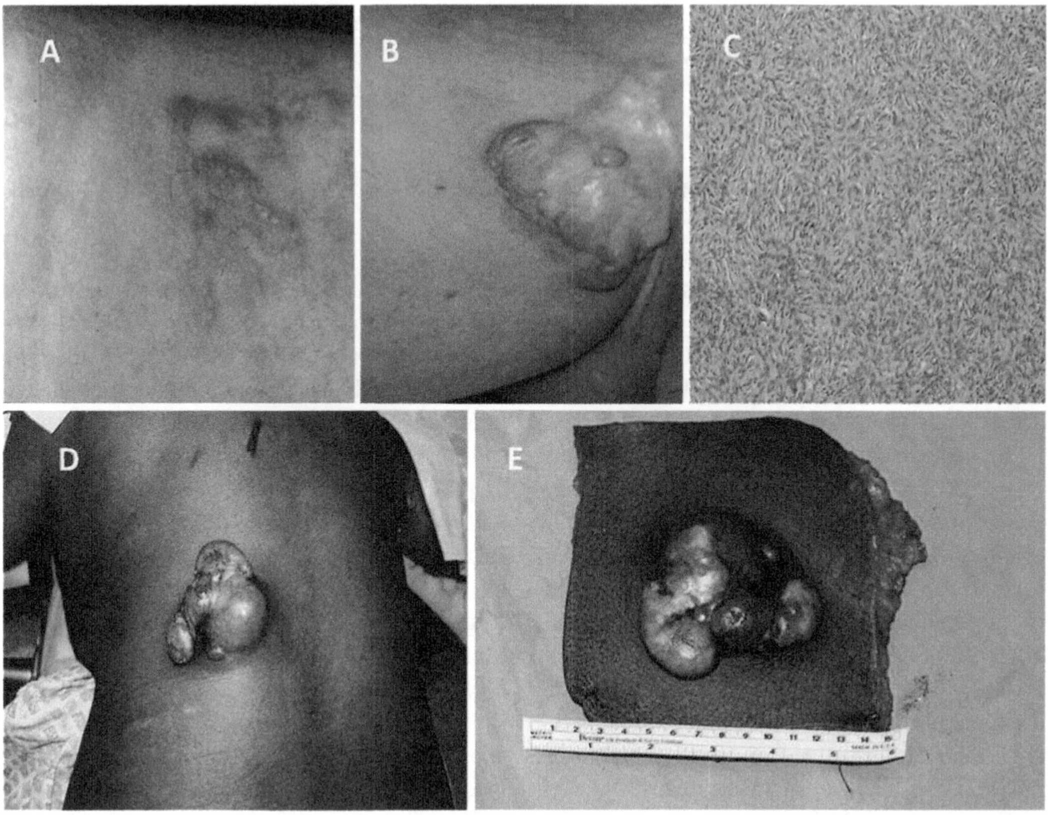

Fig. 2.6 Dermatofibrosarcoma protuberans (DFSPs) present as slow-growing firm nodules in the skin (**a**, **b**, **d**, **e**) and are the most common sarcoma of cutaneous origin. Moh's surgery can be the preferred method in select DFSP; however, larger lesions may require a surgical wide excision. (**c**) Photomicrograph showing mildly atypical spindle cells arranged in a cartwheel or storiform pattern indicative of DFSP (hematoxylin and eosin X 200) (**c**: Courtesy of Barry DeYoung, MD, Wake Forest School of Medicine; **d**, **e**: Courtesy of Quyen D. Chu, MD, MBA, FACS)

close or positive and further surgery is not feasible. If a negative margin is achieved, no adjuvant treatment is necessary.

Current recommendations include follow-up of the primary site every 6–12 months including complete history and physical to rule out metastatic disease. Imaging is rarely required except for high-risk lesions.

Angiosarcoma

Angiosarcomas (AS) are rare endothelial-derived tumors that account for 1–2 % of all soft tissue sarcomas. They can occur anywhere, but are frequently in the skin and soft tissues, most commonly in the head and neck or areas of prior RT. AS may present as blue or erythematous patches, nodules, or tumors on the skin and can occur at a median time of 7 years (3–25 years) from time of radiotherapy. When associated with radiation, AS are usually cutaneous and maybe with edema similar to inflammatory breast cancer or cutaneous infection. Their involvement is often extensive, diffuse, high grade, and can be associated with bleeding.

With an increasing number of cases reported, there is concern about radiation-induced AS in the setting of breast conserving therapy for breast cancer (Fig. 2.7). A cumulative incidence after 15 years was found to be 0.9 per 1,000 for cases receiving radiation and 0.1 per 1,000 for

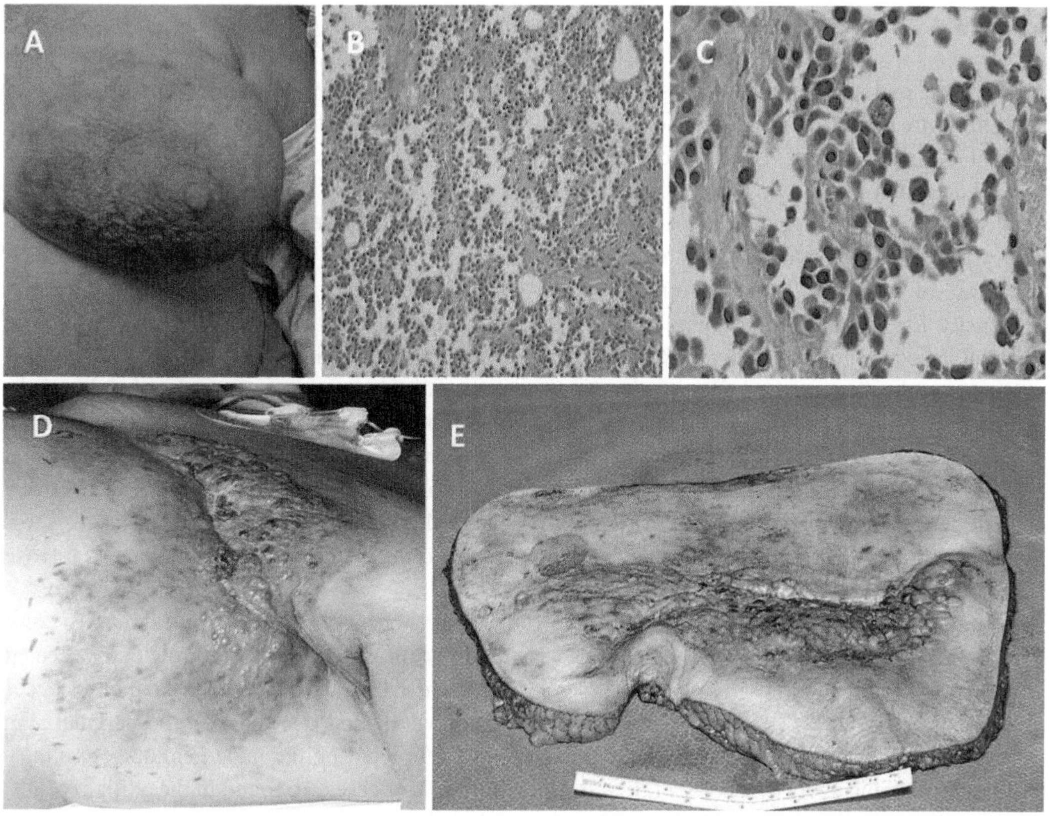

Fig. 2.7 Angiosarcomas may arise in previously irradiated skin and are increasing in frequency with the widespread use of adjuvant radiation for breast cancer (**a**, **d**, **e**). The diffuse nature and characteristic appearance of cutaneous angiosarcoma are noted on the left chest wall in the background of cutaneous radiation changes (**d**). These lesions typically necessitate an excision with wide margins due to their infiltrative nature and tendency for recurrence (**e**). Hematoxylin and eosin (H&E) sections (**b**, **c**) show a high-grade angiosarcoma with dilated vascular spaces that are dissecting and splitting tissue planes. The vascular spaces are lined and filled with highly pleomorphic malignant cells with easily identified mitosis (**a**, **d**, **e**: Courtesy of Quyen D. Chu, MD, MBA, FACS; **b**, **c**: Courtesy of Xin Gu, MD, Louisiana State University Health Sciences Center-Shreveport)

cases not receiving radiation [34]. While the occurrence of sarcoma was low, RT was associated with an increased risk of AS in or adjacent to the radiation field. The relative risk was found to be significant within 5 years of RT, but maximum risk was between 5 and 10 years.

Another variant is Stewart-Treves syndrome, also known as lymphangiosarcoma, which was first reported in a series of six patients in 1948 [35]. It is associated with chronic, long-standing lymphedema. Exogenous toxins or chemicals are also associated with AS including Thorotrast and vinyl chloride which are associated with liver angiosarcoma formation. Similarly, cutaneous angiosarcomas have been related to arsenic, radium, anabolic steroids, and gouty tophus.

Suspicious areas require a punch biopsy or a full-thickness incisional biopsy in areas of suspected AS. FNA can be performed, but are not usually definitive for the diagnosis of AS, particularly in breast cancer survivors where it can be misinterpreted as recurrent carcinoma. A correct diagnosis of this tumor requires immunohistochemical evidence of endothelial differentiation. Typical markers for AS include vimentin, factor VIII, CD31, and CD34 [36].

Surgical Considerations

Lesion size and presence of metastases often determine treatment options. Tumor imaging modalities such as CT or MRI are recommended as well as abdominal/pelvic CT and central nervous system imaging to rule out metastatic disease, which is common to the lungs and liver.

AS are biologically aggressive tumors with a propensity for metastases and being multifocal. Surgical resection with negative (R0) margins continues to be the standard for curative treatment. Wide margins are recommended which often necessitate complex reconstructions, especially when AS is RT induced. Clinically undetectable intradermal spread in addition to a high incidence of multicentricity and unclear borders results in high local recurrence rates even after R0 resections.

Other Treatments

Despite its biologic aggressiveness, a fair number of AS will respond to systemic chemotherapy. Previous literature shows a 3.8–44 % complete response rate and a 88–93 % clinical response rate with regimens using combinations of paclitaxel, doxorubicin, and gemcitabine [37]. Response rates of approximately 10 % are found with antiangiogenic agents that are mainly used for locally advanced or metastatic disease. There is limited data, but neoadjuvant chemotherapy may be useful prior to surgical excision to reduce local recurrence rates and improve recurrence-free survival.

Although seemingly counterintuitive as many AS are radiation induced, additional RT (mostly wide-field electron-beam therapy) has been found to result in regression of local skin disease and potentially prolonged survival.

Follow-Up

Patients should have a history and physical every 3–6 months for 2–3 years and then annually. Disease progression or recurrence should be managed accordingly depending on local or distant progression. Chest imaging can be considered every 6–12 months as well as primary site imaging (US, MRI, or CT).

Paget's Disease

Paget's disease is a rare cutaneous adenocarcinoma that occurs in elderly women more often than in men. It typically presents as an erythematous, scaly, eczematous plaque frequently misdiagnosed as inflammatory or infectious dermatitis. Most commonly affected sites include unilateral nipple/areola complex in mammary Paget's disease (MPD) and the vulva, perianal skin, scrotum, and penis in extramammary Paget's disease (EMPD).

EMPD occurs in apocrine-rich skin most commonly in the elderly. The most frequently affected site is the labia majora. Two thirds of cases occur on the vulva, and one third on the perianal skin and 14 % occur on the male genitalia (scrotum). Only 2 % of cases are found in the axilla, eyelids, external ear canals, trunk, and mucosal surfaces.

While most cases of MPD are associated with underlying breast carcinoma (82–92 %), EMPD is less often associated with an underlying neoplasm (9–32 %) [38]. It was therefore proposed that cases of extramammary Paget's disease can arise as epidermotropic spread from an in situ or invasive neoplasm arising in an adnexal gland within the dermis, analogous to mammary Paget's disease without a primary breast neoplasm. Of all patients with EMPD, 36 % have a strong anatomic association of internal malignancy with the EMPD site, and EMPD in the perianal area has a higher association rate (50–86 %) with an internal malignancy than those with EMPD on the labia majora (5–25 %) [39].

Several punch biopsies should be performed for diagnosis and assessment of depth of invasion. The use of immunohistochemistry may be necessary to confirm the diagnosis. For EMPD, underlying gastrointestinal or genitourinary neoplasms must be ruled out. Imaging of the abdomen and pelvis, colonoscopy, barium enema, cystoscopy, intravenous pyelogram, chest X-ray and mammogram (for the rare association of EMPD and MPD), and blood work (CEA) are all appropriate tests. FDG-PET may have utility in ruling out lymph node metastases and identifying a primary, but it is not a standard recommendation at this time.

Surgical Considerations

While there is no consensus on treatment of EMPD, surgical wide excision or Mohs micrographic surgery continues to be preferred treatments. No clear recommendations for margin width exist. Typically, wide margins up to 3 cm are recommended, but wide local excision with a 1 cm margin from the clinical border may produce negative margins and low local recurrence rates in select patients [40]. Unfortunately, multifocal and unclear borders may lead to high margin positivity. Intraoperative frozen margin assessment in addition to wide local excision and intraoperative re-excision for margin positivity is recommended. Mohs surgery can be effective and may be associated with lower rates of recurrence compared to wide local excision. Preoperative mapping biopsies to evaluate the extent of disease are often very helpful. When invasive to the subcutaneous tissues, EMPDs have a high rate of lymph node metastasis, and SLNB should be considered for staging.

Other Treatments

Trials for EMPD are few since the tumor is rare, and therefore most data for nonsurgical management consists of small series and case reports. Use of nonsurgical modalities to treat EMPD including topical imiquimod, topical 5-FU, topical bleomycin, photodynamic therapy, CO2 laser ablation, and topical retinoids has been reported with mixed results. Photodynamic therapy is not recommended for scrotal lesions or lesions <4 cm due to high recurrence rates. Radiation therapy was found effective and well tolerated for EMPD and can provide good local control. Radiation can be used to treat the primary lesion in inoperable patients or as an adjuvant for positive margins or high-risk tumors.

No optimal chemotherapy regimen for EMPD exists. Case reports for combination chemotherapy including mitomycin C and epirubicin, vincristine, cisplatin, docetaxel, and 5-FU have shown pathologic and complete responses [41]. Additionally, the overexpression of HER-2/neu in primary EMPD suggests a role for directed therapy with trastuzumab in patients with recurrent disease [42].

Follow-Up

While no clear guidelines exist, patients should have long-term follow-up with routine skin as well as regional lymph node examinations similar to other NMSC protocols. If a primary source is suspected, but not yet found, other imaging modalities as well as laboratory tests may be useful and may be repeated on a regular basis.

Eccrine Porocarcinoma

Eccrine porocarcinoma (EPC) is a rare malignancy arising from intraepidermal eccrine sweat ducts (Fig. 2.8). EPC lesions occur most commonly in the lower extremities but are also found on the head and neck. EPC may arise de novo into a malignant form but most often develops from a long-standing benign eccrine poroma that has undergone degenerative changes [43]. EPC has been reported to arise in association with extra mammary Paget's disease, sarcoidosis, chronic lymphocytic leukemia, pernicious anemia, Hodgkin's disease, HIV, and in rare cases, xeroderma pigmentosum and chronic radiation exposure.

EPC lesions present as firm, erythematous to violaceous nodules usually less than 2 cm in size. Signs and symptoms of malignant transformation include bleeding, ulceration, pain or itching, or sudden increase in size. Immunostaining is essential in establishing a diagnosis, especially to rule out the possibility of metastatic adenocarcinoma or an amelanotic melanoma. The presence of ductal structures and a PAS-positive cuticle

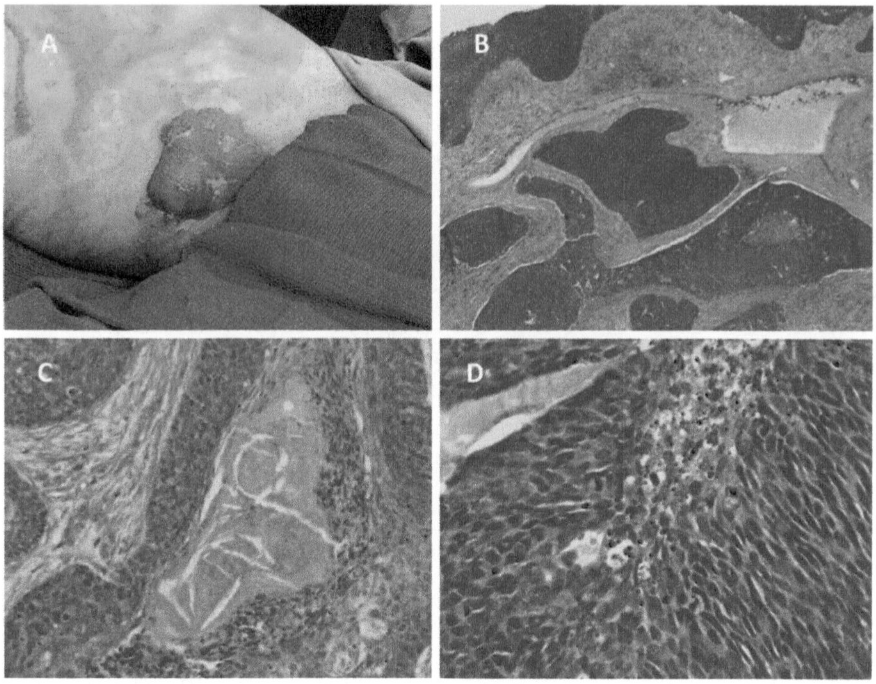

Fig. 2.8 Eccrine carcinoma occurring in a thigh (**a**). This tumor is presented in the epidermis and extends into the dermis with large cords, lobules, and islands. There is frequent central necrosis, and the tumor cells are large, hyperchromatic with marked nuclear atypia. Brisk mitosis and apoptosis are also present. The tumor shows ductal differentiation with forming PAS-positive curtile materials (**b**–**d**) (**a**: Courtesy of Roger Kim, MD, Louisiana State University Health Sciences Center-Shreveport; **b**–**d**: Courtesy of Xin Gu, MD, Louisiana State University Health Sciences Center-Shreveport)

makes metastatic adenocarcinoma less likely. Poor prognostic features include thickness >7 mm, lymphovascular invasion, and more than 14 mitoses per high power field [44].

Surgical Considerations

Primary surgical excision is the treatment of choice for EPC including either wide excision or Mohs surgery. One study reviewing 9 cases of EPC reported a curative rate of 70–80 % after excision with 2 cm margins [45]. For recurrent or metastatic EPC tumors, limited data exist. Response to radiation therapy is often partial and is reserved for palliative care. Systemic chemotherapy has also shown limited response. Therefore, early detection and definitive excision provides the highest chance of survival. Due to EPC rarity, the role of sentinel lymph node biopsy for staging EPC has not been defined, but should be considered for accurate staging.

Special Consideration: Neglected NMSC

Not uncommonly, patients will present to the surgeon with locally advanced BCC and SCC. The causes of late presentations include neglect due to patient anxiety, denial, and/or economic considerations. However, some lesions such as MCC may grow rapidly and present in a locally advanced state despite patient diligence. The standard evaluation should be performed including a thorough history and physical examination looking for signs or symptoms of distant metastatic disease. When appropriate, imaging should be obtained to rule out distant metastases. If distant metastases are found, then the treatment options should favor a systemic approach such as chemotherapy or targeted therapy. In the background of metastatic disease, surgery should be employed for the locally advanced primary lesion only for palliation of uncontrolled bleeding, pain, or infection. If no evidence of metastatic disease is identified, then an extensive surgery to obtain clear margins should be planned with the likelihood of delayed closure if all margins are free of tumor. Primary suture closure is usually not possible, so consideration for healing by secondary intention, delayed skin grafting, and/or rotational or free flaps may be necessary. Given the often extensive nature of these lesions, either neoadjuvant or adjuvant radiation therapy should also be considered.

Salient Points

- *Basal cell carcinoma (BCC)*
  - The most common type of skin cancer.
  - Treatment is wide local excision (WLE).
    - 3–5 mm margin is adequate.
    - 5–10 mm margin for infiltrative/morpheaform lesions.
  - Moh's surgery is also appropriate.
  - Nonsurgical options include PDT, topical 5-FU, imiquimod, and XRT.
  - Vismodegib: Hedgehog pathway inhibitor FDA approved for refractory locally advanced BCC or metastatic BCC.
- *Squamous cell carcinoma (SCC)*
  - The second most common type of nonmelanoma skin cancer.
  - Can arise from actinic keratosis.
  - Bowen's disease: in situ lesion.
  - Treatment is WLE with 4–6 mm margin.
  - Moh's surgery is also appropriate.
  - Sentinel lymph node biopsy (SLNBx) is an option for high-risk lesions (size>2 cm, poorly differentiated, perineural or lymphatic invasion).
  - Palpable lymph nodes require FNA for diagnosis.
  - Positive LNs require node dissection.
  - Nonsurgical options include PDT for superficial SCC but not invasive SCC, topical 5-FU, imiquimod, and XRT.
  - Topical diclofenac is indicated for actinic keratosis.
  - Cetuximab: anti-EFR approved for recurrent or metastatic SCC of the head and neck.
- *Merkel cell carcinoma*
  - Aggressive neuroendocrine tumor arises in the dermoepidermal junction.
  - Affects elderly Caucasians.
  - Associated with Merkel cell polyomavirus.
  - AEIOU features: asymptomatic, expanding rapidly, immune suppression, older than 50 years, ultraviolet-exposed site on a person with fair skin.
  - Common in immunosuppressed populations (organ transplant recipient and HIV patients).
  - Positive staining for CK-20, but negative for thyroid transcription factor 1 (TTF-1).
  - Size>2 cm in diameter portends a poor prognosis.
  - Treatment is WLE (1–2 cm margins) and SLNBx.
    - Lymphadenectomy for involved lymph nodes
  - XRT is used adjunctly for locoregional control.
  - Other treatment options: Moh's surgery.
- *Dermatofibrosarcoma protuberans (DFSP)*
  - Locally aggressive with high rates of local recurrence but low risk of metastasis.
  - The most common sarcoma of cutaneous origin.
  - Ninety percent due to chromosomal translocation resulting in PDGFB/COLIA1 fusion protein.
  - Treatment: WLE with at least 2 cm margins including the investing fascia.
  - Larger margins (3–4 cm) may be required for recurrent or extensive tumors.
  - Moh's is also an option.
  - Imatinib, sunitinib, and sorafenib have been used with mixed results.
  - XRT may be used for large tumors or when margins are close or positive, and further surgery is not feasible.
- *Angiosarcoma*
  - Highly aggressive tumor with poor outcome

- Associated with radiation, especially in the setting of breast conserving therapy for breast cancer
- Stewart-Treves syndrome (lymphangiosarcoma): variant of angiosarcoma, associated with long-standing lymphedema
- Need to rule out metastatic disease as part of the workup
- Requires wide margin of resection
- May require paclitaxel, doxorubicin, and gemcitabine

• *Paget's Disease*
  - Rare cutaneous adenocarcinoma, scaly eczematous plaque.
  - Affects nipple/areolar complex.
  - Recommended margins: 3 cm.
  - Moh's surgery may be an option.

• *Eccrine porocarcinoma*
  - Arises form intraepidermal eccrine sweat ducts.
  - Treatment is WLE with 2 cm margins.

Questions

1. All of the following characteristics regarding BCC are true *EXCEPT*:
   A. Induced by UV radiation.
   B. Frequently metastasize to distant sites.
   C. Associated with a known mutation in hedgehog signaling.
   D. Surgical therapy is often curative.
2. Regarding NMSCs, incisional biopsies or definitive wide excisions should be performed:
   A. Transversely on extremities
   B. Longitudinally on extremities
   C. With no consideration for the next step
   D. In the easiest manner to close
3. A 38-year-old, red-headed woman who has an extensive history of tanning presents with a raised, pearly white lesion on her shoulder. The immediate next step in management is:
   A. Close follow-up
   B. Wide excision with 3 mm margins
   C. Radiation therapy
   D. Full-thickness biopsy
4. Features that are associated with a worse prognosis in SCC include all of the following *EXCEPT*:
   A. Poorly differentiated histology
   B. Evidence of perineural invasion
   C. Lymph node metastasis
   D. Noninvasive or in situ disease at time of presentation
5. Which of the following is a true statement regarding MCC:
   A. Associated with Merkel cell polyomavirus
   B. Less common in immunosuppressed populations
   C. Radiation resistant
   D. Can be distinguished as cutaneous in origin by TTF-1 staining
6. DFSPs are accurately characterized by each of the following statements *EXCEPT*:
   A. Associated with a distinct chromosomal translocation.
   B. Commonly spreads to lymph nodes.
   C. Maybe treated with tyrosine kinase inhibitors.
   D. Clear surgical margins are generally curative.
7. True or False: Angiosarcomas rarely arise from previously irradiated fields.
   A. True
   B. False
8. True or False: Surgery remains the most important, curative treatment modality for NMSCs.
   A. True
   B. False

Answers

1. B
2. B
3. D
4. D
5. A
6. B
7. B
8. A

References

1. Kasper M, Jaks V, Hohl D, Toftgard R. Basal cell carcinoma – molecular biology and potential new therapies. J Clin Invest. 2012;122(2):455–63. Epub 2012/02/02.
2. Hogan DJ, To T, Gran L, Wong D, Lane PR. Risk factors for basal cell carcinoma. Int J Dermatol. 1989;28(9):591–4. Epub 1989/11/01.
3. Roewert-Huber J, Lange-Asschenfeldt B, Stockfleth E, Kerl H. Epidemiology and aetiology of basal cell carcinoma. Br J Dermatol. 2007;157 Suppl 2:47–51. Epub 2007/12/11.
4. de Zwaan SE, Haass NK. Genetics of basal cell carcinoma. Australas J Dermatol. 2010;51(2):81–92; quiz 3–4; Epub 2010/06/16.
5. Dourmishev LA, Rusinova D, Botev I. Clinical variants, stages, and management of basal cell carcinoma. Indian Dermatol Online J. 2013;4(1):12–7. Epub 2013/02/27.
6. Saldanha G, Fletcher A, Slater DN. Basal cell carcinoma: a dermatopathological and molecular biological update. Br J Dermatol. 2003;148(2):195–202. Epub 2003/02/18.
7. Edge SB, Byrd DR, Compton CC, et al. Cutaneous squamous cell carcinoma and other cutaneous carcinomas. In: AJCC cancer staging manual. 7th ed. New York: Springer; 2010. p. 523–6.
8. Gulleth Y, Goldberg N, Silverman RP, Gastman BR. What is the best surgical margin for a Basal cell carcinoma: a meta-analysis of the literature. Plast Reconstr Surg. 2010;126(4):1222–31. Epub 2010/10/05.
9. Avril MF, Auperin A, Margulis A, Gerbaulet A, Duvillard P, Benhamou E, et al. Basal cell carcinoma of the face: surgery or radiotherapy? Results of a randomized study. Br J Cancer. 1997;76(1):100–6. Epub 1997/01/01.
10. Stockfleth E. The paradigm shift in treating actinic keratosis: a comprehensive strategy. J Drugs Dermatol: JDD. 2012;11(12):1462–7. Epub 2013/02/05.
11. Rowe DE, Carroll RJ, Day Jr CL. Prognostic factors for local recurrence, metastasis, and survival rates in squamous cell carcinoma of the skin, ear, and lip. Implications for treatment modality selection. J Am Acad Dermatol. 1992;26(6):976–90. Epub 1992/06/11.
12. Brodland DG, Zitelli JA. Surgical margins for excision of primary cutaneous squamous cell carcinoma. J Am Acad Dermatol. 1992;27(2 Pt 1):241–8. Epub 1992/08/01.
13. Samarasinghe V, Madan V. Nonmelanoma skin cancer. J Cutan Aesthet Surg. 2012;5(1):3–10. Epub 2012/05/05.
14. Kwon S, Dong ZM, Wu PC. Sentinel lymph node biopsy for high-risk cutaneous squamous cell carcinoma: clinical experience and review of literature. World J Surg Oncol. 2011;9:80. Epub 2011/07/21.
15. Veness MJ. High-risk cutaneous squamous cell carcinoma of the head and neck. J Biomed Biotechnol. 2007;2007(3):80572. Epub 2007/06/02.
16. Fink-Puches R, Soyer HP, Hofer A, Kerl H, Wolf P. Long-term follow-up and histological changes of superficial nonmelanoma skin cancers treated with topical delta-aminolevulinic acid photodynamic therapy. Arch Dermatol. 1998;134(7):821–6. Epub 1998/07/29.
17. Marmur ES, Schmults CD, Goldberg DJ. A review of laser and photodynamic therapy for the treatment of nonmelanoma skin cancer. Dermatol Surg. 2004;30(2 Pt 2):264–71. Epub 2004/02/12.
18. Morton C, Horn M, Leman J, Tack B, Bedane C, Tjioe M, et al. Comparison of topical methyl aminolevulinate photodynamic therapy with cryotherapy or fluorouracil for treatment of squamous cell carcinoma in situ: results of a multicenter randomized trial. Arch Dermatol. 2006;142(6):729–35. Epub 2006/06/21.
19. Patel GK, Goodwin R, Chawla M, Laidler P, Price PE, Finlay AY, et al. Imiquimod 5% cream monotherapy for cutaneous squamous cell carcinoma in situ (Bowen's disease): a randomized, double-blind, placebo-controlled trial. J Am Acad Dermatol. 2006;54(6):1025–32. Epub 2006/05/23.
20. Uribe P, Gonzalez S. Epidermal growth factor receptor (EGFR) and squamous cell carcinoma of the skin: molecular bases for EGFR-targeted therapy. Pathol Res Pract. 2011;207(6):337–42. Epub 2011/05/03.
21. Bonner JA, Harari PM, Giralt J, Azarnia N, Shin DM, Cohen RB, et al. Radiotherapy plus cetuximab for squamous-cell carcinoma of the head and neck. N Engl J Med. 2006;354(6):567–78. Epub 2006/02/10.
22. Heath M, Jaimes N, Lemos B, Mostaghimi A, Wang LC, Penas PF, et al. Clinical characteristics of Merkel cell carcinoma at diagnosis in 195 patients: the AEIOU features. J Am Acad Dermatol. 2008;58(3): 375–81. Epub 2008/02/19.
23. Agelli M, Clegg LX. Epidemiology of primary Merkel cell carcinoma in the United States. J Am Acad Dermatol. 2003;49(5):832–41. Epub 2003/10/25.
24. Feng H, Shuda M, Chang Y, Moore PS. Clonal integration of a polyomavirus in human Merkel cell carcinoma. Science. 2008;319(5866):1096–100. Epub 2008/01/19.
25. Scott MP, Helm KF. Cytokeratin 20: a marker for diagnosing Merkel cell carcinoma. Am J Dermatopathol. 1999;21(1):16–20. Epub 1999/02/23.
26. Allen PJ, Bowne WB, Jaques DP, Brennan MF, Busam K, Coit DG. Merkel cell carcinoma: prognosis and treatment of patients from a single institution. J Clin Oncol. 2005;23(10):2300–9. Epub 2005/04/01.
27. Medina-Franco H, Urist MM, Fiveash J, Heslin MJ, Bland KI, Beenken SW. Multimodality treatment of Merkel cell carcinoma: case series and literature review of 1024 cases. Ann Surg Oncol. 2001;8(3):204–8. Epub 2001/04/21.
28. Mojica P, Smith D, Ellenhorn JD. Adjuvant radiation therapy is associated with improved survival in Merkel cell carcinoma of the skin. Journal Clin Oncol. 2007;25(9):1043–7. Epub 2007/03/21.

29. Poulsen M, Rischin D, Walpole E, Harvey J, Mackintosh J, Ainslie J, et al. High-risk Merkel cell carcinoma of the skin treated with synchronous carboplatin/etoposide and radiation: a Trans-Tasman Radiation Oncology Group Study–TROG 96:07. J Clin Oncol. 2003;21(23):4371–6. Epub 2003/12/04.
30. Sanmartin O, Llombart B, Lopez-Guerrero JA, Serra C, Requena C, Guillen C. Dermatofibrosarcoma protuberans. Actas dermo-sifiliograficas. 2007;98(2):77–87. Epub 2007/04/03.
31. Llombart B, Serra-Guillen C, Monteagudo C, Lopez Guerrero JA, Sanmartin O. Dermatofibrosarcoma protuberans: a comprehensive review and update on diagnosis and management. Semin Diagn Pathol. 2013;30(1):13–28. Epub 2013/01/19.
32. Gloster Jr HM. Dermatofibrosarcoma protuberans. J Am Acad Dermatol. 1996;35(3 Pt 1):355–74; quiz 75–6; Epub 1996/09/01.
33. Malhotra B, Schuetze SM. Dermatofibrosarcoma protuberans treatment with platelet-derived growth factor receptor inhibitor: a review of clinical trial results. Curr Opin Oncol. 2012;24(4):419–24. Epub 2012/04/19.
34. Monroe AT, Feigenberg SJ, Mendenhall NP. Angiosarcoma after breast-conserving therapy. Cancer. 2003;97(8):1832–40. Epub 2003/04/04.
35. Stewart FW, Treves N. Lymphangiosarcoma in postmastectomy lymphedema; a report of six cases in elephantiasis chirurgica. Cancer. 1948;1(1):64–81. Epub 1948/05/01.
36. Breiteneder-Geleff S, Soleiman A, Kowalski H, Horvat R, Amann G, Kriehuber E, et al. Angiosarcomas express mixed endothelial phenotypes of blood and lymphatic capillaries: podoplanin as a specific marker for lymphatic endothelium. Am J Pathol. 1999;154(2):385–94. Epub 1999/02/23.
37. DeMartelaere SL, Roberts D, Burgess MA, Morrison WH, Pisters PW, Sturgis EM, et al. Neoadjuvant chemotherapy-specific and overall treatment outcomes in patients with cutaneous angiosarcoma of the face with periorbital involvement. Head Neck. 2008;30(5):639–46. Epub 2008/01/24.
38. Lloyd J, Flanagan AM. Mammary and extramammary Paget's disease. J Clin Pathol. 2000;53(10):742–9. Epub 2000/11/07.
39. Goldblum JR, Hart WR. Perianal Paget's disease: a histologic and immunohistochemical study of 11 cases with and without associated rectal adenocarcinoma. Am J Surg Pathol. 1998;22(2):170–9. Epub 1998/03/21.
40. Murata Y, Kumano K. Extramammary Paget's disease of the genitalia with clinically clear margins can be adequately resected with 1 cm margin. Eur J Dermatol: EJD. 2005;15(3):168–70. Epub 2005/05/24.
41. Moretto P, Nair VJ, Hallani SE, Malone S, Belanger E, Morash C, et al. Management of penoscrotal extramammary Paget disease: case series and review of the literature. Curr Oncol. 2013;20(4):e311–20. Epub 2013/08/02.
42. Plaza JA, Torres-Cabala C, Ivan D, Prieto VG. HER-2/neu expression in extramammary Paget disease: a clinicopathologic and immunohistochemistry study of 47 cases with and without underlying malignancy. J Cutan Pathol. 2009;36(7):729–33. Epub 2009/06/13.
43. Penneys NS, Ackerman AB, Indgin SN, Mandy SH. Eccrine poroma: two unusual variants. Br J Dermatol. 1970;82(6):613–5. Epub 1970/06/01.
44. Robson A, Greene J, Ansari N, Kim B, Seed PT, McKee PH, et al. Eccrine porocarcinoma (malignant eccrine poroma): a clinicopathologic study of 69 cases. Am J Surg Pathol. 2001;25(6):710–20. Epub 2001/06/08.
45. Lozano Orella JA, Valcayo Penalba A, San Juan CC, Vives Nadal R, Castro Morrondo J, Tunon AT. Eccrine porocarcinoma. Report of nine cases. Dermatol Surg. 1997;23(10):925–8.
46. Compton C, Byrd D, Garcia-Aguilar J, et al. Cutaneous squamous cell carcinoma and other cutaneous carcinomas. In: Compton C, Byrd D, Garcia-Aguilar J, Kurtzman S, Olawaiye A, Washington M, editors. AJCC cancer staging atlas. 2nd ed. New York: Springer; 2012. p. 357–70.

Part II

Breast

Noninvasive Breast Cancer

3

Tania K. Arora and Harry D. Bear

Abbreviations

DCIS	Ductal carcinoma in situ
LCIS	Lobular carcinoma in situ
SEER	Surveillance, epidemiology, and end results
ADH	Atypical ductal hyperplasia
ER	Estrogen receptor
PR	Progesterone receptor
BCT	Breast-conserving therapy
NSABP	National surgical adjuvant breast & bowel project
EORTC	European Organization for Research and Treatment of Cancer
ECOG	Eastern Cooperative Oncology Group
SLNB	Sentinel lymph node biopsy
NCCN	National Comprehensive Cancer Network
MRI	Magnetic resonance imaging
STAR	Study of tamoxifen and raloxifen
PLCIS	Pleomorphic lobular carcinoma in situ

T.K. Arora, M.D.
Department of Surgery, Geisinger Health System,
100 North Academy Ave., Danville, PA 17822, USA
e-mail: tkarora@hotmail.com

H.D. Bear, M.D., Ph.D. (✉)
Department of Surgery, Virginia Commonwealth
University, P.O. Box 980011, Richmond
VA 23298-0011, USA
e-mail: hdbear@vcu.edu

Learning Objectives

After reading this chapter, you should be able to:

1. Classify noninvasive breast cancers
2. Identify risk factors
3. Describe the diagnostic workup
4. Understand pathologic characteristics
5. Describe medical and surgical therapies

Background

The two common types of noninvasive breast cancer are known as ductal carcinoma in situ (DCIS) and lobular carcinoma in situ (LCIS). In both of these lesions, abnormal cells are present within the milk ducts (DCIS) or the lining of a lobule (LCIS). "In situ" is the Latin word for "in the original position" and indicates that the abnormal cells have not invaded through the basement membrane (Fig. 3.1). These lesions have different behaviors and a different demographic profile. While neither has any potential for metastasis or death, the treatment and prevention goals for DCIS are more aggressive. In fact, LCIS, despite the word "carcinoma" in its name, should NOT be considered a malignant diagnosis. The American Cancer society estimates that 63,300 new cases of carcinoma in situ of the breast were diagnosed in the United States in 2012. The majority of in situ breast cancers are DCIS, which accounted for 83 % of in situ cases diagnosed between 2004 and 2008 [1]. The incidence of DCIS increases with age and increased

Q.D. Chu et al. (eds.), *Surgical Oncology: A Practical and Comprehensive Approach*,
DOI 10.1007/978-1-4939-1423-4_3, © Springer Science+Business Media New York 2015

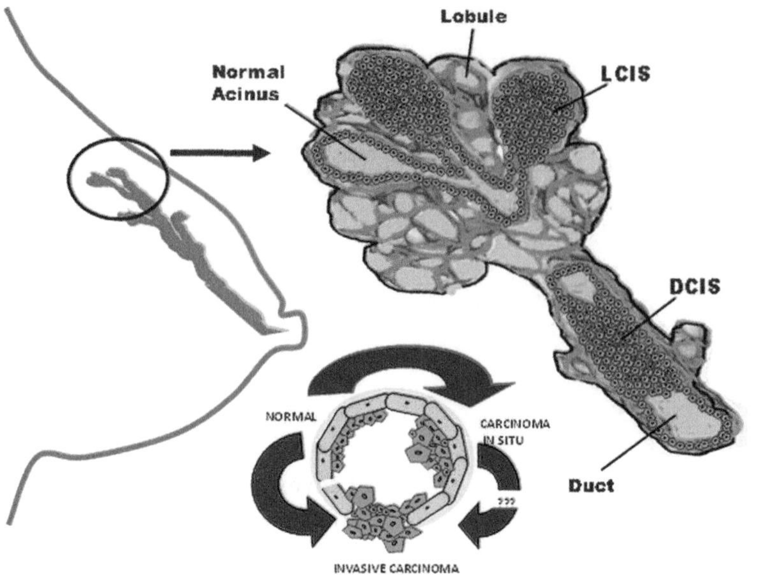

Fig. 3.1 Pathophysiology of DCIS and LCIS

from 5.8 per 100,000 women in the 1970s to a plateau of 32.5 per 100,000 women in 2004. This rise has been attributed primarily to the introduction of breast cancer screening programs [2].

Ductal Carcinoma In Situ

DCIS represents approximately 20 % of all newly diagnosed breast cancers. Risk factors for DCIS are similar to invasive breast cancer and include family history of breast cancer, increased breast density, obesity, and nulliparity or late age at first live birth. Like invasive breast cancer, DCIS is also a component of the inherited breast-ovarian cancer syndrome defined by mutations in the BRCA genes; mutation rates are low and similar to those for invasive breast cancer (about 5 % of all cases). Similar to invasive breast cancer, DCIS tends to occur at a younger age in women with inherited BRCA mutations [3, 4]. The average age of diagnosis is between 54 and 56, with the majority of cases found in postmenopausal women. According to the Surveillance, Epidemiology, and End Results (SEER) data for women diagnosed from 1984 to 1989, the risk of death from breast cancer in women with DCIS is low, estimated at 1.9 % within 10 years, and is most commonly related to an invasive recurrence in the breast [5].

Pathophysiology

DCIS is the proliferation of abnormal ductal epithelial cells that are limited to and have not invaded beyond the basement membrane. DCIS is considered a precursor of invasive carcinoma, but does not fully express the malignant phenotype. The progression to invasive breast cancer is not obligatory and cannot be reliably predicted. It is also critically important to keep in mind that the distinction between low-grade DCIS and atypical duct hyperplasia (ADH) can be difficult, even for experienced pathologists, and some have advocated a more conservative approach to these "borderline" lesions [6, 7].

Classification of DCIS into histopathological subtypes facilitates prognostication and management decisions [8]. Conventional histologic patterns include comedo, solid, cribriform, papillary, and micro-papillary. Grading of low, intermediate, and high is also assigned based on nuclear features including nuclear size, shape, chromatin texture, and mitotic activity. While papillary and cribriform patterns often have low nuclear grade, comedo tumors generally have high nuclear grade. Comedo lesions have a solid growth pattern and central necrosis with calcifications and are associated with an increased risk of local recurrence and invasion [9].

Pathologists should examine tissue specimens excised for DCIS thoroughly to exclude small foci of invasive disease. The size and overall extent of the DCIS should be reported along with the margin width – distance to the resection margin. Nuclear grade, distance to the closest margin, and extent of margin involvement should also be examined and reported. Testing the specimen for estrogen receptor (ER) and progesterone receptor (PR) is done routinely to guide management decisions. However, it is generally better to wait until the definitive resection to test for ER and PR rather than testing needle biopsy material, since any invasive component, if present, should be assessed preferentially.

Diagnosis

Ninety percent of DCIS lesions are identified radiographically by the presence of microcalcifications. Less common presentations include a palpable mass, mammographic mass, Paget's disease of the nipple, or bloody nipple discharge. Mammographic patterns that represent DCIS include punctate, linear, or branching calcifications reflecting a ductal orientation [9, 10]. All patients with newly diagnosed DCIS should have diagnostic mammographic views with magnification to fully assess morphology and extent of calcifications. Diagnosis should usually be confirmed by stereotactic core biopsy, which allows for surgical planning. When stereotactic biopsy is not possible because of depth, breast tissue that is too thin or implants, wire-localized excisional biopsy can be substituted. However, this practice should be the exception, with needle biopsy being preferred.

Silverstein and colleagues devised a prognostic index that correlated the risk of local recurrence with several pathologic features [11]. Features originally included size, margin, and grade but now also include patient age (Table 3.1).

Table 3.1 Van Nuys prognostic index

Score	Size	Margin	Pathological classification	Age (yrs)
1	<15 mm	>10 mm	Non-high-grade lesion w/o comedo necrosis (nuclear grade 1 or 2)	>60
2	16–40 mm	1–9 mm	Non-high-grade lesion w/ comedo necrosis (nuclear grade 1 or 2)	40–60
3	>41 mm	<1 mm	All high-grade lesion w/ or w/o necrosis (nuclear grade 3)	<40

Adapted from Silverstein [11]. With permission from Elsevier

Although this index was reported to be able to identify patients with such a low risk of recurrence that they might not need radiation, other studies indicate that most DCIS patients benefit from irradiation after breast-conserving surgery (see below).

Treatment

Therapeutic strategies to manage DCIS include surgery, radiation therapy, and adjuvant endocrine therapy, with the goal of preventing the development of recurrence, especially with invasive cancer. In the past, DCIS was treated with total or even modified radical mastectomy, but subsequent trials have suggested that breast-conserving surgery is safe for DCIS and that removal of lymph nodes is not beneficial. Mastectomy affords a cure rate of approximately 98 %, with local recurrence rates at approximately 1 % [12]. Mastectomy is still appropriate for some patients with large tumors (>4 cm, depending on breast size), multicentric lesions (meaning DCIS in more than one quadrant of the breast; however, this is now being challenged), inability to obtain negative margins despite multiple attempts, recurrence after breast conservation (particularly with prior radiation therapy; however, recent trials are examining the role of repeat BCT in this setting), lack of access to a radiation facility, risk of noncompliance, or patient preference. Approximately 96 % of recurrences occur in the same quadrant, implicating the presence of residual disease as the underlying cause. Women treated with mastectomy for DCIS are good candidates for immediate breast reconstruction with implants or autologous flaps, since lymph node involvement and need for radiation are unlikely.

Although mastectomy is effective, it is more aggressive than most women with DCIS require. Breast-conserving therapy (BCT) – wide excision with negative margins followed by radiation – is associated with less morbidity compared to mastectomy but has a higher risk of local recurrence. National Surgical Adjuvant Breast and Bowel Project Protocol B-17 (NSABP B-17) randomized 818 women with DCIS to excision alone versus excision followed by radiation. There was a reduction in the incidence of invasive ipsilateral recurrences from 21.1 % to 8.1 % when radiation was added, but no difference in the overall survival (86 % vs. 87 %) at 12 years. There was also a reduction in noninvasive recurrence from 18.3 to 8.9 %. At 8 years follow-up, the risk of contralateral invasive breast cancer (3.5 %) was similar to the rate in the ipsilateral (3.9 %) breasts treated with lumpectomy and irradiation [12]. At 15 years, ipsilateral invasive recurrence was also reduced with the addition of radiation compared to excision alone (8.9 % vs. 19.4 %) [13]. The European Organization for Research and Treatment of Cancer (EORTC) examined similar randomized groups (excision alone vs. excision followed by radiotherapy) in 1,111 women with DCIS detected mammographically which were <5 cm. Adequate lumpectomy, as in B-17, was defined by negative margins, meaning "no tumor on ink." Recurrence rates at 10 years for excision alone were significantly higher than for those treated with excision followed by radiation (26 % vs. 10 %). Like NASBP B-17, disease-free and overall survival was similar in the two groups [14]. These data supported the recommendation for all patients receiving breast-conserving surgery for DCIS to receive postoperative radiation. Re-excision(s) or mastectomy may be required to obtain negative margins. A negative margin – an absence of tumor at the inked surface of the specimen – is considered a minimum requirement. A margin width of 1–2 mm is usually sufficient for women who undergo radiation therapy. A wider margin, ideally 10 mm if achievable, is preferred for women considering breast-conserving surgery alone. Obtaining wider margins of excision and whether this can obviate the need for radiation is a current area of controversy [13, 15–17]. The original analysis which derived the Van Nuys Prognostic Index suggested that women with a lower score may have a low risk for recurrence and therefore not require radiation. Subsequent attempts to validate and replicate this analysis have not been consistent [18, 19]. The Eastern Cooperative Oncology Group 5194 (ECOG) also examined excision without radiation in women with DCIS. Limitations for the extent of DCIS were established for low/intermediate and high-grade lesions, and all excised specimens had a minimum surgical margin of 3 mm. Tamoxifen was allowed but not required following surgery. After a median follow-up of 6.7 years, the 5-year rate of local recurrence was 6.1 % for low/intermediate grade lesions and 15.3 % for high-grade lesions. While longer follow-up is necessary, the study suggests that carefully selected patients treated with breast-conserving surgery without radiation had low rates of local recurrence [20]. To date there is no clinical or pathologic feature that reliably predicts that excision without radiation will have no local failure, and ideal nomograms to assist in this evaluation are still to be determined [21]. Preliminary data from ECOG 5194 suggest that a gene expression profile analysis may provide further assistance in the identification of a subset of patients who may have a low enough risk of recurrence after excision that they may not have a benefit from adjuvant radiation [22]. Although this DCIS score can predict risk of recurrence without radiation, it does not truly predict the benefit or lack of benefit from the addition of radiation.

The incidence of lymph node involvement in women with DCIS is 1–2 % and likely related to a missed focus of invasion in excised specimens. Retrospective analysis of NSABP B-17 and B-24 suggests that sentinel lymph node biopsy would generally have a low yield and is unnecessary. Even when apparent cancer cells are found in axillary lymph nodes of patients who are not found to have any evidence of invasion in the breast primary, the overall outcomes of these patients do not appear to be different from other DCIS patients. There may be as much as a 20 % chance of finding an invasive cancer within an excision specimen after an initial needle biopsy diagnosis of DCIS (i.e., upstaging). The decision to perform a sentinel lymph node biopsy (SLNB) may be patient-driven in order to avoid a second operation. Relative indications to perform SLNB in patients with DCIS include those undergoing mastectomy (because of difficulty with subsequent SLNB) and risk factors for invasion such as palpability, comedo morphology, necrosis, or recurrent disease.

Adjuvant Systemic Therapy

It was the observation in patients with invasive disease that tamoxifen – a mixed estrogen agonist/antagonist – decreased contralateral breast cancer and ipsilateral recurrence that made it attractive for use in DCIS. Between 1991 and 1994 the NSABP trial B-24 randomized 1,804 women with DCIS treated with excision and radiation to either tamoxifen or placebo for 5 years. The ipsilateral breast recurrence rates for women less than age 50 were 33.3/1000 versus 20.8/1000 with placebo and tamoxifen, respectively, and for women 50 and older were 13/1000 with placebo versus 10.2/1000 with tamoxifen. At 5 years, the incidence of either subsequent invasive or noninvasive breast cancer in either breast was reduced by 37 %; the incidence of invasive breast cancer in either breast was reduced from 7.2 % to 4.1 % with tamoxifen. Nevertheless, tamoxifen had no effect on overall survival. Among women with ER-positive disease, there was a significant reduction in any breast cancer event, while in women with ER-negative disease, there appeared to be only a trend toward reduction [23, 24]. The use of aromatase inhibitors for DCIS is currently under study. For example, the NSABP B-35 trial compares tamoxifen with anastrozole for women with DCIS treated with lumpectomy + irradiation.

Lobular Carcinoma In Situ

Lobular carcinoma in situ (LCIS) is a predictor for increased risk of development of invasive breast cancer but is neither a premalignant lesion nor an anatomic marker for the site of invasive disease. The risk is conferred to both the ipsilateral and contralateral breasts. It is usually found incidentally on biopsy that is performed for another lesion. The mean age of diagnosis in many series is between 44 and 46, and more than 80 % of cases are found in premenopausal women. Because of the absence of mammographic or clinical presentation, the true incidence of LCIS is unknown. The SEER database reports the incidence as 3.19 per 100,000 women [25].

Pathophysiology

LCIS is a noninvasive abnormal proliferation of cells in the terminal duct and lobule of the breast (see Fig. 3.1). The growth of cells within the acini of the lobule often has pagetoid extension into the ducts. E-cadherin staining is used to differentiate cells of ductal and lobular origin. The immunohistochemical stain is strongly present in the membrane of DCIS specimens but is absent in LCIS [26]. Two subtypes of LCIS have been described: classic and pleomorphic (discussed below). Classic LCIS has smaller nucleoli and less frequent mitotic figures compared to pleomorphic.

The presence of LCIS is considered a risk factor for subsequent invasive cancer. Although the risk of developing invasive lobular carcinoma is higher than for the general population, the majority of women with LCIS who develop cancer develop ductal carcinoma. The time to the development of invasive cancer is generally in the range of 10–15 years [9]. In one series, after a 10-year follow-up of 4853 cases of LCIS, 7.1 % developed invasive cancer with an equal frequency of cancer occurring in both breasts [27]. The lifelong risk of developing an invasive cancer is estimated to be 1 % per year and the relative risk two-fold compared to women without LCIS. [28].

Treatment

The management of LCIS discovered on core needle biopsy is controversial. Several series between 1999 and 2008 report an underestimation of malignancy after comparing core needle biopsies with excised specimens ranging from 0 to 50 %, with an overall underestimation of malignancy of 27 %[29]. Current National Comprehensive Cancer Network (NCCN) guidelines suggest excision for all patients diagnosed with LCIS on core needle biopsy [30].

When LCIS is diagnosed or found in isolation on excisional biopsy, no further surgical intervention is required. Unlike DCIS, clear margins are not required and ipsilateral mastectomy and radiation are not indicated. There is no role for axillary lymph node biopsy or dissection in the absence of invasive disease. Local recurrences following excision, as seen with DCIS, are uncommon. If invasive carcinoma is detected in the excision specimen, then appropriate staging and treatment strategies should be initiated.

Women with LCIS should be counseled on the increased but still relatively low risk of ipsilateral or contralateral breast cancer, and the alternatives of observation, chemoprevention, and prophylactic mastectomy should be discussed. In the absence of other risk factors (family history, BRCA mutation, personal history of breast cancer), prophylactic mastectomy should be considered a drastic measure and only used if patients insist. To date there are no randomized efficacy trials comparing observation to prophylactic mastectomy. If the observation alternative is elected, careful surveillance should be continued indefinitely. Current guidelines recommend a history and physical exam every 6–12 months and annual screening mammography. LCIS places a patient at intermediate risk, and according to current guidelines, magnetic resonance imaging (MRI) is not indicated for surveillance in the absence of a strong family history [30].

Chemoprevention

In the NSABP P-1 trial 13,338 high-risk women (6 % had LCIS) were randomized to receive tamoxifen or placebo for 5 years. The risk of invasive breast cancer was reduced from 42.5/1,000 to 24.8/1,000 with tamoxifen at 7 years. For noninvasive breast cancer, the risk reduction was from 15.8/1,000 to 10.2/1,000. The rate of development of breast cancer in the tamoxifen group was 6 versus 12 in the placebo group per 1,000 women [31]. Although there were not a large number of LCIS patients in the P-1 trial, the proportional reduction in breast cancers with tamoxifen for this subset was even greater than for the trial as a whole.

Raloxifene, another selective estrogen receptor modulator, has also been evaluated in postmenopausal high-risk women, including those with LCIS. In the Study of Tamoxifen and Raloxifene (STAR) trial, over 19,000 patients (9 % had LCIS) were randomized to compare tamoxifen with raloxifene. The trial demonstrated that both agents were equally effective in reducing the incidence of invasive breast cancer. Among women with a history of LCIS, both drugs were equally effective at reducing the incidence of invasive breast cancer. Tamoxifen had reduced the incidence of DCIS and LCIS by half. Raloxifene was not quite as effective as tamoxifen against noninvasive cancer but had fewer serious side effects [32].

Pleomorphic LCIS

PLCIS is distinguished as an aggressive subtype of LCIS with larger nuclei and increased pleomorphism and is often associated with microcalcifications and central necrosis. Many of these features overlap with DCIS, making distinction difficult. Surgical excision with negative margins is recommended, but no evidence supports wide margins or radiation for this lesion [29]. Some authors recommend treating PLCIS like DCIS.

Phyllodes Tumors

Phyllodes tumors are rare breast lesions made up of stromal and epithelial components. The tumor was first described in 1838 by Johannes Muller who originally named it cystosarcoma phyllodes. For the sake of uniformity of histologic and biologic variants, the World Health Organization recommended in 1982 that the range of lesions fall under the heading of phyllodes tumors.

These lesions account for <0.5 % of all breast tumors with a median age of 40–45 [33, 34]. The majority of patients present because of a palpable breast lump that is firm, mobile, and smooth. The tumor varies in size, but in one large series of 106 patients, over 70 % were less than 5 cm at the time of diagnosis [35].

Pathophysiology

Phyllodes tumors are histologically graded into benign, borderline, or malignant tumors based on characteristic features. Some authors have noted that there is not a clear correlation between histology and clinical outcome [33, 36]. All three classifications of phyllodes recur locally, but only borderline and malignant tumors metastasize [33]. Approximately 25 % of phyllodes tumors are malignant but only about 17–22 % metastasize. The most common reported sites of metastases are in the lung, soft tissue, bone, and pleura. Histologic examination of metastases shows greater resemblance to sarcomas [33, 34].

Tumor size and the presence of necrosis, high mitotic count, stromal overgrowth, severe nuclear pleomorphism, increased mitotic index, stromal atypia, and infiltrating margins have been shown to be predictive of metastasis [33, 34, 36]. Similarly, resection margins <1 cm, increased mitotic index, tumor necrosis, and large tumor size have been identified as factors predictive of local recurrence [33].

Diagnosis

There are no radiographic features that distinguish phyllodes tumors from fibroadenomata [33, 35]. Precise diagnosis is best obtained on examination of the resected specimen; however, core biopsy of palpable lesions may reduce the number of operations on fibroepithelial lesions [37].

Microscopically, tumors are mostly fibroadenomatous and stromal elements with varying degrees of pleomorphism and necrosis [34]. Phyllodes tumors are distinguished from fibroadenomas by the presence of increased stromal cellularity [36].

Surgical Treatment

Surgical treatment for localized phyllodes consists of wide local excision, preferably with a ≥1 cm margin free of tumor, if possible. Retrospective study demonstrated improved disease-free survival and decreased local recurrence with negative margins [33]. Enucleation has had a recurrence rate of 15.8 % and is not recommended for phyllodes tumors which lack a capsule [35]. Mastectomy is recommended only if negative margins cannot be achieved with lumpectomy. As phyllodes tumors spread hematogenously and rarely spread to axillary lymph nodes, a lymph node dissection of the axilla is not recommended unless lymph nodes are clinically suspicious [33, 38]. The management of phyllodes recurrences is less clear. Some authors argue that treatment should be tailored to the tumor size, breast size, histology, age, patient desire, and extent of disease [35].

Adjuvant Therapy

In spite of complete resection for benign and malignant tumors, recurrence rates of between 5–15 % and 20–30 % are reported, respectively [33]. There are a few small series that have addressed adjuvant chemotherapy and none that demonstrate benefit. There are more promising results with adjuvant radiotherapy. One retrospective series of 37 patients with malignant phyllodes demonstrated decreased recurrence and improved survival with adjuvant radiotherapy [39]. A prospective study of 46 patients with borderline and malignant tumors and with negative margins following resection had no local recurrences after a median follow-up of 56 months [40].

Salient Points

- DCIS and LCIS represent a group of neoplastic lesions that are confined to the breast ducts and lobules (see Table 3.2).
- DCIS is a premalignant lesion and the main goal of therapy is to prevent invasive disease with surgery and radiation.
    - For ER + DCIS, adjuvant endocrine therapy should be considered.

Table 3.2 Features of DCIS and LCIS

	DCIS	LCIS
Average age	Late 50s	Late 40s
Menopausal status	Majority POST	Majority PRE
Clinical signs	Can be associated with Paget's, nipple discharge, mass	None
Mammographic signs	Microcalcifications	None
% of subsequent invasive cancer in ipsilateral breast	~99 %	~50 %
% of subsequent invasive cancer in contralateral breast	~1 %	50 %
Need for negative excision margin	Yes	No
Benefit from endocrine therapy	Yes	Yes

- Most women who undergo breast-conserving therapy for DCIS should have wide excision to achieve negative margins followed by post-operative radiation.
- Indications for mastectomy for DCIS are (1) large tumor relative to breast size, (2) multicentric disease (although this is now being challenged), (3) persistent positive margins, (4) salvage surgery for recurrence (although this also is now being challenged), (5) lack of access to radiation facility, (6) noncompliant patient, and (7) patient preference.
- Recurrence of DCIS is infrequent, can occur over decades, and usually occurs at the site of previous excision.
- Relative indications for SLNB in patients with DCIS include those undergoing mastectomy and risk factors for invasion such as palpability, mass on mammogram, comedo morphology, necrosis, or recurrent disease.
- Tamoxifen as adjuvant therapy for DCIS decreases recurrences, but has no effect on overall survival.
- LCIS is a marker which increases the risk for invasive cancer in both breasts and can be followed clinically.
- The majority of women with LCIS who develop cancer develop ductal carcinoma.
- For isolated LCIS following excisional biopsy, further surgery and obtaining clear margin are not necessary.
- Pleomorphic LCIS is an aggressive subtype of LCIS, some advocate treating it like DCIS.
- Women with LCIS may benefit from chemoprevention with tamoxifen or raloxifene.
- Phyllodes tumor is a rare lesion of the breast that is classified in three histologic forms (benign, borderline, malignant) and has a varied biologic behavior.
- Treatment of phyllodes involves wide local excision with the intent of negative margins.
- There is no need for assessing lymph nodes when treating phyllodes, unless they are clinically suspicious.
- Adjuvant radiotherapy may have a role in the treatment of borderline and malignant lesions, but further study is needed.

Questions

1. Which of the following regarding DCIS is true?
   A. DCIS accounts for 40 % of all new breast cancers in the United States.
   B. 50 % of DCIS is detected on imaging.
   C. The diagnosis of invasive cancer is less common than DCIS.
   D. Due to better screening, the incidence of DCIS is increasing.
   E. DCIS tends to occur in older women with BRCA mutations.
2. Most DCIS lesions are detected by:
   A. Screening Mammogram
   B. Palpation
   C. Skin changes
   D. MRI
   E. Ultrasound
3. Which of the following regarding DCIS is true?
   A. DCIS is categorized by the size of the lesion, nuclear grade, the presence and

extent of comedo necrosis, and to a lesser extent, architectural pattern.
B. Measured margin widths are not an important prognostic indicator for local recurrence.
C. The hallmark is stromal invasion.
D. Size has no correlation to local recurrence.
E. Postoperative radiation has increased overall survival.

4. Tamoxifen increases survival in:
   A. DCIS
   B. Invasive ductal carcinoma
   C. LCIS
   D. Phyllodes tumors
   E. Pleomorphic LCIS
5. Mastectomy is not appropriate for a 43-year-old woman with a left breast DCIS for which of the following:
   A. Patient preference
   B. Multicentric lesions
   C. Inadequate margins
   D. Recurrence after BCS
   E. Tumors that are >2 cm
6. An SLNB in a woman with DCIS on core biopsy is not a reasonable option for:
   A. Patients with histological confirmation of concurrent invasive disease
   B. Patients with recurrent invasive disease
   C. Patients undergoing mastectomy
   D. Patients with concurrent atypical ductal hyperplasia
   E. Patients with a palpable mass
7. Which of the following statements is true?
   A. Patients with LCIS require biopsy of the contralateral breast.
   B. Patients with LCIS are at an increased risk of developing breast cancer.
   C. The majority of patients with LCIS who develop cancer develop lobular cancer.
   D. E-cadherin immunohistochemical staining is strongly present in LCIS but not in DCIS.
   E. A positive margin for LCIS requires a re-excision to achieve a negative margin

8–10: Matching

8.	STAR	A. Looked at the effects of tamoxifen vs. placebo after BCT
9.	NSABP B-17	B. Compared excision alone vs. excision + radiation
10.	NSABP B-24	C. Compared the effects of tamoxifen and raloxifene in women with LCIS

11. Which of the following statements is TRUE regarding LCIS?
    A. The relative risk of developing an invasive cancer in women with LCIS is ~ threefold higher than for women without LCIS.
    B. LCIS is usually identified mammographically.
    C. Most cases occur in postmenopausal women.
    D. The absolute risk of invasive cancer is approximately 1 % per year and appears to be lifelong.
    E. LCIS is usually identified clinically.
12. Which of the following is true of phyllodes tumors?
    A. Phyllodes tumors metastasize via lymphatics.
    B. Treatment of phyllodes tumors requires hormone therapy.
    C. Phyllodes tumors have decreased stromal cellularity compared to fibroadenoma.
    D. Treatment of phyllodes tumors generally requires axillary node sampling.
    E. Phyllodes tumors have decreased recurrence with a 1 cm negative margin of excision.

Correct Answers

1. D
2. A
3. A
4. B
5. E
6. D
7. B
8. C
9. B

10. A
11. D
12. E

References

1. American Cancer Society. Breast cancer facts & figures 2011–2012. Atlanta: American Cancer Society, Inc. 2011.
2. Allegra CJ, Aberle DR, Ganschow P, Hahn SM, Lee CN, Millon-Underwood S, Pike MC, Reed SD, Saftlas AF, Scarvalone SA, Schwartz AM, Slomski C, Yothers G, Zon R. National Institutes of Health State-of-the-Science Conference Statement: Diagnosis and Management of Ductal Carcinoma In Situ September 22–24, 2009. J Natl Cancer Inst. 2010;102(3):161–69.
3. Kerlikowske K, Barclay J, Grady D, et al. Comparison of risk factors for ductal carcinoma in situ and invasive breast cancer. J Natl Cancer Inst. 1997;89:76.
4. Claus EB, Stowe M, Carter D. Family history of breast and ovarian cancer and the risk of breast carcinoma in situ. Breast Cancer Res Treat. 2003;78:7.
5. Ernster VL, Barclay J, Kerlikowske K, Wilkie H, Ballard-Barbash R. Mortality among women with ductal carcinoma in situ of the breast in the population-based surveillance, epidemiology and end results program. Arch Intern Med. 2000;160(7):953.
6. Rosen PP. Fibroepithelial neoplasms. In: Rosen PP, editor. Rosen's breast pathology. 3rd ed. Philadelphia: Lippincott Williams & Wilkins; 2009. p. 187–229.
7. Esserman LJ, Thompson Jr IM, Reid B. Overdiagnosis and overtreatment in cancer: an opportunity for improvement. JAMA. 2013;310(8):797–8.
8. Patani N, Khaled Y, Al Reefy S, Mokbel K. Ductal carcinoma in-situ: an update for clinical practice. Surg Oncol. 2011;20(1):e23–31.
9. Giuliano AE, Mabry H. Ductal and lobular carcinoma in situ of the breast. In: Cameron JL, editor. Current surgical therapy. Philadelphia: Mosby Elsevier; 2009.
10. Dershaw DD, Abramson A, Cha I, et al. Ductal carcinoma in situ: mammographic findings and clinical implications. Radiology. 1989;170:411.
11. Silverstein MJ. The University of Southern California/Van Nuys prognostic index for ductal carcinoma in situ of the breast. Am J Surg. 2003;186:337.
12. Fisher B, Land S, Mamounas E, et al. Prevention of invasive breast cancer in women with ductal carcinoma in situ: an update of the National Surgical Adjuvant Breast and Bowel Project experience. Semin Oncol. 2001;28:400.
13. Wapnir IL, Dignam JJ, Fisher B, et al. Long-term outcomes of invasive ipsilateral breast tumor recurrences after lumpectomy in NSABP B-17 and B-24 randomized clinical trials for DCIS. J Natl Cancer Inst. 2011;103:478.
14. Julien JP, Biijker N, Fentiman IS, et al. Radiotherapy in breast conserving treatment for ductal carcinoma in situ: first results of the EORTC randomized phase III trial 10853 – EORTC Breast Cancer Cooperative Group and EORTC Radiotherapy Group. Lancet. 2000;355:528–33.
15. Silverstein MJ, Lagios MD, Groshen S, et al. The influence of margin width on local control of ductal carcinoma in situ of the breast. N Engl J Med. 1999; 340:1455.
16. Bijker N, Meijnen P, Peterse JL, et al. Breast-conserving treatment with or without radiotherapy in ductal carcinoma-in-situ: ten-year results of European Organisation for Research and Treatment of Cancer randomized phase III trial 10853 – a study by the EORTC Breast Cancer Cooperative Group and EORTC Radiotherapy Group. J Clin Oncol. 2006;24(21):3381–7.
17. Holmberg L, Garmo H, Granstrand B, et al. Absolute risk reductions for local recurrence after postoperative radiotherapy after sector resection for ductal carcinoma in situ of the breast. J Clin Oncol. 2008;26(8):1247–52.
18. Boland GP, Chan KC, Kox WF, et al. Value of the Van Nuys Prognostic Index in prediction of recurrence of ductal carcinoma in situ after breast-conservation surgery. Br J Surg. 2003;90(4):426.
19. MacAusland SG, Hepel JT, Chong FK, et al. An attempt to independently verify the utility of the Van Nuys Prognostic Index for ductal carcinoma in situ. Cancer. 2007;1109120:2648.
20. Hughes LL, Wang M, Page DL, et al. Local excision alone without irradiation for ductal carcinoma in situ of the breast: a trial of the Eastern Cooperative Oncology Group. J Clin Oncol. 2009;27(32):5319–24. Epub 2009 Oct 13.
21. Yi M, Meric-Bernstam F, Kuerer HM, et al. Evaluation of a breast cancer nomogram for predicting risk of ipsilateral breast tumor recurrences in patients with ductal carcinoma in situ after local excision. J Clin Oncol. 2012;30(6):600–7. Epub 2012 Jan 17.
22. Solin LJ, Gray R, Baehner FL, Butler S, Badve S, Yoshizawa C, et al. A quantitative multigene RT-PCR assay for predicting recurrence risk after surgical excision alone without irradiation for ductal carcinoma in situ (DCIS): a prospective validation study of the DCIS score from ECOG E5194. Cancer Res. 2011;71(24):108s.
23. Allred DC, Anderson SJ, Paik S, et al. Adjuvant tamoxifen reduces subsequent breast cancer in women with estrogen receptor-positive ductal carcinoma in situ: a study based on NSABP protocol B-24. J Clin Oncol. 2012;30(12):1268–73.
24. Fisher B, Dignam J, Wolmark N, et al. Tamoxifen in treatment of intraductal breast cancer: National Surgical Adjuvant Breast and Bowel Project B-24 randomized controlled trial. Lancet. 1999;353:1993.
25. Li CI, Anderson BO, Daling JR, Moe RE. Changing incidence of lobular carcinoma in situ of the breast. Breast Cancer Res. 2002;75(3):259–68.

26. Acs G, Lawton TJ, Rebbeck TR, LiVolsi VA, Zhang PJ. Differential expressio n of E-cadherin in lobular and ductal neoplasms of the breast and its biologic and diagnostic implications. Am J Clin Pathol. 2001;115(1):85–9.
27. Chuba PJ, Hamre MR, Yap J, et al. Bilateral risk for subsequent breast cancer after lobular carcinoma-in-situ: analysis of surveillance, epidemiology, and end results data. J Clin Oncol. 2005;23:5534.
28. Page DL, Kidd Jr TE, Dupont WD, et al. Lobular neoplasia of the breast: higher risk for subsequent invasive cancer predicted by more extensive disease. Hum Pathol. 1991;22:1232.
29. Hussain M, Cunnick GH. Management of lobular carcinoma in-situ and typical lobular hyperplasia of the breast-A review. Eur J Surg Oncol. 2011;37:279–89.
30. National Comprehensive Cancer Network (NCCN) guidelines for DFSP. Available at: www.nccn.org. Accessed 1 Sept 2012
31. Fisher B, Costantino JP, Wickerham DL, et al. Tamoxifen for the prevention of breast cancer: current status of the National Surgical Adjuvant Breast and Bowel Project P-1 study. J Natl Cancer Inst. 2005; 97:1652.
32. Vogel VG, Costantino JP, Wickerham DL, et al. Effects of tamoxifen vs raloxifene on the risk of developing invasive breast cancer and other disease outcomes: the NSABP Study of Tamoxifen and Raloxifene (STAR) P-2 trial. JAMA. 2006;295:2727.
33. Khosravi-Shahi P. Management of non-metastatic phyllodes tumors of the breast: review of the literature. Surg Oncol. 2011;20:143–8.
34. Hawkins RE, Schofield JB, Fisher C, et al. The clinical and histologic criteria that predict metastases from cystosarcoma phyllodes. Cancer. 1992;69(1):141–7.
35. Chua CL, Thomas A, Ng BK. Cystosarcoma phyllodes: a review of surgical options. Surgery. 1989; 105:141–7.
36. Ward RM, Evans HL. Cystosarcoma phyllodes a clinicopathologic study of 26 cases. Cancer. 1986;58: 2282–9.
37. Komenaka IK, El-Tamer M, Pile-Spellman E, et al. Core needle biopsy as a diagnostic tool to differentiate phyllodes tumor from fibroadenoma. Arch Surg. 2003;138:987–90.
38. Barnhart GR, DeBlois GG, Kay S, Neifeld JP. Management of Cystosarcoma: a reassessment. Breast Dis Breast. 1985;11(2):17–23.
39. Pandey M, Mathew A, Kattoor J, et al. Malignant phyllodes. Breast J. 2001;7:411–6.
40. Barth RJ, Wells WA, Mitchell SE, Cole BF. A prospective, multi-institutional study of adjuvant radiotherapy after resection of malignant phyllodes. Ann Surg Oncol. 2009;16:2288–94.

Early Breast Cancers

4

Quyen D. Chu and Roger H. Kim

Learning Objectives

After reading this chapter, you should be able to:

- Recognize what constitutes early breast cancer
- Understand how to evaluate and manage patients with early breast cancer
- Appreciate the treatment paradigm of early breast cancer
- Select options for local, regional, and systemic control of the disease

Introduction

Besides skin cancer, breast cancer is the most common cancer among American women. It is also the second leading cause of cancer death in women, exceeded only by lung cancer [1]. Approximately, 1 in 8 (12 %) women in the United States will develop invasive breast cancer in her lifetime. For 2013, it is estimated that 232,340 new cases of invasive breast cancer will be diagnosed in the United States, and about 39,620 women will die of the disease. Death rates from breast cancer have declined by 34 % since 1990, and this is believed to be attributable to earlier detection and improved treatment [1].

Historically, radical and disfiguring surgery (radical mastectomy or Halsted mastectomy) was the treatment of choice for women with breast cancer. Although the cancer was removed, recurrence was unacceptably high without adjuvant therapy. A 1972 landmark study by Fisher et al. found that two-thirds (67 %) of patients who had nodal involvement had recurrences within 5 years following a definitive operation. Over half of the patients with four or more involved nodes developed metastases within 18 months of their operation [2, 3]. Clearly, surgery alone, although a necessary component of treatment, will not cure the majority of patients with breast cancer.

A multidisciplinary approach is used to treat patients with breast cancer. Depending on the resources available, at a minimum, such an approach requires a surgeon, medical oncologist, radiation oncologist, and pathologist. Other individuals include geneticist, nutritionist, social worker, plastic surgeon, patient navigator, etc.

The majority of women in the United States with breast cancer (60–70 %) will present with EBC (Stage I/II). Operable or early breast cancers are those that are small relative to the breast and are deemed resectable [Stage 1 (T1N0), Stage 2A (T0N1, T1N1, T2N0), Stage 2B (T2N1, T3N0)].

Q.D. Chu, M.D., M.B.A, FACS (✉)
Department of Surgery, Louisiana State University Health Sciences Center – Shreveport, 1501 Kings Highway, P.O. Box 33932, Shreveport, LA 71130-3392, USA
e-mail: qchu@lsuhsc.edu

R.H. Kim, M.D.
Department of Surgery, Louisiana State University Health Sciences Center – Shreveport and the Feist-Weiller Cancer Center, 1501 Kings Highway, P.O. Box 33932, Shreveport, LA 71130-3392, USA
e-mail: rkim@lsuhsc.edu

Q.D. Chu et al. (eds.), *Surgical Oncology: A Practical and Comprehensive Approach*,
DOI 10.1007/978-1-4939-1423-4_4, © Springer Science+Business Media New York 2015

Note that EBC also includes N1 disease. In this chapter, we will address management of EBC.

Patients who present with either a large neglected tumor (i.e., a fungating mass), bulky adenopathy, and/or evidence of inflammatory breast cancer (i.e., peau d'orange; see Chap. 5-Locally Advanced Breast Cancer) are considered to have clinical Stage III breast cancer. Unfortunately, a number of these patients will have metastatic disease (Stage IV), but this can only be determined after having performed a battery of tests as part of the staging work-up.

Risk Factors

Risk factors for breast cancer can be grouped into those that are modifiable and those that are not. Non-modifiable risk factors include gender, age, family history, early menarche, and late menopause. Known inherited genetic mutations such as BRCA-1 and/or BRCA-2 are also non-modifiable risk factors. Modifiable risk factors include postmenopausal obesity, use of estrogen and progestin menopausal hormones, cigarette smoking, and alcohol consumption [1]. Some of these factors carry the highest risk, while others carry an intermediate to low risk. Age, personal history of early onset breast cancer (<40 years), biopsy-confirmed atypical hyperplasia and lobular carcinoma in situ, inheriting BRCA1-1 or BRCA-2 mutations, and having two or more first-degree relatives with breast cancer diagnosed at an early age carry the highest relative risk (RR) for developing breast cancer ($RR > 4.0$) [1]. High-dose radiation to the chest (i.e., past treatment for Hodgkin lymphoma), personal history of breast cancer at age $\geq$ 40 years, high endogenous estrogen or testosterone levels (postmenopausal), and having one first-degree relative with breast cancer carry a moderate relative risk of breast cancer ($RR = 2.1$–4.0). Alcohol consumption, Ashkenazi (Eastern European) Jewish heritage, early menarche, and hormone replacement therapy increase the relative risk of breast cancer slightly ($RR = 1.1$–2.0); the cancers among women taking hormone replacement therapy tend to be of more favorable prognosis [4] (Table 4.1).

Table 4.1 Risk factors for developing breast cancer

Risk factors	Relative risk (-fold)
Age (≥65 years)	>4.0
Genetic factors: BRCA-1 and BRCA-2	>4.0
Lobular carcinoma in situ (LCIS)	7.0–11.0
Family history	
One first-degree relative	2.0
Two first-degree relatives	3.0
Personal history of breast cancer	
Early onset (<40 years)	>4.0
≥40 years	2.1–4.0
Dense breasts	>4.0
Proliferative lesions without atypia	1.5–2.0
Ductal hyperplasia	
Fibroadenoma	
Sclerosing adenosis	
Radial scar	
Papillomatosis	
Proliferative lesions with atypia	3.5–4.0
Atypical ductal hyperplasia (ADH)	
Atypical lobular hyperplasia (ALH)	
Previous chest radiation (especially for Hodgkin or non-Hodgkin lymphoma)	2.1–4.0
Early menarche (before age 12) or late menopause (>55 years)	1.1–2.0
Ashkenazi (Eastern European) Jewish heritage	1.1–2.0
Diethylstilbestrol (DES) exposure	1.1–2.0
Nulliparity, first child after age 30	1.1–2.0
Birth control pill, hormone replacement therapy	1.1–2.0
Alcohol consumption	1.1–2.0
Obesity	1.1–2.0
Inactivity	1.1–2.0
History of endometrium, ovary, or colon cancer	1.1–2.0

Gail Model of Risk Assessment

Given a set of risk factors, what is the probability that a woman will develop breast cancer during the next 5 years and by age 90 years? While there are several models such as Gail [5], Claus [6], or Tyrer-Cuzick [7] that estimate breast cancer risk, the Gail model is the more widely known. The most updated version of the Gail model has been implemented into a variety of formats, one of which is the Breast Cancer Risk Assessment Tool

(BCRAT); BCRAT is available on the National Cancer Institute (NCI) website (http://cancer.gov/bcrisktool). The BCRAT incorporates information such as patient's age, age at menarche, age at first live birth, number of 1st degree relatives with breast cancer, number of prior breast biopsies, presence of atypia on biopsy, and race/ethnicity. Such a model informs the patient and her health-care providers of her risk and allows them an opportunity to select appropriate management options to reduce such a risk.

Histologic Subtypes

The female adult breast is arranged into 15–20 lobes, with each lobe made up of many smaller lobules. The lobules are all linked by ducts, which terminates in the nipple. Adipose tissue fills the spaces between lobules and ducts (Fig. 4.1). Each breast contains a rich network of blood vessels and lymphatics, the latter drains into the axilla, supraclavicular region, internal mammary lymph nodes, as well as other parts of the body (Fig. 4.2).

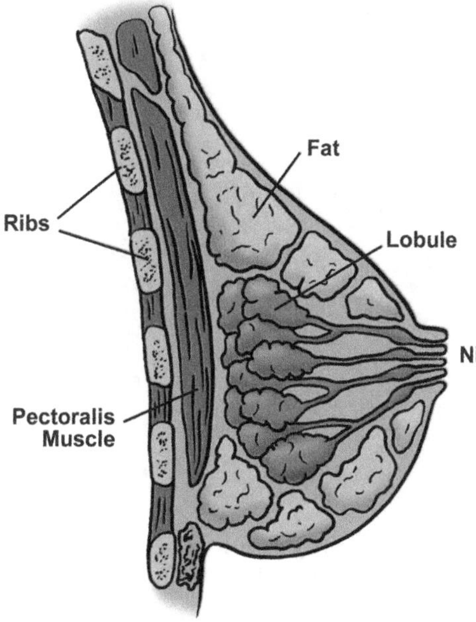

Fig. 4.1 *Female breast anatomy*: the ductal-lobule system is comprised of numerous lobules with acini. Each lobule empties into a terminal duct, which empties into a segmental duct, and finally into the collecting ducts. There are about 15–20 collecting ducts that converge under the areola (Courtesy of Quyen D. Chu, MD, MBA, FACS)

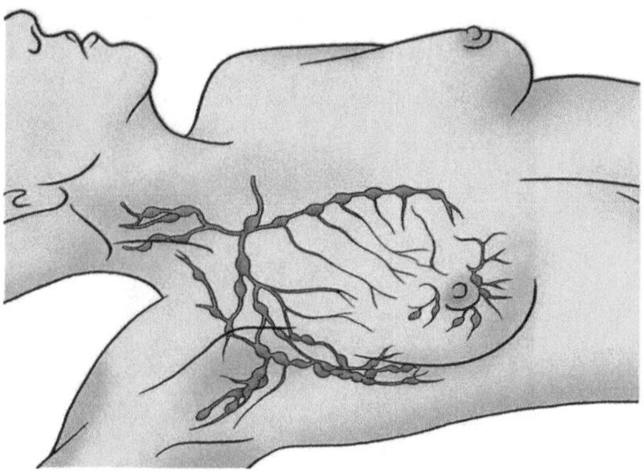

Fig. 4.2 Lymphatic system of the breast: lymphatic drainage begins from the breast lobules and flow into the axillary lymph nodes, internal mammary lymph nodes, retromammary lymph nodes, and infraclavicular and supraclavicular lymph nodes. The axillary lymph nodes receive approximately 75 % of the lymph drained from the breast. Lymphatics may also reach the sheath of the rectus abdominis, the subperitoneal and subhepatic plexuses, and the contralateral breast (Courtesy of Quyen D. Chu, MD, MBA, FACS)

Breast cancer encompasses a variety of histologies including ductal, lobular, medullary, tubular, and metaplastic. Of these, invasive ductal carcinoma (IDC) is the most common, accounting for about 80 % of the cases [8, 9] (Fig. 4.3a). Invasive lobular carcinoma (ILC) is the second most common, accounting for about 8–15 % of all invasive breast cancer [8, 10]. ILC typically arranges itself in a linear arrangement (single-file pattern), has a tendency to grow around ducts and lobules in a circumferential manner, and is associated with desmoplastic stromal reaction (Fig. 4.3b). Compared to IDC, ILC tends to be well differentiated; has a lower rate of HER-2 overexpression [11], higher rate of hormone receptor positivity [10], and higher incidence of bilaterality, multifocality, and multicentricity [12, 13]; and is more likely to harbor micrometastatic disease [14]. Other histologic types that are associated with a good prognosis are medullary, mucinous, tubular, cribriform, and adenoid cystic carcinoma of the breast, while micropapillary carcinoma and angiosarcoma are the more aggressive subtypes (Fig. 4.3c–f). Regardless of the subtypes,

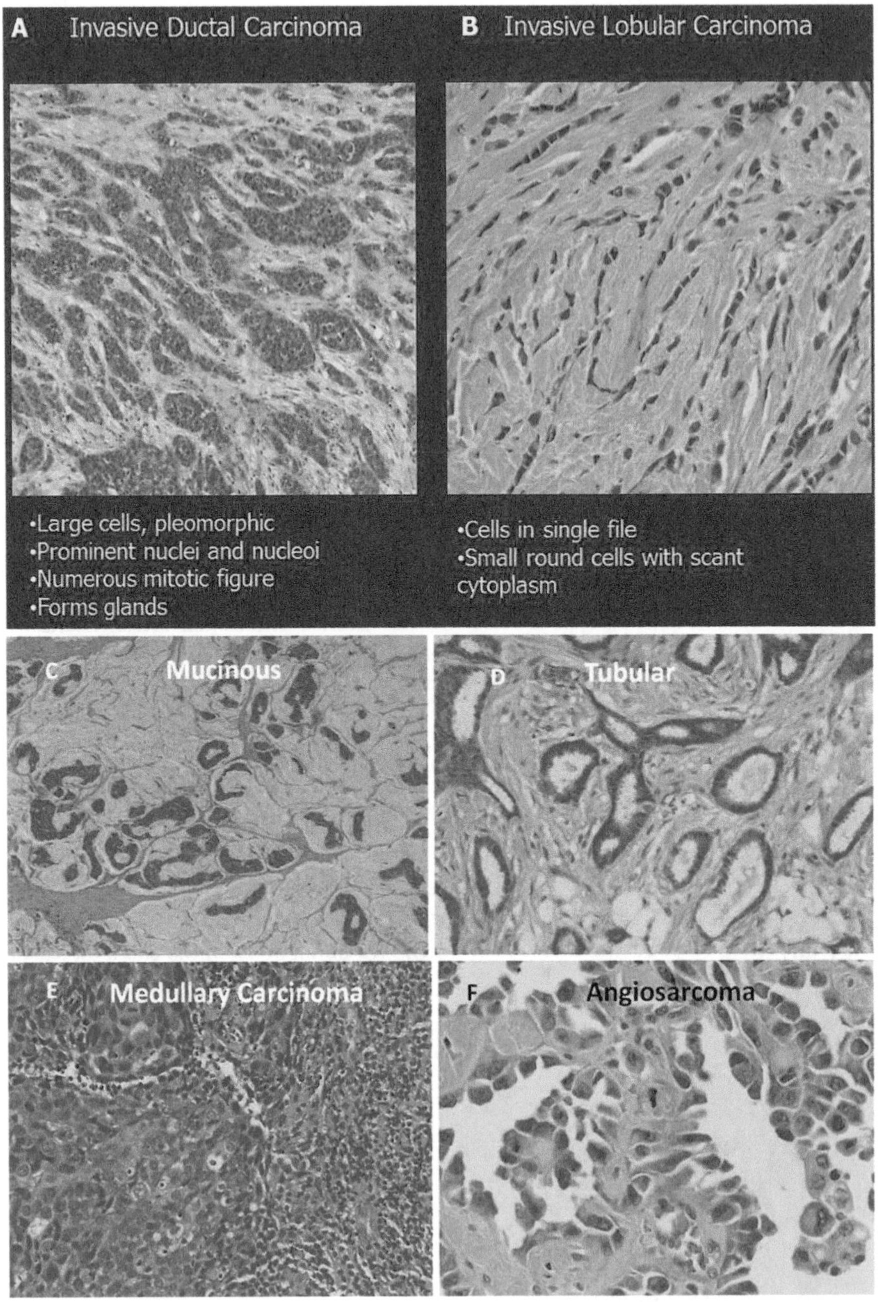

Fig. 4.3 Hematoxylin and eosin (H&E) sections of invasive ductal carcinoma (**a**) and invasive lobular carcinoma (**b**). Mucinous carcinoma is characterized by accumulation of abundant extracellular mucin around invasive tumor acini, nests, and trabeculae (**c**; low power, 40×). Tubular carcinoma (**d**; high power 100×): the glands reveal angular contours and are composed of single layer of neoplasm epithelial cells. The nuclear pleomorphism is lower grade. Stroma fibrosis and elastosis are associated with infiltrative invasion. Medullary carcinoma (**e**; high power 100×): this tumor is characterized by nodular expansion and peripheral lymphocytic infiltration. The tumor grows as syncytial sheets surrounded by a diffuse lymphocytic reaction. The tumor cells are poorly differentiated with high nuclear pleomorphism and mitotic rate. Angiosarcoma (**f**): this tumor is high grade with dilated vascular spaces that are dissecting and splitting tissue planes. The vascular spaces are lined and filled with highly pleomorphic malignant cells with easily identified mitosis (**a**–**f**: Courtesy of Quyen D. Chu, MD, MBA, FACS)

treatment is the same for all because current treatment guidelines and decision strategies are not dependent on subtypes.

Evaluation and Management of Early Breast Cancer

Once a diagnosis of breast has been made, the clinician should ask the following important questions: am I dealing with (1) an operable or early breast cancer (EBC), (2) locally advanced breast cancer (LABC) or inflammatory breast cancer (IBC), or (3) metastatic breast cancer? This is important because the answer will help guide her/him in selecting the most appropriate treatment option.

The answer to be above question is based on the clinician's initial assessment of the patient's clinical presentation. This is referred to as the *clinical stage*, which is different from the *pathologic stage*; the latter is based on the final pathology after the definitive operation. There are occasions whereby the clinician's initial impression may be discordant with the pathologic stage (i.e., clinical impression that the patient has an EBC, but in actuality, she has advanced stage breast cancer). Regardless, the initial treatment of the patient is still predicated on the initial clinical examination. An example is a woman who presents with a breast mass that measures approximately 2.5 cm (T2) and without evidence of axillary lymphadenopathy on clinical examination (N0). Her *clinical stage* at this point is Stage 2 (T2N0). After undergoing definitive surgery, the final pathology demonstrated a 2.5 cm cancer (T2) with 5 out of 15 lymph nodes involved with metastatic tumor (N2). Therefore, her *pathologic stage* is Stage 3 (T2N2).

To determine the clinical stage, the size of the tumor and the status of the axilla should be documented. For asymptomatic patients with EBC, no further metastatic work-up is necessary. However, respiratory and neurologic complaints, bone pain, etc. necessitate a metastatic work-up. The American Joint Committee on Cancer (AJCC) TNM staging system, 7th edition, is used to stage patients with EBC [15] (Table 4.2).

Table 4.2 American Joint Committee on Cancer (AJCC) TNM Staging for Breast Cancer (7th edition)

Primary tumor (T)	
TX	Primary tumor cannot be assessed
T0	No evidence of primary tumor
Tis	Carcinoma in situ
Tis (DCIS)	Ductal carcinoma in situ
Tis (LCIS)	Lobular carcinoma in situ
TIS (Paget's)	Paget's disease of the nipple NOT associated with invasive carcinoma and/or carcinoma in situ (DCIS and/or LCIS) in the underlying breast parenchyma. Carcinomas in the breast parenchyma associated with Paget's disease are categorized based on the size and characteristics of the parenchymal disease, although the presence of Paget's disease should still be noted
T1	Tumor $\leq$ 20 mm in greatest dimension
T1mi	Tumor $\leq$ 1 mm in greatest dimension
T1a	Tumor > 1 mm but $\leq$ 5 mm in greatest dimension
T1b	Tumor > 5 mm but $\leq$ 10 mm in greatest dimension
T1c	Tumor > 10 mm but $\leq$ 20 mm in greatest dimension
T2	Tumor > 20 mm but $\leq$ 50 mm in greatest dimension
T3	Tumor > 50 mm in greatest dimension
T4	Tumor of any size with direct extension to the chest wall and/or to the skin (ulceration or skin nodules). Note: invasion of the dermis alone does not qualify as T4
T4a	Extension to the chest wall, not including only pectoralis muscle adherence/invasion
T4b	Ulceration and/or ipsilateral satellite nodules and/or edema (including peau d'orange) of the skin, which do not meet the criteria for inflammatory carcinoma
T4c	Both T4a and T4b
T4d	Inflammatory carcinoma (see "Rules for Classification")

(continued)

Table 4.2 (continued)

Distant metastases (M)	
MO	No clinical or radiographic evidence of distant metastases
cMO(i+)	No clinical or radiographic evidence of distant metastases, but deposits of molecularly or microscopically detected tumor cells in circulating blood, bone marrow, or other nonregional nodal tissue that are no larger than 0.2 mm in a patient without symptoms or signs of metastases
M1	Distant detectable metastases as determined by classic clinical and radiographic means and/or histologically proven larger than 0.2 mm

Anatomic stage/prognostic groups			
Stage 0	Tis	N0	M0
Stage IA	T1*	N0	M0
Stage IB	T0	N1mi	M0
	T1*	N1mi	M0
Stage IIA	T0	N1**	M0
	T1*	N1**	M0
	T2	N0	M0
Stage IIB	T2	N1	M0
	T3	N0	M0
Stage IIIA	T0	N2	M0
	T1*	N2	M0
	T2	N2	M0
	T3	N1	M0
	T3	N2	M0
Stage IIIB	T4	N0	M0
	T4	N1	M0
	T4	N2	M0
Stage IIIC	Any T	N3	M0
Stage IV	Any T	Any N	M1

Notes
*T1 includes T1mi
**T0 and T1 tumors with nodal micrometastases only are excluded from Stage IIA and are classified Stage IB
*M0 includes M0(i+)
*The designation pM0 is not valid; any M0 should be clinical
*If a patient presents with M1 prior to neoadjuvant systemic therapy, the stage is considered Stage IV and remain Stage IV regardless of response to neoadjuvant therapy
Stage designation may be changed if postsurgical imaging studies reveal the presence of distant metastases, provided that the studies are carried out within 4 months of diagnosis in the absence of disease progression and provided that the patient has not received neoadjuvant therapy
*Postneoadjuvant therapy is designated with "yc" or "yp" prefix. Of note, no stage group is assigned if there is a complete pathologic response (CR) to neoadjuvant therapy, for example, ypT0ypN0cM0

Regional lymph nodes (N)	
Clinical	
NX	Regional lymph nodes cannot be assessed (e.g., previously removed)
N0	No regional lymph node metastases
N1	Metastases to movable ipsilateral level I, II axillary lymph node(s)
N2	Metastases in ipsilateral level I, II axillary lymph nodes that are clinically fixed or matted or in clinically detected* ipsilateral internal mammary nodes in the absence of clinically evident axillary lymph node metastases
N2A	Metastases in ipsilateral level I, II axillary lymph nodes fixed to one another (matted) or to other structures

(continued)

Table 4.2 (continued)

Regional lymph nodes (N)	
Clinical	
N2B	Metastases only in clinically detected* ipsilateral internal mammary nodes and in the absence of clinically evident axillary lymph node metastases
N3	Metastases in ipsilateral infraclavicular (level III axillary) lymph node(s) with or without level I, II axillary lymph node involvement or in clinically detected*ipsilateral internal mammary lymph node(s) with clinically evident level I, II axillary lymph node metastases or metastases in ipsilateral supraclavicular lymph node(s) with or without axillary or internal mammary lymph node involvement
N3A	Metastases in ipsilateral infraclavicular lymph node(s)
N3B	Metastases in ipsilateral internal mammary lymph node(s) and axillary lymph node(s)
N3C	Metastases in ipsilateral supraclavicular lymph node(s)
Notes	
*"Clinically detected" is defined as detected by imaging studies (excluding lymphoscintigraphy) or by clinical examination and having characteristics highly suspicious for malignancy or a presumed pathologic macrometastasis based on fine-needle aspiration biopsy with cytologic examination. Confirmation of clinically detected metastatic disease by fine-needle aspiration without excision biopsy is designated with an (f) suffix, for example, cN3a(f). Excisional biopsy of a lymph node or biopsy of a sentinel node, in the absence of assignment of a pT, is classified as a clinical N, for example, cN1. Information regarding the confirmation of the nodal status will be designated in site-specific factors as clinical, fine-needle aspiration, core biopsy, or sentinel lymph node biopsy. Pathologic classification (pN) is used for excision or sentinel lymph node biopsy only in conjunction with a pathologic T assignment	

Pathologic (PN)	
pNX	Regional lymph nodes cannot be assessed (e.g., previously removed or not removed for pathologic study)
pN0	No regional lymph node metastasis identified histologically
	Note: isolated tumor cell clusters (ITC) are defined as small clusters of cells not greater than 0.2 mm, or single tumor cells, or a cluster of fewer than 200 cells in a single histologic cross section. ITCs may be detected by routine histology or by immunohistochemical (IHC) methods. Nodes containing only ITCs are excluded from the total positive node count for purposes of N classification but should be included in the total number of nodes evaluated
pN0(i-)	No regional lymph node metastases histologically, negative IHC
pN0(i+)	Malignant cells in regional lymph node(s) no greater than 0.2 mm (detected by H&E or IHC including ITC)
pN0(mol-)	No regional lymph node metastases histologically, negative molecular findings (RT-PCR)
pN0(mol+)	Positive molecular findings (TR-PCR)**, but no regional lymph node metastases detected by histology or IHC
pN1	Micrometastases or metastases in 1–3 axillary lymph nodes and/or in internal mammary nodes with metastases detected by sentinel lymph node biopsy but not clinically detected***
pN1mi	Micrometastases (greater than 0.2 mm and/or more than 200 cells, but none greater than 2.0 mm)
pN1a	Metastases in 1–3 axillary lymph nodes, at least one metastasis greater than 2.0 mm
pN1b	Metastases in internal mammary nodes with micrometastases or macrometastases detected by sentinel lymph node biopsy but not clinically detected***
pN1c	Metastases in 1–3 axillary lymph nodes and in internal mammary lymph nodes with micrometastases or macrometastases detected by sentinel lymph node biopsy but not clinically detected***
pN2	Metastases in 4–9 axillary lymph nodes or in clinically detected****internal mammary lymph nodes in the absence of axillary lymph node metastases
pN2a	Metastases in 4–9 axillary lymph nodes (at least one tumor deposit greater than 2.0 mm)

(continued)

Table 4.2 (continued)

Pathologic (PN)	
pN2b	Metastases in clinically detected**** internal mammary lymph nodes in the absence of axillary node metastases
pN3	Metastases in 10 or more axillary lymph nodes or in infraclavicular (level III axillary) lymph nodes or in clinically detected**** ipsilateral internal mammary lymph nodes in the presence of one or more positive level I, II axillary lymph nodes or in more than three axillary lymph nodes and in internal mammary lymph nodes with micrometastases or macrometastases detected by sentinel lymph node biopsy but not clinically detected*** or in ipsilateral supraclavicular lymph nodes
pN3a	Metastases in 10 or more axillary lymph nodes (at least one tumor deposit greater than 2.0 mm) or metastases to the infraclavicular (level III axillary lymph) nodes
pN3b	Metastases in clinically detected**** ipsilateral internal mammary lymph nodes in the presence of one or more positive axillary lymph nodes or in more than three axillary lymph nodes and in internal mammary lymph nodes with micrometastases or macrometastases detected by sentinel lymph node biopsy but not clinically detected***
pN3c	Metastases in ipsilateral supraclavicular lymph nodes

Notes

*Classification is based on axillary lymph node dissection with or without sentinel lymph node biopsy. Classification based solely on sentinel lymph node biopsy without subsequent axillary lymph node dissection is designated (sn) for "sentinel node," for example, pN0(sn)

**Rt-PCR: reverse transcriptase/polymerase chain reaction

***"Not clinically detected" is defined as not detected by imaging studies (excluding lymphoscintigraphy) or not detected by clinical examination

****"Clinically detected" is defined as detected by imaging studies (excluding lymphoscintigraphy) or by clinical examination and having characteristics highly suspicious for malignancy or a presumed pathologic macrometastasis based on fine-needle aspiration biopsy with cytologic examination

Adapted from Ref. [16]. With permission from Springer Verlag

In treating patients with EBC, the clinician needs to address the following: (1) local control (the primary breast tumor and the at-risk ipsilateral breast), (2) regional control (axillary lymph nodes), and (3) distant control (systemic disease). In general, the surgeon, along with her/his radiation oncologist, is responsible for the first two considerations, while her/his medical oncology colleague is responsible for the third.

Patients often present with an abnormal mammogram or breast ultrasound, with or without a palpable mass. In addition, complaints of breast pain, nipple discharge, or a palpable breast mass may also be the reasons why a patient would seek medical counseling. The initial evaluation consists of a complete history and physical examination, focusing mainly on the risk factors for breast cancer (see above), including a gynecologic history, and thoroughly examining the breast.

If the patient has no imaging, a mammogram or an ultrasound should be ordered. The most recent imaging studies should be compared with prior studies. A thorough review of the patient's mammogram and/or breast ultrasound should be done with a radiologist. Breast ultrasound is useful for younger women (<40 years old) who tend to have denser breast tissue than older women. In some situations, both a mammogram and ultrasound might be necessary to complete the evaluation.

Classic mammographic abnormalities that are highly suggestive of a malignancy include an abnormality with irregular or spiculated borders, architectural distortion, or suspicious calcifications (linear, branching, ductally oriented, pleomorphic, clustered) (Fig. 4.4). For ultrasound, the following features are worrisome for malignancy: hypoechoic, posterior shadowing, irregular borders, nonparallel orientation, and asymmetry (Fig. 4.5).

The American College of Radiology (ACR) has developed a standardized system of describing mammographic and ultrasound readings. The system, the Breast Imaging Reporting and Data System (BI-RADS), groups the findings into categories numbering from 0 through 6. In general, BI-RADS 0 requires additional imaging, BI-RADS 1 and 2 can be observed with annual mammogram, BI-RADS 3 requires a repeat

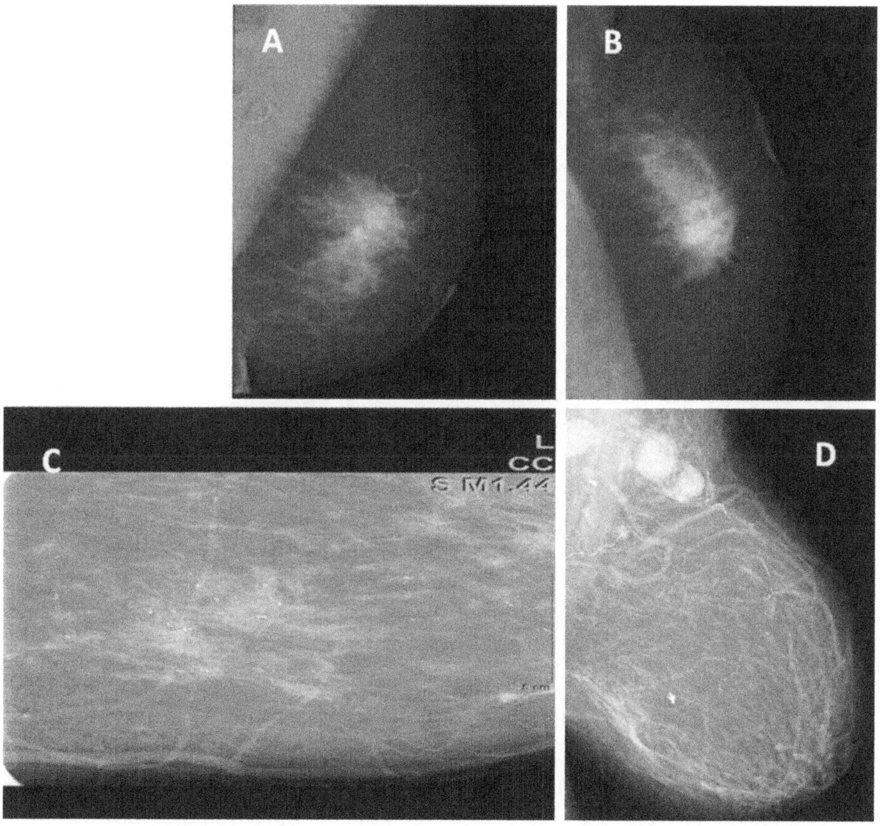

Fig. 4.4 Mammogram images (**a**) and (**b**) are views of an obscured mass in the left breast which on compression images and ultrasound was given BI-RADS 5, and pathology demonstrated an invasive ductal carcinoma. Image (**c**) depicts pleomorphic calcifications in a linear segmental distribution which is typical of DCIS. In this example, DCIS has evidence of cancer that has infiltrated the axillary lymph nodes (**d**) (Courtesy of Quyen D. Chu, MD, MBA, FACS)

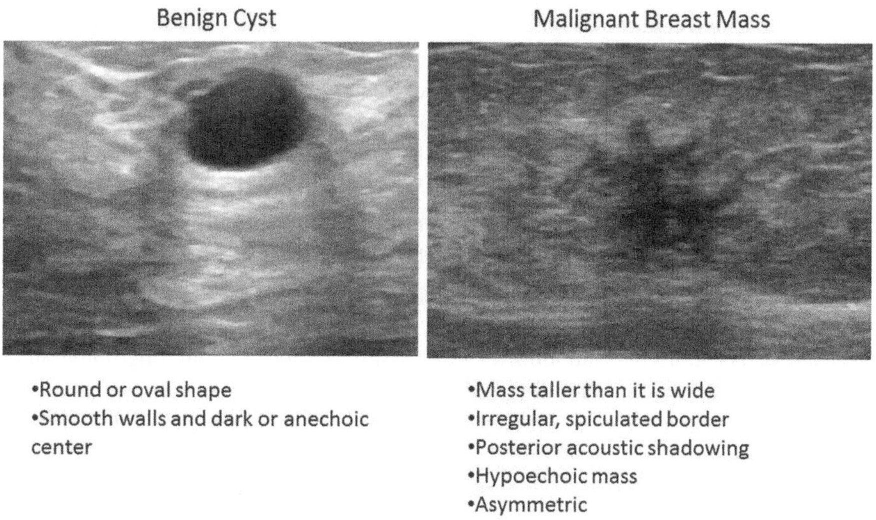

Fig. 4.5 Abnormal ultrasound (B): features that are worrisome for malignancy include an asymmetric, hypoechoic mass with irregular margins and posterior shadowing (Courtesy of Quyen D. Chu, MD, MBA, FACS)

Table 4.3 Breast imaging reporting and data system (BI-RADS)

BI-RADS readings	Implications
0	Additional imaging evaluation and/or comparison to prior mammograms is needed
1	Negative. No significant abnormality to report. Annual screening mammogram is recommended as deemed appropriate
2	Benign (noncancerous) finding. Annual screening mammogram is recommended as deemed appropriate
3	Probably benign finding. Follow-up with repeat imaging in 6 months and regularly thereafter until the finding is known to be stable (usually at least 2 years)
4	Suspicious abnormality. Biopsy should be considered
5	Highly suggestive of malignancy (95 % chance of cancer). Biopsy should be considered
6	Known biopsy. Proven malignancy

mammogram 6 months and thereafter until the finding is known to be stable (usually at least 2 years), BI-RADS 4 and 5 require a biopsy, and BI-RADS 6 is a biopsy-proven cancer (a mammogram usually obtained after a known cancer by a previous biopsy; the mammogram, in such a case, may be used to see how sensitive the cancer is to systemic therapy) (Table 4.3). Of note, mammograms have a 10 % false-negative rate. Thus, clinical suspicion should prompt the clinician to pursue a more intense investigation despite a negative mammographic reading. On occasions, there may be discordance between the BI-RADS assignments for the mammogram and ultrasound (i.e., BI-RADS 3 for mammogram and BI-RADS 4 for ultrasound). In such a situation, we recommend to err on the conservative side and proceed with the work-up based on the highest BI-RADS reading.

A brief mentioned of screening MRI of the breast is warranted. There are no randomized trials available to determine whether screening MRI reduces mortality from breast cancer. However, screening MRI is thought to be cost effective for women between ages 30 and 60 years who either carry a BRCA mutation or have a 50 % chance of carrying such a mutation [17]. The estimated cost per quality-adjusted life-year (QALY) gained in this group is approximately $55,420–$130,625 (i.e., it costs this much per additional life-year per person). Although there is no absolute QALY threshold, in the United States, it is thought to be around $50,000–$100,000 per QALY gained, while in the United Kingdom, it is approximated to be around $30,000–$45,000 [18].

The American Cancer Society (ACS), endorsed by ACR and Society of Breast Imaging (SBI) [19], recommends annual MRI screening, along with mammography, for women at high lifetime risk (≥20 %) of developing breast cancer, beginning at age 30. The lifetime risk can be calculated using the already mentioned risk estimation models, although ACS does not recommend using the Gail model because it does not incorporate family history of ovarian or breast cancer in 2nd-degree relatives [20]; high lifetime risk includes patients with known BRCA1 or BRCA2 gene mutation or who have a 1st-degree relative with a BRCA1 or BRCA2 gene mutation and history of radiation to the chest at the ages between 10 and 30 years and patients with Li-Fraumeni syndrome or Cowden syndrome or who have a 1st-degree relative with one of these syndromes [21]. For those who are at a moderate risk of developing breast cancer (15–20 % lifetime risk), it is recommended that they discuss screening MRIs with their physicians. Moderate risk group includes those who have a personal history of breast cancer, DCIS, LCIS, ADH, atypical lobular hyperplasia, or those with extremely dense breasts or unevenly dense breasts seen on mammograms. Low-risk group includes those whose lifetime risk of breast cancer is less than 15 %; routine screening MRI is not recommended [22]. Screening MRIs should be done in a facility that also has the capability of performing an MRI-guided breast biopsy (Table 4.4). It must be stressed that MRI is not meant to replace mammography and that the guidelines are not intended to replace sound clinical judgment or considered standard of care.

Routine preoperative MRI should not be used in all cancer patients since it has no significant impact on outcome. A recent meta-analysis found that preoperative MRI for staging breast cancer

Table 4.4 Recommendations for breast MRI screening

Characteristics	Time to begin screening (years)
Proven BRCA mutation carriers Annual MRI beginning at age 30	Annually by age 30 but not before age 25
1st-degree relatives of BRCA mutation carriers but have not been tested Annual MRI beginning at age 30	Annually by age 30 but not before age 25
History of chest irradiation between ages 10–30 Annual MRI beginning 8 years after radiation therapy	Annually beginning 8 years after radiation therapy but not before age 25
Lifetime risk ≥ 20–25 %, as defined by models that are dependent on family history (not the Gail model)	Annually by age 30 but not before age 25 or 10 years before the age of the youngest affected relative, whichever is later
Patients with following genetic syndromes and their first-degree relatives Li-Fraumeni Cowden Bannayan-Riley-Ruvalcaba	Annually beginning at age 30–35 years

did not reduce the risk of local ipsilateral recurrence and distant recurrence [22]. Additionally, preoperative MRI not only fails to reduce re-excisions rate [23], it increases the odds of a patient receiving a mastectomy who would otherwise be a candidate for a BCT [24].

Biopsy Techniques

Breast masses can be cystic, solid, or both. Cystic masses can be aspirated with a fine-needle aspiration (FNA), guided either by palpation or ultrasound (US). Non-bloody aspirate can be discarded unless there is a clinical or radiologic suspicion of an associated malignancy. For non-cystic abnormality, the selection of the most appropriate biopsy technique will depend on whether the abnormality is palpable or non-palpable. Excisional biopsy as the initial diagnostic tool should be avoided unless minimally invasive biopsy techniques (percutaneous image-guided biopsy or palpation-guided) are not available. In general, a percutaneous biopsy such as a core needle biopsy (CNB) with either a 12–14 gauge needle or vacuum-assisted biopsy with a 7–11 gauge needle is the preferred initial diagnostic procedure for both palpable and non-palpable lesions [25]. If the biopsy is positive for either noninvasive cancer (DCIS; see Chap. 3) or invasive cancer, the clinician can then provide the patient with an optimal plan of care, which can include a single trip to the operating room for a definitive surgery. If it is negative or nondiagnostic, then the result should be put in context with the clinical examination and radiologic imaging. If the clinical exam and radiologic imaging are in concordance with the biopsy result (triple concordance), then the likelihood of a missed malignancy is very low (accuracy ranges from 93 to 99 %). However, if there is any discordance (i.e., lesion is suspicious for malignancy based on clinical exam and/or radiologic imaging), then the lesion should be excised for a definitive diagnosis (i.e., excisional biopsy for palpable lesion, needle localization biopsy for non-palpable lesion). Curvilinear incisions following Langer's skin lines should be considered for optimal cosmesis (Fig. 4.6), and the pathologic specimen should be appropriately oriented. Specimens should be marked in a consistent manner to avoid confusion by the pathologist about the proper orientation, which could influence appropriate re-excision to achieve negative margins. Although a commonly used method calls for a short stitch be placed to designate the superior margin and a long stitch to indicate the lateral margin, this two-stitch method has been shown to be associated with an error rate of 31 % [26]. Intraoperative inking by the surgeon or placement of at least three separate marking sutures/clips for specimen orientation is recommended.

For patients with high-risk lesions such as atypical ductal hyperplasia (ADH), atypical lobular hyperplasia, lobular carcinoma in situ, and radial scars (complex sclerosing lesions) found on percutaneous biopsy, a surgical excision should be performed to assure that no occult DCIS or invasive cancer is present [25].

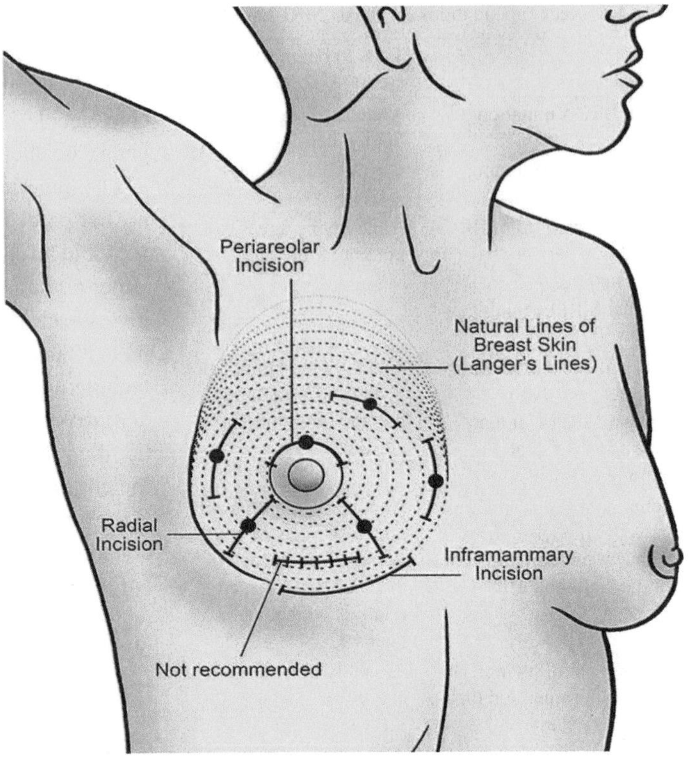

Fig. 4.6 Recommended curvilinear incisions to be used when operating on the breast (Courtesy of Quyen D. Chu, MD, MBA, FACS)

Of note, if a percutaneous biopsy will remove most or all of the abnormality, then a clip or some other imaging marker should be inserted at the time of biopsy.

Non-palpable Lesions

Besides CNB, stereotactic core biopsy or ultrasound-guided biopsy is also an acceptable modality for non-palpable lesions. For lesion ≤ 1 cm, percutaneous excision using a vacuum-assisted device is recommended [25]. In situations where more tissue is required for a definitive diagnosis, a needle or wire localization biopsy can be performed. Such specimen should be sent to the radiologist to confirm that the abnormal lesion has indeed been excised. Of note, a lesion detected on an ultrasound should be confirmed ex vivo with an ultrasound, while one that was detected on a mammogram should be confirmed ex vivo with a mammogram. If the final specimen is negative for malignancy, our practice has been to repeat the imaging in 6 months.

Palpable Lesions

Although CNB is the preferred initial procedure for palpable lesions, an FNA is also acceptable. In expert hands, the accuracy rate of an FNA ranges from 89 to 98 %. However, the advantage with CNB is that it can differentiate whether the carcinoma is intraductal or invasive, whereas FNA may not because it is limited by few loose cells. For large suspicious lesions (>5 cm), a CNB or an incisional biopsy (taking a small piece of the mass) may be performed to obtain a tissue diagnosis and for determining receptor statuses. This is especially important if neoadjuvant (chemotherapy before surgery) is being considered. Our approach is to send a small piece of the incised mass for frozen section to confirm a diagnosis of cancer before leaving the operating room.

Treatment

Local Control

Once a diagnosis of cancer has been confirmed, the surgeon will need to consider the options of obtaining **local control**. The primary goal is two-fold: (1) resect the primary tumor to negative margins and (2) address the at-risk breast. Options for local control are (1) mastectomy (see Fig. 6.1, Chap. 6) or (2) lumpectomy with negative margins, followed by breast irradiation (XRT), which is also known as breast-conserving therapy (BCT). There is a whole range of radiation options; these include external beam radiation (whole-breast radiation), accelerated partial breast irradiation, 3D conformal radiotherapy, and brachytherapy. External beam radiation is the most common and therefore, unless specified otherwise, most of the discussion on radiation implies the use of this modality.

BCT yields equivalent survival outcome as a mastectomy. The National Surgical Adjuvant Breast and Bowel Project (NSABP) B-04 was the first clinical trial that demonstrated that less radical surgery (i.e., total mastectomy or TM ± radiation) was equivalent to a Halsted radical mastectomy (i.e., removing the breast, the underlying pectoral muscles, and axillary contents) [27–30]. The trial enrolled 1,665 women, and the latest 25-year follow-up results reported in 2002 demonstrated that there were no significant differences in the disease-free survival (DFS), relapse-free survival (RFS), distant-disease-free survival (DDFS), and overall survival (OS) among TM, TM plus radiation, and RM [31] (Table 4.5).

Subsequent to the NSABP B-04 trial, the NSABP B-06 trial evaluated 1,843 women with tumors 4 cm or less and randomized them into three groups: TM and ALND (modified radical mastectomy), lumpectomy and ALND with breast irradiation, or lumpectomy and ALND without breast irradiation [33, 39]. The latest 20-year follow-up results, also reported in 2002, found no significant differences in the DFS, DDFS, or OS among the three groups [33]. However, patients who underwent a lumpectomy with breast irradiation had a significantly lower cumulative incidence of ipsilateral breast cancer recurrence (14.3 %) than those who underwent a lumpectomy without breast irradiation (39.2 %) ($P < 0.001$).

The Early Breast Cancer Trialists' Collaborative Group (EBCTCG) performed a meta-analysis of 10,801 women from 17 randomized trials of radiotherapy (XRT) versus no radiotherapy after BCT and found that XRT resulted in a 15.7 % absolute reduction in recurrence at 10 years ($2p < 0.00001$) and a 3.8 % absolute reduction in breast cancer death at 15 years ($2p = 0.00005$) compared to no XRT [40]. The magnitude was observed to be higher in node positive than node positive patients (absolute reduction in recurrence, 21.2 % versus 15.4 %, respectively, and absolute reduction in mortality, 8.5 % versus 3.3 %, respectively) [40]. Thus, NSABP B-06 and EBCTCG, along with other clinical trials, established that BCT with radiation is equally effective as a mastectomy and that BCT must be accompanied by XRT [34–36] (Table 4.5).

Role of Accelerated Partial Breast Irradiation

Accelerated partial breast irradiation (APBI) has been explored as an alternative technique to whole-breast irradiation (WBI). The rationale behind APBI is based on data that demonstrated that 80–90 % of local recurrences following a lumpectomy are within the cavity site [31, 41, 42]. Thus, by delivering an intense dose of radiation to the surgical bed, local recurrence rate should be equivalent to WBI. Another advantage with APBI is that it is administered over a shorter period of time (1–2 weeks) instead of the traditional 6-week period with WBI. This is important, especially for women who are candidates for BCT but who happen to reside in a place that is substantially far away from their nearest radiation facility.

APBI comes in different forms, including multicatheter interstitial brachytherapy, intraoperative RT (IORT), external beam conformal therapy (EBRT), and intracavitary balloon

Table 4.5 Selected trials comparing mastectomy and breast-conserving therapy for breast cancer

Trials/authors/ref	N	Mean follow-up (years)	Treatment group	Outcome
NSABP B-04/Fisher [32]	1,665	25	(1) TM (2) TM+XRT (3) RM	No significant differences in DFS, RFS, DDFS, and OS among the three groups
NSABP B-06/Fisher [33]	1,843	20	(1) MRM (2) L+ALND	No significant differences in DFS, DDFS, and OS among the three groups
			(3) L+ALND+XRT	L alone had higher cumulative incidence of ipsilateral breast cancer recurrence compared to L+XRT (39 % versus 14 %; $P<0.001$)
NCI/Jacobson [34]	247	10	(1) MRM (2) L+ALND+XRT	No significant differences in DFS, OS, or locoregional recurrence rate between the two groups
Milan/Veronesi [35]	701	20	(1) RM	No significant differences in OS, rates of contralateral breast cancers, distant metastases, or second primary cancers between the two groups
			(2) L+ALND+XRT	L group had significantly higher tumor recurrence rate than the RM group ($P<0.001$)
DBCG/Blichert-Toft [36]	793	20	(1) MRM	No significant differences in local tumor control, RFS, OS between the two groups
			(2) L+ALND+XRT	L had higher rate of new primaries, while MRM had higher rate of true tumor recurrence
EORTC/van Dongen [37]	903	NA	(1) MRM (2) L+ALND+XRT	No significant difference in DDS, local-regional recurrence, and OS between the two groups
IGR/Sarrazin [38]	179	10	(1) MRM (2) L+ALND+XRT	No significant difference in distant metastasis, local-regional recurrence, contralateral breast cancer, and OS between the two groups

NSABP National Surgical Adjuvant Breast and Bowel Project, *EBCTCG* Early Breast Cancer Trialists' Collaborative Group, *NCI* National Cancer Institute, *DBCG* Danish Breast Cancer Cooperative Group, *EORTC* European Organization for Research and Treatment of Cancer, *IGR* Institut Gustave-Roussy, *L* lumpectomy, *TM* total mastectomy, *XRT* radiation therapy, *RM* radical mastectomy, *MRM* modified radical mastectomy, *ALND* axillary lymph node dissection, *DFS* disease-free survival, *RFS* relapse-free survival, *DDFS* distant-disease-free survival, *OS* overall survival, *NA* not available

brachytherapy such as MammoSite® (Hologic, Inc., Bedford, MA, USA). The American Society of Breast Surgeons (ASBS) MammoSite® Breast Brachytherapy Registry Trial [43] recently published their final analysis on 1,449 patients with early breast cancer who were treated with BCT and MammoSite® and were followed-up for greater than 5 years. Their results, which are similar to others [44, 45], found that the 5-year actuarial ipsilateral breast tumor recurrence (IBTR) rate was 3.8 %, which is in line with historic rate of 2 % for WBI [46]. Additionally, the rate of excellent/good cosmesis at 84 months approached 91 %, and the rates of infectious and noninfectious complications were comparable to WBI historic data [43]. The limitations with this study are the potential for selection bias (surgeons might be reluctant to report complications since it is a volunteer registry), lack of long-term outcomes, and comparison against historic controls.

However, Smith et al. performed a retrospective review of over 92,000 women in the Medicare

Table 4.6 NSABP B-39/RTOG 0413 criteria for clinical trial comparing accelerated partial breast irradiation (APBI) with whole-breast radiation (WBI) in women with early breast cancer

Patients with Stage 0, I, and II breast cancer resected by lumpectomy
Tumor size ≤ 3 cm
No more than 3 histologically positive nodes

SEER database and reported that compared to WBI, women who were treated with brachytherapy had a higher mastectomy rate, more frequent infectious and noninfectious complications, and higher incidence of fat necrosis, although the 5-year OS was equivalent between WBI and APBI [47]. The limitations with this study include comparison of WBI with older form of brachytherapy with less control of radiation dose and the use of an administrative database that may be fraught with selection bias, incomplete information, and potential inaccuracy.

Whether APBI is equivalent to WBI is currently the focus of the NSABP B-39/RTOG 0413 clinical trial, a trial that randomizes patients with early stage breast cancer (Stage 0–II) to receive either WBI or APBI. Criteria include patients whose tumor is ≤ 3 cm and who possess no more than three histologically positive lymph nodes (Table 4.6). Unfortunately, results will not be known for another 5–10 years [48].

The decision to perform BCT depends on many factors, one of which is cosmesis. If the lumpectomy will result in a disfigurement of the remaining breast, it is better to opt for a mastectomy. In addition, BCT is ideal for patients who are compliant, are not pregnant, have access to a radiation facility, have no history of radiation therapy to the chest wall (i.e., history of radiation for lymphoma), and have no history of collagen vascular disease (i.e., scleroderma and systemic lupus erythematosus).

One of the tenets in breast surgery is the need to achieve a negative margin to avoid local recurrence (LR). What constitutes an adequate negative margin, however, remains an area of great interest. According to NSABP, a negative margin is defined as having no tumor at the inked surgical margin, irrespective of the distance from the nearest tumor cell. In a meta-analysis, of 21 studies and over 14,000 women with early breast cancer who underwent BCT, Houssami et al. confirmed that those with positive margins (presence of any cancer, invasive and/or DCIS at the inked margin) had a significantly higher likelihood of having LR (odds ratio of 2.42; $P<0.001$) compared to those with negative margins [49]. The margin width (1 mm versus 2 mm versus 5 mm), however, had no significant impact on the rate of LR. The authors conclude that it is reasonable to define a minimum distance of 1 mm for negative margins in women who undergo BCT for early breast cancer [49]. Finally, a panel of breast experts recently developed a guideline for defining adequate margins in the setting of BCT and adjuvant radiation therapy and concluded that no ink on tumor should suffice as adequate margin in invasive cancer [50].

To summarize this portion of the discussion, both a mastectomy and a BCT will achieve equivalent local control. In a mastectomy, the tumor and the at-risk breast are removed at the same setting, whereas in BCT, the tumor is resected and the at-risk breast is irradiated. A negative margin is a negative margin. The role of APBI will be clarified, based on the results of the NSABP B-39/RTOG 0413 clinical trial.

Regional Control

Once a local control option has been selected, the next goal is to obtain **regional control**. Although there is a rich network of lymphatics that drains the breast, surgeons generally focus their attention on the axillary lymph nodes for evidence of metastases. Lymph node status is one of the most important prognostic factors in breast cancer [51]. Options for assessing the lymph nodes are sentinel lymph node biopsy (SLNBx) or axillary lymph node dissection (ALND); the latter, when combined with a mastectomy, is a modified radical mastectomy (MRM) (Fig. 4.7a–d).

Historically, ALND was a routine component of the management of the majority of patients with early breast cancer. The procedure, however, does carry some inherent risks such as neurovascular

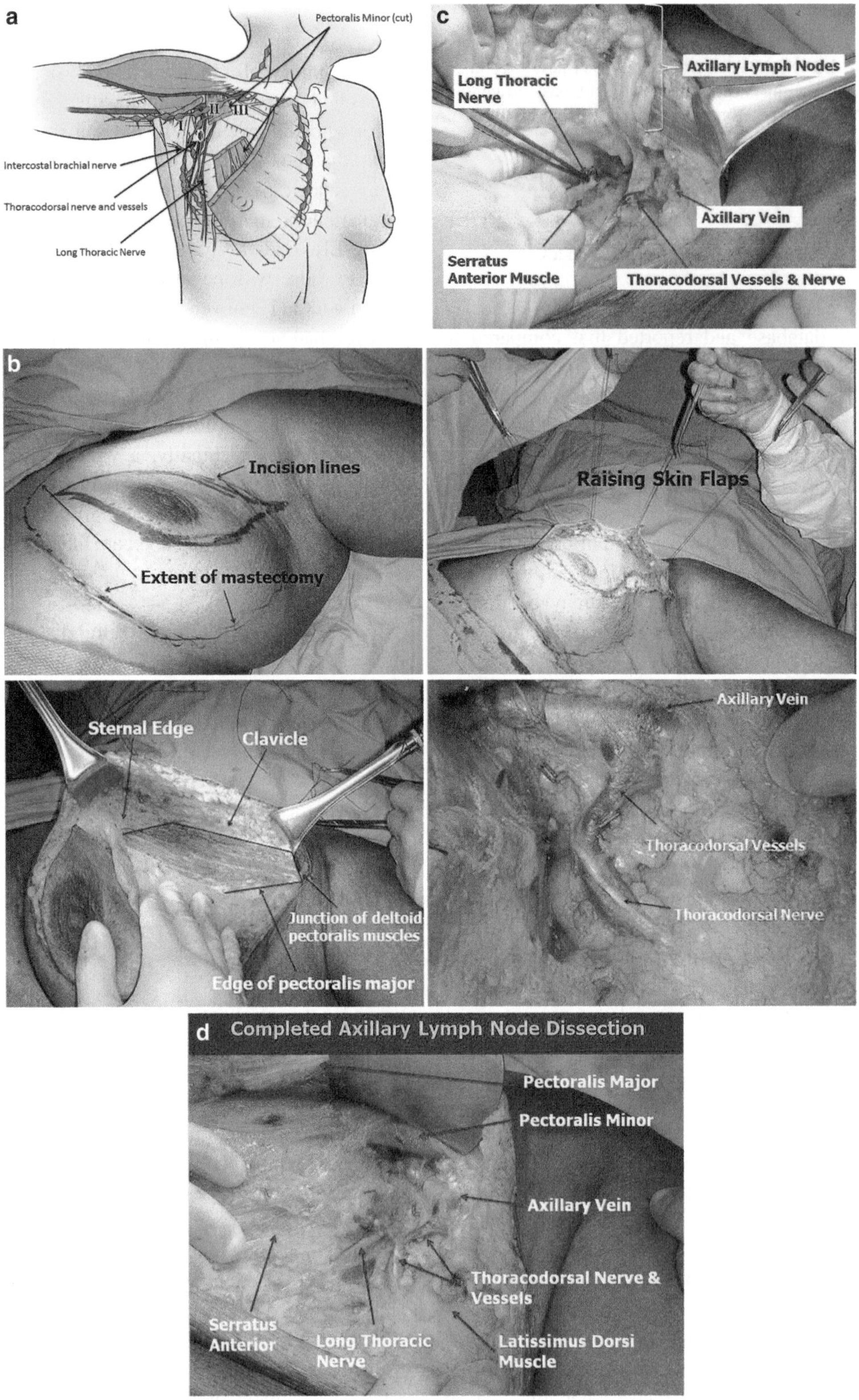

Fig. 4.7 A modified radical mastectomy (MRM) requires a thorough knowledge of breast anatomy (**a**). In general, the following nerves should be preserved: the long thoracic nerve, which innervates the serratus anterior and lies along the muscle. Injury to this nerve can result in a "winged scapula." The thoracodorsal nerve generally runs along the thoracodorsal vessels and at a right angle to the axillary vein. The nerve innervates the latissimus dorsi, and an injury to it

injury (injury to the axillary vessels or long thoracic nerve), seroma formation, decrease in range of motion in the shoulder, and chronic lymphedema. Minimizing these risks without compromising oncologic principles became a major focus of the medical community. Sentinel lymph node biopsy became an alternative technique to assess the axilla for a subset of patients. The principle behind SLNBx is that when breast cancer metastasizes to the lymph nodes, it does so in an orderly manner. Because breast cancer generally drains to the first echelon of lymph nodes before draining to the subsequent echelons of lymph nodes, the likelihood of having metastases in subsequent echelons will be low if there is no evidence of metastases in the first echelon of lymph nodes.

SLNBx removes only a small number of lymph nodes and therefore requires less dissection in the axilla. Several studies have demonstrated that SLNBx is less morbid [52, 53] and yielded equivalent outcome as an ALND [54–58] (Table 4.7). Sentinel lymph node identification rate ranges 95–98.7 %, and the false-negative rate is generally less than 10 % [55–57]. Most surgeons use both isosulfan blue (blue dye) and technetium-99 sulfur colloid (double-tracer technique) to identify the sentinel nodes (Fig. 4.8a, b). Injection can be done either peritumorally or subareolar [59], the latter being done in situation when the tumor is not palpable (Fig. 4.9). To achieve an acceptable false-negative rate (FNR) threshold of 10 %, at least two sentinel nodes should be retrieved. NSABP B-32 reported an FNR of 18 % with 1 SLN resected, 10 % with 2 SLNs resected, and 7 % with 3 SLNs resected [60]. When the sentinel node(s) cannot be identified, a standard ALND should be performed. On occasions, internal mammary lymph node(s) (IMN) may be seen on lymphoscintigraphy,

Table 4.7 Selected series comparing sentinel lymph node biopsy with axillary lymph node dissection

Author/year	# Patients	Median follow-up (mos)	Axillary recurrence rate SLNBx	Axillary recurrence rate ALND	5-year DFS SLNBx	5-year DFS ALND	5-year OS SLNBx	5-year OS ALND
Veronesi 2003/2010 [54, 55]	516	102	0 %	2 %	89.9 %	88.9 %	93.5 %	89.7 %
			$p=0.17$		$p=0.52$		$p=0.15$	
Zavagno [56]	749	56	0.29 %	0 %	87.6 %	89.9 %	94.8 %	95.5 %
(Sentinella/GIVOM) 2008			$p=$NA		$p=0.77$		$p=$NA	
Krag (NSABP-B32) [57]	5,611	95.6	0.7 %	0.4 %	88.6 %	89.0 %	95.0 %	96.4 %
2010		(mean)	$p=0.22$		$p=0.54$		$p=0.12$	
Giuliano [58]	891	76	0.9 %	0.5 %	83.9 %	82.2 %	92.5 %	91.8 %
(ACOSOG Z0011) 2011					$p=0.14$		$p=0.25$	

GIVOM Gruppo Interdisciplinare Veneto di Oncologia Mammaria, *NSABP* National Surgical Adjuvant Breast and Bowel Project, *ACOSOG* American College of Surgeons Oncology Group, *SLNB*x sentinel lymph node biopsy, *ALND* axillary lymph node dissection, *NA* not available, *DFS* disease-free survival, *OS* overall survival

Fig. 4.7 (continued) results in the patient being unable to raise the trunk with the upper limb. Finally, the intercostal brachial nerve supplies sensation to the back of the arm. Its injury can lead to a feeling of "numbness" in the upper medial aspect of the arm. The levels of the lymph nodes are named based on their relationship to the pectoralis minor muscle. Axillary lymph node dissection generally involves removal of level I lymph nodes (lateral to the pectoralis minor muscle) and level II lymph nodes (underneath/posterior to the pectoralis minor muscle). Level III lymph nodes (above and medial to the pectoralis minor muscle) are removed when they are palpable. This generally requires resecting the pectoralis minor muscle at its insertion into the coracoid process. (**b**) A modified radical mastectomy begins with an elliptical incision that incorporates the nipple/areolar complex. The superior and inferior flaps are raised and the breast tissue is removed. Note that the axillary contents are below the axillary vein and that the thoracodorsal nerve tends to run parallel to the thoracodorsal vessels. (**c**) This figure shows the major structures just before the axillary contents are removed. (**d**) Picture of a completed axillary lymph node dissection. Note the long thoracic nerve along the serratus anterior muscle (**a**–**d**: Courtesy of Quyen D. Chu, MD, MBA, FACS)

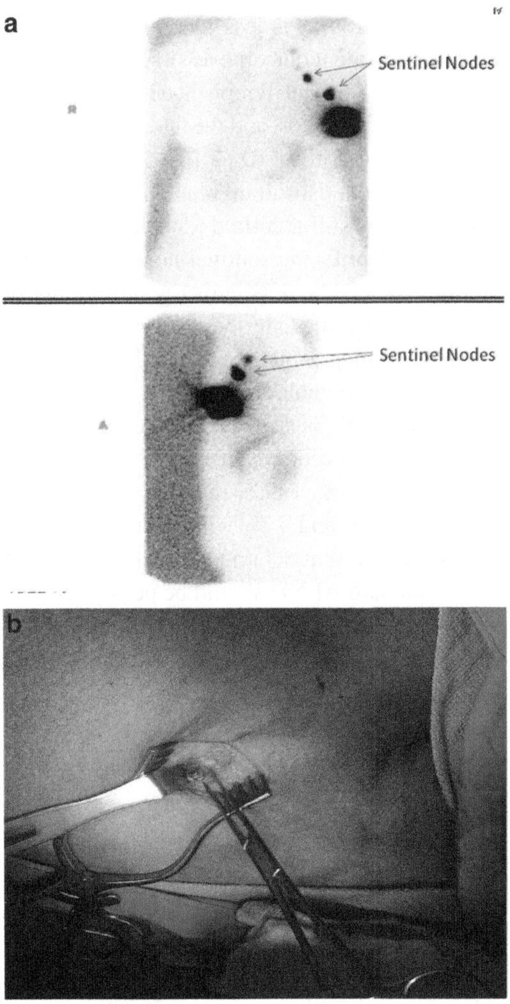

Fig. 4.8 Sentinel lymph node mapping of a breast cancer using lymphoscintigraphy (**a**). Radiotracer used was Tc-99 m sulfur colloid. Sentinel node was identified with isosulfan blue (blue dye) (**b**) (Courtesy of Quyen D. Chu, MD, MBA, FACS)

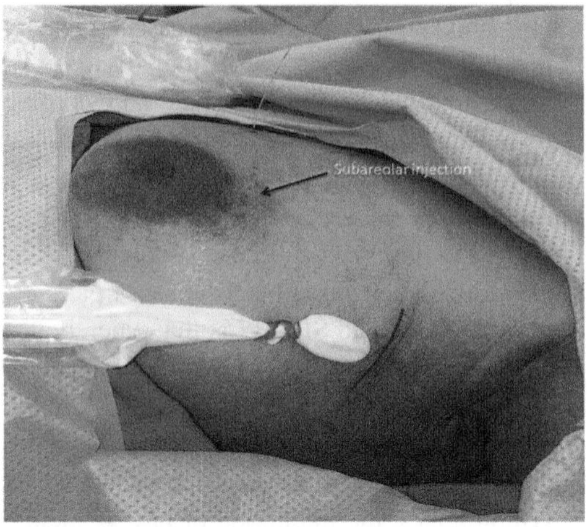

Fig. 4.9 Subareolar injection can be performed to identify sentinel nodes. This can be done in situations when the tumor is not palpable (Courtesy of Quyen D. Chu, MD, MBA, FACS)

especially for cancers located in the medial aspect of the breast. Most surgeons do not perform IMN biopsy or dissection due to the associated morbidity; instead, the IMN is generally treated with radiation.

ACOSOG Z0010 and NSABP B-32 reported that SLN disease detected on IHC has no clinical significance and, therefore, recommended that IHC staining of SLNs is unnecessary [61, 62]. Thus, hematoxylin and eosin staining of SLN is all that is needed, and given the recent ACOSOG Z0011 data, intraoperative frozen-section analysis of the SLN should be avoided for nodes that are not highly suspicious, especially if the patient meets ACOSOG Z0011 criteria.

Should a Completion ALND Be Performed for Low-Volume Axillary Disease?

Sentinel lymph node biopsy is now the standard of care for most women with invasive breast cancer and indicated for virtually any patient with clinically node-negative invasive breast cancer [63]. The American Society of Clinical Oncology (ASCO) recommends SLNBx in patients with T1 and T2 tumors and clinically node-negative disease [64]. It also supports SLNBx for those with multicentric tumors and with ductal carcinoma in situ (DCIS) who opted for a mastectomy since an SLNBx will be impossible to perform if an invasive tumor is found in the mastectomy specimen [64]. For patients who have palpable axillary lymphadenopathy or are pregnant, or for an SLNBx that cannot be identified, or if the technique is not available, an axillary lymph node dissection (ALND) should be performed (Table 4.8).

For patients with a negative SLNBx, no further surgery in the axilla is needed. However, how should a patient with positive SLNBx be managed? Traditionally, such a patient undergoes a completion ALND because the incidence of additional

Table 4.8 Indications and contraindications for sentinel lymph node biopsy

Indications: clinically negative axilla and
1. T1/T2 tumors
2 DCIS in women who opted for a mastectomy
Controversial indications
1. Multicentric tumor
2. Prior axillary surgery
3. T3/T4
Absolute contraindications
1. Clinically palpable axillary lymphadenopathy
2. Large T4 tumors
3. Inflammatory breast cancer
4. Pregnant women

disease on ALND can be as high as 53 % [65]. In the past, several predictive nomograms were developed to estimate the risk of additional positive nodes in the hope of sparing women the morbidity of unnecessary ALND [66, 67]. However, such nomograms will likely be supplanted by recent data from the American College of Surgeons Oncology Group (ACOSOG) Z0011 trial.

ACOSOG Z0011 demonstrated that a completion ALND might not be necessary in a subset of patients who have positive SLNBx [58]. ACOSOG Z0011 was a phase III non-inferiority trial that randomized 891 women who had positive sentinel lymph nodes to either observation ($N=446$) or undergo a completion ALND ($N=445$). All women had BCT, clinical T1–T2 tumor, systemic therapy as appropriate, and whole-breast irradiation (WBI) with tangential fields (TFs) which partially covers level 1 and 2 lymph nodes. At a median follow-up of 6.3 years, regional recurrence was less than 1 % with SLNBx alone, despite 27 % of patients having had additional metastases in the undissected axillary nodes (based on indirect evidence that 27 % of patients in the ALND group had nodal disease). The 5-year OS for SLNBx alone versus ALND group was 92.5 % and 91.8 %, respectively ($p=0.25$), and the 5-year DFS for SLNBx alone versus ALND group was 83.9 % and 82.2 %, respectively ($p=0.14$). On multivariate analysis, neither the number of positive SLNBx, size of SN metastasis, nor number of LNs removed was associated with locoregional recurrence. This may be due to the effectiveness of systemic therapy and TF irradiation to eliminate low-volume residual nodal disease.

Table 4.9 ACOSOG Z0011 criteria precluding the need for a completion axillary lymph node dissection in patients with positive sentinel lymph node biopsy

1. T ≤ 5 cm
2. ≤2 positive sentinel lymph nodes
3. Lumpectomy with whole-breast irradiation
4. Receiving systemic therapy

Thus, based on Z0011, SLNBx alone is adequate for patients who meet all of the following three criteria: (1) small tumor (T ≤ 5 cm), (2) two sentinel lymph nodes or fewer are positive, and (3) the patient will undergo a lumpectomy with adjuvant systemic therapy and radiation to the axilla (Table 4.9). It must be cautioned that patients who have a mastectomy or those who will not receive radiation that covers the axilla (i.e., partial breast irradiation) will still require an ALND for a positive sentinel lymph node biopsy.

The International Breast Cancer Study Group Trial 23-01 (IBCSG 23-01) also reported similar results as the Z0011 trial. IBCSG randomized 931 patients with non-palpable axilla whose tumor was ≤ 5 cm and SLNBx with one or more micrometastasis (≤2 mm) to either observation or completion ALNDs. Similar to Z0011, less than 1 % recurred in the axilla in the observation group, and there was no significant difference in either DFS or OS between the groups [68].

What Is the Role of Preoperative Ultrasound-Guided Biopsy of the Axilla?

Preoperative axillary ultrasound combined with US-guided axillary lymph node biopsy has been championed by some clinicians because it avoids having the patient undergo a two-step axillary surgery (SLNBx followed by completion ALND). However, given the recent ACOSOG Z0011 data, such a practice may be limited to a select group of patients. US evaluation may have a role in those who will undergo a mastectomy, since patients with an US-guided biopsy-proven axilla can undergo a one-step surgery (completion ALND). However, patients with a negative US-guided biopsy should undergo an SLNBx since a recent meta-analysis found that one in four women with a US-guided biopsy-proven negative axilla has a positive SLNBx [69].

Role of SLNBx in Patients Who Undergo Neoadjuvant Chemotherapy

Although SLNBx is an acceptable option for patients with clinically node-negative breast cancer who will undergo primary surgery, its role and timing for patients who undergo neoadjuvant chemotherapy is unclear. For those who present with clinically negative lymph node (cN0), the options are either SLNBx before or after neoadjuvant chemotherapy. Pooled analysis of data in the literature suggests that SLNBx after neoadjuvant chemotherapy for cN0 is an acceptable diagnostic procedure because the sentinel lymph node identification rate and false negative rate (FNR) are comparable to patients who undergo SLNBx before chemotherapy [70]. However, for patients with cN0 but a positive SLNBx who opted for neoadjuvant therapy, an ALND should be performed since the FNR for a second SLNBx following neoadjuvant chemotherapy is above 50 % [71].

What is the reliability of performing an SLNBx following neoadjuvant therapy for those who present with clinically positive nodal disease (cN+)? ACOSOG Z1071 (Alliance) [72] and SENTinel NeoAdjuvant (SENTINA) [71] evaluated patients with cN+who underwent SLNBx following neoadjuvant chemotherapy and found that the procedure resulted in a high FNR. For those that had two or more SLNBs retrieved, the FNR was 12.6 % in the ACOSOG Z1071 trial. Even if the patient's axilla was downstaged to cN(−) following neoadjuvant chemotherapy, the FNR was 18.5 %, as reported in the SENTINA trial. Thus, the results of both trials exceeded the 10 % threshold. Because of this, the authors concluded that SLNBx following neoadjuvant chemotherapy for patients with cN(+) is not a reliable alternative over ALND (Table 4.10).

Table 4.10 Trials evaluating role of sentinel lymph node biopsy after neoadjuvant chemotherapy in node-positive breast cancer

Trials/author/year/ref	N	False-negative results (based on # LNs retrieved)
ACOSOG Z1071	663	1 SLN: 31.5 %[a]
Boughey/2013 [72]		2 SLNs: 21 %
		≥ 3 SLNs: 9 %
SENTINA/Kuehn/2013 [71]	1,737	1 SLN: 24.3 %
		2 SLNs: 18.5 %
		≥ 3 SLNs: <10 %

ACOSOG American College of Surgeons Oncology Group, *SENTINA* SENTinel neoAdjuvant
[a]Based on patients with clinical N1 disease; *SLN* sentinel lymph node

Can Regional Nodal Irradiation Substitute ALND?

The European Organization for Research and Treatment of Cancer (EORTC) **A**fter **M**apping of the **A**xilla: **R**adiotherapy or **S**urgery (AMAROS) was a phase III trial comparing ALND with axillary radiation therapy (ART) in women with EBC tumor [73, 74]. Nearly 5,000 women with tumor < 3 cm and positive SLNBx were randomly assigned to either a completion ALND or ART, the latter encompasses all three levels of the axilla and the medial part of the supraclavicular fossa. Systemic therapy was given as appropriate and 80 % of patients had BCT. With a follow-up beyond 10 years, the final analysis, which was presented at the 2013 Annual Meeting of the American Society of Clinical Oncology (ASCO), found that compared to ALND, ART resulted in equivalent 5-year OS (93.27 % ALND, 92.52 % ART, $p = 0.338$) and 5-year DFS (86.9 % ALND, 82.65 ART, $p = 0.178$). The rate of regional recurrence was 0.43 % in the ALND arm and 1.19 % in the ART arm. However, lymphedema was twice as high in the ALND as in the ART arm [74]. Notwithstanding, this data makes the management of patients with positive SLNBx more complex. Should patients with a small tumor and one positive SLNBx who opted for BCT be offered conventional radiation with tangential field or nodal regional irradiation, the latter would be considered by many as overtreatment? Complications from regional nodal irradiation include pain, pneumonitis, lymphedema, brachial plexus neuropathy, malignancy, radiation dermatitis, and poor cosmetic outcome.

As an aside, both the Z0011 and AMAROS use the non-inferiority test rather than a superiority test. Such a test requires fewer patients and can often fail to detect small significant differences. Thus, longer follow-up will be necessary to understand the impact of the experimental arm.

Should Regional Nodal Irradiation Be Given to High-Risk Early Breast Cancer?

There is a group of patients with EBC who are at high risk of developing recurrent disease, despite optimal WBI. The NCIC Clinical Trials Group MA.20 (NCIC CTG MA.20) trial evaluated the role of adding regional nodal irradiation (RNI) to WBI in high-risk women who underwent BCT for EBC and received adjuvant systemic therapy. High-risk groups include node-positive patients and node-negative patients who have tumor ≥ 5 cm or if it was ≥ 2 cm and fewer than 10 lymph nodes removed, with either ER-negative, nuclear grade 3, or evidence of lymphovascular invasion [75]. Over 1,800 women were randomized to conventional WBI or WBI + RNI; RNI included the internal mammary, supraclavicular, and high axillary lymph nodes. The interim analysis found that after a median follow-up of 62 months, WBI + RNI significantly reduced locoregional recurrence from 5.5 to 3.2 % ($HR = 0.58$; $P = 0.02$) and distant recurrence from 13.0 to 7.6 % ($HR = 0.64$; $P = 0.002$). The DFS was better in the WBI + RNI group (89.7 %) than the WBI group (84 %; $P = 0.003$), although OS was not significantly different (92.3 % WBI + RNI versus 90.7 % WBI; $P = 0.07$) [75].

Given the two options for local control and two options for regional control, on any given patient, there can be up to four options for achieving locoregional control: (1) lumpectomy/XRT + SLNBx, (2) lumpectomy/XRT + ALND, (3) mastectomy + SLNBx, and (4) mastectomy + ALND, also known as a modified radical mastectomy (MRM).

Should Postmastectomy Radiation Be Given to High-Risk Early Breast Cancer?

Postmastectomy radiation (PMRT) is known to be of benefit in patients with locally advanced breast cancer and those with ≥ 4 positive LNs [76, 77]. However, its role in those with T1–2 and limited nodal disease (1–3 positive LNs) remains controversial. Retrospective data showed that among patients with T1–2 tumors and 1–3 positive axillary lymph nodes, postmastectomy radiation reduces LRR rate especially in those who are ≤ 50 years or have evidence of lymphovascular invasion (LVI) [78, 79]. PMRT can also be considered in those with 1–3 involved nodes with large tumors, extranodal extension, or inadequate axillary dissections.

Distant Control

The majority of recurrences occur during the first 2 years following treatment. The risk of recurrences averages around 4 % per year after 5 years [80]. Distant control is of utmost importance and will require the assistance of colleagues who have expertise in the field of medical oncology. Note that in managing patients with early breast cancer, the surgeons directly impact local and regional control. She/he cannot excise potential blood stream metastases with her/his scalpel. Distant control will require systemic therapy (adjuvant therapy), either in the form of chemotherapy, hormonal therapy, and/or biologic therapy. A patient with early breast cancer may be a candidate for any combination of these therapies.

Adjuvant therapy is therapy following definitive surgery, while neoadjuvant or preoperative therapy is therapy before definitive surgery. The course of therapy chosen is predicated mainly on the characteristics of the primary tumor, although other factors such as the patient's age, comorbidities, and risk of relapse also are considered in the final plan of therapy. Besides confirming the tumor histology, the pathologist will provide many key information; among them are tumor size (T status), margin status, grade, nodal status (N status) (i.e., the number of lymph nodes involved in relation to the total number of lymph nodes retrieved), and receptor statuses for estrogen receptor (ER status), progesterone receptor (PR status), and HER-2.

When evaluating the efficacy of a therapy, it is important to have a clear understanding of several important statistical concepts, mainly hazard

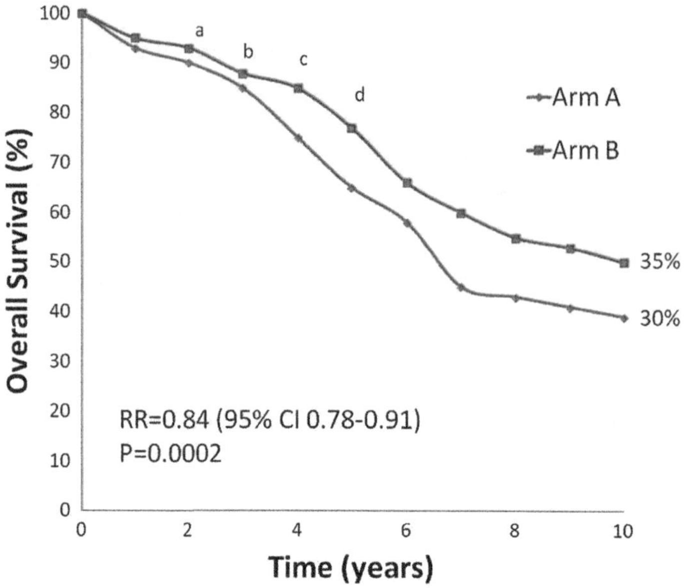

Fig. 4.10 *Absolute risk reduction, relative risk reduction (RRR), and hazard ratio (HR)*: note that arm B resulted in a significantly improved overall survival compared to arm A. Compared to arm A, treatment with arm B resulted in the absolute risk reduction of 5 % at 10 years (35–30 %) and the relative risk reduction of 16 % (RRR = 1-RR*100 or 1-0.84 * 100). Another important concept is the hazard ratio (HR), which is the time-to-event analysis or an instantaneous event rate. HR equals to the hazard in the treatment arm divided by the hazard in the control arm. HR measures the *probability* that an individual has an event (i.e., recurrence) at a particular time period. For instance, if the HR is 0.34, then the participants in the treatment arm B have a 66 % (1–0.34 × 100) reduction in having an outcome (i.e., death) compared to the control arm A at *any* particular time along the follow-up period (points a–d) (Courtesy of Quyen D. Chu, MD, MBA, FACS)

ratio (HR), absolute risk reduction (ARR), and relative risk reduction (RRR); the last is often referred to as a proportional risk reduction. All three metrics can be converted and reported as percentages. The ARR is the absolute difference between the curves at a selected time period, while the RRR is calculated as one minus the relative risk (RR) times 100 (Fig. 4.10). For instance, in the example given in Fig. 4.10, the ARR is 5 % and the RRR is 16 %. If one were to ask the uninformed individual the question of whether he/she prefers to have an ARR of 5 % or a RRR of 16 %, most would choose the latter. However, the correct answer would be that it does not matter because the two are equivalent.

Another important statistical concept is the hazard ratio (HR), which is the time-to-event analysis or an instantaneous event rate. HR equals to the hazard in the treatment arm divided by the hazard in the control arm. HR measures the *probability* that an individual has an event (i.e., recurrence) at a particular time period. For instance, if the HR is 0.34, then the participants in the treatment arm have a 66 % (1–0.34 × 100) reduction in having an outcome (i.e., recurrent disease) compared to the control arm at *any* particular time along the follow-up period. Although similar to relative risk, they are not the same. RR does not care about events along the time period, but rather measures *the total number of events at the end of the study*.

Adjuvant Chemotherapy

Adjuvant chemotherapy reduces breast cancer recurrence and mortality by approximately 30 % and 20 %, respectively [81]. The 20 % absolute improvement in survival rate was the result of small incremental improvements made over the decades, beginning with a 4 % improvement with CMF, 4 % with anthracyclines, 5 % with taxanes, and finally up to 8.8 % with trastuzumab.

Randomized trials performed prior to the era of systemic chemotherapy demonstrated a 10-year overall survival of 60 % for patients with operable breast cancer [82]. Clearly, there was room for improvement. The NSABP B-01 trial was the first to demonstrate the effectiveness of using single agent chemotherapy (thiotepa) in the adjuvant setting [83, 84]. NSABP B-05 was a confirmatory trial but used melphalan instead of thiotepa [85]. Combination regimen with cyclophosphamide, methotrexate, and fluorouracil (CMF) was first introduced by the Italian group at the Istituto Nazionale Tumori (ITA) of Milan [86] and the efficacy of polychemotherapy in patients with EBC was confirmed by many studies, including the meta-analysis by the Early Breast Cancer Trialists' Collaborative Group (EBCTCG) [87, 88]. Anthracycline-based chemotherapy (i.e., adriamycin or epirubicin) entered the scene in the early 1980s, and various anthracycline-based combinations (AC, FEC, FAC, etc.) were subsequently demonstrated to offer a significant, albeit small, advantage over non-anthracycline-based chemotherapy (CMF) [88, 89]. Compared to CMF, anthracycline-based therapy resulted in a significant reduction in recurrence and breast cancer mortality; the 10 year relative risk reduction in recurrence and mortality was 11 % and 20 %, respectively, and the absolute reduction in recurrence and breast cancer mortality was 2.6 % and 4.1 %, respectively [88].

In the early 2000s, taxanes were tested against the classic anthracycline (AC or EC) regimen in high-risk patients, mainly those with node-positive EBC. Taxanes are potent agents that bind to and stabilize microtubules, thereby preventing their depolymerization. Paclitaxel (Taxol®) and docetaxel (Taxotere®) are the two most actively tested agents. Multiple clinical trials demonstrated the superiority of adding taxanes to the regimen in high-risk early breast cancer patients [90]. A recent meta-analysis of 14 randomized phase III studies of over 25,000 patients demonstrated improved DFS and OS with docetaxel-containingregimenovernon-docetaxel-containing regimen in node-positive patients [90]. Similarly, the recent 2012 EBCTCG meta-analysis of outcomes among 100,000 women in 123 randomized trials of adjuvant chemotherapy reported that compared to non-taxane anthracycline regimen, the taxane + anthracycline regimen resulted in a significant 8-year relative risk reduction of recurrence and breast cancer mortality by 16 % and 14 %, respectively. This translates to an absolute benefit of 4.6 % and 2.8 % for breast cancer recurrence and breast cancer mortality, respectively [88].

Is Taxane Indicated in High-Risk Node-Negative Patients?

Although taxane-based adjuvant therapy is standard of care for patients with node-positive breast cancer, its use in node-negative breast cancer remains controversial [91, 92]. The Spanish Breast Cancer Research Group (GEICAM) 9805 trial randomly assigned 1,060 women with node-negative operable breast cancer who have at least one high-risk factor for recurrence according to the 1998 St. Gallen criteria (tumor size $\geq$2 cm, TNBC, grade 2 or 3, or age $<$35 years) to either standard chemotherapy (fluorouracil, doxorubicin, and cyclophosphamide-FAC) or taxane-based therapy (docetaxel, doxorubicin, and cyclophosphamide-TAC) [91]. At a median follow-up of 77 months, there was a 32 % reduction in the risk of recurrence when docetaxel was added to the standard AC regimen ($P=0.01$). However, there was no significant difference in OS between the two groups ($P=0.29$), and more significant grade 3 or 4 toxicities were observed in the docetaxel group ($P<0.001$) [91]. Similar results were also observed in a trial conducted by the European Cooperative Trial in Operable Breast Cancer [92] as well as a recent meta-analysis [90].

Should All Patients Be Offered Adjuvant Chemotherapy?

Despite its effectiveness, chemotherapy does have its inherent toxicities; approximately 1 % of patients have life-threatening toxicities [93]. Historically, the decision to offer adjuvant chemotherapy relies on clinicopathologic factors such as age, tumor size, axillary lymph node status, pathologic grade, hormone receptor status, and HER-2 status. While these factors are useful in treatment decisions, they are imperfect. Nodal status, traditionally regarded as the most powerful prognosticator in breast cancer, either overestimates or underestimates outcome in 20–30 % of patients; up to 20 % of node-negative patients may develop systemic disease whereas 30 % of node-positive patients may not [94, 95]. Molecular profiling of tumors to search for a "molecular signature" of aggressiveness may provide useful prognostic and predictive information [96, 97]. Of note, prognostic factors predict patient outcome regardless of the treatment given (i.e., tumor size, nodal status), whereas predictive factors indicate responsiveness to a specific treatment (i.e., ER/PR status) [98]. Some factors such as ER/PR and HER-2 are both prognostic and predictive. Predictive factors are complimentary to prognostic factors in that it can be used to select appropriate additional therapy for a patient when necessary.

Many prognostic studies grouped patients as either belonging to the low-risk group or high-risk group, although some also include an intermediate-risk group. In general, high risk is defined as a risk of recurrence of greater than 10 % at 5 years and include those that have nodal involvement [N (+)], HER-2-positive disease [HER-2 (+)], ER-negative disease [ER (−)], triple-negative breast cancer [TNBC or ER(−), PR(−), HER-2(−)], high grade, and high proliferation index as measured by Ki-67. Some would also consider node-negative disease with tumor measuring greater than 1 cm as belonging to the high-risk group [99], although such a low threshold might lead to overtreatment.

There are a number of prognostic indexes that separate the low-risk from the high-risk group. Three clinicopathologic indices will be highlighted, while the three major molecular profiling platforms (Oncotype DX®, MammaPrint®, Mammostrat®) will be discussed under the *Prognostic Indices to Identify Low-Risk Estrogen Receptor-Positive, Node-Negative Patients* section. All indices have their strengths and weaknesses.

The three prognostic indices that use clinicopathologic features are the Nottingham Prognostic Index (NPI) [100], Adjuvant!Online (AOL) [101], and the St. Gallen guidelines [102]. The Adjuvant!Online (AOL) is a web-based actuarial tool that incorporates four tumor characteristics (tumor size, tumor grade, nodal status, ER status) and one patient characteristic (age) in order to predict patient outcome at 10 years. The St. Gallen uses six tumor characteristics (tumor size, tumor grade, nodal status, ER/PR status, HER-2 status, degree of peritumoral vascular invasion) and one patient characteristic (age) and categorizes patients into low risk, intermediate risk, and high risk; it is commonly used in Europe. The Nottingham Prognostic Index (NPI) takes into account three tumor characteristics (tumor size, tumor grade, and nodal status), and like the AOL, it predicts the 10-year survival rate based on a score; the lower the score, the higher the survival rate. Note that all three indices incorporate tumor size, nodal status, and tumor grade (Table 4.11).

Using Subtypes as a Basis to Predict the Need for Chemotherapy

Molecular profiling of breast cancers has ushered not only a novel system of classifying tumors but also a new era of personalized medicine [96]. Genetic profiling has found that breast cancer represents a spectrum of a molecularly heterogeneous disease that can be classified into five "intrinsic" or "molecular" tumor subtypes that are characterized by similarities in gene expression patterns: (1) luminal A [high expression of hormone receptors (HR) and associated genes], (2) luminal B (moderate expression of HR and associated genes), (3) HER-2 enriched (HER-2 positive/non-luminal, but low expression of HR), (4) normal-like, and (5) basal-like (ER/PR/HER-2), the last often referred to as the triple-negative breast cancer (TNBC) [96, 97]. Of these subtypes, the HER-2 positive/non-luminal and basal-like have a more unfavorable clinical outcome but tend to be more sensitive to paclitaxel- and doxorubicin-containing preoperative chemotherapy than the luminal- and normal-like subtypes [103]. Additionally, HER-2-positive/non-luminal and basal-like subtypes are associated with higher likelihood of pathologic CR to preoperative chemotherapy [103–105].

Table 4.11 Prognostic platforms

Authors/ref	Type of indices	Platform
Adjuvant!Online (AOL)	Clinical	Tumor size
		Nodal status
		Tumor grade
		ER status
		Age
Nottingham Prognostic Index (NPI)	Clinical	Tumor size
		Nodal status
		Tumor grade
St. Gallen	Clinical	Tumor size
		Nodal status
		Tumor grade
		ER/PR status
		Age
		HER-2 Status
		Degree of peritumoral vascular invasion
Paik	Oncotype DX (RS)	Low risk: RS <18
		Intermediate risk: RS 18–30
		High risk: ≥31
Jankowitz	BCI	HOXB13:IL17BR (H:I) and 5-gene molecular grade index (MGI)
MammaPrint®	70-gene signature	Low risk
		High risk
Mammostrat®	SLC7A5, p53, HTF9C, NDRG1, CEACAM5	Low risk: (≤0)
		Moderate risk: (>0 and ≤0.7)
		High risk: >0.7
RxPONDER Trial	Oncotype DX (RS)	Node (+) (1–3 positive nodes)
		Hormone (+)
		HER-2 (−)

Because gene expression array technology is not readily available in many institutions, a simplified classification that uses IHC, which is readily available in many institutions, was proposed as an alternate to classify intrinsic subtypes of breast cancer [106]. This classification, proposed by the St. Gallen International Expert Consensus Panel, determines the expressions of ER, PR, HER-2, and Ki-67 and classified breast cancer subtypes into five categories: (1) luminal A, (2) luminal B (HER-2 negative), (3) luminal B (HER-2 positive), (4) HER-2 positive, and (5) basal-like [106, 107]. Based on such a classification, the Panel agreed that the luminal A subtype was less responsive to chemotherapy and there is no preferred chemotherapy regimen that could be defined for this subtype. Additionally, luminal A tends to have excellent prognosis, which further supports the notion that chemotherapy can be spared for patients who belong to this subtype. All the other subtypes appeared to be sensitive to chemotherapy [106]. The clinical value of this system, however, is still being evaluated. A more thorough discussion of impact of breast cancer subtypes on outcome can be found in the next chapter, Chap. 5, *Locally Advanced Breast Cancer*.

Adjuvant Hormonal Therapy (Tamoxifen and Aromatase Inhibitors)

In his reading before the Edinburgh Medico-Chirurgical Society in 1896, Beatson described the disappearance of a woman's inoperable breast cancer 8 months after performing a bilateral oophorectomy [3, 108]. The observation that certain types of breast cancer are under the influence of ovarian function eventually led to the development on an entire class of therapeutics that either block estrogen receptor (ER; tamoxifen) or reduce circulating level of estrogen (i.e., aromatase inhibitors or AIs) [3].

Postmenopausal women with hormone receptor-positive tumors are the largest group of operable breast cancer patients, representing nearly 75 % of all breast cancers [109, 110]. For these patients, 5 years of adjuvant tamoxifen was the standard of care [111, 112]. Tamoxifen, a selective estrogen receptor modulator (SERM), significantly reduces the risk of breast recurrence (both ipsilateral and contralateral) and mortality. In 2011, the Early Breast Cancer Trialists' Collaborative Group (EBCTCG) updated their meta-analysis of 20 trials of 21,457 women and, with a median follow-up of 13 years, reported that women who took 5 years of tamoxifen compared to those who did not had an almost 50 % proportional relative risk reduction of relapse during years 0–4, a 32 % relative risk reduction of relapse during years 5–9, and an almost 30 % proportional risk reduction in breast cancer mortality during the first 15 years after diagnosis [113]. Such benefits were observed, irrespective of age, nodal status, and whether or not chemotherapy was used [113].

The addition of tamoxifen to chemotherapy produces additional benefits when compared to either alone [114, 115]. The 2005 EBCTCG meta-analysis found that the estimated breast mortality rates throughout the next 15 years were halved by combination of anthracycline-based chemotherapy and tamoxifen [114]. For women taking tamoxifen and/or chemotherapy, there is no added benefit of having their ovaries ablated or suppressed by oophorectomy, ovarian irradiation, or treatment with luteinizing hormone-releasing hormone agonist such as goserelin [114, 116].

Despite a number of advantages with tamoxifen, there are limitations. Tamoxifen increases the risk of uterine cancer and thromboembolic events because of its estrogen agonistic effect. Additionally, the risk of recurrence after 5 years of tamoxifen can be as high as 2 % per year for women with node-negative disease and 4 % per year for women with node-positive disease [80, 117, 118]. Given these limitations and the historic data demonstrating a lack of efficacy of longer use of tamoxifen [119–121], investigators began searching for alternative hormonal candidates. One such candidate was the aromatase inhibitors (AI).

Table 4.12 Risk profile between tamoxifen and aromatase inhibitors

Tamoxifen	Aromatase inhibitors
Deep venous thrombosis	Ischemic cardiovascular events
Pulmonary emboli	Arthralgias
Stroke	Osteoporosis/fractures
Transient ischemic attack	Visual disturbances
Endometrial cancer	

Aromatase Inhibitors

AIs can decrease serum estrogen concentration by more than 90 %, but only in postmenopausal women [122]. Currently, the three 3rd-generation AIs in clinical use are anastrozole (Arimidex), letrozole (Femara), and exemestane (Aromasin). Both anastrozole and letrozole are reversible nonsteroidal aromatase inhibitors, and exemestane is an irreversible steroidal aromatase inactivator. All three have excellent oral bioavailability and require once a day dosing. Unlike tamoxifen, the AIs are associated with a lower risk of thromboembolic event and endometrial cancers. However, they can lead to loss of bone density due to their lack of having a partial agonist activity, but such a concern can be addressed by using bisphosphonates [123] (Table 4.12). A major disadvantage with the AIs is that, unlike tamoxifen which can be used for all women with ER-positive tumors, it cannot be used for premenopausal women because of its inability to suppress ovarian aromatase activity. However, several trials are currently evaluating the role of adjuvant AIs in combination with ovarian function suppression (i.e., luteinizing hormone-releasing hormone [LH-RH] agonist) in premenopausal women [124].

Multiple phase III randomized trials have evaluated AIs as primary adjuvant monotherapy in place of tamoxifen, sequential or switching therapy after 2–3 years of either tamoxifen or an AI, or as extended adjuvant therapy [125] (Table 4.13). In a head-to-head comparison of an AI versus tamoxifen to determine the role of AIs as primary monotherapy, the Arimidex, Tamoxifen, Alone or in Combination (ATAC) trial was the first clinical trial to demonstrate that an aromatase inhibitor was more effective than tamoxifen in prolonging disease-free survival (DFS) [126, 136]. However, ATAC did not demonstrate a significant overall survival (OS) advantage with an AI [126]. These results have also been validated by the Tamoxifen and Exemestane Adjuvant Multinational (TEAM) trial [131] and the Breast International Group 1–98 [130], although the latter did demonstrate an OS survival advantage with letrozole in its latest report [130] (Table 4.13).

For the sequential or switching strategy, there were several clinical trials that demonstrated a significant advantage of prolonging DFS by switching to an AI after 2 or 3 years of tamoxifen for a total of 5 years of endocrine therapy [127, 128]. However, other trials demonstrated no significant advantage with such a strategy [130, 132]. Besides the Intergroup Exemestane Study [128], most of the studies failed to show a significant OS advantage with such a strategy (Table 4.13).

Clinical trials evaluating the role of extending treatment using an AI for up to 5 years after 5 years of tamoxifen consistently demonstrated a significant prolongation of DFS [118, 129, 133, 135]. The National Cancer Institute of Canada Clinical Trials Group MA.17 (MA.17) randomized over 5,000 women to tamoxifen alone versus tamoxifen followed by 5 years of letrozole [118] and found a significant prolongation of DFS in the extended group. However, the OS was similar in the extended and placebo arms, although subgroup analysis demonstrated an OS advantage in the node-positive patients [3, 118]. The trial was terminated early following the first interim analysis when the data and safety monitoring committee concluded that the data was compelling enough to inform patients of the results and to give women in the placebo arm an opportunity to switch to an AI. Because of this, the long-term impact on OS may never truly be known. An updated report of MA.17 found an overall survival benefit with extended use of letrozole, but such a result was arrived at only after some complex statistical analysis [129]. However, in fairness, the authors did caution that these analyses should be considered as exploratory based on a number of strong assumptions.

Tamoxifen 5 Years Versus 10 Years

Previous trials have found that extending the duration of tamoxifen beyond 5 years provided no additional benefit compared to 5 years [119]. These trials likely lacked adequate power to detect a statistical significant difference between the two arms. The preliminary results from the global Adjuvant Tamoxifen: Longer Against Shorter (ATLAS) randomly allocated 12,894 women of all ages who had early breast cancer to either continue tamoxifen for up to 10 years or stop at 5 years and found that 10 years of tamoxifen led to a significant reduction in the risk of relapse of 30 % ($P = 0.01$) and mortality reduction of 48 % ($P < 0.0001$) [137]. Although there was an increased incidence of endometrial cancer and pulmonary embolism with the extended therapy, there was no increased incidence of stroke and a decreased incidence of ischemic heart disease. The authors believed that the benefits of 10 years of tamoxifen outweighed these risks, however.

The adjuvant Tamoxifen Treatment offers more (aTTom) trial recently reported their updated results on extending tamoxifen therapy from 5 years to 10 years, and their conclusions were similar to those in the ATLAS trial [138]. aTTom randomized nearly 7,000 women to either 5 years or 10 years of tamoxifen and found that 10 years of tamoxifen was associated with a significant 15 % reduction in the risk of recurrence (relative risk [RR] = 0.085, 95 % CI: 0.076–0.95; $P = 0.003$) and a significant 25 % reduction in the risk of breast cancer mortality at year 10 ($RR = 0.75$, 95 % CI: 0.63–0.90; $P = 0.0007$) [138]. Ten years of tamoxifen resulted in very little effect on non-breast cancer mortality, and the absolute hazard ratio of endometrial cancer was 0.5 %. Similar to the ATLAS trial, the benefits

Table 4.13 Selected trials evaluating third-generation aromatase inhibitors in the adjuvant setting

Trials/year/ reference	N	Study design	Median follow-up (months)	DFS	OS
ATAC (2010) [126]	9,366	A versus T versus Combination (primary therapy)	120	*HR*=0.86(95 % CI: 0.78–0.93) **P=0.003**	**NS**
ITA (2013) [127]	448	Switch to A after 2 or 3 years of T versus T for 5 years (sequential therapy)	128	*HR*=0.64 (95 % CI: 0.44–0.94)[a] **P=0.02**	**P=0.3**
IES (2012) [128]	4,742	Switch to E after 2 or 3 years of T versus T × 5 years (sequential therapy)	91	*HR*=0.81 (95 % CI: 0.71–0.92) **P=0.001**	*HR*=0.86 (95 % CI: 0.75–0.99) **P=0.04**
MA.17 (2012) [129]	5,187	T × 5 years versus T × 5 years → L × 5 years (extended therapy)	64	*HR*=0.52 (95 % CI: 0.45–0.61) **P<0.001**	*HR*=0.61 (95 % CI: 0.52–0.71) **P<0.001**[b]
BIG I-98 (2010) [130]	8,010	T × 5 years versus L × 5 years versus T × 2 years → L × 3 years versus L × 2 years → T × 3 years (primary therapy and sequential therapy)	97	**L versus T**: *HR*=0.82 (95 % CI: 0.74–0.92) **P=0.002** **T → L**: *HR*=1.07 (95 % CI: 0.92–1.25) **P=0.36** **L → T**: *HR*=1.06 (95 % CI: 0.91–1.23) **P=0.48**	**LversusT**: *HR*=0.79 (95 % CI: 0.69–90) **P=0.0006** **T → L**: *HR*=1.10 (95 % CI: 0.90–1.33) **P=0.36** **L → T**: *HR*=0.97 (95 % CI: 0.80–1.19) **P=0.79**
TEAM (2011) [131]	9,779	E × 5 years versus T → E (total 5 years) (monotherapy versus sequential therapy)	60	*HR*=0.97 (95 % CI: 0.88–1.08) **P=0.60**	*HR*=1 (95 % CI: 0.89–1.14) **P>0.99**
ABCSG-8 (2012) [132]	3,714	T × 5 years versus T × 2 years → A × 3 years (monotherapy versus sequential therapy)	60	RFS → *HR*=0.80 (95 % CI: 0.63–1.01) **P=0.06**	*HR*=0.87 (95 % CI: 0.64–1.16) **P=0.33**
NSABP B-33(2008) [133]	1,598	T × 5 years → E × 5 years versus T × 5 years → P × 5 years (extended therapy)	30	DFS → *RR*=0.68; **P=0.07** ‡ RFS → *RR*=0.44; **P=0.004** ‡	**NS**
MA.27 (2013) [134]	7,576	E × 5 years versus A × 5 years (primary therapy)	49	EFS → *HR*=1.02 (95 % CI: 0.87–1.18) ‡ **P=0.85**	*HR*=0.93 (95 % CI: 0.77–1.13) **P=0.46**
ABCSG-6a (2007) [135]	856	T × 5 years versus T × 5 years → A × 3 years (extended therapy)	62	*HR*=0.62 (95 % CI: 0.40–0.96) **P=0.031**	*HR*=0.89 (95 % CI: 0.59–1.34) **P=0.57**

ATAC Arimidex, Tamoxifen, Alone or in Combination, *ITA* Italian Tamoxifen Anastrozole trial, *IES* Intergroup Exemestane Study, *MA.17* National Cancer Institute of Canada Clinical Trials Group MA.17, *BIG* Breast International Group, *TEAM* Tamoxifen and Exemestane Adjuvant Multinational trial, *ABCSG* Austrian Breast and Colorectal Cancer Study Group, *NSABP* National Surgical Adjuvant Breast and Bowel Project, *A* anastrozole, *T* tamoxifen, *E* exemestane, *L* letrozole, *P* placebo, *NS* not significant, *HR* hazard ratio, *RR* relative risk, *DFS* disease-free survival, *OS* overall survival, *EFS* event-free survival, *HR* hazard ratio

[a]RFS: relapse-free survival, ‡ 4-year results

[b]Data based on complex statistical analysis after crossover was allowed (see text)

of 10 years of tamoxifen seems to outweigh the risks. Of note, both ATLAS and aTTom included premenopausal or perimenopausal women, which implies that 10 years of tamoxifen might be a viable option for these patients. However, such a decision should be made jointly by the patient and her clinicians after weighing in all the risk and benefits.

The 2010 American Society of Clinical Oncology (ASCO) guidelines on adjuvant endocrine therapy for hormone receptor-positive breast cancer recommends tamoxifen for 5 years for premenopausal or perimenopausal women, and for postmenopausal women, the following recommendations were made: (1) an AI as primary therapy for 5 years; (2) switching to an AI following tamoxifen for 2–3 years, but the total time for endocrine therapy should not be longer than 5 years; and (3) extended therapy with an AI for 5 years following 5 years of tamoxifen. It should be noted that these guidelines were published before the results of the ATLAS and aTTom, and it is anticipated that future ASCO guidelines might likely recommend 10 years of tamoxifen as an option for primary endocrine therapy (Table 4.14).

There remain several questions for which there are no clear answers. Although the data recommend switching to an AI following 2–3 years of tamoxifen, it is not known whether switching after year 1 or year 4 is equivalent to switching after year 2 or 3. Besides the BIG 1-98 trial [130], most of the data on sequential therapy analyzed the switch to occur following tamoxifen. It is unclear what the outcome is for women who experienced intolerable side effects from an AI who later switched to tamoxifen. Given the benefit of 10 years of tamoxifen, should patients who opted for an AI as primary adjuvant hormonal therapy be given a total of 10 years of an AI?

The best course of adjuvant endocrine therapy for patients with early breast cancer should reside with the treating clinician and the patients. Some of the factors such as the patient's age, tumor biology, tumor burden, and comorbidities should be taken into consideration before embarking on a specific hormonal regimen.

Table 4.14 Adjuvant endocrine therapy options for patients with hormone receptor-positive early breast cancer

Premenopausal
Tamoxifen × 5 years[a]
If tamoxifen is contraindicated or intolerable due to side effects:
Chemical oophorectomy (gonadotropin-releasing hormone agonists)
Surgical oophorectomy
Radiation oophorectomy
Postmenopausal
Primary treatment
Aromatase inhibitor (AI) × 5 years
Tamoxifen × 5 years[a]
Sequential treatment
Tamoxifen × 2–3 years, switch to AI × 2–3 years (total of endocrine therapy: 5 years)
Extended treatment
Tamoxifen × 5 years + AI × 5 years

[a]ATLAS and aTTom data support the use of tamoxifen for 10 years (see text)

Prognostic Indices to Identify Low-Risk Estrogen Receptor-Positive, Node-Negative Patients

As mentioned previously, combination of chemotherapy and endocrine therapy yielded superior outcome compared to endocrine therapy alone for patients with hormone receptor-positive tumors [114]. However, the majority of patients (75–85 %) with ER(+), LN(−) disease do just fine with hormonal therapy alone. The goal of managing patients with ER(+), LN(−) disease is to identify the 15 % who will need chemotherapy in addition to adjuvant hormonal therapy while sparing the majority of the toxicities of chemotherapy. Current predictive and prognostic indices are under development to address this issue. Most clinicians would agree that women age ≥ 35 years with hormone-positive tumors that are < 1 cm and without unfavorable microscopic features can be treated with hormonal therapy alone [102].

Oncotype DX® (Genomic Health), MammaPrint® (Agendia), and Mammostrat® (Clarient) are gene expression assays used to stratify patients with EBC into risk categories. Paik et al. developed a 21-gene recurrence score

(RS; Oncotype DX®) based on monitoring the mRNA expression levels of 16 cancer-related genes in relation to 5 reference genes on formalin-fixed, paraffin-embedded tissues (FFPE). Patients were grouped into three groups based on their RS: (1) low risk (RS < 18), (2) intermediate risk (RS 18–30), and (3) high risk (RS ≥ 31). Patients in the low-risk group derived minimal benefit from chemotherapy (absolute decrease in distant recurrence rate at 10 years of −1.1 %), while those in the high-risk group experienced a large chemotherapy benefit (absolute decrease in distant recurrence rate at 10 years of 27.6 %). Besides predicting the risk of distant recurrence, RS also predicts the risk of LRR; the LRR was 4.3 % in the low-risk group, 7.2 % in the intermediate-risk group, and 15.8 % in the high-risk group [139].

It remains unknown what the benefit is for the intermediate-risk group [140]. The TAILORx (Trial for Assigning Individualized Options for Treatment [Rx]) is a prospective trial that will enroll over 10,000 women with early breast cancer, ER(+), LN(−), to determine the value of chemotherapy for patients with intermediate RS of 12–25 [141]. Patients in this group will be randomized to hormone therapy or hormone therapy plus chemotherapy, while those in the high-risk group (RS > 25) will be given chemotherapy along with hormonal therapy, and low-risk group (RS < 11) will be followed to validate their excellent prognosis. Results are not expected until 2015.

One of the concerns with the Oncotype DX® is its diminished ability to assess risk beyond 5 years from diagnosis [142]. The Breast Cancer Index (BCI), another index that classifies ER (+), LN (−) tumors into high-risk and low-risk groups, addresses this concern [143]. Like Oncotype DX®, it measures gene expression by quantitative real-time PCR but uses different biomarkers, HOXB13:IL17BR (H:I) and the 5-gene molecular grade index (MGI). In a prospective comparison with Oncotype DX®, BCI was found to be equivalent at identifying patients who were at risk of developing early recurrences despite receiving hormonal treatment. However, BCI was better at assessing long-term recurrence risk. Such a finding is relevant since more than half of recurrences in ER-positive breast cancer happen after 5 years of hormonal therapy [143]. However, these results will need to be prospectively validated. The American Society of Clinical Oncology (ASCO) [144], the National Comprehensive Cancer Network (NCCN) [145], and the St. Gallen International Expert Consensus group [106] recommend Oncotype DX in certain situations.

The Microarray for Node-Negative Disease May Avoid Chemotherapy (MINDACT) trial under the aegis of the European Organization for Research and Treatment of Cancer compares MammaPrint®, a 70-gene prognostic signature that was approved by the US Food and Drug [146], with Adjuvant!Online. Similar to Oncotype DX®, MammaPrint® uses FFPE tumor tissue as well as fresh tissue. Patients must have tumors ≤ 5 cm, LN(−) or LN(+) disease. The primary aim was to determine whether this 70-gene signature had prognostic value independent of the best clinical risk classifications, AOL. Compared to AOL, the 70-gene signature outperformed it for all endpoints measured. A prospective, validation MINDACT trial has recently completed recruitment of 6,600 patients, and results are expected to be available around 2015.

The recent microarRAy prognoSTics in breast cancER (RASTER) study was the first prospective trial that demonstrated the feasibility of incorporating MammaPrint® in a community-based setting. It found that patients with low-risk EBC can forego adjuvant systemic therapy [147]; of the 85 % of women who were in the low-risk category who opted to forego adjuvant chemotherapy, the 5-year DFS was 97 % [147]. Of note, all of the breast cancers were node-negative and 80 % were ER(+) disease. Because recurrences in this group may not occur until 5 years or more, longer follow-up will be required to understand the impact of MammaPrint®.

The advantage with the MammaPrint® is that patients are categorized as high or low risk, thus eliminating the uncertainty of indeterminate scores as reported by Oncotype DX® and Mammostrat®. Furthermore, MammaPrint can be applied to virtually all EBC versus the other two platforms, which can only be applied to patients with hormone-positive disease. Results of both TAILORx (launched in the United States) and MINDACT (launched in Europe) will further delineate the role of genetic profiling in the clinic.

The concerns with Oncotype DX® and the MammaPrint® are that these assays are relatively expensive and technically challenging and utility is limited. The Mammostrat®, which is an immunohistochemical assay that measures the level of five proteins (SLC7A5, p53, HTF9C, NDRG1, CEACAM5), is an assay that attempts to address some of these concerns [148, 149]. Based on the expression of these proteins, a prognostic index is generated, and patients are grouped into three risk categories: low (≤0), moderate (>0 and ≤0.7), and high (>0.7) risk of recurrence [148, 150]. However, prospective trials will need to be performed before Mammostrat® can be widely used in the clinical setting.

Node-positive patients are generally considered to be the high-risk group, and almost all patients are offered adjuvant systemic therapy. However, some have recently questioned whether within this subgroup there exists a population of patients for whom systemic chemotherapy might not be of benefit [142]. Albain et al. who retrospectively analyzed data from the SWOG-8814 phase 3 trial for postmenopausal women with ER(+), LN(+) disease who were treated with tamoxifen and adjuvant chemotherapy found that patients with a low RS (Oncotype DX®) did not appear to benefit from additional anthracycline-based chemotherapy, despite having positive nodes [142]. Similar observations were also made with the 70-gene MammaPrint [151].

Finally, the SWOG RxPONDER Trial (RX for Positive Node, Endocrine Responsive Breast Cancer or protocol S1007) is a prospective clinical trial that is enrolling women with 1–3 positive nodes and hormone receptor-positive and HER-2 (−) tumors to determine whether chemotherapy can be avoided for those with RS ≤25. For now, it is safe to state that until compelling data suggest otherwise, all node-positive patients should receive systemic therapy, regardless of the results of genetic assays.

Adjuvant Target-Specific Therapy (Biologics)

Trastuzumab

The *HER2/Neu* gene encodes a tyrosine kinase receptor that is responsible for growth and differentiation of normal and transformed epithelial cells [152]. Its amplification and overexpression occurs in approximately 20–30 % of patients with breast cancer and portends a poor outcome [153]. Trastuzumab (Herceptin®) is an engineered humanized monoclonal antibody that has activity against the extracellular domain of the *HER2/Neu* receptor by blocking its function. Like many promising therapeutics, trastuzumab's efficacy was initially demonstrated in the metastatic setting [154, 155] prior to its evaluation in the adjuvant setting. Multiple well-designed clinical trials demonstrated that patients who had operable HER2-positive breast cancers benefitted from the addition of trastuzumab to the adjuvant regimen [156–161] (Table 4.15). The addition of trastuzumab for 1 year not only lowers mortality rate by 35 %, but also reduced the relative risk of recurrence by 40–50 %, a figure that has not been observed since the use of tamoxifen in hormone receptor-positive disease [161, 162]. The key point to remember is that the addition of trastuzumab to adjuvant chemotherapy for patients with HER-2 positive tumors yielded better outcome than adjuvant chemotherapy alone.

Duration of Trastuzumab

The question of whether 1 year of trastuzumab or longer duration should be standard of care was answered by the Herceptin Adjuvant (HERA) trial [163]. HERA randomized over 5,000 women with HER-2 positive breast cancer who had adjuvant chemotherapy into three arms: (1) observation, (2) trastuzumab for 1 year, and (3) trastuzumab for 2 years. With 8 years follow-up, there were no significant differences in disease-free survival and overall survival between the 1-year and 2-year regimens [163]. Thus, the recommended duration of trastuzumab is 1 year.

Cardiotoxicity such as congestive heart failure and decline in left ventricular ejection fraction is a major concern when trastuzumab is combined

Table 4.15 Selected trials evaluating adjuvant trastuzumab for operable breast cancer

Trial, year	# Patients	Study design	Median follow-up	Risk reduction in recurrence (%)[a]	Risk reduction in death[a]
Romond 2005 [157]	3,351	(1) Control: AC + T (2) Experiment: AC + T + trastuzumab × 52 weeks	2 years	52	33
Piccart-Gebhart 2005 [156]	5,081	(1) Control: C[b] (2) Experiment: C + trastuzumab × 52 weeks	1 year	51	NS
Joensuu 2006 [158]	232	(1) Control: FEC + docetaxel or vinorelbine (2) Experiment: FEC + docetaxel or vinorelbine plus trastuzumab	36 months	58	59 (NS)
Spielmann 2009 [159]	528	(1) Control: C (2) Experiment: C + trastuzumab	47	14 (NS)	NS
Slamon 2011 [160]	3,222	(1) Control: AC + T (2) Experiment 1: AC + T + trastuzumab × 52 weeks (3) Experiment 2: TCH	65 months	25–36	23–37
Moja 2012[c] [161]	11,991	(1) Control: C (2) Experiment: C + trastuzumab	NA	40	34

AC adriamycin, Cyclophosphamide, *C* chemotherapy, *T* taxol-based, *FEC* fluorouracil, epirubicin, cyclophosphamide, *NS* not significant between the trastuzumab and non-trastuzumab groups, *TCH* docetaxel, carboplatin, trastuzumab × 52 weeks, *NA* not applicable

[a]In favor of trastuzumab

[b]Patients received chemotherapy of choice, but 94 % had anthracycline-based chemotherapy

[c]Cochrane review that includes locally advanced breast cancer

with the anthracyclines (i.e., doxorubicin) [155]. An alternative solution would be to identify a non-anthracycline regimen that can be combined with trastuzumab so as to reduce the incidence of cardiotoxicity. Slamon et al. reporting for the Breast Cancer International Research Group 006 (BCIRG-006) randomized 3,222 women with HER-2-positive early stage breast cancer into three arms: (1) doxorubicin, cyclophosphamide, and docetaxel alone (AC-T); (2) the same regimen with 52 weeks of trastuzumab (AC-T plus trastuzumab); or (3) docetaxel, carboplatin, and 52 weeks of trastuzumab (TCH) [160]. Although their study was not powered to detect equivalence between the two regimens, the data demonstrated that the non-anthracycline group had similar efficacy with respect to disease-free and overall survival as the anthracycline group, but with a lower incidence of congestive heart failure (4 cases in the non-anthracycline group versus 21 cases in the anthracycline group). Future clinical trials will need to be conducted to validate these interesting results.

Given the cardiotoxicity profile of trastuzumab, a clinical trial was conducted to compare whether 6 months of trastuzumab yielded similar outcome as 12 months of trastuzumab [164]. The Protocol for Herceptin as Adjuvant therapy with Reduced Exposure (PHARE) study recruited 1,691 patients from 156 centers in France and found that although 12 months of trastuzumab resulted in more significant cardiac events than

6 months of trastuzumab, it nevertheless yielded significantly longer disease-free survival than the 6 months regimen. PHARE recommended that despite the higher cardiac events, 12 months of adjuvant trastuzumab should remain the standard of care. Impact on overall survival was not reported since the primary endpoint of the study was disease-free survival [164].

An area of controversy is the use of trastuzumab for small tumors (<1 cm). With the exception of the BCIRG-006 trial, the other large clinical trials had excluded patients with tumors < 1 cm. Although small HER-2-positive tumors have been shown to portend a poorer outcome than HER-2-negative tumors [165], there is limited evidence to support the routine use of trastuzumab in this subset of tumors. Given the uncertainties of the absolute benefit and potential cardiotoxicities associated with trastuzumab for patients with small tumors, the National Comprehensive Cancer Network (NCCN) recommends adjuvant chemotherapy, with or without trastuzumab for women with lymph node-negative tumors that are 0.6–1 cm in size and for smaller tumors that have ≤2 mm axillary lymph node metastases (pN1mi) [145].

Currently, there are no data to support the use of adjuvant trastuzumab in combination with endocrine therapy alone for women with ER-positive, HER-2-positive breast cancer. Such patients should generally be treated with adjuvant chemotherapy, trastuzumab, and endocrine therapy.

Neoadjuvant Chemotherapy

Historically, preoperative or neoadjuvant chemotherapy was reserved for patients with locally advanced breast cancer. Encouraging results in a select group of patients prompted the first clinical trial, the NSABP B-18, to evaluate the role of neoadjuvant chemotherapy (Adriamycin & Cyclophosphamide or AC) for patients with EBC. A subsequent trial, NSABP B27, investigated the role of AC followed by taxane in the neoadjuvant setting and found that this regimen doubled the rate of pathologic complete response (pCR), a surrogate for a good outcome, from 13.7 % as seen with the AC regimen to 26.1 % as seen with the AC + taxane regimen [166].

The advantage with the neoadjuvant approach is that it downstages the tumor, allowing for a modest increase in the breast conservation therapy (BCT) rate from 7 to 12 % [167, 168]. Of note, the rate of BCT did not increase with the addition of docetaxel [166]. Additionally, neoadjuvant therapy facilitates monitoring of tumor response to allow for adjustment of dose or switching to another effective drug regimen in cases of drug resistance. However, neoadjuvant chemotherapy has not been shown to improve OS over adjuvant systemic therapy, and although it is an acceptable option in select patients with EBC, postoperative adjuvant systemic therapy remains the standard of care for the majority of patients with EBC. Neoadjuvant approach is generally employed for those with tumors ≥ 2 cm and for locally advanced breast cancer.

Multiple clinical trials have used pCR as a surrogate for long-term outcomes [105, 169, 170]. Historically, novel drugs for breast cancer generally had to be approved in the metastatic setting followed by adjuvant clinical trials before they can be approved by the FDA. Such a process can take years or even decades before a potential drug can be approved. In May 2012, the FDA proposed an accelerated approval process based on pCR as an endpoint in high-risk breast cancer. Whether this translates to an improved long-term outcome remains to be proven [105]. Interpreting the literature about the impact of neoadjuvant therapy on pCR can be difficult since the standardized definition of pCR is lacking. For some, no pathologic residual tumor in the breast tumor is considered pCR, while for others, pCR included the breast tumor and axillary nodes. Still, others included the presence of focal invasive cancer or noninvasive residual tumor (i.e., DCIS) as pCR, while others consider pCR as having a complete absence of both invasive and noninvasive component [105]. Minckwitz et al. recently analyzed a large pool of over 6,000 women from seven randomized clinical trials and found that by defining pCR as having no invasive or in situ residuals in breast and nodes, they can identify those with favorable and unfavorable outcomes. Additionally, pCR is a suitable surrogate marker for patients with highly proliferative lesions such as ER-negative, HER-2 positive, and TNBC [105]. It had no prognostic value in patients with subtype luminal A (ER-positive and/or PR-positive, HER-2 negative, grade 1 or 2) tumors or subtype luminal B/HER-2-positive tumors (ER-positive and/or PR-positive, HER-2 positive, all grades). The role of neoadjuvant endocrine therapy is not as well defined as that for neoadjuvant chemotherapy. Outside of a clinical trial, neoadjuvant endocrine therapy should not be used in young women [171].

A recent randomized phase III trial, the Neoadjuvant Study of Sequential Epirubicin with Cyclophosphamide and Paclitaxel With or Without Gemcitabine (Neo-tAnGo), found that although adding gemcitabine did not improve overall survival, giving taxanes before standard anthracycline chemotherapy resulted in a significantly higher pCR than the standard anthracycline first sequence (20 % versus 15 %, $p=0.03$) [172].

Neoadjuvant Target-Specific Therapy (Dual Inhibition of HER-2 Receptors)

Although trastuzumab is effective against HER-2 positive tumors, not all patients derive equal benefit from it due to intrinsic or acquired resistance to HER-2 blockade [173]. Dual inhibition of the HER-2 receptor with a humanized monoclonal antibody (trastuzumab) with another humanized monoclonal antibody targeting a different epitope of HER-2 (pertuzumab or Perjeta®) or a tyrosine kinase inhibitor (lapatinib or Tykerb®) was found to be effective in the advanced setting [174]. This then sets the stage for its clinical testing in high-risk early stage breast cancer patients [175–180]. The clinical trials on dual inhibitors used pathologic complete response (pCR) as their endpoint, which the FDA defines as the absence of invasive cancer in the breast and lymph nodes. Such a metric is now considered as an acceptable surrogate endpoint of treatment efficacy based on data that found improved outcomes among patients who achieved a pCR status [181].

Results from multiple phase 2 and 3 clinical trials demonstrated the superiority of a dual HER-2 inhibition for patients with HER-2-positive, high-risk early breast cancer [175–180] (Table 4.16). In the Neoadjuvant Study of Pertuzumab and Herceptin in an Early Regimen Evaluation (NeoSphere) trial of 417 patients with operable breast cancer (>2 cm), LABC, or IBC, dual inhibition with trastuzumab and pertuzumab resulted in a 39 % of patients achieving pCR versus 21 % in the trastuzumab arm ($P=0.0063$) [176]. Of note, all patients received docetaxel as standard chemotherapy, and the majority of patients (61 %) had operable breast cancer. The most common grade 3 or higher toxicities in the docetaxel, trastuzumab, and pertuzumab group were neutropenia (44.9 %), febrile neutropenia (8.4 %), leukopenia (4.7 %), and diarrhea (5.6 %).

The TRYPHAENA (Trastuzumab plus Pertuzumab in Neoadjuvant HER2-Positive Breast Cancer) trial was a phase 2 trial that randomized 225 patients with operable, LABC, or IBC with a primary goal of assessing the cardiac tolerability of neoadjuvant trastuzumab and pertuzumab given along with anthracycline-containing or anthracycline-free standard chemotherapy regimen. The investigators found that the combination of pertuzumab and trastuzumab, along with standard chemotherapy regimen resulted in low rates of symptomatic left ventricular systolic dysfunction as well as high pCR rates (57–66 %) [180].

Based on the results of the NeoSphere and TRYPHAENA trials, the FDA recently granted an accelerated approval of pertuzumab (Perjeta®) to be used in combination with trastuzumab (Herceptin®) and chemotherapy in the neoadjuvant setting for patients with HER-2-positive tumors who have early breast cancer, locally advanced breast cancer, or inflammatory breast cancer. Permanent approval is possible with additional future confirmatory trials. Pertuzumab is the first one of its kind to be approved in the neoadjuvant setting for breast cancer patients.

Targeted therapies are generally administered over a 1-year period, although it remains to be

Table 4.16 Selected trials on neoadjuvant treatment with dual inhibitors against HER-2 receptors

Trials/author/year/ref	N	Types of trial	Criteria[a]	Groups	Results
NeoSphere Gianni/2012 [176]	417	Phase 2	Operable ≈ 61 % LABC ≈ 32 % IBC ≈ 7 %	**Group A**: TH + D **Group B**: P+TH+D **Group C**: P+TH **Group D**: P+D	pCR: Group A: 21.5 % Group B: 39.3 % $P = 0.0141$ *Combination of trastuzumab, pertuzumab, and docetaxel yielded highest pCR rate*
TRYPHAENA Schneeweiss/2013 [180]	225	Phase 2	Operable ≈ 69 % LABC ≈ 25 % IBC ≈ 6 %	**Arm A**: ECF + TH + P × 3 → D + TH + P × 3 (concurrent treatment) **Arm B**: ECF × 3 → D + TH + P × 3 **Arm C**: D C TH + P × 6	pCR: Group A: 61.6 % Group B: 57.3 % Group C: 66.2 % *Combination of trastuzumab, pertuzumab, and standard chemotherapy had low rates of symptomatic LVSD*
CHER-LOB Guarneri/2012 [177]	121	Phase 2	Stage IIA ≈ 31 % Stage IIB ≈ 51 % Stage IIIA ≈ 18 %	**Arm A**: C + TH **Arm B**: C + L **Arm C**: C + TH + L C: paclitaxel → ECF	pCR: Arm A: 25 % Arm B: 26.3 % Arm C: 46.7 % $P = 0.019$ *Combination of trastuzumab, pertuzumab, and standard chemotherapy yielded highest pCR rate*
NeoALTTO Baselga/2012 [178]	154	Phase 3	N0/N1 ≈ 84 % Excluded IBC	**Arm A**: C + TH **Arm B**: C + L **Arm C**: C + TH + L C: paclitaxel	pCR: Group A: 29.5 % Group B: 24.7 % Group C: 51.3 % $P = 0.0001$ between Group A & C *Combination of trastuzumab, lapatinib, and standard chemotherapy yielded highest pCR rate*
GeparQuinto, GBG 44 Untch/2012 [179]	620	Phase 3	Operable ≈ 83 % LABC/ IBC ≈ 17 %	**Group 1**: C + TH **Group 2**: C + L	*Chemotherapy with lapatinib was inferior to chemotherapy with trastuzumab*

NeoSphere Neoadjuvant Study of Pertuzumab and Herceptin in an Early Regimen Evaluation, *TRYPHAENA* Trastuzumab plus Pertuzumab in Neoadjuvant HER2-Positive Breast Cancer, *CHER-LOB* Chemotherapy, Herceptin and Lapatinib in Operable Breast cancer, *NeoALTTO* Neoadjuvant Lapatinib and/or Trastuzumab Treatment Optimisation, *GBG* German Breast Group; *LABC* locally advanced breast cancer, *IBC* inflammatory breast cancer, *pCR*: pathologic complete response, *T* taxol, *TH* trastuzumab, *L* lapatinib, *P* pertuzumab, *ECF* epirubicin, cyclophosphamide, fluorouracil, *C* carboplatin, *D* docetaxel, *LVSD* left ventricular systolic dysfunction

[a]Percentages were based on averages of the group

seen what the optimum duration should be. Given the encouraging results of the dual inhibitors in the neoadjuvant setting, it is natural to conjecture its use in the adjuvant setting. The next set of clinical trials will evaluate the combination of pertuzumab, trastuzumab, and standard chemotherapy (APHINITY;NCT01358877) or combination of lapatinib, trastuzumab, and standard chemotherapy (ALLTO;NCT00490139) in the adjuvant setting. The ALLTO trial has already finished recruitment, while the APHINITY trial is ongoing, expecting to accrue nearly 5,000 patients with HER-2-positive breast cancer.

In summary, neoadjuvant therapy is generally reserved for those with locally advanced breast cancer or tumors > 2 cm. However, in light of the improved pathologic complete response rates in patients with specific subtypes, an argument can be made that, following diagnosis of breast cancer, definitive surgery should be performed only after receptor status of the tumor is known. This will allow identification of patients who may benefit from a neoadjuvant approach to therapy.

Other Considerations

Treatment of Elderly Patients with Early ER (+) Breast Cancer

In general, standard treatment that would normally be offered to younger women should not be withheld for older women who are medically fit. However, for women age 70 years or older with clinical Stage I (T1N0M0) and ER-positive tumor, a lumpectomy and a standard course of tamoxifen can be adequate treatment [182]. Hughes et al. recently reported the 12.6 years median follow-up results of CALGB 9343 and found that women with the above criteria who were treated with lumpectomy and tamoxifen alone had no significant differences in time to mastectomy, time to distant metastasis, breast cancer-specific survival, or OS compared to those who had lumpectomy, tamoxifen, and radiation [182]. The 10-year OS was 67 % for the irradiation group and 66 % in the nonirradiated group [182]. However, there was a significant difference in the incidence of locoregional recurrence (LRR) and ipsilateral breast recurrence (IBTR); at 10 years, LRR was 8 % lower in the radiation group, and IBTR was 7 % lower in the radiation group.

Axillary lymph node dissection (ALND) was allowed but not encouraged. Of those who did have an ALND, the axillary recurrence rate was 0 %. Of those who did not have an ALND, the recurrence rate was 0 for the irradiation group and 3 % for the nonirradiated group. Of the 636 women studied, only 3 % died of breast cancer, whereas 49 % died of other causes. What this implies is that in this population of elderly women, survival is dictated by competing comorbidities rather than by breast cancer treatments. Similar results were also noted in other trials, despite the eligibility criteria being slightly different among them [32, 183–185].

Invasive Lobular Carcinoma (ILC)

A special attention is given to the surgical management of invasive lobular carcinoma (ILC). It is well recognized that ILC infiltrative growth patterns tend to be discontinuous and that there is a higher incidence of margin positivity and intra-surgical conversion to mastectomy [186]. Because of these features, there is a bias toward a more aggressive surgery such as a mastectomy and axillary lymph node dissection. However, if a clear margin can be achieved, patients with ILC can be effectively treated with BCT as well as with SLNBx [187].

Triple-Negative Breast Cancer (TNBC)

A little more than a decade ago, Perou et al. published a seminal article, outlining a novel method of classifying breast cancers based on genetic profiling [96]. Among the different subtypes of breast cancer, basal-like cancer is one of the most biologically aggressive [97, 188]. Triple-negative breast cancer (TNBC) is the lexicon often used by clinicians to describe these tumors that lack ER, PR, and HER-2 expressions. They represent approximately 17–37 % of all breast cancers and tend to be high grade [97]. TNBC are more common in younger and premenopausal African-American women, although outcome does not appear to be race/ethnicity dependent [189, 190].

Surgical, radiation treatment, and chemotherapeutic options (neoadjuvant and adjuvant) for patients with TNBC are similar to the other subtypes [191, 192]. Unlike other subtypes, there are no target-specific treatments for patients with TNBC, other than chemotherapy (mainly anthracycline and taxanes). Despite their poor prognosis, TNBCs tend to be more sensitive to chemotherapy than the other subtypes [103, 192]. This has often been referred to as the "triple-negative paradox" [192].

Impairment of the BRCA1 pathway [193] has been implicated in TNBC, and because of this, platinum-based chemotherapy and other DNA-damaging agents have been investigated as potential novel therapy. One of the DNA-damaging agents being investigated is the poly(ADP-ribose) polymerase (PARP) inhibitors (iniparib, olaparib, veliparib) [194]. In general, damaged DNA is repaired by two mechanisms: (1) base excision repair (repairs single-stranded DNA breaks) and (2) homologous recombination (repairs double-stranded DNA breaks). In patients with BRCA mutations (i.e., TNBC), the homologous recombination repair mechanism is compromised in tumor cells but not in somatic cells. Thus, tumor cells depend on the base excision repair mechanism, which requires PARP. When a PARP inhibitor is introduced, tumor cells lose their ability to repair DNA, giving rise to synthetic lethality [195] (Fig. 4.11). Although there are several PARP inhibitors currently being investigated [196, 197], none has yet demonstrated any significant impact to warrant wide clinical use.

Axillary Lymph Node Metastases Without Known Primary (Occult Breast Cancer)

On occasion, a woman may present with a palpable axillary mass that is biopsy-proven to be adenocarcinoma or poorly differentiated carcinoma and an undetectable primary breast tumor. In such a case, a diagnosis of an occult breast cancer (OBC) should be entertained. OBC represents 0.1–1.0 % of all breast cancers [198] and is considered as Stage II breast cancer (T0N1/2M0) according to the AJCC staging system [15]. Other primaries that involve the axilla include lung cancer, thyroid cancer, gastrointestinal cancers, melanomas, lymphoma, uterine, ovarian, sweat gland, sarcomas, and nonmelanoma skin cancers [199]. Confirmation of an axillary metastasis can be achieved either with an FNA, core needle biopsy, or ultrasound-guided biopsy.

A complete breast examination and a mammography should be performed as the initial work-up since up to 20 % of non-palpable occult lesions can be detected on a mammogram [200]. Histologic confirmation of the mammographically abnormal breast lesion should be performed. In the case when the biopsy is negative for cancer or when the mammogram does not reveal an abnormality, a breast MRI should be performed. Breast MRI can detect a primary breast cancer in approximately 75 % of women in such a situation [201, 202]. A chest and abdominal CT scan is also recommended as part of the work-up [145].

Certain markers such as ER/PR, mammaglobin, BRST2, CEA, CK7, ER/PR, and CA-125 are positive for breast cancer, while TTF-1 is negative for breast cancer but positive for lung cancer. Positivity on any one marker might not be sufficient to help clinch the diagnosis (i.e., ER/PR positivity can also be seen in gynecologic, stomach, and lung cancer), but rather, it is a constellation of positive markers that helps make the diagnosis.

If after completing the above work-up and the primary is still not found on the breast or elsewhere, the patient is then deemed as having an OBC; 65 % of the time, the primary source is the ipsilateral breast [203, 204]. Optimal treatment for OBC is controversial, although all patients should undergo an axillary node dissection. Whether one chooses to perform a mastectomy (MRM) or whole-breast irradiation (WBI) as definitive treatment is still an area of debate. In a series of 45 patients with OBC, Vlastos et al.

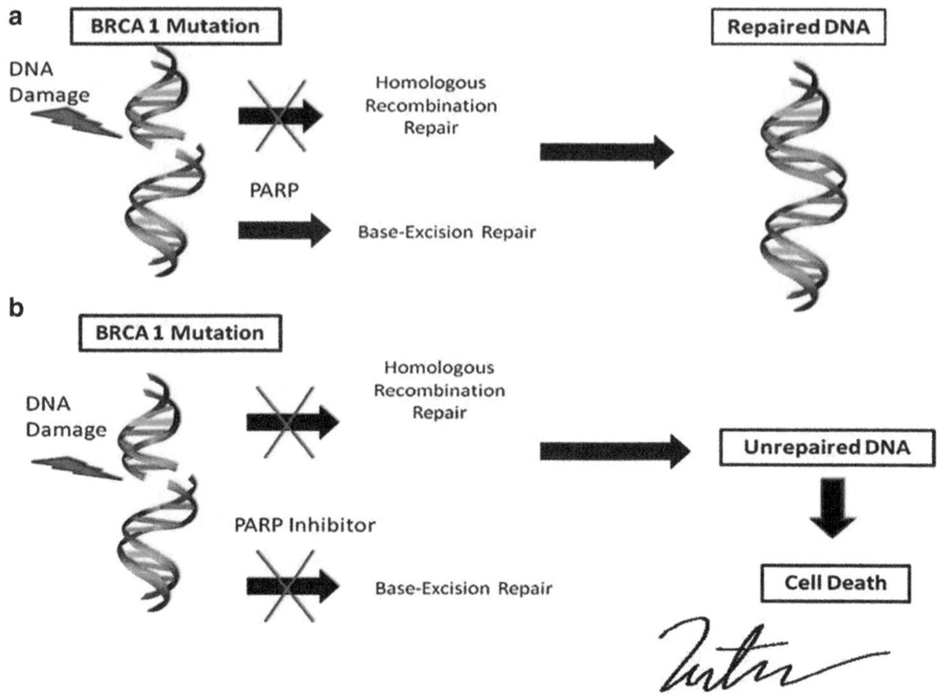

Fig. 4.11 Synthetic lethality: damaged DNAs are repaired by several major pathways. The base excision repair (BER) pathway uses the poly(ADP-ribose) polymerases (PARP) proteins to repair single-strand breaks. The homologous recombination (HR) pathway repairs double-strand breaks. In BRCA deficient tumors, the HR pathway is defective, leaving the tumor cells to use the BER as an alternative pathway for DNA repair (**a**). When PARP inhibitors are given, the BER pathway is now compromised, leading to unrepaired damaged DNA and ultimately to tumor cell death (**b**) (Courtesy of Quyen D. Chu, MD, MBA, FACS)

compared mastectomy with WBI and found no significant differences in locoregional recurrence (15 % versus 13 %), distant metastases (31 % versus 22 %), or 5-year survival (75 % versus 79 %) [205]. Thus, patients with OBC have an option of an MRM or WBI and ALND.

Adjuvant therapy for patients with OBC should follow guidelines similar to patients with Stage II breast cancer. Five-year overall survival depends on the nodal status; for those with N1 disease (1–3 positive nodes), it is 87 %, and for those with 4 or more positive lymph nodes, it is halved (42 %) [205].

Paget's Disease of the Breast

Paget's disease of the breast is a rare disease that involves the skin of the nipple/areolar complex. It is different from Paget's disease of the vulva, penis, and bone. Patients typically present with complaints of itchy, scaly, eczematous, crusty, flaky, or thickened skin on or around the nipple/areolar complex. These nonspecific symptoms are commonly seen in benign conditions, and as a result, the diagnosis of Paget's disease of the breast may be delayed. Diagnosis is made by a full thickness biopsy of the skin that demonstrates Paget cells in the epidermis.

Paget's disease of the breast is almost always associated with an underlying breast pathology (92–100 %), which can either be DCIS or invasive breast cancer [206–208]. Therefore, these patients should undergo a work-up to search for an underlying malignancy. Two-thirds of patients will have the disease within the central quadrant of the breast, and approximately 50 % of patients will have an associated palpable breast mass [209]; palpable masses tend to be invasive while non-palpable ones tend to be DCIS. When an abnormality is not detected on a mammogram or ultrasound, it is reasonable to order a breast MRI to look for an occult primary [210].

Management remains controversial since there is no level 1 data that specifically address local management of Paget's disease. Historically, a mastectomy with or without a lymph node dissection was recommended since the incidence of multicentric (36 %) and multifocal in situ and invasive carcinomas identified in mastectomy specimens is high and local excision alone resulted in a recurrence rate that can be as high as 40 % [211]. However, as mentioned in the early part of the chapter, randomized trials on the surgical treatment of early breast cancer clearly demonstrated equivalent outcomes between a mastectomy and BCT. This implies that BCT should also be a viable option for patients with Paget's disease limited to the central segment of the breast. It is recommended that if BCT is entertained, the nipple/areolar complex should be completely excised along with the underlying breast tissue (central mastectomy). Whole-breast irradiation should also be ensued. Sentinel lymph node biopsy should be performed in all patients undergoing mastectomy, those with invasive cancer undergoing central mastectomy, and those with DCIS undergoing central mastectomy who is suspected to have an occult invasive component.

The outcome is similar to that of women with other types of breast cancer. However, those with an underlying palpable breast tumor tend to have a poorer prognosis that those who do not [212].

Male Breast Cancer

Male breast cancer is rare, occurring in less than 1 % of all breast cancers [213, 214]. For 2013, it is estimated that there are 2,240 new cases and 410 deaths in the United States. The median age of onset is 67, which is 5–10 years older than female breast cancer [215]. Although BRCA1 mutation can occur in men with breast cancer, BRCA 2 mutations are more common, with 4–16 % of men with breast cancer being carriers of such a mutation. Invasive ductal carcinoma is the most common tumor pathology; however, LCIS has not been reported.

Because of its rarity, most of the clinical decision for male breast cancer is an extrapolation of studies for female breast cancer. Thus, male breast cancer shares many resembling characteristics with female breast cancers such as sharing identical AJCC/TNM staging system, having analogous prognostic factors such as tumor size and lymph node status, affording similar surgical and adjuvant treatment options, and possessing comparable overall survival stage per stage of disease.

Unlike female breast cancer, almost all male breast cancers are hormone receptor-positive; approximately 90 % express estrogen receptor and 81 % express progesterone receptor [213]. Consequently, hormonal therapy is a viable therapy, although compliance can be a problem. In a large retrospective study examining tamoxifen-related side effects among male breast cancer, it was found that almost 21 % of patients discontinued the medication due to weight gain (22 %), sexual dysfunction/loss of libido (22 %), hot flashes (13 %), neurocognitive defects (9 %), and thromboembolic events (9 %) [216].

Chemoprevention

The finding that tamoxifen had significantly reduced the incidence of contralateral breast cancer prompted the NSABP to perform a preventive trial in women without personal history of breast cancer but were deemed to be at high risk of developing cancer. The definition of high risk varies among the studies, but in general, they include women ages ≥ 60 years, Gail 5-year risk score ≥ 1.66 %, and those with a history of having atypical ductal hyperplasia, lobular hyperplasia, or lobular carcinoma in situ [217–220].

NSABP P-1 trial demonstrated that tamoxifen reduces the cumulative incidence of both invasive and noninvasive breast cancer by 50 % in high-risk premenopausal and postmenopausal women [217]. Because of the concerns of developing endometrial cancers and the side effects associated with tamoxifen, NSABP subsequently performed the Study of Tamoxifen And Raloxifene (STAR) trial, a trial that directly compares tamoxifen with raloxifene (a second-generation SERM) [218].

Similar to tamoxifen, raloxifene reduces the incidence of invasive breast cancer, although the magnitude was less than tamoxifen (38 % versus 50 %; $P=0.01$). The initial results of the STAR trial showed raloxifene to be less effective than tamoxifen at reducing the incidence of noninvasive breast cancer [218], but the latest update found no significant difference between the two agents in this area [221]. Raloxifene had a better safety profile than tamoxifen; the incidence of uterine cancer, thromboembolic events, and cataract development was significantly lower in the raloxifene group [221] (Table 4.17).

Despite the positive benefits of tamoxifen and raloxifene, compliance has been poor due to their serious toxic effects [222]. Because of this, the AIs were tested and found to be an acceptable alternative to the SERMs [219, 220]. Sponsored by the National Cancer Institute of Canada, the MAP.3 trial randomized over 4,500 postmenopausal women to either 5 years of exemestane or placebo. At a median follow-up of 35 months, those that took exemestane for approximately 5 years had a 65 % relative reduction in the annual incidence of invasive breast cancer compared to placebo ($P=0.002$). There were no serious toxic effects with exemestane (Table 4.17).

The International Breast Cancer Interventional Study II (IBIS-II) recently reported their results of anastrozole on 3,864 postmenopausal women who were considered to be at high risk of developing breast cancer and found similar results as the MAP.3 trial [220]. However, patients taking anastrozole experienced a higher frequency of musculoskeletal and vasomotor symptoms, hypertension, and gynecologic adverse events (vaginal or uterine prolapsed and vaginal pruritus) compared to placebo.

The American Society of Clinical Oncology (ASCO) Clinical Practice Guideline recently updated its key recommendations that included exemestane, along with tamoxifen and raloxifene, as an option for chemoprevention [223] (Table 4.18). Given the more recent data from the IBIS-II, it is conceivable that future ASCO recommendations will include anastrozole.

Despite a significant reduction in the incidence of invasive breast cancer, none of the four preventive trials demonstrated any significant reduction in mortality. Perhaps this fact, combined with the potential toxicity associated with the medication, may be one of the reasons why chemoprevention has not been widely embraced [224].

Salient Points

- Early Breast Cancer includes a subset of N(+) patients (T1-2N1).
- The Gail model is used to assess a woman's lifetime risk of developing breast cancer. Such assessment is useful for counseling at-risk patients regarding the risks and benefits of chemopreventive therapy (tamoxifen, raloxifene, or AIs).
- Regardless of breast cancer histologic subtypes, treatment is generally the same.
- Screening breast MRI should be used in high-risk patients, mainly those with BRCA1/2 mutations, Li-Fraumeni syndrome or Cowden syndrome, 1st-degree relative with BRCA1/2 mutation, history to radiation to the chest at a young age, or lifetime risk ≥ 20 %.
- Avoid excisional biopsy as the initial diagnostic tool. Instead, consider FNA and CNB.
- The role of accelerated partial breast irradiation is still being defined.
- A negative margin is defined as no tumor at the inked surgical margin, irrespective of the distance from the nearest tumor cell.
- SLNBx can be performed for any patient with clinically negative node.
- IHC is not necessary to assess SLNs.
- SLNBx can be performed in patients with multicentric disease and those with DCIS who opted for a mastectomy.
- For those with positive sentinel lymph nodes, an axillary lymph node dissection can be avoided as long as all of the following criteria are met:
  - Tumor ≤ 5 cm
  - ≤ 2 positive sentinel lymph nodes
  - Breast conservation therapy patients who will receive external beam radiation and adjuvant systemic therapy

Table 4.17 Selected chemoprevention clinical trials

Trials/year/reference	# Patients	Study design	Median follow-up (months)	Criteria for high risk	Outcome
NSABP P-1 (2005)/ Fisher [217]	13,388	T versus P × 5 years	74	Age ≥ 60 years	Tamoxifen reduces invasive BC by 43 %
				Gail score > 1.66 %	Tamoxifen reduces osteoporotic fractures by 32 %
				Atypia/LCIS	Tamoxifen increases risk of stroke, DVT, and cataracts
NSABP P2 (2006)/ Vogel [218, 221]	19,490	R versus T × 5 years	81	Gail score >1.66 %	Raloxifene reduces invasive BC by 38 %, while tamoxifen reduces it by 50 %
				LCIS	Tamoxifen was superior in reducing breast cancer risk Raloxifene was superior in reducing endometrial cancer, thromboembolic events, and cataracts
NCIC CTG MAP.3 (2011)/Goss [219]	4,560	E versus P × 5 years	35	Age ≥ 60 years Gail score >1.66 % Atypia/LCIS/lobular hyperplasia DCIS with mastectomy	Exemestane reduces invasive BC by 65 % No differences between E and P in incidence of skeletal fractures, cardiovascular events, other cancers, or treatment-related deaths
IBIS-II (2013)/ Cuzick [220]	3,864	A versus P × 5 years	60	Family history Atypia/LCIS Breast density	Anastrozole reduces invasive BC by 50 % Significantly more vasomotor symptoms, musculoskeletal aches and pains, and hypertension in anastrozole group

NSABP National Surgical Adjuvant Breast and Bowel Project, *NCIC CTG MAP.3* National Cancer Institute of Canada, MAP.3, *IBIS* International Breast Cancer Intervention Study, *T* tamoxifen, *R* raloxifene, *E* exemestane, *A* anastrozole, *P* placebo, *BC* breast cancer, *DVT* deep venous thrombosis, *LCIS* lobular carcinoma in situ, *DCIS* ductal carcinoma in situ

Table 4.18 Selected summary of the American Society of Clinical Oncology chemoprevention recommendations

Premenopausal women
Tamoxifen × 5 years
Postmenopausal women
Tamoxifen × 5 years
Raloxifene × 5 years
Exemestane × 5 years
Anastrozole × 5 years (not listed by ASCO but recent data demonstrated its efficacy)

Based on data from Ref. [223]

- The role of SLNBx for those undergoing neoadjuvant chemotherapy remains debatable.
- For locoregional control options for patients with EBC, see Fig. 4.12.
- Systemic treatment includes chemotherapy, hormonal therapy, and/or biologic therapy.
- AC has better outcome than CMF as adjuvant chemotherapy.
- Addition of taxanes improves outcome, but mainly for N(+) disease.
- Systemic therapy may not be beneficial to all patients: prognostic indices can help decide who will benefit from chemotherapy. These include Adjuvant!Online, Nottingham Prognostic Index, St. Gallen guidelines, Oncotype DX®, MammaPrint®, and Mammostrat®.
- Adjuvant hormonal therapy (tamoxifen or AI) improves outcome; combination of hormonal therapy and chemotherapy further improves outcome compared to either alone.

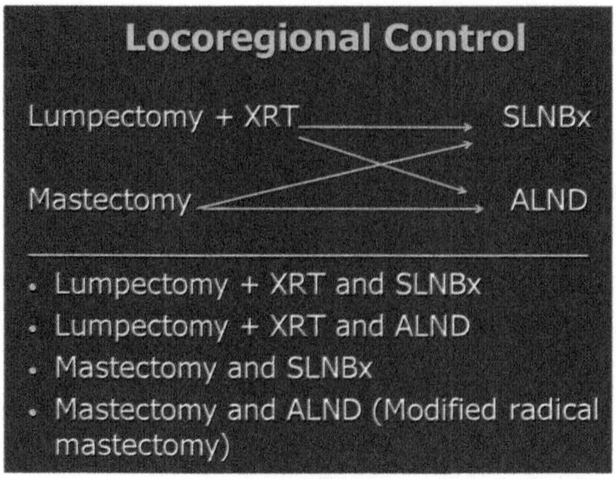

Fig. 4.12 Locoregional options for patients with EBC

- Tamoxifen increases risk of endometrial cancer and thromboembolic events. AIs increase risk of bone loss and can only be used in women with no ovarian function.
- 5 years of tamoxifen followed by 5 years of an AI improves DFS but not OS.
- 10 years of tamoxifen is better than 5 years.
- For ER(+) LN(−) patients, the decision to consider additional chemotherapy is being addressed by the use of genetic profiling platforms such as the Oncotype DX® and MammaPrint®.
  - Oncotype DX is a 21-gene platform that uses RS to group patients into three groups: low risk, intermediate risk, and high risk.
  - MammaPrint uses the 70-gene signature and groups patients into low risk and high risk.
  - Low-risk group can potentially avoid chemotherapy.
  - TAILORx trial will address what to do with the Oncotype DX intermediate-risk group.
  - RxPONDER trial evaluates whether chemotherapy is needed in ER(+), LN(+) patients with low RS.
- 1 year of Herceptin is indicated for HER-2-positive tumors.
- Neoadjuvant chemotherapy is appropriate in select patients.
  - pCR is a surrogate marker of long-term outcomes.
  - Taxanes given before standard anthracycline chemotherapy is better than standard anthracycline first therapy.
- Dual inhibition of HER-2-positive tumors (Herceptin + pertuzumab or lapatinib) improves outcomes compared to Herceptin alone.
- Women > 70 years old can undergo lumpectomy and tamoxifen (without SLNBx or irradiation) if they meet the following criteria:
  - Tumor ≤ 2 cm
  - ER (+)
- TNBC is aggressive tumor that lacks target-specific therapy.
- Options for treating occult breast cancer include:
  - MRM
  - Breast irradiation and axillary lymph node dissection
- There are five intrinsic subtypes: (1) luminal A, (2) luminal B, (3) HER-2 positive, (4) basal-like or TNBC, and (5) normal-like.
- Overview treatment of patients with EBC (see Fig. 4.13).

Questions

1. A 55-year-old woman has a 1.5 cm suspicious breast mass without evidence of lymphadenopathy. She underwent a core needle biopsy of this mass that confirmed an invasive adenocarcinoma. The next step in management is:
   A. Lumpectomy and sentinel lymph node biopsy
   B. Mastectomy
   C. Radiation
   D. Chemotherapy
   E. Hormonal therapy
2. A 65-year-old woman had a lumpectomy for a 4 cm breast cancer with negative margins. She has 1 out of 2 positive sentinel lymph nodes. Which of the following is an acceptable option?
   A. Observation
   B. Adjuvant systemic therapy and whole-breast irradiation
   C. Radiation alone
   D. Chemotherapy followed by mastectomy

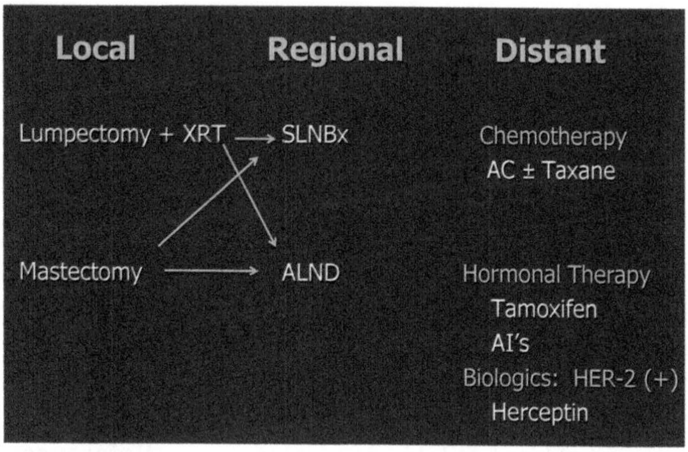

Fig. 4.13 Overview treatment of patients with EBC

E. Mastectomy

3. A 75-year-old woman with a 1.8 cm breast cancer that was excised with a negative margin. She has no clinical lymphadenopathy. Which of the following statements is true?
   A. Given her age, observation is appropriate.
   B. Hormonal therapy alone is adequate, regardless of other factors.
   C. Chemotherapy should be offered, regardless of other factors.
   D. Hormonal therapy alone is appropriate if her tumor is ER(+).
   E. Modified radical mastectomy and radiation therapy.
4. A 35-year-old woman presented with a 1.9 cm breast mass that demonstrated an invasive ductal carcinoma. She is otherwise asymptomatic. The patient elected to undergo a mastectomy. In addition to the mastectomy, the patient will need:
   A. CT scan of abdomen to rule out liver involvement
   B. Radiation therapy alone
   C. Mastectomy alone
   D. Axillary lymph node dissection and radiation
   E. Sentinel lymph node biopsy
5. A 55-year-old woman with a 3.5 cm breast cancer elected to undergo a mastectomy and a sentinel lymph node biopsy. One of two lymph nodes was involved. Her tumor is HER-2 negative. The next step in management is:
   A. Radiation
   B. Chemoradiation therapy
   C. Systemic therapy that includes 1 year of Herceptin
   D. Axillary lymph node dissection
   E. Observation
6. A 32-year-old woman presented with a 1.2 cm breast cancer with involved margins following a lumpectomy. Which of the following is the best option?
   A. Re-excision to negative margins, radiation therapy, and sentinel lymph node biopsy
   B. Re-excision to negative margins, radiation therapy and axillary lymph node dissection
   C. Mastectomy and axillary lymph node dissection
   D. Mastectomy and sentinel lymph node biopsy
   E. Re-excision to negative margins alone
7. All of the following statements are true EXCEPT:
   A. Adjuvant tamoxifen can be given for 10 years.
   B. Adjuvant aromatase inhibitors (AIs) can be given for 10 years.

   C. 10 years of adjuvant tamoxifen yields better outcome than 5 years of tamoxifen.
   D. AIs can be given for 5 years after 5 years of tamoxifen.
   E. AIs can be given 2 or 3 years after tamoxifen for a total of 5 years of endocrine therapy.

8. A 45-year-old woman presented with a 1.8 cm breast cancer with involved margins. She has palpable axillary lymphadenopathy. Which is the best treatment option?
   A. Re-excision to negative margins and sentinel lymph node biopsy
   B. Mastectomy with sentinel lymph node biopsy
   C. Re-excision to negative margins with axillary lymph node dissection
   D. Mastectomy alone
   E. Re-excision to negative margins alone

9. A 65-year-old woman presented with a palpable axillary lymphadenopathy. A mammogram and other diagnostic work-ups searching for a primary source were unhelpful. All of the following statements are true EXCEPT:
   A. Whole-breast irradiation and axillary lymph node dissection.
   B. MRM.
   C. Over 60 % has an occult breast primary cancer.
   D. She is considered to have Stage III breast cancer.
   E. TTF-1 is positive for lung primary but negative for breast primary.

10. A 60-year-old woman presented with a 3.0 cm invasive lobular carcinoma (ILC). Palpable. All of the following statements are true EXCEPT:
   A. A mastectomy is recommended because of the histology.
   B. ILC has a tendency to be discontinuous resulting in a higher incidence of margin positivity.
   C. Breast-conserving therapy is an option.
   D. Sentinel lymph node biopsy is an option.
   E. Systemic therapy regimen is the same as for invasive ductal carcinoma.

Answers

1. A
2. B
3. D
4. E
5. D
6. A
7. B
8. C
9. D
10. A

References

1. Desantis C, Ma J, Bryan L, Jemal A. Breast cancer statistics, 2013. CA Cancer J Clin. 2014; 64(1):52–62.
2. Fisher B. Surgical adjuvant therapy for breast cancer. Cancer. 1972;30(6):1556–64.
3. Chu QD, McDonald JC, Li BD. Adjuvant therapy for patients who have node-positive breast cancer. Adv Surg. 2006;40:77–98.
4. Colditz GA. Estrogen, estrogen plus progestin therapy, and risk of breast cancer. Clin Cancer Res. 2005;11(2 Pt 2):909s–17.
5. Gail MH, Brinton LA, Byar DP, et al. Projecting individualized probabilities of developing breast cancer for white females who are being examined annually. J Natl Cancer Inst. 1989;81(24):1879–86.
6. Claus EB, Risch N, Thompson WD. Autosomal dominant inheritance of early-onset breast cancer. Implications for risk prediction. Cancer. 1994;73(3): 643–51.
7. Tyrer J, Duffy SW, Cuzick J. A breast cancer prediction model incorporating familial and personal risk factors. Stat Med. 2004;23(7):1111–30.
8. Sastre-Garau X, Jouve M, Asselain B, et al. Infiltrating lobular carcinoma of the breast. Clinicopathologic analysis of 975 cases with reference to data on conservative therapy and metastatic patterns. Cancer. 1996;77(1):113–20.
9. Katz A, Saad ED, Porter P, Pusztai L. Primary systemic chemotherapy of invasive lobular carcinoma of the breast. Lancet Oncol. 2007;8(1):55–62.
10. Arpino G, Bardou VJ, Clark GM, Elledge RM. Infiltrating lobular carcinoma of the breast: tumor characteristics and clinical outcome. Breast Cancer Res. 2004;6(3):R149–56.
11. Viale G, Rotmensz N, Maisonneuve P, et al. Lack of prognostic significance of "classic" lobular breast carcinoma: a matched, single institution series. Breast Cancer Res Treat. 2009;117(1):211–4.
12. Horn PL, Thompson WD. Risk of contralateral breast cancer. Associations with histologic, clinical, and therapeutic factors. Cancer. 1988;62(2):412–24.

13. Ashikari R, Huvos AG, Urban JA, Robbins GF. Infiltrating lobular carcinoma of the breast. Cancer. 1973;31(1):110–6.
14. Gainer SM, Lodhi AK, Bhattacharyya A, Krishnamurthy S, Kuerer HM, Lucci A. Invasive lobular carcinoma predicts micrometastasis in breast cancer. J Surg Res. 2012;177(1):93–6.
15. Edge SB, Compton CC. The American Joint Committee on Cancer: the 7th edition of the AJCC cancer staging manual and the future of TNM. Ann Surg Oncol. 2010;17(6):1471–4.
16. Compton C, Byrd D, Garcia-Aguilar J, et al. Breast. In: Compton C, Byrd D, Garcia-Aguilar J, Kurtzman S, Olawaiye A, Washington M, editors. AJCC cancer staging atlas. 2nd ed. New York: Springer; 2012. p. 419–40.
17. Plevritis SK, Kurian AW, Sigal BM, et al. Cost-effectiveness of screening BRCA1/2 mutation carriers with breast magnetic resonance imaging. JAMA. 2006;295(20):2374–84.
18. McCabe C, Claxton K, Culyer AJ. The NICE cost-effectiveness threshold: what it is and what that means. Pharmacoeconomics. 2008;26(9):733–44.
19. Lee CH, Dershaw DD, Kopans D, et al. Breast cancer screening with imaging: recommendations from the Society of Breast Imaging and the ACR on the use of mammography, breast MRI, breast ultrasound, and other technologies for the detection of clinically occult breast cancer. J Am Coll Radiol. 2010;7(1):18–27.
20. Ward EM, Smith RA. Integrating tools for breast cancer risk assessment, risk reduction, and early detection. Cancer Epidemiol Biomarkers Prev. 2010;19(10):2428–9.
21. Saslow D, Boetes C, Burke W, et al. American Cancer Society guidelines for breast screening with MRI as an adjunct to mammography. CA Cancer J Clin. 2007;57(2):75–89.
22. Houssami N, Turner R, Macaskill P, et al. An individual person data meta-analysis of preoperative magnetic resonance imaging and breast cancer recurrence. J Clin Oncol. 2014;32:1–14.
23. Turnbull LW, Brown SR, Olivier C, et al. Multicentre randomised controlled trial examining the cost-effectiveness of contrast-enhanced high field magnetic resonance imaging in women with primary breast cancer scheduled for wide local excision (COMICE). Health Technol Assess. 2010;14(1):1–182.
24. Houssami N, Turner R, Morrow M. Preoperative magnetic resonance imaging in breast cancer: meta-analysis of surgical outcomes. Ann Surg. 2013;257(2):249–55.
25. Silverstein MJ, Lagios MD, Recht A, et al. Image-detected breast cancer: state of the art diagnosis and treatment. J Am Coll Surg. 2005;201(4):586–97.
26. Molina MA, Snell S, Franceschi D, et al. Breast specimen orientation. Ann Surg Oncol. 2009;16(2):285–8.
27. Fisher B, Montague E, Redmond C, et al. Comparison of radical mastectomy with alternative treatments for primary breast cancer. A first report of results from a prospective randomized clinical trial. Cancer. 1977;39(6 Suppl):2827–39.
28. Fisher B, Gebhardt MC. The evolution of breast cancer surgery: past, present, and future. Semin Oncol. 1978;5(4):385–94.
29. Fisher B, Redmond C, Fisher ER, et al. Ten-year results of a randomized clinical trial comparing radical mastectomy and total mastectomy with or without radiation. N Engl J Med. 1985;312(11):674–81.
30. Fisher B. A biological perspective of breast cancer: contributions of the National Surgical Adjuvant Breast and Bowel Project clinical trials. CA Cancer J Clin. 1991;41(2):97–111.
31. Fisher B, Jeong JH, Anderson S, Bryant J, Fisher ER, Wolmark N. Twenty-five-year follow-up of a randomized trial comparing radical mastectomy, total mastectomy, and total mastectomy followed by irradiation. N Engl J Med. 2002;347(8):567–75.
32. Fisher B, Bryant J, Dignam JJ, et al. Tamoxifen, radiation therapy, or both for prevention of ipsilateral breast tumor recurrence after lumpectomy in women with invasive breast cancers of one centimeter or less. J Clin Oncol. 2002;20(20):4141–9.
33. Fisher B, Anderson S, Bryant J, et al. Twenty-year follow-up of a randomized trial comparing total mastectomy, lumpectomy, and lumpectomy plus irradiation for the treatment of invasive breast cancer. N Engl J Med. 2002;347(16):1233–41.
34. Jacobson JA, Danforth DN, Cowan KH, et al. Ten-year results of a comparison of conservation with mastectomy in the treatment of stage I and II breast cancer. N Engl J Med. 1995;332(14):907–11.
35. Veronesi U, Cascinelli N, Mariani L, et al. Twenty-year follow-up of a randomized study comparing breast-conserving surgery with radical mastectomy for early breast cancer. N Engl J Med. 2002;347(16):1227–32.
36. Blichert-Toft M, Nielsen M, Düring M, et al. Long-term results of breast conserving surgery vs. mastectomy for early stage invasive breast cancer: 20-year follow-up of the Danish randomized DBCG-82TM protocol. Acta Oncol. 2008;47(4):672–81.
37. van Dongen JA, Bartelink H, Fentiman IS, et al. Randomized clinical trial to assess the value of breast-conserving therapy in stage I and II breast cancer, EORTC 10801 trial. J Natl Cancer Inst Monogr. 1992;11:15–8.
38. Sarrazin D, Lê MG, Arriagada R, et al. Ten-year results of a randomized trial comparing a conservative treatment to mastectomy in early breast cancer. Radiother Oncol. 1989;14(3):177–84.
39. Fisher B, Bauer M, Margolese R, et al. Five-year results of a randomized clinical trial comparing total mastectomy and segmental mastectomy with or without radiation in the treatment of breast cancer. N Engl J Med. 1985;312(11):665–73.
40. Darby S, McGale P, Correa C, et al. Effect of radiotherapy after breast-conserving surgery on 10-year

recurrence and 15-year breast cancer death: meta-analysis of individual patient data for 10,801 women in 17 randomised trials. Lancet. 2011;378(9804): 1707–16.
41. Liljegren G, Holmberg L, Bergh J, et al. 10-Year results after sector resection with or without postoperative radiotherapy for stage I breast cancer: a randomized trial. J Clin Oncol. 1999;17(8):2326–33.
42. Veronesi U, Marubini E, Mariani L, et al. Radiotherapy after breast-conserving surgery in small breast carcinoma: long-term results of a randomized trial. Ann Oncol. 2001;12(7):997–1003.
43. Shah C, Badiyan S, Ben Wilkinson J, et al. Treatment efficacy with accelerated partial breast irradiation (APBI): final analysis of the American Society of Breast Surgeons MammoSite(®) breast brachytherapy registry trial. Ann Surg Oncol. 2013;20(10): 3279–85.
44. Shah C, Antonucci JV, Wilkinson JB, et al. Twelve-year clinical outcomes and patterns of failure with accelerated partial breast irradiation versus whole-breast irradiation: results of a matched-pair analysis. Radiother Oncol. 2011;100(2):210–4.
45. Polgár C, Fodor J, Major T, et al. Breast-conserving treatment with partial or whole breast irradiation for low-risk invasive breast carcinoma–5-year results of a randomized trial. Int J Radiat Oncol Biol Phys. 2007;69(3):694–702.
46. Hughes KS, Schnaper LA, Berry D, et al. Lumpectomy plus tamoxifen with or without irradiation in women 70 years of age or older with early breast cancer. N Engl J Med. 2004;351(10):971–7.
47. Smith GL, Xu Y, Buchholz TA, et al. Association between treatment with brachytherapy vs whole-breast irradiation and subsequent mastectomy, complications, and survival among older women with invasive breast cancer. JAMA. 2012;307(17): 1827–37.
48. Smith BD, Arthur DW, Buchholz TA, et al. Accelerated partial breast irradiation consensus statement from the American Society for Radiation Oncology (ASTRO). Int J Radiat Oncol Biol Phys. 2009;74(4):987–1001.
49. Houssami N, Macaskill P, Marinovich ML, et al. Meta-analysis of the impact of surgical margins on local recurrence in women with early-stage invasive breast cancer treated with breast-conserving therapy. Eur J Cancer. 2010;46(18):3219–32.
50. Moran M, Schnitt S, Giuliano A, et al. Society of Surgical Oncology-American Society for Radiation Oncology consensus guideline on margins for breast-conserving surgery with whole-breast irradiation in stages I and II invasive breast cancer. Int J Radiat Oncol Biol Phys. 2014;88(3):553–64.
51. Fisher B, Bauer M, Wickerham DL, et al. Relation of number of positive axillary nodes to the prognosis of patients with primary breast cancer. An NSABP update. Cancer. 1983;52(9):1551–7.
52. Fleissig A, Fallowfield LJ, Langridge CI, et al. Post-operative arm morbidity and quality of life. Results of the ALMANAC randomised trial comparing sentinel node biopsy with standard axillary treatment in the management of patients with early breast cancer. Breast Cancer Res Treat. 2006;95(3):279–93.
53. Lucci A, McCall LM, Beitsch PD, et al. Surgical complications associated with sentinel lymph node dissection (SLND) plus axillary lymph node dissection compared with SLND alone in the American College of Surgeons Oncology Group Trial Z0011. J Clin Oncol. 2007;25(24):3657–63.
54. Veronesi U, Paganelli G, Viale G, et al. A randomized comparison of sentinel-node biopsy with routine axillary dissection in breast cancer. N Engl J Med. 2003;349(6):546–53.
55. Veronesi U, Viale G, Paganelli G, et al. Sentinel lymph node biopsy in breast cancer: ten-year results of a randomized controlled study. Ann Surg. 2010;251(4):595–600.
56. Zavagno G, De Salvo GL, Scalco G, et al. A Randomized clinical trial on sentinel lymph node biopsy versus axillary lymph node dissection in breast cancer: results of the Sentinella/GIVOM trial. Ann Surg. 2008;247(2):207–13.
57. Krag DN, Anderson SJ, Julian TB, et al. Sentinel-lymph-node resection compared with conventional axillary-lymph-node dissection in clinically node-negative patients with breast cancer: overall survival findings from the NSABP B-32 randomised phase 3 trial. Lancet Oncol. 2010;11(10):927–33.
58. Giuliano AE, Hunt KK, Ballman KV, et al. Axillary dissection vs no axillary dissection in women with invasive breast cancer and sentinel node metastasis: a randomized clinical trial. JAMA. 2011;305(6): 569–75.
59. Klimberg VS, Rubio IT, Henry R, Cowan C, Colvert M, Korourian S. Subareolar versus peritumoral injection for location of the sentinel lymph node. Ann Surg. 1999;229(6):860–4. discussion 864–865.
60. Krag DN, Anderson SJ, Julian TB, et al. Technical outcomes of sentinel-lymph-node resection and conventional axillary-lymph-node dissection in patients with clinically node-negative breast cancer: results from the NSABP B-32 randomised phase III trial. Lancet Oncol. 2007;8(10):881–8.
61. Hunt KK, Ballman KV, McCall LM, et al. Factors associated with local-regional recurrence after a negative sentinel node dissection: results of the ACOSOG Z0010 trial. Ann Surg. 2012;256(3): 428–36.
62. Weaver DL, Ashikaga T, Krag DN, et al. Effect of occult metastases on survival in node-negative breast cancer. N Engl J Med. 2011;364(5):412–21.
63. Surgeons ASoB. American Society of Breast Surgeons guidelines for performing sentinel lymph node biopsy in breast cancer. 2010. Accessed 2 Dec 2013.

64. Lyman GH, Giuliano AE, Somerfield MR, et al. American Society of Clinical Oncology guideline recommendations for sentinel lymph node biopsy in early-stage breast cancer. J Clin Oncol. 2005;23(30): 7703–20.
65. Kim T, Giuliano AE, Lyman GH. Lymphatic mapping and sentinel lymph node biopsy in early-stage breast carcinoma: a metaanalysis. Cancer. 2006; 106(1):4–16.
66. Katz A, Niemierko A, Gage I, et al. Can axillary dissection be avoided in patients with sentinel lymph node metastasis? J Surg Oncol. 2006;93(7):550–8.
67. Mittendorf EA, Hunt KK, Boughey JC, et al. Incorporation of sentinel lymph node metastasis size into a nomogram predicting nonsentinel lymph node involvement in breast cancer patients with a positive sentinel lymph node. Ann Surg. 2012;255(1):109–15.
68. Galimberti V, Cole BF, Zurrida S, et al. Axillary dissection versus no axillary dissection in patients with sentinel-node micrometastases (IBCSG 23–01): a phase 3 randomised controlled trial. Lancet Oncol. 2013;14(4):297–305.
69. Diepstraten SC, Sever AR, Buckens CF, et al. Value of preoperative ultrasound-guided axillary lymph node biopsy for preventing completion axillary lymph node dissection in breast cancer: a systematic review and meta-analysis. Ann Surg Oncol. 2014; 21(1):51–9.
70. van Deurzen CH, Vriens BE, Tjan-Heijnen VC, et al. Accuracy of sentinel node biopsy after neoadjuvant chemotherapy in breast cancer patients: a systematic review. Eur J Cancer. 2009;45(18):3124–30.
71. Kuehn T, Bauerfeind I, Fehm T, et al. Sentinel-lymph-node biopsy in patients with breast cancer before and after neoadjuvant chemotherapy (SENTINA): a prospective, multicentre cohort study. Lancet Oncol. 2013;14(7):609–18.
72. Boughey JC, Suman VJ, Mittendorf EA, et al. Sentinel lymph node surgery after neoadjuvant chemotherapy in patients with node-positive breast cancer: the ACOSOG Z1071 (Alliance) clinical trial. JAMA. 2013;310(14):1455–61.
73. Straver ME, Meijnen P, van Tienhoven G, et al. Role of axillary clearance after a tumor-positive sentinel node in the administration of adjuvant therapy in early breast cancer. J Clin Oncol. 2010;28(5): 731–7.
74. Rutgers E, Donker M, Straver M, et al. Radiotherapy or surgery of the axilla after a positive sentinel node in breast cancer patients. Final analysis of the EORTC AMAROS trial. J Clin Oncol. 2013;31 Suppl:abstr LBA1001.
75. Whelan T, Olivotto I, Ackerman I, et al. NCIC-CTG MA.20: an intergroup trial of regional nodal irradiation in early breast cancer. J Clin Oncol. 2011;29 Suppl:abstr LBA 1003.
76. Recht A, Edge SB, Solin LJ, et al. Postmastectomy radiotherapy: clinical practice guidelines of the American Society of Clinical Oncology. J Clin Oncol. 2001;19(5):1539–69.
77. Taylor ME, Haffty BG, Rabinovitch R, et al. ACR appropriateness criteria on postmastectomy radiotherapy expert panel on radiation oncology-breast. Int J Radiat Oncol Biol Phys. 2009;73(4): 997–1002.
78. Moo TA, McMillan R, Lee M, et al. Selection criteria for postmastectomy radiotherapy in t1-t2 tumors with 1 to 3 positive lymph nodes. Ann Surg Oncol. 2013;20(10):3169–74.
79. Truong PT, Olivotto IA, Kader HA, Panades M, Speers CH, Berthelet E. Selecting breast cancer patients with T1-T2 tumors and one to three positive axillary nodes at high postmastectomy locoregional recurrence risk for adjuvant radiotherapy. Int J Radiat Oncol Biol Phys. 2005;61(5):1337–47.
80. Saphner T, Tormey DC, Gray R. Annual hazard rates of recurrence for breast cancer after primary therapy. J Clin Oncol. 1996;14(10):2738–46.
81. Early Breast Cancer Trialists' Collaborative Group. Effects of adjuvant tamoxifen and of cytotoxic therapy on mortality in early breast cancer. An overview of 61 randomized trials among 28,896 women. N Engl J Med. 1988;319(26):1681–92.
82. Early Breast Cancer Trialists' Collaborative Group. Effects of radiotherapy and surgery in early breast cancer. An overview of the randomized trials. N Engl J Med. 1995;333(22):1444–55.
83. Fisher B, Ravdin RG, Ausman RK, Slack NH, Moore GE, Noer RJ. Surgical adjuvant chemotherapy in cancer of the breast: results of a decade of cooperative investigation. Ann Surg. 1968;168(3): 337–56.
84. Fisher B, Slack N, Katrych D, Wolmark N. Ten year follow-up results of patients with carcinoma of the breast in a co-operative clinical trial evaluating surgical adjuvant chemotherapy. Surg Gynecol Obstet. 1975;140(4):528–34.
85. Fisher B, Carbone P, Economou SG, et al. 1-Phenylalanine mustard (L-PAM) in the management of primary breast cancer. A report of early findings. N Engl J Med. 1975;292(3):117–22.
86. Bonadonna G, Brusamolino E, Valagussa P, et al. Combination chemotherapy as an adjuvant treatment in operable breast cancer. N Engl J Med. 1976; 294(8):405–10.
87. Early Breast Cancer Trialists' Collaborative Group. Polychemotherapy for early breast cancer: an overview of the randomised trials. Lancet. 1998; 352(9132):930–42.
88. Peto R, Davies C, Godwin J, et al. Comparisons between different polychemotherapy regimens for early breast cancer: meta-analyses of long-term outcome among 100,000 women in 123 randomised trials. Lancet. 2012;379(9814):432–44.
89. Eifel P, Axelson JA, Costa J, et al. National Institutes of Health Consensus Development Conference Statement: adjuvant therapy for breast cancer, November 1–3, 2000. J Natl Cancer Inst. 2001;93(13):979–89.
90. Jacquin JP, Jones S, Magné N, et al. Docetaxel-containing adjuvant chemotherapy in patients with

early stage breast cancer. Consistency of effect independent of nodal and biomarker status: a meta-analysis of 14 randomized clinical trials. Breast Cancer Res Treat. 2012;134(3):903–13.
91. Martín M, Seguí MA, Antón A, et al. Adjuvant docetaxel for high-risk, node-negative breast cancer. N Engl J Med. 2010;363(23):2200–10.
92. Gianni L, Baselga J, Eiermann W, et al. Phase III trial evaluating the addition of paclitaxel to doxorubicin followed by cyclophosphamide, methotrexate, and fluorouracil, as adjuvant or primary systemic therapy: European Cooperative Trial in Operable Breast Cancer. J Clin Oncol. 2009;27(15):2474–81.
93. Sparano JA, Wang M, Martino S, et al. Weekly paclitaxel in the adjuvant treatment of breast cancer. N Engl J Med. 2008;358(16):1663–71.
94. Weidner N, Cady B, Goodson WH. Pathologic prognostic factors for patients with breast carcinoma. Which factors are important. Surg Oncol Clin N Am. 1997;6(3):415–62.
95. Silverstein MJ, Skinner KA, Lomis TJ. Predicting axillary nodal positivity in 2282 patients with breast carcinoma. World J Surg. 2001;25(6):767–72.
96. Perou CM, Sørlie T, Eisen MB, et al. Molecular portraits of human breast tumours. Nature. 2000;406(6797):747–52.
97. Sørlie T, Perou CM, Tibshirani R, et al. Gene expression patterns of breast carcinomas distinguish tumor subclasses with clinical implications. Proc Natl Acad Sci U S A. 2001;98(19):10869–74.
98. Isaacs C, Stearns V, Hayes DF. New prognostic factors for breast cancer recurrence. Semin Oncol. 2001;28(1):53–67.
99. Tack DK, Palmieri FM, Perez EA. Anthracycline vs nonanthracycline adjuvant therapy for breast cancer. Oncology (Williston Park). 2004;18(11):1367–76. discussion 1378, 1381.
100. Todd JH, Dowle C, Williams MR, et al. Confirmation of a prognostic index in primary breast cancer. Br J Cancer. 1987;56(4):489–92.
101. Ravdin PM, Siminoff LA, Davis GJ, et al. Computer program to assist in making decisions about adjuvant therapy for women with early breast cancer. J Clin Oncol. 2001;19(4):980–91.
102. Goldhirsch A, Wood WC, Gelber RD, et al. Progress and promise: highlights of the international expert consensus on the primary therapy of early breast cancer 2007. Ann Oncol. 2007;18(7):1133–44.
103. Rouzier R, Perou CM, Symmans WF, et al. Breast cancer molecular subtypes respond differently to preoperative chemotherapy. Clin Cancer Res. 2005;11(16):5678–85.
104. Mathieu MC, Rouzier R, Llombart-Cussac A, et al. The poor responsiveness of infiltrating lobular breast carcinomas to neoadjuvant chemotherapy can be explained by their biological profile. Eur J Cancer. 2004;40(3):342–51.
105. von Minckwitz G, Untch M, Blohmer JU, et al. Definition and impact of pathologic complete response on prognosis after neoadjuvant chemotherapy in various intrinsic breast cancer subtypes. J Clin Oncol. 2012;30(15):1796–804.
106. Goldhirsch A, Wood WC, Coates AS, et al. Strategies for subtypes–dealing with the diversity of breast cancer: highlights of the St. Gallen International Expert Consensus on the Primary Therapy of Early Breast Cancer 2011. Ann Oncol. 2011;22(8):1736–47.
107. Cheang MC, Voduc D, Bajdik C, et al. Basal-like breast cancer defined by five biomarkers has superior prognostic value than triple-negative phenotype. Clin Cancer Res. 2008;14(5):1368–76.
108. Beatson G. On the treatment of inoperable cases of carcinoma of the mamma: suggestions for a new method of treatment, with illustrative cases. Lancet. 1896;2:104–7.
109. Rugo HS. The breast cancer continuum in hormone-receptor-positive breast cancer in postmenopausal women: evolving management options focusing on aromatase inhibitors. Ann Oncol. 2008;19(1):16–27.
110. Wolff AC, Dowsett M. Estrogen receptor: a never ending story? J Clin Oncol. 2011;29(22):2955–8.
111. Goldhirsch A, Wood WC, Gelber RD, Coates AS, Thürlimann B, Senn HJ. Meeting highlights: updated international expert consensus on the primary therapy of early breast cancer. J Clin Oncol. 2003;21(17):3357–65.
112. Fisher B, Dignam J, Bryant J, Wolmark N. Five versus more than five years of tamoxifen for lymph node-negative breast cancer: updated findings from the National Surgical Adjuvant Breast and Bowel Project B-14 randomized trial. J Natl Cancer Inst. 2001;93(9):684–90.
113. (EBCTCG) EBCTCG. Relevance of breast cancer hormone receptors and other factors to the efficacy of adjuvant tamoxifen: patient-level meta-analysis of randomized trials. The Lancet. 2011;378:771–84.
114. (EBCTCG) EBCTCG. Effects of chemotherapy and hormonal therapy for early breast cancer on recurrence and 15-year survival: an overview of the randomised trials. Lancet. 2005;365(9472):1687–717.
115. Fisher B, Redmond C, Legault-Poisson S, et al. Postoperative chemotherapy and tamoxifen compared with tamoxifen alone in the treatment of positive-node breast cancer patients aged 50 years and older with tumors responsive to tamoxifen: results from the National Surgical Adjuvant Breast and Bowel Project B-16. J Clin Oncol. 1990;8(6):1005–18.
116. Group ABCTC. Ovarian ablation or suppression in premenopausal early breast cancer: results from the international adjuvant breast cancer ovarian ablation or suppression randomized trial. J Natl Cancer Inst. 2007;99(7):516–25.
117. Pritchard KI. Aromatase inhibitors in adjuvant therapy of breast cancer: before, instead of, or beyond tamoxifen. J Clin Oncol. 2005;23(22):4850–2.
118. Goss PE, Ingle JN, Martino S, et al. Randomized trial of letrozole following tamoxifen as extended adjuvant therapy in receptor-positive breast cancer:

updated findings from NCIC CTG MA.17. J Natl Cancer Inst. 2005;97(17):1262–71.
119. Fisher B, Dignam J, Bryant J, et al. Five versus more than five years of tamoxifen therapy for breast cancer patients with negative lymph nodes and estrogen receptor-positive tumors. J Natl Cancer Inst. 1996; 88(21):1529–42.
120. Tormey DC, Gray R, Falkson HC, Eastern Cooperative Oncology Group. Postchemotherapy adjuvant tamoxifen therapy beyond five years in patients with lymph node-positive breast cancer. J Natl Cancer Inst. 1996;88(24):1828–33.
121. Stewart HJ, Forrest AP, Everington D, The Scottish Cancer Trials Breast Group, et al. Randomised comparison of 5 years of adjuvant tamoxifen with continuous therapy for operable breast cancer. Br J Cancer. 1996;74(2):297–9.
122. Goss PE, Strasser K. Aromatase inhibitors in the treatment and prevention of breast cancer. J Clin Oncol. 2001;19(3):881–94.
123. Reid DM, Doughty J, Eastell R, et al. Guidance for the management of breast cancer treatment-induced bone loss: a consensus position statement from a UK Expert Group. Cancer Treat Rev. 2008;34 Suppl 1:S3–18.
124. Gnant M, Mlineritsch B, Stoeger H, et al. Adjuvant endocrine therapy plus zoledronic acid in premenopausal women with early-stage breast cancer: 62-month follow-up from the ABCSG-12 randomised trial. Lancet Oncol. 2011;12(7):631–41.
125. Burstein HJ, Prestrud AA, Seidenfeld J, et al. American Society of Clinical Oncology clinical practice guideline: update on adjuvant endocrine therapy for women with hormone receptor-positive breast cancer. J Clin Oncol. 2010;28(23):3784–96.
126. Cuzick J, Sestak I, Baum M, et al. Effect of anastrozole and tamoxifen as adjuvant treatment for early-stage breast cancer: 10-year analysis of the ATAC trial. Lancet Oncol. 2010;11(12):1135–41.
127. Boccardo F, Guglielmini P, Bordonaro R, et al. Switching to anastrozole versus continued tamoxifen treatment of early breast cancer: long term results of the Italian Tamoxifen Anastrozole trial. Eur J Cancer. 2013;49(7):1546–54.
128. Bliss JM, Kilburn LS, Coleman RE, et al. Disease-related outcomes with long-term follow-up: an updated analysis of the intergroup exemestane study. J Clin Oncol. 2012;30(7):709–17.
129. Jin H, Tu D, Zhao N, Shepherd LE, Goss PE. Longer-term outcomes of letrozole versus placebo after 5 years of tamoxifen in the NCIC CTG MA.17 trial: analyses adjusting for treatment crossover. J Clin Oncol. 2012;30(7):718–21.
130. Regan MM, Neven P, Giobbie-Hurder A, et al. Assessment of letrozole and tamoxifen alone and in sequence for postmenopausal women with steroid hormone receptor-positive breast cancer: the BIG 1–98 randomised clinical trial at 8·1 years median follow-up. Lancet Oncol. 2011;12(12):1101–8.
131. van de Velde CJ, Rea D, Seynaeve C, et al. Adjuvant tamoxifen and exemestane in early breast cancer (TEAM): a randomised phase 3 trial. Lancet. 2011;377(9762):321–31.
132. Dubsky PC, Jakesz R, Mlineritsch B, et al. Tamoxifen and anastrozole as a sequencing strategy: a randomized controlled trial in postmenopausal patients with endocrine-responsive early breast cancer from the Austrian Breast and Colorectal Cancer Study Group. J Clin Oncol. 2012;30(7):722–8.
133. Mamounas EP, Jeong JH, Wickerham DL, et al. Benefit from exemestane as extended adjuvant therapy after 5 years of adjuvant tamoxifen: intention-to-treat analysis of the National Surgical Adjuvant Breast And Bowel Project B-33 trial. J Clin Oncol. 2008;26(12):1965–71.
134. Goss PE, Ingle JN, Pritchard KI, et al. Exemestane versus anastrozole in postmenopausal women with early breast cancer: NCIC CTG MA.27–a randomized controlled phase III trial. J Clin Oncol. 2013; 31(11):1398–404.
135. Jakesz R, Greil R, Gnant M, et al. Extended adjuvant therapy with anastrozole among postmenopausal breast cancer patients: results from the randomized Austrian Breast and Colorectal Cancer Study Group Trial 6a. J Natl Cancer Inst. 2007;99(24):1845–53.
136. Group AT. Anastrozole alone or in combination with tamoxifen versus tamoxifen alone for adjuvant treatment of postmenopausal women with early breast cancer: first results of the ATAC randomized trial. Lancet. 2002;359:2131–9.
137. Davies C, Pan H, Godwin J, et al. Long-term effects of continuing adjuvant tamoxifen to 10 years versus stopping at 5 years after diagnosis of oestrogen receptor-positive breast cancer: ATLAS, a randomised trial. Lancet. 2013;381(9869):805–16.
138. Gray RG, Rea D, Handley K, et al. aTTom: long-term effects of continuing adjuvant tamoxifen to 10 years versus stopping at 5 years in 6,953 women with early breast cancer. J Clin Oncol. 2013;Abstrt 5.
139. Mamounas EP, Tang G, Fisher B, et al. Association between the 21-gene recurrence score assay and risk of locoregional recurrence in node-negative, estrogen receptor-positive breast cancer: results from NSABP B-14 and NSABP B-20. J Clin Oncol. 2010;28(10):1677–83.
140. Paik S, Tang G, Shak S, et al. Gene expression and benefit of chemotherapy in women with node-negative, estrogen receptor-positive breast cancer. J Clin Oncol. 2006;24(23):3726–34.
141. Sparano JA. TAILORx: trial assigning individualized options for treatment (Rx). Clin Breast Cancer. 2006;7(4):347–50.
142. Albain KS, Barlow WE, Shak S, et al. Prognostic and predictive value of the 21-gene recurrence score assay in postmenopausal women with node-positive, oestrogen-receptor-positive breast cancer on chemotherapy: a retrospective analysis of a randomised trial. Lancet Oncol. 2010;11(1):55–65.

143. Sgroi DC, Sestak I, Cuzick J, et al. Prediction of late distant recurrence in patients with oestrogen-receptor-positive breast cancer: a prospective comparison of the breast-cancer index (BCI) assay, 21-gene recurrence score, and IHC4 in the TransATAC study population. Lancet Oncol. 2013;14(11):1067–76.
144. Harris L, Fritsche H, Mennel R, et al. American Society of Clinical Oncology 2007 update of recommendations for the use of tumor markers in breast cancer. J Clin Oncol. 2007;25(33):5287–312.
145. National Comprehensive Cancer Network (NCCN) guidelines. Available at: www.nccn.org. 2013. Accessed 23 May 2013.
146. Bogaerts J, Cardoso F, Buyse M, et al. Gene signature evaluation as a prognostic tool: challenges in the design of the MINDACT trial. Nat Clin Pract Oncol. 2006;3(10):540–51.
147. Drukker CA, Bueno-de-Mesquita JM, Retèl VP, et al. A prospective evaluation of a breast cancer prognosis signature in the observational RASTER study. Int J Cancer. 2013;133(4):929–36.
148. Ring BZ, Seitz RS, Beck R, et al. Novel prognostic immunohistochemical biomarker panel for estrogen receptor-positive breast cancer. J Clin Oncol. 2006; 24(19):3039–47.
149. Bartlett JM, Bloom KJ, Piper T, et al. Mammostrat as an immunohistochemical multigene assay for prediction of early relapse risk in the tamoxifen versus exemestane adjuvant multicenter trial pathology study. J Clin Oncol. 2012;30(36):4477–84.
150. Ross DT, Kim CY, Tang G, et al. Chemosensitivity and stratification by a five monoclonal antibody immunohistochemistry test in the NSABP B14 and B20 trials. Clin Cancer Res. 2008;14(20):6602–9.
151. Mook S, Schmidt MK, Viale G, et al. The 70-gene prognosis-signature predicts disease outcome in breast cancer patients with 1–3 positive lymph nodes in an independent validation study. Breast Cancer Res Treat. 2009;116(2):295–302.
152. Yamauchi H, Stearns V, Hayes DF. When is a tumor marker ready for prime time? A case study of c-erbB-2 as a predictive factor in breast cancer. J Clin Oncol. 2001;19(8):2334–56.
153. Slamon DJ, Clark GM, Wong SG, Levin WJ, Ullrich A, McGuire WL. Human breast cancer: correlation of relapse and survival with amplification of the HER-2/neu oncogene. Science. 1987;235(4785):177–82.
154. Vogel C, Cobleigh MA, Tripathy D, et al. First-line, single-agent Herceptin(R) (trastuzumab) in metastatic breast cancer. A preliminary report. Eur J Cancer. 2001;37 Suppl 1:25–9.
155. Slamon DJ, Leyland-Jones B, Shak S, et al. Use of chemotherapy plus a monoclonal antibody against HER2 for metastatic breast cancer that overexpresses HER2. N Engl J Med. 2001;344(11):783–92.
156. Piccart-Gebhart MJ, Procter M, Leyland-Jones B, et al. Trastuzumab after adjuvant chemotherapy in HER2-positive breast cancer. N Engl J Med. 2005;353(16):1659–72.
157. Romond EH, Perez EA, Bryant J, et al. Trastuzumab plus adjuvant chemotherapy for operable HER2-positive breast cancer. N Engl J Med. 2005;353(16): 1673–84.
158. Joensuu H, Kellokumpu-Lehtinen PL, Bono P, et al. Adjuvant docetaxel or vinorelbine with or without trastuzumab for breast cancer. N Engl J Med. 2006;354(8):809–20.
159. Spielmann M, Roché H, Delozier T, et al. Trastuzumab for patients with axillary-node-positive breast cancer: results of the FNCLCC-PACS 04 trial. J Clin Oncol. 2009;27(36):6129–34.
160. Slamon D, Eiermann W, Robert N, et al. Adjuvant trastuzumab in HER2-positive breast cancer. N Engl J Med. 2011;365(14):1273–83.
161. Moja L, Tagliabue L, Balduzzi S, et al. Trastuzumab containing regimens for early breast cancer. Cochrane Database Syst Rev. 2012;4, CD006243.
162. Hortobagyi GN. Trastuzumab in the treatment of breast cancer. N Engl J Med. 2005;353(16):1734–6.
163. Goldhirsch A, Gelber RD, Piccart-Gebhart MJ, et al. 2 years versus 1 year of adjuvant trastuzumab for HER2-positive breast cancer (HERA): an open-label, randomised controlled trial. Lancet. 2013;382(9897): 1021–8.
164. Pivot X, Romieu G, Debled M, et al. 6 months versus 12 months of adjuvant trastuzumab for patients with HER2-positive early breast cancer (PHARE): a randomised phase 3 trial. Lancet Oncol. 2013;14(8): 741–8.
165. Gonzalez-Angulo AM, Litton JK, Broglio KR, et al. High risk of recurrence for patients with breast cancer who have human epidermal growth factor receptor 2-positive, node-negative tumors 1 cm or smaller. J Clin Oncol. 2009;27(34):5700–6.
166. Bear HD, Anderson S, Brown A, et al. The effect on tumor response of adding sequential preoperative docetaxel to preoperative doxorubicin and cyclophosphamide: preliminary results from National Surgical Adjuvant Breast and Bowel Project Protocol B-27. J Clin Oncol. 2003;21(22):4165–74.
167. van der Hage JA, van de Velde CJ, Julien JP, Tubiana-Hulin M, Vandervelden C, Duchateau L. Preoperative chemotherapy in primary operable breast cancer: results from the European Organization for Research and Treatment of Cancer trial 10902. J Clin Oncol. 2001;19(22):4224–37.
168. Fisher B, Brown A, Mamounas E, et al. Effect of preoperative chemotherapy on local-regional disease in women with operable breast cancer: findings from National Surgical Adjuvant Breast and Bowel Project B-18. J Clin Oncol. 1997;15(7):2483–93.
169. Kaufmann M, Hortobagyi GN, Goldhirsch A, et al. Recommendations from an international expert panel on the use of neoadjuvant (primary) systemic treatment of operable breast cancer: an update. J Clin Oncol. 2006;24(12):1940–9.
170. Kuerer HM, Newman LA, Smith TL, et al. Clinical course of breast cancer patients with complete

pathologic primary tumor and axillary lymph node response to doxorubicin-based neoadjuvant chemotherapy. J Clin Oncol. 1999;17(2):460–9.
171. Cardoso F, Loibl S, Pagani O, et al. The European Society of Breast Cancer Specialists recommendations for the management of young women with breast cancer. Eur J Cancer. 2012;48(18):3355–77.
172. Earl HM, Vallier AL, Hiller L, et al. Effects of the addition of gemcitabine, and paclitaxel-first sequencing, in neoadjuvant sequential epirubicin, cyclophosphamide, and paclitaxel for women with high-risk early breast cancer (Neo-tAnGo): an open-label, 2×2 factorial randomised phase 3 trial. Lancet Oncol. 2014;15(2):201–12.
173. Nahta R, Esteva FJ. HER2 therapy: molecular mechanisms of trastuzumab resistance. Breast Cancer Res. 2006;8(6):215.
174. Blackwell KL, Burstein HJ, Storniolo AM, et al. Randomized study of Lapatinib alone or in combination with trastuzumab in women with ErbB2-positive, trastuzumab-refractory metastatic breast cancer. J Clin Oncol. 2010;28(7):1124–30.
175. Gianni L, Eiermann W, Semiglazov V, et al. Neoadjuvant chemotherapy with trastuzumab followed by adjuvant trastuzumab versus neoadjuvant chemotherapy alone, in patients with HER2-positive locally advanced breast cancer (the NOAH trial): a randomised controlled superiority trial with a parallel HER2-negative cohort. Lancet. 2010;375(9712):377–84.
176. Gianni L, Pienkowski T, Im YH, et al. Efficacy and safety of neoadjuvant pertuzumab and trastuzumab in women with locally advanced, inflammatory, or early HER2-positive breast cancer (NeoSphere): a randomised multicentre, open-label, phase 2 trial. Lancet Oncol. 2012;13(1):25–32.
177. Guarneri V, Frassoldati A, Bottini A, et al. Preoperative chemotherapy plus trastuzumab, lapatinib, or both in human epidermal growth factor receptor 2-positive operable breast cancer: results of the randomized phase II CHER-LOB study. J Clin Oncol. 2012;30(16):1989–95.
178. Baselga J, Bradbury I, Eidtmann H, et al. Lapatinib with trastuzumab for HER2-positive early breast cancer (NeoALTTO): a randomised, open-label, multicentre, phase 3 trial. Lancet. 2012;379(9816):633–40.
179. Untch M, Loibl S, Bischoff J, et al. Lapatinib versus trastuzumab in combination with neoadjuvant anthracycline-taxane-based chemotherapy (GeparQuinto, GBG 44): a randomised phase 3 trial. Lancet Oncol. 2012;13(2):135–44.
180. Schneeweiss A, Chia S, Hickish T, et al. Pertuzumab plus trastuzumab in combination with standard neoadjuvant anthracycline-containing and anthracycline-free chemotherapy regimens in patients with HER2-positive early breast cancer: a randomized phase II cardiac safety study (TRYPHAENA). Ann Oncol. 2013;24(9):2278–84.
181. Guarneri V, Broglio K, Kau SW, et al. Prognostic value of pathologic complete response after primary chemotherapy in relation to hormone receptor status and other factors. J Clin Oncol. 2006;24(7):1037–44.
182. Hughes KS, Schnaper LA, Bellon JR, et al. Lumpectomy plus tamoxifen with or without irradiation in women age 70 years or older with early breast cancer: long-term follow-up of CALGB 9343. J Clin Oncol. 2013;31(19):2382–7.
183. Pötter R, Gnant M, Kwasny W, et al. Lumpectomy plus tamoxifen or anastrozole with or without whole breast irradiation in women with favorable early breast cancer. Int J Radiat Oncol Biol Phys. 2007;68(2):334–40.
184. Winzer KJ, Sauerbrei W, Braun M, et al. Radiation therapy and tamoxifen after breast-conserving surgery: updated results of a 2 × 2 randomised clinical trial in patients with low risk of recurrence. Eur J Cancer. 2010;46(1):95–101.
185. Tinterri C, Gatzemeier W, Zanini V, et al. Conservative surgery with and without radiotherapy in elderly patients with early-stage breast cancer: a prospective randomised multicentre trial. Breast. 2009;18(6):373–7.
186. Yeatman TJ, Cantor AB, Smith TJ, et al. Tumor biology of infiltrating lobular carcinoma. Implications for management. Ann Surg. 1995;222(4):549–59. discussion 559–561.
187. Singletary SE, Patel-Parekh L, Bland KI. Treatment trends in early-stage invasive lobular carcinoma: a report from the National Cancer Data Base. Ann Surg. 2005;242(2):281–9.
188. van' t Veer LJ, Dai H, van de Vijver MJ, et al. Gene expression profiling predicts clinical outcome of breast cancer. Nature. 2002;415(6871):530–6.
189. Trivers KF, Lund MJ, Porter PL, et al. The epidemiology of triple-negative breast cancer, including race. Cancer Causes Control. 2009;20(7):1071–82.
190. Chu QD, Henderson AE, Ampil F, Li BD. Outcome for patients with triple-negative breast cancer is not dependent on race/ethnicity. Int J Breast Cancer. 2012;2012:764570.
191. Parker CC, Ampil F, Burton G, Li BD, Chu QD. Is breast conservation therapy a viable option for patients with triple-receptor negative breast cancer? Surgery. 2010;148(2):386–91.
192. Carey LA, Dees EC, Sawyer L, et al. The triple negative paradox: primary tumor chemosensitivity of breast cancer subtypes. Clin Cancer Res. 2007;13(8):2329–34.
193. Kennedy RD, Quinn JE, Mullan PB, Johnston PG, Harkin DP. The role of BRCA1 in the cellular response to chemotherapy. J Natl Cancer Inst. 2004;96(22):1659–68.
194. Hiller DJ, Chu QD. Current status of poly(ADP-ribose) polymerase inhibitors as novel therapeutic agents for triple-negative breast cancer. Int J Breast Cancer. 2012;2012:829315.
195. Iglehart JD, Silver DP. Synthetic lethality–a new direction in cancer-drug development. N Engl J Med. 2009;361(2):189–91.

196. Tutt A, Robson M, Garber JE, et al. Oral poly(ADP-ribose) polymerase inhibitor olaparib in patients with BRCA1 or BRCA2 mutations and advanced breast cancer: a proof-of-concept trial. Lancet. 2010;376(9737):235–44.
197. Fong PC, Boss DS, Yap TA, et al. Inhibition of poly(ADP-ribose) polymerase in tumors from BRCA mutation carriers. N Engl J Med. 2009;361(2):123–34.
198. Baron PL, Moore MP, Kinne DW, Candela FC, Osborne MP, Petrek JA. Occult breast cancer presenting with axillary metastases. Updated management. Arch Surg. 1990;125(2):210–4.
199. Copeland EM, McBride CM. Axillary metastases from unknown primary sites. Ann Surg. 1973;178(1):25–7.
200. Kyokane T, Akashi-Tanaka S, Matsui T, Fukutomi T. Clinicopathological characteristics of non-palpable breast cancer presenting as axillary mass. Breast Cancer. 1995;2(2):105–12.
201. Chen C, Orel SG, Harris E, Schnall MD, Czerniecki BJ, Solin LJ. Outcome after treatment of patients with mammographically occult, magnetic resonance imaging-detected breast cancer presenting with axillary lymphadenopathy. Clin Breast Cancer. 2004;5(1):72–7.
202. Buchanan CL, Morris EA, Dorn PL, Borgen PI, Van Zee KJ. Utility of breast magnetic resonance imaging in patients with occult primary breast cancer. Ann Surg Oncol. 2005;12(12):1045–53.
203. Rosen PP, Kimmel M. Occult breast carcinoma presenting with axillary lymph node metastases: a follow-up study of 48 patients. Hum Pathol. 1990;21(5):518–23.
204. Ellerbroek N, Holmes F, Singletary E, Evans H, Oswald M, McNeese M. Treatment of patients with isolated axillary nodal metastases from an occult primary carcinoma consistent with breast origin. Cancer. 1990;66(7):1461–7.
205. Vlastos G, Jean ME, Mirza AN, et al. Feasibility of breast preservation in the treatment of occult primary carcinoma presenting with axillary metastases. Ann Surg Oncol. 2001;8(5):425–31.
206. Kothari AS, Beechey-Newman N, Hamed H, et al. Paget disease of the nipple: a multifocal manifestation of higher-risk disease. Cancer. 2002;95(1):1–7.
207. Kollmorgen DR, Varanasi JS, Edge SB, Carson WE. Paget's disease of the breast: a 33-year experience. J Am Coll Surg. 1998;187(2):171–7.
208. Yim JH, Wick MR, Philpott GW, Norton JA, Doherty GM. Underlyingb pathology in mammary Paget's disease. Ann Surg Oncol. 1997;4(4):287–92.
209. Sakorafas GH, Blanchard K, Sarr MG, Farley DR. Paget's disease of the breast. Cancer Treat Rev. 2001;27(1):9–18.
210. Morrogh M, Morris EA, Liberman L, Van Zee K, Cody HS, King TA. MRI identifies otherwise occult disease in select patients with Paget disease of the nipple. J Am Coll Surg. 2008;206(2):316–21.
211. Dixon AR, Galea MH, Ellis IO, Elston CW, Blamey RW. Paget's disease of the nipple. Br J Surg. 1991;78(6):722–3.
212. Ling H, Hu X, Xu XL, Liu ZB, Shao ZM. Patients with nipple-areola Paget's disease and underlying invasive breast carcinoma have very poor survival: a matched cohort study. PLoS One. 2013;8(4):e61455.
213. Giordano SH, Cohen DS, Buzdar AU, Perkins G, Hortobagyi GN. Breast carcinoma in men: a population-based study. Cancer. 2004;101(1):51–7.
214. Fentiman IS, Fourquet A, Hortobagyi GN. Male breast cancer. Lancet. 2006;367(9510):595–604.
215. Nahleh ZA, Srikantiah R, Safa M, Jazieh AR, Muhleman A, Komrokji R. Male breast cancer in the veterans affairs population: a comparative analysis. Cancer. 2007;109(8):1471–7.
216. Pemmaraju N, Munsell MF, Hortobagyi GN, Giordano SH. Retrospective review of male breast cancer patients: analysis of tamoxifen-related side-effects. Ann Oncol. 2012;23(6):1471–4.
217. Fisher B, Costantino JP, Wickerham DL, et al. Tamoxifen for the prevention of breast cancer: current status of the National Surgical Adjuvant Breast and Bowel Project P-1 study. J Natl Cancer Inst. 2005;97(22):1652–62.
218. Vogel VG, Costantino JP, Wickerham DL, et al. Effects of tamoxifen vs raloxifene on the risk of developing invasive breast cancer and other disease outcomes: the NSABP Study of Tamoxifen and Raloxifene (STAR) P-2 trial. JAMA. 2006;295(23):2727–41.
219. Goss PE, Ingle JN, Alés-Martínez JE, et al. Exemestane for breast-cancer prevention in postmenopausal women. N Engl J Med. 2011;364(25):2381–91.
220. Cuzick J, Sestak I, Forbes J, et al. Anastrozole for prevention of breast cancer in high-risk postmenopausal women (IBIS-II): an international, double-blind, randomized placebo-controlled trial. The Lancet. 2013. http://dx.doi.org/10.1016/S0140-6736(13)62292-8.
221. Vogel VG, Costantino JP, Wickerham DL, et al. Update of the National Surgical Adjuvant Breast and Bowel Project Study of Tamoxifen and Raloxifene (STAR) P-2 Trial: preventing breast cancer. Cancer Prev Res (Phila). 2010;3(6):696–706.
222. Lippman SM. The dilemma and promise of cancer chemoprevention. Nat Clin Pract Oncol. 2006;3(10):523.
223. Visvanathan K, Hurley P, Bantug E, et al. Use of pharmacologic interventions for breast cancer risk reduction: American Society of Clinical Oncology clinical practice guideline. J Clin Oncol. 2013;31(23):2942–62.
224. Port ER, Montgomery LL, Heerdt AS, Borgen PI. Patient reluctance toward tamoxifen use for breast cancer primary prevention. Ann Surg Oncol. 2001;8(7):580–5.

Locally Advanced Breast Cancer (LABC)

5

Quyen D. Chu, Ernest Kwame Adjepong-Tandoh, and Rosemary Bernadette Duda

Learning Objectives
After reading this chapter, you should be able to:

- Recognize what constitutes locally advanced breast cancer (LABC).
- Understand how to evaluate and manage patients with LABC.
- Know the difference between inflammatory breast cancer (IBC) and noninflammatory locally advanced breast cancer (non-IBC LABC).
- Be cognizant of the multimodality approach to treating patients with LABC (neoadjuvant systemic therapy, surgery, and radiation).
- Appreciate the positive implication of a pathologic complete response (pCR) following neoadjuvant chemotherapy.

Q.D. Chu, M.D., M.B.A., FACS (✉)
Department of Surgery, Louisiana State University Health Sciences Center – Shreveport, 1501 Kings Highway, P.O. Box 33932, Shreveport, LA 71130-3392, USA
e-mail: qchu@lsuhsc.edu

E.K. Adjepong-Tandoh, M.Bch.B.
Department of Surgery, University of Ghana Medical School, Accra-North, P. O. Box AN-11835, 1233 Accra, Ghana
e-mail: themaconsole@yahoo.com

R.B. Duda, M.D., MPH
Department of Surgery, Beth Israel Deaconess Medical Center, Howard Medical School, 330 Brookline Ave. Stoneman 9- Surgical Oncology, Boston, MA 02215, USA
e-mail: rduda@caregroup.harvard.edu; rduda@bidmc.harvard.edu

Introduction

As mentioned in the previous chapter (Chap. 4, Early Breast Cancer), the majority of women in the United States with breast cancer (60–70 %) present with early-stage disease (Stage I/II). Unfortunately, in developing nations, up to 70 % of women have advanced stage breast cancer upon presentation (Stage III/IV) [1]. Such high incidence of advanced stage breast cancer is also seen in the underserved population of the United States.

Locally advanced breast cancer (LABC) represents a heterogeneous group of diseases with variable clinical presentations. It is associated with a 50 % or greater increased risk for distant recurrent disease compared to early breast cancer [2]. LABC encompasses two broad categories of patients: inflammatory breast cancer (IBC) and non-IBC LABC. The former is characterized by a rapid onset of symptoms and signs such as diffuse erythema and edema (peau d'orange) of the breast, often without a clinically evident underlying breast mass (Fig. 5.1) while the latter is often typified by a large, ulcerative, and fungating breast mass that is a consequence of a long-standing, neglected breast cancer (Fig. 5.2a). Although both have a high incidence of developing distant disease, they, by definition, have no evidence of metastases (M0) at the time of diagnosis. Thus they are considered as stage 3 breast cancer.

Despite their advanced stage at presentation, a considerable percentage of patients with LABC can be cured, and thus, treating physicians should aim for a curative intent when caring for these patients.

Q.D. Chu et al. (eds.), *Surgical Oncology: A Practical and Comprehensive Approach*, DOI 10.1007/978-1-4939-1423-4_5, © Springer Science+Business Media New York 2015

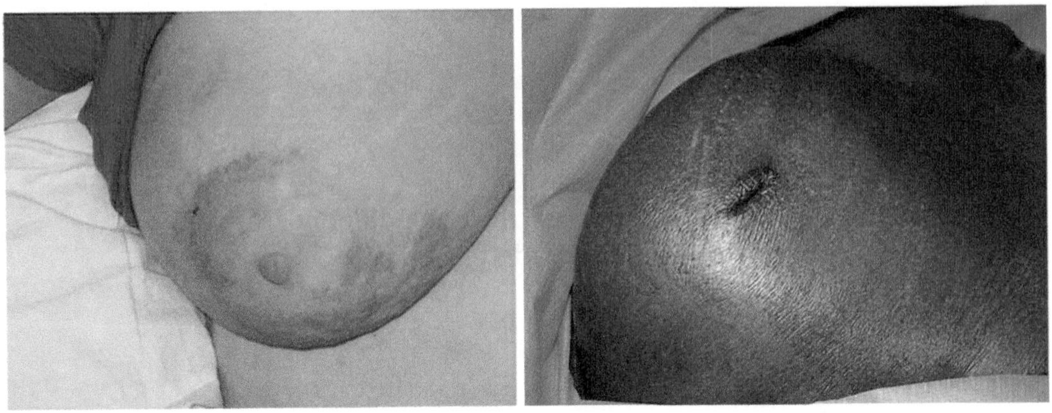

Fig. 5.1 Inflammatory breast cancer: Note the swollen breast, erythema, skin thickening, and peau d'orange. (Courtesy of Quyen D. Chu, MD, MBA, FACS)

Clinical Presentation

Inflammatory Breast Cancer (IBC)

Inflammatory breast cancer (IBC) (T4d in the American Joint Committee on Cancer staging system) represents the most aggressive variant of breast cancer, accounting for approximately 1–5 % of all breast cancers in the United States. Clinically, patients present with a *rapid* onset of breast tenderness, erythema, edema, pain, skin thickening, and breast swelling. Nipple retraction can occur when the central portion of the breast is involved (Fig. 5.2b). Nearly 55–85 % of patients with IBC have axillary lymph node involvement at presentation and about 30 % have distant disease at the time of diagnosis [3]. The clinical picture is caused by tumor blockage of the lymphatic channels. Such presentation can be mistaken for mastitis or breast abscess (Fig. 5.3), which can contribute to a delay in diagnosis and treatment. In general, mastitis occurs almost exclusively in lactating women. A trial of antibiotics for 1 week with a close follow-up is a reasonable approach for those that present with a low clinical suspicion for IBC. However, failure to have a complete resolution of signs and symptoms should prompt the clinician to proceed with further investigation to rule out IBC.

The diagnosis of IBC is primarily clinical with histologic confirmation of invasive carcinoma [4]. Histologically, IBC is diagnosed by showing evidence of tumor cells in the dermal lymphatic channels, although this pathognomonic finding is not necessarily a prerequisite for its diagnosis; dermal lymphatic invasion is found in only approximately 60 % of patients with IBC [5].

Our understanding of the behavior of IBC is limited due to the rare incidence of IBC and our lack of having a clear definition of IBC. In 2008, an international panel of experts convened and developed criteria for IBC, and they are as follows: (1) a rapid onset of breast erythema, edema and/or peau d'orange, and/or warm breast, with or without an underlying palpable mass; (2) duration of history of no more than 6 months; (3) erythema occupying at least one-third of the breast; (4) and histologic confirmation of invasive carcinoma [6].

Non-IBC Locally Advanced Breast Cancer (Non-IBC LABC)

Non-IBC LABC includes large tumors (>5 cm or T3), tumors of any size that involve skin and/or chest wall (cT4a-c or Stage IIIB), tumors with fixed or matted axillary lymph nodes or tumors clinically detected in the ipsilateral internal mammary nodes without involvement of axillary lymph nodes (N2), and tumors that involve ipsilateral infraclavicular, supraclavicular, or internal mammary lymph nodes with axillary lymph nodes involvement (cN3 or Stage IIIC).

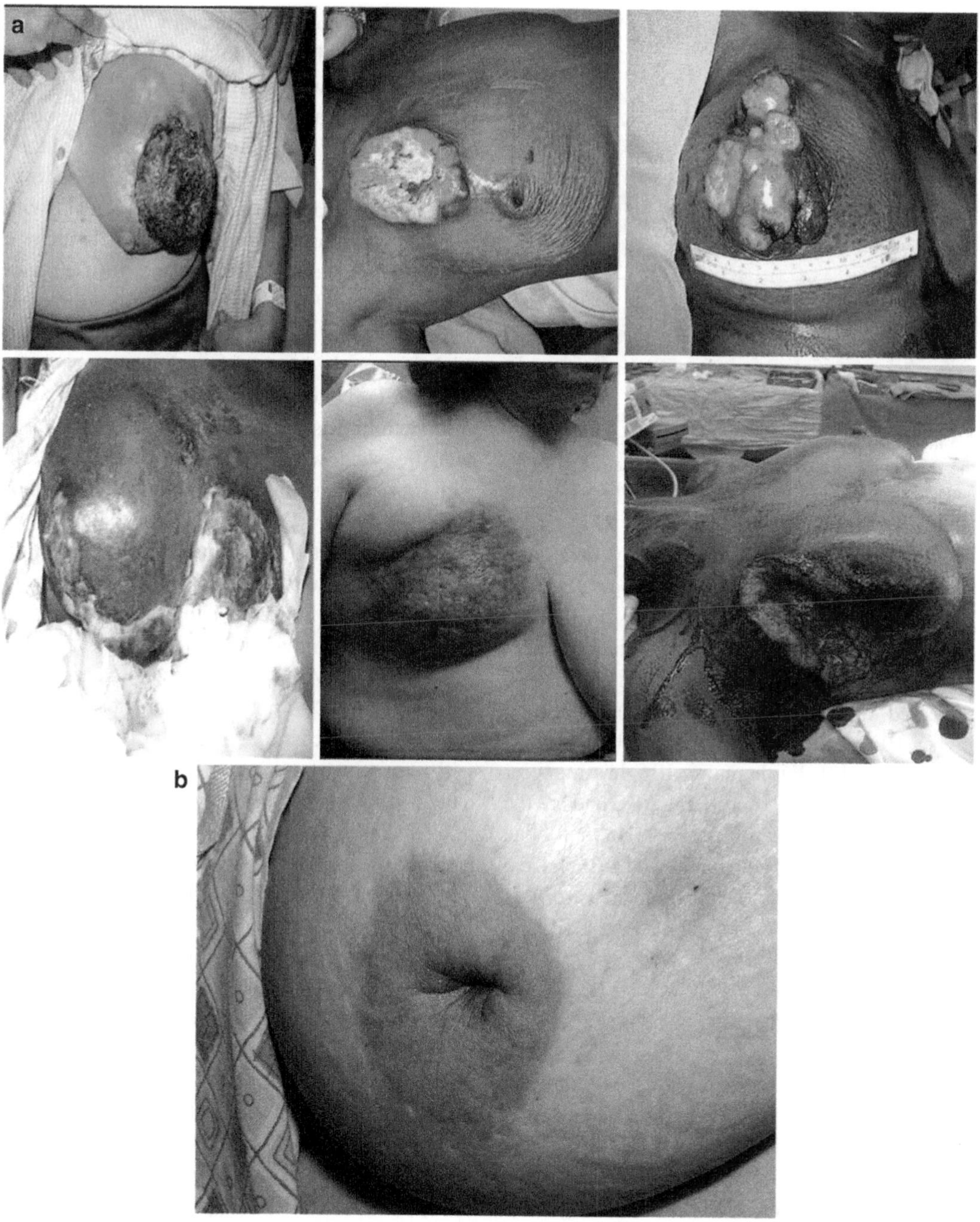

Fig. 5.2 (**a**): Pictures of patients with non-IBC LABC. (**b**): A patient with non-IBC LABC who presents with nipple retraction. (Courtesy of Quyen D. Chu, MD, MBA, FACS)

On occasion, women with non-IBC LABC can present with an inflammatory recurrence of the chest wall following a mastectomy, but such a presentation is considered as secondary IBC. This is different than primary IBC.

Although IBC and non-IBC LABC are grouped together under the LABC category, they nevertheless represent two distinct biologic entities [7–9]. In contrast to non-IBC LABC, there is a higher incidence of IBC in African-American women;

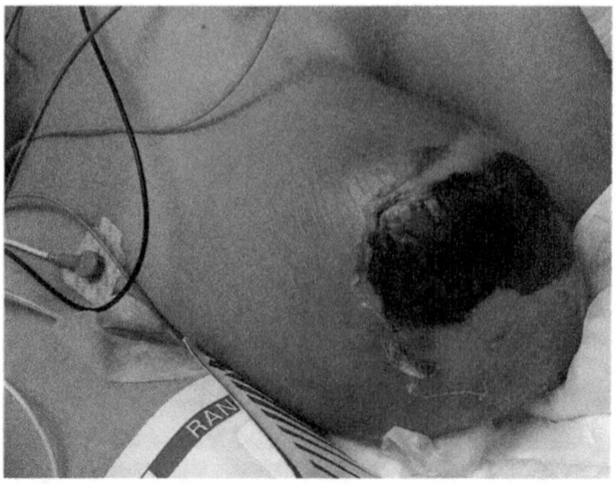

Fig. 5.3 A patient with a breast abscess that mimics IBC. An incision and drainage was performed and a biopsy of the skin and underlying tissue excluded the diagnosis of cancer. (Courtesy of Quyen D. Chu, MD, MBA, FACS)

affected women with IBC tend to be younger and have a high body mass index. Biologically, IBC possesses lower ER expression (up to 80 % of IBCs have ER-negative and/or PR-negative tumors [10]), high nuclear grade, high mitotic index, increased tumor expression of E-cadherin, and higher HER-2 expression (up to 50 % of IBC tumors) [11–13]. Furthermore, IBC has a poorer prognosis compared to non-IBC LABC and has the propensity for distant soft-tissue, brain, and bone metastases [4, 7, 8, 14]; patients with IBC have a 43 % increased risk of death from breast cancer compared to patients with non-IBC LABC [8].

Diagnosis and Staging

The initial tests for women with LABC are the same as for those with early breast cancer. A bilateral mammogram is often the first imaging study to be done to detect synchronous lesions in the ipsilateral and contralateral breast (Fig. 5.4). For patients who present with a large, fungating neglected breast carcinoma, an ipsilateral mammogram, which requires compression, may cause unnecessary discomfort for the patient. In such a situation, an ipsilateral mammogram can be avoided since a significant percentage of these patients may not be candidates for BCT. However, when a significant response is observed following neoadjuvant therapy and the patient is a candidate for BCT, a post-chemotherapy mammogram, ultrasound, or MRI should be performed.

For patients with non-IBC LABC, a mammographic abnormality such as a mass will be obvious. For those with IBC, a mass may not be present in up to 40 % of patients. The most common mammographic findings for patients with IBC are signs of inflammation, which include skin and trabecular thickening and diffuse opacity (Fig. 5.5). Ultrasound is a useful adjunct to mammography. Besides showing marked skin thickening and edema of the subcutaneous plane, evidenced by diffuse hyperechogenicity and architectural distorting with marked posterior acoustic shadowing [15], ultrasound can help with assessing nodal involvement. Ultrasound-guided biopsy of enlarged lymph nodes can be done. It is reported that ultrasound can detect up to 93 % of ipsilateral axillary nodal involvement and up to 50 % of infraclavicular, supraclavicular, and internal mammary nodal involvement [16].

The role of MRI in patients who clearly have non-IBC LABC is not well characterized. It is probably not necessary, especially for those who will require a mastectomy. However, MRI does have a role when evaluating response to induction chemotherapy in patients with non-IBC LABC (please see subsequent section below). For patients with IBC, MRI may be the most accurate test for detecting a primary breast lesion since imaging features seen in mammograms are not specific for IBC [17] (Fig. 5.6).

For the majority of patients, a core needle biopsy is all that is necessary to establish a diagnosis for patients with IBC and non-IBC LABC; often, sufficient material from the FNA is available to perform assays for hormone and HER-2 receptors according to the American Society of Clinical Oncology/College of American Pathologists guidelines [18–21]. However, if there is insufficient material to establish a diagnosis or obtain receptor statuses, an incisional biopsy may be required. For those with palpable axillary lymph nodes, an FNA can also be performed to confirm evidence of nodal disease. For patients with IBC, preferably two punch biopsies (Fig. 2.3 of Chap. 2) are needed to evaluate for evidence of tumor emboli in the dermal lymphatic channels

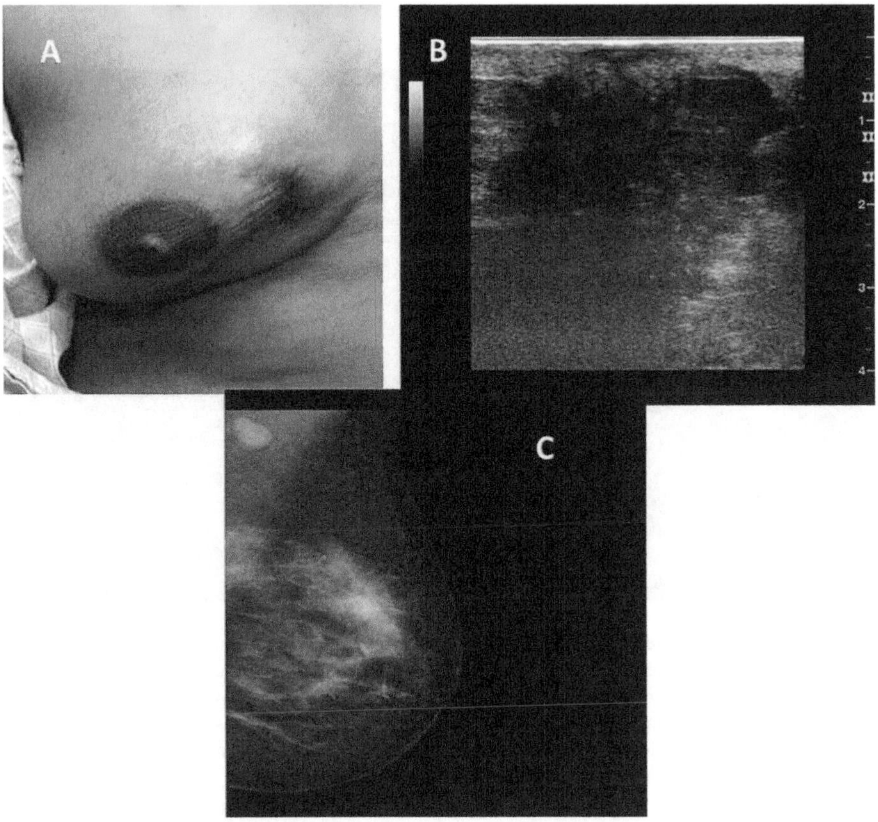

Fig. 5.4 A 60-year-old Caucasian woman with a noninflammatory locally advanced right breast cancer (**a**). Because of the extent of disease, she was not able to tolerate a right mammogram. However, a right breast ultrasound demonstrated a solid, hypoechoic mass with irregular borders and posterior acoustic shadowing (**b**). Her left mammogram demonstrated a synchronous breast cancer with an apparent nodal disease (**c**). (Courtesy of Quyen D. Chu, MD, MBA, FACS)

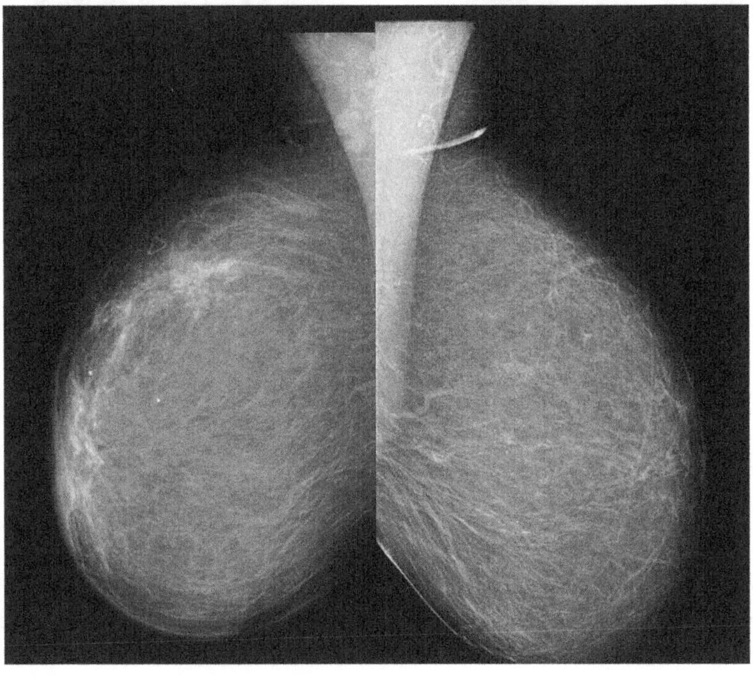

Fig. 5.5 Mammogram of a patient with IBC showing skin thickening and a breast mass (*left*) in contrast to the normal breast (*right*) (Courtesy of Stacy Lee, MD, Louisiana State University Health Sciences Center Shreveport)

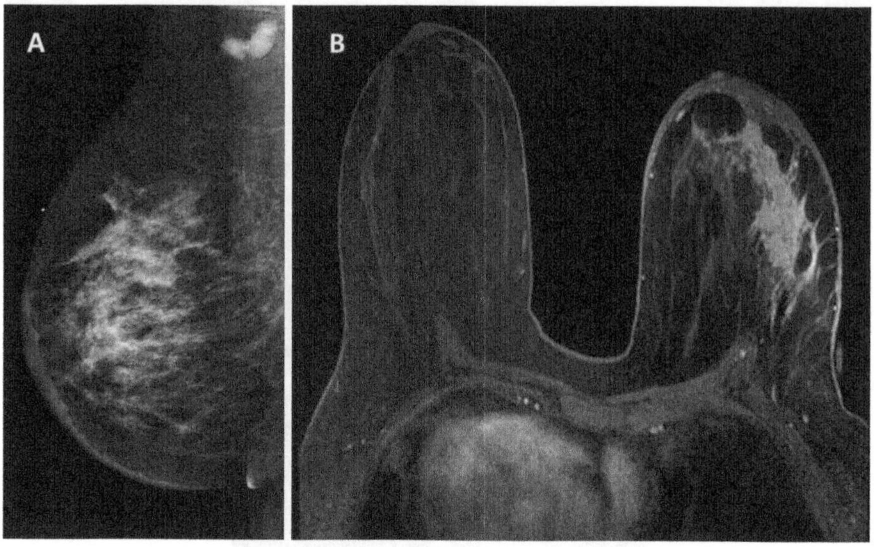

Fig. 5.6 A 48-year-old woman presenting with a three-month history of left breast heaviness. MLO view shows pleomorphic calcifications with associated trabecular and skin thickening suspicious for inflammatory breast cancer (**a**). Axial T1-weightedf fat-suppression post contrast image shows a large area of confluent enhancement with overlying skin thickening suspicious for malignancy (**b**). A core biopsy confirmed high-grade invasive ductal cancer and ductal carcinoma in situ (Courtesy of Priscilla Slanetz, MD, Beth Israel Deaconess Medical Center, Harvard Medical School)

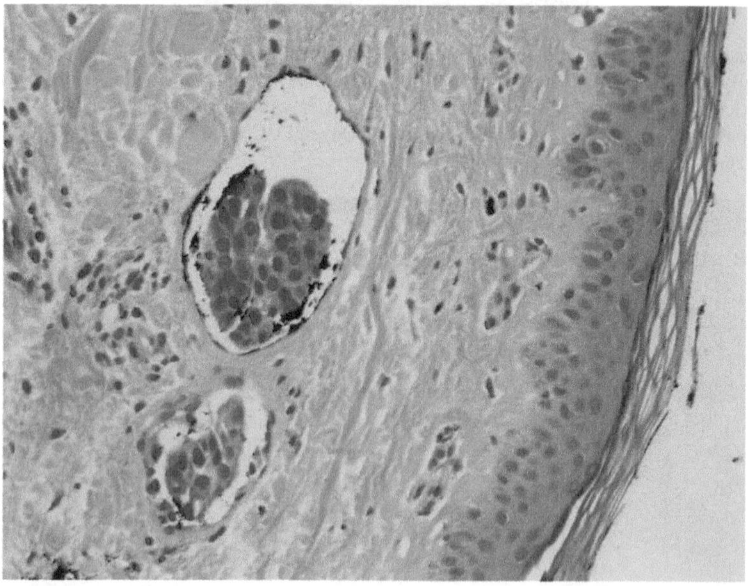

Fig. 5.7 Hematoxylin and eosin stain of an IBC specimen demonstrating dermal tumor emboli in the lymphovascular spaces. (Courtesy of Quyen D. Chu, MD, MBA, FACS)

and confirm the diagnosis of carcinoma (Fig. 5.7). This is helpful to confirm IBC and also in a situation when a core biopsy is inconclusive.

Because patients with LABC are at an increased risk of having concurrent distant disease, a metastatic work-up is often performed, which can include chest X-rays, bone scans, liver ultrasounds, abdominal CT scans, PET/CT scans, and MRI's, with the intent of identifying patients who have incurable disease and would receive palliative therapy only [22]. The National Comprehensive Cancer Network (NCCN) guidelines recommend a metastatic work-up for patients with T3N1 disease (Stage IIIA), yet for those with N2/N3 disease, a metastatic work-up is considered optional [23]. Chu et al. recently evaluated 256 patients with N2/N3 diseases and demonstrated that T stage is a useful barometer to select patients who might require additional metastatic work-up. For patients with T0, T1, or T2 diseases, the incidence of Stage IV disease was 0 %, 0 %, and 6 %, respectively. However, this incidence increases with higher T stage; 22 % for T3 and 36 % for T4 tumors [22]. Thus, the authors recommend a routine metastatic work-up for patients with N2/N3 diseases who have T3/T4 tumors. Further validation is needed to confirm such findings. A panel of international experts recommend that all patients with IBC should undergo a metastatic work-up with a CT and a bone scan [6].

The use of [18] F-FDG PET scan is considered optional in the work-up of patients with LABC (category 2B in NCCN guidelines) [23]. It is useful in situations where standard imaging studies are equivocal or suspicious [23]. PET/CT outperforms bone scanning such that a positive result on a PET/CT precludes the need to pursue a bone scan [24]. PET scan can also detect additional distant lesions that were not seen on conventional imaging [24] (Fig. 5.8). A prospective study evaluating 117 patients with LABC who underwent conventional imaging methods as well as PET/CT found that PET/CT outperformed conventional imaging methods. PET/CT revealed unsuspected lymph node involvement in 32 additional patients that were missed by conventional imaging modalities. In addition, distant metastases were detected in 43 patients using PET/CT versus 28 patients with conventional imaging modalities. PET/CT altered the stage of 61 patients (52 %), which impacted the recommended treatment for the patients [24]. Whether PET/CT impacts overall survival remains unknown.

Staging can be performed using the American Joint Committee on Cancer (AJCC) TNM staging system, 7th edition [25] (Table 4.2 of Chap. 4, Early Breast Cancer).

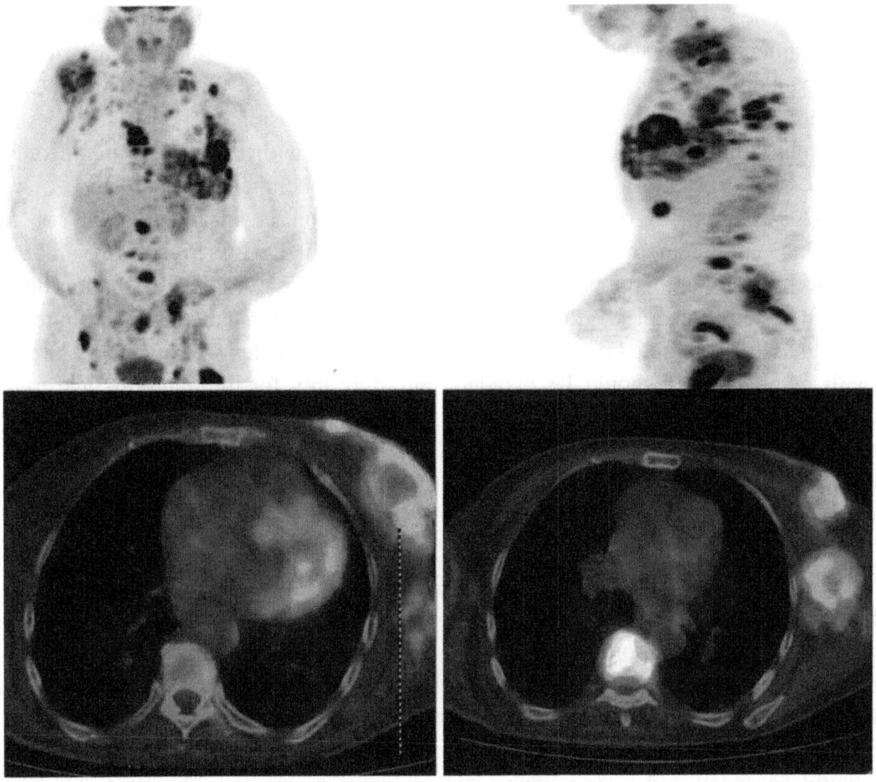

Fig. 5.8 PET/CT scan showing a *left* locally advanced breast cancer that has widespread distant metastases. (Courtesy of Quyen D. Chu, MD, MBA, FACS)

Treatment Overview: Multimodality Approach

Historically, outcome with single modality for patients with LABC has been dismal. When treated with radiation ± chemotherapy, radiation plus surgery, or combined chemoradiation therapy plus surgery, the 5-years DFS was 6 %, 24 %, and 40 %, respectively [26]. Untreated IBC can lead to the demise of more than 90 % of patients within 1 year. More recent data demonstrated that multimodality therapy comprising of chemotherapy, target-specific therapy, surgery, and radiation resulted in 5-years overall survival that can reach greater than 60 % [27].

Unlike early breast cancer, there is a paucity of phase three clinical trials on LABC. Additionally, many trials evaluating LABC grouped IBC and non-IBC LABC together, treating them as one disease rather than as distinct entity. Furthermore, randomized trials of neoadjuvant therapy often include a mix bag of patients that included patients with large operable breast cancer as well as those with IBC and/or non-IBC LABC. Finally, the duration of treatment and sequence of agents is undefined for patients with LABC. Regardless of these limitations, there are some general principles that currently hold true when managing patients with LABC. For one, neoadjuvant chemotherapy (NAC) comprising of anthracyclines (i.e., Adriamycin, epirubicin) and taxanes (i.e., paclitaxel, docetaxel) is used for both IBC and non-IBC LABC. Conventional wisdom dictates that concomitant HER-2-targeted therapy (trastuzumab) with anthracyclines should be avoided due to cardiotoxicity. If trastuzumab is to be used for those with HER-2-positive tumors, a non-anthracycline regimen of docetaxel and carboplatin has been recommended. However, recent data suggest that combination of trastuzumab and anthracycline is relatively safe and effective [28] (see section below). If trastuzumab is to be used, it should be given in conjunction with neoadjuvant chemotherapy and continued postoperatively for a total of 1 year.

Four to six cycles of preoperative systemic therapy should be considered over a course of 4–6 months before surgery [6]. For patients with IBC who had a clinical response (partial or complete) with neoadjuvant therapy, a modified radical mastectomy (MRM) should be performed, followed by postoperative radiation and hormonal therapy, if indicated [23]. Breast conserving therapy (BCT) is an option for patients with non-IBC LABC who had a clinical response. However, for those who did not respond to neoadjuvant therapy, taxane should be administered for those that are taxane naïve, and radiation should be offered prior to an MRM (Fig. 5.9). Local control rates when surgery is performed following neoadjuvant therapy for nonresponders, partial responders, and complete responders are 33 %, 68 %, and 89 %, respectively [29]. Although controversial, a delay in reconstruction in patients with LABC should be considered. However, some patients may strongly desire immediate reconstruction. Skin-sparing mastectomy is contraindicated in patients with IBC.

In general, adjuvant chemotherapy (i.e., chemotherapy following surgery) is not necessary if the patient had completed her scheduled NAC regimen. Surgery in the form BCT is an option for select patients with non-IBC LABC, while it is contraindicated for those with IBC. Although there are occasional reports of success with BCT in patients with IBC, BCT should only be performed in a clinical trial.

Radiation is an integral part of managing patients with LABC, irrespective of the degree of tumor response to NAC. Radiation fields should encompass supraclavicular and internal mammary lymph nodes for patients. Figure 5.9 shows an algorithm for the diagnosis and treatment of patients with LABC.

cCR and pCR Definition

Patients undergoing NAC are followed closely to evaluate their response to therapy. Clinical assessment of response to therapy relies on palpating the lesion to determine whether the primary tumor has decreased in size and if so, whether it is a partial clinical response (residual palpable mass) or a complete clinical response

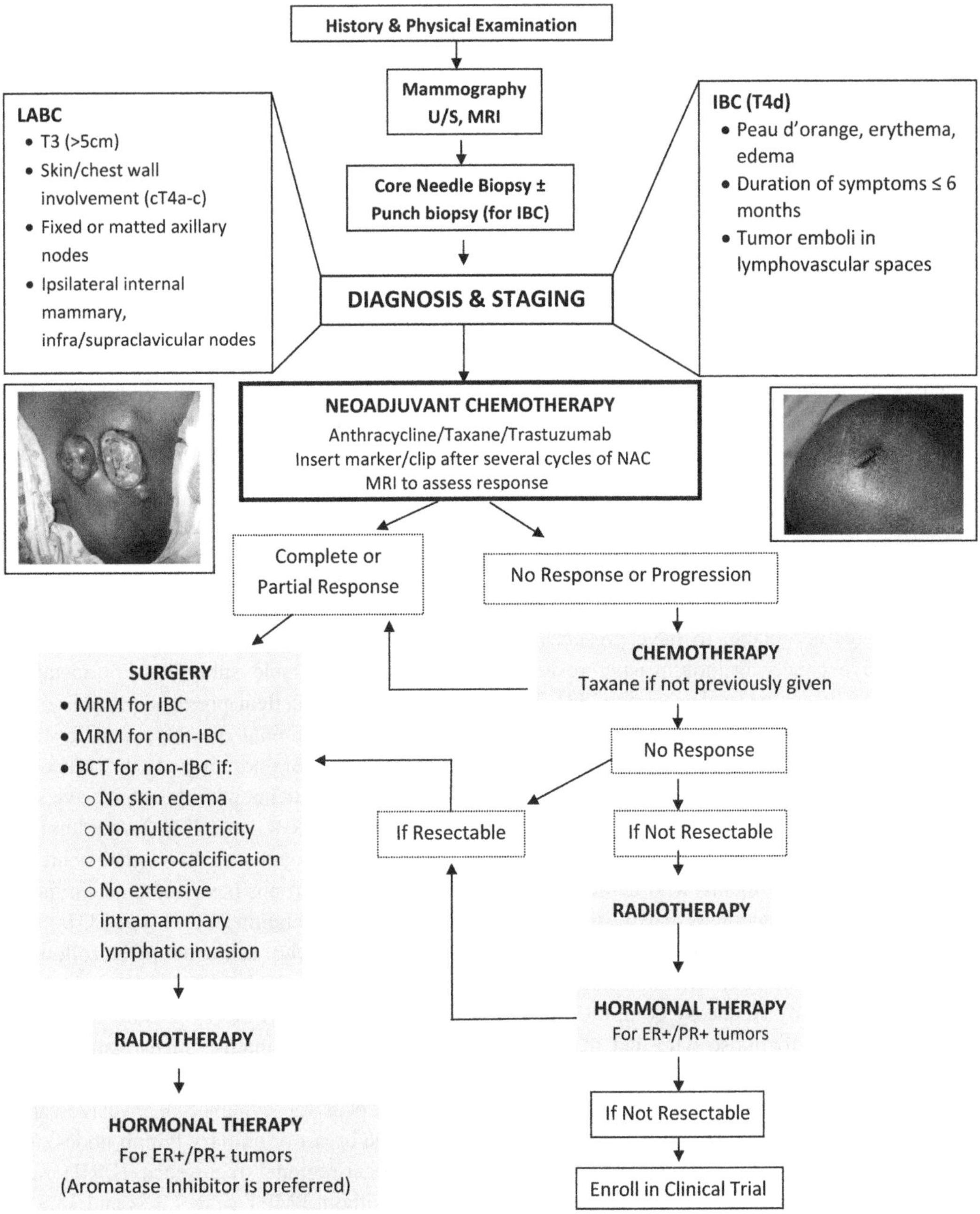

Fig. 5.9 Algorithm for the diagnosis and treatment of patients with LABC. (Courtesy of Quyen D. Chu, MD, MBA, FACS)

(cCR; no palpable mass). Although a cCR can be achieved, this does not necessary mean that there is an absence of residual tumor on the final pathologic specimen; it is possible for a tumor to achieve a cCR but not a pathologic complete response (pCR) (i.e., on pathologic sectioning, viable tumor cells are seen; this is referred to as achieving partial pathologic response or pPR). However, if there is no residual tumor seen under the microscope, the patient is deemed to have a pathologic complete response or pCR. Conversely, a patient may have an abnormality as seen on imaging or clinical exam following neoadjuvant therapy, yet has pCR. This can occur in a third of patients. What this means is that regardless of the sensitivity of imaging and clinical examination following NAC, a surgical specimen is still needed for determining the final pathologic response status.

The rates of cCR and pCR vary among the series and are dependent on the regimen used. In general, about 27 % of patients will achieve cCR and 10–26 % for pCR [30, 31]. pCR rate for anthracycline is less than 15 %, but this rate increases to 33 % with the addition of taxane and can reach up to 55 % with the addition of trastuzumab [32].

Standardized definition of pCR is lacking; pCR can mean (1) no pathologic residual tumor in the breast tumor, (2) no invasive component in the breast and axillary nodes, (3) complete absence of invasive and noninvasive component (DCIS), or (4) acceptable to have presence of focal invasive cancer or noninvasive residual tumor (i.e., DCIS) in the final specimen [33]. The American Society of Clinical Oncology guidelines define pCR as total disappearance of malignant cells, both in the breast and axillary lymph nodes [34].

pCR is a surrogate marker for long-term outcomes [31, 33–35]. Patients who achieve pCR have more favorable outcomes than those who do not. This is applicable for patients with IBC as well as noninflammatory LABC. In a study of 61 patients with IBC by Hennessy et al, the 5-year DFS was 78.6 % for those who had pCR, but dropped to 25.4 % for those with residual disease. Similarly, the 5-year OS was 82.5 % in the pCR group while it was 37.1 % in those with residual disease [36]. A recent meta-analysis of 12 randomized controlled trials of neoadjuvant systemic therapy demonstrated that pCR from both the breast and the lymph nodes was associated with improved event-free survival (HR = 0.48; $P<0.001$) and overall survival (HR = 0.36; $P<0.001$) [31]. Elevated Ki-67, a marker of proliferation, before NAC was found to be an independent predictor of pCR in LABC [37, 38]. pCR is accepted by the FDA as an endpoint for approving novel medication for patients with high-risk tumors. Whether pCR translates to an improved long-term outcome will need to be proven by randomized trials [33].

pCR status is a paradox; the more aggressive subtypes (i.e., triple-negative breast cancer or TNBC and HER-2+/nonluminal) tend to carry a poorer prognosis compared to the less aggressive subtypes (i.e., luminal A and B), yet they are more likely to achieve pCR status. In fact, a greater pCR rate is seen not only in the TNBC and HER-2+ tumors but also in those that are ER negative, poorly differentiated, and highly proliferative [31, 33]. Cortazar et al. found that pCR rates range between 7 and 16 % in hormone receptor-positive (HR+) tumors (i.e., less aggressive types), 18–30 % in HR+/HER2+ tumors, 31–50 % in HR-/HER2+ tumors, and 34 % in TNBC [31].

Although pCR is a useful prognostic marker for the more aggressive subtypes (i.e., TNBC and HER-2+), it may not play such an important role in the more favorable subtypes. For instance, because of the excellent prognosis that is often associated with luminal A subtype, pCR status has very little or no impact on outcome. Conversely, for patients with the aggressive subtypes such as TNBC or HER-2+/nonluminal, pCR is highly prognostic; those that achieved pCR in these subgroups have outcome similar to those that have the luminal A subtype [33].

For patients who achieved pCR following neoadjuvant chemotherapy, whether postmastectomy radiotherapy (PMRT) should be given remains an area of intense investigation. In a study of 106 patients (84 % had LABC) who achieved a pCR (no evidence of invasive carcinoma in the breast or axillary lymph nodes), the 10-year local-regional recurrence (LRR) rates with and without PMRT were 7.3 % and 33.3 %, respectively ($P=.04$). PMRT was associated with improved disease-specific and OS, even in those who achieved pCR [39]. However, in another study of 134 patients with Stage II–III breast cancer, PMRT did not have an impact on LRR or OS in those who achieved pathologically negative LNs following neoadjuvant chemotherapy [40]. Despite these compelling data, most clinicians would opt for PMRT for patients with LABC.

A multidisciplinary panel of expert, under the auspice of the National Cancer Institute (NCI), recommends PMRT following neoadjuvant chemotherapy for patients presenting with clinical Stage III disease or those with positive lymph nodes after neoadjuvant therapy. As an aside, for those who initially present with Stage II disease who achieved pCR following neoadjuvant therapy, there is limited data to support PMRT routine use [41]. National Surgical Adjuvant Breast and Bowel Project (NSABP) B-18 and B-27 trials showed that the 8-year risk of locoregional recurrence (LRR) after a mastectomy for patients who initially present with clinical Stage II disease is less than 10 % for those with negative LNs after preoperative chemotherapy [41].

Neoadjuvant Chemotherapy (NAC)

The two major goals of treating patients with LABC are to obtain locoregional control and eradicate occult systemic disease. Central to such goals is neoadjuvant chemotherapy. Neoadjuvant chemotherapy, also referred to as preoperative chemotherapy, induction chemotherapy, or primary chemotherapy, allows downsizing and downstaging of large inoperable primary tumors so that they can become operable. NAC also increases BCT rate, provides insight to the effectiveness of the chemotherapeutic regimen, answers research questions, and allows earlier treatment of micrometastatic disease (Fig. 5.10a, b).

The theoretical disadvantages associated with the NAC approach is that the initial tumor size and number of involved lymph nodes may not be accurately assessed. Because of bulky disease, NAC will have to treat a much greater disease burden. There is also a concern of an increased risk for surgical complications and drug resistance. Because surgery is performed later, there is a potential delay in curative local therapy should the patient not respond to NAC [42–44]. Despite these disadvantages, the advantages with the neoadjuvant approach appear to outweigh the risks. Regardless, there are no significant differences in OS or disease progression between patients

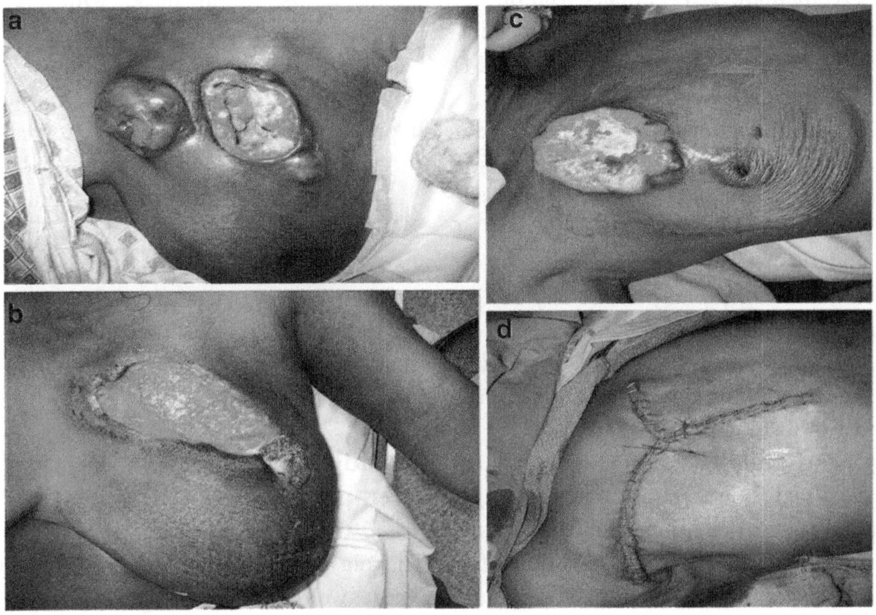

Fig. 5.10 A patient with a partial response to neoadjuvant chemotherapy (**a**, **b**). Another patient who had a minimal response after optimal NAC and radiation therapy (**c**, **d**). The patient underwent a successful modified radical mastectomy without the need for a skin or tissue flap. This was accomplished using the "Mercedes-Benz" closure (**c**). (Courtesy of Quyen D. Chu, MD, MBA, FACS)

undergoing NAC or adjuvant chemotherapy [45]. These facts were demonstrated in the NSABP B18 (4 cycles of Adriamycin and cyclophosphamide (AC) before versus after surgery) and NSABP-B27 (similar regimen as B-18, except taxane was added) trials and confirmed by a meta-analysis of nine randomized studies [45]. It should be noted that since there is no phase III data comparing NAC with adjuvant chemotherapy in patients with LABC, the assumption that NAC is comparable to adjuvant chemotherapy is based on retrospective studies [46] as well as on data extrapolated from operable breast cancer.

Most clinicians caring for patients with LABC would opt for the NAC approach rather than the adjuvant, and thus, NAC has become the standard of care for patients with LABC. Up to 90 % of patients undergoing NAC achieved major objective responses and downstaging. Following NAC, surgery alone, radiotherapy alone, or a combination of both modalities has been reported for non-IBC LABC patients. For patients with IBC, an MRM is the surgery of choice. Surgical options for non-IBC LABC include an MRM or a lumpectomy, axillary lymph node dissection, and postoperative radiotherapy. Patients who do not want the NAC approach and have resectable disease should undergo surgery (usually an MRM) followed by adjuvant chemoradiation therapy.

All patients undergoing NAC should have a fiducial clip, marker, or small coil inserted inside the tumor prior to completion of NAC. This is especially important because up to 30 % of patients undergoing NAC will have pCR, with the implication that there may not be any detectable or palpable disease to help guide the surgeon when he/she proceeds with excision. A marker may not be necessary for patients with IBC since the majority of them will receive an MRM.

For patients with LABC, multiple studies demonstrated that anthracycline-containing regimen resulted in superior response rate over non-anthracycline regimen [47]. The addition of a taxane to systemic anthracycline-based regimen further refined the neoadjuvant strategy [48–51] (Table 5.1). NSABP-B27 enrolled 2,411 patients with operable breast cancer that included clinical T1–3, N1, M0 to preoperative AC followed by surgery, AC + docetaxel followed by surgery, or AC followed by surgery, followed by docetaxel . The study demonstrated that the addition of docetaxel to the conventional AC regimen in the preoperative setting nearly doubled the percentage of patients achieving a pCR from 13.7 % to 26.1 % ($P<0.001$) and increased the percentage of patients achieving a cCR from 40.1 % to 63.6 % ($P<0.001$) [48]. Although disease-free survival (DFS) was improved, overall survival (OS) was not with the addition of docetaxel. The Aberdeen Breast Group also reported similar results in a phase III trials of 162 patients with LABC [50]. The pCR was 34 % in the docetaxel group versus 16 % ($P=0.04$) in the cyclophosphamide, vincristine, doxorubicin, prednisolone (CVAP) group, and the cCR was 94 % in the docetaxel group versus 66 % in the CVAP group ($P=0.001$). Interesting, unlike NSABP B-27, the Aberdeen group demonstrated an improved OS with the addition of docetaxel [50].

In a retrospective analysis of 240 patients with IBC, those who were treated with 5-fluorouracil, Adriamycin, cyclophosphamide (FAC) followed by paclitaxel had an objective response rate of 84 % vs 74 % in those with FAC alone. Additionally, the pCR was 25 % for those that received paclitaxel vs 10 % for those with FAC alone. The addition of paclitaxel resulted in an improvement in median OS and progression-free survival as compared to FAC alone [51].

Dose-dense chemotherapy (administration of a full dose of drugs over a shorter time period than standard) data for LABC are encouraging, but is still relegated as investigational and not recommended outside the confines of a clinical trial.

Neoadjuvant Endocrine Therapy (NET)

The role of neoadjuvant endocrine therapy (NET) is not as well defined as that for NAC. Retrospective data suggest that NET may be just as effective as neoadjuvant chemotherapy in terms of achieving clinical response and rate of breast conservation [52]. A phase III trial comparing neoadjuvant

Table 5.1 Neoadjuvant chemotherapy for inflammatory and locally advanced breast cancer (non-trastuzumab based)

Study	Year	Patients	Population	Chemotherapy regimen	pCR rate	Overall RR	5-year DFS	5-year OS
Hortobagyi [113]	1988	174	LABC	FAC	16.7 %	NR	84 % (for IIIa), 33 % (for IIIb)	84 %(for IIIa), 44 % (for IIIb)
Perloff [114]	1988	113	LABC and IBC	CAFVP	NR	72 %	NR	NR
Pierce [115] and Low [116]	1992 2004	107	LABC and IBC	CAFM	29 %	57 %	NR	61 % (for IIIa), 36 % (for IBC), 31 % (for non-IBC IIIb)
Colozza [117]	1996	31	LABC and IBC	CAP	8 %	76.7 %	29 % (6 years)	28 % (6 years)
Ueno [47]	1997	172	IBC	FAC, FACVP, FACVP±MV	NR, NR, NR	74 %	32 %	40 %
Clark [118]	1998	34	LABC	A	21 %	65 %	77 % (3 years)	88 % (3 years)
Kuerer [35]	1999	372	LABC	FAC	12 %	NR	NR	NR
Cristofanilli [119]	2001	42	IBC	FAC±T	14 %	81 %	NR	NR
Favret [120]	2001	64	LABC	FAC	NR	92 %	58 %	75 %
Smith [50] Hutcheon [121]	2002	50, 47	LABC	CVAP, CVAP+docetaxel	16 %, 34 %	66 % 94 %	77 % (3 years), 90 % (3 years)	84 % (3 years), 97 % (3 years)
Harris [122]	2003	54	IBC	CMF or FAC	30 %	52 %	49 %	56 %
McIntosh [123]	2003	166	LABC	CVAP	15 %	75 %	NR	NR
Therasse [124]	2003	448	LABC	CEF, EC+filgrastim	14 %, 20 %	79.9 %, 85.7 %	NR, NR	53 %, 51 %
Espinosa [125]	2004	51	LABC and IBC	ET	18 %	78 %	NR	NR
Ezzat [126]	2004	126	LABC	PC	16 %	91 %	63 %	85 %
Gajdos [127]	2004	138	LABC	CMF or CAF	13 %	53 %	46 %	55 %
Lebowitz [128]	2004	30	LABC	Docetaxel+capecitabine	10 %	90 %	NR	NR
de Matteis [129]	2004	30	LABC+IBC	ET	13.3 %	76.7 %	NR	NR
Shen [130]	2004	33	LABC+IBC	NR	12 %	85 %	70 %	78 %
Thomas [131]	2004	193	LABC	VACP	12.2 %	83.4 %	51 %	60 %
Erol [132]	2005	74	LABC	CMF	18.9 %	88 %	52 %	79.9 %
Gradishar [133]	2005	45	LABC	Docetaxel	10 %	49 %	NR	80 %
Kao [134]	2005	15	LABC and IBC	T+vinorelbine+XRT	46.7 %	93 %	33 % (4 years)	56 % (4 years)
Tham [135]	2005	51	LABC	Docetaxel	20 %	75 %	NR	78 % (2 years)
Veyret [136]	2006	102	IBC	FEC-HD	14.7	91.1 %	35.7 % (10 years)	41.2 % (10 years)
Ellis [137]	2006	265	LABC and IBC	AC+T, metronomic AC+T	17 %, 26 %	NR, NR	NR, NR	NR, NR
Villman [138]	2007	41	LABC and IBC	ECX	19 %	74 %	NR	NR
von Minckwitz [49]	2008	1,390	LABC and IBC	TAC	22.2 %	100 %	NR	NR
Manga [139]	2009	60	LABC and IBC	ATX	8.3 %	77 %	76 % (3 years)	90 % (3 years)

RR response rate, *DFS* disease-free survival, *OS* overall survival, *IBC* inflammatory breast cancer, *LABC* locally advanced breast cancer, *NR* not reported, *XRT* radiation therapy, *CAFVP* cyclophosphamide+doxorubicin+fluorouracil+vincristine+prednisone, *FAC* fluorouracil+doxorubicin+cyclophosphamide, *VP* vincristine+prednisone, *CMF* cyclophosphamide+methotrexate+5-fluorouracil, *CAF* cyclophosphamide+doxorubicin+5-fluorouracil, *MV* methotrexate+vinblastine, *FEC* 5-fluorouracil+epirubicin+cyclophosphamide, *A* doxorubicin, *AC* doxorubicin+cyclophosphamide, *T* paclitaxel, *CAP* cyclophosphamide+doxorubicin+cisplatin, *CAFM* cyclophosphamide+doxorubicin+5-fluorouracil+methotrexate, *CVAP* cyclophosphamide+vincristine+doxorubicin+prednisolone, *ET* epirubicin+docetaxel, *PC* paclitaxel+cisplatin, *VACP* vincristine+doxorubicin+cyclophosphamide+prednisone, *AT* doxorubicin+docetaxel, *EC* epirubicin+cyclophosphamide, *CEF* cyclophosphamide, + epirubicin+fluorouracil, *TAC* docetaxel+doxorubicin+cyclophosphamide
Reprinted from Ref. [44]. With permission from John Wiley & Sons, Inc.

Table 5.2 Selected clinical trials comparing neoadjuvant aromatase inhibitors with tamoxifen

Authors (Yr)	N	Menopause status	Response rate			BCT rate		
Ellis 2001 [55]	324	Postmenopausal	Letrozole	Tamoxifen		Letrozole	Tamoxifen	
			60 %	41 %	$P=0.004$	48 %	36 %	$P=0.036$
Eiermann 2001 [57]	337	Postmenopausal	Letrozole	Tamoxifen		Letrozole	Tamoxifen	
			55 %	36 %	$P<0.001$	45 %	35 %	$P=0.022$
Smith 2005 [60]	330	Postmenopausal	Anastrozole	Tamoxifen		Anastrozole	Tamoxifen	
IMPACT trial			58 %	22 %	$P=0.18$	44 %	31 %	$P=0.23$
Cataliotti 2006 [56]	451	Premenopausal	Anastrozole	Tamoxifen		Anastrozole	Tamoxifen	
PROACT trial			39.5 %	35.4 %[b]	$P=0.03$	43 %	30.8 %	$P=0.04$
			50.0 %	46.2 %[c]	$P=0.04$			
Masuda 2012 [58][a]	204	Premenopausal	Anastrozole	Tamoxifen		N/A		
			70.4 %	50.5 %[c]	$P=0.004$			

BCT breast conserving therapy, *IMPACT* immediate preoperative anastrozole, tamoxifen, or combined with tamoxifen *PROACT* preoperative "Arimidex" compared to tamoxifen
[a]All patients received goserelin to suppress ovarian function
[b]Based on ultrasound measurement
[c]Based on caliper measurements, *N/A* not available

chemotherapy versus tamoxifen and GnRHa in women with hormone receptor-positive, HER-2-negative, lymph node-positive, primary breast cancer in premenopausal women (NEST trial; NCT01622361) is being conducted and is expected to be completed in 2016 [53].

Preliminary studies suggest that neoadjuvant aromatase inhibitors (AIs) may be more effective than tamoxifen in decreasing tumor size and increasing breast conservation rate [54–58] (Table 5.2). Whether anastrozole, exemestane, or letrozole is the preferred neoadjuvant AI might not make much of a difference since American College of Surgeons Oncology Group (ACOSOG) Z1031 trial found that the response rates among the three agents were equivalent [59]. Recall that AIs are only effective in women without functioning ovaries (i.e., postmenopausal women) (see Chap. 4, Early Breast Cancer for more thorough explanation). Most of the NET trials were done on postmenopausal women [55–57, 60], except for one, which treated premenopausal patients with goserelin to suppress their ovarian function [58]. Of the five selected trials, only one did not find any significant difference in response rate or breast conservation rate between anastrozole and tamoxifen [58]. Outside of a clinical trial, neoadjuvant endocrine therapy should not be used in young women [61]. Hormonal therapy should only be restricted to patients with hormone receptor-positive tumors.

Although 35–50 % of patients with hormone receptor-positive breast cancer respond to NET, pCR occurs only in less than 5 % of patients. Because pCR occurs less frequently with NET and may not be an important proxy of long-term benefit, other parameters such as clinical response and proliferation rate, as measured by Ki-67 labeling index, may be more relevant surrogates of long-term benefit [62]. However, further validation studies are needed before these parameters can be accepted in the oncology community.

The average duration of treatment of NET is between 3 and 4 months [52]. Because NET is less toxic than neoadjuvant chemotherapy and that it can be given over a long period of time (up to 24 months [54]), NET may be a suitable approach for those who are considered unfit for chemotherapy or surgery (i.e., elderlies) [54, 63].

HER-2 Target-Specific Agents

As mentioned in this chapter, overexpression of HER-2 is associated with a high recurrence and low survival in patients with breast cancer. Patients with IBC are known to have an increased incidence of HER-2 overexpression [11]. The Neoadjuvant Herceptin (NOAH) trial was a phase III trial that evaluates the efficacy of adding trastuzumab (Herceptin®) to conventional chemotherapy in 235 patient with HER-2+ IBC or non-IBC LABC [28]. Patients were randomized to receive either neoadjuvant chemotherapy with trastuzumab followed by adjuvant trastuzumab or neoadjuvant chemotherapy alone. Chemotherapy consisted of doxorubicin, paclitaxel, cyclophosphamide, methotrexate, and fluorouracil. The trastuzumab group had significantly improved 3-year event-free survival (EFS; 71 % vs 56 %, HR=0.56; $p=0.013$) [28]. The most recent update with a median follow-up of 5.4 years confirmed significant improvement in EFS ($p=0.016$), breast cancer-specific survival ($p=0.023$), and a strong trend toward improved OS ($p=0.055$) [64].

Besides demonstrating the superiority of trastuzumab over standard regimen, NOAH also showed that combination of trastuzumab with an anthracycline, which historically results in a 27 % risk of cardiotoxicity [65], is relatively safe. Only two patients (2 %) had reversible congestive heart failure but remained alive at the time of the final report. Trastuzumab should be given for 1 year. Whether combination of trastuzumab and anthracycline becomes standard of care will not be known until some distant future.

Combination of lapatinib and paclitaxel as neoadjuvant systemic therapy for IBC patients with HER-2 overexpression demonstrated a 78.6 % clinical response rate and a 18.2 % pCR rate [66]. Further studies are needed to validate the above results before it can become a routine practice.

Dual Inhibition of HER-2 Receptors in the Neoadjuvant Setting

The role of targeting HER-2-positive tumors using two inhibitors has been elucidated in Chap. 4, Early Breast Cancer (see Table 4.16). This section will summarize the findings from the selected clinical trials as they relate to patients with LABC.

There are five reported clinical trials on the role of dual inhibitors against HER-2 receptors. Most demonstrated a significant rate of pCR with dual inhibitors [67–71]. Besides trastuzumab (Herceptin®), pertuzumab (Perjeta®), which, like trastuzumab, is a humanized monoclonal antibody but targets a different epitope of HER-2, and lapatinib (Tykerb®), a tyrosine kinase inhibitor, have been tested in combination with trastuzumab [67–71]. Combination of trastuzumab with pertuzumab plus standard chemotherapy regimen had resulted in a significantly high pCR rate (45.8–66 %) [67, 68] and low incidence of left ventricular systolic dysfunction [67]. Similarly, combination of trastuzumab and lapatinib demonstrated high pCR rates, ranging from 46.7 to 62.0 % [69, 70, 72]. To put things in perspective, historic pCR is around 15–20 % with conventional chemotherapy; thus, a pCR rate of nearly 50–60 % with the addition of dual inhibition of HER-2 to standard chemotherapy is a testament of progress made in the field of breast cancer.

Combination of trastuzumab and pertuzumab is the first neoadjuvant regimen for breast cancer that received FDA-accelerated approval. Permanent approval will require future confirmatory trials. It should be noted that although LABC were included in many of these trials, it represents the minority since the majority of patients had operable, early breast cancer (60–84 %). Additionally, these excellent outcomes were only seen in those with HER-2-positive tumors, a subset of breast cancers that make up of only 20 % of all breast cancers.

Other Target-Specific Therapy

Bevacizumab (Avastin®, Genentech/Roche), a recombinant humanized monoclonal anti-VEGF antibody; everolimus, an inhibitor of mammalian target of rapamycin (mTOR); trastuzumab, an inhibitor of HER-2 receptor; and lapatinib, an inhibitor of HER-2 receptor tyrosine kinase, have all been tested in combination with current chemotherapy to evaluate the feasibility, safety, and efficacy in the neoadjuvant setting [73–79]. Most of the studies, however, are small phase II clinical trials.

Monitoring Response to Neoadjuvant Chemotherapy

Compared to clinical assessment, ultrasound, and mammography, MRI is superior at assessing response to NAC [80]. The purpose of using MRI for patients who are undergoing NAC is two-folds: (1) assess tumor response during treatment, and (2) detect residual disease after treatment. Assessment of tumor response during treatment is generally done before the completion of the chemotherapy regimen and occurs after the first cycle(s) of NAC.

Because tumor shrinkage occurs late in the course of chemotherapy, physical exam alone to assess tumor response during the early course of chemotherapy is unreliable. However, tumor vascularity decreases early in responsive tumors and because contrast enhancement on MRI is related to tumor vascularity, a reduction in the degree of enhancement on breast MRI is a reliable metric to gauge tumor sensitivity to chemotherapy.

One of the arguments for using MRI during treatment is to identify responders from nonresponders so that clinicians can switch chemotherapeutic regimen for those who are the nonresponders. While this appears to be a sound argument, current data do not seem to support it [81]. Large randomized trials such as the NSABP B-27 and Aberdeen trial found that those patients who did not respond well to anthracycline-based regimen did not do well with the addition of taxane-based regimen [48, 50]. Furthermore, the GeparTrio trial reported that the rate of pCR among the nonresponders who were switched to an alternative chemotherapy regimen did not improve after the switch [49, 82]. Thus, the advantage of using MRI during treatment should be to (1) identify those who are the responders so that current therapy can be continued and (2) identify the nonresponders so as to avoid unnecessary toxicity and costs associated with the ineffective chemotherapy regimen; this latter group of patients could then be offered early surgery.

Although MRI is a good predictor of pCR in all tumor subtypes, it is more accurate in determining the actual pathologic size and residual disease in patients with HER-2+ and TNBC than the luminal subtypes [83, 84]. MRI shows a high false-negative detection rate of pCR for non-palpable IBC (21 %) [85]. In addition, it was not very accurate in determining the final tumor size following NAC [14]. MRI is suboptimal at detecting multiple islands of small residual invasive cancers that are distributed over a large region of the breast. Perhaps, this is one of the reasons why breast conserving therapy (BCT) is contraindicated in women with IBC. The role of using PET/CT to monitor response remains an area of investigation [86].

Surgery

Surgery is an integral component of therapy, irrespective of whether or not the patient achieved a complete clinical response. Surgery can be performed within 2–6 weeks of completing the last cycle of chemotherapy. BCT is a feasible option for select patients with non-IBC LABC. With neoadjuvant therapy, up to 25 % of patients with LABC can be successfully treated with BCT. Criteria for BCT following NAC include (1) complete resolution of skin edema, (2) sufficient reduction in tumor size, (3) no evidence of multicentricity (more than 2 lesions on different breast quadrants), (4) absence of extensive suspicious microcalcifications, and (5) lack of extensive intramammary lymphatic invasion. When these criteria are met, local recurrence rate and 10-year OS following BCT are equivalent to those with early, operable breast cancer [87]. Even with BCT, an axillary lymph node dissection should be part of the operation for the majority of patients with LABC because recent data demonstrated the uncertainty of performing a SLNBx for those with clinically positive lymph nodes [88, 89] (Table 4.10, Chap. 4, Early Breast Cancer). A mastectomy should be considered for those with persistent positive margins after repeat margin resection, those with multicentric disease or evidence of extensive DCIS or microcalcifications, tumors fixated to the skin or chest wall, and contraindications to radiation, such as collagen vascular disease [90]. Again, it should be reiterated that patients with IBC should undergo a modified radical mastectomy (MRM).

As mentioned earlier, a patient who achieved a complete clinical response following NAC might still harbor residual disease. Unfortunately, this will not be known without a pathologic evaluation.

Thus, even with a complete clinical response, an MRM or an excision of an abnormality as detected either on post-neoadjuvant radiologic studies or clinical exam is a must. For those with non-IBC LABC who have no evidence of any abnormality following NAC, a needle-guided localization technique that helps excise a 2 cm tissue surrounding the radiologic marker is recommended to assess for residual disease (i.e., assessment for pCR). Of note, the marker should generally be placed under ultrasound or mammographic guidance after several cycles of NAC when the tumor has shrunken to approximately 2 cm in size. Because NAC does not necessarily result in a uniform effect throughout the breast, placing the marker prior to NAC might result in it being located asymmetrically away from the epicenter of the tumor following NAC [91, 92].

On occasions, a persistent large mass will remain even after optimal NAC (Fig. 5.10c, d). In such a situation, a split thickness skin graft or rotational flap to cover the chest wall defect following a mastectomy is an option. Alternatively, the incision can be placed such that it can be closed without the need for a graft by using what we termed as the "Mercedes-Benz" closure (Figs. 5.10b and 5.11).

For patients with IBC, optimal outcome depends on whether or not pCR was achieved. For patients who had minimal or no response to NAC, a mastectomy will not have an impact on survival. Almost 90 % of such patients will develop distant metastases after a mastectomy. However, for those who had only partial response to NAC, surgery appeared to have helped some of the patients; the percentage of patients who developed distant

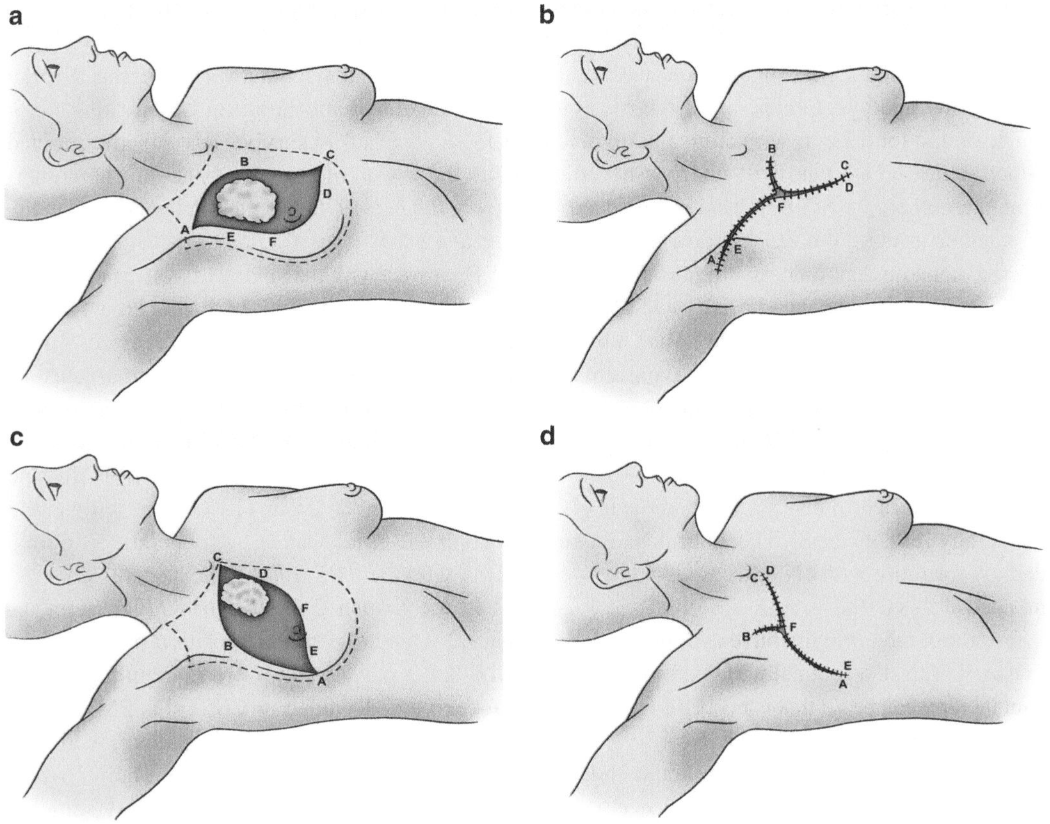

Fig. 5.11 Placement of incision and extent of a mastectomy for patients who had residual tumor following NAC. These incisions can be performed without the need for a skin or tissue flap. *Solid line* around the *red area* represents recommended incision for the mastectomy. *Dotted lines* represent extent of breast tissue to be removed. (Courtesy of Quyen D. Chu, MD, MBA, FACS)

metastasis dropped from 69 to 47 % when surgery was performed in these patients [93]. In performing a mastectomy, the surgeon should strive to achieve negative surgical margins.

For the nonresponders, second-line chemotherapy or radiation therapy should precede surgery. Palliative resections can provide symptomatic relief from a boggy tumor or for those whose wounds are a challenge to manage. In such situations, the aid from plastic and reconstructive colleagues will be beneficial in planning the operation.

Sentinel Lymph Node Biopsy for Patients Undergoing Neoadjuvant Chemotherapy

The role of sentinel lymph node biopsy (SLNBx) for patients undergoing neoadjuvant chemotherapy has been discussed in Chap. 4, Early Breast Cancer (see Table 4.10). This section will briefly reiterate the findings. In general, SLNBx is not a viable option for patients with clinically involved lymph nodes (cN+) who will undergo neoadjuvant chemotherapy [88, 89]. This is irrespective of whether or not the node was downstaged following neoadjuvant therapy. In the ACOSOG Z1071 trial of patients who initially had cN+disease, the false-negative rate (FNR) was 12.6 % in those who had 2 or more sentinel lymph nodes retrieved after neoadjuvant chemotherapy. In the Sentinel Neoadjuvant (SENTINA) trial, the FNR was 18 % in those who initially had cN+disease but was converted to cN- after neoadjuvant chemotherapy [89]. Thus, SLNBx after neoadjuvant therapy for those with cN+disease is not recommended at this point.

For those who initially have a clinically negative axilla (cN-), a sentinel node before neoadjuvant therapy can be all that is needed to assess the axilla if the SLNBx is negative. However, if the results are positive, such a patient should undergo an axillary lymph node dissection following neoadjuvant therapy because the FNR is unacceptably high with a subsequent SLNBx (>50 %) [89]. SLNBx should not be entertained for patients with IBC, irrespective of whether or not they presented initially with nodal involvement.

Postmastectomy Radiation Therapy

As mentioned previously, there are no DFS or OS differences between neoadjuvant and adjuvant chemotherapy [94]. Thus, there are instances when a patient received an appropriate modified radical mastectomy prior to chemotherapy for an operable breast cancer and is found to have advanced nodal disease (i.e., N2). Given her risk of recurrence even with optimal systemic adjuvant therapy, the patient may benefit from postoperative radiation (PMRT). PMRT, in the appropriate setting, can result in an absolute reduction in locoregional recurrence by 20–27 % and increase overall survival (OS) by 8–9 % [95–98] .

Postmastectomy radiotherapy (PMRT) was commonly employed to reduce locoregional failure (LRF) in the pre-chemotherapy era [99–102]. Although PMRT imparted a significant two-third reduction in LRF, studies such as the Early Breast Cancer Trialists' Collaborative Group (EBCTCG) that performed a meta-analysis of 36 randomized trials failed to demonstrate an OS advantage [99, 103]. Such a lack of survival advantage combined with the advent of effective systemic chemotherapy in the late 1970s resulted in the decline in the use of PMRT.

However, with the advent of systemic therapy, a subset of patients with high-risk breast cancer had extended survival and recurred local-regionally, which facilitated the reemergence of PMRT [95–98, 104–107]. Evidence of an overall survival advantage with PMRT in high-risk breast cancer patients was provided in 1997 by the British Columbia Group (BCG) [95, 96] and the Danish Breast Cancer Cooperative Group (DBCCG) [97, 98] (Table 5.3).

In the British Columbia trial, 318 premenopausal women with node-positive breast cancer who had a mastectomy were randomly assigned to receive CMF alone or CMF plus PMRT [95]. Approximately a third of the patients had four or more involved lymph nodes. Their 20-year follow-up (a median follow-up of 249 months) demonstrated a statistically significant reduction in the crude risk of isolated LRF from 26 to 10 % (RR=0.36; $p=0.002$), improved breast cancer-specific survival from 38 to 53 % (RR=0.67; $p=0.008$), and a statistically significantly improved

Table 5.3 Randomized trials demonstrating significant advantages with postmastectomy radiotherapy (PMRT)

				LRF		DFS		OS	
Trials [Ref]	# pts	% ≥ 4LN's	Median follow-up	Control	PMRT	Control	PMRT	Control	PMRT
British Columbia [95, 96][a]	318	35 %	249 mo	26 %[c]	10 % ($p=0.002$)	25 %[c]	35 % ($p=0.009$)	37 %[c]	47 % ($p=0.03$)
Danish 82b [97][b] (premenopausal)	1,708	85 %	114 mo	32 %[d]	9 % ($p<0.001$)	34 %[d]	48 % ($p<0.001$)	45 %[d]	54 % ($p<0.001$)
Danish 82c [98][b] (postmenopausal)	1,375	33 %	123 mo	35 %[e]	8 % ($p<0.001$)	24 %[e]	36 % ($p<0.001$)	36 %[e]	45 % ($p=0.03$)

Modified from Ref. [94]. With permission from Elsevier
Legend:
LRF locoregional failure, *DFS* disease-free survival, *OS* overall survival
[a]20-year follow-up results
[b]10-year follow-up results
[c]CMF 6 or 12 months
[d]CMF 9 cycles
[e]Tamoxifen 30 mg × 1 year

OS from 37 to 47 % (RR = 0.73; $p=0.03$) in the PMRT group [96].

The DBCCG conducted two concurrent trials to evaluate the role of PMRT in high-risk patients. The 82b trial studied premenopausal women for which 85 % of enrollees had ≥4 involved lymph nodes, while the 82c trial evaluated postmenopausal women with 33 % of enrollees having ≥4 involved lymph nodes [97, 98]. Both 82b and 82c trials each demonstrated an absolute 9 % overall survival advantage with PMRT and a significant absolute 23 % (82b trial) and 27 % (82c trial) reduction in LRF with PMRT (Table 5.3).

One of the critiques about the BCG and DBCG trials is the low number of axillary lymph nodes that were retrieved when compared with the other four large clinical trials that had excluded PMRT for high-risk patients [104–107]. The median numbers of lymph nodes retrieved in the BCG and DBCG trials were 11 and 7, respectively, whereas the median numbers of lymph nodes reported by the four large trials were between 15 and 17 [104–107]. Consequently, the 10-year cumulative rates of LRF in patients with 1–3 involved lymph nodes were 30 to 33 % in the BCG and DBCG trials, respectively, versus 13 to 19 % observed in the four large trials. For those with ≥4 involved lymph nodes, the 10-year cumulative rates of LRF were 42 to 46 % in the BCG and DBCG trials, versus 24 to 35 % in the four large trials [104].

Consensus statements from the National Institutes of Health Consensus Panel on Adjuvant Therapy of Operable Breast Cancer, the American Society of Therapeutic Radiology and Oncology, the American College of Radiology, the American Society of Clinical Oncology, and the Health Canada recommended PMRT for patients with four or more positive axillary nodes [108]. Although there is insufficient evidence for PMRT in patients with 1–3 positive nodes, it is reasonable to consider it in such patients who also have large tumors, extranodal extension, or inadequate axillary node dissections. The decision for PMRT should rest upon sound clinical judgment.

For patients with IBC and non-IBC LABC who underwent neoadjuvant chemotherapy followed by a mastectomy, PMRT should be given, regardless of response, as recommended by a panel of multidisciplinary experts [41].

Impact of Molecular Subtypes on Response to Postmastectomy Radiation for Patients with LABC

Molecular subtyping of breast cancer has led to the classification of breast cancer into 5 distinct subtypes: (1) luminal A, (2) luminal B, (3) HER-2 enriched (HER-2 positive), (4) normal-like, and (5) basal-like or often referred to as the triple-negative breast cancer (TNBC) [109, 110].

The basal-like and HER-2-positive subtypes are considered to be the most aggressive subtypes, while luminal A is the least aggressive; luminal B subtype carries an intermediate outcome.

Data from the Danish trials, DBCG 82b and DBCG 82c, were evaluated to assess the impact of breast cancer subtypes on PMRT response [111]. Using tissue microarray sections to stain tumors from 1,000 patients for ER, PR receptor statuses (Rec), and HER-2 expressions, Kyndi et al. constructed four subgroups that resemble their respective subtypes – (1) Rec+/HER-2- [luminal A], (2) Rec+/HER-2+ [luminal B], (3) Rec-/HER-2- [TNBC], and (4) Rec-/HER-2+ [HER-2+] – and found that OS after PMRT was seen only among patients with good prognostic markers such as hormone receptor-positive and HER-2-negative tumors [111]. Those with hormone receptor-negative tumors (i.e., TNBC) and HER-2-positive tumors had no survival advantage with PMRT.

Although these provocative data will need to be validated, they nevertheless reveal some interesting idea, mainly, that it may be possible in the future to select patients who will or will not benefit from PMRT based on biologic subtyping of their tumors.

Prognostic Factors

Prognostic factors for patients with LABC are very similar to those with early-stage breast cancer and poor prognosis include higher T stage (extent of tumor involvement), advanced N stage, high proliferation index (Ki-67), ER/PR tumors, and high grade [112]. In addition, response to NAC is an independent predictor of survival. As mentioned previously, those who achieved pCR have significant improvement in DFS and OS compared to those who did not achieve pCR.

Summary

LABC consists of two separate entities: inflammatory breast cancer (IBC) and non-IBC locally advanced breast cancer (non-IBC LABC). IBC is the most aggressive form of breast cancer. Patients with IBC present with a rapid onset of symptom and the affected breast has a typical peau d'orange appearance. Patients with non-IBC LABC typically presents with a neglected breast cancer that has grown and festered, involving the skin, underlying muscle, and occupying a large portion of the breast. Nodal involvement is common in patients with LABC. Management is multimodality and generally involves neoadjuvant systemic therapy such as anthracycline and taxane, trastuzumab for HER-2-positive tumors, and endocrine therapy (preferably an aromatase inhibitor) for hormone-positive tumors. Neoadjuvant endocrine therapy is an option, although its use has not been well established as NAC. Sentinel lymph node is contraindicated in patients with IBC and should be viewed with caution for patients with LABC. A modified radical mastectomy is the surgery of choice for patients with IBC as well as for the majority of patients with non-IBC LABC. However, in well select patients with non-IBC LABC, breast conserving therapy is a viable option. Complete pathologic response (pCR) following NAC predicts outcome for patients with LABC.

Salient Points

- LABC comprises of inflammatory breast cancer (IBC) and non-IBC LABC.
- IBC presents with a rapid onset (≤6 months) of breast swelling, tenderness erythema, and skin thickening (peau d'orange) which can be mistaken for a breast infection.
- Tumor emboli in the dermal lymphatics, along with clinical suspicion, is pathognomonic of IBC, although the presence of tumor emboli is not a prerequisite for diagnosis.
- Multimodality such as neoadjuvant systemic therapy, surgery, and radiation is the preferred approach for both IBC and non-IBC LABC.
- Neoadjuvant chemotherapy (NAC) comprises of anthracyclines and taxanes.
- Trastuzumab for 1 year is recommended for patients with HER-2-positive tumors, but it should be used cautiously when combined with an anthracycline to avoid cardiotoxicity. However, recent data suggest that combination of trastuzumab and anthracycline can be safely used together.

- Breast conserving therapy is an option for patients with non-IBC LABC, but not for patients with IBC.
- Sentinel node biopsy is contraindicated in IBC as well as in the majority of patients with non-IBC LABC.
- MRI during NAC is a useful modality to gauge for response during treatment.
- A modified radical mastectomy should be the surgery of choice for patients with IBC.
- Pathologic complete response (pCR) is a prognostic marker; those who achieved pCR tend to have better disease-free and overall survival compared to those who do not.
- pCR rate is higher among proliferative and poorly differentiated tumors and ER-negative, HER-2-positive, and triple-negative breast cancers.
- Neoadjuvant endocrine therapy (NET) is emerging as a potential option for select patients with endocrine-positive tumors.
- Aromatase inhibitors may be more effective than tamoxifen for hormone-positive tumors.
- Combination of trastuzumab and pertuzumab (dual inhibition of HER-2 receptors) is the first neoadjuvant regimen that received FDA-accelerated approval.

Questions

1. Which one of the following responses is the characteristic of the diagnosis of locally advanced breast cancer (LABC)?
   A. LABC is a homogenous type of breast cancer with a common clinical presentation that includes a large palpable mass and palpable axillary lymph nodes.
   B. LABC is the most frequent form of breast cancer in countries that lack routine breast cancer screening.
   C. LABC is rare (<5 %) in countries where breast cancer screening is common.
   D. LABC includes inflammatory and noninflammatory breast cancer, which represents one distinct biologic entity.
   E. B and C.
2. What clinical signs are consistent with inflammatory breast cancer (IBC)?
   A. Rapid onset of symptoms and signs (<6 months) including breast pain/tenderness, diffuse erythema extending over at least one-third of the breast, peau d'orange of the skin, and a breast mass that may or may not be palpable.
   B. Rapid onset of symptoms and signs including breast pain/tenderness, diffuse erythema over the entire breast, peau d'orange of the skin, and an ulcerated breast mass.
   C. Slow onset of symptoms and signs including breast pain, diffuse erythema, peau d'orange of the skin, and an ill-defined breast mass.
   D. A large, ulcerative, painful breast mass with erythema along the ulcer margins.
   E. A large, ulcerative, non-painful breast mass with erythema along the ulcer margins.
3. Which of the following statement(s) is/are true regarding IBC?
   A. IBC is the most aggressive form of breast cancer and is primarily a clinical diagnosis with histologic confirmation of malignancy.
   B. Axillary node involvement is present in approximately 45 % of patients at presentation.
   C. Lymphatic channels of the skin are obstructed by inflammatory cellular debris, resulting in the erythematous skin changes.
   D. A, B, and C.
   E. A and C.
4. The pathognomonic finding for patients with IBC is:
   A. Dermal lymphatic channels encased by tumor cells
   B. Dermal lymphatic channels obstructed by tumor cells
   C. Identified in all patients with IBC
   D. Identified in less than 10 % of patients with clinically suspicious IBC
   E. An obstruction of dermal lymphatic channels with inflammatory cellular debris.

5. Management of patients with LABC includes:
    A. Pretreatment evaluation that includes mammograms and radiographic studies to assess for metastatic disease, including a bone scan and an abdominal CT scan.
    B. Pretreatment core needle biopsy of the breast lesion to obtain sufficient tissue for diagnosis as well as hormone receptors and HER-2 receptor analysis.
    C. MRI of the breast is mandatory to assess tumor response to neoadjuvant chemoradiotherapy.
    D. A, B, and C.
    E. A and B.
6. The initial treatment of patients with LABC (IBC and non-IBC) is:
    A. Modified radical mastectomy
    B. Breast conservation therapy (partial mastectomy with radiation therapy) for patients with cancers < 5 cm
    C. Radiation treatments to the breast, axillary, supraclavicular, and infraclavicular lymph nodes
    D. Systemic therapy that includes 4–6 cycles of anthracyclines (such as Adriamycin) and taxanes (such as paclitaxel)
    E. Systemic therapy, such as tamoxifen, Arimidex or exemestane, for patients who are estrogen or progesterone receptor positive
7. Surgical management, such as a mastectomy or partial mastectomy, of patients with LABC:
    A. Is never indicated as the prognosis is too poor for a benefit
    B. Is indicated only if the patient had a complete response to systemic therapy
    C. Provides a 75 % local control rate when there is a complete response to neoadjuvant systemic therapy
    D. Has a 68 % local control rate when there is a partial response to neoadjuvant systemic therapy
    E. Should routinely include immediate reconstruction for patients undergoing a modified radical mastectomy
8. Following neoadjuvant chemotherapy, radiation therapy is administered:
    A. Only when there is no response to systemic therapy
    B. In advance of systemic therapy
    C. Following either a mastectomy or partial mastectomy
    D. Only following a partial mastectomy
    E. To axillary lymph nodes if positive for metastatic disease
9. The major goals of neoadjuvant systemic therapy include:
    A. Obtain locoregional control.
    B. Eradicate occult systemic disease.
    C. Avoid a mastectomy or a partial mastectomy.
    D. A, B, and C.
    E. A and B.
10. Neoadjuvant chemotherapy can:
    A. Downsize the primary tumor so that it is operable.
    B. Increase the rate of eligible patients for a partial mastectomy versus a total mastectomy.
    C. Obscure the accuracy of the total number of axillary nodes involved with metastatic disease.
    D. Increase the risk of postoperative surgical complications.
    E. All of the above.

Answers

1. B
2. A
3. A
4. B
5. E
6. D
7. D
8. C
9. E
10. E

References

1. Shulman LN, Willett W, Sievers A, Knaul FM. Breast cancer in developing countries: opportunities for improved survival. J Oncol. 2010;2010:595167.
2. Singletary SE, Allred C, Ashley P, et al. Revision of the American Joint Committee on Cancer staging system for breast cancer. J Clin Oncol. 2002;20(17): 3628–36.
3. Walshe JM, Swain SM. Clinical aspects of inflammatory breast cancer. Breast Dis. 2005;22: 35–44.
4. Dawood S, Ueno NT, Valero V, et al. Incidence of and survival following brain metastases among women with inflammatory breast cancer. Ann Oncol. 2010;21(12):2348–55.
5. Bonnier P, Charpin C, Lejeune C, et al. Inflammatory carcinomas of the breast: a clinical, pathological, or a clinical and pathological definition? Int J Cancer. 1995;62(4):382–5.
6. Dawood S, Merajver SD, Viens P, et al. International expert panel on inflammatory breast cancer: consensus statement for standardized diagnosis and treatment. Ann Oncol. 2011;22(3):515–23.
7. Anderson WF, Chu KC, Chang S. Inflammatory breast carcinoma and noninflammatory locally advanced breast carcinoma: distinct clinicopathologic entities? J Clin Oncol. 2003;21(12):2254–9.
8. Dawood S, Ueno NT, Valero V, et al. Differences in survival among women with stage III inflammatory and noninflammatory locally advanced breast cancer appear early: a large population-based study. Cancer. 2011;117(9):1819–26.
9. Buzdar AU, Singletary SE, Booser DJ, Frye DK, Wasaff B, Hortobagyi GN. Combined modality treatment of stage III and inflammatory breast cancer. M.D. Anderson Cancer Center experience. Surg Oncol Clin N Am. 1995;4(4):715–34.
10. Paradiso A, Tommasi S, Brandi M, et al. Cell kinetics and hormonal receptor status in inflammatory breast carcinoma. Comparison with locally advanced disease. Cancer. 1989;64(9):1922–7.
11. Parton M, Dowsett M, Ashley S, Hills M, Lowe F, Smith IE. High incidence of HER-2 positivity in inflammatory breast cancer. Breast. 2004;13(2): 97–103.
12. Charafe-Jauffret E, Tarpin C, Bardou VJ, et al. Immunophenotypic analysis of inflammatory breast cancers: identification of an "inflammatory signature". J Pathol. 2004;202(3):265–73.
13. Colpaert CG, Vermeulen PB, Benoy I, et al. Inflammatory breast cancer shows angiogenesis with high endothelial proliferation rate and strong E-cadherin expression. Br J Cancer. 2003;88(5): 718–25.
14. Cristofanilli M, Valero V, Buzdar AU, et al. Inflammatory breast cancer (IBC) and patterns of recurrence: understanding the biology of a unique disease. Cancer. 2007;110(7):1436–44.
15. Li BD, Sicard MA, Ampil F, et al. Trimodal therapy for inflammatory breast cancer: a surgeon's perspective. Oncology. 2010;79(1–2):3–12.
16. Yang WT, Le-Petross HT, Macapinlac H, et al. Inflammatory breast cancer: PET/CT, MRI, mammography, and sonography findings. Breast Cancer Res Treat. 2008;109(3):417–26.
17. Renz DM, Baltzer PA, Böttcher J, et al. Inflammatory breast carcinoma in magnetic resonance imaging: a comparison with locally advanced breast cancer. Acad Radiol. 2008;15(2):209–21.
18. Hammond ME, Hayes DF, Dowsett M, et al. American Society of Clinical Oncology/College of American Pathologists guideline recommendations for immunohistochemical testing of estrogen and progesterone receptors in breast cancer. J Clin Oncol. 2010;28(16):2784–95.
19. Hammond ME, Hayes DF, Dowsett M, et al. American Society of Clinical Oncology/College of American Pathologists guideline recommendations for immunohistochemical testing of estrogen and progesterone receptors in breast cancer (unabridged version). Arch Pathol Lab Med. 2010;134(7):e48–72.
20. Wolff AC, Hammond ME, Hicks DG, et al. Recommendations for human epidermal growth factor receptor 2 testing in breast cancer: American Society of Clinical Oncology/College of American Pathologists clinical practice guideline update. J Clin Oncol. 2013;31(31):3997–4013.
21. Wolff AC, Hammond ME, Hicks DG, et al. Recommendations for human epidermal growth factor receptor 2 testing in breast cancer: American society of clinical oncology/college of American pathologists clinical practice guideline update. Arch Pathol Lab Med. 2014;138(2):241–56.
22. Chu QD, Henderson A, Kim RH, et al. Should a routine metastatic workup be performed for all patients with pathologic N2/N3 breast cancer? J Am Coll Surg. 2012;214(4):456–61; discussion 461–452.
23. National Comprehensive Cancer Network (NCCN) guidelines. Available at: www.nccn.org (2013). Accessed 23 May 2013.
24. Groheux D, Giacchetti S, Delord M, et al. 18F-FDG PET/CT in staging patients with locally advanced or inflammatory breast cancer: comparison to conventional staging. J Nucl Med. 2013;54(1):5–11.
25. Edge SB, Compton CC. The American Joint Committee on Cancer: the 7th edition of the AJCC cancer staging manual and the future of TNM. Ann Surg Oncol. 2010;17(6):1471–4.
26. Perez CA, Fields JN, Fracasso PM, et al. Management of locally advanced carcinoma of the breast. II Inflammatory carcinoma. Cancer. 1994;74 Suppl 1:466–76.
27. Giordano SH. Update on locally advanced breast cancer. Oncologist. 2003;8(6):521–30.
28. Gianni L, Eiermann W, Semiglazov V, et al. Neoadjuvant chemotherapy with trastuzumab followed by adjuvant trastuzumab versus neoadjuvant

chemotherapy alone, in patients with HER2-positive locally advanced breast cancer (the NOAH trial): a randomised controlled superiority trial with a parallel HER2-negative cohort. Lancet. 2010;375(9712):377–84.
29. Thoms WW, McNeese MD, Fletcher GH, Buzdar AU, Singletary SE, Oswald MJ. Multimodal treatment for inflammatory breast cancer. Int J Radiat Oncol Biol Phys. 1989;17(4):739–45.
30. Fisher B, Brown A, Mamounas E, et al. Effect of preoperative chemotherapy on local-regional disease in women with operable breast cancer: findings from National Surgical Adjuvant Breast and Bowel Project B-18. J Clin Oncol. 1997;15(7):2483–93.
31. Cortazar P, Zhang L, Untch M, Mehta K, Costantino J, et al. Meta-analysis results from the Collaborative Trials in Neoadjuvant Breast Cancer. 2012 San Antonio Breast Cancer Symposium. Cancer Res. 2012;72(24 (Suppl 3)):Abstract S1–11.
32. Dawood S, Gonzalez-Angulo AM, Peintinger F, et al. Efficacy and safety of neoadjuvant trastuzumab combined with paclitaxel and epirubicin: a retrospective review of the M. D Anderson experience. Cancer. 2007;110(6):1195–200.
33. von Minckwitz G, Untch M, Blohmer JU, et al. Definition and impact of pathologic complete response on prognosis after neoadjuvant chemotherapy in various intrinsic breast cancer subtypes. J Clin Oncol. 2012;30(15):1796–804.
34. Kaufmann M, Hortobagyi GN, Goldhirsch A, et al. Recommendations from an international expert panel on the use of neoadjuvant (primary) systemic treatment of operable breast cancer: an update. J Clin Oncol. 2006;24(12):1940–9.
35. Kuerer HM, Newman LA, Smith TL, et al. Clinical course of breast cancer patients with complete pathologic primary tumor and axillary lymph node response to doxorubicin-based neoadjuvant chemotherapy. J Clin Oncol. 1999;17(2):460–9.
36. Hennessy BT, Gonzalez-Angulo AM, Hortobagyi GN, et al. Disease-free and overall survival after pathologic complete disease remission of cytologically proven inflammatory breast carcinoma axillary lymph node metastases after primary systemic chemotherapy. Cancer. 2006;106(5):1000–6.
37. Dowsett M, Smith IE, Ebbs SR, et al. Short-term changes in Ki-67 during neoadjuvant treatment of primary breast cancer with anastrozole or tamoxifen alone or combined correlate with recurrence-free survival. Clin Cancer Res. 2005;11(2 Pt 2):951s–8s.
38. Petit T, Wilt M, Velten M, et al. Comparative value of tumour grade, hormonal receptors, Ki-67, HER-2 and topoisomerase II alpha status as predictive markers in breast cancer patients treated with neoadjuvant anthracycline-based chemotherapy. Eur J Cancer. 2004;40(2):205–11.
39. McGuire SE, Gonzalez-Angulo AM, Huang EH, et al. Postmastectomy radiation improves the outcome of patients with locally advanced breast cancer who achieve a pathologic complete response to neoadjuvant chemotherapy. Int J Radiat Oncol Biol Phys. 2007;68(4):1004–9.
40. Le Scodan R, Selz J, Stevens D, et al. Radiotherapy for stage II and stage III breast cancer patients with negative lymph nodes after preoperative chemotherapy and mastectomy. Int J Radiat Oncol Biol Phys. 2012;82(1):e1–7.
41. Buchholz TA, Lehman CD, Harris JR, et al. Statement of the science concerning locoregional treatments after preoperative chemotherapy for breast cancer: a National Cancer Institute conference. J Clin Oncol. 2008;26(5):791–7.
42. Sinclair S, Swain SM. Primary systemic chemotherapy for inflammatory breast cancer. Cancer. 2010; 116 Suppl 11:2821–8.
43. Mamounas EP. Neoadjuvant chemotherapy for operable breast cancer: is this the future? Clin Breast Cancer. 2003;4 Suppl 1:S10–9.
44. Liu SV, Melstrom L, Yao K, Russell CA, Sener SF. Neoadjuvant therapy for breast cancer. J Surg Oncol. 2010;101(4):283–91.
45. Mauri D, Pavlidis N, Ioannidis JP. Neoadjuvant versus adjuvant systemic treatment in breast cancer: a meta-analysis. J Natl Cancer Inst. 2005;97(3):188–94.
46. Cunningham JD, Weiss SE, Ahmed S, et al. The efficacy of neoadjuvant chemotherapy compared to postoperative therapy in the treatment of locally advanced breast cancer. Cancer Invest. 1998;16(2):80–6.
47. Ueno NT, Buzdar AU, Singletary SE, et al. Combined-modality treatment of inflammatory breast carcinoma: twenty years of experience at M. D Anderson Cancer Center. Cancer Chemother Pharmacol. 1997;40(4):321–9.
48. Bear HD, Anderson S, Brown A, et al. The effect on tumor response of adding sequential preoperative docetaxel to preoperative doxorubicin and cyclophosphamide: preliminary results from National Surgical Adjuvant Breast and Bowel Project Protocol B-27. J Clin Oncol. 2003;21(22):4165–74.
49. von Minckwitz G, Kümmel S, Vogel P, et al. Intensified neoadjuvant chemotherapy in early-responding breast cancer: phase III randomized GeparTrio study. J Natl Cancer Inst. 2008;100(8):552–62.
50. Smith IC, Heys SD, Hutcheon AW, et al. Neoadjuvant chemotherapy in breast cancer: significantly enhanced response with docetaxel. J Clin Oncol. 2002;20(6):1456–66.
51. Cristofanilli M, Gonzalez-Angulo AM, Buzdar AU, Kau SW, Frye DK, Hortobagyi GN. Paclitaxel improves the prognosis in estrogen receptor negative inflammatory breast cancer: the M. D Anderson Cancer Center experience. Clin Breast Cancer. 2004;4(6):415–9.
52. Charehbili A, Fontein DB, Kroep JR, et al. Neoadjuvant hormonal therapy for endocrine sensitive breast cancer: a systematic review. Cancer Treat Rev. 2014;40(1):86–92.

53. clinicaltrials.gov/show/NCT01622361. Neo-adjuvant study of chemotherapy versus endocrine therapy in premenopausal patient with hormone responsive, HER2 negative, lymph node positive breast cancer (NEST). 2013. Accessed 12 Feb 2014.
54. Dixon JM, Anderson TJ, Miller WR. Neoadjuvant endocrine therapy of breast cancer: a surgical perspective. Eur J Cancer. 2002;38(17):2214–21.
55. Ellis MJ, Coop A, Singh B, et al. Letrozole is more effective neoadjuvant endocrine therapy than tamoxifen for ErbB-1- and/or ErbB-2-positive, estrogen receptor-positive primary breast cancer: evidence from a phase III randomized trial. J Clin Oncol. 2001;19(18):3808–16.
56. Cataliotti L, Buzdar AU, Noguchi S, et al. Comparison of anastrozole versus tamoxifen as preoperative therapy in postmenopausal women with hormone receptor-positive breast cancer: the preoperative "Arimidex" compared to Tamoxifen (PROACT) trial. Cancer. 2006;106(10):2095–103.
57. Eiermann W, Paepke S, Appfelstaedt J, et al. Preoperative treatment of postmenopausal breast cancer patients with letrozole: a randomized double-blind multicenter study. Ann Oncol. 2001;12(11):1527–32.
58. Masuda N, Sagara Y, Kinoshita T, et al. Neoadjuvant anastrozole versus tamoxifen in patients receiving goserelin for premenopausal breast cancer (STAGE): a double-blind, randomised phase 3 trial. Lancet Oncol. 2012;13(4):345–52.
59. Ellis MJ, Suman VJ, Hoog J, et al. Randomized phase II neoadjuvant comparison between letrozole, anastrozole, and exemestane for postmenopausal women with estrogen receptor-rich stage 2 to 3 breast cancer: clinical and biomarker outcomes and predictive value of the baseline PAM50-based intrinsic subtype - ACOSOG Z103. J Clin Oncol. 2011;29(17):2342–9.
60. Smith IE, Dowsett M, Ebbs SR, et al. Neoadjuvant treatment of postmenopausal breast cancer with anastrozole, tamoxifen, or both in combination: the Immediate Preoperative Anastrozole, Tamoxifen, or Combined with Tamoxifen (IMPACT) multicenter double-blind randomized trial. J Clin Oncol. 2005;23(22):5108–16.
61. Cardoso F, Loibl S, Pagani O, et al. The European Society of Breast Cancer Specialists recommendations for the management of young women with breast cancer. Eur J Cancer. 2012;48(18):3355–77.
62. Ellis MJ, Tao Y, Luo J, et al. Outcome prediction for estrogen receptor-positive breast cancer based on postneoadjuvant endocrine therapy tumor characteristics. J Natl Cancer Inst. 2008;100(19):1380–8.
63. Hind D, Wyld L, Beverley CB, Reed MW. Surgery versus primary endocrine therapy for operable primary breast cancer in elderly women (70 years plus). Cochrane Database Syst Rev. 2006;(1), CD004272.
64. Gianni L, Eiermann W, Semiglazov V, Manikhas A, Lluch A, et al. Follow-up results of NOAH, a randomized phase III trial evaluating neoadjuvant chemotherapy with trastuzumab (CT+H) followed by adjuvant H versus CT alone, in patients with HER2-positive locally advanced breast cancer. J Clin Oncol. 2013;31(Suppl):Abstract 503.
65. Slamon DJ, Leyland-Jones B, Shak S, et al. Use of chemotherapy plus a monoclonal antibody against HER2 for metastatic breast cancer that overexpresses HER2. N Engl J Med. 2001;344(11):783–92.
66. Boussen H, Cristofanilli M, Zaks T, DeSilvio M, Salazar V, Spector N. Phase II study to evaluate the efficacy and safety of neoadjuvant lapatinib plus paclitaxel in patients with inflammatory breast cancer. J Clin Oncol. 2010;28(20):3248–55.
67. Schneeweiss A, Chia S, Hickish T, et al. Pertuzumab plus trastuzumab in combination with standard neoadjuvant anthracycline-containing and anthracycline-free chemotherapy regimens in patients with HER2-positive early breast cancer: a randomized phase II cardiac safety study (TRYPHAENA). Ann Oncol. 2013;24(9):2278–84.
68. Gianni L, Pienkowski T, Im YH, et al. Efficacy and safety of neoadjuvant pertuzumab and trastuzumab in women with locally advanced, inflammatory, or early HER2-positive breast cancer (NeoSphere): a randomised multicentre, open-label, phase 2 trial. Lancet Oncol. 2012;13(1):25–32.
69. Guarneri V, Frassoldati A, Bottini A, et al. Preoperative chemotherapy plus trastuzumab, lapatinib, or both in human epidermal growth factor receptor 2-positive operable breast cancer: results of the randomized phase II CHER-LOB study. J Clin Oncol. 2012;30(16):1989–95.
70. Baselga J, Bradbury I, Eidtmann H, et al. Lapatinib with trastuzumab for HER2-positive early breast cancer (NeoALTTO): a randomised, open-label, multicentre, phase 3 trial. Lancet. 2012;379(9816):633–40.
71. Untch M, Loibl S, Bischoff J, et al. Lapatinib versus trastuzumab in combination with neoadjuvant anthracycline-taxane-based chemotherapy (GeparQuinto, GBG 44): a randomised phase 3 trial. Lancet Oncol. 2012;13(2):135–44.
72. Robidoux A, Tang G, Rastogi P, et al. Evaluation of lapatinib as a component of neoadjuvant therapy for HER-2+ operable breast cancer: NSABP protocol B-41. J Clin Oncol. 2012;30(18 (Suppl)):Abstract LBA506.
73. von Minckwitz G, Eidtmann H, Loibl S, et al. Integrating bevacizumab, everolimus, and lapatinib into current neoadjuvant chemotherapy regimen for primary breast cancer. Safety results of the GeparQuinto trial. Ann Oncol. 2011;22(2):301–6.
74. Wedam SB, Low JA, Yang SX, et al. Antiangiogenic and antitumor effects of bevacizumab in patients with inflammatory and locally advanced breast cancer. J Clin Oncol. 2006;24(5):769–77.
75. Greil R, Moik M, Reitsamer R, et al. Neoadjuvant bevacizumab, docetaxel and capecitabine combination therapy for HER2/neu-negative invasive breast cancer: efficacy and safety in a phase II pilot study. Eur J Surg Oncol. 2009;35(10):1048–54.

76. Yardley D, Raefsky E, Castillo R, Lahiry A, LoCicero D, et al. Results of a multicenter pilot study of weekly nab-paclitaxel, carboplatin with bevacizumab, and trastuzumab as neoadjuvant therapy in HER2+ locally advanced breast cancer with SPARC correlatives. J Clin Oncol. 2009;27(15s (Suppl)):Abstract 527.
77. Hurvitz S, Bosserman L, Leland-Jones B, Thirwell M, Allison M, et al. A multicenter, double-blind randomized phase II trial of neoadjuvant treatment with single-agent bevacizumab or placebo, followed by docetaxel, doxorubicin, and cyclophosphamide (TAC), with or without bevacizumab, in patients with stage II or stage III breast cancer. J Clin Oncol. 2008;26(15S (Suppl)):Abstract 562.
78. Overmoyer B, Silverman P, Leeming R, Shenk R, et al. Phase II trial of neoadjuvant docetaxel with or without bevacizumab in patients with locally advanced breast cancer. J Clin Oncol. 2004;22(14S (Suppl)):Abstract 727.
79. Waintraub S, Tuchman V. The role of preoperative neoadjuvant cytoreductive dose-dense bevacizumab plus docetaxel followed by bevacizumab-doxorubicin-cyclophosphamide regimen in locally advanced operable breast cancer. J Clin Oncol. 2009;27(15S (Suppl)):Abstract e11524.
80. Hylton NM, Blume JD, Bernreuter WK, et al. Locally advanced breast cancer: MR imaging for prediction of response to neoadjuvant chemotherapy–results from ACRIN 6657/I-SPY TRIAL. Radiology. 2012;263(3):663–72.
81. Prevos R, Smidt ML, Tjan-Heijnen VC, et al. Pretreatment differences and early response monitoring of neoadjuvant chemotherapy in breast cancer patients using magnetic resonance imaging: a systematic review. Eur Radiol. 2012;22(12):2607–16.
82. von Minckwitz G, Kümmel S, Vogel P, et al. Neoadjuvant vinorelbine-capecitabine versus docetaxel-doxorubicin-cyclophosphamide in early nonresponsive breast cancer: phase III randomized GeparTrio trial. J Natl Cancer Inst. 2008;100(8): 542–51.
83. McGuire KP, Toro-Burguete J, Dang H, et al. MRI staging after neoadjuvant chemotherapy for breast cancer: does tumor biology affect accuracy? Ann Surg Oncol. 2011;18(11):3149–54.
84. Loo CE, Straver ME, Rodenhuis S, et al. Magnetic resonance imaging response monitoring of breast cancer during neoadjuvant chemotherapy: relevance of breast cancer subtype. J Clin Oncol. 2011;29(6): 660–6.
85. Chen JH, Mehta RS, Nalcioglu O, Su MY. Inflammatory breast cancer after neoadjuvant chemotherapy: can magnetic resonance imaging precisely diagnose the final pathological response? Ann Surg Oncol. 2008;15(12):3609–13.
86. Avril N, Sassen S, Roylance R. Response to therapy in breast cancer. J Nucl Med. 2009;50 Suppl 1: 55S–63.
87. Chen AM, Meric-Bernstam F, Hunt KK, et al. Breast conservation after neoadjuvant chemotherapy. Cancer. 2005;103(4):689–95.
88. Boughey JC, Suman VJ, Mittendorf EA, et al. Sentinel lymph node surgery after neoadjuvant chemotherapy in patients with node-positive breast cancer: the ACOSOG Z1071 (Alliance) clinical trial. JAMA. 2013;310(14):1455–61.
89. Kuehn T, Bauerfeind I, Fehm T, et al. Sentinel-lymph-node biopsy in patients with breast cancer before and after neoadjuvant chemotherapy (SENTINA): a prospective, multicentre cohort study. Lancet Oncol. 2013;14(7):609–18.
90. Kaufmann M, von Minckwitz G, Mamounas EP, et al. Recommendations from an international consensus conference on the current status and future of neoadjuvant systemic therapy in primary breast cancer. Ann Surg Oncol. 2012;19(5):1508–16.
91. Edeiken BS, Fornage BD, Bedi DG, et al. US-guided implantation of metallic markers for permanent localization of the tumor bed in patients with breast cancer who undergo preoperative chemotherapy. Radiology. 1999;213(3):895–900.
92. Dash N, Chafin SH, Johnson RR, Contractor FM. Usefulness of tissue marker clips in patients undergoing neoadjuvant chemotherapy for breast cancer. AJR Am J Roentgenol. 1999;173(4):911–7.
93. Fleming RY, Asmar L, Buzdar AU, et al. Effectiveness of mastectomy by response to induction chemotherapy for control in inflammatory breast carcinoma. Ann Surg Oncol. 1997;4(6):452–61.
94. Chu QD, McDonald JC, Li BD. Adjuvant therapy for patients who have node-positive breast cancer. Adv Surg. 2006;40:77–98.
95. Ragaz J, Jackson SM, Le N, et al. Adjuvant radiotherapy and chemotherapy in node-positive premenopausal women with breast cancer. N Engl J Med. 1997;337(14):956–62.
96. Ragaz J, Olivotto IA, Spinelli JJ, et al. Locoregional radiation therapy in patients with high-risk breast cancer receiving adjuvant chemotherapy: 20-year results of the British Columbia randomized trial. J Natl Cancer Inst. 2005;97(2):116–26.
97. Overgaard M, Hansen PS, Overgaard J, et al. Postoperative radiotherapy in high-risk premenopausal women with breast cancer who receive adjuvant chemotherapy. Danish Breast Cancer Cooperative Group 82b Trial. N Engl J Med. 1997;337(14):949–55.
98. Overgaard M, Jensen MB, Overgaard J, et al. Postoperative radiotherapy in high-risk postmenopausal breast-cancer patients given adjuvant tamoxifen: Danish Breast Cancer Cooperative Group DBCG 82c randomised trial. Lancet. 1999; 353(9165):1641–8.
99. Effects of radiotherapy and surgery in early breast cancer. An overview of the randomized trials. Early Breast Cancer Trialists' Collaborative Group. N Engl J Med. 1995;333(22):1444–55.

100. Cuzick J, Stewart H, Peto R, et al. Overview of randomized trials comparing radical mastectomy without radiotherapy against simple mastectomy with radiotherapy in breast cancer. Cancer Treat Rep. 1987;71(1):7–14.
101. Cuzick J, Stewart H, Rutqvist L, et al. Cause-specific mortality in long-term survivors of breast cancer who participated in trials of radiotherapy. J Clin Oncol. 1994;12(3):447–53.
102. Whelan TJ, Julian J, Wright J, Jadad AR, Levine ML. Does locoregional radiation therapy improve survival in breast cancer? A meta-analysis. J Clin Oncol. 2000;18(6):1220–9.
103. Favourable and unfavourable effects on long-term survival of radiotherapy for early breast cancer: an overview of the randomised trials. Early Breast Cancer Trialists' Collaborative Group. Lancet. 2000;355(9217):1757–70.
104. Taghian A, Jeong JH, Mamounas E, et al. Patterns of locoregional failure in patients with operable breast cancer treated by mastectomy and adjuvant chemotherapy with or without tamoxifen and without radiotherapy: results from five National Surgical Adjuvant Breast and Bowel Project randomized clinical trials. J Clin Oncol. 2004;22(21):4247–54.
105. Recht A, Gray R, Davidson NE, et al. Locoregional failure 10 years after mastectomy and adjuvant chemotherapy with or without tamoxifen without irradiation: experience of the Eastern Cooperative Oncology Group. J Clin Oncol. 1999;17(6):1689–700.
106. Katz A, Strom EA, Buchholz TA, et al. Locoregional recurrence patterns after mastectomy and doxorubicin-based chemotherapy: implications for postoperative irradiation. J Clin Oncol. 2000;18(15): 2817–27.
107. Wallgren A, Bonetti M, Gelber RD, et al. Risk factors for locoregional recurrence among breast cancer patients: results from International Breast Cancer Study Group Trials I through VII. J Clin Oncol. 2003;21(7):1205–13.
108. Pierce LJ. The use of radiotherapy after mastectomy: a review of the literature. J Clin Oncol. 2005;23(8): 1706–17.
109. Perou CM, Sørlie T, Eisen MB, et al. Molecular portraits of human breast tumours. Nature. 2000;406(6797):747–52.
110. Sørlie T, Perou CM, Tibshirani R, et al. Gene expression patterns of breast carcinomas distinguish tumor subclasses with clinical implications. Proc Natl Acad Sci U S A. 2001;98(19):10869–74.
111. Kyndi M, Sørensen FB, Knudsen H, et al. Estrogen receptor, progesterone receptor, HER-2, and response to postmastectomy radiotherapy in high-risk breast cancer: the Danish Breast Cancer Cooperative Group. J Clin Oncol. 2008;26(9):1419–26.
112. Somlo G, Frankel P, Chow W, et al. Prognostic indicators and survival in patients with stage IIIB inflammatory breast carcinoma after dose-intense chemotherapy. J Clin Oncol. 2004;22(10):1839–48.
113. Hortobagyi GN, Ames FC, Buzdar AU, et al. Management of stage III primary breast cancer with primary chemotherapy, surgery, and radiation therapy. Cancer. 1988;62(12):2507–16.
114. Perloff M, Lesnick GJ, Korzun A, et al. Combination chemotherapy with mastectomy or radiotherapy for stage III breast carcinoma: a Cancer and Leukemia Group B study. J Clin Oncol. 1988;6(2):261–9.
115. Pierce LJ, Lippman M, Ben-Baruch N, et al. The effect of systemic therapy on local-regional control in locally advanced breast cancer. Int J Radiat Oncol Biol Phys. 1992;23(5):949–60.
116. Low JA, Berman AW, Steinberg SM, Danforth DN, Lippman ME, Swain SM. Long-term follow-up for locally advanced and inflammatory breast cancer patients treated with multimodality therapy. J Clin Oncol. 2004;22(20):4067–74.
117. Colozza M, Gori S, Mosconi AM, et al. Induction chemotherapy with cisplatin, doxorubicin, and cyclophosphamide (CAP) in a combined modality approach for locally advanced and inflammatory breast cancer. Long-term results. Am J Clin Oncol. 1996;19(1):10–7.
118. Clark J, Rosenman J, Cance W, Halle J, Graham M. Extending the indications for breast-conserving treatment to patients with locally advanced breast cancer. Int J Radiat Oncol Biol Phys. 1998;42(2): 345–50.
119. Cristofanilli M, Buzdar AU, Sneige N, et al. Paclitaxel in the multimodality treatment for inflammatory breast carcinoma. Cancer. 2001;92(7):1775–82.
120. Favret AM, Carlson RW, Goffinet DR, Jeffrey SS, Dirbas FM, Stockdale FE. Locally advanced breast cancer: is surgery necessary? Breast J. 2001;7(2): 131–7.
121. Hutcheon AW, Heys SD, Sarkar TK, Group AB. Neoadjuvant docetaxel in locally advanced breast cancer. Breast Cancer Res Treat. 2003;79 Suppl 1:S19–24.
122. Harris EE, Schultz D, Bertsch H, Fox K, Glick J, Solin LJ. Ten-year outcome after combined modality therapy for inflammatory breast cancer. Int J Radiat Oncol Biol Phys. 2003;55(5):1200–8.
123. McIntosh SA, Ogston KN, Payne S, et al. Local recurrence in patients with large and locally advanced breast cancer treated with primary chemotherapy. Am J Surg. 2003;185(6):525–31.
124. Therasse P, Mauriac L, Welnicka-Jaskiewicz M, et al. Final results of a randomized phase III trial comparing cyclophosphamide, epirubicin, and fluorouracil with a dose-intensified epirubicin and cyclophosphamide + filgrastim as neoadjuvant treatment in locally advanced breast cancer: an EORTC-NCIC-SAKK multicenter study. J Clin Oncol. 2003;21(5):843–50.
125. Espinosa E, Morales S, Borrega P, et al. Docetaxel and high-dose epirubicin as neoadjuvant chemotherapy in locally advanced breast cancer. Cancer Chemother Pharmacol. 2004;54(6):546–52.

126. Ezzat AA, Ibrahim EM, Ajarim DS, et al. Phase II study of neoadjuvant paclitaxel and cisplatin for operable and locally advanced breast cancer: analysis of 126 patients. Br J Cancer. 2004;90(5):968–74.
127. Gajdos C, Tartter PI, Estabrook A, Gistrak MA, Jaffer S, Bleiweiss IJ. Relationship of clinical and pathologic response to neoadjuvant chemotherapy and outcome of locally advanced breast cancer. J Surg Oncol. 2002;80(1):4–11.
128. Lebowitz PF, Eng-Wong J, Swain SM, et al. A phase II trial of neoadjuvant docetaxel and capecitabine for locally advanced breast cancer. Clin Cancer Res. 2004;10(20):6764–9.
129. de Matteis A, Nuzzo F, D'Aiuto G, et al. Docetaxel plus epidoxorubicin as neoadjuvant treatment in patients with large operable or locally advanced carcinoma of the breast: a single-center, phase II study. Cancer. 2002;94(4):895–901.
130. Shen J, Valero V, Buchholz TA, et al. Effective local control and long-term survival in patients with T4 locally advanced breast cancer treated with breast conservation therapy. Ann Surg Oncol. 2004;11(9):854–60.
131. Thomas E, Holmes FA, Smith TL, et al. The use of alternate, non-cross-resistant adjuvant chemotherapy on the basis of pathologic response to a neoadjuvant doxorubicin-based regimen in women with operable breast cancer: long-term results from a prospective randomized trial. J Clin Oncol. 2004;22(12):2294–302.
132. Erol K, Baltali E, Altundag K, et al. Neoadjuvant chemotherapy with cyclophosphamide, mitoxantrone, and 5-fluorouracil in locally advanced breast cancer. Onkologie. 2005;28(2):81–5.
133. Gradishar WJ, Wedam SB, Jahanzeb M, et al. Neoadjuvant docetaxel followed by adjuvant doxorubicin and cyclophosphamide in patients with stage III breast cancer. Ann Oncol. 2005;16(8):1297–304.
134. Kao J, Conzen SD, Jaskowiak NT, et al. Concomitant radiation therapy and paclitaxel for unresectable locally advanced breast cancer: results from two consecutive phase I/II trials. Int J Radiat Oncol Biol Phys. 2005;61(4):1045–53.
135. Tham YL, Gomez LF, Mohsin S, et al. Clinical response to neoadjuvant docetaxel predicts improved outcome in patients with large locally advanced breast cancers. Breast Cancer Res Treat. 2005;94(3):279–84.
136. Veyret C, Levy C, Chollet P, et al. Inflammatory breast cancer outcome with epirubicin-based induction and maintenance chemotherapy: ten-year results from the French Adjuvant Study Group GETIS 02 Trial. Cancer. 2006;107(11):2535–44.
137. Ellis G, Green S, Russell C, et al. SWOG 0012, a randomized phase III comparison of standard doxorubicin and cyclophosphamide followed by weekly paclitaxel versus weekly doxorubicin and daily oral cyclophosphamide plus G-CSF followed by weekly paclitaxel as neoadjuvant therapy for inflammatory and locally advanced breast cancer. J Clin Oncol. 2006;24, LBA537.
138. Villman K, Ohd JF, Lidbrink E, et al. A phase II study of epirubicin, cisplatin and capecitabine as neoadjuvant chemotherapy in locally advanced or inflammatory breast cancer. Eur J Cancer. 2007;43(7):1153–60.
139. Manga GP, Shahi PK, Ureña MM, et al. Phase II study of neoadjuvant treatment with doxorubicin, docetaxel, and capecitabine (ATX) in locally advanced or inflammatory breast cancer. Breast Cancer. 2010;17(3):205–11.

BRCA1 and BRCA2 in Breast Cancer and Ovarian Cancer

6

Michael R. Cassidy and Jane E. Méndez

Learning Objectives

After reading this chapter, you should be able to:

- Learn how to recognize patients who may harbor BRCA1/2 mutations
- Appreciate the lifetime risk of developing breast cancer and ovarian cancer for those with BRCA1/2 mutations
- Know the management options for patients with BRCA1/2 mutations
- Understand the role of prophylactic mastectomy and prophylactic bilateral oophorectomy in patients with BRCA1/2 mutations

Introduction

Familial cancer predisposition syndromes, such as BRCA1 and BRCA2, are increasingly recognized as a genetically unique subset of diseases. A developing understanding of molecular genetics, along with advances in genetic testing technologies, has allowed for the identification of underlying causative genetic mutations that confer a dramatically increased risk for cancer. Consequently, there are distinct issues of diagnosis, management, and multidisciplinary support for those at risk of inherited cancer syndromes and those already diagnosed with the predisposing gene mutation. Inherited autosomal dominant gene mutations account for 5–10 % of all cases of breast cancer [1]. Among these highly penetrant genes are BRCA1, BRCA2, TP53, and PTEN. By far, the most common inherited breast cancer predisposition syndromes are associated with the BRCA1 and BRCA2 genes. While breast cancer syndromes caused by mutations in TP53 and PTEN are significant and deserve to be acknowledged, they are rare and will not be discussed within this chapter.

Incidence of Cancer in BRCA1 and BRCA2 Mutation Carriers

A range of breast cancer risk estimates appear in the literature related to BRCA1 and BRCA2 mutations. Early studies suggested BRCA1 mutations to confer a lifetime risk of breast cancer as high as 87 %, while the risk conferred by BRCA2 was quoted as 84 %. Because these studies included only families with significant numbers of cancer diagnoses, they may have been biased toward highly penetrant gene variants [2, 3]. Since that time, a large meta-analysis by Chen et al. showed the risk of breast cancer conferred

M.R. Cassidy, M.D.
Department of Surgery, Boston University School of Medicine, Boston Medical Center, 88 East Newton Street, 02118 Boston, MA, USA
e-mail: michael.cassidy@bmc.org

J.E. Méndez, M.D., F.A.C.S. (✉)
Department of Surgery, Surgical Oncology, Boston Medical Center/Boston University School of Medicine, 820 Harrison Avenue Suite 5006, 02199 Boston, MA, USA
e-mail: jane.mendez@bmc.org; jmendez88@aol.com

Q.D. Chu et al. (eds.), *Surgical Oncology: A Practical and Comprehensive Approach*,
DOI 10.1007/978-1-4939-1423-4_6,

by BRCA1 to be between 57 % and 65 %, while the risk conferred by BRCA2 was 45 % and 49 % [4]. In patients with a known BRCA mutation already diagnosed with breast cancer, the risk of a second breast cancer has been reported to be 3 % per year [5]. In terms of ovarian cancer, the risk conferred by BRCA1 and BRCA2 mutations was 40 % and 18 %, respectively [4].

Tumor Profiles of BRCA1- and BRCA2-Associated Cancers

Specific tumor characteristics have been associated with mutations in the BRCA1 and BRCA2 genes. Patients found to have mutations of BRCA1 are likely to have breast cancers that are estrogen receptor negative, progesterone receptor negative, and Her-2/neu negative, also known as "triple-negative" breast cancers. They are more commonly high grade when compared to the general population of breast cancer patients, and they are frequently diagnosed at a young age, in the third or fourth decade of life. Medullary carcinoma of the breast, while representing only 2 % of breast cancers in the general population, has been observed in up to 13 % of BRCA1 mutation carriers [6–8].

In contrast, BRCA2-associated breast cancers more closely resemble tumor profiles of sporadic breast cancer and are most often invasive ductal carcinomas. BRCA2 mutation carriers more often have estrogen receptor-positive breast cancer, although in general the tumor characteristics are less distinct than BRCA1-associated cancers [9]. These tumors are diagnosed at a slightly older age than those associated with BRCA1 mutations.

As mentioned, BRCA1 and BRCA2 mutations both confer risk for other cancers in addition to breast cancer. Most notably, those with mutations of BRCA1 have a 40 % lifetime risk of ovarian cancer, which is generally epithelial in origin and high grade and diagnosed at an advanced stage, with an average age at diagnosis of 38. Cancers of the fallopian tube and primary peritoneal cancers may also be observed. Women with BRCA2 mutations have an 18 % lifetime risk of ovarian cancer, along with fallopian tube and primary peritoneal cancers, typically diagnosed after 50 years of age [10]. Additionally, BRCA1 mutation carriers are at increased risk for pancreas and prostate cancers, while BRCA2 carriers are at increased risk for pancreas, prostate, and colon cancers [9, 11, 12].

Genetics

BRCA1 and BRCA2 are tumor suppressor genes, with a proposed role in coding for proteins involved in DNA repair. Specific identified mutations in these two genes have been associated with dramatically increased risk for breast cancer and other cancers. Over 1,000 specific gene mutations have been identified to date; the majority of these mutations lead to truncated forms of their respective proteins. Largely they are deletions, duplications, frameshift, or nonsense mutations [13]. Classically, a "two-hit" hypothesis was thought to be required for the development of cancer in the setting of autosomal dominantly inherited susceptibility mutations. This hypothesis means that an inherited mutation in one gene allele must be accompanied by a loss of the corresponding wild-type allele in order to cause a cancer phenotype. In BRCA1- and BRCA2-associated cancers, there are conflicting data as to whether the "two-hit" hypothesis applies. Some studies have supported the idea that loss of the wild-type allele is necessary to cause cancer, while other studies have refuted that concept [14–18].

Because BRCA1 and BRCA2 mutations are inherited in an autosomal dominant fashion, carriers will pass the mutation to approximately 50 % of their offspring. While the genes are considered to be highly penetrant, the cancer risk conferred may be variable, even within families that harbor the same mutation [19]. The extent to which environmental or other genetic factors play a role in disease expression is unknown.

The BRCA1 gene is found on chromosome 17q11. It contains 22 coding exons and spans approximately 100 kilobases of DNA. Its messenger RNA is 7.8 kilobases. It encodes a protein that contains 1,863 amino acids and is thought to function in regulating transcription, cell cycle control, and DNA damage repair pathways [20–25].

The BRCA2 gene is found on 13q12–13. It contains 26 coding exons and encodes a protein that contains 3,418 amino acids but currently has an unknown biologic function. Although its role in the normal cell is yet to be completely defined, the BRCA2 protein is thought to function in a similar way to the BRCA1 protein, in regulating the cell cycle and participating in DNA damage repair.

Persons of Ashkenazi Jewish heritage deserve special mention. Mutations of BRCA1 and BRCA2 are found with higher frequency in this ethnic population than in the general population. Several "founder mutations" have been identified in Ashkenazi Jewish individuals with breast cancer – in BRCA1, the most common mutations in this cohort are 185delAG and 5382insC. These specific variants account for nearly all of the BRCA1 mutations identified in this group. 185delAG and 5382insC are found at an incidence 10 times higher in the Ashkenazi Jewish population than that in the non-Jewish population. 185delAG in particular is found in 1 % of Ashkenazi Jewish women and underlies approximately 20 % of breast cancers diagnosed before the age of 40 in that population [26]. 6174delT is a founder mutation of the BRCA2 gene also present with high frequency in this group, with a described prevalence of 1.2 %. While many Ashkenazi Jewish women with breast cancer will be found to have one of these three specific founder mutations, some will have another BRCA1 or BRCA2 mutation; therefore, full sequencing of the BRCA1 and BRCA2 may be necessary for diagnosis [23, 27]. In Icelandic and Finnish populations, an identified founder mutation of the BRCA2 gene is 999del5.

It is important to distinguish autosomal dominant familial genetic syndromes from a family history of sporadic breast cancer. Approximately 23 % of patients with breast cancer will have a family history of the disease, but the majority of these will not be associated with the highly penetrant genes [28]. Rather, most cases of breast cancer in which there is a reported family history are thought to be due to mutations with low penetrance that are largely unidentified and confer an unknown degree of increased risk. BRCA1 and BRCA2 single-gene mutations, along with the other rare single-gene mutations, are a distinct category of risk for the development of breast cancer. Therefore, while a strong family history may suggest the need for further investigation, it is statistically more likely that a single-gene variant will not be discovered. This fact has implications for screening and management, as discussed later in this chapter.

Screening and Diagnosis

Screening recommendations for BRCA1 and BRCA2 have been proposed by several organizations. The American Society of Clinical Oncology (ASCO) suggests that three criteria be met when selecting candidates for genetic testing related to breast cancer genetic syndromes. First, the patient should have a personal or family history suggestive of an inherited highly penetrant genetic syndrome. Second, the test must be performed under conditions where it can be interpreted adequately. And third, the test should be performed only if its results will inform the management of the patient or his or her family members [29] (Table 6.1). The National Comprehensive Cancer Network has published guidelines for genetic counseling referrals in regard to genetic breast cancer risk. Some of these include personal or family history of early-onset breast cancer (defined as age <50 years at diagnosis); personal or family history of ovarian, fallopian tube, or primary peritoneal cancers; persons with two or more primary breast cancers; family history of breast cancer and an additional diagnosis of thyroid cancer,

Table 6.1 ASCO recommendations for genetic counseling and testing

The individual has personal or family history features suggestive of genetic cancer susceptibility
The genetic test can be adequately interpreted
The test results will aid in the management of the patient or his/her family members

Based on data from Ref. [29]

sarcoma, adrenocortical carcinoma, endometrial cancer, pancreatic cancer, brain cancer, gastric cancer, leukemia, or lymphoma on the same side of the family; men with breast cancer; and Ashkenazi Jewish ethnicity [30, 31]. Any consideration of genetic testing for hereditary cancer syndromes requires thoughtful patient education and referral to a certified genetic counselor.

The American Society of Breast Surgeons position statement on BRCA genetic testing suggests that any of the following features should prompt education and referral to genetic counseling [32]:

- Breast cancer diagnosed before the age of 50
- Two primary breast cancers in the same person
- A family history of breast cancer diagnosed before the age of 50
- Breast cancer in a man
- Personal or family history of ovarian cancer
- Personal or family diagnosis of breast cancer in the setting of Ashkenazi Jewish heritage
- A known BRCA1 or BRCA2 mutation within the family
- Triple-negative breast cancer diagnosed before the age of 60
- Pancreatic cancer associated with family history of breast or ovarian cancer

Statistical models intended to provide a likelihood of having an underlying BRCA1 or BRCA2 mutation have been developed and incorporate the personal and family history variables described above. Available models include BRCAPRO and the Breast and Ovarian Analysis of Disease Incidence and Carrier Estimation Algorithm [33, 34].

A detailed and comprehensive family history should be obtained by the clinician considering genetic testing for any patient. In regard to testing for BRCA1 and BRCA2 breast cancer syndromes, it must be recognized that these genes carry not only increased risk for breast cancer, but for other cancers as well. As such, a three-generation family history is recommended, which should elicit details about any cancers diagnosed in relatives, with particular attention to cancers of the breast, ovaries, endometrium, thyroid, adrenal, pancreas, brain, or soft tissues. Furthermore, as BRCA1 and BRCA2 are autosomal dominant and may be inherited from either parent, both maternal and paternal family histories should be thoroughly obtained. When possible, other important details to collect in the family history include age at diagnosis of cancer, risk reduction variables including chemoprevention or prophylactic operations, exposure to carcinogens, hormone and reproductive history, and previous breast biopsies. As these details are sophisticated, verification from medical records is recommended, whenever possible [35].

There are several factors that may render the family history less informative. A small family size, or a low number of the susceptible gender for gender-specific cancers, may decrease sensitivity to detect genetic predisposition syndromes. Furthermore, prophylactic operations that remove the susceptible organs create uncertainty as to whether cancer would have developed in that family member. Deaths at an early age, before the age of onset of inherited cancer syndromes, may limit the utility of the family history. If any of these factors is present, the probability of BRCA1 or BRCA2 mutation may be underestimated [36].

When the decision has been made to pursue genetic testing based on the available personal and family history, the recommended strategy is to test a family member who has already been diagnosed with cancer. This recommendation follows from the fact that a negative test in an unaffected person is rather inconclusive. It would remain unknown whether a gene mutation exists in the family, as the tested unaffected person may simply have not inherited the gene that is indeed present in other family members. Additionally, those who undergo full BRCA1 and BRCA2 gene sequencing may have a result indicating a variant of unknown significance, which indicates a DNA mutation that may or may not confer increased cancer risk.

Furthermore, if an already diagnosed person is tested, and a mutation is revealed, it allows subsequent family members to be tested only for the specific gene mutation already identified as the culprit within the family; therefore, it saves additional family members from full genetic sequencing of BRCA1 and BRCA2. In high-risk ethnic populations, such as Ashkenazi Jewish, Icelandic, and Finnish, who in general harbor increased frequency of specific founder mutations, an accepted strategy is to first test the individual specifically for the founder mutation. If the initial test is negative, proceeding to full sequencing of the BRCA1 and BRCA2 genes is then recommended.

There are several possible outcomes of genetic testing for BRCA1 or BRCA2 mutations. First, a test may indicate the existence of a known mutation causing abnormal function of the BRCA1 or BRCA2 protein. This result indicates an increased risk of breast, ovarian, and other cancers, as discussed previously. Patients with this result should then be managed according to guidelines for those with increased risk, which will include surveillance, chemoprevention, or prophylactic operations. A negative result, indicating no identified mutation of BRCA1 or BRCA2, must be interpreted in the context of personal and family history. In a patient with a known gene mutation in the family, a negative result for that specific mutation will mean that the patient has not inherited the trait; his or her risk for cancer is then considered to be equivalent to the general population and is based on factors recognized to be associated with cancers in established risk estimation models. In a patient already diagnosed with cancer, a negative result may have one of several interpretations. It may indicate that a gene mutation is not present within the family, or that a mutation does exist, but cannot be identified with current sequencing technology. It is also possible that a BRCA mutation may exist within a family, while a tested individual with cancer has a sporadic form of cancer. Finally, genetic testing for BRCA gene mutations may have an indeterminate result. That is, there may be small mutations, located in non-critical gene domains, that have unknown consequences for the functional protein. This result confers an unknown cancer risk.

In those already diagnosed with cancer and suspected of having a genetic predisposition syndrome, testing should be considered before definitive treatment plans have been decided, according to the patient's preferences. The result of the genetic test may inform the decisions regarding treatment options. For example, a woman may use the information to decide whether to pursue breast conservation or mastectomy on the affected side and may additionally consider contralateral prophylactic mastectomy based on the results of the genetic testing. However, some patients may elect to proceed with treatment for the primary cancer without genetic testing results.

The implication of genetic testing for hereditary cancer on health insurance coverage has been a concern of patients and may contribute to anxiety surrounding the test. In general, genetic test results are protected from disclosure to health insurance providers. It is illegal in the United States to deny insurance coverage based on genetic testing results and similarly illegal to consider genetic information as a preexisting condition, owing to protections set forth in the Health Insurance Portability and Accountability Act (HIPAA) of 1996. Furthermore, the federal Genetic Information Nondiscrimination Act (GINA) of 2008 prohibits discrimination based on genetic test results. Patients can generally be reassured that there is little risk to future health insurance coverage based on genetic testing results alone; however, insurance providers may inquire about cancer diagnoses within the family and the individual.

For many years, a company known as Myriad Genetics held patents making it the exclusive provider of BRCA1 and BRCA2 genetic testing in the United States. The tests were costly, at up to $4,000, which may have restricted access for some patients. In 2013, the Supreme Court issued a ruling in *Association for Molecular Pathology v. Myriad Genetics, Inc.*, which changed the landscape of genetic testing, not only for BRCA1 and BRCA2 but with broad implications for cancer diagnostics in general. In essence, the court justices determined that human genes are not eligible for patents. Their decision was based upon the premise that DNA sequences are naturally occurring, and merely sequencing a naturally occurring phenomenon is not adequately inventive to deserve a patent. Consequently, the patent held by Myriad, which provides a result by comparing an individual's isolated BRCA1 and BRCA2 sequences to reference sequences, was invalidated. Since that decision, a number of competitors have entered the market and will offer BRCA1 and BRCA2 diagnostic genetic testing. This competition in the market will lead to lower prices for these tests and may improve access for certain patients [37, 38].

Genetic Counseling

Referral for genetic testing must be preceded by detailed counseling and informed consent. In particular, the American Society of Breast Surgeons recommends a discussion of several relevant issues. Patients must understand the possible outcomes, which may include positive, negative, and inconclusive results. It is important to understand that these results will have different implications for different patients. For example, those with a family history of a known BRCA gene mutation can interpret negative results as essentially eliminating the possibility of a genetic predisposition syndrome, while those without previously identified mutation within the family should understand that a negative result will not definitively exclude the possibility of a mutation that is not detectable but may be clinically significant. The possibility of an indeterminate result must also be discussed. Patients should be educated as to the cancer risks associated with mutations in BRCA1 and BRCA2, along with medical and surgical management options. These options will include increased surveillance, chemoprevention, and prophylactic operations. There must also be an understanding that the result of genetic testing will have implications for the patient and for his or her family. A discussion of disclosure of genetic information to family, and possible testing of family members if the result is positive, should occur before testing is pursued.

In general, any consideration of genetic testing for cancer susceptibility genes should be done with the guidance of certified genetic counselors. The critical elements of genetic counseling, as defined by the National Society of Genetic Counselors, are (1) to discuss the risks, benefits, and limitations of genetic counseling (including details about sensitivity, specificity, inconclusive results, and results of unknown clinical significance), (2) to discuss cancer prevention and management, (3) to discuss psychosocial support, and (4) to provide information tailored to each patient's level of understanding [39, 40].

In order to provide the most beneficial genetic counseling, providers must have a detailed understanding of the patient's demographic and educational background. An assessment of the psychological and emotional state of the patient is also critical. In particular, it is valuable to understand the emotional well-being of the patient by assessing for symptoms of anxiety and depression and inquiring about mental health history. The emotional response to cancer diagnoses within the family can help identify patients who may experience more distress with results of genetic testing. Understanding the coping skills and strategies of the individual may similarly provide important data. Any concerns about the psychological health of the patient may warrant involvement of a mental health professional as part of the multidisciplinary team caring for the unique set of individuals considering testing for genetic predisposition syndromes [39].

In younger patients with BRCA1 or BRCA2 gene mutations, issues of reproductive options may become a concern. Genetic counselors can provide advice and support related to reproductive options, should potential parents choose to limit their risk of passing a deleterious mutation to their children. Reproductive technologies, such as preimplantation diagnosis, are available as an option to concerned individuals [41].

Management Options for Patients with BRCA1/2 Mutations

Management of women with BRAC1 or BRCA2 mutations is based upon vigilant screening and preventive measures such as chemoprevention or prophylactic operations.

Vigilant Screening Recommendations

Screening guidelines are published by the National Comprehensive Cancer Network [31]. These guidelines apply to individuals with a known personal or family mutation of BRCA1 or BRCA2. Notably, individuals who have not undergone genetic testing but who have a family member with a known BRCA1 or BRCA2 mutation should be managed according to the guidelines for patients with a confirmed genetic mutation.

That is, even the suspicion that the patient may harbor a deleterious mutation of BRCA1 or BRCA2 is enough to pursue management as if the patient has the confirmed syndrome.

Screening for Breast Cancer

In patients with known or suspected BRCA1 or BRCA2 mutations, screening should begin at age 25 or earlier based upon the earliest age at diagnosis within the family. Breast awareness and self-exam should be taught and patients instructed to perform breast self-exam every month. Clinical breast examination is recommended every 6–12 months starting at age 25 or individualized based on the earliest age of onset in the family. Patients should also be counseled regarding the risk and benefits of prophylactic mastectomy, prophylactic bilateral salpingo-oophorectomy, and chemoprevention options for breast and ovarian cancers (Table 6.2) [31]. Mammography and breast magnetic resonance imaging (MRI) are indicated yearly [30].

The use of MRI as a screening test remains somewhat controversial. MRI is useful among younger women with dense breasts, who are particularly at risk in the setting of BRCA1 and BRCA2 mutations, which cause cancers at a younger age; in this population, the test is more sensitive to detect breast cancer than mammography, ultrasound, or clinical breast exam [42, 43]. The American Cancer Society does endorse breast MRI as a screening test in those with a genetic predisposition syndrome, since the sensitivity of mammography may be as low as 33 % in these younger women with dense breasts [44, 45]. A study of alternating mammography and breast MRI every 6 months among 73 patients with BRCA1 or BRCA2 mutations showed that 12 of 13 cancers identified on MRI were not seen on the preceding mammogram 6 months earlier [46]. Additionally, the prospectively studied efficacy of a screening protocol that includes yearly breast MRI showed the strategy to have high sensitivity to detect cancers at an early stage, with excellent long-term survival outcomes [47]. However, it must be acknowledged that MRI may detect benign lesions that cannot be easily distinguished from invasive cancer by this modality. Therefore, MRI may lead to additional biopsies if used as a screening tool.

Guidelines for men with BRCA1 or BRCA2 mutations are similar to those for women; they include monthly breast self-exam, semiannual clinical breast exam, and mammography if gynecomastia is present. Screening for prostate cancer should follow population guidelines, which recommend yearly digital rectal examination and prostate-specific antigen (PSA) serology.

Table 6.2 Vigilant screening for breast cancer in BRCA1/2 mutation carriers

Breast awareness starting at age 18 years
Starting at age 25 years, clinical breast exam every 6–12 months
Annual mammography and breast MRI starting at age 25 years or individualized based on the earliest age of onset in the family
Discuss risk-reducing mastectomy
Recommend prophylactic bilateral salpingo-oophorectomy
Consider chemoprevention options for breast and ovarian cancers

Based on data from Ref. [31]

Screening for Ovarian Cancer

Regarding the increased risk of ovarian cancers in women carrying mutations of BRCA1 or BRCA2, twice yearly pelvic examinations should be performed starting at age 30 or 5–10 years before the earliest age of first diagnosis of ovarian cancer. Along with biannual pelvic examination, CA-125 serology and transvaginal ultrasound should be performed (Table 6.3) [31]. However, because early detection is often difficult despite screening, and because of the poor prognosis associated with advanced ovarian cancer,

Table 6.3 Vigilant screening for ovarian cancer in BRAC1/2 mutation carriers in those who have not elected prophylactic bilateral salpingo-oophorectomy

Every 6 months, starting at age 30 years or 5–10 years before the earliest age of first diagnosis of ovarian cancer in the family
Pelvic examination
Transvaginal ultrasound
Serum CA-125

Based on data from Ref. [31]

prophylactic bilateral salpingo-oophorectomy is the recommended management strategy for these patients, as addressed later in this chapter.

Chemoprophylaxis

Chemoprophylaxis has been studied in the context of BRCA1 and BRCA2 mutations. In women with a personal history of breast cancer, tamoxifen has been shown to reduce contralateral breast cancer risk by 50 % in BRCA1 and BRCA2 mutation carriers. Interestingly, such risk reduction occurs regardless of the tumor's receptor status, especially given that BRCA1-associated breast cancers are more often estrogen receptor negative [48–50]. Of note, although chemoprophylaxis for BRCA1 and BRCA2 mutation carriers has been shown to potentially reduce the risk of developing contralateral breast cancer, it has not been shown to significantly reduce overall mortality.

Oral contraceptives may have some protective effect for ovarian cancer in BRCA1- and BRCA2-positive patients; some studies have suggested a risk reduction as high as 60 % with oral contraceptive use of 6 years duration [51].

Prophylactic Surgery

Contemplation of prophylactic operations for breast and ovarian cancers is of particular importance among individuals carrying mutations of BRCA1 and BRCA2. Prophylactic operations are highly effective in preventing cancer; however, surgical prevention may be considered aggressive and is associated with medical and psychosocial considerations.

The available options are prophylactic bilateral, or risk-reducing, mastectomy in patients with no cancer diagnosis [52–55], therapeutic mastectomy with contralateral prophylactic mastectomy in those with a cancer diagnosis [5, 56], and finally, prophylactic bilateral salpingo-oophorectomy (PBSO) performed alone or in addition to mastectomy in patients with or without cancer [53, 57–60]. Regardless, there is a lack of data to suggest an overall survival advantage with prophylactic bilateral mastectomy for BRCA1 and BRCA2 mutation carriers, whereas there are data that demonstrate a survival advantage with PBSO [53].

Impact of Prophylactic Bilateral Mastectomy for BRCA1 and BRCA2 Carriers

Prophylactic bilateral mastectomy significantly reduces the risk of developing breast cancer in BRCA1 and BRCA2 mutation carriers [52–55] (Table 6.4). The Prevention and Observation of Surgical Endpoints (PROSE) study is an often-quoted examination of the risk reduction afforded by prophylactic bilateral mastectomy. The study prospectively followed 105 BRCA1 or BRCA2 carriers who elected to have prophylactic bilateral mastectomy and compared these to 378 matched BRCA1 or BRCA2 carriers who did not choose prophylactic bilateral mastectomy. Mean follow-up was 6.4 years. Breast cancer was ultimately diagnosed in only two women who had prophylactic bilateral mastectomy (1.9 %), while 184 women in the conservatively managed group developed breast cancer (48.7 %). The experimental design of this study accounted for prophylactic salpingo-oophorectomy as well. The authors conclude that prophylactic bilateral mastectomy provides a relative risk reduction of 90 % in women who have ovaries and of 95 % in women who have also undergone bilateral salpingo-oophorectomy. The absolute risk reduction was 46.8 % [55].

Another long-term study of 26 women with BRCA1 or BRCA2 mutation who underwent prophylactic bilateral mastectomy showed no incidence of breast cancer after an average of 13.4 years of follow-up [54]. While the magnitude of risk reduction afforded by prophylactic bilateral mastectomy is dramatic, there have been no randomized clinical trials to further define the efficacy, utility, and risk when compared with more conservative management of high-risk patients. Therefore, consideration of prophylactic bilateral mastectomy remains a largely personal and often difficult decision for the patient.

Table 6.4 Selected series of impact of prophylactic bilateral mastectomy for BRCA1/2 mutation carriers

Authors, year, ref.	*N*	Results	Conclusions
Meijers-Heijboer, 2001 [52]	139	Incidence of breast cancer **0 %**: prophylactic group **2.5 %**: surveillance group	Prophylactic mastectomy reduces incidence of breast cancer
Hartmann, 2001[54]	26	Incidence of breast cancer **0 %**: prophylactic group	Breast cancer risk reduction in prophylactic group: **90–100 %**
Rebbeck, 2004 (PROSE) [55]	483	Incidence of breast cancer **1.9 %**: prophylactic group **49 %**: surveillance group	Breast cancer risk reduction in prophylactic group: **90 %** No impact on OS
Domchek, 2010 [53]	2,482	Incidence of breast cancer **0 %**: prophylactic group[a] **5.8–8.1 %**: surveillance group[b]	Prophylactic mastectomy reduces incidence of breast cancer

Courtesy of Quyen D. Chu, MD, MBA, FACS
PROSE Prevention and Observation of Surgical Endpoints
OS overall survival
[a]Incidence was zero for those who did and those who did not have prior or concurrent prophylactic salpingo-oophorectomy (PSO)
[b]Incidence was 8.1 % for those who have prior or concurrent PSO and 5.8 % for those who did not have prior or concurrent PSO

Domchek et al. estimated the risk and mortality reduction following prophylactic surgery by analyzing data from a prospective, multicenter cohort study of 2,482 women with BRCA1 or BRCA2 mutation [53]. For women who had prophylactic mastectomy, either with or without prophylactic salpingo-oophorectomy, the number of breast cancer events observed during the 3 years of prospective follow-up was zero. In contrast, for women who did not undergo a prophylactic mastectomy, the incidence of developing breast cancer was 8.1 % in those who had prophylactic salpingo-oophorectomy and 5.1 % in those who did not [53]. Thus, this confirms that prophylactic bilateral mastectomy was associated with a decreased risk of breast cancer in BRCA1 and BRCA2 mutation carriers.

Despite the risk reduction afforded by prophylactic bilateral mastectomy, there are no prospectively collected data to determine whether the decreased incidence of breast cancer is associated with improved overall survival. Several studies have used theoretical modeling to study long-term survival associated with prophylactic bilateral mastectomy and with prophylactic bilateral salpingo-oophorectomy. These models suggest increases in survival of 2.9–5.3 additional life years with prophylactic bilateral mastectomy, and 0.3–1.7 years with prophylactic bilateral salpingo-oophorectomy, when the prophylactic procedures are performed at the age of 30 years [61, 62]. Notably, the survival benefit of the prophylactic procedures decreases when performed later in life; in these models, there were negligible years gained from prophylactic operations after the age of 60 years.

Psychological and quality of life concerns are essential considerations when discussing prophylactic bilateral mastectomy. Studies have shown that most women are content with the decision to undergo prophylactic surgery, and satisfaction rates as high as 95 % have been reported [63]. Dissatisfaction, although rare, was more common when a physician's advice was the motivating factor to pursue prophylactic surgery, rather than the initiative of the patient [64]. Sources of anxiety in dissatisfied women were related to cosmetic outcome, reconstruction outcome, body image and sexuality, and fear of developing cancer despite the prophylactic operation. Quality of life seems to be similar when comparing women who have undergone prophylactic mastectomy

Table 6.5 Selected series of impact of contralateral mastectomy for BRCA1/2 mutation carriers with personal history of breast cancer

Authors, year, ref.	*N*	Results	Conclusions
Metcalfe, 2004 [5]	491	Incidence of developing contralateral breast cancer 0.7 %: CPM group 28.8 : surveillance group	CPM significantly reduces risk of developing contralateral breast cancer
van Sprundel, 2005 [56]	148	Overall survival 94 %: CPM group 77 %: surveillance group	CPM significantly reduces risk of developing contralateral breast cancer by 91 %, irrespective of the effect of prophylactic oophorectomy No differences in the overall survival between CPM and surveillance groups

Courtesy of Quyen D. Chu, MD, MBA, FACS
CPM contralateral prophylactic mastectomy

and those at high risk of breast cancer who have not elected prophylactic surgery. Poorer quality of life in the study subjects was self-reported and appeared unrelated to issues surrounding prophylactic mastectomy, with issues of depression and poor general health being the most important contributors [65].

Impact of Contralateral Prophylactic Mastectomy in Women with History of Invasive Breast Cancer

Women with a diagnosis of unilateral breast cancer in the setting of BRCA1 or BRCA2 gene mutations may elect to have contralateral prophylactic mastectomy. Studies have shown risk reduction for breast cancer to be similar to that afforded by bilateral prophylactic mastectomy [5, 56] (Table 6.5). One study that compared BRCA1 and BRCA2 mutation carriers with stage I–IIIa breast cancer who underwent contralateral mastectomy to those who opted for surveillance alone reported a 91 % risk reduction in the contralateral prophylactic mastectomy group [56]. However, no long-term survival benefit was evident in the contralateral prophylactic mastectomy group; rather, a survival benefit was demonstrated from bilateral salpingo-oophorectomy. The mean follow-up time was 3.5 years and the authors believed that longer follow-up is needed to have a better understanding of the effect of contralateral prophylactic mastectomy on contralateral breast cancer-specific survival.

Another study of BRCA1 and BRCA2 mutation carriers with stage I–II breast cancer who were followed for an average of 9.2 years showed that only one cancer developed among 146 women who underwent contralateral prophylactic mastectomy; this translates to a rate of 0.7 % for developing contralateral breast cancer. This was in contrast to a rate of 28.8 % for developing contralateral breast cancer in women who did not undergo contralateral prophylactic mastectomy, with 97 cancer recurrences among this group of 336 women [5].

Long-term satisfaction with contralateral prophylactic mastectomy is reported to be high [66]. Contralateral prophylactic mastectomy is considered to be cost-effective in women younger than 70 years of age when compared with screening, based upon evidence from a study that employed a Markov model analysis [67].

Options for prophylactic mastectomy, whether bilateral or contralateral, include traditional total mastectomy, skin-sparing mastectomy, or nipple-sparing or subcutaneous mastectomy. Total or simple mastectomy generally entails the removal of the breast, along with the nipple-areolar complex and a significant amount of skin overlying the breast tissue (Fig. 6.1). In a skin-sparing mastectomy, a small portion of the skin including the nipple-areolar complex is removed along with the underlying breast tissue while leaving behind a significant amount of skin for reconstruction (Figs. 6.2, 6.3, and 6.4). In the nipple-sparing mastectomy, the entire skin overlying the breast including the nipple-areolar complex is preserved while the breast tissue underneath the skin is removed (Fig. 6.2).

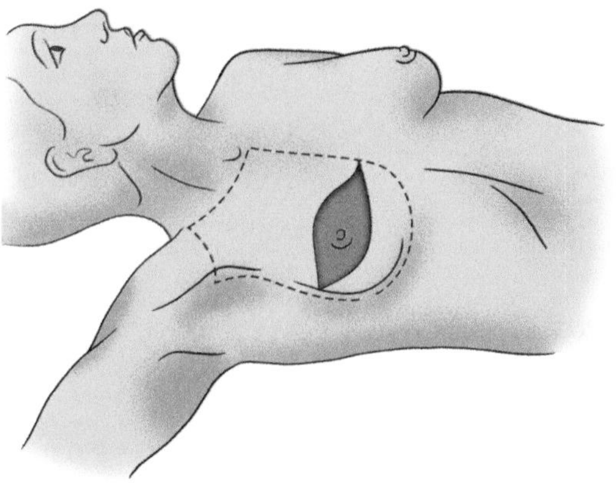

Fig. 6.1 Total or simple mastectomy: *Dotted lines* represent the extent of breast tissue to be removed. *Solid red* area represents the classic mastectomy incision, which incorporates the nipple-areolar complex and a portion of skin over the breast (Courtesy of Quyen D. Chu, MD, MBA, FACS)

Both total mastectomy and skin-sparing mastectomy are acceptable options since they have similar oncologic outcome, although the latter tend to result in a better cosmetic outcome [68]. The question of whether or not nipple-sparing mastectomy is safe and appropriate as prophylaxis in those with genetic predisposition syndromes is currently debated. A study of mastectomy specimens from BRCA1 and BRCA2 mutation carriers showed that premalignant or malignant lesions of the nipple-areolar complex occurred in 10 % of therapeutic mastectomy specimens, but in none of the prophylactic mastectomy specimens. These findings suggest that nipple-sparing mastectomy may be safe to perform as a prophylactic procedure; however, long-term outcomes are unknown and further research is needed [69].

The question of whether or not to perform sentinel lymph node biopsy at the time of prophylactic mastectomy is controversial. 3.5–5 % of all prophylactic mastectomy specimens contain occult invasive cancers [70, 71]. Once mastectomy is complete, and the opportunity to perform sentinel lymph node biopsy is lost. If sentinel lymph node biopsy is not performed during the prophylactic mastectomy and occult cancer is discovered, the only option remaining for axillary lymph node sampling is complete axillary lymph node dissection, with its attendant morbidities. Some authors have argued in favor of routine axillary lymph node biopsy at the time of prophylactic mastectomy [70], while others have suggested the procedure to be of little value in this setting [72]. Preoperative breast MRI may be a useful adjunct to identify occult cancers before proceeding with prophylactic mastectomy and may help select patients in whom sentinel lymph node biopsy should be performed [73].

Certainly, prophylactic mastectomy does afford a dramatic benefit in breast cancer prevention; it must be emphasized that even this aggressive treatment does not entirely eliminate the possibility of future breast cancer. Mastectomy cannot eliminate every breast tissue cell within the body, and any remaining breast tissue will contain the germline mutation in BRCA1 and BRCA2 carriers. There are many published accounts of breast cancer following prophylactic mastectomy [74–77]. This fact underlies the importance of continued vigilance even after risk-reducing surgery in BRCA1 and BRCA2 mutation carriers. At this time there are no generally accepted best practice guidelines for routine screening in these patients after prophylactic mastectomy; however, routine follow-up with clinical examination at least yearly is a prudent strategy [78].

The morbidity of bilateral prophylactic mastectomy is increased with immediate reconstruction. Commonly reported complications include pain, seroma, and infection. Reoperations are largely related to complications of reconstruction [79, 80].

Impact of Prophylactic Bilateral Salpingo-Oophorectomy (PBSO)

Prophylactic bilateral salpingo-oophorectomy (PBSO) is recommended for women with BRCA1 or BRCA2 mutations since there is a lack of efficacy in screening for ovarian cancer. The operation should be performed between the ages of 35 and 40 or at the conclusion of childbearing. Notably, PBSO reduces the risk of ovarian cancer by 96 %, irrespective of whether or not the patient has a personal history of breast cancer [53, 57–60] (Table 6.6). PBSO alone can provide up to 50 % breast cancer risk reduction in the setting of BRCA1 or BRCA2 mutations; such

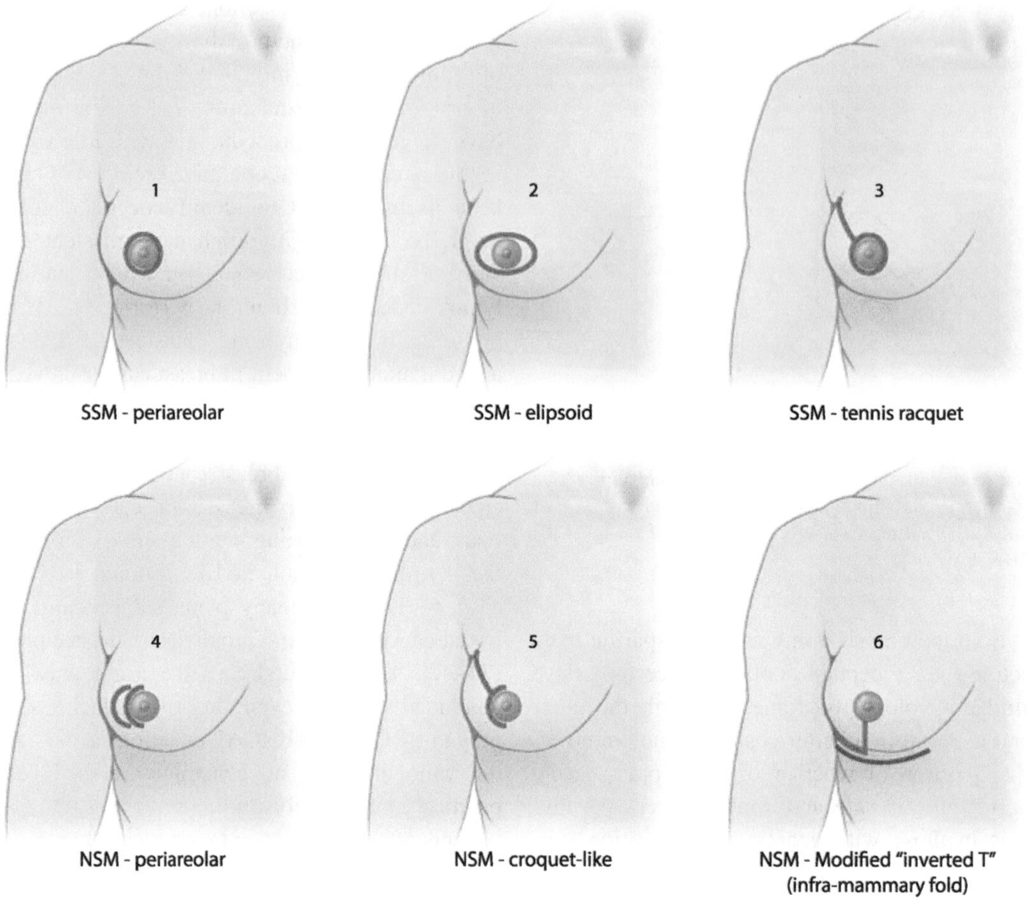

Fig. 6.2 Possible incisions for skin-sparing mastectomy (SSM) and nipple-sparing mastectomy (NSM) (Reprinted from Max Dieterich, Bernd Gerber. Patient selection and technical considerations in nipple-sparing and areola-sparing mastectomy. Current Breast Cancer Reports 2011;3(2): 79–87. from Springer Verlag)

reduction is generally observed in younger, premenopausal women [10, 60]. However, PBSO does not appear to reduce the risk of second diagnosis of primary breast cancer in patients with a personal history of breast cancer [53] (Table 6.6).

Additionally, a Markov model analysis of various prevention strategies has suggested that bilateral salpingo-oophorectomy may be associated with increased survival of 2.6 years. The addition of tamoxifen chemoprevention to bilateral salpingo-oophorectomy increased survival benefit to 4.6 years, almost as much as combined bilateral salpingo-oophorectomy and bilateral prophylactic mastectomy, which added 4.9 years of survival in this model [62]. Short-term hormone replacement in women who undergo bilateral salpingo-oophorectomy is controversial, but studies show a protective advantage of the operation even when hormone replacement therapy is used [81, 82].

In a study of 2,482 patients, Domchek et al. found that PBSO lowers all-cause mortality, irrespective of whether or not the patient has a personal history of breast cancer; however, such impact was observed mainly in women with BRCA1 mutation, although the lack of benefit in BRCA2 may be due to fewer BRCA2 participants and fewer events observed in the study [53].

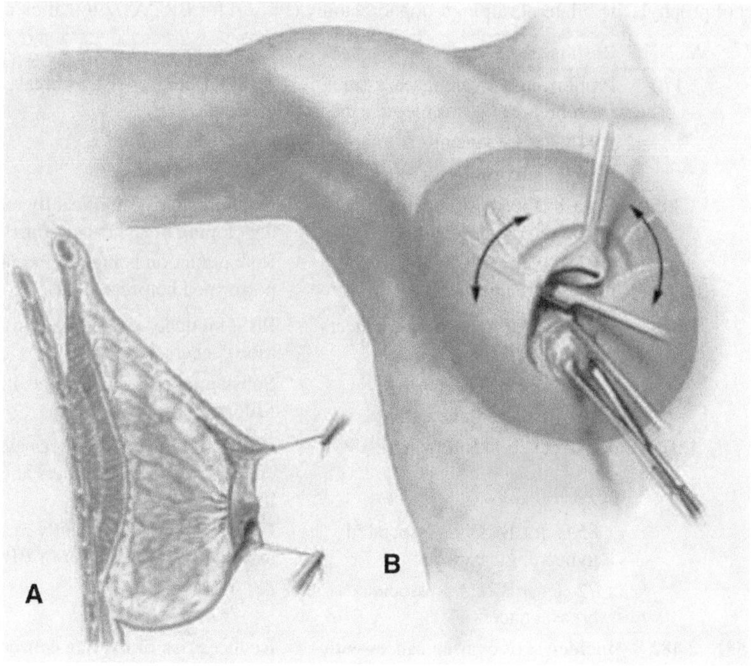

Fig. 6.3 Techniques of a skin-sparing mastectomy. The nipple-areola complex and the underlying breast tissue are included in the specimen. Skin flaps are elevated circumferentially above the breast tissue (Modified from Toth B, Daane S, Tenna S. Skin-sparing mastectomy with immediate breast reconstruction: a 10-year, single surgeon review of 105 consecutive patients. Eur J Plast Surg 2002;25:156–9. With permission from Springer Verlag)

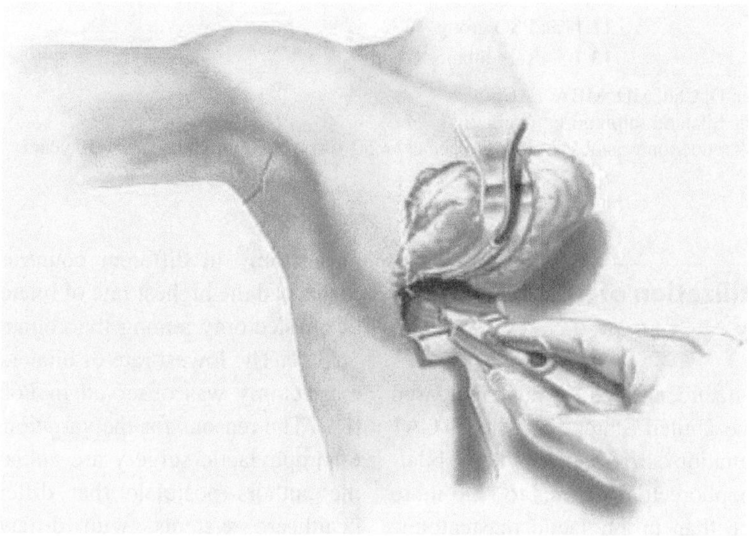

Fig. 6.4 Breast tissue is dissected away from the chest wall (Modified from Toth B, Daane S, Tenna S. Skin-sparing mastectomy with immediate breast reconstruction: a 10-year, single surgeon review of 105 consecutive patients. Eur J Plast Surg 2002;25:156–9. With permission from Springer Verlag)

Table 6.6 Impact of prophylactic bilateral salpingo-oophorectomy (PBSO) for BRCA1/2 mutation carriers

Authors, year, ref.	*N*	Results	Conclusions
Kauff, 2002 [60]	170	Proportion who are disease-free from breast or gynecologic cancers	PBSO decreases risk of breast and gynecologic cancers
		94 %: PBSO group	
		69 %: surveillance group	
Eisen, 2005 [57]	3,305	Breast cancer risk reduction following oophorectomy	Oophorectomy significantly reduces risk of developing breast cancer for BRCA1/2 carriers
		BRCA1: 56 %	Risk reduction is higher if oophorectomy was performed before age 40
		BRCA2: 46 %	
Finch, 2006 [58]	1,828	Incidence of gynecologic cancers	PBSO reduces risk of ovarian and fallopian tube cancers by 80 %
		0.22 %: PBSO group	Substantial risk for peritoneal cancer remains following PBSO
		1.0 %: surveillance group	
Kauff, 2008 [59]	1,079	Risk reduction following PBSO	PBSO significantly reduces gynecologic cancers in BRCA1 carriers and breast cancers in BRCA2 carriers
		85 % for BRCA1-associated gynecologic cancers	PBSO did not significantly impact on BRCA1-associated breast cancer or BRCA2-associated gynecologic cancers
		72 % for BRCA2-associated breast cancers	
Domchek, 2010 [53]	2,482	Incidence of ovarian cancer with no personal history of breast cancer	Reduces risk of ovarian cancer Reduces risk of breast cancer[a]
		1.3 %: PBSO group	
		5.8 %: surveillance group	
		Incidence of ovarian cancer with personal history of breast cancer	Reduces risk of ovarian cancer
		1 %: PBSO group	Does not reduce risk of second diagnosis of primary breast cancer
		6 %: surveillance group	
		Incidence of second diagnosis of primary breast cancer	
		11.1 %: PSO group	
		13.7 %: surveillance group	

Courtesy of Quyen D. Chu, MD, MBA, FACS
PBSO prophylactic bilateral salpingo-oophorectomy
[a]Breast cancer risk reduction was observed in women age < 50 years, but not in those age > 50 years

Trends in Utilization of Prophylactic Mastectomy

Rates of prophylactic mastectomy have increased over time in the United States [83]. In BRCA1 and BRCA2 mutation carriers, prophylactic bilateral salpingo-oophorectomy seems to be a more common choice than prophylactic mastectomy. However, an international analysis of prophylactic mastectomy suggests that there is a wide variation in patient acceptance of prophylactic mastectomy in different countries; the United States had the highest rate of bilateral prophylactic mastectomy among the countries studied, at 36.3 %. The lowest rate of bilateral prophylactic mastectomy was observed in Poland, at 2.7 % [84]. The reasons for the variation in acceptance of prophylactic surgery are unknown; however, the authors postulate that differences in the healthcare systems, with different access to care, may account for some of this variation. Differences in physician recommendations may also contribute to variation among countries.

Data from single institution studies have shown recent dramatic increases in women choosing both therapeutic and prophylactic mastectomies, regardless of BRCA status. In regard to prophylactic mastectomy, one study documented an increase of contralateral prophylactic mastectomy from 6.5 % in 1998 to 16.1 % in 2007, not accounting for BRCA status [85]. Carriers of the BRCA mutation are more likely than others to undergo prophylactic mastectomy [86]. Patient factors associated with increased utilization of prophylactic mastectomy are advanced education, younger age, and family history. Interestingly, increased rates of prophylactic mastectomy have been observed if the surgeon is a woman [87]. Another contributing factor may be the patient's perception of her own risk. The phenomenon of risk overestimation has been described, and many women will perceive their breast cancer risk as being higher than objective measures would indicate [88]. Similarly, women diagnosed with breast cancer will overestimate their risk of contralateral breast cancer [89]. The extent to which risk overestimation contributes to the use of prophylactic mastectomy is not known. Certainly, the decision to undergo prophylactic surgery is a complicated psychological experience, and many factors may contribute. Physicians and genetic counselors play an essential role in providing patients with the many complex details surrounding their diagnosis and risk, so that they may make an informed decision.

BRCA1 and BRCA2 in Men

As BRCA1 and BRCA2 are autosomal dominant genes, men may be carriers of gene mutations. This fact is significant both for the man who carries a BRCA gene mutation and for his family. In particular, fathers may pass BRCA gene mutations to their daughters. As in women, BRCA1 and BRCA2 mutations in men confer an increased risk of breast cancer. Men of Ashkenazi Jewish heritage are more likely to have mutations in these genes [26]. Although breast cancer is rare in general among men, a BRCA1 mutation confers a 1.8 % risk of breast cancer by age 80, compared with 0.12 % of men in the general population. BRCA2 mutations confer an even higher risk of breast cancer in men, with an 8.3 % chance of breast cancer by age 70 [90]. Additionally, when investigated by age group, the relative risk of male breast cancer among mutation carriers compared to the general population is highest at ages 30–40, indicating that BRCA1 and BRCA2 mutations are risk factors for cancer earlier in life, similar to women who carry the mutation. Guidelines for men with BRCA1 or BRCA2 mutations are similar to those for women and include monthly breast self-exam, semiannual clinical breast exam, and mammography if gynecomastia is present. BRCA1 and BRCA2 gene mutations also confer increased risk for prostate, pancreas, and colon cancers among men, a fact that has implications for screening as well.

Summary

BRCA1 and BRCA2 mutations cause familial predisposition syndromes that dramatically increase risk for breast cancer and ovarian cancer in women. Men with the mutations are also at risk for breast cancer, prostate cancer, and other cancers such as pancreatic and colon cancers. Diagnosis of a genetic predisposition syndrome includes detailed family history along with genetic testing and counseling in the appropriate settings. Patients must understand the implications of genetic testing, along with the possible outcomes and consequences of each. Management of those with BRCA1 or BRCA2 mutations includes increased surveillance or prophylactic operations, based on the preferences of the patient. Prophylactic procedures are very effective at reducing cancer risk, but do not entirely eliminate the risk of subsequent cancer. The unique needs of a patient with genetic predisposition syndromes are best met in the context of a multidisciplinary care team.

Salient Points

- BRCA1 and BRCA2 gene mutations confer increased risk for breast cancer and ovarian cancer.

- Genetic counseling and genetic testing play an important role in the management of these patients.
- Patients with known gene mutations or suspected gene mutations must be vigilantly screened and may consider prophylactic operations.
- Screening for breast cancer in mutation carriers will generally include yearly mammography and yearly breast MRI (typically alternating every 6 months) starting at age 25 or earlier based on family history.
- Screening for ovarian cancer includes biannual pelvic examination, CA-125 serology, and transvaginal ultrasound beginning at age 30 or 5–10 years before the earliest age of first diagnosis of ovarian cancer within the family; despite screening, early detection is difficult.
- For women with inherited BRCA1 or BRCA2 mutations, prophylactic mastectomy and salpingo-oophorectomy are effective at reducing the risk of breast and ovarian cancers.
- Skin-sparing mastectomy (the entire breast and nipple-areola complex is removed except for the dermis overlying the breast) is safe.
- Chemoprophylaxis (tamoxifen) potentially reduces the risk of contralateral breast cancer in women with BRCA1 and BRCA2 mutations.
- Salpingo-oophorectomy decreases risk of both breast cancer and ovarian cancer in BRCA1 and BRCA2 mutation carriers with and without a prior history of breast cancer.
- Salpingo-oophorectomy reduces risk of breast cancer mortality in BRCA1 and BRCA2 mutation carriers who have no prior history of breast cancer.
- Salpingo-oophorectomy has not been shown to reduce risk of breast cancer mortality in BRCA1 and BRCA2 mutation carriers who have prior history of breast cancer.
- Bilateral prophylactic mastectomy in BRCA1 and BRCA2 mutation carriers reduces the relative risk of breast cancer by 90 %.
- Although prophylactic mastectomy reduces risk of breast cancer in patients with inherited BRCA1 and BRCA2 mutations, it has not been shown to significantly reduce mortality.
- Prophylactic salpingo-oophorectomy reduces:
  - Risk of ovarian and fallopian tube cancers
  - Breast cancer
  - All-cause mortality (breast cancer-specific mortality and ovarian cancer-specific mortality)

Questions

1. In regard to breast cancer profiles of women with BRCA1 and BRCA2 mutations, which of the following statements is correct?
   A. Women with BRCA1-associated breast cancer have a similar rate of triple-negative breast cancers when compared to the general population.
   B. Women with BRCA2-associated breast cancer have an increased incidence of triple-negative breast cancers when compared to the general population.
   C. Women with BRCA1-associated breast cancer are more likely to have triple-negative cancers when compared to the general population
   D. Women with BRCA1-associated breast cancer have a similar rate of medullary carcinoma when compared to the general population.
2. The American Society of Breast Surgeons recommends referral to a genetic counselor for hereditary breast cancer risk assessment and testing for patients with any of the following characteristics, EXCEPT:
   A. Breast cancer diagnosed before age 50
   B. Two primary breast cancers in the same person
   C. Personal or family history of ovarian cancer
   D. Personal or family history of endometrial cancer
   E. Triple-negative breast cancer before the age 60
3. Of the following statements regarding BRCA1 and BRCA2 gene mutations, all of the following are true, EXCEPT:
   A. BRCA1 and BRCA2 gene mutations are inherited in an autosomal dominant fashion.

B. There may be variable penetrance of the gene mutation.
C. Ashkenazi Jewish, Finnish, and Icelandic populations harbor founder mutations which place them at higher risk of a BRCA1 or BRCA2 mutation than the general population.
D. BRCA1 and BRCA2 gene mutations confer a risk of breast cancer that exceeds 90 %.
E. The protein encoded by the BRCA1 gene plays a role in transcription, cell cycle control, and DNA damage repair pathways.

4. Which of the following statements regarding genetic testing for BRCA1 and BRCA2 mutations is correct?
   A. The test result may be positive, negative, or inconclusive.
   B. Full gene sequencing should always be performed, even in patients with a family member who carries a known gene mutation.
   C. Genetic testing does not require informed consent.
   D. Genetic testing results do not change management options for women already diagnosed with breast cancer.
   E. Insurance companies may consider genetic test results and deny insurance coverage based on such information.
5. The role of the genetic counselor for patients suspected of harboring a BRCA mutation is to:
   A. Arrange cancer screening for the patient
   B. Discuss the risks, benefits, and limitations of genetic testing; provide information and support
   C. Make management decisions on behalf of the patient
   D. Disclose genetic testing results to the patient's employer and insurer
6. Which of the following is true regarding screening for breast cancer in patients suspected or confirmed to carry BRCA1 or BRCA2 mutations?
   A. Yearly mammography alone should be performed beginning at age 40.
   B. There is no role for breast MRI as a screening tool.
   C. Yearly mammography along with yearly breast MRI is recommended as the preferred screening strategy.
   D. Yearly breast ultrasound is preferred over mammography for screening in younger women with dense breasts.
7. Which of the following statements about chemoprophylaxis for BRCA1 and BRCA2 mutation carriers is true?
   A. There is no role for chemoprophylaxis in the management of patients with BRCA1 or BRCA2 mutations.
   B. Oral contraceptives do not reduce the risk of ovarian cancer in patients with BRCA1 or BRCA2 mutations.
   C. Tamoxifen reduces the risk of breast cancer recurrence in patients with BRCA1 or BRCA2 mutations.
   D. Tamoxifen has no role in chemoprophylaxis for BRCA1 mutation carriers, since their tumors are more likely to be estrogen receptor negative.
8. Bilateral prophylactic mastectomy
   A. Significantly improves overall survival among BRCA1 and BRCA2 mutation carriers
   B. Significantly decreases the risk of breast cancer among BRCA1 and BRCA2 mutation carriers
   C. Is associated with high rates of dissatisfaction
   D. Totally eliminates the chances of breast cancer in the future
9. Prophylactic salpingo-oophorectomy
   A. Is unnecessary because adequate clinical screening options for ovarian cancer are available for BRCA1 and BRCA2 mutation carriers
   B. Has no role in the prevention of breast cancer among BRCA1 and BRCA2 mutation carriers
   C. Has not been demonstrated to reduce the risk of ovarian cancer in high-risk populations
   D. Significantly reduces the risk of both breast cancer and ovarian cancer among BRCA1 and BRCA2 carriers, with better protection when performed at a younger age

Answers

1. C
2. D
3. D
4. A
5. B
6. C
7. C
8. B
9. D

References

1. Margolin S, Johansson H, Rutqvist LE, Lindblom A, Fornander T. Family history, and impact on clinical presentation and prognosis, in a population-based breast cancer cohort from the Stockholm County. Fam Cancer. 2006;5(4):309–21. PubMed PMID: 16858627.
2. Ford D, Easton DF, Bishop DT, Narod SA, Goldgar DE. Risks of cancer in BRCA1-mutation carriers. Breast Cancer Linkage Consortium. Lancet. 1994;343(8899):692–5. PubMed PMID: 7907678.
3. Ford D, Easton DF, Stratton M, Narod S, Goldgar D, Devilee P, et al. Genetic heterogeneity and penetrance analysis of the BRCA1 and BRCA2 genes in breast cancer families. The Breast Cancer Linkage Consortium. Am J Hum Genet. 1998;62(3):676–89. PubMed PMID: 9497246. Pubmed Central PMCID: 1376944.
4. Chen S, Parmigiani G. Meta-analysis of BRCA1 and BRCA2 penetrance. J Clin Oncol. 2007;25(11): 1329–33. PubMed PMID: 17416853. Pubmed Central PMCID: 2267287.
5. Metcalfe K, Lynch HT, Ghadirian P, Tung N, Olivotto I, Warner E, et al. Contralateral breast cancer in BRCA1 and BRCA2 mutation carriers. J Clin Oncol. 2004;22(12):2328–35. PubMed PMID: 15197194.
6. Lakhani SR, Van De Vijver MJ, Jacquemier J, Anderson TJ, Osin PP, McGuffog L, et al. The pathology of familial breast cancer: predictive value of immunohistochemical markers estrogen receptor, progesterone receptor, HER-2, and p53 in patients with mutations in BRCA1 and BRCA2. J Clin Oncol. 2002;20(9):2310–8. PubMed PMID: 11981002.
7. Pathology of familial breast cancer: differences between breast cancers in carriers of BRCA1 or BRCA2 mutations and sporadic cases. Breast Cancer Linkage Consortium. Lancet. 1997; 349(9064): 1505–10. PubMed PMID: 9167459.
8. Thompson D, Easton DF, Breast Cancer Linkage Consortium. Cancer incidence in BRCA1 mutation carriers. J Natl Cancer Inst. 2002;94(18):1358–65.
9. Thompson D, Easton D, Breast Cancer Linkage Consortium. Variation in cancer risks, by mutation position, in BRCA2 mutation carriers. Am J Hum Genet. 2001;68(2):410–9.
10. Rebbeck TR, Lynch HT, Neuhausen SL, Narod SA, Van't Veer L, Garber JE, et al. Prophylactic oophorectomy in carriers of BRCA1 or BRCA2 mutations. N Engl J Med. 2002;346(21):1616–22. PubMed PMID: 12023993.
11. Liede A, Karlan BY, Narod SA. Cancer risks for male carriers of germline mutations in BRCA1 or BRCA2: a review of the literature. J Clin Oncol. 2004;22(4):735–42. PubMed PMID: 14966099.
12. van Asperen CJ, Brohet RM, Meijers-Heijboer EJ, Hoogerbrugge N, Verhoef S, Vasen HF, et al. Cancer risks in BRCA2 families: estimates for sites other than breast and ovary. J Med Genet. 2005;42(9): 711–9. PubMed PMID: 16141007. Pubmed Central PMCID: 1736136.
13. Walsh T, Casadei S, Coats KH, Swisher E, Stray SM, Higgins J, et al. Spectrum of mutations in BRCA1, BRCA2, CHEK2, and TP53 in families at high risk of breast cancer. JAMA. 2006;295(12):1379–88. PubMed PMID: 16551709.
14. Collins N, McManus R, Wooster R, Mangion J, Seal S, Lakhani SR, et al. Consistent loss of the wild type allele in breast cancers from a family linked to the BRCA2 gene on chromosome 13q12-13. Oncogene. 1995;10(8):1673–5. PubMed PMID: 7731724.
15. Gudmundsson J, Johannesdottir G, Bergthorsson JT, Arason A, Ingvarsson S, Egilsson V, et al. Different tumor types from BRCA2 carriers show wild-type chromosome deletions on 13q12-q13. Cancer Res. 1995;55(21):4830–2. PubMed PMID: 7585515.
16. King TA, Li W, Brogi E, Yee CJ, Gemignani ML, Olvera N, et al. Heterogenic loss of the wild-type BRCA allele in human breast tumorigenesis. Ann Surg Oncol. 2007;14(9):2510–8. PubMed PMID: 17597348.
17. Neuhausen SL, Marshall CJ. Loss of heterozygosity in familial tumors from three BRCA1-linked kindreds. Cancer Res. 1994;54(23):6069–72. PubMed PMID: 7954448.
18. Osorio A, de la Hoya M, Rodriguez-Lopez R, Martinez-Ramirez A, Cazorla A, Granizo JJ, et al. Loss of heterozygosity analysis at the BRCA loci in tumor samples from patients with familial breast cancer. Int J Cancer. 2002;99(2):305–9. PubMed PMID: 11979449.
19. Levy-Lahad E, Catane R, Eisenberg S, Kaufman B, Hornreich G, Lishinsky E, et al. Founder BRCA1 and BRCA2 mutations in Ashkenazi Jews in Israel: frequency and differential penetrance in ovarian cancer and in breast-ovarian cancer families. Am J Hum Genet. 1997;60(5):1059–67. PubMed PMID: 9150153. Pubmed Central PMCID: 1712434.
20. Gowen LC, Avrutskaya AV, Latour AM, Koller BH, Leadon SA. BRCA1 required for transcription-coupled repair of oxidative DNA damage. Science. 1998;281(5379):1009–12. PubMed PMID: 9703501.
21. Martin AM, Weber BL. Genetic and hormonal risk factors in breast cancer. J Natl Cancer Inst. 2000;92(14):1126–35. PubMed PMID: 10904085.

22. Oddoux C, Struewing JP, Clayton CM, Neuhausen S, Brody LC, Kaback M, et al. The carrier frequency of the BRCA2 6174delT mutation among Ashkenazi Jewish individuals is approximately 1 %. Nat Genet. 1996;14(2):188–90. PubMed PMID: 8841192.
23. Roa BB, Boyd AA, Volcik K, Richards CS. Ashkenazi Jewish population frequencies for common mutations in BRCA1 and BRCA2. Nat Genet. 1996;14(2):185–7. PubMed PMID: 8841191.
24. Rosen EM, Fan S, Pestell RG, Goldberg ID. BRCA1 gene in breast cancer. J Cell Physiol. 2003;196(1): 19–41. PubMed PMID: 12767038.
25. Wooster R, Weber BL. Breast and ovarian cancer. N Engl J Med. 2003;348(23):2339–47. PubMed PMID: 12788999.
26. Struewing JP, Hartge P, Wacholder S, Baker SM, Berlin M, McAdams M, et al. The risk of cancer associated with specific mutations of BRCA1 and BRCA2 among Ashkenazi Jews. N Engl J Med. 1997;336(20):1401–8. PubMed PMID: 9145676.
27. King MC, Marks JH, Mandell JB, New York Breast Cancer Study Group. Breast and ovarian cancer risks due to inherited mutations in BRCA1 and BRCA2. Science. 2003;302(5645):643–6.
28. Lynch HT, Lynch JF. Breast cancer genetics in an oncology clinic: 328 consecutive patients. Cancer Genet Cytogenet. 1986;22(4):369–71. PubMed PMID: 3731052.
29. American Society of Clinical O. American Society of Clinical Oncology policy statement update: genetic testing for cancer susceptibility. J Clin Oncol. 2003;21(12):2397–406. PubMed PMID: 12692171.
30. Daly MB, Axilbund JE, Buys S, Crawford B, Farrell CD, Friedman S, et al. Genetic/familial high-risk assessment: breast and ovarian. J Natl Compr Canc Netw. 2010;8(5):562–94. PubMed PMID: 20495085.
31. National Comprehensive Cancer Network guidelines for genetic/familial high-risk assessment: breast and ovarian. [15 Oct 2013]; Available from: http://www.nccn.org/professionals/physician_gls/pdf/genetics_screening.pdf
32. American Society of Breast Surgeons Position Statement on BRCA genetic testing for patients with and without breast cancer. [15 Oct 2013]; Available from: https://www.breastsurgeons.org/statements/PDF_Statements/BRCA_Testing.pdf
33. Antoniou AC, Hardy R, Walker L, Evans DG, Shenton A, Eeles R, et al. Predicting the likelihood of carrying a BRCA1 or BRCA2 mutation: validation of BOADICEA, BRCAPRO, IBIS, Myriad and the Manchester scoring system using data from UK genetics clinics. J Med Genet. 2008;45(7):425–31. PubMed PMID: 18413374.
34. Parmigiani G, Chen S, Iversen Jr ES, Friebel TM, Finkelstein DM, Anton-Culver H, et al. Validity of models for predicting BRCA1 and BRCA2 mutations. Ann Intern Med. 2007;147(7):441–50. PubMed PMID: 17909205. Pubmed Central PMCID: 2423214.
35. Daly MB, Axilbund JE, Bryant E, Buys S, Eng C, Friedman S, et al. Genetic/familial high-risk assessment: breast and ovarian. J Natl Compr Canc Netw. 2006;4(2):156–76. PubMed PMID: 16451772.
36. Weitzel JN, Lagos VI, Cullinane CA, Gambol PJ, Culver JO, Blazer KR, et al. Limited family structure and BRCA gene mutation status in single cases of breast cancer. JAMA. 2007;297(23):2587–95. PubMed PMID: 17579227.
37. Kesselheim AS, Cook-Deegan RM, Winickoff DE, Mello MM. Gene patenting – the supreme court finally speaks. N Engl J Med. 2013;369(9):869–75. PubMed PMID: 23841703.
38. Offit K, Bradbury A, Storm C, Merz JF, Noonan KE, Spence R. Gene patents and personalized cancer care: impact of the myriad case on clinical oncology. J Clin Oncol. 2013;31(21):2743–8. PubMed PMID: 23766521.
39. Berliner JL, Fay AM, Practice Issues Subcommittee of the National Society of Genetic Counselors' Familial Cancer Risk Counseling Special Interest Group. Risk assessment and genetic counseling for hereditary breast and ovarian cancer: recommendations of the National Society of Genetic Counselors. J Genet Couns. 2007;16(3):241–60. PubMed PMID: 17508274.
40. Trepanier A, Ahrens M, McKinnon W, Peters J, Stopfer J, Grumet SC, et al. Genetic cancer risk assessment and counseling: recommendations of the national society of genetic counselors. J Genet Couns. 2004;13(2):83–114. PubMed PMID: 15604628.
41. Offit K, Sagi M, Hurley K. Preimplantation genetic diagnosis for cancer syndromes: a new challenge for preventive medicine. JAMA. 2006;296(22):2727–30. PubMed PMID: 17164459.
42. Kriege M, Brekelmans CT, Boetes C, Besnard PE, Zonderland HM, Obdeijn IM, et al. Efficacy of MRI and mammography for breast-cancer screening in women with a familial or genetic predisposition. N Engl J Med. 2004;351(5):427–37. PubMed PMID: 15282350.
43. Warner E, Plewes DB, Hill KA, Causer PA, Zubovits JT, Jong RA, et al. Surveillance of BRCA1 and BRCA2 mutation carriers with magnetic resonance imaging, ultrasound, mammography, and clinical breast examination. JAMA. 2004;292(11):1317–25. PubMed PMID: 15367553.
44. Kuhl CK, Schrading S, Leutner CC, Morakkabati-Spitz N, Wardelmann E, Fimmers R, et al. Mammography, breast ultrasound, and magnetic resonance imaging for surveillance of women at high familial risk for breast cancer. J Clin Oncol. 2005;23(33):8469–76. PubMed PMID: 16293877.
45. Saslow D, Boetes C, Burke W, Harms S, Leach MO, Lehman CD, et al. American Cancer Society guidelines for breast screening with MRI as an adjunct to mammography. CA Cancer J Clin. 2007;57(2):75–89. PubMed PMID: 17392385.
46. Le-Petross HT, Whitman GJ, Atchley DP, Yuan Y, Gutierrez-Barrera A, Hortobagyi GN, et al. Effectiveness of alternating mammography and magnetic resonance imaging for screening women with deleterious BRCA mutations at high risk of breast cancer. Cancer. 2011;117(17):3900–7. PubMed PMID: 21365619.

47. Passaperuma K, Warner E, Causer PA, Hill KA, Messner S, Wong JW, et al. Long-term results of screening with magnetic resonance imaging in women with BRCA mutations. Br J Cancer. 2012;107(1):24–30. PubMed PMID: 22588560. Pubmed Central PMCID: 3389408.
48. Narod SA, Brunet JS, Ghadirian P, Robson M, Heimdal K, Neuhausen SL, et al. Tamoxifen and risk of contralateral breast cancer in BRCA1 and BRCA2 mutation carriers: a case–control study. Hereditary Breast Cancer Clinical Study Group. Lancet. 2000;356(9245):1876–81. PubMed PMID: 11130383.
49. Gronwald J, Jauch A, Cybulski C, Schoell B, Bohm-Steuer B, Lener M, et al. Comparison of genomic abnormalities between BRCAX and sporadic breast cancers studied by comparative genomic hybridization. Int J Cancer. 2005;114(2):230–6. PubMed PMID: 15540206.
50. Phillips KA, Milne RL, Rookus MA, Daly MB, Antoniou AC, Peock S, et al. Tamoxifen and risk of contralateral breast cancer for BRCA1 and BRCA2 mutation carriers. J Clin Oncol. 2013;31(25):3091–9. PubMed PMID: 23918944. Pubmed Central PMCID: 3753701.
51. Narod SA, Risch H, Moslehi R, Dorum A, Neuhausen S, Olsson H, et al. Oral contraceptives and the risk of hereditary ovarian cancer. Hereditary Ovarian Cancer Clinical Study Group. N Engl J Med. 1998;339(7):424–8. PubMed PMID: 9700175.
52. Meijers-Heijboer H, van Geel B, van Putten WL, Henzen-Logmans SC, Seynaeve C, Menke-Pluymers MB, et al. Breast cancer after prophylactic bilateral mastectomy in women with a BRCA1 or BRCA2 mutation. N Engl J Med. 2001;345(3):159–64. PubMed PMID: 11463009.
53. Domchek SM, Friebel TM, Singer CF, Evans DG, Lynch HT, Isaacs C, et al. Association of risk-reducing surgery in BRCA1 or BRCA2 mutation carriers with cancer risk and mortality. JAMA. 2010;304(9):967–75. PubMed PMID: 20810374. Pubmed Central PMCID: 2948529.
54. Hartmann LC, Sellers TA, Schaid DJ, Frank TS, Soderberg CL, Sitta DL, et al. Efficacy of bilateral prophylactic mastectomy in BRCA1 and BRCA2 gene mutation carriers. J Natl Cancer Inst. 2001;93(21):1633–7. PubMed PMID: 11698567.
55. Rebbeck TR, Friebel T, Lynch HT, Neuhausen SL, Van 't Veer L, Garber JE, et al. Bilateral prophylactic mastectomy reduces breast cancer risk in BRCA1 and BRCA2 mutation carriers: the PROSE Study Group. J Clin Oncol. 2004;22(6):1055–62.
56. van Sprundel TC, Schmidt MK, Rookus MA, Brohet R, van Asperen CJ, Rutgers EJ, et al. Risk reduction of contralateral breast cancer and survival after contralateral prophylactic mastectomy in BRCA1 or BRCA2 mutation carriers. Br J Cancer. 2005;93(3):287–92. PubMed PMID: 16052221. Pubmed Central PMCID: 2361560.
57. Eisen A, Lubinski J, Klijn J, Moller P, Lynch HT, Offit K, et al. Breast cancer risk following bilateral oophorectomy in BRCA1 and BRCA2 mutation carriers: an international case–control study. J Clin Oncol. 2005;23(30):7491–6. PubMed PMID: 16234515.
58. Finch A, Beiner M, Lubinski J, Lynch HT, Moller P, Rosen B, et al. Salpingo-oophorectomy and the risk of ovarian, fallopian tube, and peritoneal cancers in women with a BRCA1 or BRCA2 Mutation. JAMA. 2006;296(2):185–92. PubMed PMID: 16835424.
59. Kauff ND, Domchek SM, Friebel TM, Robson ME, Lee J, Garber JE, et al. Risk-reducing salpingo-oophorectomy for the prevention of BRCA1- and BRCA2-associated breast and gynecologic cancer: a multicenter, prospective study. J Clin Oncol. 2008;26(8):1331–7. PubMed PMID: 18268356. Pubmed Central PMCID: 3306809.
60. Kauff ND, Satagopan JM, Robson ME, Scheuer L, Hensley M, Hudis CA, et al. Risk-reducing salpingo-oophorectomy in women with a BRCA1 or BRCA2 mutation. N Engl J Med. 2002;346(21):1609–15. PubMed PMID: 12023992.
61. Schrag D, Kuntz KM, Garber JE, Weeks JC. Decision analysis–effects of prophylactic mastectomy and oophorectomy on life expectancy among women with BRCA1 or BRCA2 mutations. N Engl J Med. 1997;336(20):1465–71. PubMed PMID: 9148160.
62. Grann VR, Jacobson JS, Thomason D, Hershman D, Heitjan DF, Neugut AI. Effect of prevention strategies on survival and quality-adjusted survival of women with BRCA1/2 mutations: an updated decision analysis. J Clin Oncol. 2002;20(10):2520–9. PubMed PMID: 12011131.
63. Borgen PI, Hill AD, Tran KN, Van Zee KJ, Massie MJ, Payne D, et al. Patient regrets after bilateral prophylactic mastectomy. Ann Surg Oncol. 1998;5(7):603–6. PubMed PMID: 9831108.
64. Frost MH, Schaid DJ, Sellers TA, Slezak JM, Arnold PG, Woods JE, et al. Long-term satisfaction and psychological and social function following bilateral prophylactic mastectomy. JAMA. 2000;284(3):319–24. PubMed PMID: 10891963.
65. Geiger AM, Nekhlyudov L, Herrinton LJ, Rolnick SJ, Greene SM, West CN, et al. Quality of life after bilateral prophylactic mastectomy. Ann Surg Oncol. 2007;14(2):686–94. PubMed PMID: 17103066.
66. Koslow S, Pharmer LA, Scott AM, Stempel M, Morrow M, Pusic AL, et al. Long-term patient-reported satisfaction after contralateral prophylactic mastectomy and implant reconstruction. Ann Surg Oncol. 2013;20(11):3422–9. PubMed PMID: 23720070.
67. Zendejas B, Moriarty JP, O'Byrne J, Degnim AC, Farley DR, Boughey JC. Cost-effectiveness of contralateral prophylactic mastectomy versus routine surveillance in patients with unilateral breast cancer. J Clin Oncol. 2011;29(22):2993–3000. PubMed PMID: 21690472. Pubmed Central PMCID: 3157962.
68. Ueda S, Tamaki Y, Yano K, Okishiro N, Yanagisawa T, Imasato M, et al. Cosmetic outcome and patient satisfaction after skin-sparing mastectomy for breast cancer with immediate reconstruction of the breast. Surgery. 2008;143(3):414–25. PubMed PMID: 18291263.

69. Reynolds C, Davidson JA, Lindor NM, Glazebrook KN, Jakub JW, Degnim AC, et al. Prophylactic and therapeutic mastectomy in BRCA mutation carriers: can the nipple be preserved? Ann Surg Oncol. 2011;18(11):3102–9. PubMed PMID: 21947588.
70. Dupont EL, Kuhn MA, McCann C, Salud C, Spanton JL, Cox CE. The role of sentinel lymph node biopsy in women undergoing prophylactic mastectomy. Am J Surg. 2000;180(4):274–7. PubMed PMID: 11113434.
71. Peralta EA, Ellenhorn JD, Wagman LD, Dagis A, Andersen JS, Chu DZ. Contralateral prophylactic mastectomy improves the outcome of selected patients undergoing mastectomy for breast cancer. Am J Surg. 2000;180(6):439–45. PubMed PMID: 11182394.
72. Soran A, Falk J, Bonaventura M, Keenan D, Ahrendt G, Johnson R. Is routine sentinel lymph node biopsy indicated in women undergoing contralateral prophylactic mastectomy? Magee-Womens Hospital experience. Ann Surg Oncol. 2007;14(2):646–51. PubMed PMID: 17122987.
73. McLaughlin SA, Stempel M, Morris EA, Liberman L, King TA. Can magnetic resonance imaging be used to select patients for sentinel lymph node biopsy in prophylactic mastectomy? Cancer. 2008;112(6):1214–21. PubMed PMID: 18257089.
74. Eldar S, Meguid MM, Beatty JD. Cancer of the breast after prophylactic subcutaneous mastectomy. Am J Surg. 1984;148(5):692–3. PubMed PMID: 6496863.
75. Goodnight Jr JE, Quagliana JM, Morton DL. Failure of subcutaneous mastectomy to prevent the development of breast cancer. J Surg Oncol. 1984;26(3):198–201. PubMed PMID: 6330460.
76. Willemsen HW, Kaas R, Peterse JH, Rutgers EJ. Breast carcinoma in residual breast tissue after prophylactic bilateral subcutaneous mastectomy. Eur J Surg Oncol. 1998;24(4):331–2. PubMed PMID: 9725003.
77. Ziegler LD, Kroll SS. Primary breast cancer after prophylactic mastectomy. Am J Clin Oncol. 1991;14(5):451–4. PubMed PMID: 1951182.
78. Allain DC, Sweet K, Agnese DM. Management options after prophylactic surgeries in women with BRCA mutations: a review. Cancer Control. 2007;14(4):330–7. PubMed PMID: 17914333.
79. Barton MB, West CN, Liu IL, Harris EL, Rolnick SJ, Elmore JG, et al. Complications following bilateral prophylactic mastectomy. J Natl Cancer Inst Monogr. 2005;35:61–6. PubMed PMID: 16287887.
80. Zion SM, Slezak JM, Sellers TA, Woods JE, Arnold PG, Petty PM, et al. Reoperations after prophylactic mastectomy with or without implant reconstruction. Cancer. 2003;98(10):2152–60. PubMed PMID: 14601084.
81. Eisen A, Lubinski J, Gronwald J, Moller P, Lynch HT, Klijn J, et al. Hormone therapy and the risk of breast cancer in BRCA1 mutation carriers. J Natl Cancer Inst. 2008;100(19):1361–7. PubMed PMID: 18812548. Pubmed Central PMCID: 2556701.
82. Rebbeck TR, Friebel T, Wagner T, Lynch HT, Garber JE, Daly MB, et al. Effect of short-term hormone replacement therapy on breast cancer risk reduction after bilateral prophylactic oophorectomy in BRCA1 and BRCA2 mutation carriers: the PROSE Study Group. J Clin Oncol. 2005;23(31):7804–10. PubMed PMID: 16219936.
83. Tuttle TM, Habermann EB, Grund EH, Morris TJ, Virnig BA. Increasing use of contralateral prophylactic mastectomy for breast cancer patients: a trend toward more aggressive surgical treatment. J Clin Oncol. 2007;25(33):5203–9. PubMed PMID: 17954711.
84. Metcalfe KA, Birenbaum-Carmeli D, Lubinski J, Gronwald J, Lynch H, Moller P, et al. International variation in rates of uptake of preventive options in BRCA1 and BRCA2 mutation carriers. Int J Cancer. 2008;122(9):2017–22. PubMed PMID: 18196574. Pubmed Central PMCID: 2936778.
85. Jones NB, Wilson J, Kotur L, Stephens J, Farrar WB, Agnese DM. Contralateral prophylactic mastectomy for unilateral breast cancer: an increasing trend at a single institution. Ann Surg Oncol. 2009;16(10):2691–6. PubMed PMID: 19506956.
86. Stucky CC, Gray RJ, Wasif N, Dueck AC, Pockaj BA. Increase in contralateral prophylactic mastectomy: echoes of a bygone era? Surgical trends for unilateral breast cancer. Ann Surg Oncol. 2010;17 Suppl 3:330–7. PubMed PMID: 20853055.
87. Arrington AK, Jarosek SL, Virnig BA, Habermann EB, Tuttle TM. Patient and surgeon characteristics associated with increased use of contralateral prophylactic mastectomy in patients with breast cancer. Ann Surg Oncol. 2009;16(10):2697–704. PubMed PMID: 19653045.
88. Iglehart JD, Miron A, Rimer BK, Winer EP, Berry D, Shildkraut MJ. Overestimation of hereditary breast cancer risk. Ann Surg. 1998;228(3):375–84. PubMed PMID: 9742920. Pubmed Central PMCID: 1191495.
89. Abbott A, Rueth N, Pappas-Varco S, Kuntz K, Kerr E, Tuttle T. Perceptions of contralateral breast cancer: an overestimation of risk. Ann Surg Oncol. 2011;18(11):3129–36. PubMed PMID: 21947590.
90. Tai YC, Domchek S, Parmigiani G, Chen S. Breast cancer risk among male BRCA1 and BRCA2 mutation carriers. J Natl Cancer Inst. 2007;99(23):1811–4. PubMed PMID: 18042939. Pubmed Central PMCID: 2267289.

Breast Cancer During Pregnancy

7

Roger H. Kim and Quyen D. Chu

Learning Objectives

After reading this chapter, you should be able to:

- Describe the evaluation and workup of patients with pregnancy-associated breast cancer
- Identify the therapeutic modalities that are contraindicated in pregnancy-associated breast cancer
- Select the appropriate options for local, regional, and systemic therapy for pregnancy-associated breast cancer

Background/Epidemiology

The management of breast cancer that arises during pregnancy presents unique challenges for the physician. Pregnancy-associated breast cancer (PABC) is defined as breast cancer that is either diagnosed during pregnancy or within the first postpartum year. Breast cancer occurs in about 1.3 cases per 10,000 live births [1]. Approximately 0.2–3.8 % of breast cancers in women under the age of 50 are diagnosed during pregnancy; this number increases to 10–20 % in women 30 years of age or younger [2].

R.H. Kim, M.D., F.A.C.S. (✉)
Q.D. Chu, M.D., M.B.A., F.A.C.S.
Department of Surgery, Louisiana State University Health Sciences Center – Shreveport and the Feist-Weiller Cancer Center, 1501 Kings Highway, P.O. Box 33932, Shreveport, LA 71130-3392, USA
e-mail: rkim@lsuhsc.edu; qchu@lsuhsc.edu

Due to physiologic changes during pregnancy, including enlargement and engorgement of the breast, there is often a delay in diagnosis of breast cancer that is estimated at 5–10 months [3]. This delay is thought to be the primary cause for the advanced stage at which PABC often presents. In spite of this, a recent large cohort study revealed no difference in overall or disease-free survival for PABC when compared to nonpregnant patients with breast cancer, after adjusting for known prognostic factors [4].

This chapter will highlight some of the issues regarding the management of PABC and outline the appropriate treatment strategy for PABC. A suggested treatment algorithm for PABC is shown in Fig. 7.1.

Imaging

Mammography is not contraindicated in pregnancy and can still be obtained with proper abdominal shielding for fetal protection. Exposure to the fetus from mammography is estimated at 0.004 Gy, significantly lower than the recommended limit of 0.05 Gy [2, 3, 5]. However, the sensitivity of mammography is decreased in the pregnant breast, to about 70 % [2, 3]. Because of this, ultrasound is generally the first modality utilized for evaluation of a breast mass. If the mass has suspicious features on ultrasound, bilateral mammograms should be obtained.

Q.D. Chu et al. (eds.), *Surgical Oncology: A Practical and Comprehensive Approach*,
DOI 10.1007/978-1-4939-1423-4_7, © Springer Science+Business Media New York 2015

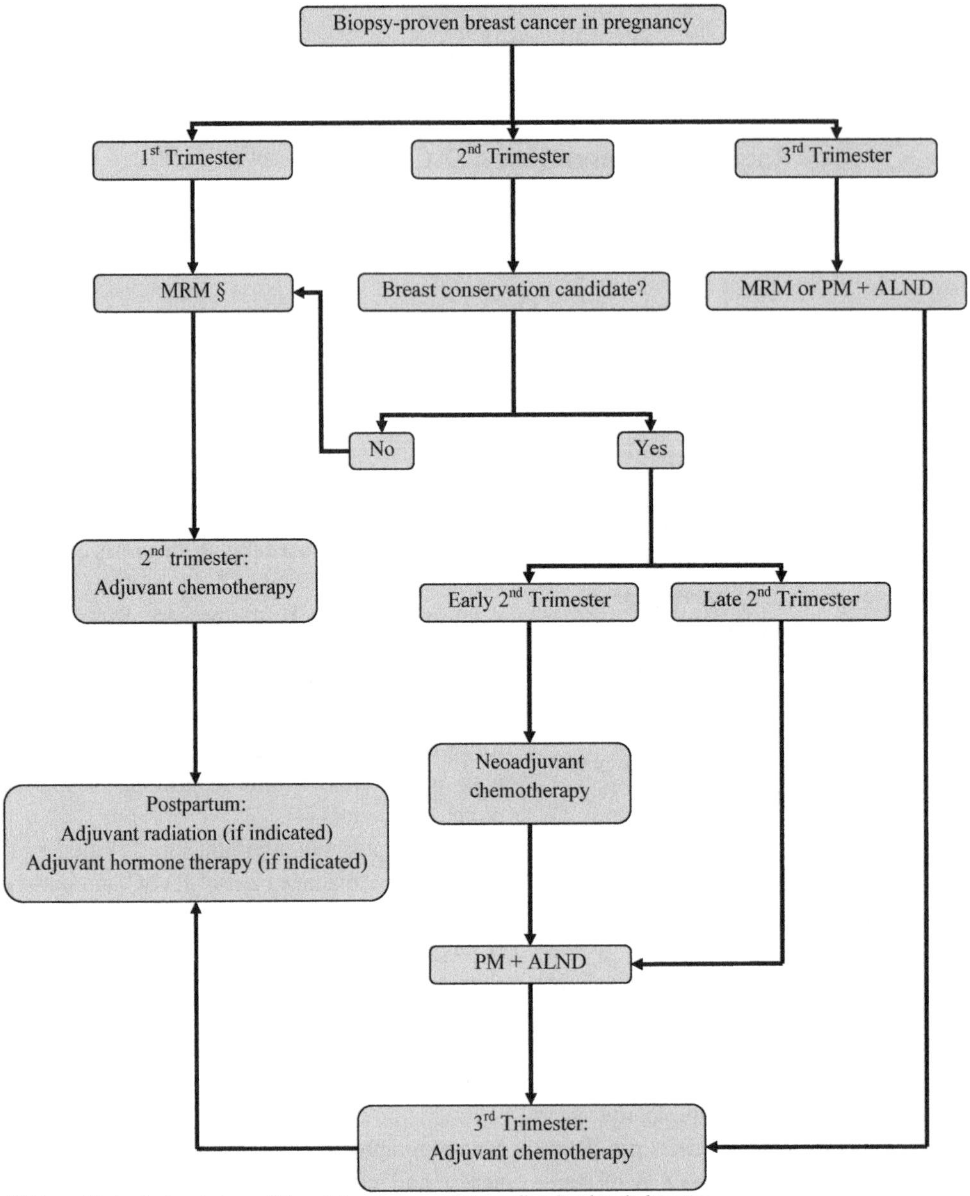

MRM: modified radical mastectomy; PM: partial mastectomy; ALND: axillary lymph node dissection
§ XRT may be an option for selected patients, although it is recommended that the patient should have a thorough discussion of the risks and benefits with her health care team.

Fig. 7.1 Algorithm for management of pregnancy-associated breast cancer (Courtesy of Roger H. Kim, MD, FACS and Quyen D. Chu, MD, MBA, FACS)

Breast magnetic resonance imaging (MRI) has not been widely utilized in PABC, due to concerns regarding gadolinium contrast, which has been shown to cross the placenta and is associated with fetal abnormalities in animal studies [2, 3].

Biopsy

Biopsy of suspicious lesions should be performed. Fine-needle aspiration (FNA) cytology is more difficult to interpret in pregnancy due to physiologic changes in the breast that mimic atypia [2, 3]. For this reason, the pathologist should be informed of the pregnancy or lactation status of patients who undergo FNA. Core needle biopsy can be obtained safely under local anesthesia during pregnancy. Excisional biopsy may also be performed under local anesthesia for tissue diagnosis.

Surgery

Surgery for breast cancer can be safely performed at any stage of pregnancy. There are multiple reports that demonstrate there is no increase in fetal abnormalities for pregnant patients undergoing general anesthesia [6, 7]. The miscarriage rates for pregnant patients undergoing non-obstetric surgery are 5.8 % overall and 10.5 % during the first trimester, which are roughly equivalent to the background miscarriage rate for all recognized pregnancies not undergoing surgery [8, 9]. Both mastectomy and breast-conservation therapy are options for PABC. Breast conservation can be safely considered if adjuvant radiation therapy will not be delayed beyond 12 weeks. If necessary, neoadjuvant chemotherapy can be given during pregnancy to allow breast-conservation therapy to be done later in pregnancy or after delivery.

Axillary staging in PABC is generally performed with axillary lymph node dissection (ALND), rather than sentinel lymph node biopsy (SLNB). The safety concern with SLNB is twofold: fetal radiation exposure from the use of Tc-99m for lymphoscintigraphy and the use of blue dye. The potential fetal exposure from Tc-99m has been calculated to be no more than 0.043 Gy and falls under the recommended limit [10]. However, the use of lymphazurin blue is contraindicated due to its unknown fetal effects as well as the risk of anaphylaxis, which increases the risk of fetal harm. Methylene blue is also contraindicated in pregnancy due to its known teratogenic effects [11]. In addition, the sensitivity and specificity of SLNB in PABC has not yet been established. There are some small series that have demonstrated safety and accuracy of SLNB in PABC [11, 12]. The role of SLNB in PABC should be considered investigational at this time.

Radiation

The indications for adjuvant radiation therapy remain the same in PABC as in the nonpregnant patient. However, it is advisable that radiation should be given after delivery for women with PABC. During the first 8 weeks of gestation, fetal doses greater than 0.05 Gy have been shown to cause malformations, intrauterine growth retardation, and mental retardation. Fetal exposure during the first trimester has been measured at 0.038 Gy [13], but the risk of spontaneous abortion is considered to be too high for safe administration of radiation therapy. During the second and third trimesters, fetal exposure levels increase due to the rising fetal position in the abdomen; fetal exposure in late gestation has been estimated at up to 2 Gy [13]. In addition, external shielding does not protect the fetus from internal scatter from within the mother's body.

Because radiation can be given 12 weeks or less after breast-conservation therapy, it remains a viable option for women who are diagnosed with PABC in the late second or third trimester. Additionally, women with PABC who are undergoing neoadjuvant treatment during the first and early second trimesters might also be candidate for breast-conservation therapy because the timing may make it safe to delay radiation until after delivery. The dilemma of giving radiation therapy to patients with PABC is for the subset of patients who are in their first and second trimester who are not undergoing neoadjuvant therapy. There is a paucity of data on the safety of administering radiation in this subset of patients. An international expert panel released a consensus statement in 2010, which states that radiotherapy is a relatively safe treatment option during the first and second trimester, although such decision should be made after a thorough discussion of the available data between the patient, her family members, and the health-care team [14].

Systemic Therapy

First trimester chemotherapy in PABC is contraindicated due to the risk of fetal malformations of up to 19 % [14, 15]. This risk drops during the second and third trimesters to 1.3 %, which is no different than the risk for fetuses without chemotherapy exposure. However, methotrexate carries high risk of teratogenesis and spontaneous abortion and is therefore contraindicated in pregnancy [15]. The CMF (cyclophosphamide, methotrexate, and 5-fluorouracil) regimen is often modified to CAF (cyclophosphamide, adriamycin, and 5-fluorouracil) because of this. There is limited data on the use of taxanes (paclitaxel and docetaxel) during pregnancy. At the present time, their use is limited to postdelivery.

There are several reports of anhydramnios with the use of trastuzumab (Herceptin), along with reversible renal failure in one fetus [3, 4]. The administration of trastuzumab in PABC is recommended only in the postpartum period.

Hormone therapy with tamoxifen is contraindicated in PABC due to reports of up to 20 % risk of fetal malformations [16]. Tamoxifen has also been associated with vaginal bleeding and spontaneous abortion. Tamoxifen, if indicated, should be delayed until postdelivery. Aromatase inhibitors are not indicated in premenopausal women and therefore have no role in the treatment of PABC.

Regardless of the type of systemic therapy protocol selected for PABC, its administration should be discontinued approximately 3 weeks prior to labor, to allow for correction of myelosuppression in both the mother and the fetus [3, 4].

Termination of Pregnancy

Elective abortion has not been shown to improve prognosis in PABC [17]. Termination of pregnancy can be considered for advanced PABC presenting during the first trimester, especially in cases where survival may be expected to be shorter than the duration of the pregnancy [5].

Salient Points

- Ultrasound is the imaging modality of first choice for a breast mass during pregnancy.
- Surgery can be performed during any trimester of pregnancy.
- Breast conservation is generally not recommended during the first trimester.
- Breast conservation is an option if adjuvant radiation will not be delayed beyond 12 weeks.
- Axillary staging is generally performed with axillary lymph node dissection.
- Chemotherapy is contraindicated during the first trimester.
- The following are contraindicated during pregnancy:
  - Methotrexate
  - Taxanes
  - Trastuzumab
  - Tamoxifen
  - Aromatase inhibitors
  - Sentinel lymph node biopsy (relative contraindication)

Questions

1. A 35-year-old woman in her 16th week of an uncomplicated pregnancy presents with a new left breast mass during a routine prenatal visit. On physical examination, there is a 3 cm palpable mass, at the 4 o'clock position of the left breast. There are no palpable lymph nodes in the left axilla. The most appropriate next step of management is:
   A. Diagnostic mammography
   B. Breast ultrasound
   C. Excisional biopsy of the mass
   D. Observation until third trimester
   E. Breast MRI
2. A 33-year-old woman in her 19th week of an uncomplicated pregnancy develops a right breast mass that measures 2 cm, at the 2 o'clock position. Imaging reveals a suspicious mass in the same area and is categorized as BIRADS 4. There are no palpable lymph nodes in the right axilla. The most appropriate next step of management is:

A. Modified radical mastectomy (MRM)
B. Observation until postpartum
C. Core needle biopsy of the mass
D. Excisional biopsy of the mass
E. Partial mastectomy (PM) and sentinel lymph node biopsy (SLNB)

3. A 30-year-old woman in her 10th week of an uncomplicated pregnancy presents with a new 2 cm right breast mass that is biopsy-proven infiltrating ductal carcinoma. There are no palpable lymph nodes in the axilla. Imaging reveals no other lesions in either breast. The most appropriate next step of management is:
   A. MRM
   B. Neoadjuvant chemotherapy, followed by MRM
   C. Neoadjuvant chemotherapy, followed by PM + axillary lymph node dissection (ALND)
   D. PM followed by external beam radiation (XRT)
   E. PM + SLNB, followed by adjuvant chemotherapy
4. A 34-year-old woman in her 20th week of an uncomplicated pregnancy develops an infiltrating ductal carcinoma of the left breast that is 3.5 cm in size. There are no other lesions in either breast on imaging. There is a palpable lymph node in the left axilla. She is interested in preserving her breast. The most appropriate next step of management is:
   A. MRM
   B. MRM followed by XRT
   C. Termination of pregnancy
   D. SLNB
   E. Neoadjuvant chemotherapy
5. A 35-year-old woman who developed left breast cancer during pregnancy has been treated with PM + ALND. The tumor size was 2.3 cm; surgical margins were negative; 2/15 lymph nodes were involved with tumor. The tumor was ER+/PR+/Her-2-. She is now in her 30th week of pregnancy. The fetus is doing well. The most appropriate sequence of adjuvant therapy is:

A.	XRT	CMF	Tamoxifen
B.	Tamoxifen	AC + T	XRT
C.	XRT	Tamoxifen	CAF
D.	CAF	XRT	Tamoxifen
E.	AC + T	XRT	Tamoxifen

XRT: external beam radiation
CMF: cyclophosphamide + methotrexate + 5-FU
CAF: cyclophosphamide + adriamycin + 5-FU
AC + T: adriamycin + cyclophosphamide + paclitaxel

6. For the patient from question #5, which of the following is the most appropriate management?
   A. Early induction of labor.
   B. Termination of pregnancy.
   C. Cessation of chemotherapy 3 weeks prior to labor.
   D. Cesarean section should be performed instead of vaginal delivery.
   E. Number of cycles of chemotherapy should be halved during pregnancy.
7. Regarding the use of sentinel lymph node biopsy during pregnancy, which of the following is true?
   A. Sentinel lymph node biopsy is contraindicated.
   B. The accuracy of sentinel lymph node biopsy during pregnancy is unknown.
   C. Lymphazurin blue is safe.
   D. Methylene blue is safe.
   E. Technetium-99m is contraindicated.
8. Which of the following adjuvant therapies is safe during pregnancy?
   A. Tamoxifen
   B. Methotrexate
   C. Paclitaxel
   D. Trastuzumab
   E. Cyclophosphamide

Answer Key

1. B.
2. C.
3. A.
4. E.
5. D.
6. C.
7. B.
8. E.

References

1. Smith LH, Dalrymple JL, Leiserowitz GS, Danielsen B, Gilbert WM. Obstetrical deliveries associated with maternal malignancy in California, 1992 through 1997. Am J Obstet Gynecol. 2001;184(7):1504–12; discussion 1512–1503.
2. Litton JK, Theriault RL. Breast cancer during pregnancy and subsequent pregnancy in breast cancer survivors. In: Harris JRLM, Morrow M, Osborne CK, editors. Diseases of the breast. Philadelphia: Lippincott Williams & Wilkins; 2010. p. 808–16.
3. Guidroz JA, Scott-Conner CE, Weigel RJ. Management of pregnant women with breast cancer. J Surg Oncol. 2011;103(4):337–40.
4. Amant F, von Minckwitz G, Han SN, et al. Prognosis of women with primary breast cancer diagnosed during pregnancy: results from an international collaborative study. J Clin Oncol. 2013;31(20):2532–9.
5. Navrozoglou I, Vrekoussis T, Kontostolis E, et al. Breast cancer during pregnancy: a mini-review. Eur J Surg Oncol. 2008;34(8):837–43.
6. Duncan PG, Pope WD, Cohen MM, Greer N. Fetal risk of anesthesia and surgery during pregnancy. Anesthesiology. 1986;64(6):790–4.
7. Mazze RI, Källén B. Reproductive outcome after anesthesia and operation during pregnancy: a registry study of 5405 cases. Am J Obstet Gynecol. 1989; 161(5):1178–85.
8. Cohen-Kerem R, Railton C, Oren D, Lishner M, Koren G. Pregnancy outcome following non-obstetric surgical intervention. Am J Surg. 2005;190(3):467–73.
9. Avalos LGC, Li D. A systematic review to calculate background miscarriage rates using life table analysis. Birth Defects Res A Clin Mol Teratol. 2012;94:417–23.
10. Keleher A, Wendt R, Delpassand E, Stachowiak AM, Kuerer HM. The safety of lymphatic mapping in pregnant breast cancer patients using Tc-99m sulfur colloid. Breast J. 2004;10(6):492–5.
11. Khera SY, Kiluk JV, Hasson DM, et al. Pregnancy-associated breast cancer patients can safely undergo lymphatic mapping. Breast J. 2008;14(3):250–4.
12. Mondi MM, Cuenca RE, Ollila DW, Stewart JH, Levine EA. Sentinel lymph node biopsy during pregnancy: initial clinical experience. Ann Surg Oncol. 2007;14(1):218–21.
13. Antypas C, Sandilos P, Kouvaris J, et al. Fetal dose evaluation during breast cancer radiotherapy. Int J Radiat Oncol Biol Phys. 1998;40(4):995–9.
14. Amant F, Deckers S, Van Calsteren K, et al. Breast cancer in pregnancy: recommendations of an international consensus meeting. Eur J Cancer. 2010;46(18): 3158–68.
15. Doll DC, Ringenberg QS, Yarbro JW. Antineoplastic agents and pregnancy. Semin Oncol. 1989;16(5): 337–46.
16. Ring AE, Smith IE, Ellis PA. Breast cancer and pregnancy. Ann Oncol. 2005;16(12):1855–60.
17. Nugent P, O'Connell TX. Breast cancer and pregnancy. Arch Surg. 1985;120(11):1221–4.

Part III

Gastrointestinal

Esophageal Cancer

8

John H. Park, Peter J. DiPasco, Joaquina C. Baranda, and Mazin F. Al-Kasspooles

Learning Objectives

After reading this chapter, you should be able to:

- Understand the epidemiologic trends
- Appreciate the importance of anatomy, workup, and proper staging
- Gain knowledge of the available treatment modalities for patients with esophageal cancer

Background

Esophageal cancer is a very aggressive disease with a 5-year relative survival rate of 19 % and an overall case fatality rate of 90 % [1, 2]. It is estimated that in 2012, there will be 17,460 new cases diagnosed with 15,070 deaths from esophageal cancer [1]. The disease affects mostly males (13,950 male vs. 3,510 female) and is the seventh leading cause of cancer death among all males and fifth among males between 40 and 79 [1]. The two major histologic variants of esophageal cancer are adenocarcinoma and squamous cell carcinoma, and it has been recognized that these represent two distinct disease entities [3].

The incidence of adenocarcinoma has dramatically risen over the past two to three decades in the United States because among white males, the incidence of esophageal adenocarcinoma has increased 463 % from the 1970s to 2000s [4] with a white to black ratio of 3:1 [5]. In contradistinction, squamous cell carcinoma has a higher predilection in the black population with a black to white ratio of 5:6 [5]. The predominant risk factors besides race and gender for the development of the two diseases also differ. A history of gastroesophageal reflux disease (GERD), Barrett's esophagus, and obesity contribute to the development of adenocarcinoma, which most often occurs in the lower third of the esophagus and gastroesophageal junction (GEJ), while a history of smoking and alcohol use are more closely associated with the development of squamous cell carcinoma that mostly effects the upper third and middle esophagus [6]. Other risks factors for the development of esophageal cancer include nitrate consumption, diet (high calorie, high fat, low intake of raw vegetables and fruit), tylosis, Plummer-Vinson syndrome, achalasia, caustic injuries, previous malignancy, and previous irradiation [2, 7].

J.H. Park, M.D.
Radiation Oncology, University of Kansas Medical Center, 3901 Rainbow Blvd, Mailstop 4033, Kansas City, KS 66160, USA
e-mail: jpark320@gmail.com

P.J. DiPasco, M.D. • M.F. Al-Kasspooles, M.D. (✉)
Department of General Surgery, Section of Surgical Oncology, University of Kansas Medical Center, 3901 Rainbow Blvd, Mailstop 2005, Kansas City, KS 66160, USA
e-mail: pdipasco@kumc.edu; mal-kasspooles@kumc.edu

J.C. Baranda, M.D.
Internal Medicine, University of Kansas Medical Center, 2330 Shawnee Mission Parkway, Westwood, KS 66205, USA
e-mail: jbaranda@kumc.edu

Q.D. Chu et al. (eds.), *Surgical Oncology: A Practical and Comprehensive Approach*,
DOI 10.1007/978-1-4939-1423-4_8, © Springer Science+Business Media New York 2015

Anatomy and Pathology

The esophagus is a hollow viscous organ that starts in the neck at the cricopharyngeus muscle, traverses the thorax, and ends at the GEJ. Tumors whose midpoint is in the lower thoracic esophagus, GEJ, or within the proximal 5 cm of the stomach that extend into the esophagus or GEJ are now classified as esophageal tumors [8, 9]. The esophagus is further subdivided into the cervical (15–18 cm from the incisors), upper thoracic (18–24 cm), middle thoracic (24–32 cm), and lower thoracic (32–40 cm) esophagus. Knowledge of the lymphatic drainage patterns for each section is important in order to properly treat and stage the patients. The cervical esophagus drains to the neck and supraclavicular nodes. The upper thoracic esophagus drains to the nodes on the innominate artery and ligamentum arteriosum, paraesophageal, and paratracheal nodes. The middle thoracic esophagus drains to the tracheobronchial, paraesophageal, and pulmonary hilar nodes. The lower thoracic esophagus drains to the paraesophageal and diaphragmatic nodes. Finally, the GEJ drains to the nodes on left gastric, celiac, common hepatic, and splenic arteries, as well as the paracardiac and lesser curvature nodes.

The surface of the esophageal wall is covered with an epithelial layer followed by the basement membrane, lamina propria, muscularis mucosae, submucosa, muscularis propria, and adventitia. Since the esophagus lacks a true serosa, tumors are able to spread to adjacent organs without having to traverse an anatomic barrier. Adjacent structures at risk to direct extension include the lung, bronchi, heart, pericardium, corresponding pleuras, diaphragm, mediastinum, aorta, trachea, vertebral bodies, and the recurrent laryngeal nerve.

Squamous cell carcinoma arises from a background of chronic esophagitis, usually from chronic irritation from smoking and alcohol use, which in turn leads to increased epithelial cell turnover, dysplasia, the development of carcinoma in situ, and finally invasive malignancy [3]. Molecular genetic underpinnings include alterations of p53 and p16 and CpG island methylation at CDKN2A/p16INK4a [10]. The pathogenesis of adenocarcinoma is closely tied with those patients whose chronic GERD causes Barrett's metaplasia, also called intestinal metaplasia, because the squamous epithelium of the esophagus is gradually replaced by columnar cells containing goblet cells [11]. This in turn leads to dysplasia and invasive malignancy [3]. Patients with GERD have 7.7 times the risk of developing esophageal adenocarcinoma, and those with longstanding GERD and severe symptoms have 43.5 times the risk [12]. Likewise, those with Barrett's esophagus have 30–60 times the risk of developing esophageal adenocarcinoma [13]. Molecular genetics of adenocarcinoma include the loss of heterozygosity of Rb, p53, and CDKN2A/p16INK4a [10].

Staging

The American Joint Committee on Cancer (AJCC) TNM classification and stage groupings are directly related to prognosis and are updated as new and emerging data arises [14, 15].

Recent changes from the 6th the 7th edition of the AJCC TNM tumor classification include separate staging for squamous cell carcinoma and adenocarcinoma (reflecting that they are distinct entities), T4 staging subclassified into resectable versus unresectable, the inclusion of tumor location and grade, downgrading celiac nodes to regional nodes [16], and that the number of lymph nodes is more prognostic than if they are regional [17–21] (Table 8.1). Stage groupings for squamous cell carcinoma and adenocarcinoma of the esophagus are different and are shown in Table 8.1. Figures 8.1 and 8.2 show examples of early stage and locally advanced cancers, respectively.

The overall survival by the previous staging system (as long-term follow up is currently unavailable for the current staging system) is approximately as follows: [22]

- Stage 0: 100 %
- Stage I: 30–40 %
- Stage IIA: 30–40 %
- Stage IIB: 10–30 %
- Stage III: 10–15 %
- Stage IV: 0–5 %

Table 8.1 American Joint Committee on Cancer (AJCC) TNM staging for esophageal carcinomas (7th edition)

Primary tumor (T)*	
TX	Primary tumor cannot be assessed
T0	No evidence of primary tumor
Tis	High-grade dysplasia**
T1	Tumor invades lamina propria, muscularis mucosae, or submucosa
T1a	Tumor invades lamina propria or muscularis mucosae
T1b	Tumor invades submucosa
T2	Tumor invades muscularis propria
T3	Tumor invades adventitia
T4	Tumor invades adjacent structures
T4a	Resectable tumor invading pleura, pericardium, or diaphragm
T4b	Unresectable tumor invading other adjacent structures such as aorta, vertebral body, trachea, etc.

*At least maximal dimension of the tumor must be recorded and multiple tumors require the T(m) suffix

**High-grade dysplasia includes all noninvasive neoplastic epithelial that was formerly called carcinoma in situ, a diagnosis that is no longer used for columnar mucosae anywhere in the GIT

Regional lymph nodes (N)*	
NX	Regional lymph nodes cannot be assessed
N0	No regional lymph nodes metastasis
N1	Metastasis in 1–2 regional lymph nodes
N2	Metastasis in 3–6 regional lymph nodes
N3	Metastasis in ≥7 regional lymph nodes

*Number must be recorded for the total number of regional nodes sampled and total number of reported with metastases

Distant metastasis (M)	
M0	No distant metastasis
M1	Distant metastasis

Adapted with permission from AJCC: Esophagus and Esophagogastric Junction. In: Compton C, Byrd D, Garcia-Aguilar J, Kurtzman S, Olawaiye A, Washington M, eds.: AJCC Cancer Staging Atlas. 2nd ed. New York, NY: Springer, 2012, pp 129

Anatomic stage/prognostic groups

Squamous cell carcinoma*

Stage	T	N	M	Grade	Tumor location**
0	Tis (HGD)	N0	M0	1, X	Any
IA	T1	N0	M0	1, X	Any
IB	T1	N0	M0	2–3	Any
	T2-3	N0	M0	1, X	Lower, X
IIA	T2-3	N0	M0	1, X	Upper, middle
	T2-3	N0	M0	2–3	Lower, X
IIB	T2-3	N0	M0	2–3	Upper, middle
	T1-2	N1	M0	Any	Any
IIIA	T1-2	N2	M0	Any	Any
	T3	N1	M0	Any	Any
	T4a	N0	M0	Any	Any
IIIB	T3	N2	M0	Any	Any
IIIC	T4a	N1-2	M0	Any	Any
	T4b	Any	M0	Any	Any
	Any	N3	M0	Any	Any
IV	Any	Any	M1	Any	Any

(continued)

Table 8.1 (continued)

*Or mixed histology including a squamous component or NOS

**Location of primary cancer site is defined by the position of the upper (proximal) edge of the tumor in the esophagus

Adenocarcinoma

Stage	T	N	M	Grade
0	Tis (HGD)	N0	M0	1, X
IA	T1	N0	M0	1–2, X
IB	T1	N0	M0	3
	T2	N0	M0	1–2, X
IIA	T2	N0	M0	3
IIB	T3	N0	M0	Any
	T1-2	N1	M0	Any
IIIA	T1-2	N2	M0	Any
	T3	N1	M0	Any
	T4a	N0	M0	Any
IIIB	T3	N2	M0	Any
IIIC	T4a	N1-2	M0	Any
	T4b	Any	M0	Any
	Any	N3	M0	Any
IV	Any	Any	M1	Any

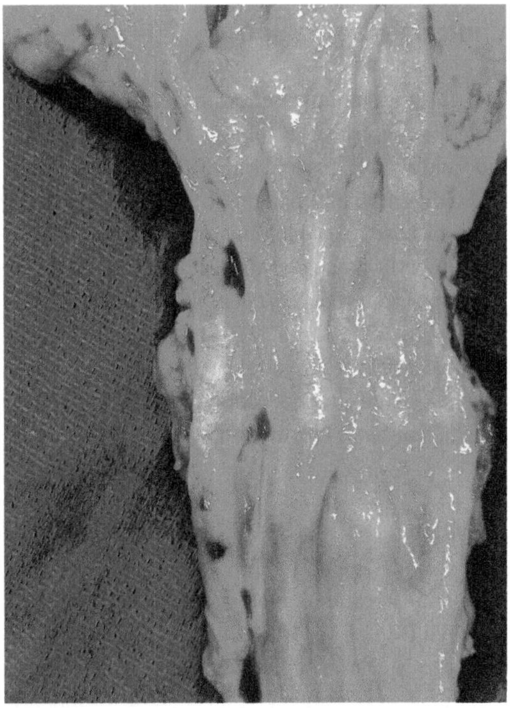

Fig. 8.1 An early stage distal esophageal adenocarcinoma contained within the adventitia

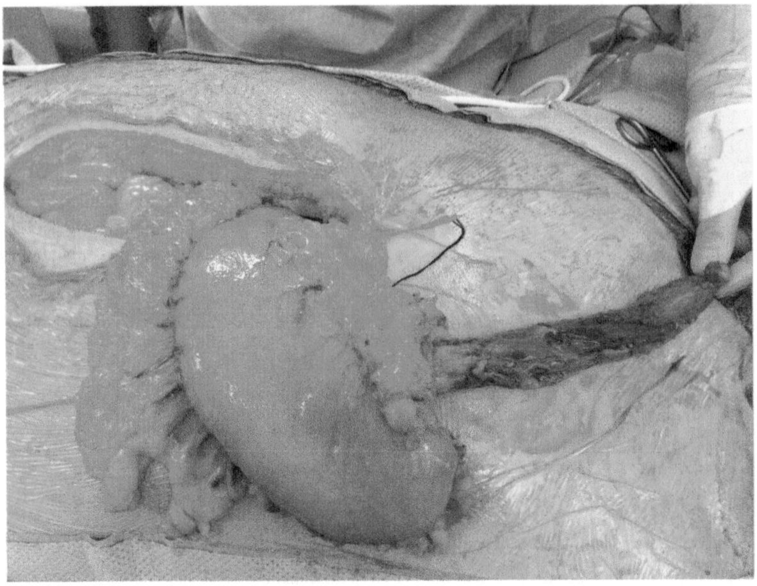

Fig. 8.2 A locally advanced gastroesophageal junction lesion with involvement of the lesser curvature of the stomach

Overall prognosis can also be thought in terms of localized, regional, or distant disease with 5-year relative survival rates of 37 %, 18 %, and 3 %, respectively [23].

Clinical Presentation

The most common symptoms on presentation include progressive dysphagia from solids to liquids and weight loss. These often come on slow and indolently, and patients often present late in their disease. Association of symptoms with more locally advanced disease includes hoarseness from recurrent laryngeal nerve involvement, chest pain from thoracic and mediastinal invasion, back pain from vertebral body invasion, and dyspnea from tracheoesophageal or bronchoesophageal fistula formation.

Workup

Historically, patients received a barium swallow with plain films (esophagography) to detect the presence of an esophageal mass. Nowadays, additional confirmatory tests include esophagogastroduodenoscopy (EGD) for direct visualization of the upper GI tract and determination of the extent of longitudinal spread and biopsy confirmation (Fig. 8.3). This is then followed by an endoscopic ultrasound (EUS) with a fine needle aspiration (FNA). EUS is the ideal imaging modality to assess depth of tumor invasion with a T-stage sensitivity of 81–90 % and specificity of about 99 % and an N-stage sensitivity of 96.7 % and specificity of 95.5 % with FNA [24]. Additional tests include a computed tomography (CT) scan and an integrated positron emission tomography and CT scan (PET/CT).

CT scans allows anatomic visualization of the extent of spread, lymphadenopathy, and relations with adjacent structures that assists surgeons in determining feasibility and extent of resection, as well as assists radiation oncologists in determining the extent of their treatment fields. CT detection of nodal metastases has an accuracy rate of 68–96 %, sensitivity rate of 8–75 %, and specificity rate of 77–94 % [25]. These rates are variable because they depend on the location of the nodal groups. For example, the sensitivity rate for detecting cervical paraesophageal nodes is 75 %, whereas it is 8 % for lesser curvature nodes.

PET/CT scans allow the visualization of metabolic activity to enhance identification of distant metastases and can change patient

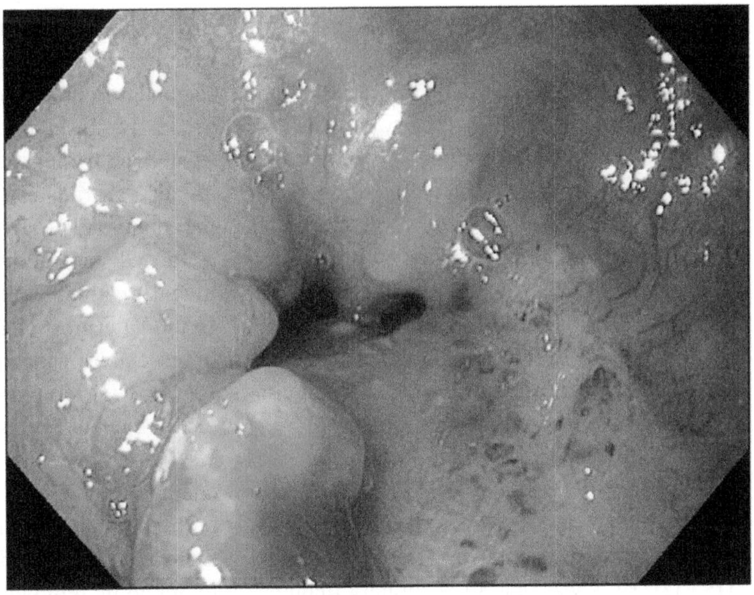

Fig. 8.3 An endoscopic picture of a distal esophageal adenocarcinoma (Courtesy of Quyen D. Chu, MD, MBA, FACS)

management up to 20 % of the cases [26]. PET/CT sensitivity to detect locoregional metastases is 51 % with a specificity of 84 %, and its sensitivity for detecting distant metastases is 67 % with a specificity of 97 % [26]. Pre- and post-treatment standardized uptake values (SUV) from PET may also have prognostic significance [27]. Additional workup for tumors above the carina without evidence of metastatic disease includes bronchoscopy and optional laparoscopy for GEJ tumors without evidence of metastatic disease [9].

Treatment

A multimodality approach is essential for the treatment of esophageal cancer, as treatment options vary widely according to stage. Table 8.2 demonstrates basic outline of treatment recommendations.

For carcinoma in situ (high-grade dysplasia) or lesions limited to the lamina propria and muscularis mucosa (Tis–T1a), a superficial approach is an option since these lesions have a low risk of spread and a cancer mortality of only 5 %. However, invasion into the *submucosa* dramatically increases the risk of spread and has a mortality risk of 40 %; hence superficial treatments are recommended only for stages Tis–T1a.

Table 8.2 Treatment recommendations by stage

Stage	Treatment
Tis–T1a	Endoscopic mucosal resection, photodynamic therapy, radiofrequency ablation, or esophagectomy alone
T1b	Esophagectomy alone
T2–T4, node positive	Neoadjuvant chemoradiation followed by esophagectomy
Distant metastasis	Palliative chemotherapy, radiation, or chemoradiation, esophageal dilation and stenting

The three main superficial approaches include endoscopic mucosal resection (EMR), photodynamic therapy (PDT), and radiofrequency ablation (RFA). EMR involves a submucosal injection of fluid to separate the lesion from the muscular layer of the esophagus to allow complete resection of the lesion [2]. Photodynamic therapy (PDT) uses monochromatic light to excite a photosensitizing agent that is selectively concentrated into malignant tissues causing the production of superoxide and hydroxyl radicals that lead to apoptosis, necrosis, vascular occlusion, and activation of the immune response [28]. RFA involves the use of ablation catheters inside a cylindrical balloon that is placed adjacent to lesions to ablate tissues using heat via an electrical current [2, 11]. Since RFA heating requires an electrically conductive path, it results in heating of tissues just next to the catheter [29].

A study by the University of Pennsylvania found that the sensitivity, specificity, and positive and negative predictive values of preoperative EUS for submucosal invasion were 100 %, 94 %, 83 %, and 100 %, respectively [30]. An Italian study found lower rates of accuracy with sensitivity, specificity, and positive and negative predictive values of 88 %, 63 %, 67 %, and 86 %, respectively; however, the authors still conclude that EUS is an extremely useful tool when considering nonsurgical treatment options [31].

A prospective single institutional study was performed examining the role of EMR for mucosal lesions showing high-grade dysplasia or early cancer in Barrett's esophagus after diagnosis by EUS [32]. EUS was able to accurately diagnose 85 % of the lesions (1 patient overstaged and 6 understaged). A meta-analysis of the staging accuracy of esophageal cancer by EUS found the sensitivity and specificity for T1 lesions to be 81.6 % and 99.4 %, respectively [24]. These studies provide further support that EMR is an acceptable treatment option after diagnosis by EUS. Nevertheless, the incidence of occult adenocarcinoma in high-grade dysplasia has been reported to be as high as 40 %, and if the lesion has characteristics that are worrisome for a predilection for lymph node metastases such as lymphovascular space invasion, neural invasion, tumor size > 2 cm, or multifocality, an esophagectomy, especially in the era of minimally invasive techniques, still warrants consideration [33–35]. The morbidity from such a procedure for early stage disease is acceptable as the University of Pittsburgh's review of their T1 esophagectomy patients found that on their Gastroesophageal Reflux Disease-Health Related Quality of Life (GERD-HRQOL) questionnaire, 89 % and 10.6 % of patients had excellent and satisfactory HRQOL scores, respectively [35].

Surgery

After clinical staging is completed, treatment of esophageal cancers is relegated to three broad categories: immediate surgical therapy, surgical therapy following chemotherapy with or without radiation therapy, and nonsurgical management. Esophageal precancerous lesions such as high-grade dysplasia or very early cancers can be treated with the aforementioned strategies, but are also candidates for immediate resection. For the majority of esophageal cancers, however, advanced stage at diagnosis will mandate neoadjuvant treatment followed by surgical resection. In the lattermost category are the metastatic and unresectable cancers (i.e., those that locally invade vital structures such as the aorta or tracheobronchial tree) – these are not offered surgical resection, but rather offered palliative chemoradiotherapy. As the esophagus traverses both the thoracic and the abdominal cavities, there are understandably several approaches to facilitate its removal. Despite these variations, a few constants hold true which follow below.

In concordance with all other solid organ resections for malignancy, a minimum number of lymph nodes retrieved are recommended to constitute adequate diagnostic and therapeutic benefit. Based upon consensus statement by the National Comprehensive Cancer Network's esophageal cancer work group, this number has been established at 15 nodes [36]. For upper and middle esophageal lesions, this mainly comprises the adventitial tissue surrounding the esophagus within the posterior mediastinum. For distal esophageal lesions, this represents paraesophageal nodes from the hiatal region and those along the course of the left gastric artery. In regard to surgical margins, obtaining a longitudinal esophageal margin is generally attainable considering the generous length of the organ; for upper third or low cervical tumors, however, this can sometimes require a partial or total laryngectomy with pharyngogastric reconstruction. It should be mentioned though that historically, due to poor function and survival outcomes, many experts feel that definitive chemoradiation therapy is more appropriate for proximal esophageal cancers.

The gastric margin, conversely, can become a concern in particular with lesions found at the gastroesophageal junction, which is an area frequently involved in western series [37]. In this situation, obtaining a comfortable margin of (preferably) five centimeters sometimes cannot be achieved while still preserving enough proximal stomach to fashion a suitable conduit for esophageal reconstruction (Figs. 8.4 and 8.5).

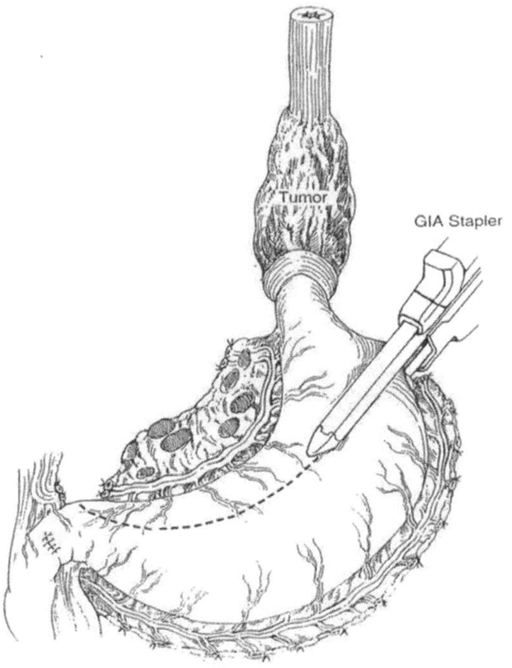

Fig. 8.4 Resecting the distal lesion of the esophagus and creating a gastric conduit. The stomach is mobilized after ligating all vessels supplying the stomach except for the right gastroepiploic vessel. Note that the lymph nodes along the lesser curvature are included in the specimen (Reprinted from Ref. [40]. With permission from Elsevier)

In that instance, an alternate conduit is required such as colon or jejunum in selected circumstances (Fig. 8.6).

All patients undergoing esophageal resection will have several days of nil per os (NPO) status, and this period can increase substantially if there are any untoward complications such as anastomotic leak. Therefore, enteral access by routine placement of a jejunal feeding tube is highly recommended. This tube remains in place for roughly 1 month after surgery and is removed once the patient has demonstrated that adequate caloric intake and stabilization of postoperative weight loss can be achieved by oral diet alone. Another distinct advantage of a routine jejunostomy tube placement is that if the patient develops troubles with oral nutrition in the future, whether due to stricture, recurrence, or simply failure to thrive, the jejunostomy site can be percutaneously cannulated by an interventional radiologist and immediate enteral feedings can commence without difficulties [38]. In our practice, we have found this to be of great use even years after the initial surgery. For those patients who are plagued by continued weight loss or radiation-induced esophagitis preventing oral nutrition during the neoadjuvant phase of their treatment, it is sometimes necessary to have enteral access placed before esophagectomy. For these purposes, we have found either percutaneously

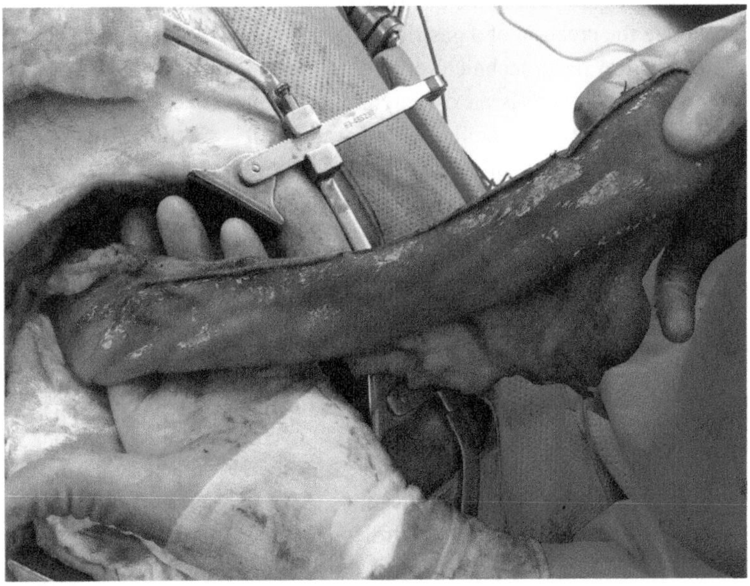

Fig. 8.5 A reconstructed esophagus using a gastric conduit

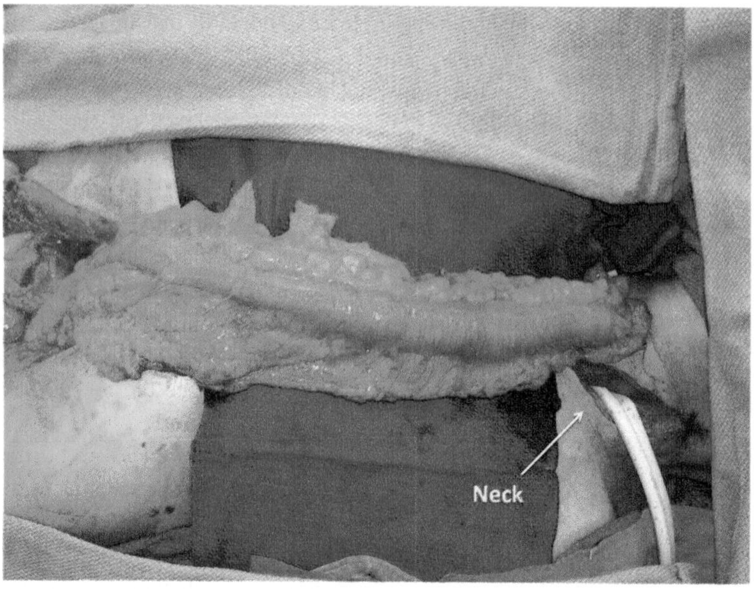

Fig. 8.6 *Colonic interposition using the right colon.* Blood supply is based on the inferior mesenteric artery (Courtesy of Quyen D. Chu, MD, MBA, FACS)

placed gastrostomy tubes by interventional radiology or traditional surgical jejunostomy tube placement to be superior to percutaneous endoscopy gastrostomy (PEG) tubes. The benefit of the former preferred tube is that the footprint of a 14–16 French Cook-type catheter on the gastric wall is considerably smaller than the common 20–24 French PEG-style tube. A small catheter gastrostomy can be easily oversewn and imbricated frequently with one or two sutures, whereas the PEG style tubes often produce a more pronounced disfigurement of the gastric wall and can jeopardize the creation of a gastric tube.

Aside from these technical considerations of esophagectomy, there is an overarching concept that can differentiate overall success of surgical management: volume. In a recent meta-analysis comprising nearly 28,000 patients, the overall surgical mortality significantly decreased in proportion to the number of esophagectomy cases performed by the given institution per year [39]. Undoubtedly, as the expertise of the surgeon, surgical team, and postoperative care team increases, so does patient safety. One major aspect of this relationship is likely related to the resources available in high-volume centers in the arena of rescue therapies for postoperative complications. After a surgery of this magnitude, regardless of the approach, several significant complications can arise that require adjunctive procedures to remedy, such as percutaneous drain placements, complex endoscopic interventions, and sophisticated cardiopulmonary team care. Furthermore, the aptitude of experienced nursing personnel in identifying these potential complications in an early phase may allow more swift resolution before progression. In a center where only a small number of these cases occur annually, these resources may not have the level of expertise or readiness to rescue an ailing patient who is rapidly deteriorating.

Esophagectomy Techniques

Transhiatal

As its name implies, a transhiatal esophagectomy is constituted by dissecting the middle and distal thirds of the esophagus through the diaphragmatic hiatus without the need for thoracotomy (Fig. 8.7) [40]. A cervical exposure is used to dissect the proximal third and complete the dissection in continuity with the abdominal approach. A long gastric tube is created and then drawn through the posterior mediastinum until it reaches

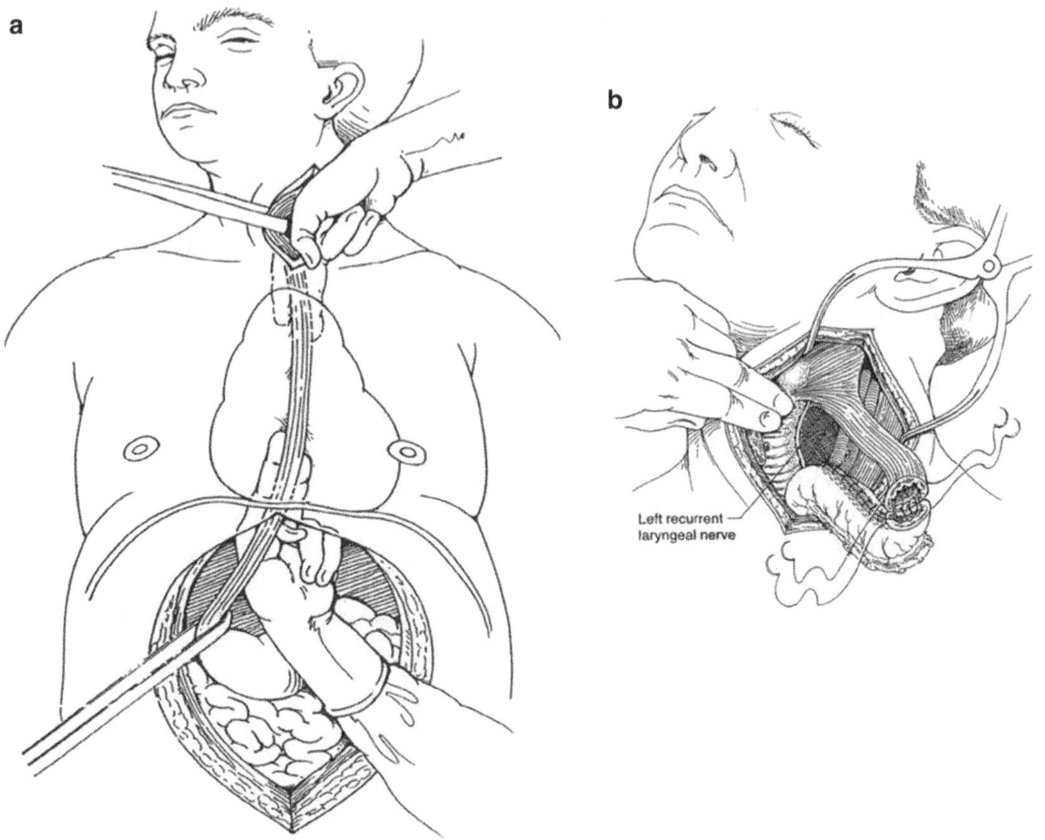

Fig. 8.7 Transhiatal esophagectomy technique. (**a**) The esophagus is bluntly dissected away from the surrounding structure with the fingers, taking care to not injure the membranous portion of the trachea. A left neck incision is also made to further mobilize the cervical esophagus. Care is taken to avoid injury to the left recurrent laryngeal nerve. (**b**) A cervical esophagogastrostomy anastomosis is performed in the left neck (Reprinted from Ref. [40]. With permission from Elsevier)

the skin level of the neck. An anastomosis between the cervical esophagus and this neo-esophagus is then created. Tumors located anywhere along the entire length of the esophagus to the gastric cardia can be resected equally with adequate margins. Advantages of this technique include the avoidance of entering the thorax, lower mortality from a leak at the cervical anastomosis, compared to a leak in the thorax from a transthoracic approach and the ability to remove the entire length of the esophagus when the consideration of long-segment Barrett's or margins is of concern. Without a thoracotomy, the pulmonary complications often plaguing esophageal resection are generally mitigated, which has been substantiated in the literature by a decreased length of ICU stay for the transhiatal technique [41]. Cervical anastomoses are created outside the radiated field of the mediastinum, and leaks in this locale generally will fistulize to the cervical skin without even fever or abscess formation. Near uniform closure of these fistulas will follow with cessation of oral intake alone, in great contrast to the 4–10 % need for reoperation that follows a thoracic duct leak. Disadvantages to this technique include the limited ability to dissect middle esophageal tumors, a questionable completeness of radical lymphadenectomy in the posterior mediastinum, thoracic duct leak at the level of the left neck, higher anastomotic leak rate compared to the transthoracic approach, and the increased risk of inadvertent injury to the tracheobronchial tree or azygos vein during blunt dissection of the proximal esophagus. Additionally, in the absence of direct visualization, the recurrent laryngeal nerves are at increased risk of injury when compared to esophagectomy via thoracotomy. A jejunal feeding tube is placed in all patients to bolster nutritional intake.

Transthoracic

Arguably the most commonly employed method of esophagectomy, resection via a right thoracotomy and laparotomy (Ivor-Lewis) remains the gold standard method of resecting any esophageal tumor of the middle and distal third as well as those extending to the gastric cardia [40, 42] (Fig. 8.8). Unlike a transhiatal approach, the advantage of direct dissection of the posterior mediastinum and the peri-esophageal tissue allows a more deliberate and thorough lymphadenectomy. The esophagus is divided at or above the level of the azygos vein, and a gastric tube similar to that created in the transhiatal procedure is anastomosed at that location. Advantages also include the ability to carefully preserve the membranous portions of the tracheobronchial tree and lower locoregional recurrences when compared to transhiatal esophagectomy. Disadvantages include the severe morbidity and mortality associated with anastomotic leak into the thorax or mediastinum, thoracic duct leak, an overall higher incidence of pulmonary complications, and the occasional necessity to expand to a cervical exposure if a proximal margin cannot be cleared [42]. This final addition constitutes a so-called "three-field" esophagectomy (i.e., McKeown), effectively combining the advantages

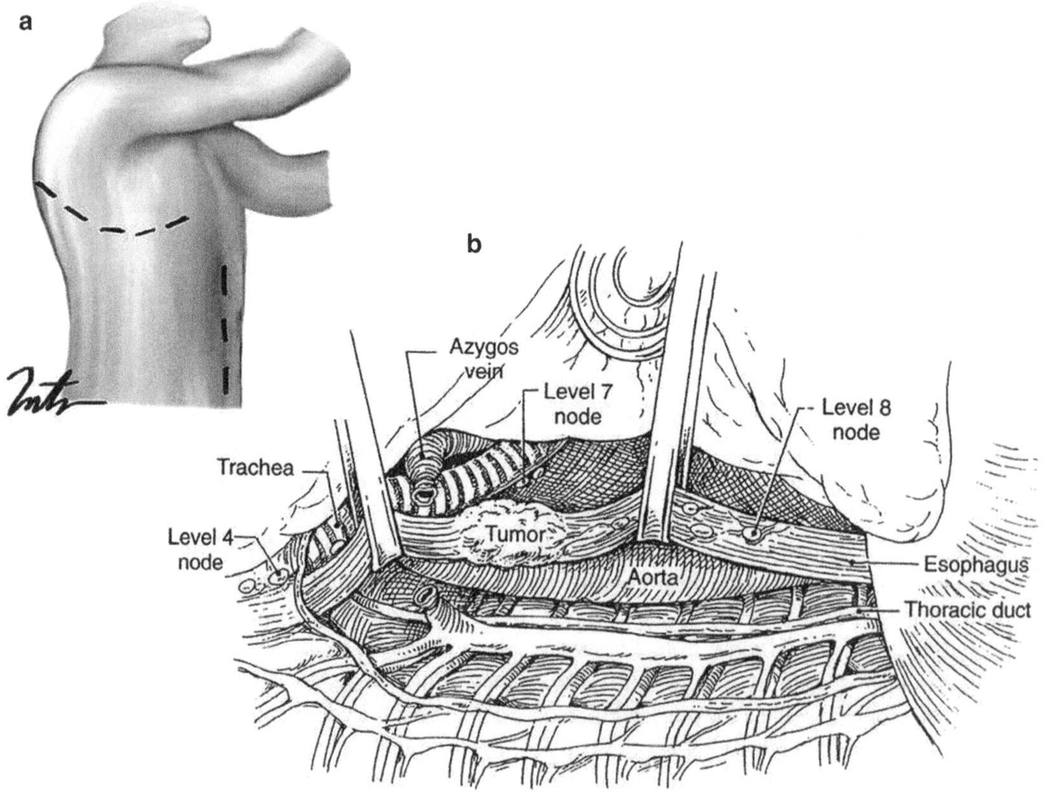

Fig. 8.8 (**a**) An Ivor-Lewis approach includes an abdominal and a right thoracic incision (Courtesy of Thuy-Tien Chu). (**b**) The azygos vein is ligated, the thoracic esophagus is mobilized, and the mediastinal lymph nodes are retrieved (Reprinted from Ref. [40]. With permission from Elsevier)

of both approaches. Perhaps counterintuitively, however, the safety profile of this third resection technique is actually inferior to either prior method, likely due to its application in only the most challenging tumors from a surgical standpoint. Again, as in all types of esophagectomy, a feeding jejunostomy is placed in all patients.

On occasion, a left thoracotomy instead of a right thoracotomy is performed for GEJ and cancer involving the cardia of the stomach. In such a situation, esophagogastric anastomosis is performed just superior to the inferior pulmonary veins. The disadvantage with this approach is the presence of the aortic arch, which limits the surgeon's ability to perform a higher anastomosis, although some have advocated tunneling the conduit behind the aortic arch. The left thoracotomy approach is not as widely performed as the other approaches, and it is mentioned here only for completeness.

Minimally Invasive Techniques

As with the adaptation of many oncologic resections from traditional open approaches to minimally invasive methods, esophagectomy has been well documented in the literature as a feasible and oncologically sound undertaking [43, 44]. Preserving the steps and general architecture of the original operation, minimally invasive esophagectomy (MIE) can be performed with or without thoracoscopic dissection of the intrathoracic esophagus. Though no prospective randomized trials to compare MIE and open techniques exist, several series have indicated that MIE is safe and effective, allowing an oncologically sound resection (evidenced by extent of lymphadenectomy and margin clearance) with a comparably safe risk profile when compared to historical standards [45]. Similar to the advantages afforded by minimally invasive techniques employed in other operations, decreased postoperative pain, faster return of bowel function, and improved cosmesis have been achieved in comparison to the traditional open methods [45]. This is especially true in the avoidance of thoracotomy provided by thoracoscopic resection and reconstruction.

Extent of Lymphadenectomy

Completeness of lymphadenectomy has been long considered the obligate partner to the successful resection of primary tumors, and this concept has been the subject of some scrutiny over the preceding years. With the refinement of neoadjuvant therapies, there has been a general sense of devaluation placed upon radical lymphadenectomies so prevalent in historical view. Driving this scrutiny is the inherent difference between the operative approaches in regard to emphasis placed on accessibility to lymph nodes; several studies have indicated that the transthoracic approach allows a more thorough lymphadenectomy, and indeed, the number of lymph nodes retrieved is often higher compared to the transhiatal approach. Surgeons who endorse the transhiatal approach despite the reproducibly lower number of lymph nodes harvested submit the supporting literature that long-term outcome is not influenced by the number of nodes removed at surgery [46, 47].

Alternate Methods of Reconstruction

Occasionally, either due to tumor- or anatomic-related considerations, the stomach is not a suitable candidate for esophageal reconstruction. In these instances, the most commonly employed conduit is an interposition of a segment of the colon either in the posterior mediastinum or the anterior mediastinum [48, 49] (Figs. 8.6 and 8.9). Similarly, an isolated jejunal segment can also be used to provide the necessary hollow viscus to reconstitute the upper digestive tract. In the case of the former, special preparation in the preoperative phase is required to verify the integrity of the colon for eventual use. Colonoscopy to ensure the absence of neoplasms and mesenteric angiography to evaluate the vascular inflow of the future pedicle are necessary steps if such a reconstruction is planned. As for the former, several techniques of improving the vascular supply of what is often a free graft have been described. These often involve augmenting arterial inflow to the

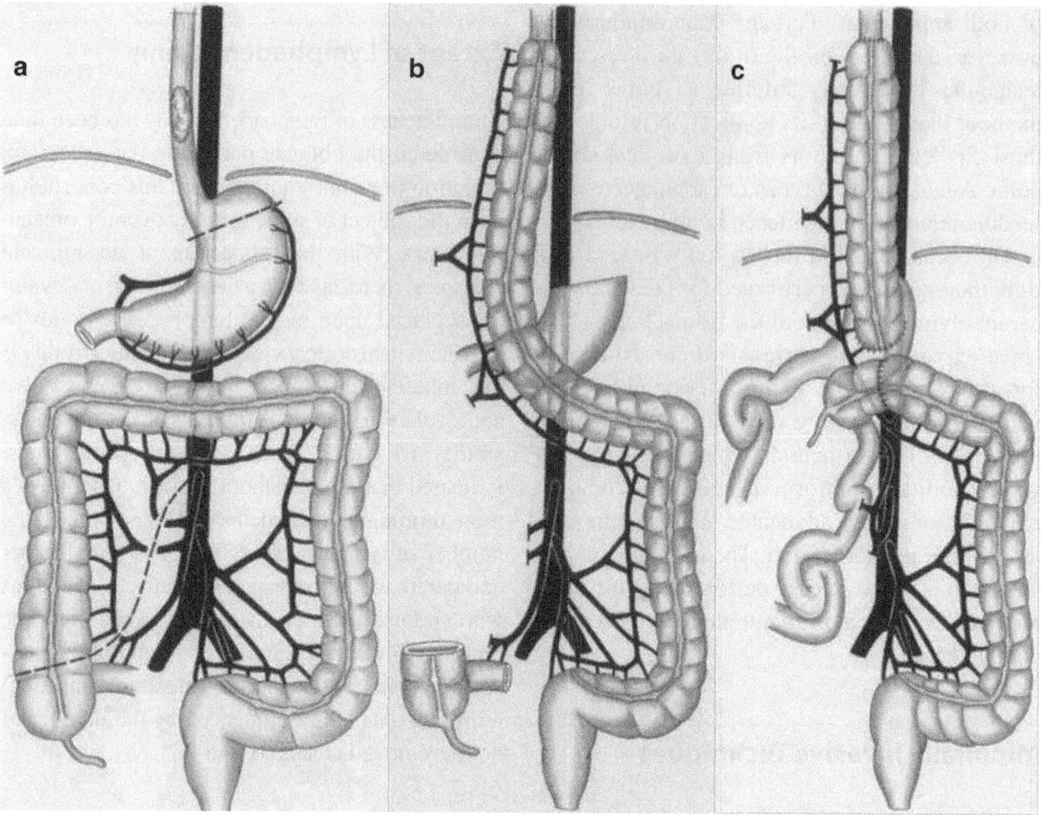

Fig. 8.9 Technique of using the right colon as an alternative conduit (Reprinted from Ref. [49]. With permission from Wolters Kluwer Health)

intestinal mesentery by direct arterial anastomosis to the common carotid artery. Though quality of life is somewhat limited by these alternate reconstruction techniques, they do offer a preferable alternative to lifelong intestinal discontinuity and the presence of a cervical esophagostomy or "spit fistula."

Radiation

The rationale for radiation therapy is for the definitive management for unresectable cases or to sterilize microscopic disease near the primary tumor and in regional lymph nodes as part of a neoadjuvant regimen. The use of chemoradiation for nonsurgical candidates was established by the Radiation Therapy Oncology Group (RTOG) 8501 trial where radiation alone was compared to concurrent chemoradiation [50]. The trial showed a dismal 5-year overall survival rate of 0 % versus 27 % for the concurrent arm.

Given the relatively low definitive radiation dose, several trials have investigated the role of radiation dose escalation to improve outcomes. The intergroup 0213 trial randomized patients to receive 64.8 Gy versus 50.4 Gy [51]. The results of this trial found no significant difference between the two arms in median survival (13.0 vs. 18.1 months), 2-year overall survival (31 % vs. 40 %), or locoregional failure (56 % vs. 52 %). This trial has been criticized as 7 of the 11 treatment-related deaths occurred prior to receiving 50.4 Gy.

RTOG 9207 was a phase I/II study of concurrent chemotherapy followed by a brachytherapy boost [52]. Brachytherapy is a radiation technique that uses a point source of radioactive material that is brought close to the tumor. These sources have a limited range and are often used to deliver high conformal doses while sparing normal tissues. Unfortunately, a 12 % incidence of fistula formation was found from this technique and thus has not been readily adopted. Although efforts to dose escalate radiation have failed, it is important to note that approximately a quarter of unresectable patients can be cured with definitive chemoradiation.

For surgical candidates, there is some controversy regarding the benefit of neoadjuvant chemoradiation over surgery alone as several clinical trials failed to demonstrate an advantage with the neoadjuvant approach (Univ. of Michigan [53], European Organisation for Research and Treatment of Cancer (EORTC) [54], Univ. of Ulsan in Korea [55], and the combined Trans Tasman Radiation Oncology Group (TROG) and Australasian Gastro-Intestinal Trials Group (AGITG [56])). In contradistinction, an older study by Walsh et al. at St. James Hospital (Ireland) found an advantage with chemoradiation [57], and several recent studies including the Cancer and Leukemia Group B (CALGB) 9781 [58], the Chemoradiotherapy for Oesophageal Cancer Followed by Surgery Study (CROSS) trial [59], as well as a meta-analysis [60] found a significant survival advantage to trimodality therapy.

The CROSS trial was a landmark trial that randomized 366 patients to neoadjuvant carboplatin and paclitaxel with radiation therapy versus surgery alone. Seventy-five percent of these patients had adenocarcinoma. The results showed that the trimodality approach significantly doubled median survival from 24.0 to 49.4 months with a 5-year overall survival of 47 % in the trimodality group versus 34 % in the surgery-alone group ($p=0.003$). Trimodality approach is now the preferred treatment for locally advanced esophageal cancers at many centers.

There also have been several trials examining the role of surgery in the context of chemoradiation. A German trial from the University Clinic of Tubingen randomized high-risk esophageal cancer patients, after receiving induction chemotherapy, to either concurrent chemoradiation followed by surgery or to chemoradiation alone [61]. The Fédération Francophone de Cancérologie Digestive (FFCD) in France also performed a similar trial where all patients initially received chemoradiation and where responders were randomized to surgery [62]. The results from both trials found no difference in overall survival and an increase in treatment-related mortality in the surgery groups. It is important to note that both trials showed local control benefits to the surgery arm. The German trial found a 2-year progression free survival benefit of 76.5 % in the surgery arm versus 64.3 % in the chemoradiation alone arm, while the FFCD trial found a 2-year locoregional control benefit of 66 % in favor of surgery versus 56 % in the nonsurgical arm.

Histology was also a factor in the two studies. All patients in the German trial and 89 % of patients in the FFCD trial had squamous cell carcinomas (SCC). Such histology is not what is generally observed in the United States since most US patients have adenocarcinoma. Furthermore, SCCs tend to respond better to chemoradiation than adenocarcinomas; in the CROSS trial, patients who had SCC had a complete response rate of 49 % compared to 23 % in the adenocarcinoma group [59]. The German trial also hinted at a late nonsignificant survival benefit after 3 years for the surgery arm. The FFCD trial may not have shown a survival benefit in the surgery arm because they only randomized patients who responded to chemoradiation. It is important to remember that approximately half of the patients undergoing definitive chemoradiation will fail locally, further highlighting the need for surgical intervention [51].

GEJ tumors are now treated similarly with neoadjuvant chemotherapy and radiation followed surgical resection, especially in the United States; however, other treatment strategies for GEJ and distal esophageal tumors include perioperative (neoadjuvant and adjuvant) chemotherapy based on the Medical Research Council Adjuvant Gastric Infusional Chemotherapy (MAGIC) trial that showed a benefit to this regimen over surgery alone [63]. This will be expounded in more detail in the chemotherapy section. In the past, some have also treated GEJ tumors postoperatively with 5-FU and leucovorin before, during, and after radiation based on the Intergroup 0116 that found a benefit to postoperative chemoradiation versus surgery alone [64].

Cervical esophageal cancer is treated similarly to a primary squamous cell carcinoma of the head and neck. Primary surgical resection for cervical esophageal cancer has been done historically, but the outcomes are poor and patients often require adjuvant chemoradiation [65–67]. More institutions are moving toward definitive chemoradiation for organ preservation, as the hypopharynx, larynx, and esophagus must be removed using a pharyngo-laryngo-esophagectomy and definitive chemoradiation has similar efficacy in comparison to those patients receiving surgical resection [65–67].

The current standard chemoradiation regimen consists of 50.4 Gy in 1.8 Gy fractions concurrently with a fluoropyrimidine or taxane-based regimen for definitive and neoadjuvant chemoradiation patients. Radiation therapy is delivered daily Monday through Friday. Prior to treatment, the esophageal tumor is contoured on a CT scan and typically a 5 cm longitudinal margin with a 1–2 cm radial margin is used to encompass not only the tumor, but microscopic spread and to account for daily organ motion and patient setup errors. In addition, normal structures such as the heart, lungs, liver, and spinal cord are also contoured. This creates a 3D model that is placed into an advanced computer algorithm that allows the radiation oncologist to see the dose to the target, while minimizing dose to surrounding normal structures. Typically three to four radiation fields are used to encompass the target volume. Variations in treatment planning include treating the initial volume at risk to 45 Gy followed by a reduced field to the gross disease only to 50.4 Gy. Given the distribution of esophageal lymphatics, paraesophageal lymph nodes will naturally be included when targeting the primary disease with a margin. Tumors proximal to the carina also have the bilateral supraclavicular nodes treated, whereas for distal and GEJ tumors, the celiac axis nodes are included in the radiation portal. A typical AP field can be seen in Fig. 8.10.

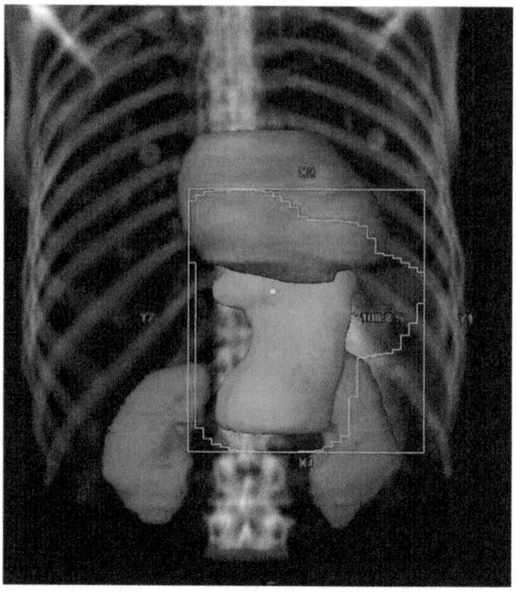

Fig. 8.10 A typical anterior posterior (AP) field for radiation therapy: the heart is in red, kidneys in magenta, and the planning treatment volume (PTV) in cyan

Chemotherapy

The preceding sections discussed the role of local regional therapies for esophageal cancer in patients without evidence of distant metastasis. The goal of primary therapy is for cure. Adjuvant therapy is given in addition to primary treatment with the aim of reducing recurrence and improving cure rate. Neoadjuvant therapy is adjuvant therapy administered prior to the established or standard therapy. With the exception of early esophageal cancer (Tis and T1 disease), the cure rates are low with surgery alone. Sixty-five to eighty percent of patients who undergo surgery for esophageal cancer will fail in distant sites such as the liver, lung, bone, retroperitoneum, and brain. For these reasons, chemotherapy has been incorporated in the treatment of localized disease. The rationale for the use of systemic cytotoxic agents in this disease is twofold. One is to control micrometastasis and secondly to potentiate the therapeutic effects of radiation therapy. Definitive therapy using systemic chemotherapy concurrently given with radiation therapy is a reasonable treatment option for patients who have localized or locally advanced disease who have comorbidities precluding surgical resection of their esophageal cancer as described previously. The goal in the treatment of advanced esophageal cancer is for palliation of symptoms as well as prolongation of life. Chemotherapy is an effective form of palliation in advanced esophageal cancer. In this section, we will discuss the data on the role of chemotherapy in localized, locally advanced, and metastatic esophageal cancer.

Localized/Resectable Disease: Neoadjuvant Therapy

Complete pathologic response is associated with better outcome. A number of randomized clinical trials address the benefit of neoadjuvant chemotherapy prior to surgery versus surgery alone in patients with localized esophageal cancer (Table 8.3) [68, 69, 63]. These trials were associated with low complete pathologic response rates. Four trials fail to show benefit while three showed improvement in survival associated with neoadjuvant chemotherapy. Among the three trials shown in Table 8.3, it is the MAGIC trial reported by Cunningham that is perhaps cited the most [63]. The patients who received perioperative chemotherapy (three preoperative and three postoperative cycles of intravenous epirubicin, cisplatin, and fluorouracil or ECF) had higher overall survival rate with a hazard ratio of 0.75 compared to the surgery-alone arm. The 5-year survival rate (36 % vs. 23 %) was statistically significantly better in favor of the perioperative arm. It is important to note, however, that 62 % of the patients had adenocarcinoma and almost three-quarters had gastric cancer. A meta-analysis was performed using 11 trials comparing surgery alone to neoadjuvant chemotherapy followed by surgery in esophageal and GE junction tumors [70]. The results suggest an absolute survival benefit of 5 % in 2 years in favor of the neoadjuvant chemotherapy followed by the surgery group.

Several randomized clinical trials and meta-analyses have demonstrated the benefit of a tri-modality approach in improving survival compared to surgery alone. Neoadjuvant treatment with chemotherapy and radiation is associated with a complete pathologic response rate of 16–40 % [53, 56–59, 71, 72]. Combined chemotherapy and radiation therapy, given before surgery, is also associated with an improvement in local control compared to surgery alone. Table 8.4 demonstrates selected trials of neoadjuvant combined chemotherapy and radiation followed by surgery versus surgery alone.

Table 8.3 Selected phase III randomized trials of neoadjuvant chemotherapy followed by surgery in esophageal cancer

Study/year	Phase	*N*	Histology	Location	Treatment	pCR (%)	Median survival (mos)
Kelsen [68] 1998	III	440	Squamous: 46 % Adenoca: 54 %	Esophagus: N/A GEJ: N/A	5FU/Cis x 3	3	CT/S: 14.9 S: 16.1 $P=0.53$
MRC [69] 2002	III	100	Squamous: 31 % Adenoca: 66 %	Esophagus: 90 % Cardia: 10 %	5FU/Cis x 2	4	CT/S: 16.8 S: 13.3 $P=0.004$
Cunningham [63] or MAGIC trial 2006	III	503	Squamous: 37 % Adenoca: 62 %	Esophagus:15 % GEJ: 11 % Stomach: 74 %	ECF	0	5-years survival CT/S: 36 % S: 23 % $P=0.009$

pCR pathologic complete response, *Adenoca* adenocarcinoma, *GEJ* gastroesophageal junction, *5FU* 5-fluorouracil, *Cis* cisplatin, *CT* chemotherapy, *XRT* radiation therapy, *S* surgery, *mos* months, *ECF* epirubicin, cisplatin, 5-fluorouracil, *MAGIC* Medical Research Council Adjuvant Gastric Infusional Chemotherapy, *MRC* Medical Research Council, *N/A* not available

Table 8.4 Selected trials of neoadjuvant combined chemotherapy and radiation and their results

Study/year	Phase	*N*	Histology	Location	Treatment	pCR (%)	Median survival (mos)
Walsh [57] 1996	III	113	Adenoca: 100 %	Esophagus: 65 % Cardia: 35 %	5FU/Cis x 2 XRT 40 Gy	25	CT/XRT/S: 16 S: 11 *P*=0.01
Urba [53] 2001	III	100	Squamous: 25 % Adenoca: 75 %	Esophagus: 100 %	5FU/Cis/vinblastine x 2 45 Gy	28	CT/XRT/S: 16.9 S: 17.6 *P*=0.15
Burmeister [56] 2005	III	256	Squamous: 37 % Adenoca: 62 %	Esophagus: 100 %	5FU/Cis x 1 35 Gy	16	CT/XRT/S: 22.2 S: 19.3 *P*=0.57
Tepper [58] 2008	III	56	Squamous: 25 % Adenoca: 75 %	Esophagus GEJ	5FU/Cis x 2 50.4 Gy	40	CT/XRT/S:54 S: 21 *P*=0.002
Mariette [71] 2010	III	195	Squamous: 70 % Adenoca: 29 %	Esophagus: 100 %	5FU/Cis x 2 45 Gy	29	CT/XRT/S: 31.8 S: 43.8 *P*=0.66
Leichman [72] 2011	II	93	Adenoca: 100 %	Esophagus: 60 % GEJ: 40 %	Oxaliplatin/5FU 45 Gy Oxaliplatin/5FU	28	CT/XRT/S/CT: 28.3
Van Hagen [59] 2012	III	368	Squamous: 23 % Adenoca: 75 %	Esophagus: 73 % GEJ: 24 %	Carboplatin/paclitaxel 41.4 Gy	29	CT/XRT/S: 49.4 S: 24 *P*=0.003

Adenoca adenocarcinoma, *5FU* 5-fluorouracil, *Cis* cisplatin, *CT* chemotherapy, *S* surgery, *mos* months, *GEJ* gastroesophageal junction, *XRT* radiation therapy

Metastatic Disease

The goal of therapy for advanced disease is primarily for palliation although there may be potential for prolongation in life with therapy. The most common symptoms which need palliation are malignant dysphagia and poor nutrition. Endoscopic palliation with esophageal dilation and stent placement as well as PEG tube placement may improve the quality of life of these patients. Treatment options include endoscopic ablation (laser, cryotherapy, and PDT), dilation, and surgery; however, the most commonly used approaches are endoluminal stenting and radiation +/– chemotherapy [73]. Careful patient selection is imperative, but because of the favorable response rate, full doses of concurrent chemoradiation are often used given the poor quality of life and nutritional status of these patients [74].

As in systemic therapy for localized disease, there is not just one standard but a number of standard chemotherapy regimens that may be used in patients with metastatic esophageal cancer. Combination therapy is generally associated with a better chance of benefit compared to a single agent; however, for elderly patients and those with a poor performance status, single agent chemotherapy or best supportive care are appropriate alternatives. The list below represents a sample of chemotherapeutic regimens used in advanced disease:

- Trastuzumab, capecitabine, cisplatin (for HER2/neu + tumors)
- FOLFOX6 or 7 (oxaliplatin, 5FU/LV)
- FOLFIRI (irinotecan, 5FU/LV)
- DCF/mDCF (docetaxel, cisplatin, 5FU)
- EOX (epirubicin, oxaliplatin, capecitabine)
- ECF (epirubicin, cisplatin, 5FU)
- ECX (epirubicin, cisplatin, capecitabine)
- Irinotecan, cisplatin
- Paclitaxel, carboplatin
- Paclitaxel, cisplatin
- Docetaxel, irinotecan

The combination of epirubicin, cisplatin, and 5-fluorouracil is a standard chemotherapy regimen that is also used in the advanced disease of the GEJ and the stomach. Cisplatin is associated with significant side effects such as emesis, nephrotoxicity, and neuropathy. These side effects can be ameliorated when oxaliplatin is used instead of cisplatin. 5-fluorouracil (5-FU) is given as continuous infusion requiring central venous access. Because of potential complications associated with central venous access (thrombosis, infection), an oral substitute such as capecitabine appears to be an attractive alternative to 5-FU. In an effort to determine the non-inferiority of oxaliplatin to cisplatin and of capecitabine, an oral fluoropyrimidine alternative to 5-FU, the investigators of the Randomized ECF for Advanced and Locally Advanced Esophagogastric Cancer 2 (REAL-2) trial enrolled more than a 1,000 patients and showed that capecitabine and oxaliplatin are just as effective as fluorouracil and cisplatin, respectively, in patients with previously untreated, unresectable, or metastatic esophagogastric cancer [75].

Given that approximately 22 % of patients with gastroesophageal junction (GEJ) and gastric cancer have HER-2 overexpression, a clinical trial to assess the efficacy of trastuzumab, a monoclonal antibody against human epidermal growth factor receptor 2, against HER-2 positive GEJ and gastric tumors would appear to be the next logical step [76]. In fact, this was the case. The Trastuzumab for Gastric or Gastro-Oesophageal Junction Cancer (ToGA) trial conducted an open-label, international, phase III, randomized controlled trial in 122 centers in 24 countries. In this trial, 594 patients with inoperable locally advanced, recurrent, or metastatic HER-2 positive gastric or GEJ tumors were randomly assigned to receive capecitabine plus cisplatin with or without trastuzumab [77]. Of note, 17–20 % were GEJ tumors while 80 % were gastric cancer. The addition of trastuzumab to chemotherapy was associated with improvement of median overall survival of 13.8 months compared with 11.1 months in those assigned to chemotherapy alone. The rates of overall grade 3 or 4 adverse and cardiac adverse events were not different between the two groups.

Although there are some improvements in the outcome of patients with esophageal cancer, therapy remains unsatisfactory. Survival remains dismal particularly for those patients with unresectable and metastatic disease. We continue to treat patients empirically without much information as to prognostic and predictive factors that may help personalize their therapy. The Southwest Oncology group has a trial that is actively enrolling patients seeking to assign patients into therapy based on biologic markers and predictors or response. Novel agents targeting proteins in signal transduction are currently being tested either as single agent or in combination with conventional cytotoxic drugs in order to identify improved and effective therapy for advanced esophageal and GEJ cancers.

Salient Points

- There has been an epidemiologic shift in the past two to three decades as most cases of esophageal cancer are now adenocarcinoma instead of squamous cell carcinoma.
- Esophageal squamous cell carcinoma and adenocarcinoma represent two distinct diseases.
- Smoking and alcohol use are closely tied with squamous cell carcinoma, whereas obesity, GERD, and Barrett's esophagus are associated with adenocarcinoma.
- The basic divisions of the esophagus include the cervical, thoracic (divided into upper, middle, and lower thirds), and the gastroesophageal junction.
- The esophagus lacks a serosa; thus tumors do not have an anatomic barrier inhibiting spread to adjacent structures.
- Recent staging changes include separate staging for squamous cell carcinoma and adenocarcinoma, T4 subclassification, inclusion of tumor location and grade, celiac nodes as regional disease (for lower esophageal tumors), and N stage based on the number of positive nodes.
- Symptoms often come on slow and indolently, and patients often present late in their disease.
- Imaging techniques work in conjunction to accurately stage the patient and direct therapy including the type and extent of surgical resection and radiation field planning.
- Lesions limited to the lamina propria (Tis) and muscularis mucosa (T1a) have limited potential for spread and low cancer mortality of 5 %, but with invasion into the submucosa, the risk of spread increases and mortality rises to 40 %. This is the rationale behind the use of EMR, PDT, and ablation for Tis and T1a, but not T1b lesions.
- High volume centers have significantly decreased surgical mortality.
- A transhiatal esophagectomy is constituted by dissecting the middle and distal thirds of the esophagus through the diaphragmatic hiatus without the need for thoracotomy.
- Advantages of a transhiatal esophagectomy technique include the avoidance of entering the thorax, improved safety of a cervical anastomosis, and the ability to remove the entire length of the esophagus when the consideration of long-segment Barrett's or margins is of concern.
- Disadvantages to a transhiatal esophagectomy include the limited ability to dissect middle esophageal tumors, a questionable completeness of radical lymphadenectomy in the posterior mediastinum, and the increased risk of inadvertent injury to the tracheobronchial tree during blunt dissection of the proximal esophagus.
- A transthoracic esophagectomy via a right thoracotomy and laparotomy remains the gold standard method of resecting any esophageal tumor of the middle and distal thirds as well as those extending to the gastric cardia.
- Advantages to a transthoracic esophagectomy include a more deliberate and thorough lymphadenectomy, preservation of the membranous portions of the tracheobronchial tree, and lower locoregional recurrences.
- Disadvantages to a transthoracic esophagectomy include the severe morbidity and mortality associated with anastomotic leak into the thorax or mediastinum, an overall higher incidence of pulmonary complications, and the occasional necessity to expand to a cervical exposure if a proximal margin cannot be cleared.

- Minimally invasive techniques are now commonly employed methods of esophagectomy and is safe and effective with a comparably safe risk profile when compared to historical standards.
- There is a controversy regarding trimodality therapy, but recent studies and a meta-analysis support the use of neoadjuvant chemoradiation versus surgery alone.
- GEJ tumors can be treated with neoadjuvant chemoradiation or perioperative chemotherapy.
- Cervical esophageal tumors are often treated with definitive chemoradiation for organ preservation.
- The supraclavicular fossae are included in the radiation field for tumors above the carina, and the celiac axis is covered for distal and GEJ tumors, given the pattern of lymphatic drainage.
- The backbone of chemotherapy consists of fluoropyrimidine or taxane-based regimens.
- There is a shift toward less toxic and more convenient alternative chemotherapy agents in oxaliplatin and capecitabine (oral form of 5-FU) over cisplatin and 5-FU.
- Biomarkers and their targeted agents play an important role in the modern era of cancer treatment. The use of trastuzumab in combination with chemotherapy for HER2-positive GEJ tumors is now the preferred treatment for metastatic disease.
- Although a patient may have metastatic disease, the palliation of malignant dysphagia is important and can be aggressively treated with full dose concurrent chemoradiation.

Questions

1. In the United States, the preferred treatment regimen for resectable stage II–III esophageal cancer:
   A. Surgery alone
   B. Concurrent chemoradiation
   C. Surgery followed by concurrent chemoradiation
   D. Neoadjuvant chemoradiation followed by surgery
   E. Neoadjuvant chemotherapy followed by surgery and maintenance trastuzumab
2. A 68-year-old male with stage T4N0M0 unresectable esophageal cancer is seen by you in consultation. The recommended treatment is:
   A. Chemotherapy followed by radiation therapy alone
   B. Chemotherapy followed by concurrent chemoradiation
   C. Dose-escalated radiation using external beam or brachytherapy
   D. Concurrent chemoradiation to standard doses
   E. Chemotherapy alone
3. Adenocarcinoma and squamous cell carcinoma of the esophagus represent:
   A. One disease with the same etiologic factors and treatments
   B. A strong case can be made that they represent different diseases, but with the same treatment options
   C. A strong case can be made that they represent different diseases, with different treatment options
   D. Etiologic factors and epidemiologic trends have not been clearly identified for esophageal cancer
4. A 55-year-old obese female with a recent diagnosis of a clinical T2 adenocarcinoma of the gastroesophageal junction is found to have a single left supraclavicular lymph node with an SUV of 7.6 on PET/CT. What is her nodal stage?
   A. N0
   B. N1
   C. N2
   D. N3
   E. The supraclavicular lymph node represents metastatic disease
5. A 75-year-old male with asymptomatic metastatic adenocarcinoma is scheduled to undergo chemotherapy with cisplatin and continuous infusion 5-FU. He asks if there are any other therapies he should be considering and you recommend:
   A. Trastuzumab, a monoclonal antibody against HER2/neu
   B. Cetuximab, a monoclonal antibody against EGFR
   C. Everolimus, an mTOR inhibitor

   D. Bevacizumab, a monoclonal antibody against VEGF
   E. Neoadjuvant concurrent chemoradiation followed by esophagectomy to optimize local control
6. The lymphatic drainage of the esophagus is listed correctly below EXCEPT:
   A. The cervical esophagus drains to the neck and supraclavicular nodes
   B. The upper thoracic esophagus drains to the nodes on the innominate artery and ligamentum arteriosum, paraesophageal, and paratracheal nodes
   C. The middle thoracic drains to the tracheobronchial, paraesophageal, and pulmonary hilar nodes
   D. The lower thoracic esophagus drains to the paraesophageal, diaphragmatic, and pancreaticoduodenal nodes
   E. GEJ drains to the nodes on the left gastric, celiac, common hepatic, and splenic arteries, as well as the paracardiac and lesser curvature nodes
7. Which of the following is NOT an ideal method for enteral access for nutrition?
   A. Percutaneously placed gastrostomy tubes by interventional radiology
   B. Traditional surgical jejunostomy tube placement
   C. Using the traditional 20–24 French PEG-style tube
   D. Using a 14–16 French Cook-type catheter
8. Advantages of a transhiatal esophagectomy include all the following EXCEPT:
   A. Avoidance of a thoracotomy
   B. Improved safety of a cervical anastomosis
   C. Decreased pulmonary complications
   D. Completeness of lymphadenectomy
9. Which of the following surgical techniques can be technically challenging when resecting a cT3N1 squamous cell carcinoma of the esophagus measured at 24 cm from the incisors?
   A. Transhiatal esophagectomy
   B. Transthoracic esophagectomy
   C. Three-field esophagectomy
   D. Ivor-Lewis esophagectomy

Answers

1. D
2. D
3. C
4. B
5. A
6. D
7. C
8. D
9. A

References

1. Siegel R, Naishadham D, Jemal A. Cancer statistics, 2012. CA Cancer J Clin. 2012;62(1):10–29.
2. Posner MC, Minsky BD, Ilson DH. Cancer of the esophagus. In: Devita VTL, Lawrence TS, Rosenberg SA, editors. Rosenberg's cancer: principles & practice of oncology. 9th ed. Philadelphia: Lippincott Williams & Wilkins; 2011. p. 887.
3. Siewert JR, Ott K. Are squamous and adenocarcinomas of the esophagus the same disease? Semin Radiat Oncol. 2007;17(1):38–44.
4. Brown LM, Devesa SS, Chow WH. Incidence of adenocarcinoma of the esophagus among white Americans by sex, stage, and age. J Natl Cancer Inst. 2008;100(16):1184–7.
5. Blot WJ, Devesa SS, Kneller RW, Fraumeni Jr JF. Rising incidence of adenocarcinoma of the esophagus and gastric cardia. JAMA. 1991;265(10):1287–9.
6. Holmes RS, Vaughan TL. Epidemiology and pathogenesis of esophageal cancer. Semin Radiat Oncol. 2007;17(1):2–9.
7. Minsky BD, Goodman K, Warren R. Cancer of the esophagus. In: Hoppe RTP, Phillips TL, Roach M, editors. Leibel and Phillips textbook of radiation oncology. Philadelphia: Elsevier Saunders; 2010. p. 772.
8. Akiyama H, Tsurumaru M, Kawamura T, Ono Y. Principles of surgical treatment for carcinoma of the esophagus: analysis of lymph node involvement. Ann Surg. 1981;194(4):438–46.
9. National Comprehensive Cancer Network. NCCN guidelines version 1.2012: esophageal and esophagogastric junction cancers. 2012. www.nccn.org. Accessed 21 May 2012.
10. Kleinberg L, Brock MV, Jagannath SB, Forastiere AA. Cancer of the esophagus. In: Abeloff MD, Armitage JO, Niederhuber JE, Kastan MB, McKenna WG, editors. Abeloff's clinical oncology. 4th ed. Philadelphia: Churchill Livingston Elsevier; 2008. p. 1402.
11. Shaheen NJ, Sharma P, Overholt BF, et al. Radiofrequency ablation in Barrett's esophagus with dysplasia. N Engl J Med. 2009;360(22):2277–88.

12. Lagergren J, Bergström R, Lindgren A, Nyrén O. Symptomatic gastroesophageal reflux as a risk factor for esophageal adenocarcinoma. N Engl J Med. 1999;340(11):825–31.
13. Cossentino MJ, Wong RK. Barrett's esophagus and risk of esophageal adenocarcinoma. Semin Gastrointest Dis. 2003;14(3):128–35.
14. Hsu PK, Wu YC, Chou TY, Huang CS, Hsu WH. Comparison of the 6th and 7th editions of the American Joint Committee on Cancer tumor-node-metastasis staging system in patients with resected esophageal carcinoma. Ann Thorac Surg. 2010;89(4):1024–31.
15. Esophagus and esophagogastric junction. In: Edge SB, Byrd DR, Compton CC, et al. editors. AJCC Cancer Staging Manual. 7th ed. New York: Springer; 2010. pp. 103–11.
16. Hofstetter W, Correa AM, Bekele N, et al. Proposed modification of nodal status in AJCC esophageal cancer staging system. Ann Thorac Surg. 2007;84(2):365–73; discussion 374–75.
17. Peyre CG, Hagen JA, DeMeester SR, et al. The number of lymph nodes removed predicts survival in esophageal cancer: an international study on the impact of extent of surgical resection. Ann Surg. 2008;248(4):549–56.
18. Rizk N, Venkatraman E, Park B, Flores R, Bains MS, Rusch V. The prognostic importance of the number of involved lymph nodes in esophageal cancer: implications for revisions of the American Joint Committee on Cancer staging system. J Thorac Cardiovasc Surg. 2006;132(6):1374–81.
19. Greenstein AJ, Litle VR, Swanson SJ, Divino CM, Packer S, Wisnivesky JP. Effect of the number of lymph nodes sampled on postoperative survival of lymph node-negative esophageal cancer. Cancer. 2008;112(6):1239–46.
20. Greenstein AJ, Litle VR, Swanson SJ, Divino CM, Packer S, Wisnivesky JP. Prognostic significance of the number of lymph node metastases in esophageal cancer. J Am Coll Surg. 2008;206(2):239–46.
21. Han K, Basran PS, Cheung P. Comparison of helical and average computed tomography for stereotactic body radiation treatment planning and normal tissue contouring in lung cancer. Clin Oncol (R Coll Radiol). 2010;22(10):862–7.
22. Lin SH, Zhongxing L. Esophageal cancer. In: Lu JJ, Brady LW, editors. Decision making in radiation oncology. Berlin: Springer; 2011. p. 337.
23. Survival rates for esophagus cancer by stage. 2012. http://www.cancer.org/Cancer/EsophagusCancer/DetailedGuide/esophagus-cancer-survival-rates. Accessed 29 May 2012.
24. Puli SR, Reddy JB, Bechtold ML, Antillon D, Ibdah JA, Antillon MR. Staging accuracy of esophageal cancer by endoscopic ultrasound: a meta-analysis and systematic review. World J Gastroenterol. 2008;14(10):1479–90.
25. Chandawarkar RY, Kakegawa T, Fujita H, Yamana H, Hayabuthi N. Comparative analysis of imaging modalities in the preoperative assessment of nodal metastasis in esophageal cancer. J Surg Oncol. 1996;61(3):214–7.
26. van Westreenen HL, Westerterp M, Bossuyt PM, et al. Systematic review of the staging performance of 18F-fluorodeoxyglucose positron emission tomography in esophageal cancer. J Clin Oncol. 2004;22(18):3805–12.
27. Swisher SG, Erasmus J, Maish M, et al. 2-Fluoro-2-deoxy-D-glucose positron emission tomography imaging is predictive of pathologic response and survival after preoperative chemoradiation in patients with esophageal carcinoma. Cancer. 2004;101(8):1776–85.
28. Weinberg BD, Allison RR, Sibata C, Parent T, Downie G. Results of combined photodynamic therapy (PDT) and high dose rate brachytherapy (HDR) in treatment of obstructive endobronchial non-small cell lung cancer (NSCLC). Photodiagnosis Photodyn Ther. 2010;7(1):50–8.
29. Lubner MG, Brace CL, Hinshaw JL, Lee Jr FT. Microwave tumor ablation: mechanism of action, clinical results, and devices. J Vasc Int Radiol. 2010;21(8 Suppl):S192–203.
30. Scotiniotis IA, Kochman ML, Lewis JD, Furth EE, Rosato EF, Ginsberg GG. Accuracy of EUS in the evaluation of Barrett's esophagus and high-grade dysplasia or intramucosal carcinoma. Gastrointest Endosc. 2001;54(6):689–96.
31. Rampado S, Bocus P, Battaglia G, Ruol A, Portale G, Ancona E. Endoscopic ultrasound: accuracy in staging superficial carcinomas of the esophagus. Ann Thorac Surg. 2008;85(1):251–6.
32. Larghi A, Lightdale CJ, Memeo L, Bhagat G, Okpara N, Rotterdam H. EUS followed by EMR for staging of high-grade dysplasia and early cancer in Barrett's esophagus. Gastrointest Endosc. 2005;62(1):16–23.
33. Pennathur A, Awais O, Luketich JD. Minimally invasive esophagectomy for Barrett's with high-grade dysplasia and early adenocarcinoma of the esophagus. J Gastrointest Surg. 2010;14(6):948–50.
34. Luna RA, Gilbert E, Hunter JG. High-grade dysplasia and intramucosal adenocarcinoma in Barrett's esophagus: the role of esophagectomy in the era of endoscopic eradication therapy. Curr Opin Gastroenterol. 2012;28(4):362–9.
35. Pennathur A, Farkas A, Krasinskas AM, et al. Esophagectomy for T1 esophageal cancer: outcomes in 100 patients and implications for endoscopic therapy. Ann Thorac Surg. 2009;87(4):1048–54; discussion 1054–55.
36. Rizk NP, Ishwaran H, Rice TW, et al. Optimum lymphadenectomy for esophageal cancer. Ann Surg. 2010;251(1):46–50.
37. Strong VE, Song KY, Park CH, et al. Comparison of gastric cancer survival following R0 resection in the United States and Korea using an internationally validated nomogram. Ann Surg. 2010;251(4):640–6.
38. Morrison JJ, McVinnie DW, Suiter PA, de Quadros NM. Percutaneous jejunostomy: repeat access at the healed site of prior surgical jejunostomy with US and

fluoroscopic guidance. J Vasc Int Radiol. 2012;23(12): 1646–50.
39. Markar SR, Karthikesalingam A, Thrumurthy S, Low DE. Volume-outcome relationship in surgery for esophageal malignancy: systematic review and meta-analysis 2000–2011. J Gastrointest Surg. 2012;16(5): 1055–63.
40. Bolton JS, Fuhrman GM, Richardson WS. Esophageal resection for cancer. Surg Clin North Am. 1998;78(5): 773–94.
41. Orringer MB, Sloan H. Esophagectomy without thoracotomy. J Thorac Cardiovasc Surg. 1978;76(5): 643–54.
42. Stiles BM, Altorki NK. Traditional techniques of esophagectomy. Surg Clin North Am. 2012;92(5): 1249–63.
43. Verhage RJ, Hazebroek EJ, Boone J, Van Hillegersberg R. Minimally invasive surgery compared to open procedures in esophagectomy for cancer: a systematic review of the literature. Minerva Chir. 2009;64(2):135–46.
44. Santillan AA, Farma JM, Meredith KL, Shah NR, Kelley ST. Minimally invasive surgery for esophageal cancer. J Natl Compr Cancer Netw. 2008;6(9): 879–84.
45. Levy RM, Trivedi D, Luketich JD. Minimally invasive esophagectomy. Surg Clin North Am. 2012;92(5):1265–85.
46. Chang AC, Ji H, Birkmeyer NJ, Orringer MB, Birkmeyer JD. Outcomes after transhiatal and transthoracic esophagectomy for cancer. Ann Thorac Surg. 2008;85(2):424–9.
47. Nystrom B. Surveillance of hospital-associated infections. Infection. 1989;17(1):43–5.
48. Motoyama S, Kitamura M, Saito R, et al. Surgical outcome of colon interposition by the posterior mediastinal route for thoracic esophageal cancer. Ann Thorac Surg. 2007;83(4):1273–8.
49. Fürst H, Hartl WH, Löhe F, Schildberg FW. Colon interposition for esophageal replacement: an alternative technique based on the use of the right colon. Ann Surg. 2000;231(2):173–8.
50. Cooper JS, Guo MD, Herskovic A, et al. Chemoradiotherapy of locally advanced esophageal cancer: long-term follow-up of a prospective randomized trial (RTOG 85-01). Radiation Therapy Oncology Group. JAMA. 1999;281(17):1623–7.
51. Minsky BD, Pajak TF, Ginsberg RJ, et al. INT 0123 (Radiation Therapy Oncology Group 94-05) phase III trial of combined-modality therapy for esophageal cancer: high-dose versus standard-dose radiation therapy. J Clin Oncol. 2002;20(5):1167–74.
52. Gaspar LE, Winter K, Kocha WI, Coia LR, Herskovic A, Graham M. A phase I/II study of external beam radiation, brachytherapy, and concurrent chemotherapy for patients with localized carcinoma of the esophagus (Radiation Therapy Oncology Group Study 9207): final report. Cancer. 2000;88(5):988–95.
53. Urba SG, Orringer MB, Turrisi A, Iannettoni M, Forastiere A, Strawderman M. Randomized trial of preoperative chemoradiation versus surgery alone in patients with locoregional esophageal carcinoma. J Clin Oncol. 2001;19(2):305–13.
54. Bosset JF, Gignoux M, Triboulet JP, et al. Chemoradiotherapy followed by surgery compared with surgery alone in squamous-cell cancer of the esophagus. N Engl J Med. 1997;337(3):161–7.
55. Lee JL, Park SI, Kim SB, et al. A single institutional phase III trial of preoperative chemotherapy with hyperfractionation radiotherapy plus surgery versus surgery alone for resectable esophageal squamous cell carcinoma. Ann Oncol. 2004;15(6):947–54.
56. Burmeister BH, Smithers BM, Gebski V, et al. Surgery alone versus chemoradiotherapy followed by surgery for resectable cancer of the oesophagus: a randomised controlled phase III trial. Lancet Oncol. 2005;6(9): 659–68.
57. Walsh TN, Noonan N, Hollywood D, Kelly A, Keeling N, Hennessy TP. A comparison of multimodal therapy and surgery for esophageal adenocarcinoma. N Engl J Med. 1996;335(7):462–7.
58. Tepper J, Krasna MJ, Niedzwiecki D, et al. Phase III trial of trimodality therapy with cisplatin, fluorouracil, radiotherapy, and surgery compared with surgery alone for esophageal cancer: CALGB 9781. J Clin Oncol. 2008;26(7):1086–92.
59. van Hagen P, Hulshof MCCM, van Lanschot JJB, et al. Preoperative chemoradiotherapy for esophageal or junctional cancer. N Engl J Med. 2012;366(22): 2074–84.
60. Gebski V, Burmeister B, Smithers BM, Foo K, Zalcberg J, Simes J. Survival benefits from neoadjuvant chemoradiotherapy or chemotherapy in oesophageal carcinoma: a meta-analysis. Lancet Oncol. 2007;8(3):226–34.
61. Stahl M, Stuschke M, Lehmann N, et al. Chemoradiation with and without surgery in patients with locally advanced squamous cell carcinoma of the esophagus. J Clin Oncol. 2005;23(10):2310–7.
62. Bedenne L, Michel P, Bouche O, et al. Chemoradiation followed by surgery compared with chemoradiation alone in squamous cancer of the esophagus: FFCD 9102. J Clin Oncol. 2007;25(10):1160–8.
63. Cunningham D, Allum WH, Stenning SP, et al. Perioperative chemotherapy versus surgery alone for resectable gastroesophageal cancer. N Engl J Med. 2006;355(1):11–20.
64. Smalley SR, Benedetti JK, Haller DG, et al. Updated analysis of SWOG-directed intergroup study 0116: a phase III trial of adjuvant radiochemotherapy versus observation after curative gastric cancer resection. J Clin Oncol. 2012;30(19):2327–33.
65. Wang S, Liao Z, Chen Y, et al. Esophageal cancer located at the neck and upper thorax treated with concurrent chemoradiation: a single-institution experience. J Thorac Oncol. 2006;1(3):252–9.
66. Burmeister BH, Dickie G, Smithers BM, Hodge R, Morton K. Thirty-four patients with carcinoma of the cervical esophagus treated with chemoradiation therapy. Arch Otolaryngol Head Neck Surg. 2000; 126(2):205–8.

67. Tong DK, Law S, Kwong DL, Wei WI, Ng RW, Wong KH. Current management of cervical esophageal cancer. World J Surg. 2011;35(3):600–7.
68. Kelsen DP, Ginsberg R, Pajak TF, et al. Chemotherapy followed by surgery compared with surgery alone for localized esophageal cancer. N Engl J Med. 1998; 339(27):1979–84.
69. Group MRCOCW. Surgical resection with or without preoperative chemotherapy in oesophageal cancer: a randomised controlled trial. Lancet. 2002;359: 1727–33.
70. Sjoquist KM, Burmeister BH, Smithers BM, et al. Survival after neoadjuvant chemotherapy or chemoradiotherapy for resectable oesophageal carcinoma: an updated meta-analysis. Lancet Oncol. 2011;12(7): 681–92.
71. Mariette C. Surgery alone versus chemoradiotherapy followed by surgery for localized esophageal cancer. J Clin Oncol. 2010;28:4005.
72. Leichman LP, Goldman BH, Bohanes PO, et al. S0356: a phase II clinical and prospective molecular trial with oxaliplatin, fluorouracil, and external-beam radiation therapy before surgery for patients with esophageal adenocarcinoma. J Clin Oncol. 2011; 29(34):4555–60.
73. Hanna WC, Sudarshan M, Roberge D, et al. What is the optimal management of dysphagia in metastatic esophageal cancer? Curr Oncol. 2012;19(2):e60–6.
74. Ahmad NR, Goosenberg EB, Frucht H, Coia LR. Palliative treatment of esophageal cancer. Semin Radiat Oncol. 1994;4(3):202–14.
75. Cunningham D, Starling N, Rao S, et al. Capecitabine and oxaliplatin for advanced esophagogastric cancer. N Engl J Med. 2008;358(1):36–46.
76. Yano T, Doi T, Ohtsu A, et al. Comparison of HER2 gene amplification assessed by fluorescence in situ hybridization and HER2 protein expression assessed by immunohistochemistry in gastric cancer. Oncol Rep. 2006;15(1):65–71.
77. Bang YJ, Van Cutsem E, Feyereislova A, et al. Trastuzumab in combination with chemotherapy versus chemotherapy alone for treatment of HER2-positive advanced gastric or gastro-oesophageal junction cancer (ToGA): a phase 3, open-label, randomised controlled trial. Lancet. 2010;376(9742): 687–97.

Gastric Cancer

9

Elizabeth P. Ketner, Quyen D. Chu,
Martin S. Karpeh Jr., and Nikhil I. Khushalani

Learning Objectives

After reading this chapter, you should be able to:

- Recognize what constitutes early gastric cancer
- Understand how staging dictates treatment and prognosis of gastric cancer
- Know the surgical options for patients with gastric cancer
- Appreciate the impact of adjuvant chemoradiotherapy and perioperative chemotherapy for "curative" surgery
- Select options for local, regional, and systemic control of the disease

Background

Gastric cancer is one of the leading causes of cancer death worldwide, second only to lung cancer. Despite the decreasing incidence of gastric cancer due to changes in diet and food preparation, prognosis is still poor with overall 5-year survival rates ranging from 5 to 15 % in the USA and other Western countries. In Japan where gastric cancer is endemic, the introduction of mass screening in the 1970s has led to early diagnosis with dramatic improvement in the 5-year survival rate. In the USA however, stomach cancer still occurs at more advanced stages. It is diagnosed more frequently in men with an incidence ratio of approximately 2:1 and a peak incidence in the seventh decade in men, with a slightly later peak incidence in women [1].

Advances in nonoperative staging techniques including endoscopic ultrasound (EUS) have enabled more accurate staging of gastric cancer which is critical to distinguish locoregional (or operable) from distant (non-operable) disease. Similar to many other cancers, staging at the time of diagnosis highly impacts both the treatment plan and prognosis for patients. Because early gastric cancer is often asymptomatic or causes vague, nonspecific symptoms, such as pain unrelieved by eating and weight loss, most patients are diagnosed with advanced disease. Even after a "curative" gastrectomy, up to 80 % of patients may experience disease recurrence and require treatment beyond surgery.

Pathology

Malignant gastric neoplasms are comprised of several histologic subtypes including adenocarcinoma, lymphoma, carcinoid tumors, gastrointestinal

E.P. Ketner, M.D. • M.S. Karpeh Jr., M.D.
Department of Surgery, Mount Sinai Beth Israel Medical Center, New York, NY, USA
e-mail: eketner@chpnet.org; siehk934@gmail.com

Q.D. Chu, M.D., M.B.A., F.A.C.S.
Department of Surgery, LSU Health Sciences Center-Shreveport, Shreveport, LA, USA
e-mail: qchu@lsuhsc.edu

N.I. Khushalani, M.D. (✉)
Department of Medicine, Roswell Park Cancer Institute, Elm and Carlton Streets, Buffalo, NY, USA 14263
e-mail: nikhil.khushalani@roswellpark.org

Q.D. Chu et al. (eds.), *Surgical Oncology: A Practical and Comprehensive Approach*,
DOI 10.1007/978-1-4939-1423-4_9,

stromal tumors, and leiomyosarcoma. Approximately 95 % of all malignant gastric tumors are adenocarcinomas. Further discussion in this chapter will focus on this histology.

There are two classifications, the World Health Organization (WHO) and the Lauren classification. WHO classifies gastric cancer into four types: papillary, tubular, mucinous, and signet ring cell. The Lauren classification divides gastric carcinoma into the intestinal and diffuse subtypes [2]. These variants differ in pathologic, epidemiologic, etiologic, and prognostic features. The intestinal subtype is usually found in the distal stomach, more common in elderly and found in conjunction with atrophic gastritis. Diffuse adenocarcinoma is mostly found in the cardia (but can arise in any part of the stomach), occurs more frequently in young patients without any predisposing condition, and prognosis is worse. Hereditary diffuse gastric cancer has been associated with germline mutations in the E-cadherin (*CDH1*) gene and/or hypermethylation in both inherited and sporadic forms; prophylactic gastrectomy should be considered for young adults harboring this mutation [3, 4].

H. pylori infection has been linked to both intestinal and diffuse subtypes of adenocarcinoma, conferring a three times greater risk of gastric cancer, regardless of age, sex, or race [5]. The treatment principles for the two histologic subtypes are the same and dictated by the tumor node metastases (TNM) staging at time of diagnosis as well as pathologic staging after surgery.

Human epidermal growth factor receptor-2 (HER-2) overexpression is observed in up to 23 % of patients with gastric cancer [6, 7]. However, its clinical significance in resectable cancer is unknown. The current recommendation is to obtain HER-2 expression for those with metastatic disease, but not for resectable disease [8].

Diagnosis and Staging

Abdominal pain, early satiety, nausea, vomiting, bloating, anorexia, and weight loss are the most common clinical symptoms in gastric cancer. Anemia, from occult gastrointestinal bleeding, may also be a presenting feature prompting a diagnostic esophagogastroduodenoscopy (EGD) (Fig. 9.1).

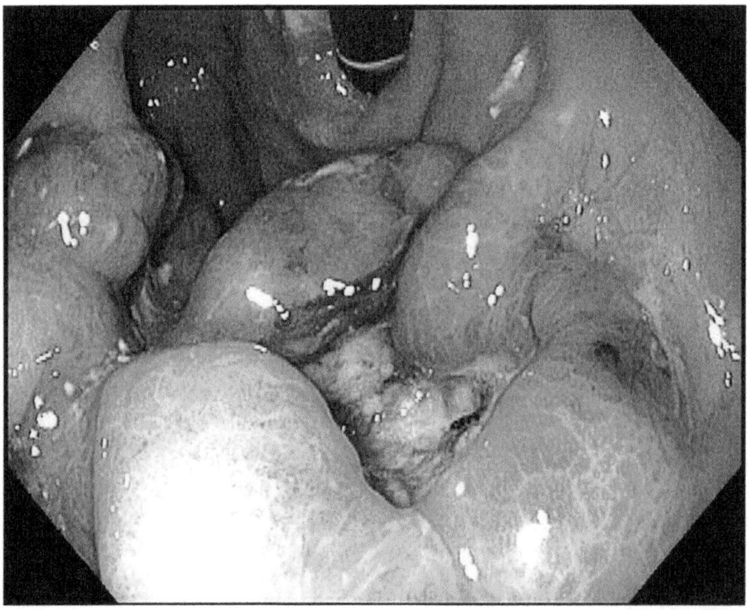

Fig. 9.1 EGD picture of a 51-year-old man with a large gastric fundus adenocarcinoma (Courtesy of Quyen D. Chu, MD, MBA, FACS)

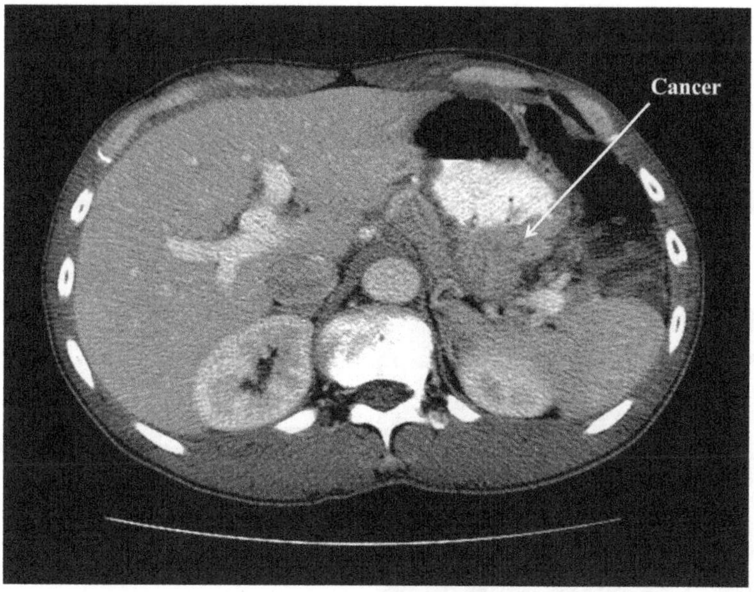

Fig. 9.2 CT scan of the same gentleman who has a large gastric fundus adenocarcinoma. There was no evidence of nodal disease on CT scan (Courtesy of Quyen D. Chu, MD, MBA, FACS)

Ascites and bowel obstruction secondary to peritoneal metastases are clinical indicators of advanced stage disease where the goal of therapy is typically palliative. Similarly, the presence of palpable lymph nodes in the left supraclavicular basin (Virchow's node), in the left axillary region (Irish node), or in the periumbilical area (Sister Mary Joseph node) essentially precludes a curative attempt at surgery. The clinical evaluation in gastric cancer must also include pelvic and rectal examination to exclude the presence of ovarian metastases (Krukenberg's tumor) and cul-de-sac metastases (Blumer's shelf), respectively.

While an EGD confirms the pathologic diagnosis in most cases, it is important to recognize cases that may lack an obvious mucosal component. These tumors often result in poor gastric distensibility (*linitis plastica*) secondary to diffuse submucosal infiltration and require deeper biopsies for diagnosis. Typical staging studies include contrast-enhanced computed tomography (CT) of the chest, abdomen, and pelvis (Fig. 9.2). While this modality provides excellent definition of nodal and visceral metastases, it has low sensitivity for identifying metastases to the peritoneum. The presence of distant metastases on CT imaging essentially precludes the need for any additional staging procedures. For those patients with radiographically localized disease, EUS can provide useful information about the depth of invasion, especially in early gastric cancer [9]. Its role in predicting nodal involvement, however, is less reliable, especially when the nodal stations are further away from the probe.

The role of 18-fluoro-deoxyglucose positron emission tomography (FDG-PET) in the staging of gastric cancer is evolving (Fig. 9.3). While it can serve as an adjunct to CT imaging in the detection of occult metastatic disease [10], its use as a stand-alone staging tool is limited by a high false-negative rate in tumors of low metabolic uptake and those that have a low expression of *SLC2A1*, a transmembrane transporter of FDG [11, 12].

A diagnostic laparoscopy (DL) with lavage to exclude peritoneal metastases is utilized at many institutions prior to surgery with curative intent or the delivery of planned neoadjuvant therapy. A positive laparoscopy, including positive cytology from washings, is considered as M1 disease, which portends a poor prognosis and alters the treatment plan in a substantial number of patients, including avoidance of a laparotomy [13, 14].

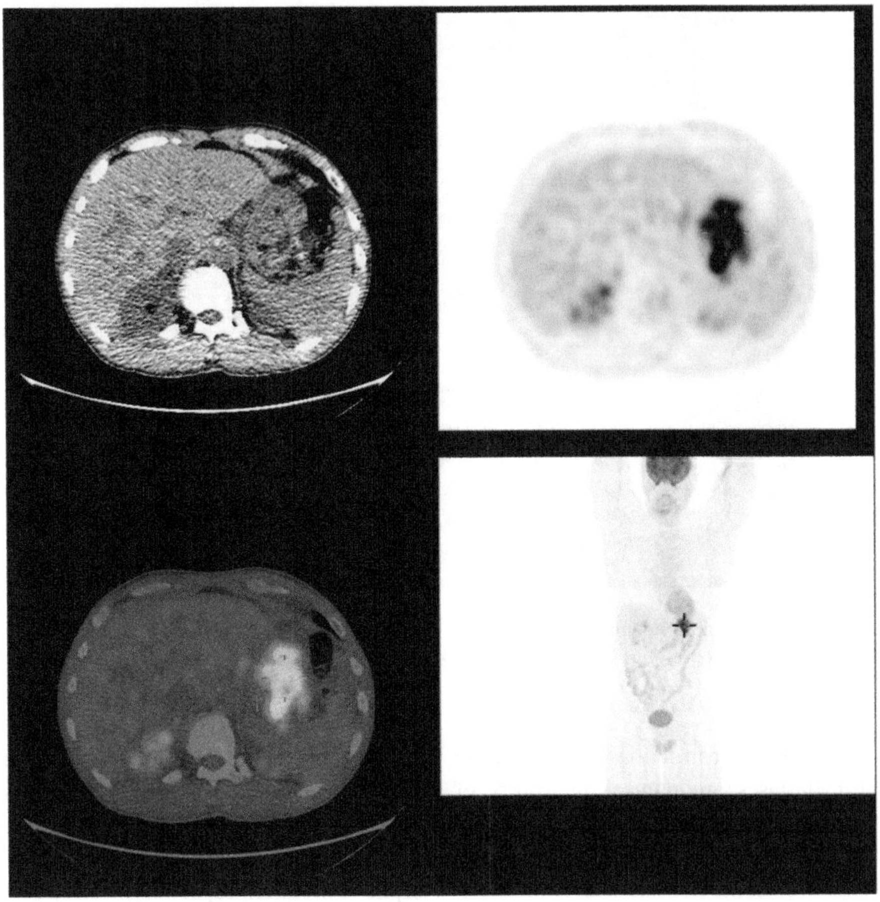

Fig. 9.3 PET/CT of the same gentleman who has a large gastric fundus adenocarcinoma. There was evidence of markedly intense FDG uptake in an area of gastric fundus extending to greater curvature consistent with aggressive neoplasm. There was no evidence of locoregional or distant disease. The patient underwent a total gastrectomy and splenectomy (due to tumor extending into the splenic hilum) with a D2 dissection. Final pathology demonstrated a moderately differentiated T4 adenocarcinoma (9 cm maximal diameter) with 11 out of 26 positive lymph nodes. The closest margin was 5 cm from the tumor. Adjuvant chemoradiation was given (Courtesy of Quyen D. Chu, MD, MBA, FACS)

DL is useful in situations where the patient is at risk of harboring distant disease (i.e., T3 or N1 disease identified on preoperative imaging). However, DL is limited in detecting disease in the perigastric lymph nodes as well as small intraparenchymal liver metastases.

Adenocarcinoma of the gastroesophageal junction (GEJ) has been considered as either esophageal or gastric cancer. In 1987, Siewert et al. classified these tumors into three types [15]. Type 1 tumors are those with the epicenter 1–5 cm proximal to the GEJ (adenocarcinoma of the distal esophagus), type II are those with epicenter 1 cm proximal to the GEJ and 2 cm distal to GEJ (true cardiac cancer), and type III are those with the epicenter 2–5 cm distal to the GEJ (inferior cardiac cancer) (Fig. 9.4).

There are two staging systems that are widely used in clinical practice and research, the American Joint Committee on Cancer (AJCC/TNM) staging system according to the 7th edition (Table 9.1) and the Japanese staging system. The Japanese staging system is based on the anatomic involvement of the nodal stations [17]. The AJCC/TNM staging directly affects the potential success of an R0 resection [8].

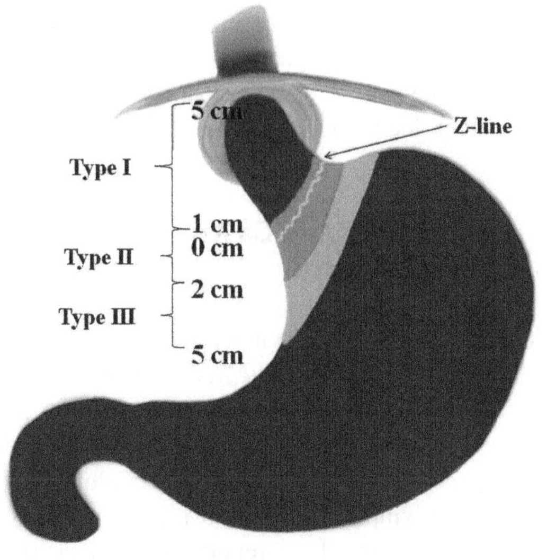

Fig. 9.4 *Siewert classification of adenocarcinoma of the gastroesophageal junction*: type I (esophageal adenocarcinoma) is from 5 to 1 cm above the Z line, type II (cardia cancer) is from 1 cm over to 2 cm below the Z line, and type III is from 2 cm below to 5 cm below the Z line (Courtesy of Quyen D. Chu, MD, MBA, FACS)

In 2010, the AJCC made three important changes to the staging of gastric cancer. First, only tumors arising more than 5 cm distal to the gastroesophageal junction (GEJ) would be staged as gastric cancers; those at the GEJ and those within 5 cm of the GEJ with involvement of the GEJ (Siewert types I–III GEJ tumors) would be classified and staged as esophageal carcinoma. Siewert type III is considered gastric cancer only if the esophagus is not infiltrated. Secondly, the T3 category was changed from "*invading the serosa*" to "*invading through the muscle into the subserosal connective tissue.*" Tumors invading the serosa are now classified as T4 along with invasion into adjacent structures. This second change was implemented in an effort to align the staging of gastric cancers with tumors of the rest of the gastrointestinal tract (esophagus, small and large intestine). Thirdly, the T1 stage was subdivided into T1a (lamina propria or muscularis mucosa confined) and T1b (submucosal involvement) for data collection purposes [18].

Superior outcomes among the Japanese surgeons have been attributed to many reasons, one of which is the Will Rogers phenomenon.

Table 9.1 American Joint Committee on Cancer (AJCC) TNM staging for stomach carcinomas (7th edition)

Primary tumor (T)	
TX	Primary tumor cannot be assessed
T0	No evidence of primary tumor
Tis	Carcinoma in situ: intraepithelial tumor without invasion of the lamina propria
T1	Tumor invades lamina propria, muscularis mucosae, or submucosa
T1a	Tumor invades lamina propria or muscularis mucosae
T1b	Tumor invades submucosa
T2	Tumor invades muscularis propria*
T3	Tumor penetrates subserosal connective tissue without invasion of visceral peritoneum or adjacent structures **, ***
T4	Tumor invades serosa (visceral peritoneum) or adjacent structures**, ***
T4a	Tumor invades serosa (visceral peritoneum)
T4b	Tumor invades adjacent structures

*Note: A tumor may penetrate the muscularis propria with extension into the gastrocolic or gastrohepatic ligaments, or into the greater or lesser omentum, without perforation of the visceral peritoneum covering these structures. In this case, the tumor is classified T3. If there is perforation of the visceral peritoneum covering the gastric ligaments or the omentum, the tumor should be classified T4

**The adjacent structures of the stomach include the spleen, transverse colon, liver, diaphragm, pancreas, abdominal wall, adrenal gland, kidney, small intestine, and retroperitoneum

***Intramural extension to the duodenum or esophagus is classified by the depth of the greatest invasion in any of these sites, including the stomach

Anatomic stage/prognostic groups			
Group	T	N	M
Stage 0	Tis	N0	M0
Stage IA	T1	N0	M0
Stage IB	T2	N0	M0
	T1	N1	M0
Stage IIA	T3	N0	M0
	T2	N1	M0
	T1	N2	M0
Stage IIB	T4a	N0	M0
	T3	N1	M0
	T2	N2	M0
	T1	N3	M0
Stage IIIA	T4a	N1	M0
	T3	N2	M0
	T2	N3	M0

(continued)

Table 9.1 (continued)

Anatomic stage/prognostic groups			
Group	T	N	M
Stage IIIB	T4b	N0	M0
	T4b	N1	M0
	T4a	N2	M0
	T3	N3	M0
Stage IIIC	T4b	N2	M0
	T4b	N3	M0
	T4a	N3	M0
Stage IV	Any T	Any N	M1

Regional lymph nodes (N)[†]	
NX	Regional lymph nodes cannot be assessed
N0	No regional lymph nodes metastasis*
N1	Metastasis in 1–2 regional lymph nodes
N2	Metastasis in 3–6 regional lymph nodes
N3	Metastasis in ≥ 7 regional lymph nodes
N3a	Metastasis in 7–15 regional lymph nodes
N3b	Metastasis in ≥ 16 regional lymph nodes

[†]Retropancreatic, para-aortic, portal, retroperitoneal, and mesenteric nodes are considered M1-disease.

*A designation of pN0 should be used if all examined lymph nodes are negative, regardless of the total number removed and examined.

Distant metastasis (M)	
M0	No distant metastasis
M1	Distant metastasis

Adapted from Compton et al. [16]. With permission from Springer Verlag

Will Rogers was a comedian who was believed to have made a comment about the plight of people during the 1930s Great Depression. He commented that "when the Okies left Oklahoma and moved to California, they raised the average intelligence level in both states." How this applies to gastric staging is that when Japanese surgeons perform extended nodal dissection, they tend to more accurately stage their patients than surgeons from the USA, the majority of whom do not perform extended node dissection and therefore potentially understage their patients. Thus, patients who are stage II cancers in the USA may actually be stage III (stage migration), which may account for a lower survival in the USA than the Japanese data, stage for stage. This phenomenon is referred to as stage migration and suggests that the differences in outcomes between the two groups of surgeons were not due to more surgery (i.e., more extensive nodal dissection), but rather due to more accurate staging.

Treatment of Early Gastric Cancer and Local Control

Tumors confined to the mucosa and submucosa (T1) are referred to as *early gastric cancers* (EGC) regardless of lymph node status. Overall, these patients do very well, experiencing cure rates exceeding 80–90 % after surgery alone. The number of lymph node metastasis is an important prognostic factor. In a report from Japan, the 5-year survival rate was intimately linked to nodal disease burden, which decreases from 85 % for N0 disease to 61 % for N1 involvement, 31 % for N2 disease, 10 % for N3 disease, and only 2 % for N4 disease [19].

Despite the changes in incidence, screening, and diagnosis, the paradigm that guides operative management for gastric cancer has not changed over the last century – complete surgical resection is the only potentially curative treatment for localized disease. An important change occurred in the early 1990s when reports from large series from Japan showed the efficacy of using local resection techniques such as an endoscopic mucosal resection (EMR) without a lymphadenectomy or gastrectomy for a select group of patients who were at very low risk of having nodal metastases. The proposed selection criteria include: (1) the tumor is small (≤3 cm in diameter), (2) well differentiated and without lymphovascular invasion, and (3) superficially elevated and/or depressed but without ulceration or definitive submucosal invasion [20, 21]. Given the low likelihood of identifying such lesions in a Western population, its applicability to this cohort appears to be limited. Furthermore, long-term outcome with EMR is lacking. Thus, EMR should only be performed under the auspice of a clinical trial or be limited to medical centers that are highly experienced with such a technique.

If the tumor has spread into the submucosa, the incidence of lymph node metastasis increases,

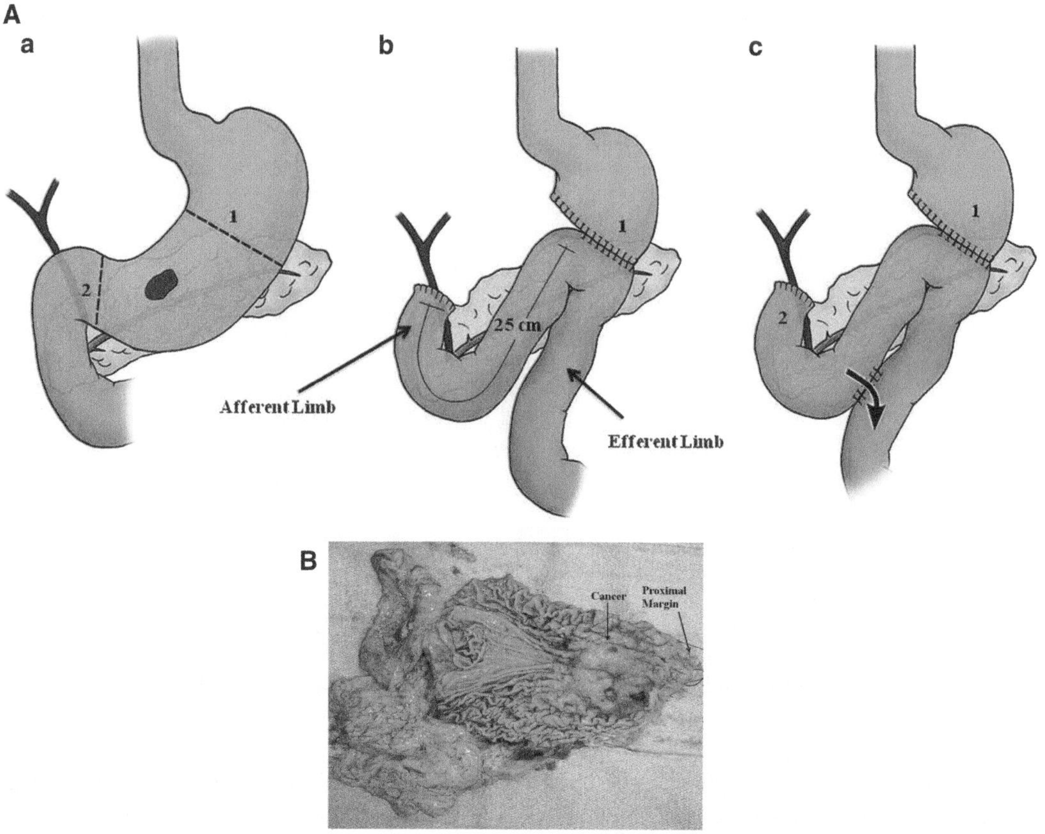

Fig. 9.5 *Partial gastrectomy with a Billroth II (BII) gastrojejunostomy reconstruction.* The "classic" BII gastrojejunostomy reconstruction is shown in Panel B. Panel C represents a BII gastrojejunostomy with a Braun enteroenterostomy (**a**). Afferent loop syndrome may occur if the afferent limb is made too long (>25 cm). In some instances, a patient may have prolonged gastroparesis following a subtotal gastrectomy and a BII reconstruction. A Braun enteroenterostomy can be used to address these complications and should be created approximately 25 cm distal to the BII gastrojejunostomy to divert contents of the afferent limb (bile) from the stomach. Figure 9.5b shows a large distal gastric adenocarcinoma that was resected with negative margins ((**a**, **b**): Courtesy of Quyen D. Chu, MD, MBA, FACS)

and more definitive surgery (i.e., gastrectomy) must be performed to ensure an R0 resection. A subject of great controversy in the past was whether all gastric cancer patients should have a total gastrectomy or a subtotal gastrectomy. Two prospective randomized trials, one from France and a second from Italy conducted over two decades ago, concluded the following: both procedures have similar 5-year survival rates, but a subtotal gastrectomy is a technically easier operation, is associated with less perioperative morbidity and mortality, allows for better postoperative nutritional status and quality of life, and hence is preferred over total gastrectomy, when feasible [22, 23]. Therefore, our current practice is to perform a subtotal gastrectomy for tumors of the distal stomach and body (Fig. 9.5a–b), depending on the tumor size and margin status and a total gastrectomy for most cancers of the proximal stomach and large tumors in the fundus. A Billroth II gastrojejunostomy (BII) is the preferred method of reconstruction with a caveat that the afferent limb should not be longer than 25 cm in order to avoid the acute afferent loop syndrome (ALS), a potentially serious condition that usually requires emergent surgical intervention (Fig. 9.5a).

As an aside, patients who underwent a subtotal gastrectomy with a BII reconstruction may have a number of gastric motility disorders postoperatively. Two worth mentioning include gastroparesis

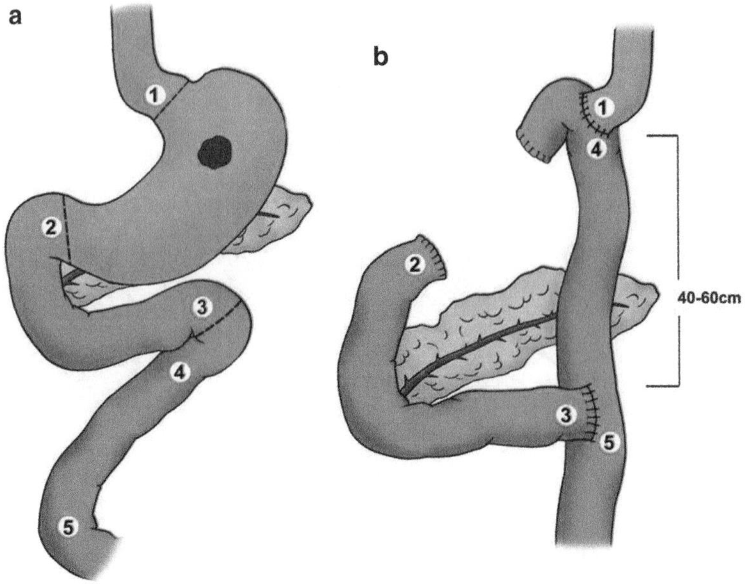

Fig. 9.6 *Total gastrectomy with a Roux-En-Y esophagojejunostomy reconstruction.* Note that the proximal jejunal "Y" limb should be anastomosed to the distal jejunal "Roux" limb approximately 40–60 cm from the esophagojejunostomy anastomoses to avoid symptomatic bile reflux (Courtesy of Quyen D. Chu, MD, MBA, FACS)

and afferent loop syndrome. Symptoms for both include upper abdominal pain, nausea and vomiting, early satiety, and anorexia, although ALS tends to present with an acute abdomen. Patients are unable to tolerate per oral intake and require long-term nasogastric tube resulting in a prolonged post-operative recovery time and hospital stays. The causes of postoperative gastroparesis are unclear but may be related to damage of the gastric electrical pacemaker, gastrointestinal dysfunction, and vagus resection following subtotal gastrectomy [24]. As mentioned above, ALS is due to an obstruction of the afferent limb and is mainly due to technical errors (i.e., creation of a long afferent limb), but also due to twisting or kinking of the afferent limb or swelling at the anastomosis of the afferent limb to the stomach. Regardless, the solution to the above two conditions is to create a Braun entero-enterostomy (Fig. 9.5a), either at the time of the initial operation or when these complications occur. The Braun enteroenterostomy helps to divert contents of the afferent limb (bile) to the distal bowel.

For cancers in the proximal stomach, a total gastrectomy with a Roux-en-Y reconstruction is performed (Fig. 9.6), although a subtotal gastrectomy can still be considered if a negative margin can be achieved. The distance between the esophagojejunostomy anastomoses and the jejunojejunostomy anastomoses should be 40–60 cm in order to avoid symptomatic bile reflux.

For the majority of gastric cancers, 5 cm is considered a safe proximal margin. The presence of a microscopic positive margin should be managed in the context of the extent of disease being treated. In patients without significant lymph node metastasis (≤5 positive lymph nodes out of 15 pathologically examined), survival is significantly decreased by leaving a positive margin. However, if patients that have five or more positive lymph nodes, the presence of a positive margin will have little influence on disease-related survival [25]. This brings us to our next consideration in the operative management of gastric tumors – regional control and the extent of lymph node resection.

Regional Control

In order to accurately depict a tumor as N0 within the AJCC/TNM classification, a minimum of 15 lymph nodes is required to be examined by pathology. The Japanese Research Society for the Study of Gastric Cancer has defined a standard for the extent of lymph node dissection and labeled them D1-4 (Fig. 9.7). D-dissection should be distinguished from R-resection; D-dissection describes the extent of lymphadenectomy, while R-resection describes the degree of residual tumor left behind after resection. An R0 resection is a complete resection without evidence of gross or microscopic disease; an R1 is one that has no gross disease, but has evidence of microscopic residual disease, and an R2 is one that has gross residual disease.

A D1 dissection includes a subtotal or total gastrectomy and removal of only the perigastric nodes along the lesser and greater curvature of the stomach (Stations 1–6). A D2 dissection adds the removal of nodes along the left gastric artery, common hepatic artery, celiac trunk, and splenic artery and hilum (Stations 7–12). With some proximal T4 tumors, resection of the spleen and pancreatic tail is necessary to achieve adequate nodal clearance along the splenic artery and hilum, but in most cases the spleen and distal pancreas can and should be preserved (Fig. 9.8). Given the distinction between D-dissection and R-resection, one can see how it is possible to have an R1 resection (microscopic disease) with a D2 dissection.

Prophylactic distal pancreatectomy and splenectomy should not be routinely performed; a splenectomy should only be done when the hilum is involved. D3 and D4 resections involve resecting more distant and periaortic nodes, and recent data has shown that this extent of lymphadenectomy does not improve survival over a D2 dissection [26, 27].

Just as total gastrectomy (in comparison to subtotal) is associated with greater postoperative morbidity and mortality, so can a more extensive

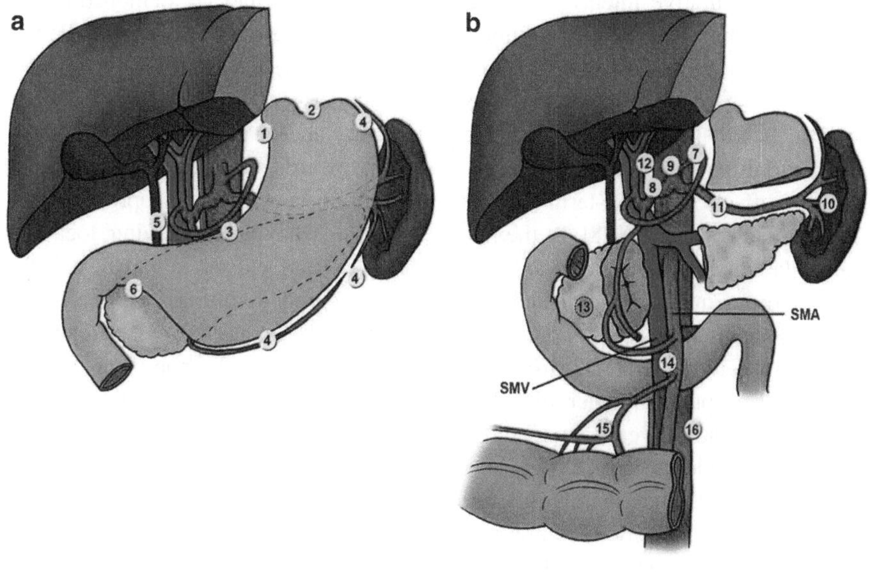

Fig. 9.7 *Gastric cancer nodal stations*: station *1* right paracardial; station *2* left paracardial; station *3* lesser curvature of the stomach, along left and right gastric arteries; station *4* greater curvature of the stomach, along left and right gastroepiploic arteries and short gastric arteries; station *5* suprapyloric, along right gastric artery; station *6* infrapyloric, along right gastroepiploic artery; station *7* trunk of left gastric artery; station *8* common hepatic artery; station *9* celiac artery; station *10* splenic hilum; station *11* splenic artery; station *12* hepatoduodenal ligament, along proper hepatic artery, common bile duct, and portal vein; station *13* posterior surface of pancreatic head; station *14* superior mesenteric vein; station *15* middle colic vessels; station *16* para-aortic. D1 dissection: stations 1–6; D2 dissection: stations 1–12 (Courtesy of Quyen D. Chu, MD, MBA, FACS)

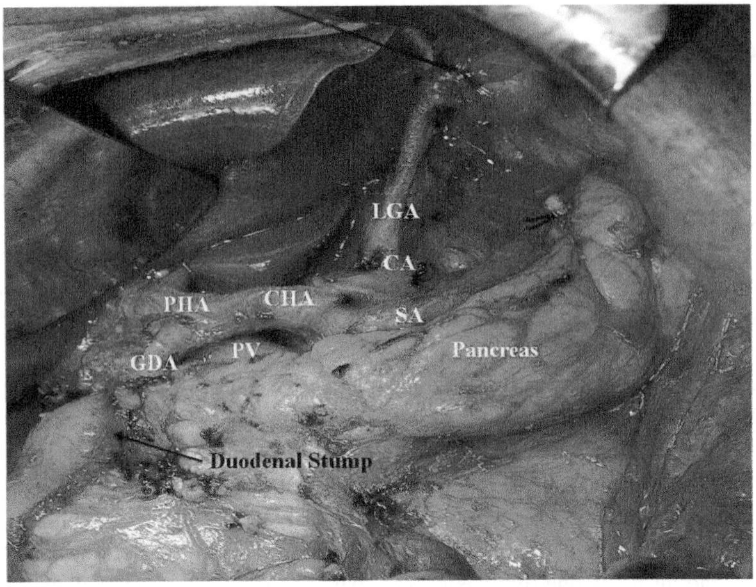

Fig. 9.8 Intraoperative picture of a modified D2 dissection for distal gastric cancer. The distal pancreas and spleen were preserved. *LGA* left gastric artery, *CA* celiac axis, *SA* splenic artery, *CHA* common hepatic artery, *PV* portal vein, *PHA* proper hepatic artery, *GDA* gastroduodenal artery (Courtesy of Quyen D. Chu, MD, MBA, FACS)

lymph node dissection [25]. A randomized Dutch trial of 1,078 patients with gastric cancer (711 patients treated with curative intent), for which the majority had pathologic T1 to T3 tumors, found no long-term overall survival benefit from an extended D2 versus conventional D1 lymph node dissection. It was thought that the higher postoperative mortality rate associated with a D2 dissection likely offsets the long-term survival advantage with a D2 dissection [28]. In the final report from this landmark trial, which was exemplified by the rigorous quality control including training of Dutch surgeons by an expert counterpart from Japan in performing a D2 dissection, the overall survival for patients undergoing a D1 dissection was 30 % at 11 years compared to 35 % for those who underwent a D2 dissection ($P=0.53$) [26]. However, when the investigators stratified patients postoperatively by lymph node stage, those with N2 disease who had a D2 resection had a statistically significant improvement in 11-year survival rates of 21 % compared with 0 % in the D1 group. At a median follow-up of 15 years, there was a lower locoregional recurrence rate in the D2 lymphadenectomy group than the D1 group, though this group had a higher rate of postoperative morbidity, mortality, and reoperation [29]. A meta-analysis of 12 randomized trials comparing D1 and D2 demonstrated no significant difference in OS (HR = 0.92, 95 % CI, 0.77–1.10, $P=0.36$), but a subgroup analysis of patients who underwent a D2 dissection without a splenectomy and/or pancreatectomy demonstrated a trend towards OS benefit [30]. Therefore, D2 resection is a reasonable approach when the likelihood of the patient having locally advanced nodal disease exists. In Japan, a D2 dissection is considered a routine practice. However, D2 should only be performed by experienced and trained surgeons. To complete the operation, a feeding jejunostomy should be considered for postoperative feeding.

Laparoscopic techniques have become an integral part of surgical practice over the past several decades. For gastric cancer, multiple retrospective studies have reported the advantages of laparoscopic gastrectomy (LG) over open gastrectomy (OG) [31–34]. A recent meta-analysis of 15 nonrandomized comparative studies has also shown that although LG had a longer operative time than OG, it was associated with lower intraoperative blood loss, overall complication rate, fewer wound-related complications, quicker recovery of gastrointestinal motility with shorter time to first flatus and oral intake, and shorter hospital stay [34]. A randomized prospective trial comparing laparoscopic assisted with open subtotal gastrectomy reported that LG had a significantly lower blood loss (229 ± 144 ml versus 391 ± 136 ml; $P<0.001$), shorter time to resumption of oral intake (5.1 ± 0.5 days versus 7.4 ± 2 days; $P<0.001$), and earlier discharge from hospital (10.3 ± 3.6 days versus 14.5 ± 4.6 days; $P<0.001$) [35] (Table 9.2).

Laparoscopic subtotal gastrectomy appears to offer similar oncologic outcomes as open subtotal gastrectomy as reported in multiple retrospective studies [34, 41–44] as well as in six randomized controlled trials [35–40] (Table 9.2). As an aside, there are no clinical trials comparing laparoscopic total gastrectomy with open total gastrectomy. Unfortunately, most of these clinical trials had small number of patients; the highly quoted study by Huscher et al. reported only 59 patients [35]. To address the concern of insufficient power, the Korean Laparoscopic Gastrointestinal Surgery Study (KLASS) Group is conducting a large, multicenter phase III trial of 1,415 patients from 12 institutions to compare overall survival, disease survival, morbidity, mortality, quality of life, inflammatory and immune responses, and cost-effectiveness between laparoscopic distal gastrectomy and open distal gastrectomy on early stage gastric cancer (cT1N0M0-cT2aN0M0) (Clinical Trials.gov ID: NCT00452751) [40]. A separate trial comparing laparoscopic surgery with open surgery in advanced gastric cancer is also underway (KLASS 02). Results of these studies will not be available until the distant future.

LG is an option for early distal gastric cancer, but should only be performed by surgeons who are adept and competent with the technique.

Distant Control

Adjuvant Chemoradiation Therapy

Despite curative attempts with surgery, many patients with gastric cancer experience disease recurrence, both locoregionally and at distant sites. Patients with serosal involvement or diffuse/signet ring cell histology have a high risk of peritoneal relapse [45, 46]. Postoperative nomograms have attempted to define a group who is at risk of relapse following surgery [47, 48]. The patterns of failure have led to extensive efforts to incorporate multimodality therapy such as chemotherapy and radiation in the management of resectable gastric cancer. Permutations of trials using exclusively postoperative therapy (adjuvant), preoperative treatment (neoadjuvant), or a combination thereof (perioperative) have resulted in the evolution of geographical paradigms of management across continents. A summary of the major trials in this regard is outlined in Table 9.3. In general, options for patients with resectable gastric cancer include (1) *adjuvant chemoradiation therapy*, (2) *perioperative chemotherapy* (*ECF, followed by surgery, followed by ECF*), or (3) *adjuvant chemotherapy such as oral S-1* (*tegafur, a 5-FU prodrug plus gimeracil and oteracil*) *or capecitabine and oxaliplatin*. Studies conducted throughout the 1990s that compare surgery alone versus surgery plus either adjuvant chemotherapy alone (older agent) or radiation therapy alone have yielded disappointing results. However, recent data with newer agents (S-1, capecitabine and oxaliplatin) rekindled interest in the role of adjuvant chemotherapy alone.

Based on small studies demonstrating benefit to postoperative radiotherapy with or without 5-fluorouracil (5-FU) + leucovorin (LV) and the efficacy of this strategy as definitive treatment of locally advanced, unresectable gastric cancer, Macdonald et al. initiated a large randomized trial comparing adjuvant 5-FU-based chemoradiation (CRT) to surgery alone in 556 patients who had undergone resection of stage Ib–IV (M0) gastric cancer (based on the 1988 AJCC staging). In this landmark Intergroup 0116 (INT 0116) study, which was initiated in 1991 and reported in 2001, the median overall survival (OS) improved from 27 months in the surgery alone group to 36 months in the surgery plus CRT cohort (HR for death 1.35, 95 % CI 1.09, 1.66; $p=0.005$) [49]. The corresponding 3-year survivals were 41 % and 50 %, respectively. An updated analysis of this data with more than 10 years of follow-up validated the benefit of adjuvant CRT,

Table 9.2 Trials comparing laparoscopic subtotal gastrectomy with open subtotal gastrectomy

Author, year	N	Average # LNs retrieved	Mortality	Morbidity	5-year OS	5-year DFS	Comments
Fujii, 2003 [36]	20	N/A	OG=0 % LG=0 % *P*=NS	OG=20 % LG=20 % *P*=NS	N/A	N/A	LG had Longer operative time
Hayashi, 2005 [37]	28	OG=27 ± 10 LG=28 ± 14 *P*=.85	N/A	N/A	N/A	N/A	LG had Longer operative time Earlier oral intake Shorter LOS
Lee, 2005 [38]	47	OG=38.1 ± 15.9 LG=31.8 ± 13.5 N=0.406	N/A	N/A	N/A	N/A	LG had Longer operative time Lower pulmonary complications
Huscher, 2005 [35]	59	OG=33.4 ± 17.4 LG=30.0 ± 14.9 *P*=NS	OG=6.7 % LG=3.3 % *P*=NS	OG=27.6 % LG=26.7 % *P*=NS	OG=55.7 % LG=54.8 % *P*=NS	OG=58.9 % LG=57.3 % *P*=NS	LG had Lower EBL Earlier oral intake Shorter LOS
Kim, 2008 [39]	164	OG=45.1 ± 13.8 LG=39.0 ± 11.9 *P*<0.05	N/A	OG=5 % LG=0 % N/A	N/A	N/A	LG had Longer operative time Lower EBL Shorter LOS Better QOL
Kim, 2010 [40]	342	OG=71 % had D2 LG=67 % had D2 *P*=0.48	OG=0 % LG=1.1 % *P*=0.497	OG=14.7 % LG=10/5 % *P*=0.137	N/A	N/A	No differences in morbidity or mortality between OG and LG

OG open gastrectomy, *LG* laparoscopic Gastrectomy, *NS* not significant, *OS* overall Survival, *DFS* disease-free Survival, *LOS* length of hospital Stay, *QOL* quality of Life, *N/A* not available

Table 9.3 Seminal adjuvant, perioperative, and neoadjuvant trials in gastric cancer

Study Author, year	Strategy	N	Treatment	5-year survival	Comments
INT-0116 [49]	Adjuvant	277	S	41 % (3-year OS)	Establishes role of adjuvant chemoXRT
MacDonald, 2001		282	S + CRT (F/L)	50 % (3-year OS)	
MAGIC [50]	Perioperative	253	S	23 %	Establishes role of perioperative chemotherapy
Cunningham, 2006		250	ECF→S→ECF	36 %	
ACTS-GT [51]	Adjuvant	530	S	72 %[a]	Establishes role of adjuvant chemotherapy, but S-1 is not available in the USA
Sakuramoto, 2007		529	S + S −1	61 %[a]	
EORTC 40954 [52]	Neoadjuvant	72	S	70 % (2-year OS)	Neoadjuvant chemotherapy alone was not better than surgery alone
Schuhmacher, 2010		72	CFL→S	73 % (2-year OS) $p = 0.466$	
CALGB 80101 [53]	Adjuvant	267	S + CRT (F/LV)	50 % (3-year OS)	Establishes 5-FU/LV is just as effective as ECF for adjuvant chemoXRT regimen
Fuchs, 2011		279	S + CRT (ECF)	52 % (3-year OS) $p = 0.8$	
FNCLCC/FFCD [54]	Perioperative	111	S	24 %	Outcomes similar to MAGIC trial
Ychou, 2011		113	CF→S→CF	38 %	
ARTIST [55]	Adjuvant	228	S→XC	74 % (3-years DFS)	Subset analysis of N + group demonstrated significant 3 years DFS for patients receiving capecitabine-based chemoXRT
Lee, 2012		230	S→CRT (XC)	78 % (3-years DFS) $p = 0.862$	
CLASSIC [56, 57]	Adjuvant	515	S	69 %[b]	Establishes role of adjuvant chemotherapy
Noh, 2013		520	S + XO	78 %[b]	

All survival comparisons significant unless otherwise stated

[a]Updated 5-year survival reported in 2011

[b]Updated 5-year survival reported in 2013 in abstract form

INT Intergroup trial, *MAGIC* Medical Research Council Adjuvant Gastric Infusional Chemotherapy, *ACTS-GT* Adjuvant Chemotherapy Trial of TS-1 for Gastric Cancer, *EORTC* European Organisation for Research and Treatment of Cancer, *CALGB* Cancer and Leukemia Group B, *FNCLCC/FFCD* Fédération Nationales des Centres de Lutte Contre le Cancer and Fédération Francophone de Cancérologie Digestive, *ARTIST* Adjuvant Chemoradiation Therapy in Stomach Cancer, *CLASSIC* Capecitabine and Oxaliplatin Adjuvant Study in Stomach Cancer, *OS* overall survival, *S* surgery, *CRT* chemoradiation, *F* 5-fluorouracil, *L* leucovorin, *E* epirubicin, *C* cisplatin, *S-1* tegafur, *X* capecitabine, *O* oxaliplatin demonstrating similar and significant hazard ratios for relapse and survival as the original analysis [58].

The initial valid criticisms of the INT 0116 trial include a low percentage of patients (10 %) who had the recommended D2 dissection (54 % received less than the recommended D2 dissection), which could possibly contribute to the inferior survivorship in the surgery-only arm, and that postoperative CRT was simply used to compensate for an inadequate operation. However, the updated analysis found that this was not to be the case; among patients in the CRT group, there was no survival differences based on the extent of nodal dissection. INT 0116 established postoperative 5-FU-based CRT as the standard of care in the USA for resectable gastric cancer. This is a category 1 recommendation in the guidelines of the National Comprehensive Cancer Network (NCCN) for gastric cancer patients with pathologic T3 or T4 disease or any node-positive disease provided no preoperative therapy was administered [8].

Although 5-FU and leucovorin (LV) was effective, the successor to the INT 0116, CALGB 80101, questioned whether more intensive adjuvant combination chemotherapy ECF (epirubicin, cisplatin, infusion 5-FU) can replace 5-FU and LV. The studied population was similar to that of INT 0116. Preliminary results reported in 2011 found that among the 546 patients who were accrued over 6 years, there was no difference in the median disease-free survival (DFS) (30 months for 5-FU+RT versus 28 months for ECF+RT; HR 1.00, 95 % CI 0.79, 1.27, p=0.99) or OS (37 months for 5-FU+RT versus 38 months for ECF+RT; HR 1.03, 95 % CI 0.8, 1.34, $p=0.80$) between the two groups [53]. Remarkably, the 3-year OS in the control arm of this trial (50 %) was identical to the 5-FU+RT arm of INT 0116, thus reaffirming the real-world validity of the results from these trials. Of note, patients in the 5-FU arm experienced greater grade 4 toxicity (40 % versus 26 %, $p<0.001$).

Capecitabine, an oral prodrug of 5-FU, is commonly used as an oral alternative to intravenous 5-FU in gastrointestinal cancer without compromising the efficacy and with a toxicity profile that mimics continuous infusion 5-FU. In the ARTIST (Adjuvant Chemoradiation Therapy in Stomach Cancer) trial from Korea, the efficacy of adding radiation to adjuvant chemotherapy was evaluated against adjuvant chemotherapy alone. Adjuvant capecitabine plus cisplatin (XP) for six cycles (chemotherapy only arm) was compared to four cycles of this regimen plus capecitabine-based CRT sandwiched in between (XP plus RT) [55]. Eligibility included patients with pathologic stage II or higher gastric cancer who had undergone at least a D2 gastric dissection with curative intent. A D1 dissection, the presence of microscopically positive margins, and distant nodal involvement (beyond the N2 echelon) were exclusion criteria. Although there was no significant difference in the 3-year DFS between the two arms at a median follow-up of 53.2 months (78.2 % in the XP+RT arm versus 74.2 % in the XP only arm; $p=0.0862$), and the patterns of relapse (locoregional and systemic) were similar between the two arms, there was a survival difference among node-positive patients, a population that made up approximately 87 % of the study population; the 3-year DFS for the XP+RT group was 77.5 % compared to 72.3 % for XP alone ($p=0.0365$) [55]. At the time of reporting, OS was not analyzed secondary to lack of adequate events. Thus, adjuvant CRT was effective even among patients who had adequate nodal clearance (D2 dissection). Based on this subset analysis of the ARTIST trial, the proposed ARTIST-2 trial will compare postoperative adjuvant chemotherapy alone with adjuvant chemoradiotherapy in patients with node-positive gastric cancer.

Adjuvant Chemotherapy Alone

While radiation appears to be an integral component of adjuvant therapy in gastric cancer in North America, a contrasting adjuvant paradigm without this modality exists in Japan. In 2007, the largest adjuvant trial to date was reported by the Japanese ACTS-GC (Adjuvant Chemotherapy Trial of TS-1 for Gastric Cancer) investigators. These trialists compared 12 months of oral S-1 alone in 529 patients following D2 dissection for stage II and III gastric cancer. An interim analysis demonstrated survival benefit for the S-1-treated patients at 3 years (80.1 % versus 70.1 %) which was subsequently confirmed at 5 years as well (71.7 % versus 61.1 %; HR, 0.669; 95 % CI, 0.540, 0.828) [51, 59]. While adjuvant S-1 is standard in Japan, its utility in a Western population is not known, and it is not available for use in the USA except within the aegis of a clinical study.

More recently, combination capecitabine plus oxaliplatin (CAPOX) was studied in 1035 stage II–IIIb gastric cancer patients in East Asia (South Korea, China, and Taiwan) following D2 resection (Capecitabine and Oxaliplatin Adjuvant Study in Stomach Cancer trial or the CLASSIC trial) [56]. In this randomized trial, 520 patients received up to eight cycles of adjuvant CAPOX (oral capecitabine at 1,000 mg/m^2 twice daily on days 1–14, plus IV oxaliplatin at 130 mg/m^2 on day one in a 21-day cycle), while 515 patients were scheduled to have surgery as a sole modality of treatment. In an intent-to-treat 3-year DFS analysis, CLASSIC showed superiority in the postoperative CAPOX (74 %, 95 % CI 69, 79) group compared to surgery alone (59 %, 95 % CI 53, 64; HR 0.56, 95 % CI 0.44–0.72; $p<0.0001$). In the 2013 update presented in abstract form, the 5-year OS also favored the adjuvant chemotherapy arm (78 % versus 69 %; HR 0.66, 95 % CI 0.51, 0.85, $p=0.0029$) [57]. It is important to note that nearly a third of patients assigned to chemotherapy were unable to complete all planned treatment with nearly all patients requiring chemotherapy dose attenuation. Of note, patients in the above two studies had D2 dissection, a technique that is widely employed in Asia but not in the USA. Thus efficacy of adjuvant chemotherapy alone among patients who had a D0 or D1 dissection remains uncertain.

The above trials of postoperative therapy in gastric cancer demonstrate the diverse options available for patients with resected disease. While transcontinental approaches differ, a unifying theme has clearly emerged through these investigations, mainly that surgery alone is inadequate therapy except in very early stage tumors. In addition, the delivery of postoperative chemotherapy and/or CRT is difficult, especially in the setting of nutritional compromise. This has led to the consideration of giving systemic therapy up front prior to any planned surgery for localized gastric cancer. Many phase II trials in the 1980s showed that neoadjuvant chemotherapy could be given safely without increasing peri- or postoperative morbidity and mortality. Modern trials testing this approach are discussed in more detail in the next section.

Perioperative Chemotherapy in Gastric Cancer

A landmark trial published by the Medical Research Council Adjuvant Gastric Infusional Chemotherapy (MAGIC trial) in 2006 studied 503 patients in the UK and reported the efficacy of using perioperative chemotherapy in patients with gastric cancer. It compared preoperative chemotherapy, surgical resection, and postoperative chemotherapy composed of epirubicin, cisplatin, and fluorouracil (ECF) to surgery alone and found 5-year OS of 36.3 % and 23.0 % ($P=0.009$) for the two groups, respectively [50]. Patients treated with ECF were found to have a statistically significant decrease in the size of tumor resected, less advanced nodal disease, as well as a greater percentage of patients actually receiving the adjuvant treatment compared to historic postoperative approaches.

Further evidence supporting the perioperative chemotherapy approach comes from the French collaborative groups, the Fédération Nationales des Centres de Lutte Contre le Cancer and Fédération Francophone de Cancérologie Digestive (FNCLCC/FFCD) Collaborative Groups. FNCLCC/FFCD randomized 224 patients using perioperative cisplatin plus infusion 5-FU. The trial demonstrated improved outcomes compared to surgery alone [54]. The 5-year survival for the chemotherapy-surgery group was 38 % compared to 24 % for surgery alone (HR for death: 0.69; 95 % CI, 0.50–0.95; $P=.02$) [54]. However, the vast majority of patients on this trial had EGJ tumors (64 %) with only 25 % having pure gastric cancers, reflecting a distinct change in the anatomic distribution of adenocarcinoma of the upper gastrointestinal tract. Regardless, the MAGIC and the French trials established that perioperative chemotherapy is a viable option for patients with resectable gastric cancer who underwent a curative surgery with limited D0 or D1 dissection. Whether perioperative chemotherapy is even necessary for patients who had a D2 dissection is not known.

Unlike the MAGIC and the French trials that included adjuvant chemotherapy, EORTC (European Organization for Research and Treatment of Cancer) 40954 trial eliminated the adjuvant chemotherapy component and instead compared purely preoperative chemotherapy followed by surgery versus surgery alone using cisplatin and 5-FU/LV [52]. The 2-year OS for the neoadjuvant chemotherapy group (73 %) and surgery alone group (70 %) was not statistically different ($P=0.47$). Unfortunately, the trial was underpowered and was terminated early for poor accrual because only 144 of the intended 360 patients were enrolled.

To summarize, both INT 0116 and MAGIC trials are acceptable approaches to patients with resectable non-metastatic gastric cancer. There are new phase III trials on the horizon. TOPGEAR (Trial of Preoperative Therapy for Gastric and Esophageal Junction Adenocarcinoma; NCT0 1924819) trial will compare preoperative CRT with preoperative chemotherapy, while the CRITICS (ChemoRadiotherapy after Induction Chemotherapy in Cancer of the Stomach; NCT00407186) trial will compare adjuvant CRT with adjuvant chemotherapy; both arms will receive neoadjuvant chemotherapy. Additionally, a number of phase III trials are assessing the efficacy of adding targeted agents like trastuzumab and bevacizumab to existing neoadjuvant chemotherapy.

Many phase II studies of neoadjuvant chemotherapy on locally advanced gastric cancer have demonstrated down-staging, but predicting response remains a clinical challenge. Neither current imaging nor molecular markers can reliably predict response to chemotherapy in the early course of treatment for gastric cancer. Measuring metabolic uptake on FDG-PET imaging has been studied in order to predict response and prognosticate in certain gastric cancers. Ott et al. conducted a study with 44 consecutive patients with locally advanced gastric carcinomas by FDG-PET before and 14 days after initiation of cisplatin-based polychemotherapy [60]. Tumors with a reduction of uptake by more than 35 % were considered to be "responders." Patients with a metabolic response had a 2-year survival rate of 90 % (median survival had not been reached), compared to 25 % in nonresponders (median survival for nonresponders was 18.9 months; $p=0.002$). However, about 30 % of gastric tumors are not FDG avid and thus cannot be visualized, and this is mostly the case with the diffuse type with signet cells and mucinous content. Interestingly, these tumors seem to be similar to nonresponders, suggesting that the lack of uptake may infer that the tumors are biologically unfavorable [60, 61].

Palliative Treatment

The goal for treating patients who have stage IV disease or those who cannot tolerate surgery should be palliation that will optimize the patients' quality of life. Surgical intervention should be reserved in patients who fulfill the "IHOP" criteria: *I*ntractable pain, acute *H*emorrhage, *O*bstruction not amenable to nonoperative interventions, and *P*erforation. Non-life-threatening bleeding can be addressed with endoscopic tumor ablative techniques and support with appropriate blood products. Endoluminal stenting is a viable option for tumors obstructing the GEJ tumor or those causing gastric outlet obstruction (GOO). However, for well-fit patients with a reasonable expectation of prolonged life who have GOO, a gastric bypass, either open or laparoscopic approach, is preferred over endoluminal stenting. Malnourished patients may require a feeding jejunostomy, which can be performed percutaneously (percutaneous endoscopic jejunostomy or PEJ) or as either open or laparoscopically with minimal surgical risk to the patients.

Surveillance

Seventy-four percent of recurrences occurred within 2 years after surgery, and less than 4 % occurred after 5 years following surgery [62]. Follow-up includes a complete history and physical examination every 3–6 months for 1–2 years, every 6–12 months for 3–5 years, and then annually thereafter [8]. Routine imaging and laboratory values should be avoided unless patients have signs and symptoms that necessitate a workup. Vitamin B12 and iron deficiency should be monitored and treated for patients who had a gastrectomy.

Summary

Over two decades of appropriately powered clinical trials have now established several acceptable options for the management of locoregional gastric carcinoma. While paradigms of perioperative therapy vary across continents, the emphasis on the multidisciplinary management of a patient with gastric cancer cannot be overstated. The North American clinicians prefer adjuvant CRT, and the UK and European clinicians use perioperative combination chemotherapy (ECF), while the Southeast Asian clinicians use adjuvant chemotherapy (Japanese clinicians rely on adjuvant S1; South Korea, China, and Taiwan use capecitabine and oxaliplatin). All are reasonable options for T3/T4 or node-positive patients with gastric cancer. As outlined previously, an underlying theme has emerged from these investigations. In 2014, surgery alone cannot be endorsed as a sole modality of therapy except in very early stage tumors. A multipronged approach with early involvement of the medical oncologist, radiation oncologist, and surgeon is essential if we are to build on the existing platform towards cure in resectable disease. On the other hand, the prognosis of advanced disease remains poor. Only a concerted effort in understanding the molecular biology of this disease will permit further enhancements in the clinical arena.

Salient Points

- The prognosis of gastric cancer in Western countries is better than worldwide, but it is still very poor.
- In Western countries, poor prognosis is due to vague symptoms leading to advanced disease at presentation.
- H. pylori infection and chronic gastritis are the leading causes of gastric cancer.
- Hereditary diffuse gastric cancer is associated with decreased intracellular adhesion due to E-cadherin mutation and/or hypermethylation in both inherited and sporadic forms.
- There are two histologic classifications: WHO and Lauren classification.
- HER-2 is overexpressed in up to 25 % of gastric cancer. Its clinical significance in resectable gastric cancer is unknown, but is useful in patients with metastatic disease.
- Endoscopic ultrasound is used for initial diagnosis and can stage depth of invasion but not extent of regional lymph node metastasis.
- Diagnostic laparoscopic is useful to rule out peritoneal metastases.
- Siewert classification is used to classify GEJ tumors.
  - Type I: epicenter 1–5 cm proximal to GEJ
  - Type II: epicenter 1 cm proximal to GEJ and 2 cm distal to GEJ
  - Type III: epicenter 2–5 cm distal to the GEJ
- Treatment options for local control include endoscopic mucosal resection and subtotal and total gastrectomy.
- Endoscopic mucosal resection (EMR) is generally done for tumors:
  - Less than 3 cm in diameter
  - Well or moderately differentiated
  - Superficially elevated and/or depressed without ulceration or submucosal invasion
  - However, EMR should be regarded as investigational at this point.
- Total gastrectomy should only be done for very proximal gastric tumors.
- 5 cm is recommended gastric margin for surgical resection.

- R-resection nomenclature:
  - R0: No residual gross or microscopic tumor left behind
  - R1: No gross tumor, but residual microscopic tumor left behind
  - R2: Gross tumor left behind
- Recommended number of lymph nodes to be retrieved: 15
- Although D1 lymph node resection is considered the standard of care for regional control of most locally advanced tumors, a D2 resection may provide some benefit for patients with T3 or T4 disease and those likely to have 3 or more positive nodes.
- Prophylactic splenectomy and distal pancreatectomy are not recommended.
- D2 should only be done by well-trained surgeons.
- Six clinical trials compared laparoscopic gastrectomy (LG) with open gastrectomy (OG) for distal gastric cancer.
  - LG had longer operative time.
  - LG: lower EBL, complication rate, quicker GI recovery, shorter length of hospital stay.
  - LG appears to offer similar oncologic outcomes as OG.
  - KLASS trial of over 1,400 patients might be able to definitively answer the question of whether LG is oncologically equivalent to OG.
- Recurrence both locally and distally occurs in up to 80 % of patients, and thus most patients are offered:
  - *Adjuvant chemoradiation therapy* (INT 0116 or Macdonald trial)
  - *Perioperative chemotherapy*: 3 cycles ECF→>surgery→>3 cycles ECF (MAGIC trial)
  - *Adjuvant chemotherapy*
    - (S-1): given in Japan, but is not available in the USA
    - Capecitabine and oxaliplatin: mainly in South Korea, China, and Taiwan
- FDG-PET can predict response and prognosis of gastric tumors.
- 75 % of recurrences occur within the first 2 years following resection.
- 30 % of gastric tumors do not uptake FDG and have a similarly poor prognosis to those that do not respond to chemotherapy.
- In select patients who have metastatic disease and gastric outlet obstruction but have good performance status, a gastric bypass, either done laparoscopically or open, is better than endoluminal stenting.
- Indications for surgical intervention in patients with metastatic disease are "IHOP":
  - Intractable pain
  - Hemorrhage
  - Obstruction
  - Perforation

Questions

1. Which of the following tumors can be treated with EMR?
   A. A 2 cm poorly differentiated tumor without ulceration
   B. A 2.5 cm with ulceration and submucosal invasion
   C. A 3 cm moderately differentiated tumor that is superficially elevated
   D. A 2.5 cm moderately differentiated tumor with ulceration
   E. None of the above
2. Which of the following is NOT true in differentiating diffuse- and intestinal-type cancers?
   A. Diffuse type is usually found in the cardia but can arise anywhere in the stomach.
   B. Intestinal type carries a worse prognosis.
   C. H. pylori is linked to both intestinal and diffuse subtypes of cancers.
   D. Intestinal type is usually found in older patients and associated with atrophic gastritis.
   E. None of the above.
3. What is the minimum number of lymph nodes needed for pathology in order to accurately stage a tumor N0?
   A. 8
   B. 10
   C. 12
   D. 15
   E. 20
4. Which of the following statements concerning gastric adenocarcinoma is TRUE?
   A. Predisposition is primarily genetic rather than environmental.
   B. Incidence peaks at age 40.

C. Approximately 40 % of patients present with an *early* lesion (no invasion of the muscularis propria).
D. *H. pylori*, chronic gastritis, and gastric adenomatous polyps are all risk factors for the development of gastric adenocarcinoma.
E. Gastric cancer is more common in women than men.

5. A 66-year-old male with a distant history of gastric ulcers comes to your office complaining of vague abdominal pain and a 5 pound weight loss over the last month. He takes over-the-counter Nexium which usually controls his heartburn. What would your *initial* work up entail?
A. Reassurance and follow-up in 6 months as long as he has no family history of gastric cancer
B. Instruction to continue his PPI and avoid salted and chemically preserved foods with follow-up in 6 months
C. Outpatient CT scan of the abdomen and pelvis with PO and IV contrast
D. Outpatient EGD, endoscopic ultrasound with biopsy
E. Noninvasive abdominal ultrasound to look for any obvious masses

6. The most common cause of gastric outlet obstruction in adults is:
A. Hypertrophic pyloric stenosis
B. Duodenal stricture secondary to peptic ulceration
C. Gastric adenocarcinoma
D. Gastric lymphoma
E. Iatrogenic stricture after gastric bypass (weight loss) surgery

7. For tumors of the distal stomach, a subtotal gastrectomy is preferred over total gastrectomy for all of the following reasons EXCEPT:
A. Subtotal gastrectomy confers a significantly better 5-year survival rate.
B. Total gastrectomy is a technically more difficult surgery.
C. Subtotal gastrectomy allows for a better nutritional status.
D. There is less perioperative morbidity and mortality.
E. Subtotal gastrectomy results in a better quality of life than total gastrectomy.

8. A 61-year-old woman has a partial gastrectomy with a D2 dissection and is found to have a pathologic staging of T2N1M0 (Stage IIA). Which of the following is the best postoperative management for this patient?
A. Screening endoscopy and CT abdomen pelvis every 6 months to check for recurrence.
B. Chemotherapy before and after surgery or adjuvant chemoradiation therapy.
C. Screening PET scan every 6 months to check for recurrence and/or distant metastasis.
D. Postoperative radiation alone.
E. The patient is considered cured since she had an extensive D2 dissection.

9. A 48-year-old man was diagnosed with cT3N1 adenocarcinoma of the distal stomach. Staging CT imaging did not reveal any evidence of distant metastases. A diagnostic laparoscopy confirmed the absence of peritoneal spread. Which of the following is the best treatment strategy for this patient?
A. D2 gastric resection followed by 5FU/LV-based chemoradiation.
B. Preoperative chemotherapy with epirubicin, cisplatin, and 5-FU (ECF) X 3 cycles followed by surgery followed by 3 more cycles of ECF.
C. D2 gastric resection followed by 1 year of oral S-1 where available.
D. Enrollment in a clinical trial examining preoperative chemotherapy plus postoperative chemoradiation.
E. All of the above are appropriate options.

10. Which of the following is true regarding D2 dissection in gastric cancer?
A. Removal of nodes along the lesser and greater curvatures of the stomach
B. Removal of (a) plus para-aortic nodes
C. Removal of (a) plus nodes along the left gastric artery, common hepatic artery, celiac trunk, and splenic artery and hilum
D. Removal of (a) plus left supraclavicular nodes

Answers

1. C
2. B
3. D
4. D
5. D
6. C
7. A
8. B
9. E
10. C

References

1. Karpeh M, Kelsen D, Tepper J. Cancer of the stomach. In: DeVita JV, Hellman S, Rosenberg S, editors. Cancer: principles & practice of oncology, vol. 1. 6th ed. Philadelphia: Lippincott-Williams-Wilkin; 2001. p. 1092–126.
2. Lauren P. The two histological main types of gastric carcinoma: diffuse and so-called intestinal-type carcinoma. An attempt at a histo-clinical classification. Acta Pathol Microbiol Scand. 1965;64: 31–49.
3. Machado JC, Oliveira C, Carvalho R, et al. E-cadherin gene (CDH1) promoter methylation as the second hit in sporadic diffuse gastric carcinoma. Oncogene. 2001;20(12):1525–8.
4. Grady WM, Willis J, Guilford PJ, et al. Methylation of the CDH1 promoter as the second genetic hit in hereditary diffuse gastric cancer. Nat Genet. 2000; 26(1):16–7.
5. Parsonnet J, Friedman GD, Vandersteen DP, et al. Helicobacter pylori infection and the risk of gastric carcinoma. N Engl J Med. 1991;325(16):1127–31.
6. Tanner M, Hollmén M, Junttila TT, et al. Amplification of HER-2 in gastric carcinoma: association with Topoisomerase IIalpha gene amplification, intestinal type, poor prognosis and sensitivity to trastuzumab. Ann Oncol. 2005;16(2):273–8.
7. Yan B, Yau EX, Bte Omar SS, et al. A study of HER2 gene amplification and protein expression in gastric cancer. J Clin Pathol. 2010;63(9):839–42.
8. Ajani JA, Bentrem DJ, Besh S, et al. Gastric cancer, version 2.2013: featured updates to the NCCN guidelines. J Natl Compr Canc Netw. 2013;11(5): 531–46.
9. Polkowski M, Palucki J, Wronska E, Szawlowski A, Nasierowska-Guttmejer A, Butruk E. Endosonography versus helical computed tomography for locoregional staging of gastric cancer. Endoscopy. 2004;36(7): 617–23.
10. Smyth E, Schoder H, Strong VE, et al. A prospective evaluation of the utility of 2-deoxy-2-[(18) F]fluoro-D-glucose positron emission tomography and computed tomography in staging locally advanced gastric cancer. Cancer. 2012;118(22):5481–8.
11. Yamada A, Oguchi K, Fukushima M, Imai Y, Kadoya M. Evaluation of 2-deoxy-2-[18F]fluoro-D-glucose positron emission tomography in gastric carcinoma: relation to histological subtypes, depth of tumor invasion, and glucose transporter-1 expression. Ann Nucl Med. 2006;20(9):597–604.
12. Ilson DH, Minsky BD, Ku GY, et al. Phase 2 trial of induction and concurrent chemoradiotherapy with weekly irinotecan and cisplatin followed by surgery for esophageal cancer. Cancer. 2012;118(11): 2820–7.
13. Leake PA, Cardoso R, Seevaratnam R, et al. A systematic review of the accuracy and indications for diagnostic laparoscopy prior to curative-intent resection of gastric cancer. Gastric Cancer. 2012;15 Suppl 1:S38–47.
14. Bentrem D, Wilton A, Mazumdar M, Brennan M, Coit D. The value of peritoneal cytology as a preoperative predictor in patients with gastric carcinoma undergoing a curative resection. Ann Surg Oncol. 2005;12(5):347–53.
15. Siewert JR, Hölscher AH, Becker K, Gössner W. Cardia cancer: attempt at a therapeutically relevant classification. Chirurg. 1987;58(1):25–32.
16. Compton C, Byrd D, Garcia-Aguilar J, et al. Stomach. In: Compton C, Byrd D, Garcia-Aguilar J, Kurtzman S, Olawaiye A, Washington M, editors. AJCC cancer staging atlas. 2nd ed. New York: Springer; 2012. p. 143–53.
17. Kajitani T. The general rules for the gastric cancer study in surgery and pathology. Part I. Clinical classification. Jpn J Surg. 1981;11(2):127–39.
18. Washington K. 7th edition of the AJCC cancer staging manual: stomach. Ann Surg Oncol. 2010;17(12): 3077–9.
19. Maruyama K, Okabayashi K, Kinoshita T. Progress in gastric cancer surgery in Japan and its limits of radicality. World J Surg. 1987;11(4):418–25.
20. Yamao T, Shirao K, Ono H, et al. Risk factors for lymph node metastasis from intramucosal gastric carcinoma. Cancer. 1996;77(4):602–6.
21. Gotoda T, Yanagisawa A, Sasako M, et al. Incidence of lymph node metastasis from early gastric cancer: estimation with a large number of cases at two large centers. Gastric Cancer. 2000;3(4):219–25.
22. Bozzetti F, Marubini E, Bonfanti G, Miceli R, Piano C, Gennari L. Subtotal versus total gastrectomy for gastric cancer: five-year survival rates in a multicenter randomized Italian trial. Italian Gastrointestinal Tumor Study Group. Ann Surg. 1999;230(2):170–8.
23. Gouzi JL, Huguier M, Fagniez PL, et al. Total versus subtotal gastrectomy for adenocarcinoma of the gastric antrum. A French prospective controlled study. Ann Surg. 1989;209(2):162–6.
24. Hasler WL. Gastroparesis: pathogenesis, diagnosis and management. Nat Rev Gastroenterol Hepatol. 2011;8(8):438–53.

25. Kim HJ, Karpeh MS. Surgical approaches and outcomes in the treatment of gastric cancer. Semin Radiat Oncol. 2002;12(2):162–9.
26. Hartgrink HH, van de Velde CJ, Putter H, et al. Extended lymph node dissection for gastric cancer: who may benefit? Final results of the randomized Dutch gastric cancer group trial. J Clin Oncol. 2004; 22(11):2069–77.
27. Sasako M, Sano T, Yamamoto S, et al. D2 lymphadenectomy alone or with para-aortic nodal dissection for gastric cancer. N Engl J Med. 2008;359(5):453–62.
28. Bonenkamp JJ, Hermans J, Sasako M, et al. Extended lymph-node dissection for gastric cancer. N Engl J Med. 1999;340(12):908–14.
29. Songun I, Putter H, Kranenbarg EM, Sasako M, van de Velde CJ. Surgical treatment of gastric cancer: 15-year follow-up results of the randomised nationwide Dutch D1D2 trial. Lancet Oncol. 2010;11(5): 439–49.
30. Jiang L, Yang KH, Guan QL, Zhao P, Chen Y, Tian JH. Survival and recurrence free benefits with different lymphadenectomy for resectable gastric cancer: a meta-analysis. J Surg Oncol. 2013;107(8):807–14.
31. Adachi Y, Suematsu T, Shiraishi N, et al. Quality of life after laparoscopy-assisted Billroth I gastrectomy. Ann Surg. 1999;229(1):49–54.
32. Adachi Y, Shiraishi N, Shiromizu A, Bandoh T, Aramaki M, Kitano S. Laparoscopy-assisted Billroth I gastrectomy compared with conventional open gastrectomy. Arch Surg. 2000;135(7):806–10.
33. Goh PM, Alponat A, Mak K, Kum CK. Early international results of laparoscopic gastrectomies. Surg Endosc. 1997;11(6):650–2.
34. Xiong JJ, Nunes QM, Huang W, et al. Laparoscopic vs open total gastrectomy for gastric cancer: a meta-analysis. World J Gastroenterol. 2013;19(44):8114–32.
35. Huscher CG, Mingoli A, Sgarzini G, et al. Laparoscopic versus open subtotal gastrectomy for distal gastric cancer: five-year results of a randomized prospective trial. Ann Surg. 2005;241(2):232–7.
36. Fujii K, Sonoda K, Izumi K, Shiraishi N, Adachi Y, Kitano S. T lymphocyte subsets and Th1/Th2 balance after laparoscopy-assisted distal gastrectomy. Surg Endosc. 2003;17(9):1440–4.
37. Hayashi H, Ochiai T, Shimada H, Gunji Y. Prospective randomized study of open versus laparoscopy-assisted distal gastrectomy with extraperigastric lymph node dissection for early gastric cancer. Surg Endosc. 2005; 19(9):1172–6.
38. Lee JH, Han HS. A prospective randomized study comparing open vs laparoscopy-assisted distal gastrectomy in early gastric cancer: early results. Surg Endosc. 2005;19(2):168–73.
39. Kim YW, Baik YH, Yun YH, et al. Improved quality of life outcomes after laparoscopy-assisted distal gastrectomy for early gastric cancer: results of a prospective randomized clinical trial. Ann Surg. 2008;248(5): 721–7.
40. Kim HH, Hyung WJ, Cho GS, et al. Morbidity and mortality of laparoscopic gastrectomy versus open gastrectomy for gastric cancer: an interim report–a phase III multicenter, prospective, randomized Trial (KLASS Trial). Ann Surg. 2010;251(3):417–20.
41. Kitano S, Shiraishi N, Uyama I, Sugihara K, Tanigawa N, Group JLSS. A multicenter study on oncologic outcome of laparoscopic gastrectomy for early cancer in Japan. Ann Surg. 2007;245(1):68–72.
42. Song J, Lee HJ, Cho GS, et al. Recurrence following laparoscopy-assisted gastrectomy for gastric cancer: a multicenter retrospective analysis of 1,417 patients. Ann Surg Oncol. 2010;17(7):1777–86.
43. Hwang SH, Park DJ, Jee YS, et al. Actual 3-year survival after laparoscopy-assisted gastrectomy for gastric cancer. Arch Surg. 2009;144(6):559–64.
44. Pak KH, Hyung WJ, Son T, et al. Long-term oncologic outcomes of 714 consecutive laparoscopic gastrectomies for gastric cancer: results from the 7-year experience of a single institute. Surg Endosc. 2012; 26(1):130–6.
45. Schwarz RE, Zagala-Nevarez K. Recurrence patterns after radical gastrectomy for gastric cancer: prognostic factors and implications for postoperative adjuvant therapy. Ann Surg Oncol. 2002;9(4):394–400.
46. Roviello F, Marrelli D, de Manzoni G, et al. Prospective study of peritoneal recurrence after curative surgery for gastric cancer. Br J Surg. 2003;90(9): 1113–9.
47. Kattan MW, Karpeh MS, Mazumdar M, Brennan MF. Postoperative nomogram for disease-specific survival after an R0 resection for gastric carcinoma. J Clin Oncol. 2003;21(19):3647–50.
48. Marrelli D, Roviello F. Prognostic score in gastric cancer patients. Ann Surg Oncol. 2007;14(2):362–4.
49. Macdonald JS, Smalley SR, Benedetti J, et al. Chemoradiotherapy after surgery compared with surgery alone for adenocarcinoma of the stomach or gastroesophageal junction. N Engl J Med. 2001;345(10): 725–30.
50. Cunningham D, Allum WH, Stenning SP, et al. Perioperative chemotherapy versus surgery alone for resectable gastroesophageal cancer. N Engl J Med. 2006;355(1):11–20.
51. Sakuramoto S, Sasako M, Yamaguchi T, et al. Adjuvant chemotherapy for gastric cancer with S-1, an oral fluoropyrimidine. N Engl J Med. 2007;357(18): 1810–20.
52. Schuhmacher C, Gretschel S, Lordick F, et al. Neoadjuvant chemotherapy compared with surgery alone for locally advanced cancer of the stomach and cardia: European Organisation for Research and Treatment of Cancer randomized trial 40954. J Clin Oncol. 2010;28(35):5210–8.
53. Fuchs C, Tepper J, Niedzwiecki D, et al. Postoperative adjuvant chemoradiation for gastric or gastroesophageal junction (GEJ) adenocarcinoma using epirubicin, cisplatin, and infusional (CI) 5-FU (ECF) before and after CI 5-FU and radiotherapy (CRT) compared with bolus 5-FU/LV before and after CRT: intergroup trial CALGB 80101. J Clin Oncol. 2011;29(256s):Abstr 4003.

54. Ychou M, Boige V, Pignon JP, et al. Perioperative chemotherapy compared with surgery alone for resectable gastroesophageal adenocarcinoma: an FNCLCC and FFCD multicenter phase III trial. J Clin Oncol. 2011;29(13):1715–21.
55. Lee J, Lim DH, Kim S, et al. Phase III trial comparing capecitabine plus cisplatin versus capecitabine plus cisplatin with concurrent capecitabine radiotherapy in completely resected gastric cancer with D2 lymph node dissection: the ARTIST trial. J Clin Oncol. 2012; 30(3):268–73.
56. Bang YJ, Kim YW, Yang HK, et al. Adjuvant capecitabine and oxaliplatin for gastric cancer after D2 gastrectomy (CLASSIC): a phase 3 open-label, randomised controlled trial. Lancet. 2012;379(9813):315–21.
57. Noh S, Park S, Yang H, Chung H, Chung I, et al. Adjuvant capecitabine and oxaliplatin (Xelox) for gastric cancer after D2 gastrectomy: final results from the CLASSIC trial. Ann Oncol. 2013;24 Suppl 4:iv14.
58. Smalley SR, Benedetti JK, Haller DG, et al. Updated analysis of SWOG-directed intergroup study 0116: a phase III trial of adjuvant radiochemotherapy versus observation after curative gastric cancer resection. J Clin Oncol. 2012;30(19):2327–33.
59. Sasako M, Sakuramoto S, Katai H, et al. Five-year outcomes of a randomized phase III trial comparing adjuvant chemotherapy with S-1 versus surgery alone in stage II or III gastric cancer. J Clin Oncol. 2011; 29(33):4387–93.
60. Ott K, Fink U, Becker K, et al. Prediction of response to preoperative chemotherapy in gastric carcinoma by metabolic imaging: results of a prospective trial. J Clin Oncol. 2003;21(24):4604–10.
61. Ott K, Herrmann K, Krause BJ, Lordick F. The value of PET imaging in patients with localized gastroesophageal cancer. Gastrointest Cancer Res. 2008; 2(6):287–94.
62. Marrelli D, De Stefano A, de Manzoni G, Morgagni P, Di Leo A, Roviello F. Prediction of recurrence after radical surgery for gastric cancer: a scoring system obtained from a prospective multicenter study. Ann Surg. 2005;241(2):247–55.

Small Bowel Cancer

10

David Gleason, Kimberly E. Miller-Hammond, and John F. Gibbs

Learning Objectives

After reading this chapter, the reader should be able to:

- Identify the most common types of small bowel cancer
- Describe the demographics and risk factors associated with small bowel cancers
- Understand the current pathogenesis of small bowel cancers
- Describe the various diagnostic techniques for identifying small bowel cancers
- Counsel the patient about the surgical treatments of small bowel cancers
- Apply knowledge to patient prognosis and basic chemotherapy regimens

D. Gleason, M.D. • K.E. Miller-Hammond, M.D.
Department of Surgery, Kaleida Health/Buffalo General Medical Center, State University of New York at Buffalo, 100 High St. Buffalo, 14203 NY, USA
e-mail: dfgleason4@gmail.com; kimmil83@gmail.com

J.F. Gibbs, M.D. (✉)
Department of Surgery, Jersey Shore University Medical Center/Meridian Heath, 1945 State Highway 33, 4 Floor Ackerman Neptune, 07753 NJ, USA
e-mail: jgibbs@meridianhealth.com

Introduction

Historically, small intestine cancers were predominately adenocarcinoma; however, carcinoid has eclipsed adenocarcinoma by a fourfold increased incidence to become the most frequently diagnosed subtype [1]. This chapter's focus will be on the epidemiology, incidence, risk factors, treatment, and staging of adenocarcinoma and lymphoma, as well as for the most common types of metastatic disease. A brief discussion about small bowel carcinoid and Gastrointestinal Stromal Tumors (GISTs) will be mentioned, but their treatment is covered in other chapters (Carcinoid Tumors, Chap. 26; GISTs, Chap. 28).

Epidemiology

Cancer of the small intestine comprises less than 5 % of all gastrointestinal cancers. The American Cancer Society estimates 8,810 newly diagnosed cases and 1,170 deaths from small bowel cancer in 2013 [1]. A review by Bilimoria et al. of the National Cancer Data Base (NCDB, 1985–2005) and Surveillance Epidemiology and End Results (SEER, 1973–2004) of 67,843 patients has shown that the incidence of all primary small bowel cancers is on the rise [2]. The median age of diagnosis was 67 years old (interquartile range 56–76 years) with a slight preponderance toward

Q.D. Chu et al. (eds.), *Surgical Oncology: A Practical and Comprehensive Approach*,
DOI 10.1007/978-1-4939-1423-4_10,

Table 10.1 Summary of the most common small bowel cancer characteristics

Type of cancer	Incidence rate	Common site	Risk factors	5-year survival
Carcinoid	37–44 %	Ileum (44 %)	MEN1[a]	60–75 %
Adenocarcinoma	33–36 %	Duodenum (55 %), jejunum (30 %), ileum (11 %)	Crohn's disease, celiac, FAP[b]	26–39 %
Lymphoma	15–17 %	Ileum (66 %), jejunum (20 %)	Celiac, AIDS[c], EBV[d]	25–40 %
GIST[e]	7–9 %	Jejunum		40 %
Metastasis	Melanoma (42 %), breast (16 %), lung (12 %)	Melanoma in jejunum and ileum	Primary cancer	Solitary lesion with good prognosis

[a]*MEN* multiple endocrine neoplasia
[b]Familial adenomatous polyposis
[c]*AIDS* acquired immune deficiency syndrome
[d]Epstein-Barr virus
[e]Gastrointestinal stromal tumor

men (54 %) compared to women (46 %) [1]. Although there is no racial preponderance for the development of small intestinal cancers, there seems to be a worse prognosis for African Americans, patients>55 years old, T4 tumors, distant metastasis, or poorly differentiated tumors.

A rising incidence rate has not been matched with an improved survival rate. An observed 5-year survival was 64 % in carcinoid, 32.5 % in adenocarcinoma, 39 % in stromal tumors, and 49.6 % lymphomas [2]. Small bowel adenocarcinoma has an overall survival (OS) of 12 months when all stages were analyzed.

The distribution of cancers within the small bowel is most commonly in the proximal portion for adenocarcinoma in the duodenum and jejunum. Duodenal small bowel adenocarcinoma (SBA) carries an increased mortality risk. In small bowel lymphoma, the most common site is the ileum followed by the jejunum [2] (Table 10.1).

Etiology and Pathogenesis

The small bowel comprises the majority of the gastrointestinal tract but has a very low cancer incidence. The low risk of developing SBA is likely due to a number of factors including rapid transit of contents, decreased amount of exposure of carcinogenic substances, high amount of lymphoid tissue, high amount of IgA secretion, rapid turnover of cells, and the alkaline nature of the small bowel contents [3, 4]. The most common modifiable risk factors appear to be cigarette smoking and alcohol consumption when compared to nontobacco users and nondrinkers. There are some underlying conditions that may increase the risk of small bowel cancer. Patients with celiac disease and Crohn's disease have an increased risk of both adenocarcinoma and lymphoma. Familial adenomatous polyposis (FAP) patients will have risk of duodenal and periampullary adenocarcinoma. Patients with hereditary non-polyposis colorectal cancer (HNPCC) develop adenocarcinomas of the small intestine at younger ages than the general population.

The low incidence rate and lack of screening modalities have led to a delay in diagnosis and more advanced disease at the time of presentation. The primary presenting symptoms are nonspecific and include abdominal pain, gastrointestinal bleeding, jaundice, weight loss, abdominal distention, nausea, vomiting, and anemia. The nonspecificity of the symptoms leads to a delay in diagnosis and treatment, ranging from 2 months to 12 months [5]. For this reason, 30–50 % of small intestine cancers are associated with nodal or distal metastases at the time of presentation. The median survival time of patients diagnosed of small bowel cancer is 13–20 months with a 5-year OS ranging from 0 to 28 % for adenocarcinoma,

14–30 % for lymphoma, and 60 % for carcinoid [5]. Several poor prognostic factors are age>75 years, duodenal site, TNM staging, nodal involvement, and positive surgical margins [6].

Diagnostic Tools

Historically, the diagnostic difficulty of evaluating the small bowel adequately leads to delays in diagnosis and risk for more advanced disease. This has encouraged new innovation in the evaluation of small intestine cancers. The most appropriate diagnostic modality includes a combination of noninvasive imaging and endoscopy with biopsy capability. Barium enteroclysis was, historically, the most common imaging offered to evaluate the small bowel. This was time consuming, poorly tolerated by the patient, and still not able to accurately depict mural and extramural extent of disease. Improvements in computed tomography (CT) and magnetic resonance imaging (MRI) modalities and improved small bowel enteroscopy with capsule endoscopy or double-balloon endoscopy add to the surgeon's armamentarium.

Computed topography and MRI enteroclysis are other modalities of imaging the small bowel. These radiographic modalities require the patient to fast the day prior to the study. The patient is asked to consume an oral agent to allow for optimal small intestine distention prior to the study. The diagnostic yield for both CT and MRI is similar. The advantages of CT scanning include more hospitals are equipped with CT and the patient procedural time is much less. MR imaging avoids radiation and bowel distention can be monitored dynamically to achieve the best imaging.

Various endoscopic techniques are employed for evaluating small bowel tumors. Traditional endoscopy is the gold standard for evaluating the gastrointestinal tract because of its imaging, diagnostic, and potential therapeutic capabilities. Lesions in the small bowel proximal to the ligament of Treitz are usually viewed and biopsied by conventional endoscopy. Push endoscopy is another endoscopic technique for evaluating the duodenum and 50–70 cm past the ligament of Treitz. More distal lesions are now visualized with the evolution of capsule endoscopy (CE) and double-balloon enteroscopy (DBE). With CE, the patient swallows the capsule and a signal is sent to a recording device that the patient wears on their belt. DBE, also known as push-and-pull enteroscopy, enables visualization of the entire small bowel.

Capsule endoscopy and DBE have opened new avenues for imaging small intestine cancers and as an alternative diagnostic option. The CE is a highly effective way to image the entire length of the small bowel but is limited to mucosal lesions and does not have biopsy capability. Double-balloon endoscopy is suggested if a suspicious lesion is identified on CE to obtain tissue diagnosis. The disadvantage of DBE is that it requires specialized instruments and a gastroenterologist who is trained in performing the procedure. Kopacova et al. reviewed a series of DBE of 303 procedures in 179 patients in which 74 small bowel tumors were discovered. In this series CE preceded DBE in 21 patients. They were able to detect a suspicious lesion in 20 cases (one tumor missed by CE) [7].

Intestinal Neuroendocrine Tumors (Carcinoid Tumor)

The incidence of intestinal neuroendocrine tumors (iNETs), also known as carcinoid tumors, has increased significantly over the past three decades. This section will focus on the small intestine manifestations of neuroendocrine tumors. Discussions of lung, appendiceal, pancreatic, rectal, and stomach tumors are located in other chapters of the book (Chap. 24, Pancreatic Neuroendocrine Tumors (PNETs); Chap. 26, Carcinoid Tumors). The reason for the increase in diagnosis is poorly understood but may be related to incidental findings secondary to better imaging. Neuroendocrine tumors arise from the enterochromaffin cells in the crypts of Lieberkuhn and produce vasoactive peptides, mainly serotonin. These tumors cause a significant desmoplastic reaction, causing obstructive symptoms or bowel ischemia if the mesenteric vessels are involved (Fig. 10.1; Table 10.1). Surgical resection

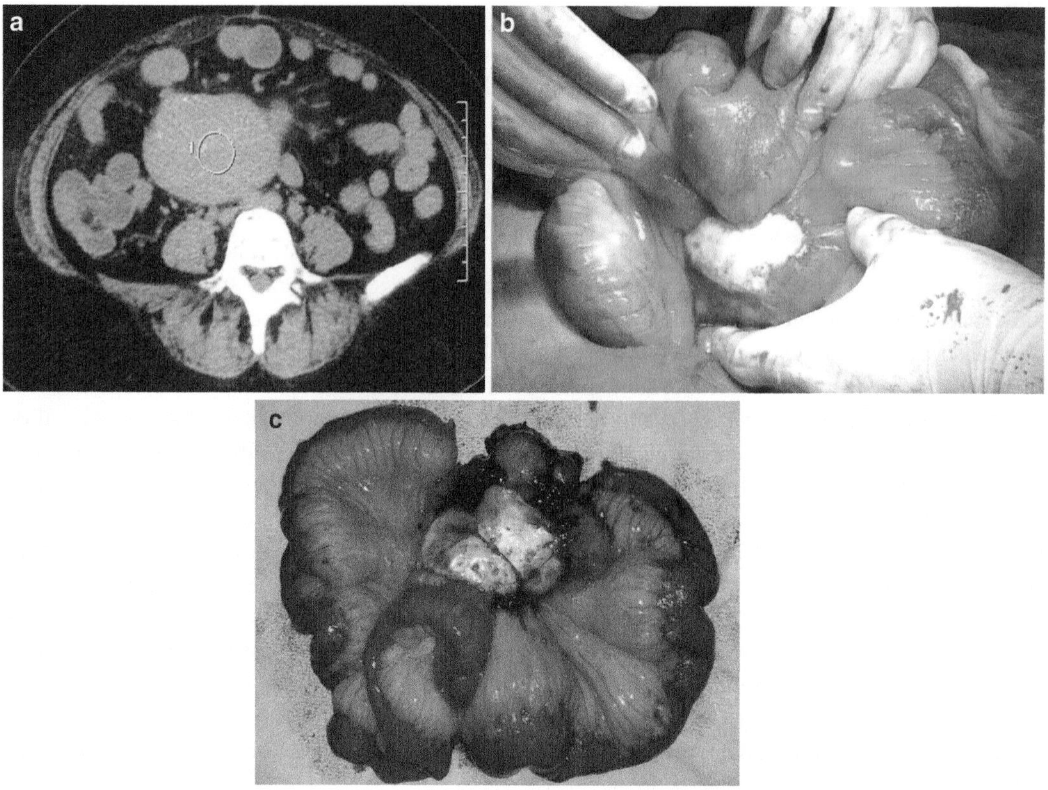

Fig. 10.1 *Small bowel carcinoid*: noncontrast CT shows a large intra-abdominal mesenteric-based mass (**a**). Intraoperative the lesion had significant desmoplastic involvement of the small bowel mesentery (**b**, **c**). (Courtesy of Gazi B. Zibari, MD, FACS)

and lymphadenectomy is the mainstay of curative treatment. Somatostatin and somatostatin analogs are key in the treatment of symptomatic or metastatic disease, but other chemotherapy agents have evolved. Overall prognosis of regional intestinal neuroendocrine tumors is 60–75 % over 5 years [1].

Neuroendocrine tumors often have an indolent growth pattern compared to similar carcinomas, and early detection can lead to curative treatment. Most small intestine tumors are located within 60 cm of the ileocecal valve but may be present anywhere in the gastrointestinal tract. Conventional CT scans with oral and IV contrast are usually sufficient to detect a primary lesion. However, carcinoids are characterized by a high potential to metastasize to other areas of the intestine or the small bowel mesentery. Synchronous tumor may be found in up to 40 % of patients at the time of laparotomy for the primary lesion. Midgut neuroendocrine tumors retain their expression of somatostatin receptors which bind octreotide. Somatostatin receptor scintigraphy with indium-111 pentetreotide has an 86–95 % sensitivity for detecting extrahepatic foci or distant metastases [8, 9]. Scintigraphy is indicated in patients for staging purposes and determination of receptor status. Somatostatin receptor (sst) expression, particularly sst2 receptor, has been correlated with better response to analog therapy and confers a better prognosis[8, 9]. Small bowel imaging with endoscopy and chest CT scan may be helpful preoperatively to further plan surgical resection and metastasis.

Patients with liver or lung metastasis are prone to the development of the carcinoid syndrome, a constellation of symptoms which includes flushing, diarrhea, and valvular heart disease. The carcinoid syndrome is caused by secretion of serotonin and other vasoactive substances into the systemic circulation. Serum chromogranin A is produced by all neuroendocrine tumors and has 86 % specificity and 68 % sensitivity. Twenty-four-hour urine collection for 5-hydroxyindolacetic acid (5-HIAA), a common metabolite of serotonin, can be used in the diagnosis and postoperative follow-up. Patients with carcinoid syndrome should have a 2D echocardiogram prior to any surgical procedure to evaluate cardiac function and valvular fibrosis [10].

Surgery is the cornerstone in the treatment of neuroendocrine tumors, but the location of the tumor is critical in surgical planning. Jejunal and ileal regional disease is commonly treated with bowel resection and lymphadenectomy. The goal of the lymph node resection is to have>12 nodes present for evaluation. Cholecystectomy is indicated during the initial surgical resection due to possible future long-term somatostatin analogue therapy and an increased risk of biliary symptoms. Duodenal tumors<10 mm and limited to the submucosal layer may undergo endoscopic submucosal dissection with low risk of perforation or bleeding [11]. Larger tumors (>10 mm) of the duodenum or involvement of the ampulla may require pancreaticoduodenectomy to obtain surgical margins (Fig. 10.2). These patients should be followed every 3–12 months with repeat 24 h urine 5-HIAA and chromogranin A tests with serial abdominal and pelvic CT scan [10].

More aggressive surgical approaches in patients with metastatic disease have emerged over the past decade. In concordance with the most recent NCCN guidelines, cytoreductive surgery may be indicated in patients with local symptoms; localized tumor metastasis or>90 % of tumor burden can be resected or ablated [12]. The United Kingdom and Ireland Neuroendocrine Tumor Society (UKI NETS) study conducted evaluated 360 patients with midgut neuroendocrine tumors with hepatic metastasis and found resection of primary lesion and metastasis had a median survival of 11.26 years compared to 5.50 years in patients without surgical intervention [13]. Hepatic radiofrequency ablation or arterial embolization can be considered for multifocal disease that is not amenable to surgical resection. Complete or partial response for symptomatic improvement, tumor markers, and imaging occurred in 70–100 %, 50–90 %, and 30–50 % of patients, respectively [14].

Medical treatment options for metastatic unresectable iNETs have expanded in recent years but are not considered curative. The goal of medical therapy is antisecretory effects and antiproliferation of the existing tumor. Of particular importance has been the development of somatostatin-analogue therapies. Somatostatin analogues were originally introduced for palliation of the carcinoid syndrome; however, recent clinical trials have demonstrated that they can exert an inhibitory effect on tumor growth. Common systemic chemotherapy regimens have been modeled after the PROMID (**P**lacebo Controlled, Double-blinded, Prospective, **R**andomized Study of the Effect of **O**ctreotide LAR in the Control of Tumor Growth in Patients with Metastatic Neuroendocrine **MID**gut tumors) study with octreotide long-acting release (LAR) and the **C**ontrolled Study of **L**anreotide **A**ntiproliferative **R**esponse in **NET** (CLARINET) trial. Current recommendations suggest first-line agents of somatostatin analogues (SSA) of octreotide or lanreotide every 4 weeks for patients with low volume stable disease. If symptoms occur or worsen, the dose of SSA can be increased and alpha interferon or an mTOR inhibitor, everolimus, may be added. Nonresponders to these agents may proceed to systemic chemotherapy with 5-flurouracil, capecitabine, and oxaliplatin. Third-line therapy includes the antiangiogenic targeting agents sunitinib or bevacizumab, which have shown evidence of improving progression-free survival [12].

Overall survival (OS) and progression-free survival (PFS) have improved in the past three decades with better surgical technique, understanding of tumor biology, and development of SSAs. The overall 5-year survival of an iNET is 60–75 %. Progression-free survival at 5 and 10 years for AJCC/UICC has been shown as 100 % stage I (5 years), 100 % stage II (5 years), 86 and 63 % stage III, and 64 % and 19 % for stage IV disease [15]. Unfavorable prognostic factors

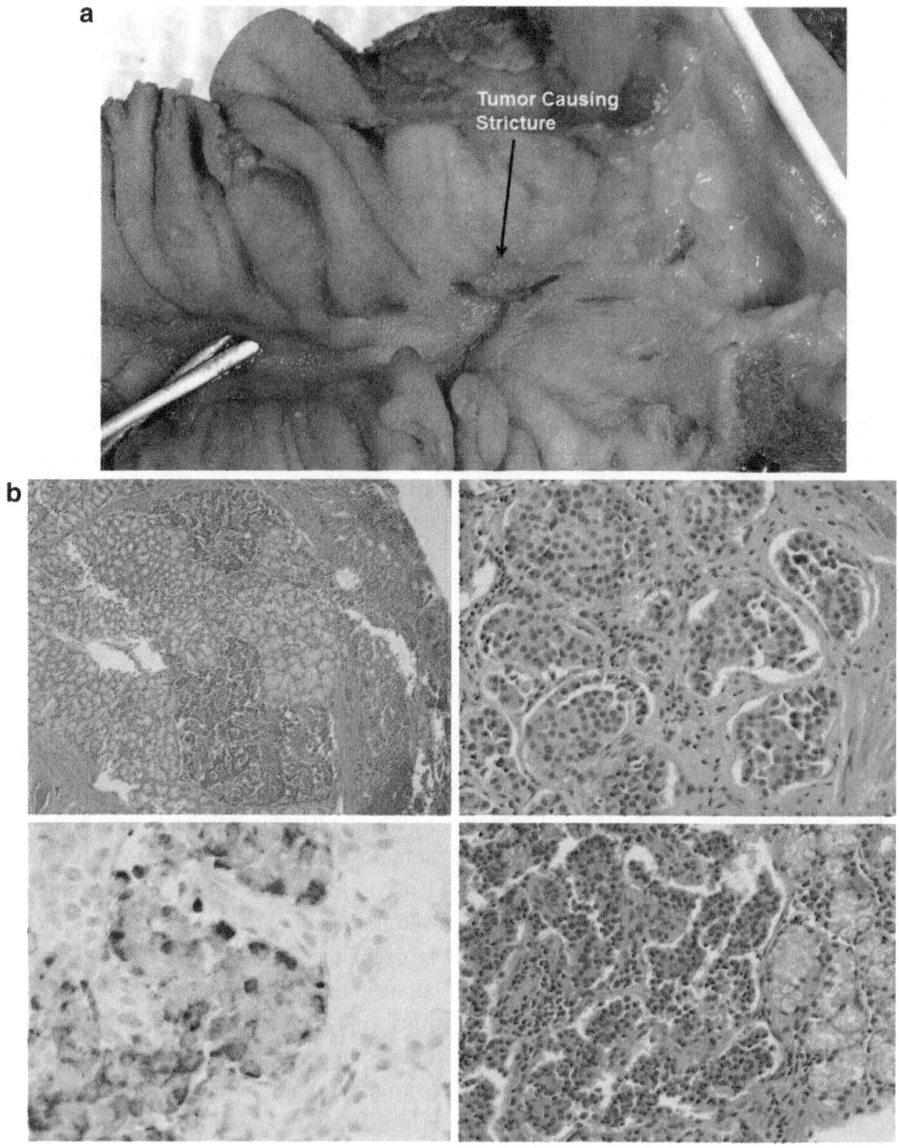

Fig. 10.2 *Neuroendocrine tumor of the small bowel*: a 61-year-old man presented with nausea and vomiting; an upper endoscopy demonstrated a tight stricture at the second portion of the duodenum. The CT scan of the abdomen demonstrated no mass or abnormality in the head of the pancreas or biliary system. He underwent a pancreaticoduodenectomy and tight stricture that was caused by a neuroendocrine tumor of the duodenum was found (**a**). H&E stain demonstrates "small blue cell tumors" that have scant, pink granular neoplasm, and round to oval stippled nucleus (**b**). The tumor stained positively for gastrin. CD31 immunostain highlights scattered vessels. Ki68 proliferation index was <2 % and was low grade, and the final stage was pT1pN1. (Courtesy of Quyen D. Chu, MD, MBA, FACS)

impacting survival include high mitotic rate, high Ki67, distant metastasis, and advanced age. Octreotide scintigraphy avidity suggests that even with hepatic metastasis, avid uptake of the nuclear marker has a better prognosis than those that had low or no uptake.

Adenocarcinoma

Small bowel adenocarcinoma (SBA) is the second most common type of cancer in the small intestine. This cancer has a tendency to present late in the course with 50 % of patients having advanced disease at the time of presentation. The adenocarcinoma sequence similar to colon cancer is thought to play a role but has not been fully elucidated yet. Patients may be at an increased risk due to a higher consumption of animal fat and protein in the Western diet or diagnosed with HNPCC, FAP, or Crohn's disease. The duodenum is the most common site of involvement (55 %) followed by jejunum (18 %) and ileum (13 %) (Table 10.1). Ileal adenocarcinoma is increased in Crohn's patients. Patients with periampullary tumors present with nausea, vomiting, and obstructive jaundice. Ampullary tumors are biologically and morphologically distinct and have a more favorable prognosis compared to pancreatic and bile duct cancers. Tumors in the jejunum and ileum commonly present with obstruction, weight loss, and frequently have lymph node involvement.

Surgery is the mainstay for curative treatment of patients with SBA (Fig. 10.3); unfortunately, many patients (32 %) have evidence of metastasis at the time of resection. Typically, adenocarcinomas are staged according to the AJCC TMN staging system in Table 10.2 based on tumor invasion, node status, and metastasis. Lymph node status and distant metastasis implicates a poorer prognosis and is associated with a decreased 5-year relative survival rate with localized disease 80.5 %, regional with lymph node involvement 68.5 %, and distant metastasis 41.5 %. The number of lymph nodes required for R0 resection was

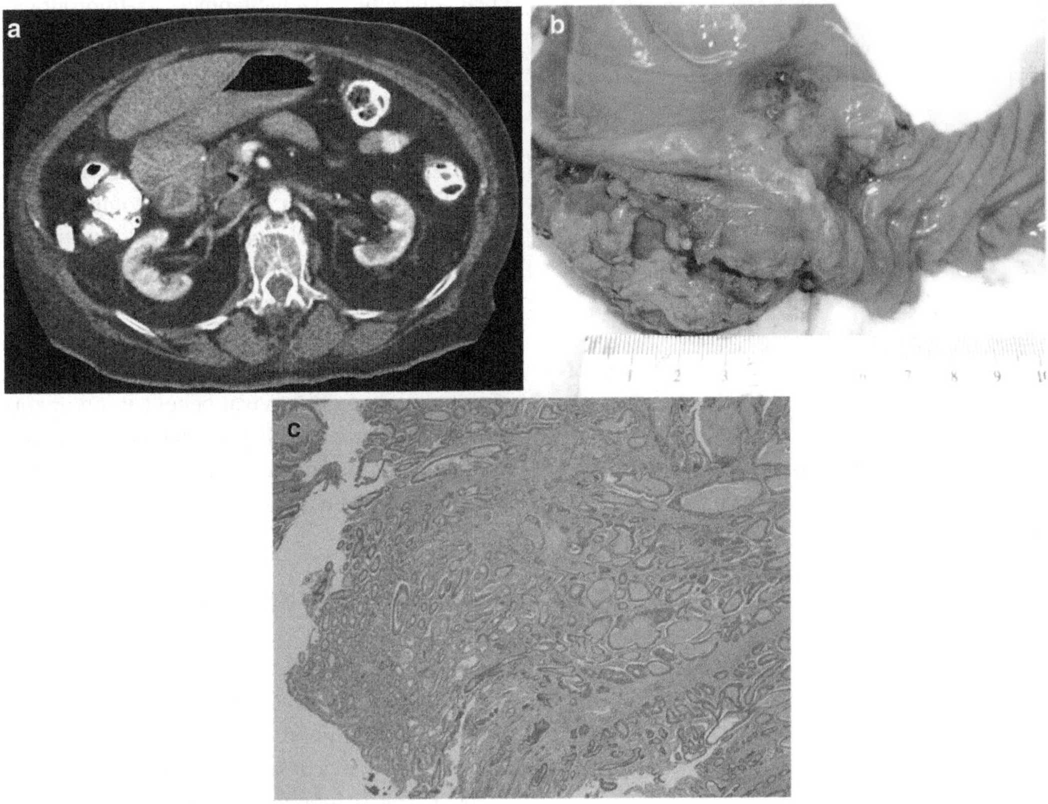

Fig. 10.3 Small bowel adenocarcinoma. A 65-year-old woman presented with a duodenal obstructing mass. On CT there is evidence of a tumor partially occluding the duodenal lumen (**a**). On gross pathologic inspection following a pancreaticoduodenectomy, the mass is felt to arise from either the duodenal or the ampulla (**b**). Final pathology revealed both duodenal and ampullary dysplasia with associated invasive adenocarcinoma. Although pathology favored ampullary adenocarcinoma, they could not definitely rule out a duodenal source. The photomicrograph of a separate patient demonstrates small bowel adenocarcinoma arising from a background of dysplasia (**c**) (Courtesy of John F. Gibbs and Joyce Paterson)

Table 10.2 American Joint Committee on Cancer (AJCC) TNM staging for small intestine cancer (7th edition)

Primary tumor (T)	
TX	Primary tumor cannot be assessed
T0	No evidence of primary tumor
Tis	Carcinoma in situ
T1a	Tumor invades lamina propria
T1b	Tumor invades submucosa*
T2	Tumor invades muscularis propria
T3	Tumor invades through muscularis propria into the subserosa or into the nonperitonealized perimuscular tissue (mesentery or retroperitoneum) with extension 2 cm or less*
T4	Tumor perforates the visceral peritoneum or directly invades other organs or structures (include other loops of small intestine, mesentery, or retroperitoneum >2 cm, and abdominal wall by way of serosa; for duodenum only, invasion of pancreas or bile duct)

*The nonperitonealized perimuscular tissue is, for jejunum and ileum, part of the mesentery and, for duodenum in areas where serosa is lacking, part of the interface with the pancreas

Regional lymph nodes (N)	
NX	Regional lymph nodes cannot be assessed
N0	No regional lymph node metastasis
N1	Metastases in 1–3 regional lymph nodes
N2	Metastases in ≥4 regional lymph nodes

Distant metastasis (M)	
M0	No distant metastasis
M1	Distant metastasis

Anatomic stage/prognostic groups			
Group	T	N	M
Stage 0	Tis	N0	M0
Stage I	T1-T2	N0	M0
Stage IIA	T3	N0	M0
Stage IIB	T4	N0	M0
Stage IIIA	Any T	N1	M0
Stage IIIB	Any T	N2	M0
Stage IV	Any T	Any N	M1

Adapted from Compton et al. [34]. With permission from Springer Verlag

reviewed by Gibbs in 2004; the current consensus of obtaining ≥10 lymph nodes is adequate without adding increase morbidity [16]. Factors that may predict a worse outcome are male sex, patients older than 55, tumor size, and poorly differentiated tumor or with positive margins. In our review of 13 published papers from 2000 to 2011 patients with SBA, the efficacy of adjuvant treatment after curative intent surgery did not improve overall survival. Table 10.3 displays the characteristics of the populations studied listed by the author and year [17–28]. In these papers curative surgery was either bowel resection including lymphadenectomy or pancreaticoduodenectomy (Whipple procedure) with negative margins. Distant metastasis after surgical resection is the most common pattern of relapse and adequate adjuvant therapy is needed. Table 10.4 shows 5-year OS and median survival time for patients with SBA.

Review of adjuvant chemotherapy regimens for SBA is largely unimpressive with results from single institutions studies showing no survival benefit. Gemcitabine, 5-fluorouracil (5-FU), and platinum-based chemotherapy were the most commonly used treatments for SBA. Zaanan et al. reviewed a population of 93 patients and found FOLFOX (5-FU, leucovorin LV, oxaliplatin) regimen to be superior to LV/5-FU [29]. Newer agents and combinations are being evaluated for improved treatment. Oxaliplatin and capecitabine and the cell surface endothelial growth receptor (EGFR) antibody drugs cetuximab and panitumumab have been effective in metastatic disease. One study reported an overall survival benefit in preoperative chemotherapy with postoperative radiation in duodenal adenocarcinoma, but this is not applicable to the entire bowel.

Gastrointestinal Stromal Tumors (GISTs)

Small bowel gastrointestinal stromal tumors (GISTs) are diagnosed in 7–9 % of patients, even though the stomach is the most common site affected. This section focuses on the small intestinal manifestations of GIST with a more detailed discussion that can be found in Chap. 28, Gastrointestinal Stromal Tumors (GISTs). These tumors arise from the interstitial cells of Cajal and are likely to be found in the jejunum (Table 10.1). Clinical presentation varies, depending on the

Table 10.3 Characteristics of studies reviewed for small bowel adenocarcinoma

Author, year	N	Mean age range	Male %	Stage breakdown I	II	III	IV	Grade definition
Ojha, A. 2000	33	57.5	64	I–III 24		IV 9		n/a
North, J. 2000	68	15–89	70	n/a				n/a
Fishman, P. 2006	113	58.2	59		30	41	32	Poor vs. well
Agarwal, S. 2007	64	17–87	57	1	14	21		n/a
Kelsey, C. 2007	32	32–77	72	3	18	2	1	Poor vs. mod and well
Chaiyasate, K. 2008	27	50–70	33		7	14	6	Poor vs. mod vs. well
Hong, S. 2009	53	26–84	55	4	12	15	22	n/a
Halfdanarson, T. 2010	491	24–97	62	40	143	138	171	Grade 1–2 vs. 3–4
Moon, Y. 2010	100	23–84	67	4	22	28	46	Poor and undiff vs. well
Han, S 2010	61	23–79	n/a	n/a				n/a
Overman, M. 2010	54	31–79	62	8	20	26		Poor vs. mod and well
Chung, W. 2011	30	30–90	n/a	3	5	9	14	Poor vs. non poor diff
Koo, D. 2011	52	26–79	59	8	20	24		Poor vs. mod vs. well diff

Table 10.4 Survival

	5-year % survival by stage				Median OS for stage (months)			
	I	II	III	IV	I	II	III	IV
Ojha, A. 2000	n/a				All stages: 9			
North, J. 2000	90	78	55	35	n/a			
Fishman, P. 2006	n/a				All stages: 17			
Agarwal, S. 2007	All stages: 21				–	–	–	5
Kelsey, C. 2007	All stages: 48				n/a			
Chaiyasate, K. 2008	All stages: 30				–	78	36	10
Hong, S. 2009	n/a				–	–	–	4
Halfdanarson, T. 2010	78	44	25	2	137	46	25	11
Moon, Y. 2010	39		10	3	–	–	11	7
Han, S 2010	All stages: 16				n/a			
Overman, M. 2010	100	87	59	–	n/a			
Chung, W. 2011	n/a				n/a			
Koo, D. 2011	100	81	28	–	n/a			
Overall					12.23 (13.9–20.5)			

anatomical location of the tumor, but in general, signs and symptoms are nonspecific which can include abdominal pain, a palpable mass, or gastrointestinal bleeding (Fig. 10.4). Preoperative evaluation of GIST should include CT scan with contrast of the abdomen and pelvis. Biopsy of the lesion is critical in planning surgical resection versus preoperative chemotherapy. The GIST is a submucosal lesion, and some series have shown a low yield to biopsy, but multiple biopsies should be taken to "unroof" the mucosa. Immunohistochemistry of GIST tumors expressing a tyrosine receptor kinase (c-Kit or CD117) mutation and platelet-derived growth factor receptor-alpha (PDGFRA) mutation is fundamental to the preoperative workup. Recent studies have shown the importance of genetic testing of the KIT mutation to determine expression of exon 9 or exon 11 within the tumor [30].

Surgery with complete resection is the standard of care in patients with a primary tumor, but recurrence to the liver and peritoneum is seen in

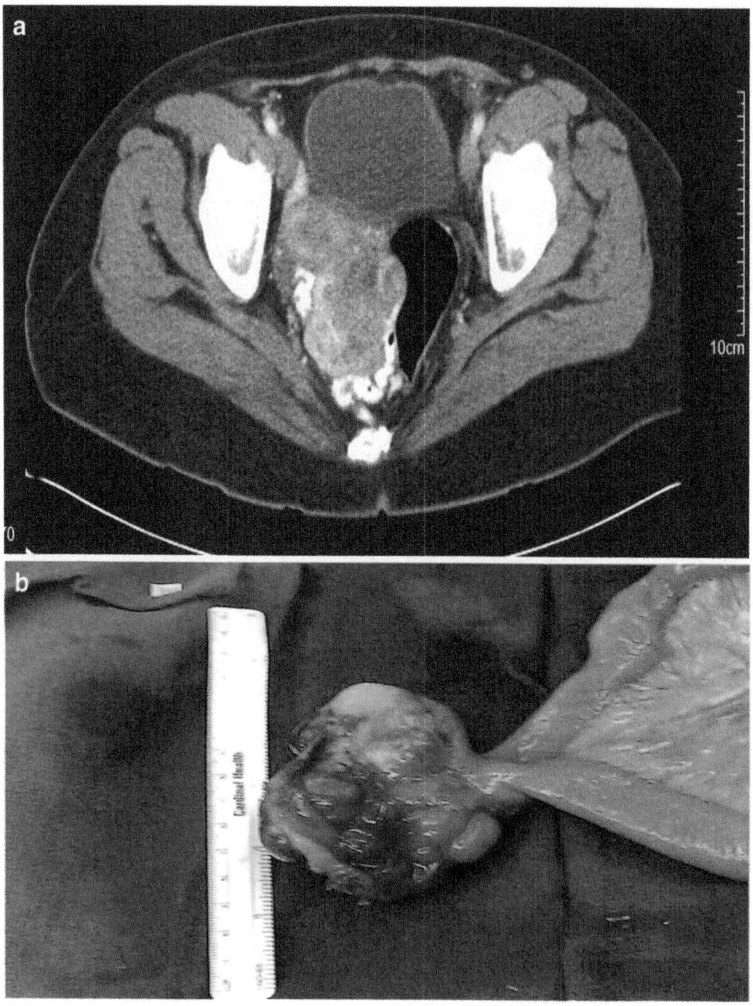

Fig. 10.4 Small bowel GIST presenting with deep pelvic pain with the CT revealing a solid lobulated echogenic mass is noted adjacent to the uterus measuring 2.7×6.0×6.1 cm (**a**). The lesion was segmentally resected (**b**) (Courtesy of John F. Gibbs)

as many of 50 % of patients [30]. The surgical goals should strive to achieve 1–2 cm negative margins without violating the pseudocapsule. There is no need to perform a lymphadenectomy since the risk of lymphatic spread is low. Patients who are on imatinib therapy can stop taking the medication just prior to surgery and can resume taking it when tolerating oral medications. However, sunitinib should be withheld for 1 week prior to a planned surgical resection. Many studies have reported the safety of laparoscopic resection with a low risk of tumor spillage, but the choice of the procedure should be decided based on a case-by-case basis and surgeon's level of comfort. Duodenal GIST poses a dilemma in planning a large surgical resection [31]. Table 10.5 shows our experience with segment duodenectomy versus pancreaticoduodenectomy. Segmental duodenectomy is a reasonable option with lower morbidity depending on the location and similar survivability compared to pancreaticoduodenectomy (Fig. 10.5; Table 10.5).

The 5-year OS is approximately 40 % for all stages with median time to resection of 2 years. Mitotic rate is the dominant pathological predictor of outcome in patients treated

Table 10.5 GIST of patients treated with local resection vs. Whipple procedure

Patient	Age	Presentation	Surgery	Tumor location	Tumor size (cm)	Mitosis/50hpf	Recurrence	Status	DFS (months)	OS (months)
1	68	GI bleeding	Local excision	D2	4.5	25	Liver	Dead	40	52
2	49	GI bleeding	Whipple	D2/D3/D4	8.5	5	Liver	Dead	25	35
3	72	Mass	Whipple	D2	10	16	Liver	Alive	23	52
4	79	Mass	Local excision	D3/D4	8	5	None	Alive	50	50
5	57	GI bleeding	Whipple	D2	4.5	1	None	Alive	46	46
6	77	Obstruction	Whipple	D2	19	205	Liver, peritoneum	Dead	5	6
7	56	GI bleeding	Local excision	D3	3.2	5	None	Alive	30	30
8	63	GI bleeding	Whipple	D3/D4	3	1	None	Alive	13	13
9	67	GI bleeding	Whipple	D2/D3	2	1	None	Alive	10	10
10	61	Incidental	Local excision	D3	4.5	1	None	Alive	8	8
11	51	GI bleeding	Local excision	D2	2	1	None	Alive	1	1

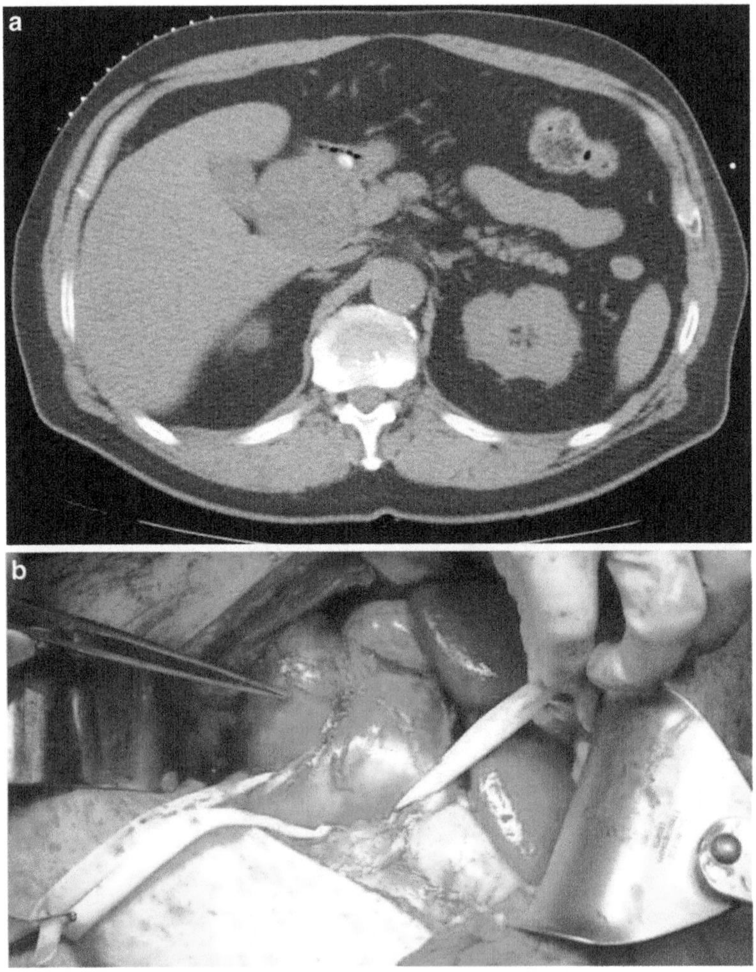

Fig. 10.5 Gastrointestinal stromal tumor (GIST) involving the first and proximal second portion of the duodenal on CT (**a**) and managed by segmental duodenectomy (**b**) (Courtesy of John F. Gibbs)

with surgery alone [32]. Patients should be followed up postoperatively every 3–6 months with CT scan of the abdomen and pelvis for the first 5 years then annually. Imatinib therapy should be continued at the discretion of the surgeon, and resection is feasible for limited recurrence with or without therapy.

Lymphoma

Primary intestinal lymphomas comprise 30–40 % of the extranodal form of lymphoma comprising 15–17 % of primary intestinal malignancy [33]. The most common site for lymphoma is the stomach followed by ileum, cecum, and then colon. These malignancies arise from the submucosal lymphoid aggregates of the ileum and can cause obstruction or become a lead point for intussusception. Mucosa-associated lymphoid tissue (MALT) lymphoma and diffuse large B-cell lymphoma are the most common types of gastrointestinal malignancies. Small intestine non-Hodgkin's lymphomas are diagnosed by evidence of small intestine lesions without peripheral or mediastinal lymphadenopathy, normal white count, and without evidence of liver or splenic involvement. Enteropathy-associated

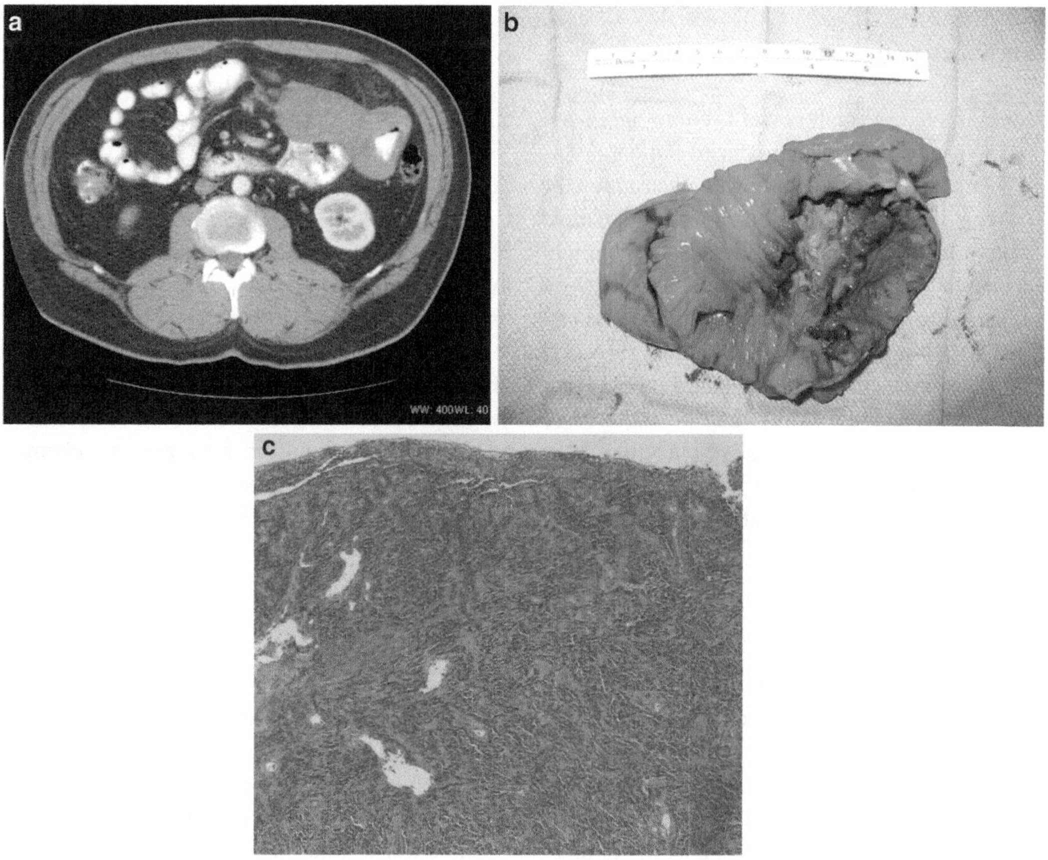

Fig. 10.6 *Lymphoma of the small bowel*: a 58-year-old male presents with weight loss and abdominal complaints, and a CT scan demonstrated a mass arising from the jejunum (**a**). He underwent an exploratory laparotomy and was found to have a mass in the proximal jejunum for which a segmental resection was performed (**b**). Pathologic diagnosis of a diffuse large B-cell non-Hodgkin's lymphoma was made (**c**). Low-power view reveals small intestinal mucosa with necrosis of superficial epithelium. The mucosa and submucosa are diffusely infiltrated with malignant small blue cells (Courtesy of Quyen D. Chu, MD, MBA, FACS)

T cell lymphoma (EATL) commonly arises in the jejunum and ileum commonly and is seen in patients with celiac sprue [33]. Patients with AIDS may develop a diffuse B-cell lymphoma, and young patients are at risk for Burkitt's lymphoma due to Epstein-Barr virus [33].

Patients with lymphoma of the small intestine are especially difficult to diagnose because of the periluminal disease and mesentery involvement. Tissue biopsy of the submucosa is important to establish diagnosis due to lack of mucosal involvement. Surgery may be required for biopsy confirmation, localized disease, hemorrhage, perforation, obstruction, or refractory to chemotherapy (Fig. 10.6). Treatment is mainly chemotherapy based with variable responses depending on the type of the lymphoma. Concern for perforation during chemotherapy as the tumor lysis response occurs. Our institutional experience has shown that patients may need multiple operations during their chemotherapy. Radiation therapy is mainly used for local control of symptoms. In case of a surgical emergency, these patients will require a multidisciplinary team. Patients that typically have a poor prognosis are men, age older than 75, black, and Hispanic. Survival is specific for the types of lymphoma: EATL and anaplastic with 8–20 % 5-year survival and MALT lymphoma with 75–80 % eradication [33].

Metastatic Disease

Metastasis to the small bowel is commonly from melanoma, breast, or lung cancer. Patients typically present with small bowel obstruction or bleeding (Table 10.1). Melanoma is the most common type of cancer to involve the jejunum and ileum (Fig. 10.7). Approximately 50 % of melanoma will have synchronous distant metastasis at the time of diagnosis. Surgical resection of metastatic lesions is the standard therapy, but gastrostomy and/or ostomy may be required to relieve obstruction for palliative purpose. There is no survival benefit with systemic chemotherapy for patients with metastatic melanoma.

Conclusion

Small bowel malignancy has a relatively low but increasing incidence when compared with other forms of cancer. Each malignancy has a different prognosis, pattern of growth, and multiple treatment options depending on the pathology. Metastatic disease is common at the time of diagnosis due to the vague abdominal symptoms or occult gastrointestinal bleeding. The surgeon should attempt to determine the tumor histology, if possible, prior to planning an operation. Emergent operation should be reserved for evidence of perforation, unrelieved obstruction, or hemorrhage. Newer endoscopy and enteroscopy techniques are better at visualizing and retrieving biopsy samples in the distal small intestine. The combination of capsule endoscopy and double-balloon endoscopy has excellent results in discovering small distal small bowel lesions.

The majority of small bowel malignancies are intestinal neuroendocrine tumors (carcinoid), adenocarcinoma, gastrointestinal stromal tumors, lymphoma, and metastatic melanoma. The incidence of carcinoid tumor has surpassed adenocarcinoma in the past few years, but the reason for this is unclear. The overall survival of patients diagnosed with small bowel malignancy ranges from 40 to 60 %. Surgery remains the mainstay of curative therapy. Newer chemotherapy regimens have improved survival of iNETs, lymphomas, and GISTs, but there is not an effective regimen for adenocarcinoma. Patients should be discussed in a multidisciplinary setting once diagnosed with small bowel malignancy for possible preoperative and/or postoperative chemotherapy. Patients will need frequent follow-up to detect tumor recurrence or metastasis.

Salient Points

- Vague abdominal pain, obstruction, and gastrointestinal bleeding are the most common signs of small bowel malignancy.
- Small bowel malignancy incidence is on the rise with intestinal neuroendocrine tumors most frequently diagnosed.
- Low rate of cancer in small intestine due to rapid transit time, secretion of IgA, high alkaline nature of the succus, and high turnover of intestinal lining.
- Age>60, celiac disease, Crohn's disease, and cigarette smoking are common risk factors for small bowel malignancies.
- Metastasis is common in 30 % of all small intestinal malignancy due to the vague symptom and delay in diagnosis.
- Carcinoid tumors can metastasize to the liver and cause carcinoid syndrome with flushing, diarrhea, and wheezing.
- 24 h urine testing for 5-HIAA, chromogranin A, and octreotide scanning are important for preoperative workup of carcinoid tumors.

Fig. 10.7 (continued) small bowel, consistent with a small bowel obstruction (**a**). He underwent a segmental resection of the small bowel (**b**). Low power shows normal small intestinal mucosa (*left*) and a protruding tumor nodule (*right*) that has destroyed the mucosa and submucosa (**c**). High power reveals diffuse infiltrating growth of malignant melanocytes. These cells are discohesive with rich eosinophilic cytoplasm, large nuclei, and prominent nucleoli. There is prominent nuclear pleomorphism, and many cells also contain dark-brown granular melanin pigments (**d**). The final pathology was a metastatic melanoma (**c** and **d**) (**a**-**b**: Courtesy of Quyen D. Chu, MD, MBA, FACS) (**c**-**d**: Courtesy of Xin Gu, MD)

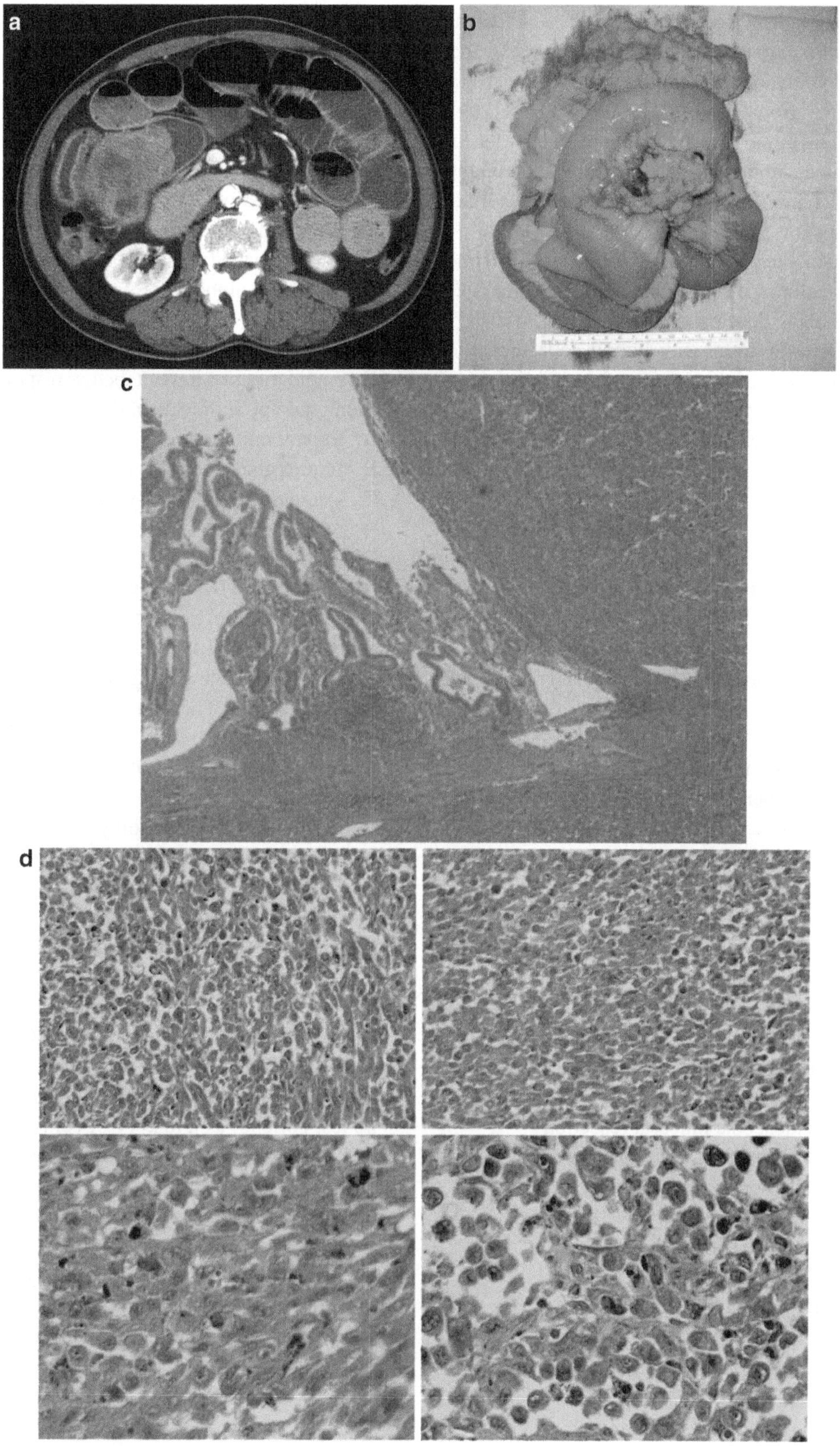

Fig. 10.7 *Malignant melanoma*: a 68-year-old gentleman with a known history of malignant melanoma presented with a small bowel obstruction. CT scan demonstrated a right lower quadrant mass and dilated

- Long-acting somatostatin and somatostatin analogs are first-line therapy in metastatic carcinoid to control symptoms and reduce overall tumor growth.
- Small bowel adenocarcinoma mainly occurs in the duodenum and jejunum and requires full lymph node dissection at the of surgical resection.
- Chemotherapy for SBA follows the regimen for colorectal cancer, but new chemotherapies are being developed.
- GISTs do not require lymph node dissection but may need preoperative imatinib for tumor reduction prior to resection.
- GIST newer genetic testing for exon 9 and exon 11 has shown tumors more responsive to imatinib.
- Lymphoma of the small intestine should undergo chemotherapy first unless surgery is needed for biopsy or rare localized disease.
- Metastatic disease is common for melanoma and breast cancer, and palliative operations should be done for obstruction and perforation.

Questions

1. A 65-year-old man presents with GI bleeding to the emergency department (Hgb 6.8 mg/dL) and is slightly tachycardic. After initial resuscitation and blood transfusion, the vital signs improve and repeat hemoglobin is 8.6 mg/dL. Endoscopy revealed a 0.9 cm submucosal lesion noted in the third portion of the duodenum. Biopsy reveals carcinoid tumor and staging CT scan is negative for liver metastasis. The surgical plan should include?
   A. Pancreaticoduodenectomy
   B. Endoscopic mucosal resection
   C. Duodenectomy with primary anastomosis
   D. LAR somatostatin therapy
2. The factors that decrease the risk of malignancy in the small bowel include:
   A. Slow transit time
   B. Decreased IgA secretion
   C. High pH (alkaline) of contents
   D. Low amount of lymphoid tissue
3. Small bowel malignancy is on the rise and the most frequently diagnosed cancer is:
   A. Adenocarcinoma
   B. Lymphoma
   C. GIST
   D. Intestinal neuroendocrine tumors
4. First-line chemotherapy in metastatic intestinal neuroendocrine tumors is:
   A. LAR somatostatin
   B. Interferon alpha
   C. Imatinib
   D. Sunitinib
5. Carcinoid tumors have a better response to chemotherapy if they display:
   A. Exon 9 mutation
   B. Expression of the sst2 receptor
   C. Decreased uptake of indium-111 pentetreotide scan
   D. Have a high Ki67
6. An 86-year-old woman with a 3 cm GIST tumor of the third portion of the duodenum, and CT scan shows small lesion of the liver. The patient is having mild midepigastric pain and early satiety. The next step in the patient's care would be:
   A. Surgical resection of the lesion with lymphadenectomy
   B. Pancreaticoduodenectomy with postoperative imatinib for liver metastasis
   C. Preoperative imatinib and follow-up for response for surgical planning
   D. Imatinib therapy alone and surgery for palliation as needed
7. A 54-year-old woman presents with chronic abdominal pain and weight loss. CT scan shows thickening of the ileum and mesentery with enlargement of para-aortic lymph nodes. Patient has a history of celiac disease and has been on a gluten-free diet for 10 years. Biopsy of the nodes reveals small bowel lymphoma. The next surgical plan should be:
   A. Ileocolonic resection with primary anastomosis with postoperative chemotherapy
   B. Ileal resection for disease with full lymph node dissection

C. Radiation therapy preoperative
D. Multidisciplinary evaluation with preoperative chemotherapy and surgical consult for complications

8. A 48-year-old woman recently relocated from Florida presents with cramping abdominal pain, nausea, and vomiting. CT scan shows multiple areas of lesions involving the mesentery of the small bowel concerning for metastatic disease. The most common metastasis to small bowel is:
A. Breast
B. Melanoma
C. Lung
D. Colorectal

Answer

1. B
2. C
3. D
4. A
5. B
6. C
7. D
8. B

References

1. American Cancer Society Facts and Figures 2013. Atlanta. http://www.cancer.org/acs/groups/content/@epidemiologysurveilance/documents/document/acspc-036845.pdf. Accessed on 13 May 2014.
2. Bilimoria KY, Bentrem DJ, Wayne JD, Ko CY, Bennett CL, Talamonti MS. Small bowel cancer in the United States. Ann Surg 2009;249(1): 63–71.
3. Speranza G, Doroshow JH, Kummar S. Adenocarcinoma of the small bowel: changes in the landscape? Curr Opin Oncol. 2010;22:387–93.
4. Cheung DY, Choi MG. Current advances in small bowel tumors. Clin Endosc. 2011;44:13–21.
5. Anzidei M, Napoli A, Zini C, Kirchin MA, Catalano C, Passariello R. Malignant tumours of the small intestine: a review of histopathology, multidetector CT and MRI aspects. Br J Radiol. 2011;84:677–90.
6. Agrawal S, McCarron EC, Gibbs JF, Nava HR, Wilding GE, Rajput A. Surgical management and outcome in primary adenocarcinoma of the small bowel. Ann Surg Oncol. 2007;14(8):2263–9.
7. Kopacova M, Rejchrt S, Bures J, Tacheci I. Small Intestinal Tumours. Gastroenterol Res Pract; 2013; 2013: 702536. doi: 10.1155/2013/702536
8. Asnacios A, Courbon F, Rochaix P, Bauvin E, Cances-Lauwers V, Susini C, Schulz S, Boneu A, Guimbaud R, Buscail L. Indium-111-pentetreotide scintigraphy and somatostatin receptor subtype 2 expression: new prognostic factors for malignant well differentiated endocrine tumors. J Clin Oncol. 2008;26(6):963–70.
9. Balon HR, Brown TLY, Goldsmith SJ, Silberstein EB, Krenning EP, Lang O, Dillehay GD, Tarrance J, Johnson M, Stabin MG. The SNM practice guideline for somatostatin receptor scintigraphy with in-111-pentetreotide. Version 2.0. J Nucl Med Technol. 2011;39(4):317–24.
10. Neuroendocrine Tumors. NCCN guidelines Version 2.2014 http://www.nccn.org/professionals/physician_gls/pdf/neuroendocrine.pdf. Accessed on 13 May 2014.
11. Kobara H, Mori H, Kazi R, Fujihara S, Nishiyama N, Ayaki M, Yachida T, Tani J, Miyoshi H, Kamada H, Morishita A, Oryu M, Tsutsui K, Haba R, Masaki T. Indications for endoscopic submucosal dissection for symptomatic benign gastrointestinal subepithelial or carcinoid tumors originating in the submucosa. Mol Clin Oncol. 2013;1:1002–8.
12. Strosberg JR, Fisher GA, Benson AB, Malin JL, GEPNET consensus panel, Cherepanov D, Broder MS. Systemic treatment in unresectable metastatic well-differentiated carcinoid tumors. Pancreas. 2013;42(3):397–404.
13. Ahmed A, Turner G, King B, Jones L, Culliford D, McCance D, Ardill J, Johnston BT, Poston G, Rees M, Buxton-Thomas M, Caplin M, Ramage JK. Midgut neuroendocrine tumours with liver metastases: results of the UKINETS study. Endocr Relat Cancer. 2009; 16:885–94.
14. Oberg K, Knigge U, Kwekkeboom D, Perren A. Neuroendocrine gastro-entero-pancreatic tumors: ESMO clinical practice guidelines for diagnosis, treatment and follow up. Ann Oncol. 2012;23(7):124–30.
15. Araujo PB, Cheng S, Mete O, Serra S, Morin E, Asa S, Ezzat S. Evaluation of the WHO 2010 grading and AJCC/UICC staging systems in prognostic behavior of intestinal neuroendocrine tumors. PLoS One. 2013;8(4):e61538. doi:10.1371/journal.pone.0061538.
16. Gibbs J. Duodenal adenocarcinoma: is total lymph node sampling predictive of outcome? Ann Surg Oncol. 2004;11(4):354–5.
17. Moon YW, Rha SY, Shin SJ, Chang J, Shim HS, Roh JK. Adenocarcinoma of the small bowel at a single Korean institute: management and prognosticators. J Cancer Res Clin Oncol. 2010;136(3):387–94.
18. Halfdanarson TR, McWillliams RR, Donohue JH, Quevedo JF. A single-institution experience with 491 cases of small bowel adenocarcinoma. Am J Surg Oncol. 2007;14(8):797–803.
19. Ojha A. Primary small bowel malignancies: single center results of three decades. J Clin Gastroenterol. 2000;30(3):289–93.
20. Overman MJ, Kopetz S, Lin E, Abbruzzese JL, Wolff RA. Is there a role for adjuvant therapy in resected

adenocarcinoma of the small intestines. Acta Oncol. 2010;49(4):474–9.
21. Chung WC, Paik CN, Jung SH. Prognostic factors associated with survival in patients with primary duodenal adenocarcinoma. Korean J Intern Med. 2011; 26(1):34–40.
22. Chaiyasate K. Prognostic factors in primary adenocarcinoma of the small intestine: 13 year single institution experience. World J Surg Oncol. 2008;6(1):12.
23. Kelsey CR, Nelson JW, Willett CG. Duodenal adenocarcinoma: patterns of failure after resection and role of chemotherapy. Int J Radiat Oncol Biol Phys. 2007;69(5):1436–41.
24. Fishman PN, Pond GR, Moore MJ. Natural history of chemotherapy effectiveness for advanced adenocarcinoma of the small bowel; a retrospective review of 113 cases. Am J Clin Oncol. 2006;29(3):225–31.
25. Overman MJ, Varadhachary GR, Kopetz S. Phase II study of capecitabine and oxaliplatin for advanced adenocarcinoma of the small bowel and ampulla of Vater. J Clin Oncol. 2009;27(16):2598–603.
26. Koo DH, Yun SC, Hong YS, Ryu MH, Lee JL, Chang HM, Kang YK, Kim SC, Han DJ, Lee YJ, Kim TW. Adjuvant chemotherapy for small bowel adenocarcinoma after curative surgery. Oncology. 2011;80(3–4): 208–13.
27. North JH, Pack MS. Malignant tumors of the small intestine: a review of 144 cases. Am Surg. 2000;66(1):46–51.
28. Hong SH, Koh YH, Rho SY, Byun JH, Oh ST, Im KW, Kim EK, Chang SK. Primary adenocarcinoma of the small intestine: presentation, prognostic factors and clinical outcome. Jpn J Clin Oncol. 2009;39(1):54–61.
29. Zaanan A, Costes L, Gauthier M, Malka M, Locher C, Mitry E, Tougeron D, Lecomte T, Gornet JM, Sobhani I, Moulin V, Afchain P, Taieb J, Bonnetain F, Aparicio T. Chemotherapy of advanced small bowel adenocarcinoma: a multicenter AGEO study. Ann Oncol. 2010;21:1786–93.
30. DeMatteo RP, Ballman KV, Antonescu CR, Corless C, Kolesnikova V, Mehren M, McCarter MD, Norton J, Maki RG, Pisters PW, Demetri GD, Brennan MF, Owzar K. Long-term results of adjuvant imatinib mesylate in localized, high-risk, primary gastrointestinal stromal tumor. ACOSOG Z9000 (Alliance) intergroup phase 2 trial. Ann Surg. 2013;258(3): 46–52.
31. Alassas M, Ong ES, Kane JM, Gibbs J. Duodenal gastrointestinal stromal tumors: a diagnostic and surgical challenge. Ann Surg. 2008;15:SK2.
32. DeMatteo RP, Gold JS, Saran L, Gönen M, Liau KH, Maki RG, Singer S, Besmer P, Brennan MF, Antonescu CR. Tumor mitotic rate, size, and location independently predict recurrence after resection or primary gastrointestinal stromal tumor. Cancer. 2008;112:608–15.
33. Bautista-Quach MA, Ake CD, Chen M, Wang J. Gastrointestinal lymphomas: morphology, immunophenotype and molecular features. J Gastrointest Oncol. 2012;3(3):209–25.
34. Compton C, Byrd D, Garcia-Aguilar J, et al. Small Intestine. In: Compton C, Byrd D, Garcia-Aguilar J, Kurtzman S, Olawaiye A, Washington M, editors. AJCC cancer staging atlas. 2nd ed. New York: Springer; 2012. p. 155–67.

Gallbladder Cancer

11

Bas Groot Koerkamp and William R. Jarnagin

Learning Objectives
After reading this chapter, you should know how to manage patients with:

- A gallbladder polyp found on imaging
- Gallbladder cancer incidentally found at pathologic review after a cholecystectomy for cholelithiasis
- Gallbladder cancer suspected during cholecystectomy for cholelithiasis
- A gallbladder and/or liver mass found on imaging suspicious for gallbladder cancer

Background

Gallbladder cancer (GBC) is the most common biliary cancer: in the USA, each year about 6,000 patients are newly diagnosed with GBC [1]. Historically, surgery for GBC was rare because patients typically presented with advanced disease when symptoms develop. Only 5 % of GBC patients underwent surgical resection in a series of MD Anderson between 1940 and 1976 [2]. Nowadays, GBC patients are often diagnosed at an early (asymptomatic) stage, typically on pathologic review after laparoscopic cholecystectomy for cholelithiasis (i.e., incidental GBC). Also, surgical management of GBC improved with the introduction of ultrasound (US), computed tomography (CT), and magnetic resonance imaging (MRI) to determine the extent of disease. Currently, a cholecystectomy with en bloc liver resection of segments 4b and 5 with lymph node dissection of the hepatoduodenal ligament is recommended for most medically fit patients with resectable GBC [3]. Improvements in both anesthesia and surgery have reduced the postoperative morbidity and mortality [4].

The focus of this chapter is the surgical management of GBC patients. We first discuss risk factors, anatomy, and staging of GBC. The core of this chapter is structured based on the patient's presentation. The patient may present to the surgical oncologist with:

- A gallbladder polyp found on imaging (US, CT, or MRI)
- Incidental GBC found at pathologic review after cholecystectomy, typically for cholelithiasis
- Incidental GBC suspected during cholecystectomy, typically for cholelithiasis
- A gallbladder and/or liver mass found on imaging suspicious for GBC

Next, we describe the surgical procedures for GBC, postoperative care and complications, and adjuvant and palliative treatments. Because of the low incidence of GBC, no randomized controlled trials (RCTs) have been performed to evaluate surgical management. Guidelines are therefore based on anatomic studies, retrospective case

B.G. Koerkamp, M.D., Ph.D.
W.R. Jarnagin, M.D. (✉)
Hepatopancreatobiliary Service, Memorial Sloan-Kettering Cancer Center, 1275 York Avenue, New York 10065, NY, USA
e-mail: b.grootkoerkamp@erasmusmc.nl; jarnagiw@mskcc.org

Q.D. Chu et al. (eds.), *Surgical Oncology: A Practical and Comprehensive Approach*,
DOI 10.1007/978-1-4939-1423-4_11, © Springer Science+Business Media New York 2015

series, and registries. RCTs evaluating adjuvant and palliative treatments typically randomize patients with any biliary cancer: conclusions regarding GBC patients are drawn from subgroup analyses or based on the assumptions that biliary cancers are similar.

Risk Factors

Chronic inflammation of the mucosa of the gallbladder is associated with GBC. GBC patients typically have coexisting cholelithiasis (90 %). However, by contrast, only about 1 % of patients with cholelithiasis are diagnosed with GBC. Cholelithiasis may cause chronic inflammation resulting in malignant transformation, or cholelithiasis and GBC may share pathogenetic features. Less common causes of chronic inflammation are pancreaticobiliary maljunction (especially in Asia), typhoid infection, and biliary-enteric fistula. These causes of chronic inflammation confer increased risks of GBC up to 10-fold.

Geography is an important risk factor for GBC: while in the Western world the incidence is 1–2 per 100,000, the incidence in India, Pakistan, Japan, Korea, and Ecuador is up to 20-fold higher [5]. In the USA, women are about twice as likely to develop GBC as men. Familial GBC is rare.

The progression of adenoma to carcinoma appears less important in the pathogenesis of GBC than in the pathogenesis of colorectal cancer. Adenomatous polyps are rare and typically do not harbor GBC unless very large; however, severe dysplasia is often found adjacent to GBC.

Anatomy and Staging

Understanding guidelines and controversies for surgical management of GBC requires knowledge regarding the relation of the gallbladder to surrounding structures, as well as patterns of lymphatic and venous drainage of the gallbladder. The gallbladder is located at the undersurface of segment 4b and segment 5 of the liver (Fig. 11.1a–c). In 60 % of GBC patients, the tumor is found in the fundus, 30 % in the body, and 10 % in the neck of the gallbladder [6]. Tumors in the gallbladder neck are more likely to involve the bile ducts because of the neck's close proximity to the right hepatic duct and the biliary confluence [7].

The intraperitoneal portion of the gallbladder is covered with (visceral) peritoneum or serosa (Fig. 11.1d). If the cancer extends beyond the serosa of the gallbladder, it may involve surrounding organs such as the stomach, duodenum, pancreas, or transverse colon (Fig. 11.1c). The part of the gallbladder facing the liver has no peritoneal covering: only a layer of perimuscular connective tissue called the cystic plate separates the muscularis of the gallbladder from the liver parenchyma (Fig. 11.1d). A simple cholecystectomy involves dissection between the muscularis of the gallbladder and the cystic plate. Consequently, if GBC is discovered at pathologic review after a simple cholecystectomy, the resection margin is likely involved, unless the tumor did not invade the muscularis and is limited to the lamina propria (T1a).

GBC typically arises in the mucosa of the gallbladder, with adenocarcinoma or its variants (adenosquamous, squamous) found in 98 % of all patients. Rare histologies of the gallbladder include neuroendocrine tumors, sarcomas, or metastatic diseases such as melanoma. The most common infiltrative subtype invades the entire gallbladder in the subserosal plane, followed by invasion of the liver and the porta hepatis. The nodular subtype forms a more circumscribed lesion; the papillary type forms polypoid lesions and is less invasive.

Dye studies have demonstrated the route of lymph flow from the gallbladder first to the cystic duct node and the nodes around the bile duct, then to nodes around the hepatic vessels and posterior to the pancreas, and finally to the aortocaval nodes near the left renal vein (Fig. 11.2) [8]. In some patients, additional lymphatics are found connecting regional lymph nodes directly to aortocaval nodes. Positive lymph nodes beyond the hepatoduodenal ligament (i.e., periaortic, pericaval, superior mesenteric artery, and/or celiac artery lymph nodes) are considered stage IV disease since the seventh edition of the American Joint Committee on Cancer (AJCC) TNM classification for GBC [9].

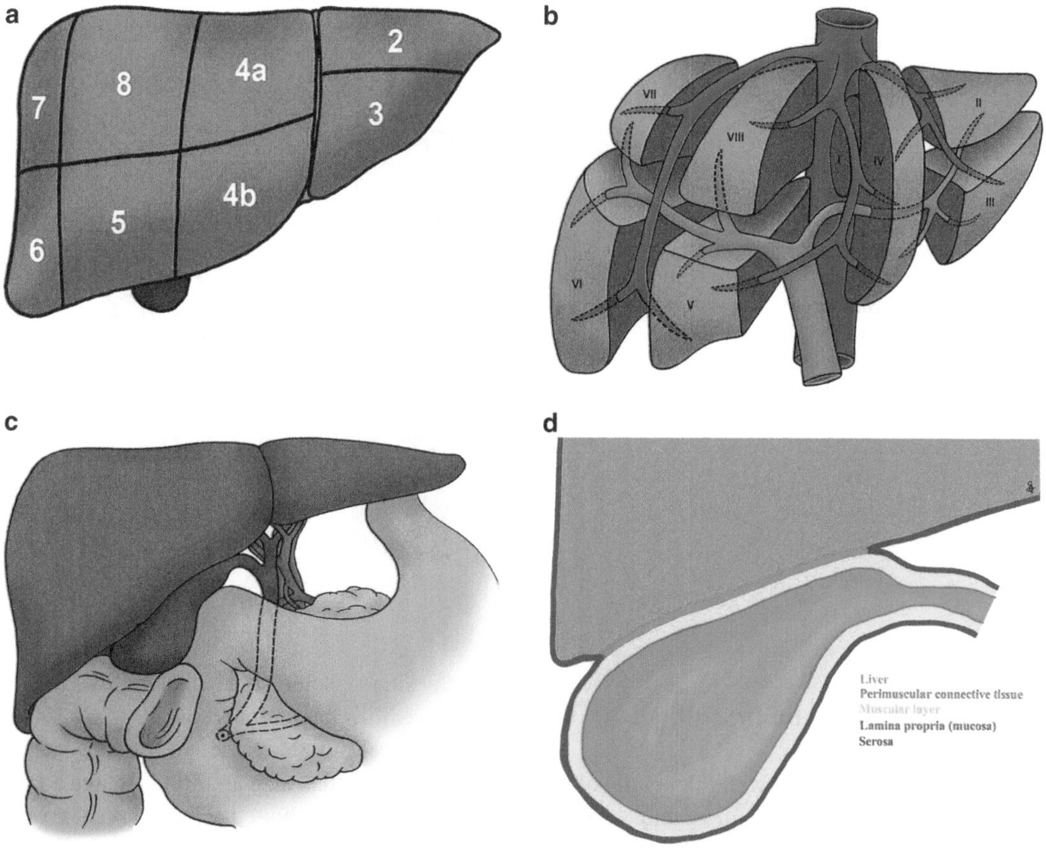

Fig. 11.1 (**a**) The gallbladder (*green*) is contiguous with segments 4b and 5 of the liver. Segment 1 (caudate lobe) is not shown. (**b**) Couinaud classification of the liver divides the liver into eight segments. (**c**) Illustration of the close relationship of the gallbladder to surrounding organs: the liver, duodenum, and transverse colon. Moreover, the cystic duct and neck of the gallbladder are in close proximity to the structures in the hepatoduodenal ligament: the common bile duct (*green*), portal vein (*blue*), and hepatic artery (*red*). (**d**) Layers of the gallbladder wall: the portion facing the liver is indicated in *red*, and the portion facing the peritoneal cavity is indicated in *blue* (Courtesy of Quyen D. Chu, MD, MBA, FACS)

Although lymphatic spread is important for staging, spread to distant sites occurs mainly through hematogenous dissemination, either directly or associated with invasion into the liver parenchyma [10]. When indocyanine green is injected in the cystic artery of GBC patients, the dye extends up to 4 cm into the parenchyma of segments 4b and 5 of the liver [11]. In an immunohistochemical study of liver resections for GBC, intrahepatic portal vein invasion was detected in more than half of the patients, up to 12 mm beyond the border of direct invasion. Metastatic nodules were found in 26 % of GBC patients, on average 16 mm beyond the border of direct invasion [12].

Table 11.1 presents the AJCC seventh edition guideline for staging of GBC, which is based on the anatomical considerations described above, as well as prognostic research [9]. Figure 11.3a presents overall survival of more than 10,000 patients with GBC diagnosed in the years 1989–1996 [9]. These data are from the National Cancer Data Base. Figure 11.3b presents overall survival of patients with GBC who had surgery, stratified by T stage and N stage [13]. These data are from the Surveillance, Epidemiology, and End Results (SEER) program, representing 26 % of the US population for the period 1991–2005. Patients with metastatic disease and stage T4 at the time of surgery were excluded [13].

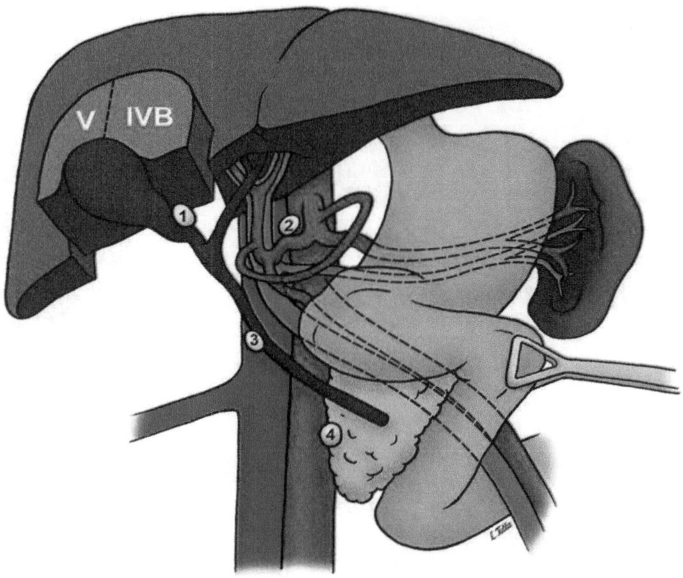

Fig. 11.2 Regional lymphadenectomy for gallbladder cancer includes lymph nodes in porta hepatis, hepatoduodenal and gastrohepatic ligament, and retroduodenal regions *Lymph Node Stations for Gallbladder Cancer* **1: Cystic duct lymph node 2: Common hepatic artery lymph node 3: Portocaval lymph nodes 4: Common bile duct lymph nodes (Courtesy of Quyen D. Chu, MD, MBA, FACS)**

Gallbladder Polyp on Imaging

Polypoid lesions and focal wall thickening of the gallbladder are found on ultrasound (US) in 3–7 % of healthy adults [14–16]. Their incidence has increased with more frequent use and improved resolution of US. Only rarely do they cause symptoms by obstructing the gallbladder outlet. Although most of these lesions are benign, some are premalignant (adenomatous polyps), and rarely GBC is found. The risk of malignant transformation of gallbladder polyps, while possible, is extremely low for small lesions (<1 cm) and appears to be lower than previously reported for larger lesions (>1 cm). Additionally, it should be recognized that small polypoid lesions are very often nonneoplastic.

Ultrasound cannot reliably distinguish premalignant polyps from pseudopolyps such as cholesterol polyps. The size of the polyp is an important predictor of malignancy. Based on a study in 1982, surgical resection has been recommended for polyps of at least 10 mm, because GBC was found only in polyps larger than 12 mm [17]. More recent studies confirmed that malignancy is extremely rare, if found at all, in polyps smaller than 10 mm, except in patients with primary sclerosing cholangitis (PSC) [18–20]. Of all polyps found on US, 7–29 % are larger than 10 mm. Risk factors for malignancy of polyps other than size and PSC are age above 50 years, Indian ethnic background, a sessile polyp, a single polyp, and the presence of gallstones [14, 19]. In patients with polyps smaller than 5 mm on US, no polyp or mass is found on pathologic examination in up to 83 %; for polyps larger than 20 mm, cancer may be present in up to 59 % [19]. Cholecystectomy for polyps of at least 10 mm remains a valid guideline based on recent series. In addition, cholecystectomy for polyps of more than 5 mm in patients with PSC appears justified, given the much higher risk of malignancy in that setting.

The resolution of conventional US is insufficient to distinguish the layers of the gallbladder wall (Fig. 11.1d). Therefore, US has a poor diagnostic accuracy for detecting a polyp that harbors GBC invading into or just beyond the lamina propria. Although CT can detect invasion of the liver parenchyma (T3) and distant metastases, its diagnostic accuracy for depth of invasion is also poor. Diagnostic accuracy for depth of invasion appears better for high-resolution US (63 %) and endoscopic ultrasound (56 %) [21]. In patients with a high likelihood of GBC

Table 11.1 American Joint Committee on Cancer (AJCC) TNM staging for gallbladder cancer (seventh edition)

Primary tumor (T)	
TX	Primary tumor cannot be assessed
T0	No evidence of primary tumor
Tis	Carcinoma in situ
T1a	Tumor invades lamina propria
T1b	Tumor invades muscular layer
T2	Tumor invades perimuscular connective tissue; no extension beyond serosa or into liver
T3	Tumor perforates the serosa (visceral peritoneum) and/or directly invades the liver and/or one extrahepatic organ or structure*
T4	Tumor invades main portal vein or hepatic artery or invades two or more extrahepatic organs or structures*

*Extrahepatic organs or structures include the stomach, duodenum, colon, pancreas, omentum, and extrahepatic bile ducts

Regional lymph nodes (N)	
NX	Regional lymph nodes cannot be assessed
N0	No regional lymph node metastasis
N1	Metastases to nodes along the cystic duct, common bile duct, hepatic artery, and/or portal vein
N2	Metastases to the periaortic, pericaval, superior mesenteric artery, and/or celiac artery lymph nodes

Distant metastasis (M)	
M0	No distant metastasis
M1	Distant metastasis

Anatomic stage/prognostic groups			
Group	T	N	M
Stage 0	Tis	N0	M0
Stage I	T1	N0	M0
Stage II	T2	N0	M0
Stage IIIA	T3	N0	M0
Stage IIIB	T1-3	N1	M0
Stage IVA	T4	N0-1	M0
Stage IVB	Any T	N2	M0
	Any T	Any N	M1

Adapted from Compton et al. [84]. With permission from Springer Verlag

(e.g., polyps larger than 15 mm), but no invasion on conventional US, a preoperative high-resolution US or endoscopic US may alter surgical management.

A simple cholecystectomy is sufficient for polyps and early (i.e., T1a) GBC (see below). Cholecystectomy can be performed open or laparoscopically. Bile spillage should be avoided because, if GBC cells are present in the bile, they can cause peritoneal or port-site metastases. The incidence of bile spillage during laparoscopic cholecystectomy for incidental GBC was about 20 % in a Japanese series of 498 patients and was associated with a higher recurrence rate of 27 % versus 14 % if no spillage occurred [22]. Other series showed that port-site or incisional recurrences occurred at least twice as often in laparoscopic versus open cholecystectomy for GBC [23, 24]. Even for in situ carcinoma, peritoneal dissemination has been described after gallbladder perforation [25]. A low threshold for conversion to open cholecystectomy is therefore recommended. A bag should be used for laparoscopic removal of the gallbladder. For patients with an increased risk of malignancy (e.g., polyp larger than 15 mm), open cholecystectomy should be considered because of the increased risk of bile spillage and peritoneal dissemination with laparoscopic resection. A simple cholecystectomy may not result in clear margins if GBC with invasion beyond the lamina propria is found. Frozen section of the gallbladder could be obtained to rule out GBC, if expertise is available for immediate liver resection (segments 4b and 5) and lymphadenectomy, but there is a high risk of sampling error in this setting. If the GBC is limited to the lamina propria (i.e., stage T1a), additional resection is not required [3].

Regarding polyps smaller than 10 mm that are not resected, the question arises whether follow-up is necessary. A study from 1962 found no GBC during a 15-year follow-up of patients with gallbladder polyps [26]. In a recent study, a follow-up US was available for 149 patients, 2–12 years after the initial US: increase in size was noted in only 1 polyp (from 3 to 5 mm, not clinically relevant), and two thirds of these small polyps were undetected at follow-up [27]. In another recent series, growth was seen in 8 out of 143 patients during follow-up, but no cancer developed [18]. On the other hand, in a small series of patients with gallbladder polyps, rapid growth was found on repeat US in the months before surgery in five patients who eventually had GBC demonstrated [28]. Because of the conflicting data, follow-up at 6- to 12-month intervals for 2 years is generally recommended.

Several other gallbladder wall lesions can be found on imaging or during surgery. Calcification of the gallbladder wall, or porcelain gallbladder, appears to increase the risk of malignant transformation. However, the risk appears to be lower than was suggested based on older studies and also seems to be related to the nature of the calcifications (i.e., diffuse versus discontiguous or selective). In a number of studies, patients with diffuse calcification of the gallbladder had no GBC identified on histopathologic analysis [29–31]. However, one study of more than 25,000 resected gallbladders found GBC in 2 out of 27 patients with selective mucosal calcification of the gallbladder wall [30]. Cholecystectomy for patients with selective mucosal calcification is therefore recommended.

Adenomyomatosis of the gallbladder is characterized by focal thickening of the gallbladder wall with cystic-appearing spaces (Rokitansky-Aschoff sinuses) that are identified with high accuracy on US. Because these lesions are invariably benign and asymptomatic, they need no surgical management or follow-up [32].

Xanthogranulomatous cholecystitis is an uncommon inflammatory disease of the gallbladder with extensive fibrosis that can present with wall thickening, mass formation, and infiltration of the liver and other adjacent organs [33]. Typical findings on imaging include diffuse gallbladder wall thickening, hypo-attenuating intramural nodules, continuous mucosal line enhancement, and the presence of gallstones [34]. However, accuracy of these findings is often insufficient to rule out GBC, and xanthogranulomatous cholecystitis is typically diagnosed at pathologic review after extended cholecystectomy (i.e., segment 4b and 5 resection en bloc with gallbladder). In a series from India comprising 198 patients resected for presumed GBC, 16 % was found to have xanthogranulomatous cholecystitis [35].

Incidental Gallbladder Cancer at Pathologic Review

Incidental GBC is found on pathologic review of about 1 % of laparoscopic cholecystectomy specimens [36–38]. These patients comprise about two thirds of all patients with potentially curable GBC. In most of these cases, the gallbladder is resected for presumed symptomatic cholelithiasis, and GBC was not suspected on preoperative imaging or during surgery. Many of these patients benefit from reoperation and definitive resection. Re-resection may be beneficial if residual cancer is limited to the liver bed, cystic stump, common bile duct, or lymph nodes in the absence of distant metastasis. A large Western study showed that 14 % of these incidental GBC patients had disseminated disease on re-exploration, and 73 % of re-resected patients had residual disease on final pathology [39, 40].

The probability of both distant metastases and local residual cancer increases with the depth of invasion (i.e., T stage). In a Japanese nationwide survey of 498 patients with incidentally found GBC, 34 % had stage T1a, 14 % T1b, 41 % T2, 8 % T3, and 2 % T4 [22]. Table 11.2 presents the probability of residual disease in the liver or

Table 11.2 Residual disease found at re-resection for incidental GBC

T stage	Number of patients	Percentage of all stages (%)	Residual disease – any[a] (%)	Residual disease – liver (%)	Residual disease – nodes (%)
T1	8	8	38	0	13
T2	67	68	57	10	31
T3	22	22	77	36	46
All stages	97	100	59	15	33

[a]Also includes disease at the cystic duct margin and trocar sites (Reprinted from Pawlik et al. [41]. With permission from Springer Verlag)

regional lymph nodes stratified by T stage, found in re-resected patients with incidental GBC [41]. In another large Western series, the median survival time was 15 months if residual disease was found (73 % of patients), compared with 72 months if no residual disease was found [40]. The National Comprehensive Cancer Network (NCCN) guideline recommends re-resection for non-metastatic patients with T1b to T3 GBC [3]. Appropriate re-resection should include, at a minimum, resection of the liver segments contiguous with the gallbladder (segments 4b and 5) and regional lymphadenectomy, with selective bile duct resection (Fig. 11.2). The surgical procedures are described in more detail below.

Many studies have evaluated the benefit of a re-resection in patients with pT1a and pT1b GBC. A systematic review of T1 GBC identified 29 retrospective studies representing 1,266 patients [42]. T1a GBC was found in 56 % of all T1 GBC patients, of whom 16 % underwent re-resection. T1b was found in 44 %, of whom 33 % underwent re-resection. Patients with T1a GBC had lymph node metastases in 2 % and patients with T1b in 11 %. Eight patients (1 %) with T1a GBC died of recurrence. Fifty-two patients (9 %) of all patients with T1b died of recurrence: 13 % recurred after simple cholecystectomy alone and 3 % recurred after definitive re-resection. In a German prospective registry, 23 of 72 patients with T1b GBC underwent a re-resection [43], and this was associated with a 3-fold lower recurrence rate and a 5-year overall survival of 79 versus 42 months for simple cholecystectomy only ($P=0.03$). In a study of more than 1,000 T1 GBC patients in the Surveillance, Epidemiology, and End Results (SEER) database, 80 % of both T1a and T1b patients underwent only a simple cholecystectomy [44]. For T1b patients, survival was better when combined with a liver resection and/or lymphadenectomy; for T1a patients, survival was similar with more extensive surgery (Fig. 11.3c). The NCCN guideline therefore recommends re-resection after an incidentally found T1b GBC [3]. For T1a GBC, the recurrence rate of a simple cholecystectomy alone is similar to the postoperative mortality rate for re-resection (approximately 1.5 %) [42]. Re-resection after an incidentally found T1a GBC is, therefore, not recommended.

Patients with T2 and T3 GBC may appear more likely to benefit from re-resection, because they are more likely to harbor residual disease than T1 GBC. However, they are also more likely to harbor occult distant metastatic disease, in which case re-resection is of no benefit. Several studies have suggested a benefit of re-resection for both T2 and T3 GBCs, using data from the SEER cancer registry [13, 45, 46]. In 781 patients with T2 GBC, the median survival time and the 5-year survival rate were 53 months and 37 %, respectively, after re-resection compared with 16 months and 21 % after cholecystectomy alone (Fig. 11.3d). In 1,118 patients with T3 GBC, the median survival and the 5-year survival rate were 11 months and 13 %, respectively, after re-resection compared with 8 months and 8 % with cholecystectomy alone (Fig. 11.3d) [13]. The benefit of re-resection persisted in node-positive patients with T1b or T2 tumors, but a benefit was not detected in node-positive patients with T3 tumors. In a German registry of 200 patients with incidental T2 GBC, 85 patients underwent re-resection, resulting in a 5-year survival of 55 % versus 35 % for patients subjected to a simple cholecystectomy [47]. In the same registry, of the 85 patients with T3 GBC, 32 underwent re-resection, but this did not result in an obvious improvement in the 5-year survival, which was only 18 %. Single institution series are smaller than these registries, but also found better survival after re-resection, especially for T2 tumors [48, 49]. The survival benefit found in these nonrandomized studies could be at least partly due to selection bias. In other words, there may well have been a good reason to exclude certain patients from re-resection that is not reflected in or is impossible to assess in retrospective analyses. Re-resection after incidentally found T2 and T3 GBCs is recommended, although the benefit is probably small for T3 GBC, and patients with node-positive T3 GBC may not benefit at all from re-resection. Unfortunately, nodal status is typically unknown after simple cholecystectomy and may not be known with certainty until the final histological analysis is complete. Table 11.3 summarizes the management of GBC patients based on T stage.

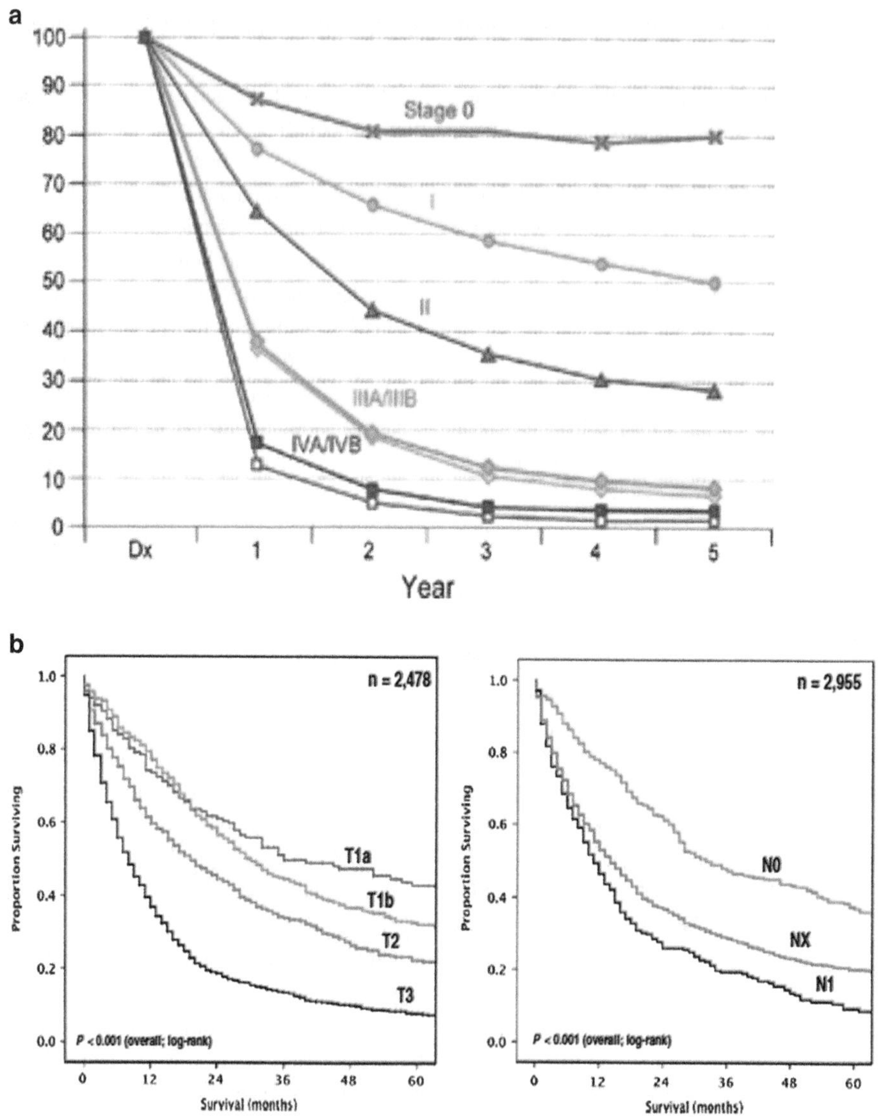

Fig. 11.3 (**a**) Overall survival of more than 10,000 patients with GBC diagnosed in the years 1989–1996. Data from the National Cancer Data Base [9]. (**b**) Overall survival for patients with gallbladder cancer who had surgery, stratified by T stage ($p<0.001$) and N stage ($P<0.001$). Data from the SEER database, representing 26 % of the US population, for the period 1991–2005. Patients with metastatic disease and stage T4 at the time of surgery were excluded. (**c**) Overall survival in patients with stage T1a ($n=300$) and T1b ($n=536$) GBC, stratified by type of surgery. C+LN, cholecystectomy with any lymph node dissection; RC, radical (i.e., extended) cholecystectomy including liver resection and regional lymph node dissection. Data from the SEER database, representing 26 % of the US population, for the period 1988–2008. (**d**) Overall survival in patients with stage T2 and T3 GBCs, further stratified by type of surgery. Radical, radical (i.e., extended) cholecystectomy including liver resection; simple, simple cholecystectomy [13]. Data from the SEER database, representing 26 % of the US population, for the period 1991–2005 ((**a**) Reprinted from Edge [9]. With permission from Springer Verlag. (**b**) Reprinted from Mayo et al. [13]. With permission from Springer Verlag. (**c**) Reprinted from Hari et al. [44]. With permission from John Wiley & Sons, Inc. (**d**) Reprinted from Mayo et al. [13]. With permission from Springer Verlag)

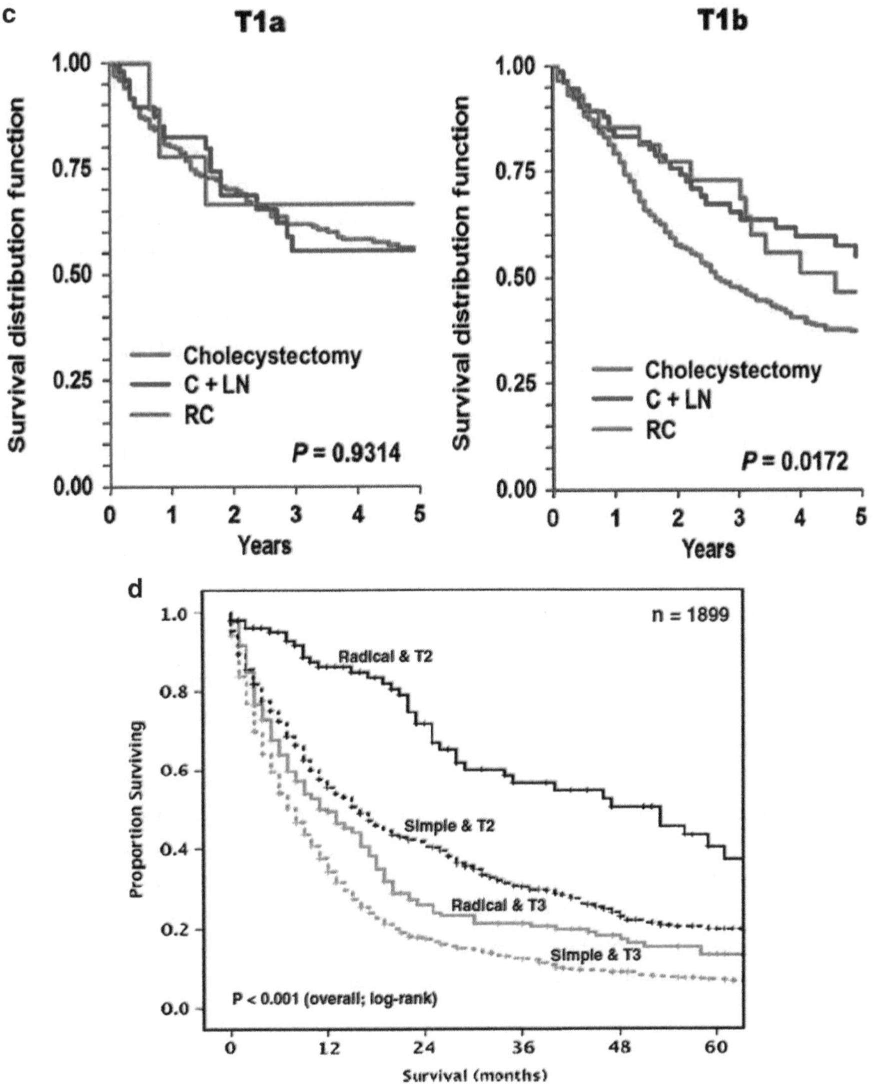

Fig. 11.3 (continued)

Before embarking on re-resection, distant metastases should be ruled out using abdominal CT or MRI and imaging of the chest. Positron-emission tomography (PET) may be of some benefit in avoiding futile surgery by detecting metastatic disease not found on cross-sectional imaging [50]. In one study, PET found distant metastasis in 3 out of 23 patients with incidental GBC [51]. As part of the work-up, it is important to review the initial imaging before cholecystectomy, the operative note, and the pathology report. These may inform on the precise location of the tumor within the gallbladder (on the peritoneal or liver side; near the fundus or near the cystic duct), inadvertent perforation of the gallbladder, and margin status at the cystic duct. If the cystic duct margin is positive for invasive cancer or high-grade dysplasia, bile duct resection is recommended to obtain clear margins. However, this information is often not included in routine histologic assessment for cholecystectomy performed for presumed benign disease. In a Western series, 8 out of 19 patients with a positive cystic duct margin had residual disease in the common bile duct [41]. Alternatively, re-resection of the cystic duct stump with frozen section could be considered [52].

Table 11.3 Management of GBC patients based on T stage

T stage	Recommendation
T1a	Simple cholecystectomy
T1b–T2	Cholecystectomy with en bloc liver resection of segments 4b and 5 (anatomical or wedge) with lymph node dissection of the hepatoduodenal ligament
T3	As for T1b–T2 but GBC in the gallbladder neck or the cystic duct may require right hepatectomy extended to segment 4b and/or bile duct resection with hepaticojejunostomy to obtain clear margins. To ensure negative margins, any adherent organ or structure[a] should also be resected
T4	As for T3, resection of two or more adherent organs or structures[a] can be considered. Palliative care if involvement of main portal vein or proper hepatic artery. Most patients in this category are not candidates for resection or will not benefit from resection even if feasible technically

[a]Adherent organs or structures other than liver include the stomach, duodenum, colon, pancreas, omentum, and extrahepatic bile ducts

Staging laparoscopy may prevent an unnecessary exploratory laparotomy if disseminated disease is found. The incidence of metastatic disease at re-exploration for GBC is 14–24 % [39, 41]. Of 46 patients undergoing staging laparoscopy in a Western series, 10 (22 %) had metastatic disease that was identified laparoscopically in only two patients, whereas in the other eight it was found at laparotomy [39]. Peritoneal metastasis is more likely in patients with poorly differentiated or T3 tumors, or after perforation of the gallbladder at cholecystectomy. The yield of staging laparoscopy would appear to be greater in such high-risk patients, and it is reasonable to use it routinely in these settings.

Incidental Gallbladder Cancer Found at Surgery

GBC is sometimes suspected during surgery, typically during laparoscopic cholecystectomy for cholelithiasis. If peritoneal or hepatic lesions are found and frozen section demonstrates GBC, the patient has metastatic disease and will not benefit from resection. If the diagnosis of GBC is suspected based on macroscopic assessment of the gallbladder and no expertise in GBC is available, it is probably best to not perform any resection and refer the patient to a specialized hepatobiliary center where the disease can be staged fully and the tumor resected in a single definitive procedure observing oncologic principles. Studies that report no difference in survival between patients undergoing two resections or a single definitive resection likely suffer from selection bias, since patients who develop disseminated disease prior to the second procedure are excluded [48, 53].

GBC may also be suspected after cholecystectomy by macroscopic assessment of the gallbladder mucosa. If the mucosa appears abnormal, then the gallbladder can be sent for frozen section histology, and definitive resection may be undertaken at that time.

Mass Found on Imaging, Suspicious for GBC

GBC is typically asymptomatic until advanced stages, when involvement of the liver and other surrounding structures occurs. At this stage, patients may present with constant right upper quadrant pain, weight loss, and nausea with vomiting. About 40 % of patients are jaundiced at presentation, an ominous finding [54]. At an advanced stage, US often demonstrates a heterogeneous mass in the gallbladder. Sometimes a diffuse thickening of the gallbladder wall is seen that can be difficult to distinguish from cholecystitis. Complete cross-sectional imaging, usually in the form of CT of the chest, abdomen, and pelvis, is recommended as the next step. PET scan may be justified in selected patients, to assess suspicious findings at distant sites, but is probably not helpful as a routine study [51].

The NCCN guideline has the same recommendations for these patients, as for patients in whom GBC was incidentally found [3]. In summary, most non-metastatic patients are expected to benefit from surgical resection. Exceptions are patients with positive lymph nodes beyond the hepatoduodenal ligament (i.e., the periaortic, pericaval, superior mesenteric artery, and/or celiac artery lymph nodes), which is considered stage IV disease according to the seventh edition of the AJCC TNM classification. Moreover, patients with T4 tumors are unlikely to benefit from surgery even if their disease is amenable to resection. T4 tumors are locally advanced and include those that invade or encase the main portal vein and the hepatic artery or involve at least two extrahepatic organs or structures (e.g., the duodenum, pancreas, and transverse colon). If a patient has substantial comorbidities, a trade-off should be made between the expected postoperative morbidity and mortality and the long-term oncologic benefits of surgery.

The prognosis of symptomatic (non-incidental) GBC patients remains poor, even after liver segment 4b and 5 resection with lymphadenectomy of the hepatoduodenal ligament. In a Western series including 54 patients with non-incidental GBC, 48 patients underwent surgical exploration of which only 11 underwent a liver resection. The median survival was only 8 months [53].

Controversies in Surgical Management

In the absence of data from prospective, controlled trials, many issues pertaining to the treatment of patients with GBC remain unresolved. This section highlights three common controversies: the extent of liver resection, indications for extrahepatic bile duct resection, and the benefit of laparoscopic port-site resection.

The first controversy concerns whether GBC patients should undergo a liver wedge resection of 1–5 cm, an anatomic resection of segments 4b and 5, or an extended right hepatectomy. In 1954, Glenn and Hays first proposed a liver resection for GBC: the gallbladder was resected en bloc with a 1 cm wedge of liver parenchyma [55]. Since then, wider liver resections have been recommended to obtain clear margins, eliminate micrometastases in the liver, and ultimately avoid recurrence in the liver [56]. The results of histological studies support an anatomic resection of segments 4b and 5 (see section on anatomy) [12, 57]. However, in a Japanese multicenter series of 485 R0 T2/3 patients, no difference in survival or local recurrence was found between wedge resection, anatomical segmental resection, or extended right hepatectomy [58]. Metastases in the liver beyond segments 4b and 5 represent stage IV disease, and survival beyond 1 year is rare; extended hepatectomy appears futile for this indication. Moreover, the postoperative mortality of extended liver resections was between 9 and 18 % in several series [59–61]. Postoperative mortality occurred mainly in the setting of liver failure due to the extensive resection in combination with obstructive jaundice in 45–100 % of these patients. Therefore, most surgeons perform a wedge resection of about 2 cm liver parenchyma (en bloc with the gallbladder, if still in situ) or an anatomic liver resection of segments 4b and 5. An extended right hepatectomy (extended to segment 4b, with or without 4a and 1) could be considered in medically fit patients with GBC arising in the gallbladder neck, Hartmann's pouch, or the cystic duct. These tumors are close to the right hepatic pedicle at an early stage, and a conventional segment 4b and 5 liver resection is likely to result in a positive margin (see section on anatomy) [49].

The second controversy concerns resection of the extrahepatic bile duct (EBD) for patients with GBC. Involvement of the EBD often results in jaundice. EBD resection for jaundiced GBC patients was traditionally performed as a matter of routine, although enthusiasm has waned with the publication of poor outcomes [62]; however, this practice is still recommended by some Asian surgeons [60, 62]. In a Western series of 82 GBC patients who presented with jaundice, 55 were explored of whom 6 were resected (including EBD resection), of whom 4 had an R0 resection [62]. All six resected patients died or recurred within 6 months. The median survival of all jaundiced GBC patients was 6 months and all patients died before 28 months. Of the 82 jaundiced patients, only three patients had node-negative disease. Because of these poor outcomes, the NCCN guideline recommends to consider resection only in node-negative jaundiced GBC patients, at an experienced center; however, definitive determination of nodal status prior to operation can be difficult [3]. Jaundice may be an early event in patients with GBC arising from the gallbladder neck, Hartmann's pouch, or the cystic duct. In theory, this small subgroup may benefit from resection. These patients have likely involvement of the right portal pedicle and require a combined extended right hepatectomy, EBD resection, and regional lymphadenectomy to obtain clear margins.

In the absence of jaundice, EBD resection in GBC patients is recommended to obtain clear margins for a positive cystic duct margin after a previous cholecystectomy. In one study, 8 of 19 patients (42 %) with a positive cystic duct margin had residual disease in the resected EBD [41]. Routine EBD resection for every GBC patient, even without evidence of tumor involvement, is recommended by some Japanese surgeons [63]. This approach is supported by a histological study that found cancer cells in the EBD in 19 of 44 (43 %) non-jaundiced patients with T2/3 GBC [64]. On the other hand, EBD resection and preservation were compared in a retrospective nationwide Japanese study including 838 T2–4 GBC patients [65]. These patients had no macroscopic involvement of the hepatoduodenal ligament and underwent an R0 resection with or without EBD resection. No difference was found in survival between EBD resection and preservation for any subgroup of T stage or N stage. A theoretical advantage of routine EBD resection is that it facilitates regional lymphadenectomy and avoids ischemia of the EBD. However, no difference in lymph node count was found between patients with and without bile duct resection [66]. Although the actual benefit of routine EBD resection remains disputed, the high complication rate is well established in both Western and Asian series. In a series of 104 GBC patients, 33 % of the patients undergoing an EBD resection had a complication that required re-intervention or resulted in permanent disability or death, versus 13 % of patients who had no EBD resection [66]. A postoperative biliary anastomotic leak may result in sepsis and death. In the long term, biliary strictures and recurrent cholangitis render the patient a "biliary cripple"[67]. The weight of evidence would support resection of the EBD only if involved with tumor or it is otherwise unavoidable in order to achieve an R0 resection.

The third controversy concerns the excision of laparoscopic port sites, simultaneous with definitive resection for incidental GBC, to avoid port-site recurrence. After spillage of bile, GBC has the unique ability to cause tumor implants on peritoneum, in biopsy tracts, and in abdominal wounds including port sites, as has been described as early as 1955 [56]. In a series of 113 patients with incidental GBC, 69 patients underwent port-site resection of which 13 (19 %) had port-site metastasis [68]. The presence of port-site metastasis was associated with a worse median survival (17 versus 42 months), but no difference in survival was detected between patients with and without port-site resection. Moreover, all 13 patients with resected port-site metastasis either had an R2 resection or recurred within 24 months. Consequently, port-site resection mainly has a role in staging and prognosis, rather than in prolonging survival, and appears to be the clinical equivalent of peritoneal metastasis. Because port-site resection can be a disfiguring operation, it is not recommended as part of the definitive operation for incidental GBC.

Description of Surgical Procedure for GBC

Before proceeding with surgery, medical evaluation and optimization is required, in particular for patients with coexisting cardiopulmonary disease. Blood products should be available because of potential blood loss associated with liver resection, although the likelihood of transfusion has decreased to low levels over the past several years [69]. The anesthesiologist should pursue low central venous pressure, which has been shown to reduce blood loss during parenchymal transection [70].

Staging laparoscopy should be considered in patients with an increased risk of disseminated disease. This includes patients with poor differentiation, T3 level of invasion, and perforation of

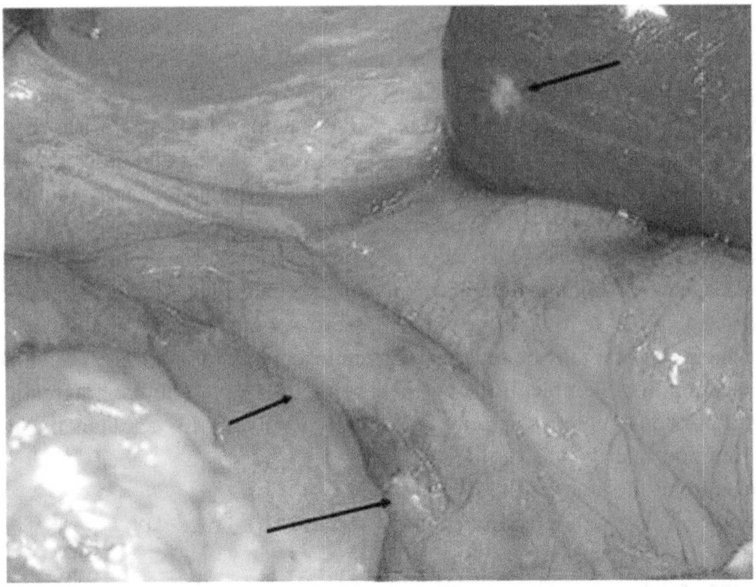

Fig. 11.4 Peritoneal metastases (*arrows*) found at re-exploration in patient with incidental gallbladder cancer (Reprinted from Hueman et al. [83]. With permission from Springer Verlag)

the gallbladder at previous cholecystectomy or symptomatic (non-incidental) GBC patients. The finding of peritoneal or hepatic metastasis (Fig. 11.4) signifies advanced, incurable disease and should terminate the procedure in nearly all cases. A right subcostal (Kocher) incision provides adequate exposure and can be extended to the left into a bilateral subcostal (chevron) incision. Alternatively, an inverted L (hockey stick) incision can be used. The teres ligament is divided and pulled upward to expose the undersurface of the liver and hepatoduodenal ligament. On inspection of the abdominal cavity, disseminated disease is often found that remained undetected at staging laparoscopy [39]. Exploration should include a Kocher maneuver to assess for suspicious retroperitoneal or aortocaval lymph nodes. If aortocaval, retropancreatic, or celiac lymph nodes are positive, the patient has the equivalent of stage IV disease and resection is futile [9].

If a single adjacent organ such as the transverse colon or duodenum is adherent to the gallbladder, en bloc resection is required to ensure clear margins. In a subgroup of 20 patients undergoing en bloc resection for adherence to the gallbladder, 10 patients had histological involvement of the organ adherent to the gallbladder [66]. If more than one adjacent organ is involved (stage T4), patients are less likely to benefit from resection, even if a complete resection can be achieved.

Regional lymphadenectomy should include the lymph nodes within the porta hepatis, gastrohepatic ligament, and retroduodenal regions [3] (Fig. 11.2). The right gastric artery is ligated, and the portal vein, hepatic artery, and common bile ducts are dissected free of surrounding lymphatic tissue, sweeping it upward toward the liver hilum. If during lymphadenectomy involvement of the main portal vein or common hepatic artery is found, the patient has T4 disease and resection is probably futile.

The segment 4b and 5 liver resection is commenced with opening of the umbilical fissure on the right side of the teres ligament. The inflow vessels to segment 4b are dissected and divided. The cystic duct is divided at the common bile duct. Next, the line of transection is marked on the liver capsule with electrocautery. Stay sutures are placed adjacent to the transection line at the anterior edge of the liver. A crushing technique is used for the parenchymal transection, and vessels are either clipped or ligated. Other parenchymal transection techniques can be used if preferred. The Endo-GIA vascular stapler is used to control large intrahepatic vessels. Transection begins medially, where first the middle hepatic vein and then the segment 5 pedicle will be encountered and divided. The main anterior pedicle and the pedicle to segment 8 are at risk for inadvertent injury during parenchymal transection, and caution must be taken. Hemostasis is achieved with the argon beam coagulator. Abdominal drainage is not necessary [71].

En bloc bile duct resection may be required to obtain an R0 resection, for example, if the cystic duct margin of a previous cholecystectomy was positive. The common bile duct is divided just above the duodenum at the start of the regional lymphadenectomy. This will facilitate the lymphadenectomy and the assessment of involvement of the portal vein and hepatic artery. However, bile duct resection did not result in an increased lymph node yield [72]. The common hepatic duct is transected at its confluence. After the resection, a Roux-en-Y limb is created for a hepaticojejunostomy. We refer the reader to other textbooks for an illustrated description of the procedure [73, 74].

Postoperative Care and Complications

Postoperative care for GBC patients after a liver segment 4b and 5 resection with lymphadenectomy of the hepatoduodenal ligament is similar to the care for other patients after liver resection. The care focuses on minimizing the risk of cardiopulmonary and thromboembolic complications by effective pain relief, pulmonary toilet, early ambulation, thrombosis prophylaxis, maintaining fluid balance (avoiding fluid overload), and early enteral diet as tolerated.

Liver resections are considered major surgery, associated with cardiopulmonary complications and a postoperative mortality of 1 % or less in high-volume centers. Liver failure is the most serious complication specific to liver resections. Fortunately, in GBC patients without cirrhosis, the risk of liver failure is very low for the conventional resection of liver segments 4b and 5. The few resected jaundiced GBC patients and those who undergo an extended liver resection are at risk for liver failure. Bile leaks after resection of liver segments 4b and 5 arise mostly from the liver parenchyma and are self-limiting with percutaneous drainage, rarely requiring endoscopic sphincterotomy and/or stent placement. Inadvertent injuries to the right anterior bile duct, segment 8 bile duct, or extrahepatic bile ducts are more serious complications that likely require endoscopic and/or surgical management. A subhepatic or right subdiaphragmatic abscess typically resolves with percutaneous drainage.

Adjuvant Therapy

After a potentially curative resection for GBC, the median overall survival for patients in the SEER database was 16 months, and the 5-year survival rate was 21 % [13]. At a median follow-up of 24 months, 66 % of the patients with resected GBC had recurred. Of all patients that recur, 85 % will present with metastatic disease with or without locoregional recurrence [75]. As a result, there is interest in investigating the role of adjuvant therapies. While there is no good prospective data, many retrospective studies have evaluated whether adjuvant chemotherapy can reduce the recurrence rate and improve survival. A phase 3 randomized controlled trial (RCT) from Japan analyzed 112 patients with GBC and found an 8 % absolute increase ($P=0.02$) in 5-year disease-free survival in GBC patients receiving adjuvant mitomycin C and 5-fluorouracil (5-FU). The NCCN guideline recommends adjuvant treatment with 5-FU or gemcitabine, which is mainly based on RCTs in the palliative setting (see below) [3, 76, 77]. Addition of cisplatin or oxaliplatin could be considered in high-risk patients (T4, N1, or R1), although it has not been demonstrated that benefits observed in the palliative setting translate to the adjuvant setting.

About 15 % of patients will present with a locoregional recurrence without metastatic disease. These patients may have benefited from adjuvant radiotherapy. No phase 3 RCT has evaluated the benefit of adjuvant radiotherapy in

GBC. Adjuvant radiotherapy has been evaluated in about 4,000 GBC patients in the SEER database [78]. Radiotherapy was associated with 15-month overall survival (versus 8 months), but overall survival after 2 years was the same. Because of the retrospective nature of this study, the difference found may be partially or entirely attributed to patient selection; furthermore, this analysis did not take into account the adequacy of resection, and the benefits may extend only to those subjected to an inadequate resection. Adjuvant radiotherapy could be considered in particular in node-negative GBC patients with a positive margin.

Palliative Therapy

Most GBC patients will eventually undergo palliative treatment. Many patients are not eligible for surgical resection at the time of diagnosis: they either have distant metastases, have locally advanced disease (e.g., involvement of portal vein or hepatic artery), or are not medically fit to undergo a liver resection. Even after potentially curative surgery, the majority of patients will recur. A phase 3 RCT including 410 patients with biliary cancer demonstrated a 3.6-month improvement in median overall survival in patients who received gemcitabine with cisplatin versus gemcitabine alone [76]. In the subgroup of 149 patients with GBC, overall survival was also significantly better with a hazard ratio of 0.61 (95 % confidence interval: 0.42–0.89). More recently, several clinical studies evaluating targeted treatments in biliary cancer found improved response rates but have failed to demonstrate a survival benefit [79, 80]. The NCCN recommends the combination of gemcitabine and cisplatin as palliative treatment [3]. Alternatively, other gemcitabine-based or 5-FU-based regimens could be considered. Radiotherapy may have benefit in GBC patients with locally advanced disease, although no randomized data are available.

Locally advanced disease often causes obstruction of the intra- and extrahepatic bile ducts. The resulting jaundice and pruritus can be palliated with drainage. Optimal biliary drainage is also important to decrease the risk of biliary sepsis. Biliary drainage can be obtained with endoscopic or percutaneous interventions. In an RCT, endoscopic and percutaneous drainage were compared in 44 GBC patients with obstructive jaundice. Successful drainage was better in the percutaneous group (89 % versus 41 %, $P<0.001$), and early cholangitis was higher in the endoscopic group (48 % versus 11 %, $P=0.002$) [81]. However, both drainage approaches are associated with high morbidity. Patients undergoing percutaneous biliary drainage for malignant bile duct obstruction were found to have a 58 % rate of major complications and a median survival of only 5 months [82]. Therefore, biliary drainage is only recommended for symptomatic relief and not preemptively, or to allow for chemotherapy.

Future Perspective

The outcomes of patients with GBC remain poor. Improvements in outcomes for patients with GBC are possible in several ways: early detection, more effective systemic treatment, better patient selection for surgery, reduced mortality and morbidity of surgery, and better adherence to guidelines. Early detection or screening for GBC is unlikely to be effective anytime soon, since the prevalence is very low even in patients with increased risk, and no test is available other than imaging, which will mainly detect late-stage GBC. Most patients with GBC will eventually die of metastatic disease, regardless of the extent of surgery. Analysis of data from a prospective registry of GBC patients may improve selection of patients that are most likely to benefit from surgical resection. Postoperative mortality and morbidity are low in high-volume hepatopancreaticobiliary (HPB) centers; regionalization of care for these complex problems may further improve outcome. Randomized comparisons of systemic treatments for patients with GBC are also challenging, because of the rarity of the disease and heterogeneity among patients with GBC. Therefore, trials for systemic treatments often combine GBC patients with other biliary cancers [76]. Several studies that used SEER data have shown that the compliance with the NCCN guideline for GBC is very poor [13, 45, 46]. In the most recent evaluated period (2003–2005), a liver resection was performed in only 16 % and a lymphadenectomy in only 5 % of all patients with non-metastatic GBC, stage T1b-3. At a population level, a substantial health gain for patients with GBC is anticipated by simply adhering to national guidelines regarding the indication for surgical resection. Finally, further molecular genetic studies will likely provide insights into disease pathogenesis and reveal novel targets for therapeutic intervention.

Salient Points

- Cholecystectomy is appropriate for patients with a gallbladder polyp larger than 10 mm.
- Open cholecystectomy is recommended for gallbladder polyps with an increased risk of malignancy (e.g., >15 mm): it decreases the chance of bile spillage and associated peritoneal seeding.
- Patients with gallbladder cancer diagnosed at pathologic review after cholecystectomy for cholelithiasis should undergo a (wedge) resection of segments 4b and 5 of the liver with lymphadenectomy of the hepatoduodenal ligament. Exceptions are patients with metastatic disease and nodal involvement beyond the hepatoduodenal ligament, patients with 2 or more extrahepatic organs involvement or invading or encasing the main portal vein and the hepatic artery or T4, and patients who are unfit for surgery.
- A staging laparoscopy prior to definitive resection is recommended in gallbladder cancer patients with an increased risk of peritoneal disease: poorly differentiated or T3 tumors, patients with bile spillage during the cholecystectomy, and patients with non-incidental (symptomatic) gallbladder cancer.
- If gallbladder cancer is suspected during surgery for cholelithiasis and no expertise is available in gallbladder cancer, it is appropriate to refer the patient to a specialized center for staging and a single definitive resection.
- Patients presenting with a mass in the gallbladder suspicious for gallbladder cancer should undergo staging including cross-sectional imaging of the chest, abdomen, and pelvis.
- A biopsy is not recommended before proceeding to surgery in a patient with a gallbladder mass suspicious for gallbladder cancer: the biopsy may cause peritoneal or abdominal wall seeding.
- A 2–3 cm wedge resection of segments 4b and 5 of the liver is sufficient for most patients with gallbladder cancer. Larger liver resections may be justified in some patients.
- Extrahepatic bile duct resection is recommended for patients with a positive margin at the cystic duct after cholecystectomy for presumed benign disease.
- Gallbladder cancer patients presenting with jaundice have a median survival of 6 months and are very unlikely to benefit from surgery.
- Extrahepatic bile duct resection in patients without macroscopic involvement of the extrahepatic bile duct does not improve survival and increases postoperative morbidity and mortality.
- Resection of laparoscopic port sites in patients with gallbladder cancer is not recommended because it does not improve survival.
- After a potentially curative resection for gallbladder cancer, the median overall survival for patients in the SEER database was 16 months, and the 5-year survival rate was 21 %.
- At a median follow-up of 24 months, 66 % of the patients with resected gallbladder cancer had recurred. Of all patients that recur, 85 % will present with metastatic disease with or without locoregional recurrence.
- Adjuvant treatment for gallbladder cancer is recommended with 5-FU or gemcitabine. Addition of cisplatin or oxaliplatin could be considered in high-risk patients.
- Adjuvant radiotherapy could be considered in particular in node-negative gallbladder cancer patients with a positive margin.
- As palliative treatment, the combination of gemcitabine and cisplatin is recommended, based on a large randomized controlled trial.

- Biliary drainage in the palliative setting is only recommended for symptomatic relief and not preemptively, or to allow for chemotherapy. Percutaneous drainage is more likely to be successful and less associated with cholangitis than endoscopic drainage.

Questions

1. A 55-year-old woman is found to have an abnormal gallbladder on ultrasound. Which abnormality does NOT require surgical management?
   A. A gallbladder polyp of 14 mm
   B. Selective mucosal calcification of the gallbladder wall
   C. A gallbladder polyp of 8 mm in a patient with primary sclerosing cholangitis
   D. Adenomyomatosis of the gallbladder wall
   E. A gallbladder mass invading the liver
2. A 69-year-old man is found to have a T3 gallbladder cancer on pathologic review after cholecystectomy for cholelithiasis. What is the next step in management?
   A. Liver resection of segments 4b and 5
   B. Staging laparoscopy
   C. Liver resection of segments 4b and 5 with lymphadenectomy of the hepatoduodenal ligament
   D. Imaging of abdomen and chest
3. A 67-year-old woman is found to have a T1a gallbladder cancer with a negative lymph node at the cystic duct on pathologic review after cholecystectomy for cholelithiasis. What is the next step in management?
   A. Liver resection of segments 4b and 5 with lymphadenectomy of the hepatoduodenal ligament.
   B. Liver resection of segments 4b and 5 without lymphadenectomy.
   C. Lymphadenectomy of the hepatoduodenal ligament without liver resection.
   D. No further surgery is recommended.
4. After introduction of the camera for a planned laparoscopic cholecystectomy in a 72-year-old woman with symptomatic cholelithiasis, the surgeon is concerned that the gallbladder looks suspicious for gallbladder cancer. What is the best next step in management?
   A. Liver resection of segments 4b and 5 en bloc with the gallbladder and bile duct with lymphadenectomy of the hepatoduodenal ligament.
   B. Abort the procedure and refer the patient to a specialized center for staging and a single definitive resection.
   C. Perform a laparoscopic cholecystectomy and refer the patient to a specialized center if pathologic review finds gallbladder cancer.
   D. Liver resection of segments 4b and 5 en bloc with the gallbladder.
5. A 75-year-old woman presents with constant right upper quadrant pain, weight loss, nausea, and vomiting. On ultrasound, she appears to have a large mass in her gallbladder. With which finding on CT of the chest, abdomen, and pelvis is she most likely to benefit from surgery?
   A. Encasement of the main portal vein
   B. Multiple bilateral pulmonary nodules ranging from 1 to 3 cm in diameter
   C. Involvement of the liver parenchyma contiguous with the gallbladder
   D. Enlarged lymph nodes at the root of the celiac artery of which biopsy shows adenocarcinoma
6. A 69-year-old man presents with a large mass in the gallbladder invading the liver on ultrasound. What is the next step in management?
   A. A laparoscopic cholecystectomy.
   B. Perform a percutaneous biopsy of the mass to distinguish gallbladder cancer from xanthogranulomatous cholecystitis.
   C. Perform a CT of the chest, abdomen, and pelvis.
   D. A (wedge) resection of segments 4b and 5 of the liver with lymphadenectomy of the hepatoduodenal ligament.
7. A 62-year-old woman was found to have a T2 gallbladder cancer on pathologic review after laparoscopic cholecystectomy for cholelithiasis. Which of the following procedures is an essential part of the definitive resection?
   A. Resection of the extrahepatic bile duct to clear disease in the submucosal lymphatics of the common bile duct

B. Resection of the port sites because patients often develop port-site metastasis
C. Lymphadenectomy of the hepatoduodenal ligament
D. Right hemihepatectomy because patients often have intrahepatic metastases beyond the segments contiguous with the gallbladder

8. Which patient with gallbladder cancer is most likely to benefit from an extrahepatic bile duct resection?
A. A 67 year-old man presenting with severe jaundice is noted on CT scan to have a gallbladder mass that has invaded the hepatoduodenal ligament
B. A 58-year-old woman presenting with a T1b gallbladder cancer incidentally found at pathologic review after cholecystectomy for cholelithiasis with a positive margin of the cystic duct
C. An 81-year-old woman presenting with a T3 gallbladder cancer incidentally found at pathologic review after cholecystectomy for cholelithiasis with a positive lymph node at the cystic duct
D. A 63-year-old man presenting with constant right upper quadrant pain and nausea and on CT a large mass in the fundus of his gallbladder invading the liver

9. Which of the following findings during an exploratory laparotomy for presumed gallbladder cancer is NOT a justification to refrain from a resection?
A. A single small peritoneal nodule on the anterior abdominal wall demonstrating adenocarcinoma on frozen section
B. A superficial nodule in segment 8 of the liver demonstrating adenocarcinoma on frozen section
C. Adherence of the gallbladder to the transverse colon suspicious for involvement of the transverse colon
D. A slightly enlarged aortocaval lymph node demonstrating adenocarcinoma on frozen section
E. Encasement of the proper hepatic artery

10. A 64-year-old woman presents with right upper quadrant pain without jaundice and on CT a large mass in the fundus of the gallbladder with multiple large pulmonary lesions suspicious for metastatic disease. What is the next step in management?
A. Endoscopic biliary drainage to prevent biliary obstruction
B. A palliative resection to prevent biliary obstruction
C. Percutaneous biliary drainage to prevent biliary obstruction
D. Biopsy of the pulmonary lesions, followed by systemic chemotherapy
E. Palliative radiotherapy to prevent biliary obstruction

Answers
1. D
2. D
3. D
4. B
5. C
6. C
7. C
8. B
9. C
10. D

References

1. Siegel R, Naishadham D, Jemal A. Cancer statistics, 2013. CA Cancer J Clin. 2013;63(1):11–30. PubMed PMID: 23335087.
2. Do Carmo M, Perpetuo MO, Valdivieso M, Heilbrun LK, Nelson RS, Connor T, et al. Natural history study of gallbladder cancer: a review of 36 years experience at M. D Anderson Hospital and Tumor Institute. Cancer. 1978;42(1):330–5. PubMed PMID: 667804.
3. NCCN. Hepatobiliary cancers 2012. 2013. Available from: http://www.nccn.org/professionals/physician_gls/pdf/hepatobiliary.pdf. Cited 27 Feb 2013.
4. Cunningham JD, Fong Y, Shriver C, Melendez J, Marx WL, Blumgart LH. One hundred consecutive hepatic resections. Blood loss, transfusion, and operative technique. Arch Surg. 1994;129(10):1050–6.
5. Randi G, Franceschi S, La Vecchia C. Gallbladder cancer worldwide: geographical distribution and risk factors. Int J Cancer. 2006;118(7):1591–602. PubMed PMID: 16397865.

6. Reid KM, Ramos-De la Medina A, Donohue JH. Diagnosis and surgical management of gallbladder cancer: a review. J Gastrointest Surg. 2007;11(5):671–81. PubMed PMID: 17468929.
7. Yamaguchi K, Chijiiwa K, Shimizu S, Yokohata K, Tsuneyoshi M, Tanaka M. Anatomical limit of extended cholecystectomy for gallbladder carcinoma involving the neck of the gallbladder. Int Surg. 1998;83(1):21–3. PubMed PMID: 9706510.
8. Shirai Y, Yoshida K, Tsukada K, Ohtani T, Muto T. Identification of the regional lymphatic system of the gallbladder by vital staining. Br J Surg. 1992;79(7):659–62. PubMed PMID: 1643479.
9. Edge SB. AJCC cancer staging manual. 7th ed. New York: Springer; 2009.
10. Chaffer CL, Weinberg RA. A perspective on cancer cell metastasis. Science. 2011;331(6024):1559–64. PubMed PMID: 21436443.
11. Tsuji T, Kanemitsu K, Hiraoka T, Takamori H, Toyama E, Tanaka H, et al. A new method to establish the rational extent of hepatic resection for advanced gallbladder cancer using dye injection through the cystic artery. HPB. 2004;6(1):33–66. PubMed PMID: 18333043. Pubmed Central PMCID: 2020642.
12. Wakai T, Shirai Y, Sakata J, Nagahashi M, Ajioka Y, Hatakeyama K. Mode of hepatic spread from gallbladder carcinoma: an immunohistochemical analysis of 42 hepatectomized specimens. Am J Surg Pathol. 2010;34(1):65–74. PubMed PMID: 19956061.
13. Mayo SC, Shore AD, Nathan H, Edil B, Wolfgang CL, Hirose K, et al. National trends in the management and survival of surgically managed gallbladder adenocarcinoma over 15 years: a population-based analysis. J Gastrointest Surg. 2010;14(10):1578–91. PubMed PMID: 20824371.
14. Aldouri AQ, Malik HZ, Waytt J, Khan S, Ranganathan K, Kummaraganti S, et al. The risk of gallbladder cancer from polyps in a large multiethnic series. Eur J Surg Oncol. 2009;35(1):48–51. PubMed PMID: 18339513.
15. Jorgensen T, Jensen KH. Polyps in the gallbladder. A prevalence study. Scand J Gastroenterol. 1990;25(3):281–6. PubMed PMID: 2320947.
16. Segawa K, Arisawa T, Niwa Y, Suzuki T, Tsukamoto Y, Goto H, et al. Prevalence of gallbladder polyps among apparently healthy Japanese: ultrasonographic study. Am J Gastroenterol. 1992;87(5):630–3. PubMed PMID: 1595653.
17. Kozuka S, Tsubone N, Yasui A, Hachisuka K. Relation of adenoma to carcinoma in the gallbladder. Cancer. 1982;50(10):2226–34. PubMed PMID: 7127263.
18. Ito H, Hann LE, D'Angelica M, Allen P, Fong Y, Dematteo RP, et al. Polypoid lesions of the gallbladder: diagnosis and followup. J Am Coll Surg. 2009;208(4):570–5. PubMed PMID: 19476792.
19. Konstantinidis IT, Bajpai S, Kambadakone AR, Tanabe KK, Berger DL, Zheng H, et al. Gallbladder lesions identified on ultrasound. Lessons from the last 10 years. J Gastrointest Surg. 2012;16(3):549–53.
20. Zielinski MD, Atwell TD, Davis PW, Kendrick ML, Que FG. Comparison of surgically resected polypoid lesions of the gallbladder to their pre-operative ultrasound characteristics. J Gastrointest Surg. 2009;13(1):19–25. PubMed PMID: 18972168.
21. Jang JY, Kim SW, Lee SE, Hwang DW, Kim EJ, Lee JY, et al. Differential diagnostic and staging accuracies of high resolution ultrasonography, endoscopic ultrasonography, and multidetector computed tomography for gallbladder polypoid lesions and gallbladder cancer. Ann Surg. 2009;250(6):943–9. PubMed PMID: 19855259.
22. Ouchi K, Mikuni J, Kakugawa Y, Organizing Committee TtACotJSoBS. Laparoscopic cholecystectomy for gallbladder carcinoma: results of a Japanese survey of 498 patients. J Hepatobiliary Pancreat Surg. 2002;9(2):256–60.
23. Lundberg O, Kristoffersson A. Open versus laparoscopic cholecystectomy for gallbladder carcinoma. J Hepatobiliary Pancreat Surg. 2001;8(6):525–9. PubMed PMID: 11956903.
24. Whalen GF, Bird I, Tanski W, Russell JC, Clive J. Laparoscopic cholecystectomy does not demonstrably decrease survival of patients with serendipitously treated gallbladder cancer. J Am Coll Surg. 2001;192(2):189–95. PubMed PMID: 11220719.
25. Wibbenmeyer LA, Wade TP, Chen RC, Meyer RC, Turgeon RP, Andrus CH. Laparoscopic cholecystectomy can disseminate in situ carcinoma of the gallbladder. J Am Coll Surg. 1995;181(6):504–10. PubMed PMID: 7582223.
26. Eelkema HH, Hodgson JR, Stauffer MH. Fifteen-year follow-up of polypoid lesions of the gall bladder diagnosed by cholecystography. Gastroenterology. 1962;42:144–7. PubMed PMID: 13889335.
27. Corwin MT, Siewert B, Sheiman RG, Kane RA. Incidentally detected gallbladder polyps: is follow-up necessary? – Long-term clinical and US analysis of 346 patients. Radiology. 2011;258(1):277–82. PubMed PMID: 20697115.
28. Kubota K, Bandai Y, Noie T, Ishizaki Y, Teruya M, Makuuchi M. How should polypoid lesions of the gallbladder be treated in the era of laparoscopic cholecystectomy? Surgery. 1995;117(5):481–7. PubMed PMID: 7740417.
29. Kim JH, Kim WH, Yoo BM, Kim JH, Kim MW. Should we perform surgical management in all patients with suspected porcelain gallbladder? Hepatogastroenterology. 2009;56(93):943–5. PubMed PMID: 19760916.
30. Stephen AE, Berger DL. Carcinoma in the porcelain gallbladder: a relationship revisited. Surgery. 2001;129(6):699–703. PubMed PMID: 11391368.
31. Towfigh S, McFadden DW, Cortina GR, Thompson Jr JE, Tompkins RK, Chandler C, et al. Porcelain gallbladder is not associated with gallbladder carcinoma. Am Surg. 2001;67(1):7–10. PubMed PMID: 11206901.
32. Kim JH, Jeong IH, Han JH, Kim JH, Hwang JC, Yoo BM, et al. Clinical/pathological analysis of gallbladder adenomyomatosis; type and pathogenesis. Hepatogastroenterology. 2010;57(99–100):420–5. PubMed PMID: 20698201.
33. Houston JP, Collins MC, Cameron I, Reed MW, Parsons MA, Roberts KM. Xanthogranulomatous cholecystitis. Br J Surg. 1994;81(7):1030–2. PubMed PMID: 7922056.

34. Zhao F, Lu PX, Yan SX, Wang GF, Yuan J, Zhang SZ, et al. CT and MR features of xanthogranulomatous cholecystitis: an analysis of consecutive 49 cases. Eur J Radiol. 2013;82:1391–7. PubMed PMID: 23726123.
35. Agarwal AK, Kalayarasan R, Javed A, Sakhuja P. Mass-forming xanthogranulomatous cholecystitis masquerading as gallbladder cancer. J Gastrointest Surg. 2013;17(7):1257–64. PubMed PMID: 23615807.
36. Darmas B, Mahmud S, Abbas A, Baker AL. Is there any justification for the routine histological examination of straightforward cholecystectomy specimens? Ann R Coll Surg Engl. 2007;89(3):238–41. PubMed PMID: 17394706. Pubmed Central PMCID: 1964718.
37. Frauenschuh D, Greim R, Kraas E. How to proceed in patients with carcinoma detected after laparoscopic cholecystectomy. Langenbeck's Arch Surg/Deutsche Gesellschaft fur Chirurgie. 2000;385(8):495–500. PubMed PMID: 11201004.
38. Kwon AH, Imamura A, Kitade H, Kamiyama Y. Unsuspected gallbladder cancer diagnosed during or after laparoscopic cholecystectomy. J Surg Oncol. 2008;97(3):241–5. PubMed PMID: 18095299.
39. Butte JM, Gonen M, Allen PJ, D'Angelica MI, Kingham TP, Fong Y, et al. The role of laparoscopic staging in patients with incidental gallbladder cancer. HPB. 2011;13(7):463–72. PubMed PMID: 21689230. Pubmed Central PMCID: 3133713.
40. Duffy A, Capanu M, Abou-Alfa GK, Huitzil D, Jarnagin W, Fong Y, et al. Gallbladder cancer (GBC): 10-year experience at Memorial Sloan-Kettering Cancer Centre (MSKCC). J Surg Oncol. 2008;98(7):485–9. PubMed PMID: 18802958.
41. Pawlik TM, Gleisner AL, Vigano L, Kooby DA, Bauer TW, Frilling A, et al. Incidence of finding residual disease for incidental gallbladder carcinoma: implications for re-resection. J Gastrointest Surg. 2007;11(11):1478–86. discussion 86–7. PubMed PMID: 17846848.
42. Lee SE, Jang JY, Lim CS, Kang MJ, Kim SW. Systematic review on the surgical treatment for T1 gallbladder cancer. World J Gastroenterol. 2011;17(2):174–80. PubMed PMID: 21245989. Pubmed Central PMCID: 3020370.
43. Goetze TO, Paolucci V. Immediate re-resection of T1 incidental gallbladder carcinomas: a survival analysis of the German Registry. Surg Endosc. 2008; 22(11):2462–5. PubMed PMID: 18247090.
44. Hari DM, Howard JH, Leung AM, Chui CG, Sim MS, Bilchik AJ. A 21-year analysis of stage I gallbladder carcinoma: is cholecystectomy alone adequate? HPB. 2013;15(1):40–8. PubMed PMID: 23216778. Pubmed Central PMCID: 3533711.
45. Coburn NG, Cleary SP, Tan JC, Law CH. Surgery for gallbladder cancer: a population-based analysis. J Am Coll Surg. 2008;207(3):371–82. PubMed PMID: 18722943.
46. Jensen EH, Abraham A, Habermann EB, Al-Refaie WB, Vickers SM, Virnig BA, et al. A critical analysis of the surgical management of early-stage gallbladder cancer in the United States. J Gastrointest Surg. 2009;13(4):722–7. PubMed PMID: 19083068.
47. Goetze TO, Paolucci V. Benefits of reoperation of T2 and more advanced incidental gallbladder carcinoma: analysis of the German registry. Ann Surg. 2008;247(1):104–8. PubMed PMID: 18156929.
48. Fong Y, Jarnagin W, Blumgart LH. Gallbladder cancer: comparison of patients presenting initially for definitive operation with those presenting after prior noncurative intervention. Ann Surg. 2000;232(4):557–69. PubMed PMID: 10998654. Pubmed Central PMCID: 1421188.
49. Reddy SK, Marroquin CE, Kuo PC, Pappas TN, Clary BM. Extended hepatic resection for gallbladder cancer. Am J Surg. 2007;194(3):355–61. PubMed PMID: 17693282.
50. Petrowsky H, Wildbrett P, Husarik DB, Hany TF, Tam S, Jochum W, et al. Impact of integrated positron emission tomography and computed tomography on staging and management of gallbladder cancer and cholangiocarcinoma. J Hepatol. 2006;45(1):43–50. PubMed PMID: 16690156.
51. Corvera CU, Blumgart LH, Akhurst T, DeMatteo RP, D'Angelica M, Fong Y, et al. 18F-fluorodeoxyglucose positron emission tomography influences management decisions in patients with biliary cancer. J Am Coll Surg. 2008;206(1):57–65. PubMed PMID: 18155569.
52. Bickenbach KA, Shia J, Klimstra DS, DeMatteo RP, Fong Y, Kingham TP, et al. High-grade dysplasia of the cystic duct margin in the absence of malignancy after cholecystectomy. HPB. 2011;13(12):865–8. PubMed PMID: 22081921. Pubmed Central PMCID: 3244625.
53. Shih SP, Schulick RD, Cameron JL, Lillemoe KD, Pitt HA, Choti MA, et al. Gallbladder cancer: the role of laparoscopy and radical resection. Ann Surg. 2007;245(6):893–901. PubMed PMID: 17522515. Pubmed Central PMCID: 1876959.
54. Grobmyer SR, Lieberman MD, Daly JM. Gallbladder cancer in the twentieth century: single institution's experience. World J Surg. 2004;28(1):47–9. PubMed PMID: 14639492.
55. Glenn F, Hill Jr MR. Primary gallbladder disease in children. Ann Surg. 1954;139(3):302–11. PubMed PMID: 13149075. Pubmed Central PMCID: 1609429.
56. Pack GT, Miller TR, Brasfield RD. Total right hepatic lobectomy for cancer of the gallbladder; report of three cases. Ann Surg. 1955;142(1):6–16. PubMed PMID: 14388606. Pubmed Central PMCID: 1465049.
57. Endo I, Shimada H, Takimoto A, Fujii Y, Miura Y, Sugita M, et al. Microscopic liver metastasis: prognostic factor for patients with pT2 gallbladder carcinoma. World J Surg. 2004;28(7):692–6. PubMed PMID: 15175901.
58. Araida T, Higuchi R, Hamano M, Kodera Y, Takeshita N, Ota T, et al. Hepatic resection in 485 R0 pT2 and pT3 cases of advanced carcinoma of the gallbladder: results of a Japanese Society of Biliary Surgery survey – a multicenter study. J Hepatobiliary Pancreat Surg. 2009;16(2):204–15. PubMed PMID: 19219399.
59. Nagino M, Kamiya J, Nishio H, Ebata T, Arai T, Nimura Y. Two hundred forty consecutive portal vein embolizations before extended hepatectomy for biliary cancer: surgical outcome and long-term follow-up. Ann Surg. 2006;243(3):364–72. PubMed PMID: 16495702. Pubmed Central PMCID: 1448943.

60. Nishio H, Ebata T, Yokoyama Y, Igami T, Sugawara G, Nagino M. Gallbladder cancer involving the extrahepatic bile duct is worthy of resection. Ann Surg. 2011;253(5):953–60. PubMed PMID: 21490453.
61. Ogura Y, Mizumoto R, Isaji S, Kusuda T, Matsuda S, Tabata M. Radical operations for carcinoma of the gallbladder: present status in Japan. World J Surg. 1991;15(3):337–43. PubMed PMID: 1853612.
62. Hawkins WG, DeMatteo RP, Jarnagin WR, Ben-Porat L, Blumgart LH, Fong Y. Jaundice predicts advanced disease and early mortality in patients with gallbladder cancer. Ann Surg Oncol. 2004;11(3):310–5.
63. Kohya N, Miyazaki K. Hepatectomy of segment 4a and 5 combined with extra-hepatic bile duct resection for T2 and T3 gallbladder carcinoma. J Surg Oncol. 2008;97(6):498–502. PubMed PMID: 18314875.
64. Shimizu Y, Ohtsuka M, Ito H, Kimura F, Shimizu H, Togawa A, et al. Should the extrahepatic bile duct be resected for locally advanced gallbladder cancer? Surgery. 2004;136(5):1012–7. discussion 8. PubMed PMID: 15523394.
65. Araida T, Higuchi R, Hamano M, Kodera Y, Takeshita N, Ota T, et al. Should the extrahepatic bile duct be resected or preserved in R0 radical surgery for advanced gallbladder carcinoma? Results of a Japanese Society of Biliary Surgery Survey: a multicenter study. Surg Today. 2009;39(9):770–9. PubMed PMID: 19779773.
66. D'Angelica M, Dalal KM, DeMatteo RP, Fong Y, Blumgart LH, Jarnagin WR. Analysis of the extent of resection for adenocarcinoma of the gallbladder. Ann Surg Oncol. 2009;16(4):806–16. PubMed PMID: 18985272.
67. Shukla PJ, Barreto SG. Systematic review: should routine resection of the extra-hepatic bile duct be performed in gallbladder cancer? Saudi J Gastroenterol. 2010;16(3):161–7. PubMed PMID: 20616410. Pubmed Central PMCID: 3003211.
68. Maker AV, Butte JM, Oxenberg J, Kuk D, Gonen M, Fong Y, et al. Is port site resection necessary in the surgical management of gallbladder cancer? Ann Surg Oncol. 2012;19(2):409–17. PubMed PMID: 21698501.
69. Jarnagin WR, Gonen M, Fong Y, DeMatteo RP, Ben-Porat L, Little S, et al. Improvement in perioperative outcome after hepatic resection: analysis of 1,803 consecutive cases over the past decade. Ann Surg. 2002;236(4):397–406. discussion -7. PubMed PMID: 12368667. Pubmed Central PMCID: 1422593.
70. Melendez JA, Arslan V, Fischer ME, Wuest D, Jarnagin WR, Fong Y, et al. Perioperative outcomes of major hepatic resections under low central venous pressure anesthesia: blood loss, blood transfusion, and the risk of postoperative renal dysfunction. J Am Coll Surg. 1998;187(6):620–5. PubMed PMID: 9849736.
71. Fong Y, Brennan MF, Brown K, Heffernan N, Blumgart LH. Drainage is unnecessary after elective liver resection. Am J Surg. 1996;171(1):158–62. PubMed PMID: 8554132.
72. Ito H, Ito K, D'Angelica M, Gonen M, Klimstra D, Allen P, et al. Accurate staging for gallbladder cancer: implications for surgical therapy and pathological assessment. Ann Surg. 2011;254(2):320–5. PubMed PMID: 21617582.
73. Lillemoe KD, Jarnagin W. Hepatobiliary and pancreatic surgery. J.E. F, editor. Philadelphia: Wolters Kluwer; 2013.
74. Clavien PA, Sarr MG, Fong Y. Atlas of upper gastrointestinal and hepato-pancreato-biliary surgery. Berlin: Springer; 2007.
75. Jarnagin WR, Ruo L, Little SA, Klimstra D, D'Angelica M, DeMatteo RP, et al. Patterns of initial disease recurrence after resection of gallbladder carcinoma and hilar cholangiocarcinoma: implications for adjuvant therapeutic strategies. Cancer. 2003;98(8):1689–700. PubMed PMID: 14534886.
76. Valle J, Wasan H, Palmer DH, Cunningham D, Anthoney A, Maraveyas A, et al. Cisplatin plus gemcitabine versus gemcitabine for biliary tract cancer. N Engl J Med. 2010;362(14):1273–81. PubMed PMID: 20375404.
77. Sharma A, Dwary AD, Mohanti BK, Deo SV, Pal S, Sreenivas V, et al. Best supportive care compared with chemotherapy for unresectable gall bladder cancer: a randomized controlled study. J Clin Oncol. 2010; 28(30):4581–6. PubMed PMID: 20855823.
78. Wang SJ, Fuller CD, Kim JS, Sittig DF, Thomas Jr CR, Ravdin PM. Prediction model for estimating the survival benefit of adjuvant radiotherapy for gallbladder cancer. J Clin Oncol. 2008;26(13):2112–7. PubMed PMID: 18378567.
79. Gruenberger B, Schueller J, Heubrandtner U, Wrba F, Tamandl D, Kaczirek K, et al. Cetuximab, gemcitabine, and oxaliplatin in patients with unresectable advanced or metastatic biliary tract cancer: a phase 2 study. Lancet Oncol. 2010;11(12):1142–8. PubMed PMID: 21071270.
80. Lee J, Park SH, Chang HM, Kim JS, Choi HJ, Lee MA, et al. Gemcitabine and oxaliplatin with or without erlotinib in advanced biliary-tract cancer: a multicentre, open-label, randomised, phase 3 study. Lancet Oncol. 2012;13(2):181–8. PubMed PMID: 22192731.
81. Saluja SS, Gulati M, Garg PK, Pal H, Pal S, Sahni P, et al. Endoscopic or percutaneous biliary drainage for gallbladder cancer: a randomized trial and quality of life assessment. Clin Gastroenterol Hepatol. 2008;6(8):944–50. e3. PubMed PMID: 18585976.
82. Robson PC, Heffernan N, Gonen M, Thornton R, Brody LA, Holmes R, et al. Prospective study of outcomes after percutaneous biliary drainage for malignant biliary obstruction. Ann Surg Oncol. 2010;17(9):2303–11. PubMed PMID: 20358300.
83. Hueman MT, Vollmer Jr CM, Pawlik TM. Evolving treatment strategies for gallbladder cancer. Ann Surg Oncol. 2009;16(8):2101–15. PubMed PMID: 19495882.
84. Compton CC, Byrd DR, Garcia-Aguilar J, et al. Gallbladder. In: Compton CC, Byrd DR, Garcia-Aguilar J, et al., editors. AJCC cancer staging atlas. New York: Springer; 2012. p. 259–68.

12 Cholangiocarcinoma

Parham Mafi, Quyen D. Chu, Richard R. Smith, and John F. Gibbs

Learning Objectives

After reading this chapter, you should be able to:

- Recognize the risk factors and presentation of cholangiocarcinoma.
- Understand the classification and staging of intrahepatic/extrahepatic cholangiocarcinoma.
- Be familiar with the diagnosis of cholangiocarcinoma and assessment of resectability.
- Understand the current trends for medical and surgical management of cholangiocarcinoma.
- Recognize the areas for potential future research and development

Background

Cholangiocarcinoma (CCA) is a rare but lethal cancer arising from the bile duct epithelium. As a whole, CCA accounts for approximately 3 % of all gastrointestinal cancers. It is an aggressive disease with a high mortality rate. Unfortunately, a significant proportion of patients with CCA present with either unresectable or metastatic disease. In a retrospective review of 225 patients with hilar cholangiocarcinoma, Jarnagin et al. reported that 29 % of patients had either unresectable disease were unfit for surgery [1].

CCA can be classified as being intrahepatic cholangiocarcinoma (ICC) or extrahepatic cholangiocarcinoma (ECC), based on the location of the tumor. ECC is divided into perihilar and distal cholangiocarcinoma (Fig. 12.1). By definition, perihilar ECC are those that arise above the confluence of cystic and common hepatic duct, mid-bile duct are those that arise between the confluence of cystic duct and common bile duct and the upper border of the duodenum, and distal CCA are those located in the duodenal and intrapancreatic portion of bile duct up to the ampulla of Vater. Intrahepatic cholangiocarcinoma (ICC) is variably defined as arising from the second or more distal branches of the intrahepatic bile ducts or involving the intrahepatic ducts not extending into the hepatic hilum [2–4]. Regardless of its classification, CCA is characterized by late diagnosis and poor outcomes.

P. Mafi, M.D.
Department of Surgery, SUNY Buffalo,
100 High St., Buffalo, NY 14203, USA
e-mail: Mafi.Parham@gmail.com

Q.D. Chu, M.D., MBA, FACS
Department of Surgery, LSU Health Sciences Center-Shreveport, 1501 Kings Hwy,
P.O. Box 33932, Shreveport, LA 71130-3932, USA
e-mail: qchu@lsuhsc.edu

R.R. Smith, M.D.
Department of Surgery, Tripler Army Medical Center,
1 Jarrett White Rd., Honolulu, HI 96859, USA
e-mail: rsmith5874@yahoo.com

J.F. Gibbs, M.D. (✉)
Department of Surgery, Jersey Shore University Medical Center/Meridian Heath,
1945 State Highway 33, 4 floor Ackerman,
Neptune, NJ 07753, USA
e-mail: jgibbs@meridianhealth.com

Q.D. Chu et al. (eds.), *Surgical Oncology: A Practical and Comprehensive Approach*,
DOI 10.1007/978-1-4939-1423-4_12, © Springer Science+Business Media New York 2015

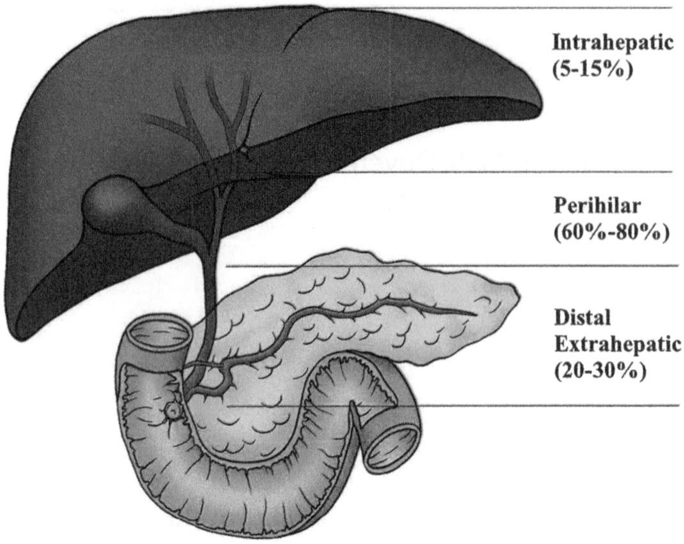

Fig. 12.1 *Anatomic location of cholangiocarcinoma subtypes*: CCA can be classified as being intrahepatic cholangiocarcinoma (ICC) or extrahepatic cholangiocarcinoma (ECC), based on the location of the tumor. ECC is divided into perihilar and distal cholangiocarcinoma. By definition, perihilar ECC are those that arise above the confluence of cystic and common hepatic duct, mid-bile duct are those that arise between the confluence of cystic duct and common bile duct and the upper border of the duodenum, and distal CCA are those located in the duodenal and intrapancreatic portion of bile duct up to the ampulla of Vater. Intrahepatic cholangiocarcinoma (ICC) is variably defined as arising from the second or more distal branches of the intrahepatic bile ducts or involving the intrahepatic ducts not extending into the hepatic hilum (Courtesy of Quyen D. Chu, MD, MBA, FACS)

Although ICC and ECC are often histologically indistinguishable, they are distinct from one another in their presentation, prognostic factors, and growth characteristics [5, 6]. Patients with ICC typically present with abdominal pain and an intrahepatic mass, whereas patients with ECC present with painless jaundice [7]. CCA should be considered in any patient who presents with obstructive jaundice. This review will focus on the surgical treatments and management of both ECC and ICC.

Incidence

CCA is an uncommon tumor with an overall incidence about 1 in 100,000 people annually in the United States. The majority of these tumors occur at the hepatic duct bifurcation (60–80 %). ICC is the second most common primary hepatic malignancy representing 5–15 % of all tumors [5, 8]. There is a marked geographic variability in the incidence of cholangiocarcinoma, the highest occurring in the Far East. The incidence of ICC in the United States and the United Kingdom has risen recently, in contrast to ECC, which appears to be decreasing [9, 10]. The rise in ICC incidence may be related to better awareness of the disease and improved diagnosis with immunohistochemistry techniques. Another factor that may contribute to ICC rising incidence is the increased immigration from high prevalent regions of the world [9, 11].

Etiology

A number of risk factors have been linked to CCA, and they are parasitic infections (e.g., *Clonorchis sinensis* and *Opisthorchis viverrini*) which are endemic in Japan and Southeast Asia, hepatolithiasis, diabetes, smoking, cirrhosis, hepatitis C virus (HCV), prior biliary-enteric anastomosis, and congenital choledochal cyst [4, 12, 13]. Other predisposing conditions include primary sclerosing cholangitis (PSC), Caroli's disease, and exposure to the contrast-medium thorotrast [4, 7, 14]. Chronic inflammation and/or injury to the bile duct epithelium are a common theme in

Table 12.1 Comparison of preexisting medical conditions among patients with extrahepatic cholangiocarcinoma, intrahepatic cholangiocarcinoma, and controls

	ECC ($n=549$)			ICC ($n=535$)			Controls ($n=102,782$)	
Condition	*N*	%	*P* value[a]	*N*	%	*P* value[a]	*N*	%
Bilary tract conditions/operations								
Choledochal cysts	27	4.9	<0.001	21	3.9	<0.001	108	0.1
Cholangitis	50	9.1	<0.001	67	12.5	<0.001	201	0.2
Biliary cirrhosis	<5	<0.9	0.003	5	0.9	<0.001	53	0.1
Cholelithiasis	202	36.8	<0.001	172	32.1	<0.001	4,273	4.2
Choledocholithiasis	87	15.8	<0.001	59	11	<0.001	543	0.5
Cholecystitis	42	7.7	<0.001	29	5.4	<0.001	973	0.9
Cholecystectomy	87	15.8	<0.001	41	7.7	<0.001	1,649	1.6
Chronic liver diseases								
Alcoholic liver disease	8	1.5	<0.001	5	0.9	0.008	310	0.3
Nonspecific cirrhosis	10	2 8	<0.001	17	3.2	<0.001	359	0.3
Hemochromatosis	<5	<0.9	0.25	<5	<0.9	0.05	282	0.3
Chronic nonalcoholic liver disease	<5	<0.9	0.08	5	0.9	0.03	353	0.3
HCV infection	<5	<0.9	0.36	<5	<0.9	0.03	142	0.1
Endocrine disorders								
Diabetes mellitus type II	165	30.1	<0.001	177	33.1	<0.001	22,764	22.1
Thyrotoxicosis	30	5.5	0.04	27	5	0.12	3,864	3.8
Digestive disorders								
IBD	10	1.8	0.03	18	3.4	<0.001	936	0.9
Crohn's disease	6	1.1	0.02	5	0.9	0.06	419	0.4
Ulcerative colitis	5	0.9	0.11	13	2.4	<0.001	595	0.6
Duodenal ulcer	20	3.6	0.001	34	6.4	<0.001	1,836	1.8
Chronic pancreatitis	13	2.4	<0.001	8	1.5	<0.001	272	0.3
Miscellaneous conditions								
Smoking	12	2.2	0.03	12	2.2	0.02	1,212	1.2
Obesity	16	2.9	0.79	23	4.3	0.12	3,201	3.1

Reprinted from Welzel et al. [13]. With permission from W.B. Saunders Co.
ECC extrahepatic cholangiocarcinoma, *HCV* hepatitis C virus, *IBD* inflammatory bowel disease, *ICC* intrahepatic cholangiocarcinoma
[a]Fisher exact test used to compute *p* value when $n<5$

all of these conditions (Table 12.1). The most common predisposing condition associated with CCA in the Western hemisphere is PSC, with a reported lifetime incidence of CCA between 6 and 10 % [7, 15].

Presentation, Diagnosis, and Assessment of Resectability

Painless jaundice is the most common presentation of ECC (i.e., perihilar or distal tumors). Patients with ICC typically present with abdominal pain, fever/chills, or an incidental liver mass found on imaging studies during a work-up for something else [5]. There are no specific blood tests or tumor markers that are diagnostic for CCA. However, a CA 19-9 level greater than 100 U/ml has been reported to predict the likelihood of malignancy in patients with PSC (sensitivity: 75–89 %; specificity: 80–86 %) and risk of recurrence after surgical resection [16]. When such a rise in CA 19-9 occurs in a patient without a history of PSC, the sensitivity decreases to 53–68 % but specificity increases up to 87 % [17, 18].

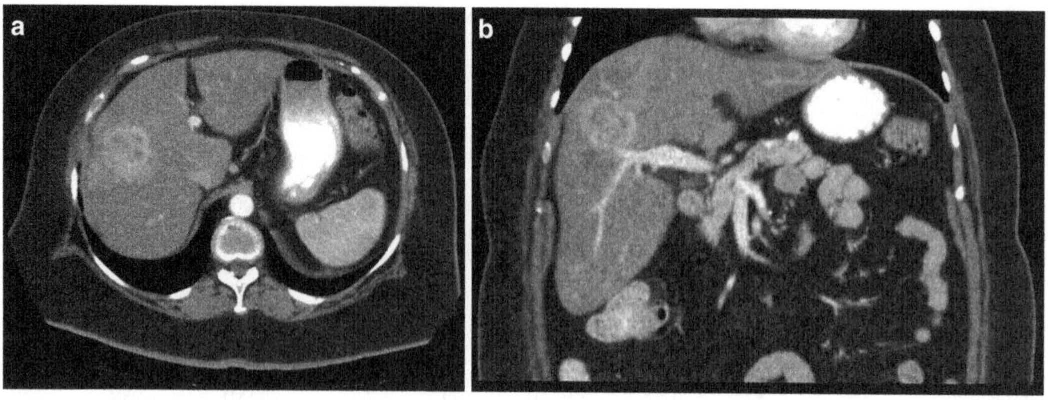

Fig. 12.2 A 72-year-old woman with an intrahepatic cholangiocarcinoma of the right lobe of the liver (**a**) axial and (**b**) coronal CT images. She underwent a successful right hepatectomy (Courtesy of Gazi B. Zibari, MD, FACS)

Carcinoembryonic antigen (CEA) is commonly monitored along with CA 19-9 when the diagnosis of cholangiocarcinoma is being entertained. Elevation of either CA 19-9 or CEA in isolation is not helpful, but in the proper clinical setting, it may increase the accuracy of diagnosing CCA. A Ramage score, which combines CA 19-9 and CEA, when elevated in a patient with PSC has a sensitivity and specificity of 71 % and 91 %, respectively [19].

Typically at the time of presentation, patients with ECC tend to have a total serum bilirubin above 10 mg/dL. An elevated alkaline phosphatase level higher than 5 times normal usually accompanies the elevated bilirubin levels, although these values are not specific enough for making the diagnosis. Patients can present with symptoms associated with cholestasis, such as pruritus, cholangitis, pale stool, and weight loss [20].

Radiologic evaluation includes ultrasound (U/S), computed tomography (CT), magnetic resonance imaging (MRI) and/or multi-detector-row computed tomography (MDCT), and magnetic resonance cholangiopancreatography (MRCP). Data on positron-emission tomography (PET) is limited. Ultrasound (U/S) has limited utility in diagnosis CCA, although it is often the first test performed. U/S is helpful in patients with obstructive jaundice so as to exclude the diagnosis of cholelithiasis and choledocholithiasis, since these conditions are more common than ECC.

In many centers, triphasic CT scan is the diagnostic test of choice to visualize the cancer and assess its relationship with adjacent vascular structures. CT is also useful to stage the patient since it could detect distant metastases. ICC typically shows hyperattenuation on delayed intravenous contrast images because of interstitial uptake of contrast medium in the tumor [21, 22] (Figs. 12.2 and 12.3). The percentage of tumor volume showing delayed uptake has been shown to correlate with increased fibrous stroma, perineural invasion, and worse prognosis [23]. On CT scans, both ICC and metastatic colorectal cancers have central hypointensity, but ICC typically has peritumoral biliary dilatation.

A hilar cholangiocarcinoma will have a picture of dilated intrahepatic biliary tree, with normal or collapsed gallbladder and extrahepatic biliary tree. Distal tumors present with dilation of the gallbladder and both the extra- and intrahepatic biliary tree. In other centers, MRI is the diagnostic imaging of choice. MRI is very accurate in delineating the longitudinal and lateral spread of extrahepatic cholangiocarcinoma and determining resectability. MRCP has also been utilized in evaluating patients with CCA (Fig. 12.4). It is accurate in defining the biliary tree, determining the site of obstruction, and is comparable to endoscopic retrograde cholangiopancreatography (ERCP) [24]. Both MRI and MRCP are the diagnostic of choice for perihilar cholangiocarcinoma.

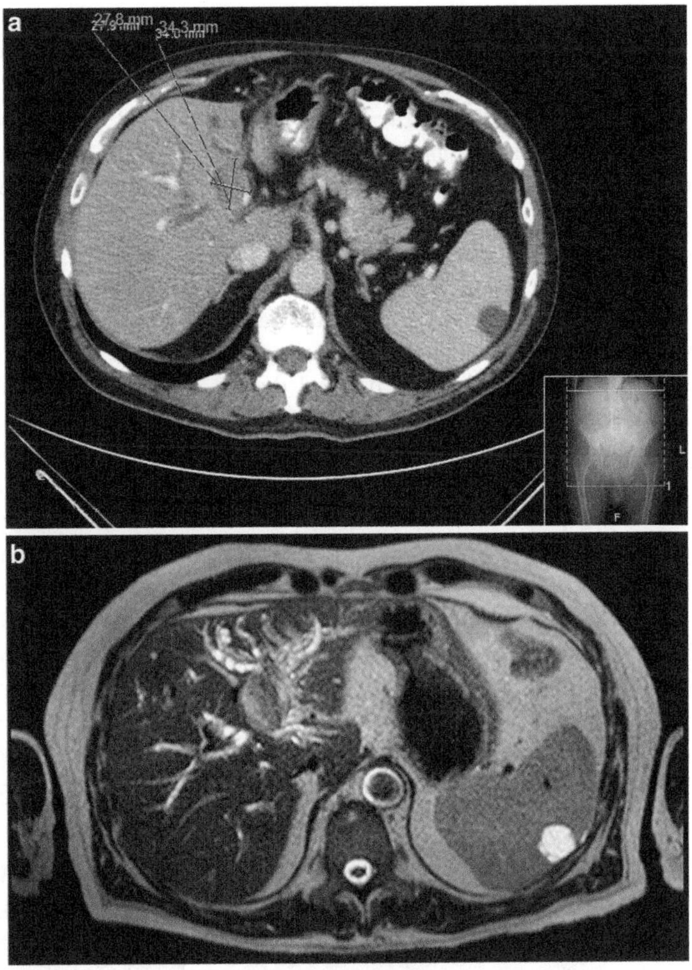

Fig. 12.3 A 73-year-old man with intrahepatic cholangiocarcinoma of the left lobe of the liver. (**a**) CT scan, (**b**) MRI. He underwent a successful left hepatectomy (Courtesy of Gazi B. Zibari, MD, FACS)

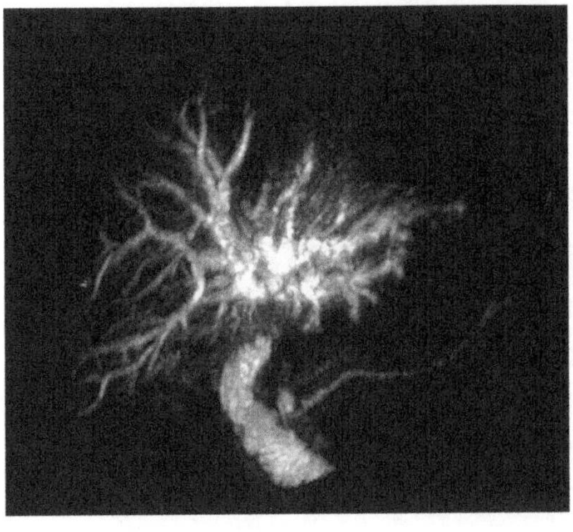

Fig. 12.4 MRCP of a patient with Klatskin's tumor (Courtesy of Gazi B. Zibari, MD, FACS)

As already mentioned, ICC generally presents as a solid liver mass. As such, a preoperative tissue diagnosis is often not necessary. The mass represents either a metastatic lesion (which is a more common situation) or a primary liver tumor. Diagnostic work-up for such a mass generally entails a search for a primary which includes a colonoscopy and upper endoscopy to rule out a gastrointestinal source, review of a chest X-ray to rule-out primary lung, and for women, a mammogram and examination of the breast to exclude breast cancer. In addition, a careful review of CT scans, preferably with a radiologist, is essential not only to characterize the liver lesion but also to evaluate the pancreas and other solid organs as possible primary tumors that give rise to the liver lesion.

It is not uncommon for the surgeon to be asked to evaluate a patient who already had a liver biopsy of a solid mass and the pathology reveals an adenocarcinoma. In such a case, the possibility of an ICC should be entertained if there is no obvious primary tumor. Because it is difficult to differentiate ICC adenocarcinoma from metastatic adenocarcinoma, a panel of immunohistochemistry stainings can be helpful. Although there is no specific stain for ICC, a particular pattern of stains can assist at making the diagnosis (positive, CK7+, CK20- with biliary epithelial dysplasia, AE1/AE3; negative, TTF1, CDX2, DPC4) [25]. Regardless, the majority of patients with liver masses should be considered for surgical resection after a proper work-up has been performed. ICC is generally diagnosed after the surgery.

For patients with extrahepatic cholangiocarcinoma, a preoperative tissue diagnosis is also not necessary for surgical intervention. Patients who present with jaundice and dilated biliary tree but have no evidence of biliary stones or intrinsic hepatic disease should be considered to have a malignancy unless proven otherwise. Most hilar strictures are cholangiocarcinoma although 10–15 % of patients may have alternative diagnosis such as gallbladder cancer, Mirizzi syndrome, and idiopathic benign focal stenosis [26]. Gallbladder cancer generally presents with a thickened, irregular, and distended gallbladder, whereas hilar cholangiocarcinoma generally presents with a shrunken gallbladder. Mirizzi syndrome is a benign condition whereby a large gallstone that is impacted in the cystic duct or neck of the gallbladder causes extrinsic compression against the common hepatic duct [27].

Benign biliary strictures at the hepatic duct confluence are rare and can often mimic malignancy. Unfortunately, there is no diagnostic test that accurately distinguishes biliary strictures from malignancy. Thus, a negative biopsy does not necessarily rule out the possibility of a cancer, and therefore, surgeons should be cognizant of this and carefully weigh the risk and benefits of observation versus resection. As a general rule, in the absence of a clear contraindication, all hilar strictures/lesions should be considered for surgical exploration (Fig. 12.5).

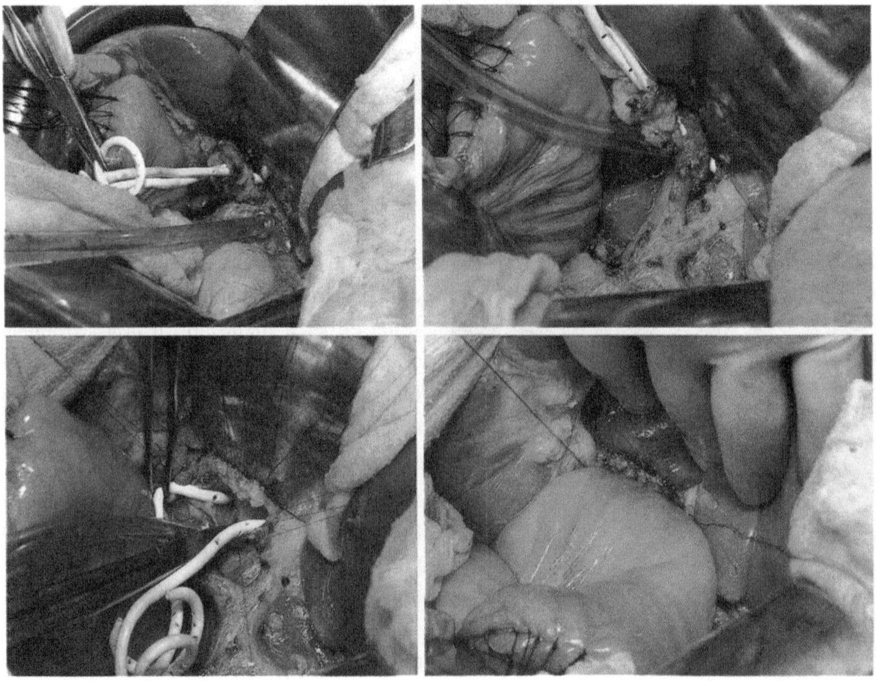

Fig. 12.5 A patient with biliary stricture at the hepatic duct bifurcation. Preoperative work-up was nondiagnostic. She underwent resection and a Roux-en-Y hepaticojejunostomy. The final pathology was a benign lesion (Courtesy of Gazi B. Zibari, MD, FACS)

For patients with obstructive jaundice without evidence of a hilar stricture or a mass in the head of the pancreas, the possibility of distal cholangiocarcinoma should be considered. Endoscopic ultrasound with biopsy can be helpful, although a negative biopsy does not exclude carcinoma and/or alter management in those who have no contraindications for surgery.

Staging and Classification

Staging of Intrahepatic Cholangiocarcinoma

Several staging and classification systems are currently being used for ICC, but the American Joint Committee on Cancer (AJCC/International) Union against Cancer (UICC) TNM classification system is the one that is widely used in the United States (Table 12.2). Historically, the staging systems for ICC and hepatocellular carcinoma were identical. However, the latest 7th edition of (AJCC/UICC) separated ICC into a separate entity based on data involving nearly 600 patients from the Surveillance, Epidemiology, and End Results (SEER) database as well as other international multicenter data [29–31]. Note that tumor size has no prognostic impact in ICC.

The Liver Cancer Study Group of Japan (LCSGJ) developed a classification system from more than 240 resected cases of ICC that is specifically based on macroscopic appearance: mass forming (MF), periductal infiltrating (PI), and intraductal growth (IG) [32] (Fig. 12.6). MF type forms a definite mass within the liver parenchyma. The PI type extends mainly longitudinally along the bile duct and often resulting in dilatation of the peripheral bile duct. The IG type proliferates toward the lumen of the bile duct papillarity or like a tumor thrombus [32]. Tumors can have more than one macroscopic appearance and in such cases, they are described with the predominant type mentioned first followed by the subordinate type separated by a "+" (i.e., mass forming + periductal infiltrating).

Table 12.2 American Joint Committee on Cancer (AJCC) TNM staging for intrahepatic bile ducts (7th edition)

Primary tumor (T)	
TX	Primary tumor cannot be assessed
T0	No evidence of primary tumor
Tis	Carcinoma in situ (intraductal tumor)
T1	Solitary tumor without vascular invasion
T2a	Solitary tumor with vascular invasion
T2b	Multiple tumors, with or without vascular invasion
T3	Tumor perforating the visceral peritoneum or involving the local extrahepatic structures by direct invasion
T4	Tumor with periductal invasion

Regional lymph nodes (N)	
NX	Regional lymph nodes cannot be assessed
N0	No regional lymph node metastasis
N1	Regional lymph node metastasis present

Distant metastasis (M)	
M0	No distant metastasis
M1	Distant metastasis present

Anatomic stage/prognostic groups			
Group	T	N	M
Stage 0	Tis	N0	M0
Stage 1	T1	N0	M0
Stage II	T2	N0	M0
Stage III	T3	N0	M0
Stage IVA	T4	N0	M0
Stage IVB	Any T	N1	M0
	Any T	Any N	M1

Adapted from Compton et al. [28]. With permission from Springer Verlag

MF is the most common subtype, representing approximately 60–80 % of ICC. PI and IG make up 15–35 % and 8–29 % of ICC, respectively. The macroscopic appearance of the disease reflects tumor cells with different biologic behavior. The biologic difference of these types is underscored by the differences in the 1-year overall survival (OS) rate of patients with ICC. MF has the best prognosis while MF+PI has the worst; the 1-year OS for MF, PI, and MF+PI are 80 %, 69, and 39 %, respectively ($P=0.0072$) [33].

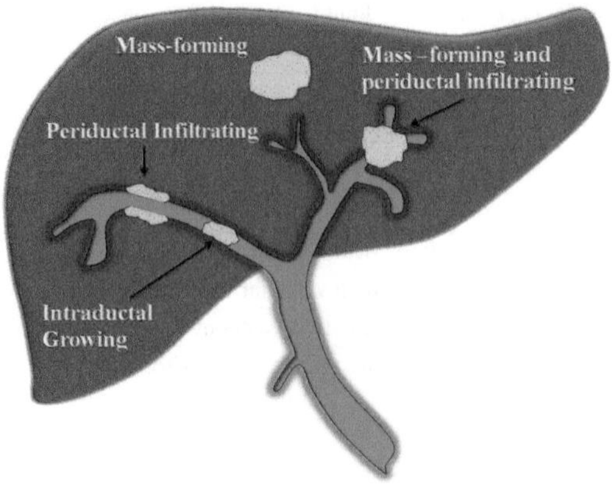

Fig. 12.6 The Liver Cancer Study Group of Japan (LCSGJ) developed a classification system of ICC: mass forming (MF), periductal infiltrating (PI), and intraductal growth (IG). MF type forms a definite mass within the liver parenchyma. The PI type extends mainly longitudinally along the bile duct and often resulting in dilatation of the peripheral bile duct. The IG type proliferates toward the lumen of the bile duct papillarity or like a tumor thrombus. Tumors can have more than one macroscopic appearance, and in such cases, they are described with the predominant type mentioned first followed by the subordinate type separated by a "+" (i.e., mass forming + periductal infiltrating) (Courtesy of Quyen D. Chu, MD, MBA, FACS)

Staging of Extrahepatic Cholangiocarcinoma

Perihilar cholangiocarcinomas are also staged according to the AJCC/UICC TNM system (Table 12.3), although they are more commonly classified according to their anatomic location and extent of ductal infiltration based on the Bismuth-Corlette classification (Fig. 12.7). Such a classification is useful because it approaches perihilar cholangiocarcinomas from a surgical perspective; the location and extent of disease determines how one surgically approach and resect the tumor. Type I tumors are limited to or confined to the common hepatic duct, type II involve the confluence of the right and left hepatic ducts, and types IIIa and IIIb are tumors of common hepatic duct that extend to either the right (IIIa) or left hepatic duct (IIIb). Type IV tumors involve both the secondary bile ducts on both right and left hepatic duct [35, 36]. For types I–IIIa Bismuth-Corlette hilar cholangiocarcinoma, an extended right hepatectomy is the procedure of choice, whereas a left or extended left hepatectomy is used for type IIIb hilar cholangiocarcinoma [37].

Distal cholangiocarcinoma is staged using the AJCC/UICC TNM classification system (Table 12.4).

Table 12.3 American Joint Committee on Cancer (AJCC) TNM staging for perihilar bile ducts (7th edition)

Primary tumor (T)	
TX	Primary tumor cannot be assessed
T0	No evidence of primary tumor
Tis	Carcinoma in situ
T1	Tumor confined to the bile duct, with extension up to the muscle layer or fibrous tissue
T2a	Tumor invades beyond the wall of the bile duct to surrounding adipose tissue
T2b	Tumor invades adjacent hepatic parenchyma
T3	Tumor invades unilateral branches of the portal vein or hepatic artery
T4	Tumor invades main portal vein or its branches bilaterally; or the common hepatic artery; or the second-order biliary radicals bilaterally; or unilateral second-order biliary radicals with contralateral portal vein or hepatic artery involvement

Regional lymph nodes (N)	
NX	Regional lymph nodes cannot be assessed
N0	No regional lymph node metastasis
N1	Regional lymph node metastasis (including nodes along the cystic duct, common bile duct, hepatic artery, and portal vein)
N2	Metastasis to periaortic, pericaval, superior mesenteric artery, and/or celiac artery lymph nodes

Distant metastasis (M)	
M0	No distant metastasis
M1	Distant metastasis present

Anatomic stage/prognostic groups			
Group	T	N	M
Stage 0	Tis	N0	M0
Stage 1	T1	N0	M0
Stage II	T2a-b	N0	M0
Stage IIIA	T3	N0	M0
Stage IIIB	T1-3	N1	M0
Stage IVA	T4	N0-1	M0
Stage IVB	Any T	N2	M0
	Any T	Any N	M1

Adapted from Compton et al. [34]. With permission from Springer Verlag

Type	Bismuth-Corlette Classification of Perihilar Tumors
I	Tumor involves common hepatic duct
II	Tumor involves bifurcation of the common hepatic duct
IIIa	Tumor involves the right hepatic duct
IIIb	Tumor involves the left hepatic duct
IV	Tumor involves both right and left hepatic ducts

Fig. 12.7 Bismuth-Corlette classification for hilar cholangiocarcinoma

Table 12.4 American Joint Committee on Cancer (AJCC) TNM staging for distal bile duct (7th edition)

Primary tumor (T)	
TX	Primary tumor cannot be assessed
T0	No evidence of Primary tumor
Tis	Carcinoma in situ
T1	Tumor confined to the bile duct histologically
T2	Tumor invades beyond the wall of the bile duct
T3	Tumor invades the gallbladder, pancreas, duodenum, or other adjacent organs without involvement of the celiac axis, or the superior mesenteric artery
T4	Tumor involves the celiac axis, or the superior mesenteric artery

Regional lymph nodes (N)	
NX	Regional lymph nodes cannot be assessed
N0	No regional lymph node metastasis
N1	Regional lymph node metastasis

Distant metastasis (M)	
M0	No distant metastasis
M1	Distant metastasis present

(continued)

Anatomic stage/prognostic groups			
Group	T	N	M
Stage 0	Tis	N0	M0
Stage IA	T1	N0	M0
Stage IB	T2	N0	M0
Stage IIA	T3	N0	M0
Stage IIB	T1	N1	M0
	T2	N1	M0
	T3	N1	M0
Stage III	T4	Any N	M0
Stage IV	Any T	Any N	M1

Adapted from Compton et al. [38]. With permission from Springer Verlag

Treatment

Curative resection offers the best chance for long-term survival. Whereas palliation with surgical bypass was once the preferred surgical procedure even for resectable disease, aggressive surgical resection is now the standard. Despite a thorough preoperative radiologic evaluation to identify

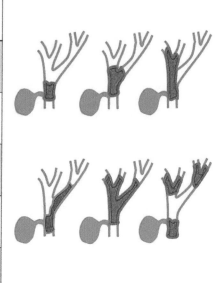

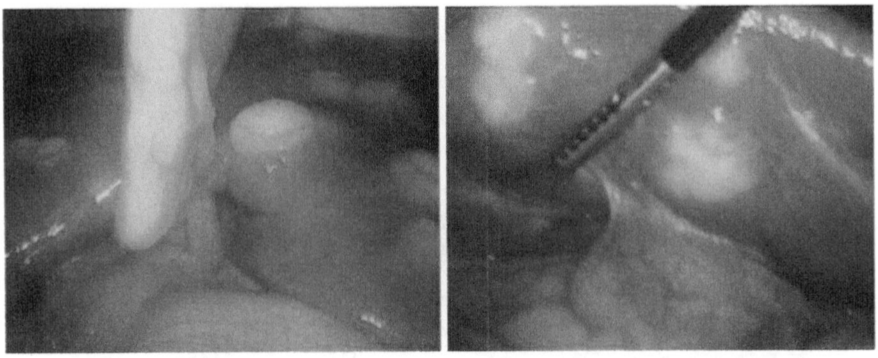

Fig. 12.8 A 65-year-old woman with multiple hepatic lesions that were suspicious for intrahepatic cholangiocarcinoma. Preoperative biopsy was nondiagnostic. She underwent a diagnostic laparoscopy and was found to have satellite lesions (Courtesy of John F. Gibbs, MD, FACS)

resectable disease, the rate of patients found to have unresectable disease at laparotomy remains 14–38 % [39–42]. Because of the relatively high rate of unresectability and the fact that survival of patients with incomplete resection is the same as those who were palliated conservatively, diagnostic laparoscopy has been used by several institutions as part of the staging process (Fig. 12.8). For patients who are known to have unresectable disease preoperatively, biliary endoprosthesis (i.e., endoscopic or percutaneous stenting) has supplanted the need for a surgical bypass.

The role for preoperative biliary decompression with a stent for patients with resectable disease is controversial. For those who have asymptomatic biliary obstruction who will undergo surgery within 1–2 weeks, a stent is not advisable. For symptomatic patients or those who will undergo chemotherapy before surgery, a stent is advisable.

Intrahepatic Cholangiocarcinoma (ICC)

Intrahepatic cholangiocarcinoma (ICC) is the second most common primary liver tumor. Surgical management of intrahepatic cholangiocarcinoma includes consideration for portal vein embolization (PVE), lymphadenectomy, extended hepatic resection with or without vascular resection, and orthotopic liver transplantation.

Resection of ICC follows the basic principles of anatomic liver resection for malignant neoplasm. The understanding of hepatic anatomy began in 1654 with Glisson's description of the liver capsule. This was followed by Cantlie's description of the division of the liver into functional halves in 1897. Finally, Couinaud defined the segmental anatomy of the liver in 1957 [43] (Fig. 12.9). The anatomic division of the liver into right and left halves is based on Cantlie's line, which is an imaginary line that extends from the gallbladder fossa to the left of the vena cava. Anatomically this is defined by the middle hepatic vein. Each half of the liver is then divided into four other segments based on the venous drainage, portal venous inflow, and arterial inflow. The caudate lobe (segment I) is separate from the left and right hepatic lobes. A thorough understanding of the hepatic segmental anatomy increases the safety of the liver resection and an anatomic resection has been shown to result in increased survival [44].

Table 12.5 shows one of the largest reported series in the literature examining outcome with hepatectomy for ICC. The 5-year overall survival is 23–40 % for resected patients [2–4, 39–41, 47, 49, 50, 52, 54–56]. The OS for an R0 resection is 36–63 % at 5 years and the postoperative mortality rate is 0–8 % [2, 3, 52]. In series with multivariate analysis, the most frequently cited significant negative prognostic factors are positive margin, satellite lesions, lymph node metastasis, lymphatic invasion, and vascular invasion. Of these, lymphatic

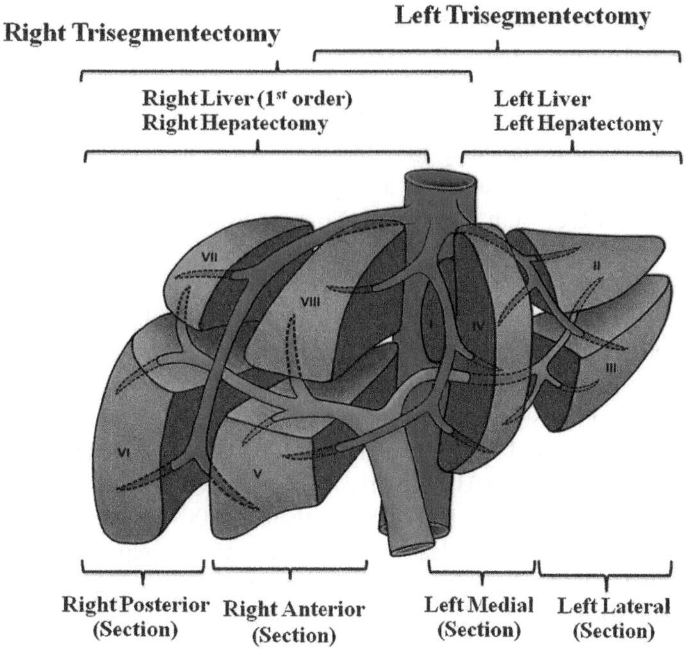

Fig. 12.9 *Couinaud's anatomic/segmental divisions of the liver and types of liver resection.* The anatomic divisions of the liver according to the Brisbane 2000 terminology, including first-order divisions (hemilivers), second-order divisions (sections), and third-order divisions (segments) (Courtesy of Quyen D. Chu, MD, MBA, FACS)

Table 12.5 Outcomes after resection for intrahepatic cholangiocarcinoma

Study	Year	N	Postop mortality (%)	Median survival (mos)	Median survival RO (mos)	1–year OS (%)	3-year OS (%)	5-year OS (%)	5-year OS RO (%)
Jan [4]	1996	41	0	12	22	54	37	26	44
Casavilla [45]	1997	34			38	60	37	31	45
Chu [46]	1999	48		16		60	30	22	
Valverde [42]	1999	30	3	28		86	22		
Weimann [47]	2000	95	5	18		64	31	21	
Inoue [48]	2000	52		18		63	36	36	55
Shimada [49]	2001	49	4	26		66			
Okabayashi [50]	2001	60	5	20	21	68	35	29	39
Ohtsuka [39]	2002	48	8	26		62	38	23	
Weber [51]	2001	33	3		46	83	55	31	
Morimoto [2]	2003	49	4			68	44	32	41
Nakagawa [41]	2005	46	6			66	38	26	
Miwa [52]	2006	41	0			79	36	29	36
DeOliveira [3]	2007	44	4	28	80			4	63

Reprinted from Smith and Gibbs [53]. With permission from Demos Publishing
RO microscopic negative resection, *OS* overall survival

and microvascular invasions are not helpful in selecting patients for resection because they cannot readily be determined preoperatively.

The influence of surgical margin on outcome is controversial. Morimoto et al. found that a positive surgical margin had a relative risk (RR) of death of 2.7 on multivariate analysis ($p=0.02$) and a 3-year OS of 12 % versus 56 % when the margin was negative [2]. Similarly, Casavilla et al. found that margin status was an independent predictor of outcome; the median OS for margin positive and margin negative was 7 months and 38 months, respectively ($p = > 0.0001$) [45]. However, Tamandl reported on 74 patients with ICC and found no difference in disease-free survival (DFS) or OS between R0 and R1 resection [57]. Regardless, the operating surgeon should strive to achieve a negative margin, although the width of the negative margin may not matter [58].

Satellite lesions are identifiable preoperatively and appear to be a particularly poor prognostic factor. Ohtsuka et al. performed a multivariate analysis on 36 patients with MF tumors who underwent resection and found that satellite lesions increased the relative risk of dying by a factor of 3.9 ($p = 0.03$). This risk was exceeded only by a CA 19-9 level greater than 10,000 units/L in predicting death following resection [39]. Similarly, Suzuki et al. examined 19 patients with MF tumor types who underwent resection and found that satellite lesions had the greatest impact on survival with an RR of dying 11.3 times greater than patients without satellite lesion; there were no 3-year survivors in the group that had satellite lesions [56]. Finally, Nakagawa et al. examined 28 patients who had resection for ICC and found that the RR of dying was 2.2 times higher for patients with satellite lesions than those without; there were no 3-year survivors [41]. Given the existing literature, we believe that the presence of multiple tumors (satellite lesions) should be considered as a relative contraindication to surgery. When the index of suspicion for satellite lesions is high even when radiologic examination states otherwise, a diagnostic laparoscopy may be of use (Fig. 12.8).

Extended Resection

Intrahepatic cholangiocarcinoma typically reaches large size prior to their recognition due to their intrahepatic location. This then leads to a delay in diagnosis. ICC often invades contiguous structures, which often necessitates an extended hepatectomy [58]. Roayaie et al. performed hepatic resection on 16 patients with ICC and reported that 88 % of them had tumors within 1.5 cm of the vena cava [59]. Extended hepatectomy is defined as resection of greater than 4 Couinaud segments, and this is often required in 7–54 % of ICCs in large series [2, 4, 39, 42, 50, 51] (Table 12.6). Extended resection of contiguous vascular structures and/or extrahepatic ducts in conjunction with hepatectomy is not uncommon. Extrahepatic bile duct resection has been combined with hepatic resection in 27–74 % as reported in some large series [2, 39, 41, 42, 51, 56, 58]. Vascular resection of the portal vein or IVC was necessary in 4–37 % as reported in many of these series (Table 12.7).

Table 12.6 Incidence of extended resection in hepatectomy for intrahepatic cholangiocarcinoma

Author	Year	Total resections	Extended resections N (%)	1-year OS (%)	3-year OS (%)	5-year OS (%)	Median OS (mos)	Postoperative mortality (%)
Casavilla [45]	1997	34	15 (44)	60	37	31		6
Chu [46]	1997	39	8 (21)	57	24	16	12	
Roayaie [59]	1998	16	11 (69)	86	64	21	43	12
Yamamoto [60]	1999	83	27 (33)			23		2
Valverde [42]	1999	30	16 (53)	86	22		28	3
Inoue [48]	2000	52	23 (44)	63	36	36	18	
Weber [51]	2001	33	15 (45)	83	55	31	37	3
Ohtsuka [39]	2002	48	26 (54)	62	38	23	25	8
Morimoto [2]	2003	51	15 (29)	68	44	32		4
Lang [58]	2005	27	27 (100)	69	55			6

Reprinted from Smith and Gibbs [53]. With permission from Demos Publishing
OS overall survival

Table 12.7 Incidence of vascular resection combined with hepatectomy in intrahepatic cholangiocarcinoma

Author	Year	Total resections	Vascular resections N (%)	1-year OS (%)	3-year OS (%)	5-year OS (%)	Median OS (mos)	Postoperative mortality (%)
Nakagawa [41]	2005	46	4 (9)	66	38	26	21	6
Chu [46]	1997	39		57	24	16	12	
Roayaie [59]	1998	16	2 (13)	86	64	21	43	12
Yamamoto [60]	1999	83	21 (25)			23		2
Valverde [42]	1999	30	2 (7)	86	22		28	3
Inoue [48]	2000	52		63	36	36	18	
Ohtsuka [39]	2002	48	12 (25)	62	38	23	25	8
Morimoto [2]	2003	51	2 (4)	68	44	32		4
Lang [58]	2005	27	11 (41)	69	55			6

Reprinted from Smith and Gibbs [53]. With permission from Demos Publishing
OS overall survival

Lang et al. examined 50 patients with locally advanced ICC undergoing surgical exploration. These patients were determined by preoperative evaluation to require extended hepatectomy. A total of 27 (54 %) patients underwent attempted curative resection; 16 (59 %) of these resection required hepatectomy combined with vascular resection, diaphragmatic resection, and extrahepatic biliary tract resection. The postoperative morbidity was 45 % in the standard resection group and 56 % in the combined resection group. The median survival for the R0 resection group was 46 months for the entire group with 3-year OS of 82 %. The median survival in the R1 group (no gross tumor but residual microscopic tumor) was 5 months compared to 7 months in the explored only group [58].

Yamamoto and associates examined 83 patients with ICC undergoing resection [60]. Fifty-six patients underwent a standard hepatectomy with or without extrahepatic bile duct resection. These were compared to 27 patients undergoing extended hepatectomy or standard hepatectomy combined with vascular resection and/or pancreatectomy. Perioperative mortality in the extended surgery group was significantly higher at 7 % compared to the standard resection with 0 % mortality ($p=0.04$). The 1-year OS was also significantly lower in the extended resection group at 22 % compared to 61 % in the standard resection group ($p=0.001$). The difference in survival may be related to a significantly higher rate of local recurrence and disseminated peritoneal recurrence. However, long-term survival was seen in patients undergoing extended surgery, with 3 of 27 patients surviving greater than 5 years. Two of the three patients had MF tumor and one had IG tumor. No patients with PI or MF+PI tumors had long-term survival [60]. Weber and associates performed hepatic resection in 33 patients with ICC. Forty-six percent of patients required resection of the extrahepatic biliary tree. In the total patient group, vascular invasion was the only factor that was significantly associated with poor outcome ($p=0.0007$). The median OS with vascular invasion was 15 months compared to 61 months when vascular invasion was absent [51].

There are a number of studies that evaluated the feasibility of combined vascular resection and hepatectomy. Hemming et al. described 22 patients who underwent combined hepatic and inferior vena cava (IVC) resection. The patients had a variety of primary and metastatic liver tumors, of which five were CCA. The majority of the patients were able to be approached in the standard lateral to medial approach to mobilizing the liver and exposing the IVC. In seven patients, an anterior approach to the IVC was used. A variety of IVC clamping techniques were utilized depending on the portion of the IVC involved with tumor. Perioperative mortality was

9 % with R0 resection rate of 91 %. Actuarial 1-, 3-, and 5-year OS was 85 %, 60 %, and 33 %, respectively [61]. From these studies, one can surmise that only select patients with advanced tumor stages will benefit from an aggressive surgical resection, which may include cava resection.

Extended hepatectomy can be achieved with acceptable morbidity and mortality, and survival appears to be comparable to standard hepatectomy if an RO resection is obtained. Regarding combining extrahepatic resection with hepatectomy, long-term survival appears possible, but only in a small number of patients, and OS is significantly worse than for patients who had less extensive disease.

Portal Vein Embolization

Hepatic insufficiency due to inadequate future liver remnant (FLR) is a serious complication following hepatic resection. Portal vein embolization (PVE) prior to hepatectomy is used to address this issue [62]. The portal venous system is accessed transhepatically with the blood flow to the ipsilateral portal vein occluded leading to hypertrophy of the contralateral hepatic lobe [63]. The indication for PVE varies and depends on the patient's underlying liver function. For patients with liver dysfunction and FLR less than 50 %, PVE should be considered [64]. Because of the risk for liver failure, patients with obstructive jaundice (>10 mg/dL) should undergo biliary decompression prior to PVE. PVE should be performed when the bilirubin is less than 5 mg/dL. Radical surgery would typically be performed 3–4 weeks later when the FLR has hypertrophied and the bilirubin is less than 2 mg/dl [65].

Nagino and associates described 240 consecutive patients with biliary tract cancer undergoing PVE prior to extended hepatectomy [66]. Twenty percent of patients had progressive disease following PVE and were not offered resection. Of the remaining 80 % of patients who underwent PVE followed by extended hepatectomy, the perioperative mortality was 4.5 %, which was comparable to a mortality rate of 3.7 % for a contemporary cohort that had less than 50 % hepatectomy but without PVE. The FLR increased significantly from 33 to 43 %, and the 3- and 5-year OS rates were 41.7 % and 26.8 %, respectively [66].

Abdalla et al. examined 42 patients undergoing extended hepatectomy for hepatobiliary malignancies [63]. The median FLR increases from baseline 18 % to 26 % following PVE, which is an 8 % increase in the median FLR (50). With PVE, the OS for the group of patients who initially had marginal FLR (FLR <25 %) was comparable to patients who had adequate preoperative FLR. Thus, PVE facilitates safe resection in patients with marginal FLR who might otherwise be precluded from resection.

Lymph Node Dissection

The rate of positive lymph nodes when routine radical lymphadenectomy was performed is 31–59 % [2, 39, 41, 49, 60, 67, 68]. Most series show positive lymph nodes to be an independent predictor of poor survival [2, 3, 6, 42, 47, 49, 50, 52]. Despite a few report of long-term survivors [2, 39, 41, 50, 56], most studies reported no long-term survival for patients with positive lymph node [42, 49, 50, 65, 69]. There is no evidence that routine lymphadenectomy confers any survival advantage.

There is no consensus on whether lymph node dissection should be performed in patients with ICC. Although some recommend lymphadenectomy along with surgical resection in patients with grossly positive nodal disease, given the overall poor outcome, the appropriateness of extensive surgery or the need for lymph node dissection as standard treatment for ICC is questionable at the present time.

Hilar Cholangiocarcinoma

Hilar cholangiocarcinoma arises from the main left or right hepatic ducts or the confluence of the two. It is also referred to as a Klatskin's tumor, which is named after Dr. Gerald Klatskin, the first person to describe this less recognized entity of his time in his landmark paper on hilar cholangiocarcinoma [54].

Diagnosing hilar cholangiocarcinoma remains a challenging task even in the hands of the most skilled surgeons and gastroenterologists. Histological confirmation without surgery remains very difficult as percutaneous or endoscopic biopsies have very low yield and are unable to delineate vascular anatomy or vascular invasion [55]. Multidetector-row computed tomography (MDCT) has been used for diagnosing hilar cholangiocarcinoma. It accurately detects portal vein or arterial invasion in up to 90 % of cases [70, 71]. MRI/MRCP are also modalities that are utilized. Endoscopic approaches including endoscopic retrograde cholangiopancreatography (ERCP), ERCP with cholangioscopy, ERCP with intraductal ultrasound, endoscopic ultrasound, and confocal laser endomicroscopy have diagnostic and therapeutic roles [62].

Since surgical resection remains the sole curative treatment for hilar CCC, patients need to be evaluated and optimized for potential surgery. In cases of obstructive jaundice, it is difficult to use the standard clinical laboratory scoring systems, such as the Child-Turcotte-Pugh or Model for End-Stage Liver Disease (MELD) score to determine a patient's capacity to tolerate major surgery that might involve liver resection. In this subset of population, a volumetric study of the FLR is very useful [72]. If it is thought that there would be insufficient volume of FLR after a curative resection, the surgeon may utilize portal vein embolization of the diseased liver to increase the size of the FLR [73]. A more thorough discussion of FLR can be found in Chapter 19, *Management of Metastatic Liver Metastasis from Colorectal Cancer.*

Hilar cholangiocarcinoma is relatively resistant to radiation and chemotherapy. Hence, surgical resection remains the only therapy that offers a possibility of cure. Unfortunately, because of the intimate location of the extrahepatic duct to the nearby structures (portal vein, hepatic artery, caudate lobe, and segments 4 and 5 of the liver), duct excision alone is not always sufficient.

Surgical management of perihilar cholangiocarcinoma depends on the Bismuth-Corlette classification (Fig. 12.7). This staging system allows the surgeon to determine the extent of resection depending on the level of biliary tree involvement. However, it does not account for portal and vascular involvement. A new staging system has been proposed that addresses the size of the tumor, the extent of biliary system, involvement of portal vein and hepatic artery, distant metastasis, lymph node involvement, and the volume of putative remnant liver after resection [74]. Other staging systems including the AJCC/TNM and Memorial Sloan Kettering Cancer Center (MSKCC) have been proposed, but Bismuth-Corlette classification, despite its limitations, is the more widely recognized and accepted system.

For type I tumors that are limited or confined to the common hepatic duct and type II which involve the confluence of the right and left hepatic ducts, an en bloc resection of the extrahepatic bile ducts with 5–10 mm margins, lymphadenectomy, cholecystectomy, and a Roux-en-y hepaticojejunostomy is the procedure of choice (Fig. 12.5). In addition, many studies have recommended a caudate lobectomy as well because of the high rate of involvement of the ducts of the caudate lobe (Fig. 12.10). Type III and type IV CCA may be amendable to curative surgical resection in highly specialized centers which may involve extended hepatectomy and vascular resection. For type II and IIIa, an extended right hepatectomy may be preferred since the right hepatic duct is short, which makes it difficult to achieve negative margins (Fig. 12.11). Additionally, the left hepatic duct tends to be long and its extrahepatic location makes it ideal for reconstruction [37]. Unlike ICC, resection of N1 nodes (hepatic hilar nodes including those along the cystic duct, common bile duct, hepatic artery, and portal vein) should be routine in any curative surgical resection of hilar cholangiocarcinoma (Fig. 12.12). However, more extensive lymph node dissection beyond the hepatoduodenal ligament (N2, which is defined as metastases to periaortic, pericaval, superior mesenteric artery, and/or celiac artery lymph nodes) is questionable since the 5-year survival is extremely low.

Several series have described the outcome after combined vascular resection and hepatectomy for patients with hilar CCA. Centrally

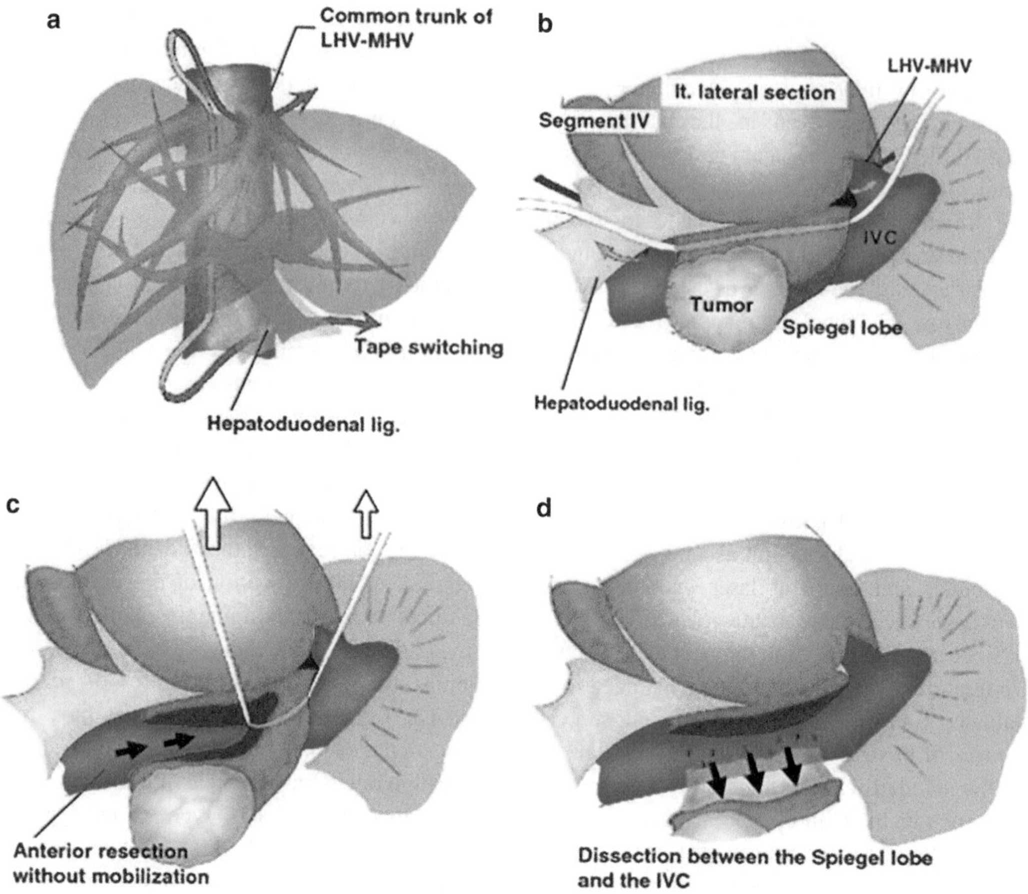

Fig. 12.10 *Isolated anterior resection of the Spiegel lobe*. (**a**) Both ends of the tape are passed between the retrohepatic inferior vena cava (IVC) and the liver parenchyma and repositioned to the left behind the common trunk of the left hepatic vein-middle hepatic vein (LHV-MHV) and the hepatoduodenal ligament. (**b**) The left lateral section is dissected and bent upwards to expose the anterior surface of the Spiegel lobe. Then, the isolated suspension of the Spiegel lobe is achieved. (**c**) With the aid of the suspending tape, the Spiegel lobe is transected through an isolated anterior approach without mobilization. (**d**) After the resection, the left wall of the IVC is fully exposed (Reprinted from Shindoh et al. [75]. With permission from Springer Verlag)

located ICCs can often present in a very similar manner to hilar CCA. Nimura et al. examined 142 patients undergoing resection for hilar CCA [76]. Ninety-nine patients had a standard resection and 43 patients had a standard resection with a vascular resection. The survival at 3 and 5 years was significantly worse for patients who had portal vein resection at 18 % and 6 % compared to standard resection at 37 % and 27 % respectively ($p = <0.0001$). The survival of the patients with portal vein resection, however, was still significantly better than patients with no resection ($p = <0.003$) [76].

Miyazaki et al. examined 161 patients who underwent resection of hilar CCA [77]. Forty-three patients underwent combined hepatectomy and vascular resection. In this study, patients undergoing portal vein resection had similar operative morbidity and mortality to patients not undergoing vascular resection. However, those who had hepatic artery resection had a significantly higher postoperative mortality rate than those who did not ($p < 0.01$). OS at 1, 3, and 5 years was significantly worse for patients undergoing portal vein resection than those with no vascular resection ($p < 0.001$). Five-year OS

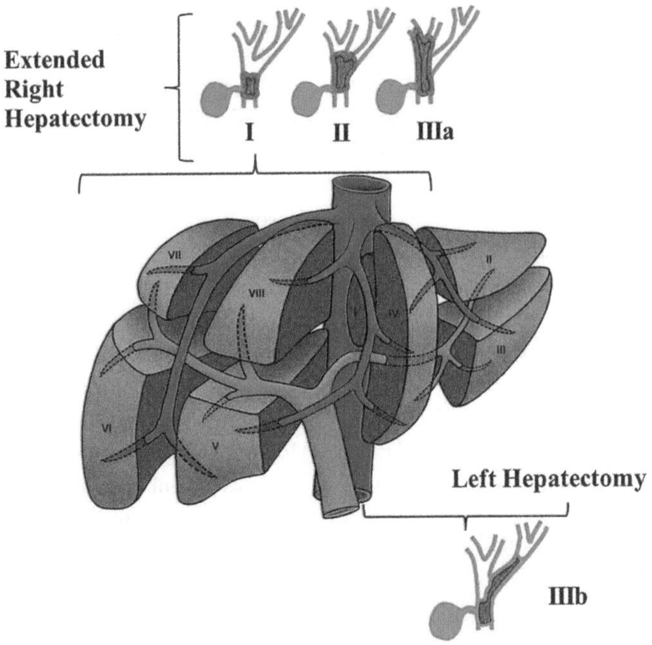

Fig. 12.11 *Type of resections for Klatskin's tumor*. An extended right hepatectomy should be considered for types I–IIIa and a left hepatectomy should be performed for type IIIb (Redrawn by Quyen D. Chu based on data from Ref. [37])

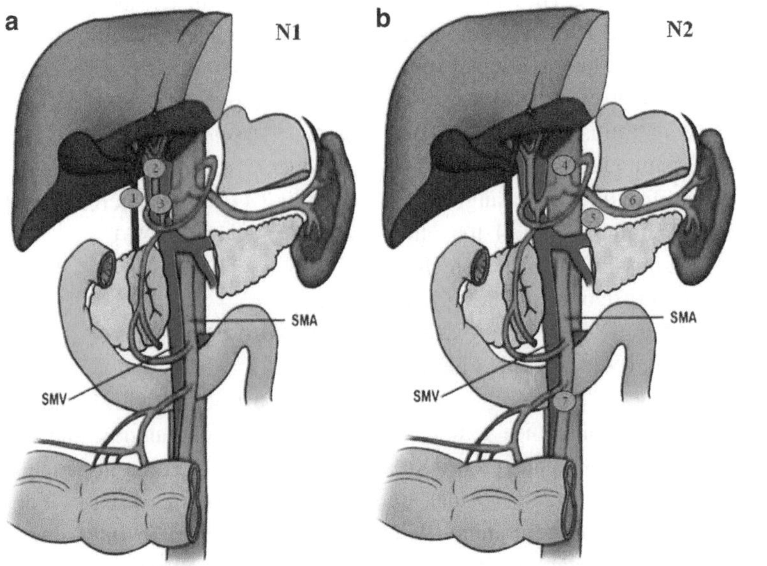

Fig. 12.12 *Nodal Stations for perihilar cholangiocarcinoma*. N1 includes nodes in the hepatoduodenal ligament (#1–3 cystic duct, common bile duct, hepatic artery, and portal vein). N2 includes nodes in the periaortic, pericaval, superior mesenteric artery, and/or celiac artery lymph nodes (#4–7) (Courtesy of Quyen D. Chu, MD, MBA, FACS)

for the portal vein resection group was 16 % compared to 30 % in the group that did not have vascular resection. Survival for hepatic artery resection was particularly poor, with no 3-year survivor and only 11 % alive at one year [77].

In general, criteria for unresectability include: (1) distant metastases, (2) lymph node metastases beyond hepatoduodenal ligament, (3) bilateral intrahepatic bile duct spread to secondary or segmental biliary radicals, (4) involvement of the main trunk of the portal vein (or common hepatic artery) proximal to its bifurcation, (5) bilobar involvement of hepatic arterial and/or portal venous branches, (6) a combination of unilateral hepatic arterial involvement with cholangiographic evidence of extensive contralateral duct spread, (7) lobar atrophy with involvement of contralateral secondary (or segmental) biliary radicles, and (8) lobar atrophy with involvement of contralateral portal vein or hepatic artery [78, 79].

Distal Cholangiocarcinoma

Distal cholangiocarcinoma or lower ducts CCA arise from the common bile duct or intrapancreatic portion of the biliary tree (from the cystic duct to the ampulla of Vater). They are distinct from ampullary carcinoma. They are more commonly in close proximity to major vascular structures and have a tendency of rapid spread. The most common presentation is painless jaundice, pruritus, abdominal pain, and weight loss. When evaluating a patient for distal cholangiocarcinoma, one should be mindful of all the other differential diagnostic possibilities. These include pancreatic head tumors, duodenal tumors, and benign biliary strictures. Distal cholangiocarcinoma is managed similarly to any other periampullary tumors.

The surgical procedure of choice remains a pancreaticoduodenectomy (Whipple procedure). A small percentage of tumors (2–8 %) that are located in the mid-portion of the common bile duct that do not involve vascular structures (i.e., portal vein) can be treated with segmental bile duct resection, followed by Roux-en-Y hepaticojejunostomy reconstruction [80, 81]. Intraoperative margins assessment should be performed prior to reconstruction. The criteria for unresectability include patients who are unfit to undergo surgery; evidence of distant metastases or lymph node involvement beyond the hepatic, portal, and peripancreatic regions; and involvement of the great vessels (i.e., superior mesenteric vessels, portal vein, and celiac axis) [82]. The prognostic factors that determine the success and survival rate after surgery are dependent on nodal involvement and tumor invasion. To avoid understaging, resection of at least 11 lymph nodes is recommended for appropriate staging based on a series from Memorial Sloan Kettering Cancer Center [83].

Neoadjuvant chemoradiation (neoCRT) has been proposed to treat patients with ECC. Such a strategy was extrapolated from experience with pancreatic adenocarcinoma but has never been tested in a phase 3 clinical trial. Despite the lack of level 1 evidence, neoCRT appears to be a reasonable approach, especially for patients who are at high risk of having positive margins, involved nodes, or early recurrence [84, 85].

A large single-center study from Johns Hopkins Hospital reviewed 239 patients from 1973 to 2004 with distal CCC, of which 96 % of the patients underwent pancreaticoduodenectomy or bile duct resection with lymphadenectomy. The study showed that patients with distal CCC had the lowest perioperative mortality rate (3 %) compared to those with hilar or intrahepatic cholangiocarcinoma [3]. The most common postoperative complications were delayed gastric emptying (10 %), pancreatic leak (13 %), and wound infection (11 %).

Palliative Procedures

Biliary obstruction with its attendant symptoms (i.e., pruritus, cholangitis, and pain) is the major reason for intervention in patients with unresectable or metastatic disease. For asymptomatic patients, the need to intervene has been questioned by many. Endobiliary stenting has supplanted the need for surgical palliation for biliary obstruction. Because surgical bypass has not been demonstrated to be superior to stenting, the latter is the preferred approach. Biliary obstruction is much less common with ICC compared to hilar CCA, but when it happens, it typically occurs as a late event as the tumor encroaches on the hilum from either the liver parenchyma or by extrinsic compression from bulky adenopathy.

Biliary obstruction can often be palliated by percutaneous transhepatic biliary drainage or endoscopic placement of an endobiliary stent. Metal stents are preferred over plastic ones for patients whose life expectancy exceeds 6 months because they are associated with fewer complications [86]. Photodynamic therapy (PDT) generates oxygen-free radicals to kill cancer cells and has been utilized via endoscopic or transhepatic techniques to relieve biliary obstruction in patients who are found to have unresectable CCA [87, 88]. When this fails or is not possible, surgical bypass can be considered. This can have durable patency and effective palliation, but is not without significant morbidity and mortality.

When surgical bypass is necessary, the most common procedure employs either a segment III or segment IV hepatic duct bypass. In most instances, a unilateral bypass may suffice even when there is no communication between the right and left biliary systems [89]. Most often, segment III bypass is typically employed because it is technically easier to perform and the location of the duct is more constant than that of segment IV [90] (Fig. 12.13)

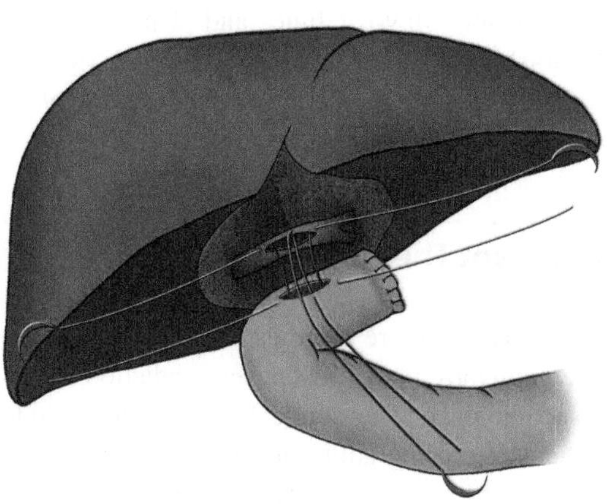

Fig. 12.13 Segment 3 cholangiojejunostomy for unresectable cholangiocarcinoma (Courtesy of Quyen D. Chu, MD, MBA, FACS)

Liver Transplantation

Given the less than ideal outcome of surgical resection, a number of centers began investigating the role of liver transplantation. Many of the reported transplantation series combine ICC and hilar CCA as a single entity. The Cincinnati Transplant Tumor Registry collected data from transplant centers worldwide and identified 207 patients with CCA who received liver transplant [91]. Twenty-one percent of CCA were incidentally found. The postoperative mortality rate was 10 %, and the median time to recurrence was 9.7 months. Interestingly, 47 % of recurrences occurred in the transplanted liver. There was also no difference in the recurrence rates between patients with known CCA and those that were incidentally found. The OS at 1, 2, and 5 years were 72, 48, and 23 %, respectively. The investigators concluded that long-term survival was possible, but only in a small number of patients, and that there were no identifiable preoperative variables to predict which patient will benefit from transplantation [91].

Ghadi and colleagues identified 10 patients in Canada who were found to have incidental CCA. Patients had stage I/II diseases without nodal metastasis. Eight of 10 patients (80 %) recurred and the median time to recurrence was 26 months with a 3-year OS of 30 % [92]. The authors also noted that, although their median time to recurrence was longer than most studies, it is likely due to lead time bias since their studies only included early stage disease. Regardless, the overall survival of 3 years remains suboptimal. Based on their findings, up-front liver transplantation for CCA is contraindicated in Canada, and this philosophy is also embraced by many other centers worldwide.

The Spanish transplantation experience with 59 patients (36 hilar and 23 peripheral) who had hilar cancer and ICC reported a 1-, 3-, and 5-year OS in the ICC patients to be 77 %, 65 %, and 42 %, respectively [93]. These survivals were better than most previously reported, but the authors recognized that they were still below the survival rates for transplantation of nonmalignant diseases. Given the limited number of donated organs available, the indication for liver transplantation for CCA has been questioned [93].

Based on the high recurrence rate after up-front transplantation, several transplantation programs began a novel approach of administering neoadjuvant chemoradiation prior to transplantation for unresectable hilar CCA. The Mayo Clinic and the University of Nebraska studies have revitalized interest in the role of transplantation for CCA through this approach. These institutions have limited their technique to hilar CCA because of the ability to deliver brachytherapy directly to the tumor in the bile duct. The Mayo Clinic transplantation division developed a protocol utilizing external beam radiation therapy (EBRT) plus bolus 5-fluorouracil (5-FU) followed by bradytherapy plus infusion 5-FU and subsequent liver transplantation in patients with unresectable stages I and II hilar CCA [94, 95]. Inclusion criteria required that the patients had no evidence of nodal, intrahepatic, or distant metastases. Two to 6 weeks following transcatheter brachytherapy, patients underwent an exploratory laparotomy to evaluate for extrahepatic disease. At laparotomy, those who were deemed to have stage I/II disease were placed on the United Network for Organ Sharing (UNOS) list and subsequently transplanted. Seventy-one patients presenting with CCA were eligible for the study and underwent the above treatment with 38 patients (54 %) who were successfully transplanted. No residual tumor was seen in 16 of 38 patients (42 %) in the explanted livers. One, 3-, and 5-year recurrence rates were 0 %, 5 %, and 12 %, respectively, with a mean time to recurrence of 40 months. Overall survival rates at 1, 3, and 5 years were 92 %, 82 %, and 82 %, respectively. The survival rate in the Mayo Clinic series approaches seen with liver transplant for nonmalignant indications. The authors concluded that neoadjuvant therapy followed by liver transplantation appears to have greater efficacy than resection for selected patients [94, 95].

The University of Nebraska utilized a similar protocol as the Mayo Clinic's but with a higher dose of brachytherapy and eliminated EBRT. Continuous 5-FU was started at the time of brachytherapy and continued until transplant. Seventeen patients were enrolled in the trial, 11 of whom completed the brachytherapy and proceeded to transplantation without progressive disease. The median OS of the transplanted patients was 25 months. Five patients (45 %) were alive without recurrence at 2.8 years to 14.5 years posttransplant [10].

What can be surmised from these studies is that up-front transplantation alone for CCA resulted in suboptimal outcome because despite having the diseased liver removed and a new donor liver transplanted, a significant number of patients will recur, half of which recurred within the new liver. By giving neoadjuvant chemoradiation therapy prior to transplantation and selecting patients carefully (i.e., stage I/II diseases), significant improvement can be achieved with transplantation. Strict inclusion criteria for transplantation for CCA include unresectable stage I/II perihilar cholangiocarcinoma 3 cm or less in radial diameter without intrahepatic or extrahepatic metastases [96].

Even with these improvements, the majority of patients with CCA will have recurrent disease with limited treatment options. Perhaps a better understanding of the risk factors for recurrence could help address recurrent disease, and the use of living-related transplantation could temper the ethical decision of using the limited resources of cadaveric livers in this population. The experience from Mayo Clinic and University of Nebraska has also prompted some investigators to begin applying neoadjuvant chemoradiation to standard hepatic resection for CCA.

Adjuvant Therapy

Currently, there are no trials comparing adjuvant chemotherapy, radiation, or chemoradiation versus resection only. The surgical series that include patients receiving adjuvant therapy do not delineate the indications, and the regimens are variable. The University of Pittsburgh group found no difference in survival between patients receiving adjuvant therapy and those who did not; the median OS was 7.2 months for those with adjuvant therapy versus 18.3 months for those without adjuvant therapy [45]. The John Hopkins University group also found no significant difference in survival between patients receiving adjuvant therapy and those who did not [3]. Currently, there is no level 1 evidence to support postsurgical adjuvant therapy [97–99]. More recently, combination therapy, including the addition of cisplatin, epirubicin, and or gemcitabine to standard 5-FU regimens, was used in unresectable cases, and the response rates of up to 40 % have been achieved [99–101]. Unfortunately, median survival is still approximately 9 months with chemotherapy [102]. This has been increased in some series up to 13.3 months when radiation is combined with hepatic intra-arterial chemotherapy, suggesting that the improved survival is due to external beam radiation therapy (EBRT) [102, 103]. The improved response of combination chemotherapy and possibly the use of intensity-modulated radiation therapy (IMRT) offer opportunities for the design of future trials.

Conclusion

Throughout this chapter, we discussed a series of studies that discussed the most appropriate method of evaluation and surgical resection of intrahepatic, hilar, and distal cholangiocarcinoma. CCA is an aggressive disease with a high mortality rate. Surgery remains the mainstay of treatment, and surgical management of CCA remains complex. Resection often includes extended hepatectomy, resection of the bile duct, and/or vascular resection. Morbidity and mortality is significantly increased with extended resections. What seems to be most important to any resection is the need to obtain a microscopically negative margin (RO resection). Patients with CCA and incomplete resection seem to fare as poorly as patients without resection. Neoadjuvant therapy prior to transplantation of early disease has revived interest in the role of transplantation for patients with CCA. The role of adjuvant and neoadjuvant therapy for CCA remains elusive.

Salient Points

- Cholangiocarcinoma (CCA) is an uncommon but lethal cancer arising from bile duct epithelium.
- There are a number of risk factors linked to cholangiocarcinoma, the most common predisposing condition associated with CCA in the Western Hemisphere is primary sclerosing cholangitis (PSC)
- Cholangiocarcinoma can be classified as intrahepatic or extrahepatic. Extrahepatic is further divided as perihilar and distal cholangiocarcinoma.
- Painless jaundice is the most common presentation of perihilar or distal tumors. Patients with intrahepatic cholangiocarcinoma typically present with abdominal pain, fever/chills, or an incidental liver mass.
- Several staging and classification systems are currently used for cholangiocarcinoma: TNM classification, Bismuth-Corlette classification, and macroscopic appearance of tumor in ICC.
- Bismuth-Corlette classification is useful for perihilar or Klatskin's tumor
- The macroscopic appearance of the disease reflects tumor cells with different biologic behavior. Mass-forming lesions have the best outcome whereas mass-forming plus periductal infiltrating lesions have the worst outcome
- The radiologic evaluation includes US, CT, MRI, MRCP, and/or multi-detector-row computed tomography (MDCT).
- Cholangiocarcinomas are better visualized using triphasic CT scan which can also be used to assess vascular involvement.
- Cholangiocarcinoma is relatively resistant to radiation and chemotherapy. Hence, surgical resection remains the only therapy that offers a curative management.
- Curative resection with microscopically negative margin (R0 resection) and thorough nodal dissection is critical in providing the most favorable outcome for extrahepatic cholangiocarcinoma
- The role of node dissection
  - For ICC: controversial.
  - For hilar cholangiocarcinoma: dissection of N1 nodes is recommended but not N2 nodes.

- For distal cholangiocarcinoma: resection of at least 11 lymph nodes is recommended for appropriate staging.

- There is a relatively high rate of unresectability and the fact that survival of patients with incomplete resection is the same as for patients palliated conservatively, diagnostic laparoscopy has been used by several institutions as part of the staging process.
- Endobiliary prosthesis such as percutaneous transhepatic cholangiography (PTHC) or endoscopic placement of endobiliary prosthesis is preferred over surgical bypass.
- Intrahepatic cholangiocarcinoma typically reaches large size prior to presentation due to their intrahepatic location. As such, they often invade contiguous structures and require extended hepatectomy.
- Extended hepatectomy is defined as resection of greater than 4 Couinaud segments. Extended resection of contiguous vascular structures and/or extrahepatic ducts in conjunction with hepatectomy is not uncommon.
- Portal vein embolization (PVE) is designed to increase the proposed functional liver remnant (FLR) prior to hepatectomy, thereby decreasing the risk of postoperative liver failure in extended hepatectomy.
- Neoadjuvant chemotherapy followed by liver transplantations is an option for patients with unresectable stage I/II extrahepatic cholangiocarcinoma.

Questions

1. Which of the following ICC macroscopic appearance based on the LCSGJ system has the worst survival rate?
   A. Mass forming (MF)
   B. Intraductal growth (IG)
   C. Periductal infiltrating (PI)
   D. MF+PI
   E. IG+PI
2. Intrahepatic cholangiocarcinoma typically presents with abdominal pain, whereas those with extrahepatic cholangiocarcinoma present with obstructive jaundice
   A. True
   B. False
3. There are number of risk factors that have been linked to cholangiocarcinoma. What is the most common predisposing condition associated with CCA in the Western Hemisphere?
   A. Smoking
   B. Diabetes
   C. HCV
   D. Primary sclerosing cholangitis
   E. Cirrhosis
4. Resection margin status influences the overall survival after resection. Patients with R0 resection have a significantly improved outcome and improved 5-year survival. What does it mean to have R0 resection?
   A. Microscopically margin-negative resection
   B. Microscopically margin- positive resection
   C. Resection with grossly visible tumor to the naked eye at the margin
   D. Resection with at least 11 surrounding lymph nodes
5. Perihilar cholangiocarcinoma is often classified according to their anatomic location and extent of ductal infiltration on the Bismuth-Corlette Classification. What is the classification of type II perihilar tumor?
   A. Tumor which involves the common hepatic duct
   B. Tumor which involves the bifurcation of the common hepatic duct
   C. Tumor which involves the right hepatic duct
   D. Tumor which involves the left hepatic duct
   E. Tumor which involves both the right and left hepatic ducts
6. Hilar cholangiocarcinoma is relatively resistant to radiation and chemotherapy. Hence, surgical resection remains the only therapy that offers a curative management. All of the following criteria listed below would make the tumor considered unresectable, *except*:
   A. Functional liver remnant (FLR) of 55 percent
   B. Lymph node metastases beyond hepatoduodenal ligament
   C. Metastases to other organs
   D. Involvement of superior mesenteric vessels
   E. Medically unfit patient

7. The role of surgical palliation for biliary obstruction has decreased with the improvement in endobiliary prosthesis. However, when surgical bypass is necessary, which procedure is preferred?
   A. Segment III hepatic duct bypass
   B. Common hepatic duct bypass
   C. Segment V hepatic duct bypass
   D. Segment VI hepatic duct bypass
   E. Segment II hepatic duct bypass
8. Mayo clinic transplant division developed a protocol for neoadjuvant chemotherapy followed with liver transplantations for patients with cholangiocarcinoma. Their inclusion criteria included all of the following, *except*:
   A. No evidence of nodal or distant metastasis
   B. No intrahepatic metastasis
   C. Unresectable stage I/II disease
   D. Must be hilar cholangiocarcinoma
   E. Must be distal cholangiocarcinoma
9. Patients with perihilar or distal cholangiocarcinoma typically will have elevated bilirubin levels and have symptoms of cholestasis. All of the following are symptoms of cholestasis, *except:*
   A. Pale stools
   B. Malabsorption
   C. Cholangitis
   D. Dark urine
   E. Abdominal pain
10. Surgical procedure of choice for distal cholangiocarcinoma remains to be a pancreaticoduodenectomy (PD). All of the following are common postoperative complication from this surgery, *except:*
   A. Delayed gastric emptying
   B. Pancreatic leak
   C. Wound infection
   D. Bile leak

Answers

1. D
2. A
3. D
4. A
5. B
6. A
7. A
8. E
9. E
10. D

References

1. Jarnagin WR, Fong Y, DeMatteo RP, et al. Staging, resectability, and outcome in 225 patients with hilar cholangiocarcinoma. Ann Surg. 2001;234(4):507–17; discussion 517–509.
2. Morimoto Y, Tanaka Y, Ito T, et al. Long-term survival and prognostic factors in the surgical treatment for intrahepatic cholangiocarcinoma. J Hepatobiliary Pancreat Surg. 2003;10(6):432–40.
3. DeOliveira ML, Cunningham SC, Cameron JL, et al. Cholangiocarcinoma: thirty-one-year experience with 564 patients at a single institution. Ann Surg. 2007;245(5):755–62.
4. Jan YY, Yeh CN, Yeh TS, Chen TC. Prognostic analysis of surgical treatment of peripheral cholangiocarcinoma: two decades of experience at Chang Gung Memorial Hospital. World J Gastroenterol. 2005;11(12):1779–84.
5. Chen MF. Peripheral cholangiocarcinoma (cholangiocellular carcinoma): clinical features, diagnosis and treatment. J Gastroenterol Hepatol. 1999;14(12):1144–9.
6. Hanazaki K, Kajikawa S, Shimozawa N, et al. Prognostic factors of intrahepatic cholangiocarcinoma after hepatic resection: univariate and multivariate analysis. Hepatogastroenterology. 2002;49(44):311–6.
7. Yoon JH, Gores GJ. Diagnosis, staging, and treatment of cholangiocarcinoma. Curr Treat Options Gastroenterol. 2003;6(2):105–12.
8. The general rules for the clinical and pathological study of primary liver cancer. The Liver Cancer Study Group. General rules for the clinical and pathological study of primary liver cancer. 2nd Engl. Edn. Tokyo: Kanehara 2003. *Jpn J Surg*. 1989;19(1):98–129.
9. Patel T. Increasing incidence and mortality of primary intrahepatic cholangiocarcinoma in the United States. Hepatology. 2001;33(6):1353–7.
10. Taylor-Robinson SD, Toledano MB, Arora S, et al. Increase in mortality rates from intrahepatic cholangiocarcinoma in England and Wales 1968–1998. Gut. 2001;48(6):816–20.
11. Monson JR, Donohue JH, Gunderson LL, Nagorney DM, Bender CE, Wieand HS. Intraoperative radiotherapy for unresectable cholangiocarcinoma–the Mayo Clinic experience. Surg Oncol. 1992;1(4):283–90.
12. Franko J, Nussbaum ML, Morris JB. Choledochal cyst cholangiocarcinoma arising from adenoma: case report and a review of the literature. Curr Surg. 2006;63(4):281–4.
13. Welzel TM, Graubard BI, El-Serag HB, et al. Risk factors for intrahepatic and extrahepatic cholangiocarcinoma in the United States: a population-based

case–control study. Clin Gastroenterol Hepatol. 2007;5(10):1221–8.
14. Sudan D, DeRoover A, Chinnakotla S, et al. Radiochemotherapy and transplantation allow long-term survival for nonresectable hilar cholangiocarcinoma. Am J Transplant. 2002;2(8):774–9.
15. Miros M, Kerlin P, Walker N, Harper J, Lynch S, Strong R. Predicting cholangiocarcinoma in patients with primary sclerosing cholangitis before transplantation. Gut. 1991;32(11):1369–73.
16. Chalasani N, Baluyut A, Ismail A, et al. Cholangiocarcinoma in patients with primary sclerosing cholangitis: a multicenter case–control study. Hepatology. 2000;31(1):7–11.
17. John AR, Haghighi KS, Taniere P, Esmat ME, Tan YM, Bramhall SR. Is a raised CA 19-9 level diagnostic for a cholangiocarcinoma in patients with no history of sclerosing cholangitis? Dig Surg. 2006; 23(5–6):319–24.
18. Patel AH, Harnois DM, Klee GG, LaRusso NF, Gores GJ. The utility of CA 19-9 in the diagnoses of cholangiocarcinoma in patients without primary sclerosing cholangitis. Am J Gastroenterol. 2000; 95(1):204–7.
19. Lindberg B, Arnelo U, Bergquist A, et al. Diagnosis of biliary strictures in conjunction with endoscopic retrograde cholangiopancreaticography, with special reference to patients with primary sclerosing cholangitis. Endoscopy. 2002;34(11):909–16.
20. Johnson SR, Kelly BS, Pennington LJ, Hanto DW. A single center experience with extrahepatic cholangiocarcinomas. Surgery. 2001;130(4):584–90; discussion 590–582.
21. Lacomis JM, Baron RL, Oliver JH, Nalesnik MA, Federle MP. Cholangiocarcinoma: delayed CT contrast enhancement patterns. Radiology. 1997;203(1):98–104.
22. Slattery JM, Sahani DV. What is the current state-of-the-art imaging for detection and staging of cholangiocarcinoma? Oncologist. 2006;11(8):913–22.
23. Asayama Y, Yoshimitsu K, Irie H, et al. Delayed-phase dynamic CT enhancement as a prognostic factor for mass-forming intrahepatic cholangiocarcinoma. Radiology. 2006;238(1):150–5.
24. Fernández-Esparrach G, Ginès A, Sánchez M, et al. Comparison of endoscopic ultrasonography and magnetic resonance cholangiopancreatography in the diagnosis of pancreatobiliary diseases: a prospective study. Am J Gastroenterol. 2007;102(8):1632–9.
25. Dodson RM, Weiss MJ, Cosgrove D, et al. Intrahepatic cholangiocarcinoma: management options and emerging therapies. J Am Coll Surg. 2013;217(4):736–750.e734.
26. Wetter LA, Ring EJ, Pellegrini CA, Way LW. Differential diagnosis of sclerosing cholangiocarcinomas of the common hepatic duct (Klatskin tumors). Am J Surg. 1991;161(1):57–62; discussion 62–53.
27. Witte CL. Choledochal obstruction by cystic duct stone. Mirizzi's syndrome. Am Surg. 1984;50(5):241–3.
28. Compton C, Byrd D, Garcia-Aguilar J, et al. Intrahepatic bile ducts. In: Compton C, Byrd D, Garcia-Aguilar J, et al., editors. AJCC cancer staging atlas. 2nd ed. New York: Springer; 2012. p. 251–8.
29. Nathan H, Aloia TA, Vauthey JN, et al. A proposed staging system for intrahepatic cholangiocarcinoma. Ann Surg Oncol. 2009;16(1):14–22.
30. de Jong MC, Nathan H, Sotiropoulos GC, et al. Intrahepatic cholangiocarcinoma: an international multi-institutional analysis of prognostic factors and lymph node assessment. J Clin Oncol. 2011;29(23): 3140–5.
31. Farges O, Fuks D, Le Treut YP, et al. AJCC 7th edition of TNM staging accurately discriminates outcomes of patients with resectable intrahepatic cholangiocarcinoma: By the AFC-IHCC-2009 study group. Cancer. 2011;117(10):2170–7.
32. Yamasaki S. Intrahepatic cholangiocarcinoma: macroscopic type and stage classification. J Hepatobiliary Pancreat Surg. 2003;10(4):288–91.
33. Sano T, Kamiya J, Nagino M, et al. Macroscopic classification and preoperative diagnosis of intrahepatic cholangiocarcinoma in Japan. J Hepatobiliary Pancreat Surg. 1999;6(2):101–7.
34. Compton C, Byrd D, Garcia-Aguilar J, et al. Perihilar bile ducts. In: Compton C, Byrd D, Garcia-Aguilar J, Kurtzman S, Olawaiye A, Washington M, editors. AJCC cancer staging atlas. 2nd ed. New York: Springer; 2012. p. 269–76.
35. Bismuth H, Nakache R, Diamond T. Management strategies in resection for hilar cholangiocarcinoma. Ann Surg. 1992;215(1):31–8.
36. Bismuth H, Corlette MB. Intrahepatic cholangioenteric anastomosis in carcinoma of the hilus of the liver. Surg Gynecol Obstet. 1975;140(2):170–8.
37. Parikh AA, Abdalla EK, Vauthey JN. Operative considerations in resection of hilar cholangiocarcinoma. HPB (Oxford). 2005;7(4):254–8.
38. Compton C, Byrd D, Garcia-Aguilar J, et al. Distal bile duct. In: Compton C, Byrd D, Garcia-Aguilar J, et al., editors. AJCC cancer staging atlas. 2nd ed. New York: Springer; 2012. p. 277–86.
39. Ohtsuka M, Ito H, Kimura F, et al. Results of surgical treatment for intrahepatic cholangiocarcinoma and clinicopathological factors influencing survival. Br J Surg. 2002;89(12):1525–31.
40. Weber SM, Jarnagin WR, Klimstra D, DeMatteo RP, Fong Y, Blumgart LH. Intrahepatic cholangiocarcinoma: resectability, recurrence pattern, and outcomes. J Am Coll Surg. 2001;193(4):384–91.
41. Nakagawa T, Kamiyama T, Kurauchi N, et al. Number of lymph node metastases is a significant prognostic factor in intrahepatic cholangiocarcinoma. World J Surg. 2005;29(6):728–33.
42. Valverde A, Bonhomme N, Farges O, Sauvanet A, Flejou JF, Belghiti J. Resection of intrahepatic cholangiocarcinoma: a Western experience. J Hepatobiliary Pancreat Surg. 1999;6(2):122–7.
43. Couinaud C. Le Foie: Etudes anatomiques et chirurgicales. Paris: Masson; 1957.

44. Wakai T, Shirai Y, Sakata J, et al. Anatomic resection independently improves long-term survival in patients with T1-T2 hepatocellular carcinoma. Ann Surg Oncol. 2007;14(4):1356–65.
45. Casavilla FA, Marsh JW, Iwatsuki S, et al. Hepatic resection and transplantation for peripheral cholangiocarcinoma. J Am Coll Surg. 1997;185(5):429–36.
46. Chu KM, Lai EC, Al-Hadeedi S, et al. Intrahepatic cholangiocarcinoma. World J Surg. 1997;21(3):301–5; discussion 305–306.
47. Weimann A, Varnholt H, Schlitt HJ, et al. Retrospective analysis of prognostic factors after liver resection and transplantation for cholangiocellular carcinoma. Br J Surg. 2000;87(9):1182–7.
48. Inoue K, Makuuchi M, Takayama T, et al. Long-term survival and prognostic factors in the surgical treatment of mass-forming type cholangiocarcinoma. Surgery. 2000;127(5):498–505.
49. Shimada M, Yamashita Y, Aishima S, Shirabe K, Takenaka K, Sugimachi K. Value of lymph node dissection during resection of intrahepatic cholangiocarcinoma. Br J Surg. 2001;88(11):1463–6.
50. Okabayashi T, Yamamoto J, Kosuge T, et al. A new staging system for mass-forming intrahepatic cholangiocarcinoma: analysis of preoperative and postoperative variables. Cancer. 2001;92(9):2374–83.
51. Weber DC, Kurtz JM, Allal AS. The impact of gap duration on local control in anal canal carcinoma treated by split-course radiotherapy and concomitant chemotherapy. Int J Radiat Oncol Biol Phys. 2001;50(3):675–80.
52. Miwa S, Miyagawa S, Kobayashi A, et al. Predictive factors for intrahepatic cholangiocarcinoma recurrence in the liver following surgery. J Gastroenterol. 2006;41(9):893–900.
53. Smith RR, Gibbs JF. Surgical management of intrahepatic biliary tract cancer. In: Thomas CR, Fuller CD, editors. Biliary tract and gallbladder cancer; 2008. Demos Medical Publishing, New York pp. 181–194
54. Klatskin G. Adenocarcinoma of the hepatic duct at its bifurcation within the porta hepatis. An unusual tumor with distinctive clinical and pathological features. Am J Med. 1965;38:241–56.
55. Nishio H, Kamiya J, Nagino M, et al. Value of percutaneous transhepatic portography before hepatectomy for hilar cholangiocarcinoma. Br J Surg. 1999;86(11):1415–21.
56. Suzuki S, Sakaguchi T, Yokoi Y, et al. Clinicopathological prognostic factors and impact of surgical treatment of mass-forming intrahepatic cholangiocarcinoma. World J Surg. 2002;26(6):687–93.
57. Tamandl D, Herberger B, Gruenberger B, Puhalla H, Klinger M, Gruenberger T. Influence of hepatic resection margin on recurrence and survival in intrahepatic cholangiocarcinoma. Ann Surg Oncol. 2008;15(10):2787–94.
58. Lang H, Sotiropoulos GC, Frühauf NR, et al. Extended hepatectomy for intrahepatic cholangiocellular carcinoma (ICC): when is it worthwhile? Single center experience with 27 resections in 50 patients over a 5-year period. Ann Surg. 2005; 241(1):134–43.
59. Roayaie S, Guarrera JV, Ye MQ, et al. Aggressive surgical treatment of intrahepatic cholangiocarcinoma: predictors of outcomes. J Am Coll Surg. 1998;187(4):365–72.
60. Yamamoto M, Takasaki K, Yoshikawa T. Extended resection for intrahepatic cholangiocarcinoma in Japan. J Hepatobiliary Pancreat Surg. 1999;6(2):117–21.
61. Hemming AW, Reed AI, Langham MR, Fujita S, Howard RJ. Combined resection of the liver and inferior vena cava for hepatic malignancy. Ann Surg. 2004;239(5):712–9; discussion 719–721.
62. Anderson MA, Appalaneni V, Ben-Menachem T, et al. The role of endoscopy in the evaluation and treatment of patients with biliary neoplasia. Gastrointest Endosc. 2013;77(2):167–74.
63. Abdalla EK, Hicks ME, Vauthey JN. Portal vein embolization: rationale, technique and future prospects. Br J Surg. 2001;88(2):165–75.
64. Kokudo N, Makuuchi M. Current role of portal vein embolization/hepatic artery chemoembolization. Surg Clin North Am. 2004;84(2):643–57.
65. Shirabe K, Shimada M, Harimoto N, et al. Intrahepatic cholangiocarcinoma: its mode of spreading and therapeutic modalities. Surgery. 2002;131(1 Suppl):S159–64.
66. Nagino M, Kamiya J, Nishio H, Ebata T, Arai T, Nimura Y. Two hundred forty consecutive portal vein embolizations before extended hepatectomy for biliary cancer: surgical outcome and long-term follow-up. Ann Surg. 2006;243(3):364–72.
67. Uenishi T, Hirohashi K, Kubo S, et al. Histologic factors affecting prognosis following hepatectomy for intrahepatic cholangiocarcinoma. World J Surg. 2001;25(7):865–9.
68. Yamamoto M, Takasaki K, Otsubo T, Katsuragawa H, Katagiri S. Recurrence after surgical resection of intrahepatic cholangiocarcinoma. J Hepatobiliary Pancreat Surg. 2001;8(2):154–7.
69. Uenishi T, Hirohashi K, Kubo S, et al. Clinicopathologic features in patients with long-term survival following resection for intrahepatic cholangiocarcinoma. Hepato-gastroenterology. 2003;50(52):1069–72.
70. Lee HY, Kim SH, Lee JM, et al. Preoperative assessment of resectability of hepatic hilar cholangiocarcinoma: combined CT and cholangiography with revised criteria. Radiology. 2006;239(1):113–21.
71. Okumoto T, Sato A, Yamada T, et al. Correct diagnosis of vascular encasement and longitudinal extension of hilar cholangiocarcinoma by four-channel multidetector-row computed tomography. Tohoku J Exp Med. 2009;217(1):1–8.
72. Lau SH, Lau WY. Current therapy of hilar cholangiocarcinoma. Hepatobiliary Pancreat Dis Int. 2012;11(1):12–7.
73. Hemming AW, Reed AI, Howard RJ, et al. Preoperative portal vein embolization for extended hepatectomy. Ann Surg. 2003;237(5):686–91. discussion 691–683.

74. Deoliveira ML, Schulick RD, Nimura Y, et al. New staging system and a registry for perihilar cholangiocarcinoma. Hepatology. 2011;53(4):1363–71.
75. Shindoh J, et al. Isolated sling suspension during resection of the Spiegel lobe of the liver: a safe alternative technique for difficult cases. J Hepatobiliary Pancreat Sci. 2010;17(3):359–64.
76. Nimura Y, Kamiya J, Kondo S, et al. Aggressive preoperative management and extended surgery for hilar cholangiocarcinoma: Nagoya experience. J Hepatobiliary Pancreat Surg. 2000;7(2):155–62.
77. Miyazaki M, Kato A, Ito H, et al. Combined vascular resection in operative resection for hilar cholangiocarcinoma: does it work or not? Surgery. 2007; 141(5):581–8.
78. Vauthey JN, Blumgart LH. Recent advances in the management of cholangiocarcinomas. Semin Liver Dis. 1994;14(2):109–14.
79. Zaydfudim V, Rosen C, Nagorney D. Hilar cholangiocarcinoma. In: Pawlik T, editor. Biliary tract and primary liver tumors, vol. 23(2). Philadelphia: Elsevier; 2014. p. 247–63.
80. Fong Y, Blumgart LH, Lin E, Fortner JG, Brennan MF. Outcome of treatment for distal bile duct cancer. Br J Surg. 1996;83(12):1712–5.
81. Wade TP, Prasad CN, Virgo KS, Johnson FE. Experience with distal bile duct cancers in U.S. Veterans Affairs hospitals: 1987–1991. J Surg Oncol. 1997;64(3):242–5.
82. Schulick RD. Criteria of unresectability and the decision-making process. HPB (Oxford). 2008; 10(2):122–5.
83. Ito K, Ito H, Allen PJ, et al. Adequate lymph node assessment for extrahepatic bile duct adenocarcinoma. Ann Surg. 2010;251(4):675–81.
84. McMasters KM, Tuttle TM, Leach SD, et al. Neoadjuvant chemoradiation for extrahepatic cholangiocarcinoma. Am J Surg. 1997;174(6):605–8; discussion 608–609.
85. Nelson JW, Ghafoori AP, Willett CG, et al. Concurrent chemoradiotherapy in resected extrahepatic cholangiocarcinoma. Int J Radiat Oncol Biol Phys. 2009;73(1):148–53.
86. Khan SA, Davidson BR, Goldin R, et al. Guidelines for the diagnosis and treatment of cholangiocarcinoma: consensus document. Gut. 2002;51 Suppl 6:VI1–9.
87. Fuks D, Bartoli E, Delcenserie R, et al. Biliary drainage, photodynamic therapy and chemotherapy for unresectable cholangiocarcinoma with jaundice. J Gastroenterol Hepatol. 2009;24(11):1745–52.
88. Harewood GC, Baron TH, Rumalla A, et al. Pilot study to assess patient outcomes following endoscopic application of photodynamic therapy for advanced cholangiocarcinoma. J Gastroenterol Hepatol. 2005;20(3):415–20.
89. Baer HU, Rhyner M, Stain SC, et al. The effect of communication between the right and left liver on the outcome of surgical drainage for jaundice due to malignant obstruction at the hilus of the liver. HPB Surg. 1994;8(1):27–31.
90. Suzuki S, Kurachi K, Yokoi Y, et al. Intrahepatic cholangiojejunostomy for unresectable malignant biliary tumors with obstructive jaundice. J Hepatobiliary Pancreat Surg. 2001;8(2):124–9.
91. Meyer CG, Penn I, James L. Liver transplantation for cholangiocarcinoma: results in 207 patients. Transplantation. 2000;69(8):1633–7.
92. Ghali P, Marotta PJ, Yoshida EM, et al. Liver transplantation for incidental cholangiocarcinoma: analysis of the Canadian experience. Liver Transpl. 2005; 11(11):1412–6.
93. Robles R, Figueras J, Turrión VS, et al. Spanish experience in liver transplantation for hilar and peripheral cholangiocarcinoma. Ann Surg. 2004; 239(2):265–71.
94. Heimbach JK, Gores GJ, Haddock MG, et al. Liver transplantation for unresectable perihilar cholangiocarcinoma. Semin Liver Dis. 2004;24(2):201–7.
95. Rea DJ, Heimbach JK, Rosen CB, et al. Liver transplantation with neoadjuvant chemoradiation is more effective than resection for hilar cholangiocarcinoma. Ann Surg. 2005;242(3):451–8; discussion 458–461.
96. Rosen CB, Heimbach JK, Gores GJ. Liver transplantation for cholangiocarcinoma. Transpl Int. 2010;23(7):692–7.
97. Yamamoto M, Ariizumi S. Intrahepatic recurrence after surgery in patients with intrahepatic cholangiocarcinoma. J Gastroenterol. 2006;41(9):925–6.
98. Benson AB, Bekaii-Saab T, Ben-Josef E, et al. Hepatobiliary cancers. Clinical practice guidelines in oncology. J Natl Compr Cancer Netw. 2006; 4(8):728–50.
99. Thongprasert S, Napapan S, Charoentum C, Moonprakan S. Phase II study of gemcitabine and cisplatin as first-line chemotherapy in inoperable biliary tract carcinoma. Ann Oncol. 2005;16(2):279–81.
100. Knox JJ, Hedley D, Oza A, et al. Combining gemcitabine and capecitabine in patients with advanced biliary cancer: a phase II trial. J Clin Oncol. 2005;23(10):2332–8.
101. Park SH, Park YH, Lee JN, et al. Phase II study of epirubicin, cisplatin, and capecitabine for advanced biliary tract adenocarcinoma. Cancer. 2006;106(2): 361–5.
102. Ben-Josef E, Normolle D, Ensminger WD, et al. Phase II trial of high-dose conformal radiation therapy with concurrent hepatic artery floxuridine for unresectable intrahepatic malignancies. J Clin Oncol. 2005;23(34):8739–47.
103. Cantore M, Mambrini A, Fiorentini G, et al. Phase II study of hepatic intraarterial epirubicin and cisplatin, with systemic 5-fluorouracil in patients with unresectable biliary tract tumors. Cancer. 2005; 103(7): 1402–7.

Pancreatic Adenocarcinoma

13

Jillian K. Smith, Quyen D. Chu, and Jennifer F. Tseng

Learning Objectives

After reading this chapter, you should be able to:

- Describe the epidemiology of pancreatic adenocarcinoma.
- Identify risk factors associated with the development of pancreatic cancer.
- Understand the factors contributing to the high mortality rate associated with pancreatic adenocarcinoma.
- Describe the development and progression of pancreatic adenocarcinoma.
- Identify the pathologic characteristics of pancreatic adenocarcinoma.
- Understand the diagnosis and staging of pancreatic adenocarcinoma.
- Identify the appropriate treatment strategies for pancreatic adenocarcinoma.

J.K. Smith, M.D., M.P.H.
Department of Surgery, University of Massachusetts Medical School, 55 Lake Avenue North, 01605 Worcester, MA, USA
e-mail: jkennedysmith@gmail.com

Q.D. Chu, M.D., M.B.A, F.A.C.S.
Department of Surgery, LSU Health Sciences Center-Shreveport, 1501 Kings Hwy, P.O. Box 33932, 71130-3932 Shreveport, LA, USA
e-mail: qchu@lsuhsc.edu

J.F. Tseng, M.D., M.P.H. (✉)
Department of Surgery, Beth Israel Deaconess Medical Center and Harvard Medical School, 330 Brookline Ave, Stoneman 913, 02459 Boston, MA, USA
e-mail: jftseng@bidmc.harvard.edu

Introduction

There are many forms of pancreatic cancer; these cancers arise from the exocrine or endocrine systems of the pancreas. The more common forms are the exocrine pancreatic cancers, which represent 95 % of all pancreatic cancers. Of these, the most common and the most aggressive form of pancreatic cancer is ductal adenocarcinoma, which will be the main focus of this chapter. Ductal adenocarcinoma is a solid exocrine neoplasm that comprises approximately 90 % of all solid pancreatic tumors. Pancreatic adenocarcinoma is known for its poor prognosis with the incidence of new cases roughly equaling its mortality each year. It was estimated for the year 2013 that there would be 45,220 new cases of pancreatic cancer in the United States and that 38,460 would die of the disease [1]. This makes pancreatic cancer the tenth leading cancer diagnosed and the fourth leading cause of cancer deaths in the United States [1]. Despite increasing trends in the use of guideline-directed care, overall survival for pancreatic cancer has not been significantly impacted [2].

Surgical resection represents the only potential for cure. However, a major factor in the lethality of pancreatic cancer remains its generally advanced stage at diagnosis. This is due in large part to the lack of adequate screening techniques. Therefore, the majority of patients with pancreatic cancer present with metastatic disease at the time of initial presentation. At this point, resection offers little or

Q.D. Chu et al. (eds.), *Surgical Oncology: A Practical and Comprehensive Approach*,
DOI 10.1007/978-1-4939-1423-4_13, © Springer Science+Business Media New York 2015

no significant oncologic benefit. Long-term outcomes are therefore primarily a reflection of the underlying malignant process.

Data from the Surveillance Epidemiology and End Results (SEER) database demonstrate a sobering 5-year survival rate of 1.8 % among patients with distant (metastatic) disease and 8.7 % for regional disease [3]. A population-based study examining patients in the National Cancer Data Base from 1992 to 1998 revealed a median survival of only 3.5 months for patients with unresectable pancreatic cancer (and only 6.8 months for patients with unresected Stage IA disease). Even with guideline-directed care, multimodality therapy including neoadjuvant or adjuvant chemoradiation with surgery, outcomes are dismal, likely due to chemo- and radiation-resistant biology of these aggressive cancers. Therefore, novel therapeutics and further investigations into the biomarkers and evolution of pancreatic adenocarcinoma are continually being developed to improve the outcome of patients with this deadly disease.

Etiology

Although several risk factors have been implicated in the development of pancreatic cancer, the etiology of pancreatic cancer remains poorly understood. Among the most commonly cited risk factors are smoking and chronic pancreatitis. Combined data from various studies have shown an odds ratio of 2.2 for the development of pancreatic cancer among smokers compared to nonsmokers and an odds ratio of 1.2 among ex-smokers [4]. Other lifestyle factors associated with pancreatic adenocarcinoma include alcohol intake, smoking, and dietary factors (high consumption of meat and fat as well as general high caloric consumption leading to obesity). Preexisting disorders of the pancreas, such as diabetes and chronic pancreatitis, have also been linked to an increased risk of pancreatic cancer. Patients with diabetes over 10 years have a demonstrated 30–40 % risk of developing pancreatic cancer [5]. As for chronic pancreatitis, studies have found an odds ratio of 2.7 for pancreatic cancer patients with antecedent chronic pancreatitis [4]. Certain patient characteristics have also been associated with increased risk of pancreatic adenocarcinoma; these include increasing age, male sex, and non-O blood group.

Familial patterns of pancreatic cancer, although rare, also exist and are the subject of ongoing investigations into the genetics of pancreatic cancer. It is estimated that while the majority are sporadic and acquired with advancing age, approximately 5–10 % of pancreatic adenocarcinomas have a familial basis. Familial inheritance patterns that have been identified include individuals in families that carry the following mutations: BRCA-2, p16INK4a, STK11/LKB1 (Peutz-Jeghers syndrome), PALB2, ataxia telangiectasia mutated (ATM), and some possible associations with mismatch repair gene mutations seen in Lynch syndrome [6].

Progression/Histopathology

As is the case for most invasive carcinomas, in the development of pancreatic cancer, there is a progression from normal epithelium to noninvasive precursor lesions identified within the ducts to invasive carcinoma. The most important and most common precursor lesions of invasive pancreatic carcinoma are termed pancreatic intraepithelial neoplasias, or PanINs. These are classified into three grades: (1) PanIN-1A (flat lesion) and PanIN-1B (micropapillary pattern) are early lesions that show minimal cytological and architectural atypia; (2) PanIN-2 lesions show mild to moderate atypia with frequent papillary formation; and (3) PanIN-3 lesions, also termed "carcinoma in situ," demonstrate severe cytological and architectural atypia with a predominantly papillary pattern but may also demonstrate a flat or cribriform pattern [7]. Through this epithelial-mesenchymal transition, the epithelial change progresses from these PanIN stages to invasive carcinoma (Fig. 13.1). Other precursor lesions include intraductal papillary mucinous neoplasia (IPMN) and mucinous cystic neoplasia (MCN).

The proposed progression model involves telomere shortening and mutations of the oncogene KRAS that occur in the early stages, followed

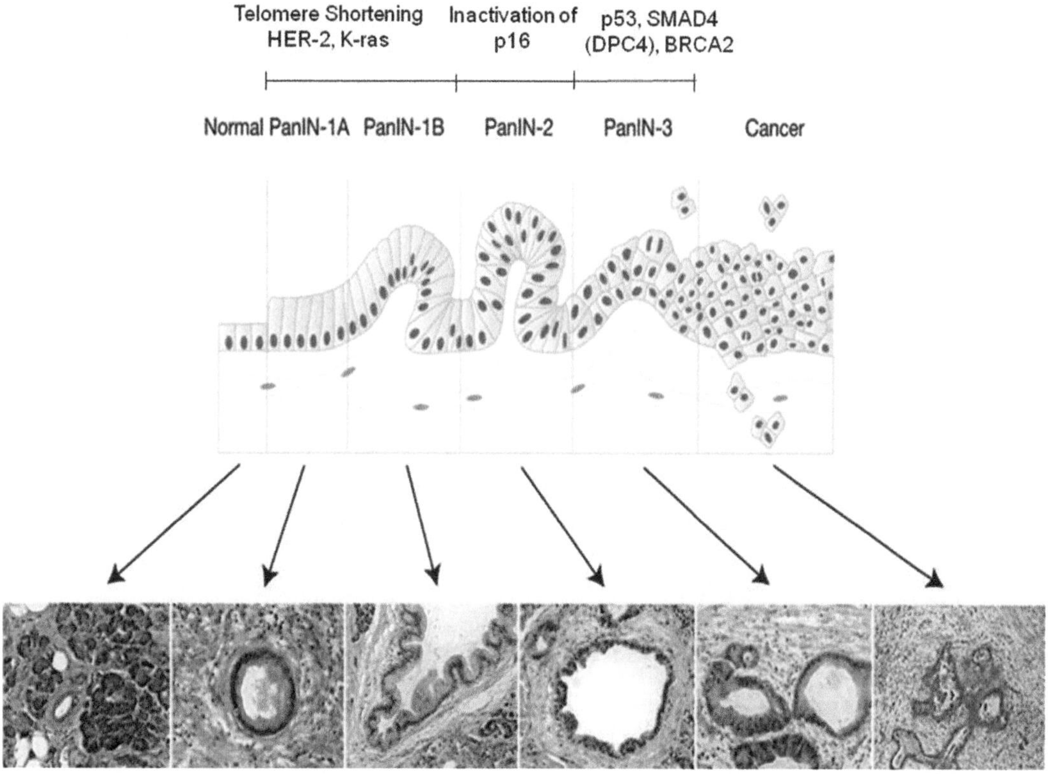

Fig. 13.1 **Proposed progression model for pancreatic cancer.** The majority of pancreatic cancer is believed to involve telomere shortening and mutations of the oncogene KRAS occurring in early stages, followed by the inactivation of the p16 tumor suppressor gene intermediately and, finally, the inactivation of the p53, SMAD4 (DPC4), and BRCA-2 tumor suppressor genes at late stages (Modified from Chang DK, Merrett ND, Biankin AV. Improving outcomes for operable pancreatic cancer: Is access to safer surgery the problem? J Gastro Hepatol 2008;23:1036–45 with permission from John Wiley & Sons, Inc.)

by the inactivation of the p16 tumor suppressor gene in the intermediate stages and, finally, the inactivation of the p53, SMAD4 (DPC4), and BRCA-2 tumor suppressor genes at late stages [8] (Fig. 13.1).

The histology of ductal adenocarcinoma is of poorly differentiated tubular structures or cell clusters; aggressive, infiltrative growth; and dense stromal fibrosis (Fig. 13.2).

Diagnosis

Signs and Symptoms

The signs and symptoms, if any, of a patient presenting with pancreatic adenocarcinoma are related to the location of the cancer within the pancreas, mainly differentiated between carcinomas of the head of the pancreas and the body or tail of the pancreas. Many patients with pancreatic head carcinomas present with weight loss and obstructive jaundice, and occasionally, there is an associated deep abdominal or back pain. Because pancreatic body-tail carcinomas are further from the bile duct, they rarely present with jaundice and may present only with weight loss and abdominal pain. Regardless of the location, the diagnosis of pancreatic cancer can be extremely difficult due to the vague presenting symptoms.

Unfortunately, no definitive early warning signs have been established [9]. The classic description of pancreatic cancer presentation is that of a patient with painless jaundice. Painless jaundice can result from obstruction at the level of the ampulla. Causes include tumors from the

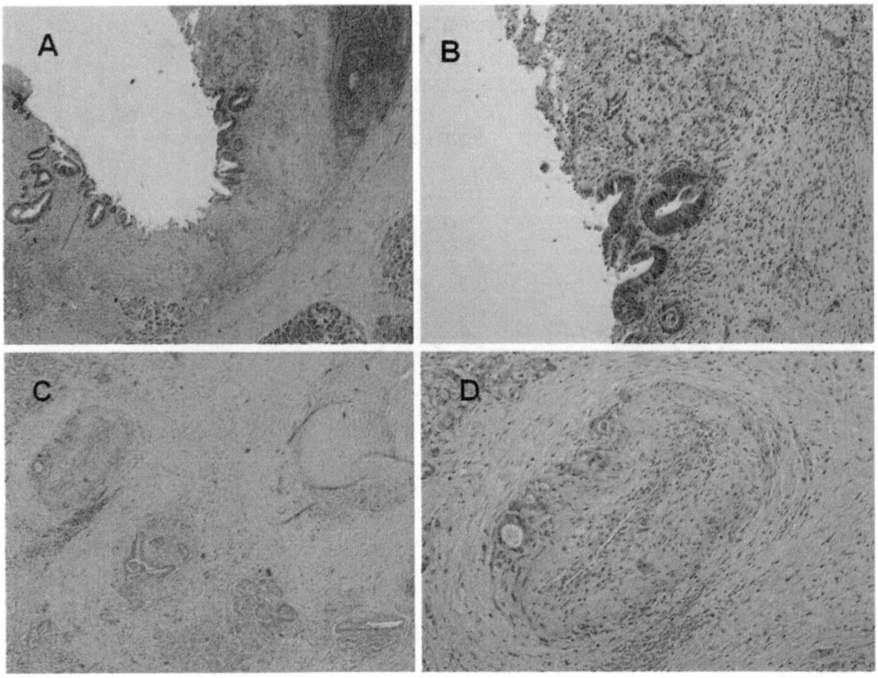

Fig. 13.2 Histology of pancreatic adenocarcinoma (Fig. 13.1a, b) with evidence of perineural and periarterial invasion (Fig. 13.1c, d) (Courtesy of Quyen D. Chu, MD, MBA, FACS)

duodenum (i.e., duodenal tumors), bile duct (i.e., cholangiocarcinoma), or pancreas (pancreatic head tumors). Patients with pancreatic head tumors have less abdominal pain than patients with body-tail tumors. Approximately one-quarter of pancreatic cancer patients have no pain at all at the time of diagnosis [10].

One study of patients diagnosed with exocrine pancreatic cancer found that the most common presenting symptoms are fatigue, weight loss, anorexia, and abdominal pain. Jaundice, hepatomegaly, right upper quadrant mass, and cachexia are among the most common presenting signs. Changes in urine and stool are also common; choluria (dark urine) occurs in approximately 60 % of pancreatic cancer patients, and hypocholia (clay-colored stool) occurs in approximately 54 %. Additionally, Courvoisier's sign (enlarged, non-tender, palpable gallbladder in a patient with jaundice) and migratory thrombophlebitis are also well-recognized signs associated with pancreatic cancer; these have been found in 13 % and 3 %, respectively, of patients diagnosed with pancreatic cancer [11]. Unfortunately, there is no screening test for pancreatic cancer, and as a result, most patients with pancreatic cancer have advanced disease by the time of diagnosis.

Laboratory Data

In a patient with an obstructed bile duct, elevated alkaline phosphatase and bilirubin levels are often present. Levels of the tumor marker CA19-9 are also elevated in patients with pancreatic cancer; unfortunately, this test is not sensitive enough to screen for and diagnose pancreatic cancer. It is usually used in follow-up after treatment.

Imaging Studies

Computed Tomography (CT Scan)

Computed tomography (CT scan) is a primary imaging modality and gold standard for evaluating pancreatic cancer. It is used for diagnosing primary pancreatic malignancy, assessing resectability, and

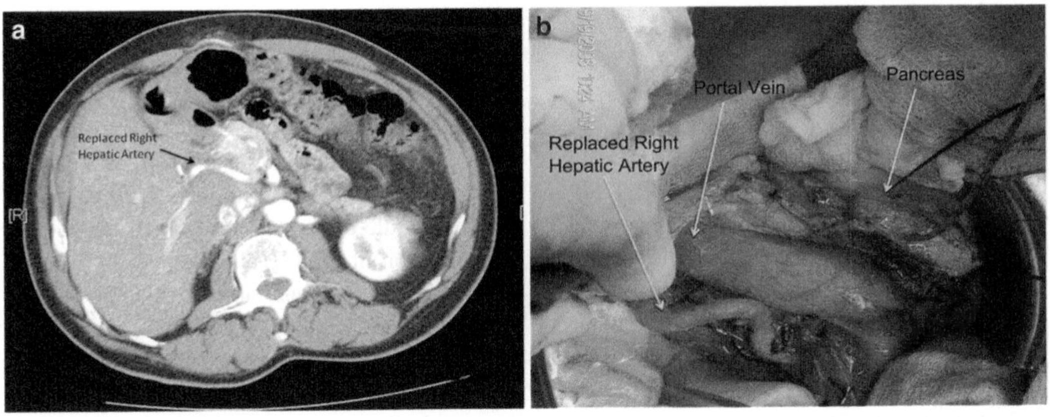

Fig. 13.3 CT scan demonstrated a replaced right hepatic artery originating from the superior mesentery artery (**a**) and an intraoperative picture of the same patient with a replaced right hepatic artery (**b**). Note that this arterial anomaly can occur in 25 % of patients (A-B: Courtesy of Quyen D. Chu, MD, MBA, FACS)

evaluating for metastases. In addition, CT scans can show anatomic anomalies such as a replaced right hepatic artery, which generally originates from the superior mesenteric artery (SMA) in 25 % of patients (Fig. 13.3).

Due to the widespread availability and the fast, relatively simple acquisition of images, CT scan is the most frequently used imaging modality to detect pancreatic abnormalities. Although it is the most cost-effective imaging modality and provides excellent anatomic detail, it may be limited in its ability to detect small tumors or peritoneal metastases. CT scan should be performed according to a defined pancreas protocol that includes multiphase technique (arterial, parenchymal, portal venous) and thin slices (3 mm or less) through the abdomen.

Magnetic Resonance Imaging (MRI)

Magnetic resonance imaging (MRI) is an alternate imaging modality. However, it is no more accurate than CT in the diagnosis or evaluation of pancreatic cancer. Furthermore, it is not as widely used due to the decreased availability and slower acquisition of images. However, MRI benefits patients in that it avoids additional radiation exposure if further imaging is needed. An additional benefit is that it can be performed along with a cholangiopancreatography (MRCP) to provide more detailed views of the pancreatic and biliary ducts.

Endoscopic Ultrasound (EUS)

Endoscopic ultrasound (EUS) can be used for closer examination, biopsy, or staging of lesions in the vicinity of the head of the pancreas. Also, it may be complementary to CT for staging and is especially helpful in detecting small tumors, which are not always visible with other imaging modalities. EUS-directed fine-needle aspiration (FNA) is preferable to CT-guided FNA for resectable disease; this is due to the improved diagnostic yield, better safety profile, and lower risk of peritoneal seeding as compared with the percutaneous approach [9].

Endoscopic Retrograde Cholangiopancreatography (ERCP)

Endoscopic retrograde cholangiopancreatography (ERCP) can be used when a mass lesion cannot be identified by the above imaging modalities in a patient who requires further evaluation and sampling of the pancreatic duct for the workup of pain, jaundice, and/or pancreatitis.

Positron Emission Tomography (PET)

Positron emission tomography (PET) is a functional imaging modality. The role of PET/CT in pancreatic imaging is still evolving and, as such, is not widely used at this time for the diagnosis or follow-up of pancreatic cancers. It is not a substitute for high-quality, contrast-enhanced CT. However, PET/CT scans may be considered after formal pancreatic CT protocol in high-risk patients to detect metastases (Fig. 13.4).

Diagnostic/Staging Laparoscopy

Recent improvement in the quality of CT imaging has decreased the utility of routine diagnostic laparoscopy (DL). However, laparoscopy is still used in many institutions prior to surgery or chemoradiation to rule out metastases, which may not be identified on imaging. This is especially true for lesions in the body and tail for which 50 % have evidence of peritoneal disease. DL is also helpful in selected cases, such as those that are at high risk for having disseminated disease (i.e., borderline resectable disease, patients with markedly elevated

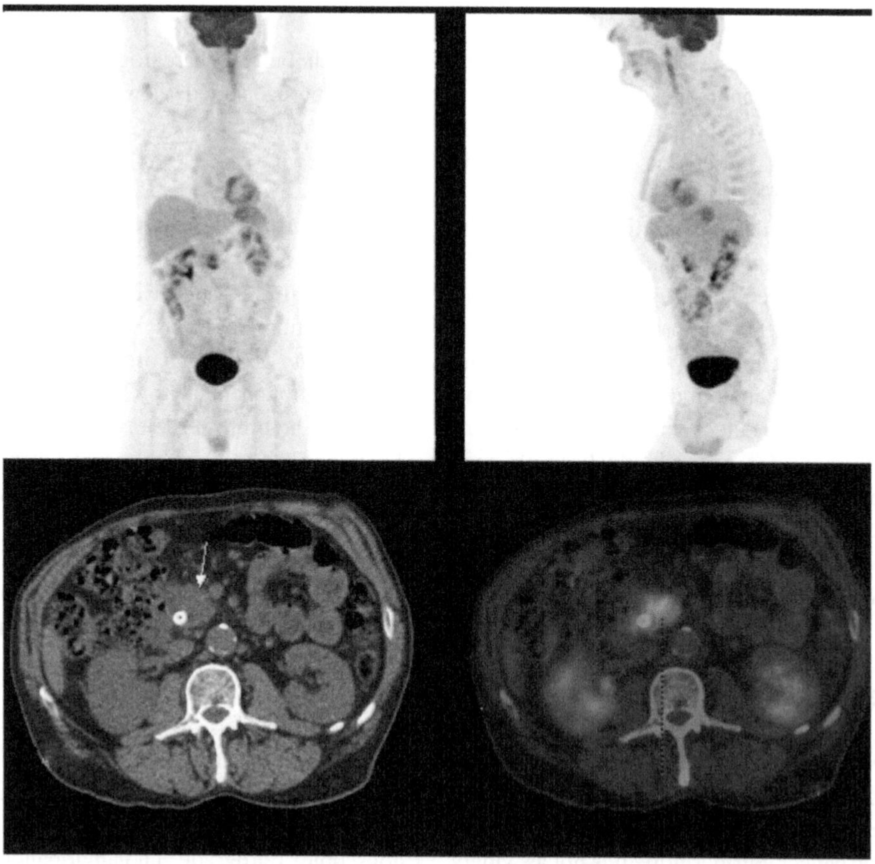

Fig. 13.4 A PET/CT scan of a 68-year-old male who presented with painless jaundice and a 3.0 cm mass in the head of the pancreas. There is a heterogeneously intense FDG avid mass involving the head of the pancreas that was suspicious for malignancy. There was no other FDG uptake identified elsewhere. The patient underwent a successful Whipple operation and the final pathology demonstrated a 4.0 cm pancreatic adenocarcinoma with 5/18 positive lymph nodes with evidence of cancer extending into portal vein. All margins, including the proximal and distal margin of the resected vein, were negative (Courtesy of Quyen D. Chu, MD, MBA, FACS)

CA19-9 level, large primary tumors, or enlarged regional lymph nodes) [9]. DL identifies occult metastatic disease that is not otherwise detected by multiple imaging modalities. Progression of disease can be identified in up to 30 % of patients with diagnostic laparoscopy [12, 13].

Staging

There are two well-recognized staging systems for pancreatic adenocarcinoma: the first, and most commonly used, is the American Joint Committee on Cancer (AJCC), also known as the TNM staging system (Table 13.1); the second staging system is the National Comprehensive Cancer Network (NCCN). The AJCC/TNM staging system is also used by the Union for International Cancer Control (UICC) for clinical, surgical, and pathologic staging, as well as for following response after treatment. The NCCN criteria classify pancreatic adenocarcinoma on the basis of surgical resectability and as such are useful as a pretreatment staging system. NCCN guidelines were adopted and modified from an expert consensus statement spearheaded by pancreatic surgical societies including the American Hepato-Pancreato-Biliary Association (AHPBA), the Society for Surgery of the Alimentary Tract (SSAT), and the Society of Surgical Oncology (SSO) (Table 13.2).

Table 13.1 American Joint Committee on Cancer (AJCC) TNM staging for pancreatic cancer (7th edition)

Primary tumor (T)	
TX	Primary tumor cannot be assessed
T0	No evidence of primary tumor
Tis	Carcinoma in situ*
T1	≤2, limited to pancreas
T2	>2, limited to pancreas
T3	Beyond pancreas, but without involvement of the celiac axis or the superior mesenteric artery
T4	Tumor involves the celiac axis or the superior mesenteric artery (unresectable primary tumor)

*This also includes the "PanInIII" classification

Regional lymph nodes (N)	
NX	Regional lymph nodes cannot be assessed
N0	No regional lymph node metastasis
N1	Regional lymph node metastasis

Distant metastasis (M)	
M0	No distant metastasis
M1	Distant metastasis

Anatomic stage/prognostic groups			
Group	T	N	M
Stage 0	Tis	N0	M0
Stage IA	T1	N0	M0
Stage IB	T2	N0	M0
Stage IIA	T3	N0	M0
Stage IIB	T1-3	N1	M0
Stage III	T4	Any N	M0
Stage IV	Any T	Any N	M1

Adapted from Compton et al. [105]. With permission from Springer Verlag

NCCN criteria defining resectability status separate pancreatic tumors into three categories: (1) localized and clearly resectable, (2) borderline resectable, and (3) locally advanced or unresectable. The specific criteria for each category are listed in Table 13.2 [9]. Of note, the borderline resectable category was not introduced until 2006.

Treatment

The management of patients with pancreatic cancer requires a multidisciplinary approach that includes participation of medical, surgical, and radiation oncologists. This also requires the expertise of radiologists and pathologists. Proper initial evaluation of a patient presenting with a pancreatic mass includes a complete history and physical examination, along with a review of laboratory and imaging studies.

In order for the treatment of pancreatic cancer to be potentially curative, guideline-directed care includes both surgical resection and chemotherapy and chemoradiation as important modalities. The first step in surgical management of pancreatic cancer is appropriate selection of surgical candidates. A patient is considered to be a surgical candidate if all of the following criteria are met: (1) the patient has a surgical disease, (2) the disease is potentially curable (i.e., no evidence of distant disease), (3) the lesion is resectable (i.e., no encasement of the superior mesenteric artery (SMA), and (4) the patient has a good performance status.

Table 13.2 The National Comprehensive Cancer Network (NCCN) and the American Hepato-Pancreato-Biliary Association (AHPBA)/Society of Surgical Oncology (SSO)/Society for Surgery of the Alimentary Tract (SSAT) pre-treatment staging system of pancreatic adenocarcinoma

Classification	Presurgical imaging criteria	Treatment recommended
Localized and clearly resectable	Absence of distant metastases Clear fat planes around the CA, HA, and SMA No SMV/PV distortion	Surgery followed by adjuvant chemoradiation or preoperative chemoradiation followed by surgery
Borderline resectable	Absence of distant metastases *SMV/PV*: Distortion or narrowing Occlusion but with suitable vessel proximal and distal, allowing for safe resection and replacement *CHA*: Abutment or short segment encasement *CA*: No abutment or encasement *SMA*: Abutment ≤ 180^0 of artery circumference *GDA*: Encasement up to HA	Neoadjuvant therapy
Locally advanced or unresectable	Absence of distant metastases *Head*: SMA encasement exceeding >180° CA abutment Unreconstructable SMV/PV occlusion Aortic or IVC invasion or encasement *Body*: SMA or CA encasement >180° Unreconstructable SMV/PV occlusion Aortic invasion *Tail*: SMA or CA encasement >180° *Nodal status*: metastases to lymph node beyond the field of resection	Chemoradiation
Metastatic	Any evidence of distant metastases	Palliative treatment: non-operative, if possible

CA celiac axis, *CHA* common hepatic artery, *SMA* superior mesentery artery, *GDA* gastroduodenal artery, *SMV* superior mesentery vein, *PV* portal vein, *IVC* inferior vena cava
(Courtesy of Quyen D. Chu, MD, MBA, FACS)

Performance status can be determined using either the Karnofsky Performance Status (KPS) scale [14] or the ECOG/Zubrod Performance Status scale [15]; the latter is less cumbersome than the former. The ECOG/Zubrod scale ranges from 0 to 5 and is as follows: (1) Zubrod 0, asymptomatic; (2) Zubrod 1, symptomatic, fully ambulatory; (3) Zubrod 2, symptomatic, in bed less than 50 % of the day; (4) Zubrod 3, symptomatic, in bed more than 50 % of the day, but not bedridden; (5) Zubrod 4, bedridden; and (6) Zubrod 5, dead. The lower the ECOG/Zubrod scale, the lower the morbidity and mortality will be from surgery. In general, surgical candidates should have an ECOG/Zubrod 0–2.

On occasions, a patient may present with obstructive jaundice with or without a definitive lesion/mass in the periampullary/head of the pancreas region. If the patient has met all of the criteria to be a surgical candidate, a preoperative tissue biopsy by percutaneous means (i.e., CT-guided biopsy) should be avoided because of the risk of cancer seeding from the needle track. However, a preoperative endoscopic ultrasound-guided biopsy of the pancreas is an acceptable modality that carries a sensitivity and specificity reaching 90 % and 100 %, respectively [16]. Percutaneous biopsy such as a CT-guided biopsy can be considered if the patient is not a surgical candidate, and a tissue biopsy is required for further management counseling or if the patient is being considered for neoadjuvant therapy.

The definitions of resectability and borderline resectability are ever evolving, but as described above, current guidelines define resectable tumors as those characterized by the absence of distant metastases and possess clear fat planes around the celiac axis, hepatic artery, and SMA and no radiologic evidence of SMV or portal vein involvement [17] (Fig. 13.5). Pancreatic tumors are considered borderline resectable if there is partial involvement of the SMV or portal vein that would allow for safe resection and reconstruction, involvement of the GDA up to the hepatic artery with either only short segment encasement or direct abutment of the hepatic artery without extension to the celiac axis, and/or tumor abutment to the SMA not exceeding 180° of vessel wall circumference (Fig. 13.6).

Standard management includes surgical resection first, followed by postoperative chemoradiation (adjuvant therapy) for those that are localized and clearly resectable. Chemoradiation is required because despite surgical resection, 80 % of patients have positive lymph nodes on pathology after a pancreatectomy, indicating that pancreatic cancer is often a *systemic* disease. For patients with borderline resectable disease, i.e., no clear margin between the tumor and the blood vessels, neoadjuvant treatment, which means chemoradiation first, followed by surgery if the tumor then becomes resectable, is often recommended. Increasingly complex vascular reconstructions and neoadjuvant therapies are increasing the boundaries of resectability; however, this must be taken in the context of the primary goal of surgical resection which is to completely remove any malignant cells. Patients left with residual disease at the time of operation have far worse outcomes than those patients with complete resections [18].

Surgical Resection

Early pancreatic resections were undertaken by surgical pioneers such as Trendelenburg, Billroth, Codivilla, Halsted, and Kausch in the late

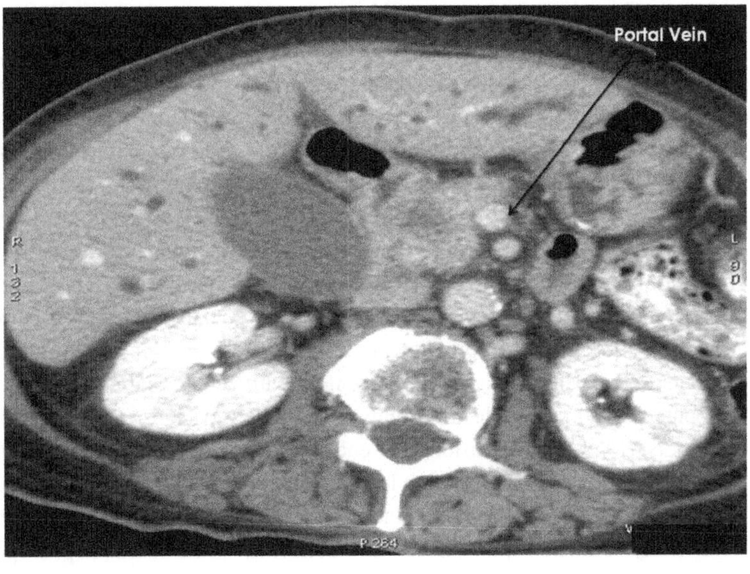

Fig. 13.5 CT scan of a patient with a mass in the head of the pancreas that is localized and easily resectable. Note a nice fat plane between the mass and the portal vein. A Whipple procedure demonstrated an adenocarcinoma of the head of the pancreas (Courtesy of Quyen D. Chu, MD, MBA, FACS)

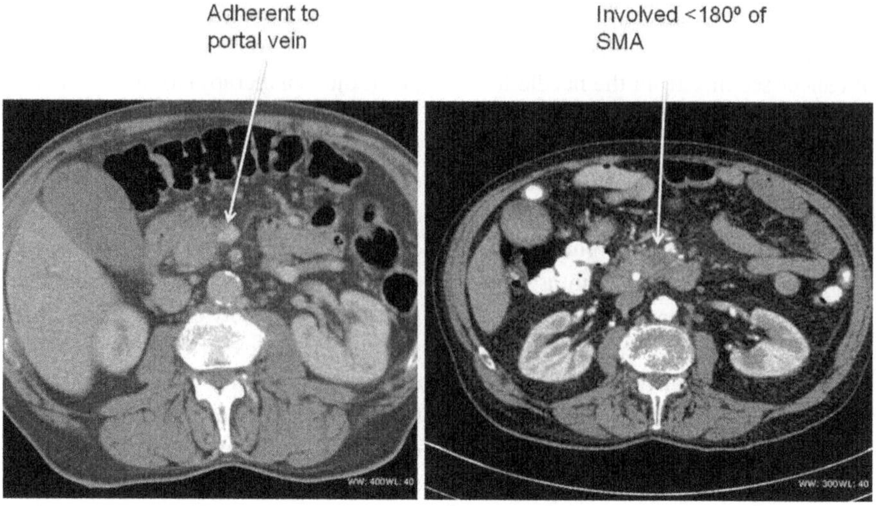

Fig. 13.6 CT scans of patients with borderline resectable pancreatic cancer. Both patients underwent neoadjuvant therapy prior to a successful Whipple operation (Courtesy of Quyen D. Chu, MD, MBA, FACS)

nineteenth and early twentieth centuries [19]. However, with perioperative mortality rates often exceeding 50 %, these operations were risky and often required multistage procedures. Operative indications and strategies were refined over the subsequent decades, culminating in the first one-stage pancreaticoduodenectomy with antrectomy performed by Dr. Allen Whipple in 1940 [20] and first total pancreatectomy by Dr. Eugene Rockey in 1942 [21]. Modest improvements in outcomes followed as surgical techniques improved over the ensuing decades, but perioperative mortality rates remained high, often exceeding 20 %, into the 1970s. However, the last 40 years has been marked by profound improvements in short-term (30-day) perioperative mortality. Mortality rates are closely associated with the extent of resection, with the highest risk occurring after a total pancreatectomy, the lowest risk occurring after a distal pancreatectomy, and an intermediate risk occurring after a pancreaticoduodenectomy (PD) [22].

Despite more recent improvements in surgical outcomes, especially at high-volume centers with perioperative mortality rates dropping below 2 % in some series [23], the historical trend of poor outcomes weighs heavy. This often leads to a nihilistic approach to the treatment of pancreatic cancer with many patients and physicians believing that the risks of pancreatic surgery outweigh the potential benefit.

Contradicting this viewpoint, recent literature suggests that as surgical techniques, patient selection, and high-volume centers continue to improve, so do surgical outcomes. Data from the Nationwide Inpatient Sample (NIS) demonstrated that the in-hospital mortality rate for all pancreatic cancer resections in the United States was 7.8 % in 1998, which was reduced to 4.6 % by 2003 [22]. Across the entire time frame of this study, the overall in-hospital mortality rate for distal pancreatectomy was 3.5 %, 6.6 % for PD, and 8.3 % for total pancreatectomy. There was a demonstrable persistent improvement in outcomes based on center volume, with a 2.4 % in-hospital mortality rate for high-volume hospitals versus 9.2 % for low-volume centers.

Despite steady gains in reducing perioperative mortality, pancreatic resections remain technically complex operations and therefore do still carry risks of significant complications including pancreatic fistula, anastomotic leak, delayed gastric emptying, infectious complications, bleeding, deep vein thrombosis, and cardiovascular events. Analysis of nationally representative discharge data from 1998 to 2006 identified a 22.7 % rate of major postoperative complications during the index hospitalization [24]. This rate remained stable, despite declining operative mortality.

As previously discussed, morbidity and mortality rates are closely correlated to the extent of the resection. Therefore, it is important to understand not only the technical aspects of each type of pancreatic resection but also the best approach for each patient with pancreatic cancer.

Pancreaticoduodenectomy

Also known as a Whipple procedure, pancreaticoduodenectomy is the most common curative resection performed for pancreatic adenocarcinoma confined to the head of the pancreas, including ampullary cancers. In this procedure, the head of the pancreas, the first and second portions of the duodenum, distal stomach, proximal jejunum, a portion of the common bile duct, the gallbladder, and the surrounding lymph nodes are removed (Fig. 13.7a, b). The reconstruction for gastrointestinal continuity includes connection of the jejunum to the remaining pancreatic duct (pancreaticojejunostomy), the bile duct (hepaticojejunostomy), and stomach (gastrojejunostomy) ("classic Whipple"; Fig. 13.7c).

"Classic" Versus Pylorus-Sparing Whipple Procedure

In comparison to the above-described "classic" Whipple procedure, the pylorus-sparing procedure does, as the name implies, preserve the stomach and pylorus. Instead, the very proximal portion of the duodenum is resected and the jejunum is then anastomosed to the duodenum (duodenojejunostomy) (Fig. 13.7d).

The debate surrounding the type of pancreaticoduodenectomy argues for pylorus-sparing on the basis of preserved gastric emptying on the one hand but, on the other hand, raises concerns about the oncologic resection, especially for larger tumors, thus advocating for the "classic" approach. Studies, however, have demonstrated no significant differences in outcomes between the two variations of this procedure. Tran et al. examined patients undergoing resection for suspected pancreatic or periampullary cancers and found no differences in median blood loss ($p=0.70$), duration of the operation ($p=0.10$), incidence of delayed gastric emptying, or overall survival between the "classic" approach and pylorus-sparing approach [25]. In a similar randomized study, Seiler et al. found that morbidity, long-term survival, quality of life, and weight gain were identical between these two variations of the procedure [26].

Total Pancreatectomy

Depending on the extent of the cancer, total pancreatectomy may be required for complete resection (Fig. 13.8). In this procedure, the entire pancreas and spleen are removed. Removing the entire pancreas, and thereby all of the insulin-producing islet cells, renders the patient to be a brittle diabetic after this procedure. Completion total pancreatectomy is often an option for patients who are septic from severe disruption of the pancreaticojejunostomy anastomosis following an elective Whipple procedure or life-threatening hemorrhage that is not amenable to conservative treatment [27].

Distal Pancreatectomy

For tumors confined to the body or tail of the pancreas, distal pancreatectomy may be performed. This procedure can be performed with or without splenectomy; most commonly it is performed with splenectomy given the overlapping blood supply and lymphatic drainage (Fig. 13.9a–b). Appropriate vaccines covering encapsulated bacteria such as *Haemophilus influenzae*, *Streptococcus pneumoniae*, and *Neisseria meningitidis* or meningococcus should be given at least 2 weeks prior to surgical resection.

The common hepatic artery, the origin of the splenic artery, and/or the celiac axis can often be involved with locally advanced cancer following neoadjuvant therapy. Although controversial, in such a patient who has no evidence of distant disease, some surgeons would perform a modified

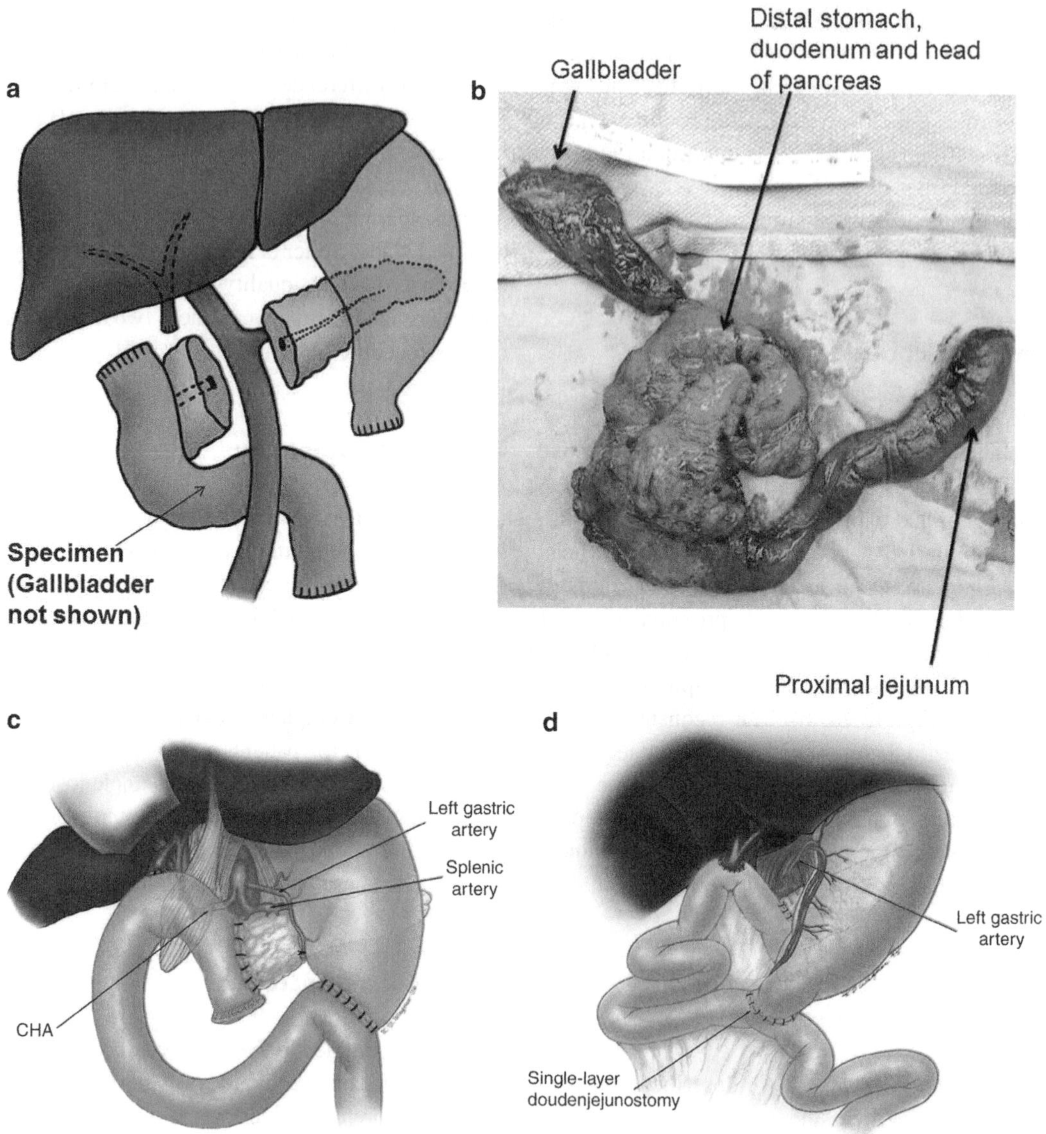

Fig. 13.7 Organs that are removed in a pancreaticoduodenectomy: a pancreaticoduodenectomy or a Whipple procedure removes the head of the pancreas, the first and second portions of the duodenum, a portion of the common bile duct, the gallbladder, and the surrounding lymph nodes. Reconstruction is achieved by performing a pancreaticojejunostomy, hepaticojejunostomy, and a gastrojejunostomy, "classic Whipple" (Figure 13. Alternatively, a pylorus-sparing reconstruction can also be performed) (A, B. Courtesy of Quyen D. Chu, MD, MBA, FACS) (C, D. Courtesy of Douglas B. Evans, MD, FACS)

Appleby procedure. The original Appleby procedure was described in the 1950s in a patient with advanced gastric cancer who underwent a total gastrectomy, distal pancreatectomy/splenectomy, and celiac axis resection [28]. The modified Appleby excludes gastrectomy. Following ligation of the celiac axis, flow to the liver is established via retrograde flow from the gastroduodenal artery (Fig. 13.9c). The procedure, although rarely done, is mentioned only to provide the readers with a better appreciation of the anatomy of the region.

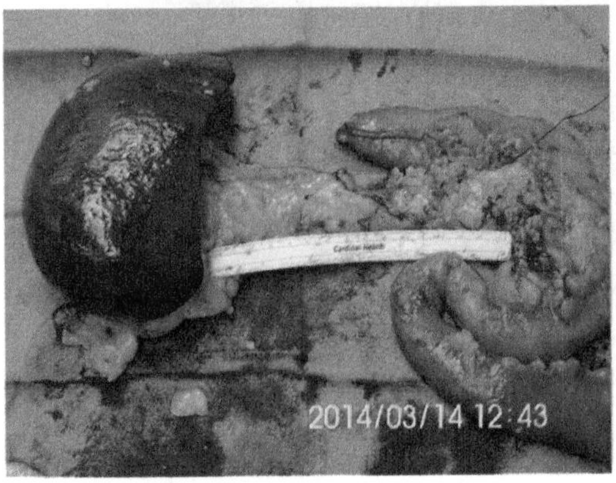

Fig. 13.8 **Total pancreatectomy**: a 56-year-old Caucasian man presented with a significant family history of pancreatic cancer. He insisted on having a screening CT scan, which revealed two separate lesions in the tail and head of the pancreas. Despite multiple counseling, he opted for a prophylactic total pancreatectomy. Final pathology demonstrated both lesions to be intraductal papillary mucinous neoplasms (IPMN) (Courtesy of Gazi Zibari, MD, FACS)

Surgical Considerations

Portal Vein Reconstruction

For cases in which the pancreatic tumor involves the superior mesenteric vein (SMV), portal vein (PV), or both, SMV/PV resection may be necessary to achieve negative margins (Fig. 13.10a, b). This should only be undertaken in special circumstances in which it is believed that R0 (microscopically negative) or R1 (grossly negative, but microscopically positive) margins can be achieved. It should also only be performed by experienced surgeons. Additional criteria for performing such a complex endeavor require that the patient has adequate inflow and outflow of the reconstructed veins and lacked any involvement of the superior mesenteric artery (SMA) and hepatic artery [29].

Extended Lymphadenectomy

This technique is currently debated as there is no definitive evidence that extended lymphadenectomy, which involves resection of retroperitoneal lymph nodes, improves survival [30]. Retrospective reports and smaller randomized trials have suggested some increase in survival, but this is not a consistent finding. Therefore, it is generally recommended, except for rare instances, such as part of a clinical trial or in the case of a large tumor that requires extended lymphadenectomy as part of an en bloc resection, that routine extended lymphadenectomy should not be performed [31].

Preoperative Biliary Drainage/Stent

Often patients with pancreatic cancer, especially those with pancreatic head tumors, present with obstructive jaundice. Symptoms of obstructive jaundice can range from mild to severe and may cause such complications as hepatic dysfunction, coagulopathy, pruritus, and cholangitis [32, 33]. In cases of severe symptoms and/or such complications, decompression of the biliary system may be required, which can successfully be accomplished with either endoscopic or percutaneous biliary stent placement. In more mild cases, the routine use of biliary drainage/stenting in the preoperative setting remains controversial. The initial rationale for decompression in these cases arose from early clinical experience that jaundiced patients undergoing surgical resection were at risk for developing postoperative complications such as infection, bleeding, and renal failure [34]. However, a more recent multicenter, randomized trial comparing preoperative biliary drainage with surgery alone for patients with cancer of the head of the pancreas found that the preoperative biliary drainage group had a significantly higher complication rate (74 %) than the surgery-only group (39 %; $p<0.001$) [35]. Therefore, current recommendations for consideration of preoperative biliary drainage/stent include patients with the following symptoms/complications—cholangitis, severe intractable pruritus, and coagulopathy—and those who will not undergo immediate surgical resection [32, 33]. Self-expanding metallic stents are preferred over plastic ones [36].

Postoperative Pancreatic Fistulas (POPF)

Although mortality after a pancreaticoduodenectomy is acceptably low (0–5 %), morbidity remains substantial, ranging from 32 % to 52 % [37–39].

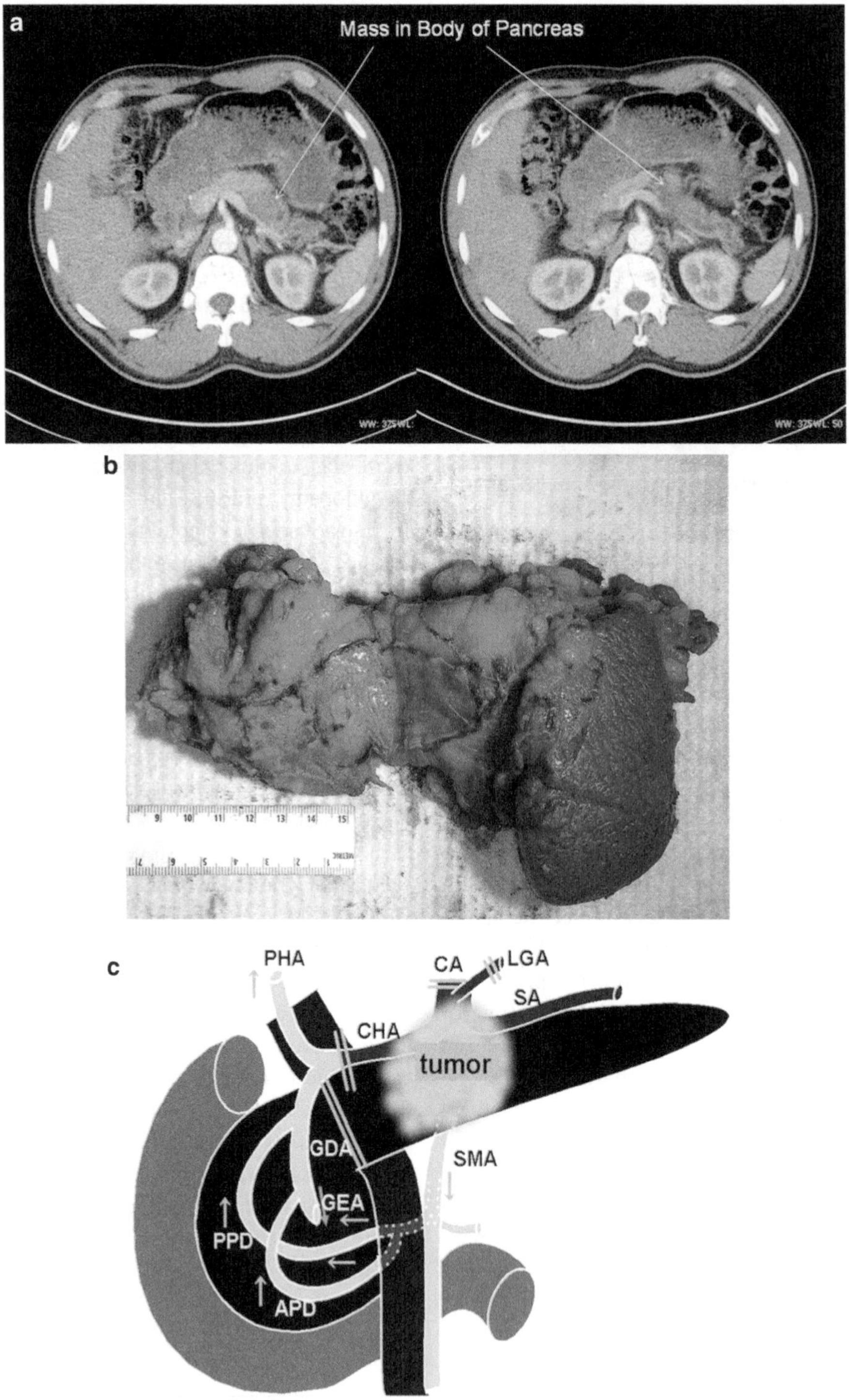

Fig. 13.9 CT scan of a patient with a mass in the body of the pancreas (**a**). The patient underwent a distal pancreatectomy and a splenectomy, which demonstrated an adenocarcinoma (**b**). The tumor measured 4.0 cm in maximal diameter with 2 out of 35 involved lymph nodes. Margins of resection were all negative. Schematic drawing of tumor involving the body of the pancreas and the celiac axis that requires a distal pancreatectomy/splenectomy and resection of the celiac axis (Appleby operation) (Fig. 13.9c). Note that retrograde flow to the proper hepatic artery (*PHA*) is via the gastroduodenal artery (GDA). *APD* anterior pancreaticoduodenal arcade, *CA* celiac axis, *CHA* common hepatic artery, *GEA* right gastroepiploic artery, *LGA* left gastric artery, *PHA* proper hepatic artery, *PPD* posterior pancreaticoduodenal arcade, *SA* splenic artery, *SMA* superior mesenteric artery (A–B. Courtesy of Quyen D. Chu, MD, MBA, FACS) (C. Reprinted from Hirano S, et al. Distal pancreatectomy with en bloc celiac axis resection for locally advanced pancreatic body cancer: Long-term results. Ann Surg 2007;246 (1):46–51 with permission from Lippincott Williams & Wilkins)

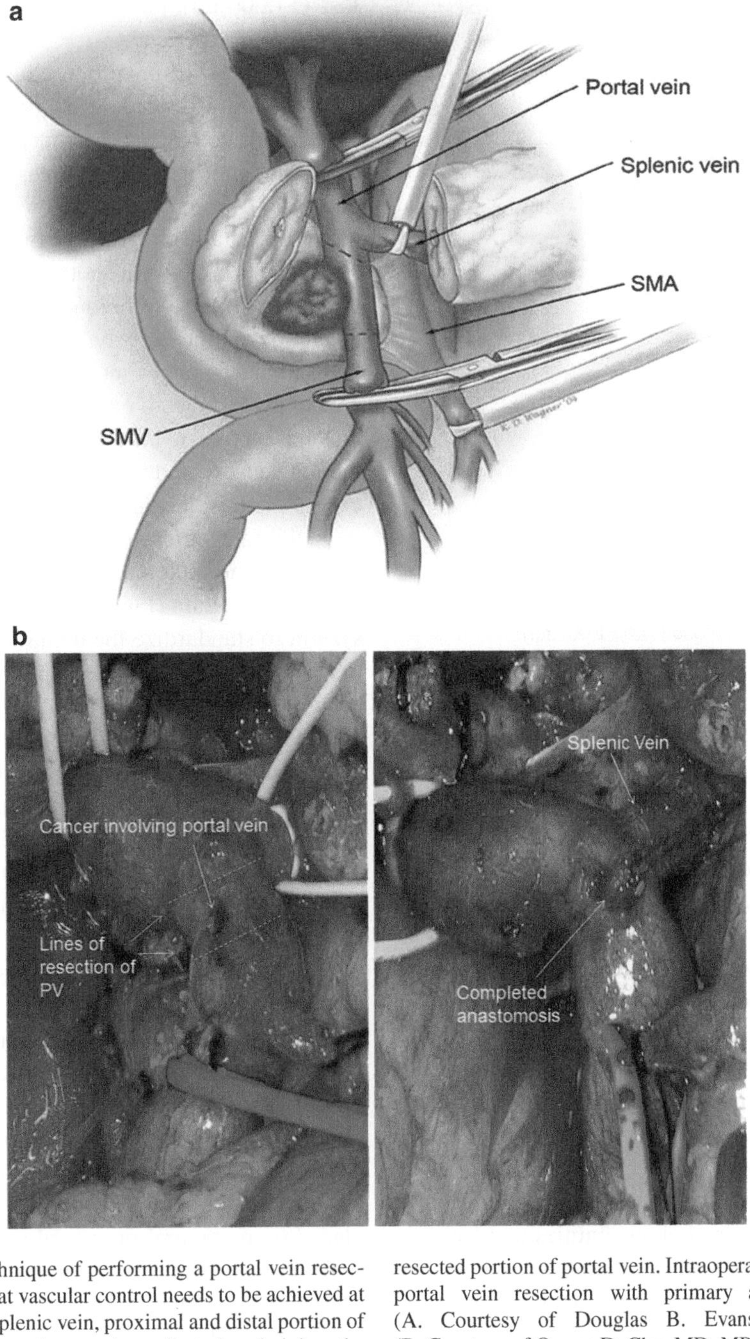

Fig. 13.10 Technique of performing a portal vein resection (**a**). Note that vascular control needs to be achieved at the level of the splenic vein, proximal and distal portion of the portal vein, and any other tributaries draining the resected portion of portal vein. Intraoperative pictures of a portal vein resection with primary anastomosis (**b**) (A. Courtesy of Douglas B. Evans, MD, FACS) (B. Courtesy of Quyen D. Chu, MD, MBA, FACS)

Of the complications, postoperative pancreatic leak/fistula (POPF) is one of the most dreaded. Depending on how one defines POPF, leakage rate varies from 0 % to 25 % [40]. Sequelae of this serious complication includes delayed gastric emptying (DGE), abdominal hemorrhage, and abscess, the latter two can result in a mortality rate of 40 % or more [41, 42].

There are many different ways of managing the pancreatic stump following a pancreaticoduodenectomy (i.e., pancreatic duct occlusion, trans-anastomotic stenting, somatostatin, etc.),

Table 13.3 Risk factors for developing pancreatic fistula following a Whipple procedure

Organ/disease-related factors
Soft pancreatic parenchyma
Duct ≤ 3 mm diameter
Pancreatic pathologies
Ampullary or duodenal carcinoma
Distal cholangiocarcinoma
Intraductal papillary mucinous neoplasia (IPMN)
Pancreatic cystadenomas
Benign islet cell tumors
Duodenal adenomas
Patient-related factors
Male gender
> 70 years of age
Prolonged jaundice
Creatinine clearance abnormality
High intraoperative blood loss (>1,000 ml)
Coronary artery disease
Operative-related factors
High intraoperative blood loss (>1,000 ml)
Prolonged operative time
Surgeon's inexperience

(Courtesy of Quyen D. Chu, M.D., M.B.A., F.A.C.S.)

although there is no consensus on any one best way. Risk factors associated with pancreatic leak following a Whipple procedure can be categorized into those that are disease-related, patient-related, and operative-related (Table 13.3).

Examples of disease-related factors include a soft pancreas because, unlike a fibrotic pancreas, pancreaticojejunostomy anastomosis is more difficult to perform. Other disease-related factors include a pancreatic duct less than or equal to 3 mm in diameter, absence of parenchymal fibrosis, fatty infiltration of the pancreatic parenchyma, and resection of pathologic entities that lacked a fibrotic pancreas such as ampullary or duodenal cancer, intraductal papillary mucinous neoplasia, cystadenomas, benign islet tumors, duodenal adenomas, and distal cholangiocarcinoma [43].

Patient-related risk factors include male gender, age > 70 years, high body mass index (BMI), coronary artery disease, prolonged jaundice, and creatinine clearance abnormality. Operative-related factors include high intraoperative blood loss (>1,000 ml), prolonged operative time, and surgeon's inexperience.

Some investigators proposed that a pancreaticogastrostomy instead of a pancreaticojejunostomy and a duct to mucosa rather than invagination of the jejunum into the pancreas are factors that decrease the rate of POPF. However, there is no definitive data to suggest that one reconstructive technique is better than another, and the selection of a reconstructive technique should be left at the discretion of the surgeon. Of interest, diabetes mellitus and neoadjuvant chemoradiation therapy appear to be protective against POPF. The mechanism is unknown, but it is thought that chemoradiation causes a reduction in pancreatic exocrine excretion, thus, leading to a lower rate of POPF.

POPF rate varies, depending on how POPF is defined. The International Study Group of Pancreatic Fistula (ISGPF) developed a grading system to standardize the definition of POPF so that surgical experiences among centers can accurately be compared [44] (Table 13.4). PFs are defined as high amylase content from the abdominal drain (>3 times the upper normal serum value) at any time on or after the third postoperative day and are grouped into grade A, B, or C based on nine clinical criteria. Grade A fistula is the most common and often referred to as a "transient fistula"; it is a biochemical leak without clinical significance and is self-limited that does not require significant intervention. However, grades B and C are clinically relevant fistulae that may require significant intervention. Grade B fistula can be associated with fever, leukocytosis, and abdominal pain. The patient's abdominal drain is left in place for a prolonged period while he/she is generally placed on parenteral or enteral nutrition. Grade C fistula can result in a life-threatening event. These patients may suffer multiorgan system failure, despite aggressive conservative management. Patients who decompensate from a significant POPF may require a reoperation to undergo a conversion of a pancreaticojejunostomy to pancreaticogastrostomy, a repair of the leak with wide peripancreatic drainage, or a completion total pancreatectomy [44, 45].

Table 13.4 International Study Group of Pancreatic Fistula (ISGPF) grading of postoperative pancreatic fistula (POPF)

Criteria	Grade A fistula	Grade B fistula	Grade C fistula
Drain amylase level	>3 times normal serum amylase	>3 times normal serum amylase	>3 times normal serum amylase
Clinical conditions	Well	Often well	Ill appearing/bad
Specific treatment[a]	No	Yes/no	Yes
US/CT (if obtained)	Negative	Negative/positive	Positive
Persistent drainage (>3weeks)[b]	No	Usually yes	Yes
Reoperation	No	No	Yes
Death related to POPF	No	No	Possibly yes
Signs of infection	No	Yes	Yes
Sepsis	No	No	Yes
Readmission	No	Yes/no	Yes/no

[a]Partial (peripheral) or total parental nutrition, antibiotics, enteral nutrition, somatostatin analogue, and/or minimal invasive drainage
[b]With or without a drain in situ
(Adapted from Bassi et al. 106]. With permission from Elsevier.)

Role of Prophylactic Somatostatin

Concerns about pancreatic fistula have prompted several investigators to evaluate the efficacy of prophylactic somatostatin in reducing such a dreaded complication. The use of prophylactic somatostatin analogues to reduce POPF remains controversial. It has not been shown to reduce mortality, and recently, a number of investigators are cautioning against its routine use. At least three meta-analyses were performed on the role of prophylactic somatostatin, one of which demonstrated no benefit in preventing clinical anastomotic leak [46–48]. A recent Cochrane analysis of 21 trials found that although the overall postoperative complication rate was significantly lower in the prophylactic somatostatin group, there were no significant differences in the reoperation rate, length of hospital stay, incidence of clinically significant fistula, or mortality rate between the somatostatin group and the controlled group [48]. In a group of patients who underwent a pancreaticoduodenectomy for malignancy, there was no significant difference in the pancreatic leak rate between the groups that received octreotide and the group that did not [49]. The differences in the conclusions of the meta-analyses may be due to publication selection biases and heterogeneity in endpoints. Somatostatin might be useful in selective cases such as those that are at risk for developing a POPF (i.e., soft gland, small duct, excessive intraoperative blood loss) [41]. Prophylactic somatostatin did not appear to have an impact on grade A fistulas [41].

Trans-anastomotic Pancreatic Duct Stenting

Trans-anastomotic pancreatic duct stenting has been proposed as a method to reduce the incidence of POPF. The theoretical advantage with stenting is that it diverts pancreatic juice away from the pancreaticojejunal anastomosis to avoid a leak. A randomized trial comparing external stenting versus no stenting found that the former had a significantly lower POPF rate (26 % vs 42 %; $P=0.034$), morbidity rate (42 % vs 62 %; $P=0.01$), and delayed gastric emptying rate (7.8 % vs 27 %; $P=0.001$), although mortality was not impacted (3.7 % vs 3.9 %; $P=0.37$) [50]. A recent meta-analysis of seven trials comparing externalized stent versus no stenting confirmed the above findings [51]. The same meta-analysis also found that when comparing internal stenting to no stenting, there was no significant difference between the two groups in postoperative complication rate. However, two randomized trials found equivalent outcomes between external and internal stenting, suggesting the role for internal stenting [52, 53].

Table 13.5 International Study Group of Pancreatic Fistula (ISGPF) grading of delayed gastric emptying

DGE	Nasogastric tube required	Unable to tolerate solid oral intake by POD	Vomiting/ gastric distension	Use of prokinetics
A	4–7 days or reinsertion > POD 3	7	±	±
B	8–14 days or reinsertion > POD 7	14	+	+
C	>14 days or reinsertion > POD 14	21	+	+

DGE delayed gastric emptying, *POD* postoperative day
(Reprinted from Giuseppe et al. [107]. With permission from Springer Verlag.)

The design of the clinical trials was very different (i.e., some perform a duct-to-mucosa pancreaticojejunostomy, while others do not) such that it is difficult to draw a definitive conclusion on the role of stenting. The decision of whether or not to stent and the choice of stenting technique are best left to the operating surgeon.

Delayed Gastric Emptying

Postoperative delayed gastric emptying (DGE) occurs when the patient is unable to tolerate per oral diet after a certain postoperative time period. Although there is no uniform definition for it, some defined DGE as occurring after the seventh, tenth, or fourteenth postoperative day. DGE is a common postoperative complication after a pancreaticoduodenectomy and is believed to be associated with major intra-abdominal complications such as POPF, biliary fistulas, and infected collections [54, 55]. DGE is observed to be more common in patients who underwent a pylorus-preserving pancreaticoduodenectomy (PPPD) compared to the classical Whipple procedure [25, 56]. ISGPS also developed a classification for DGE and reported that their grading system correlates well with the clinical course of DGE [55] (Table 13.5).

Routine Placement of an Intraoperative Intra-abdominal Drain

The routine use of intraoperative drain placement following a Whipple procedure remains controversial. Recent studies suggest that prophylactic drainage after a Whipple procedure or distal pancreatectomy does not necessarily decrease the incidence of pancreatic fistula, length of hospitalization, readmission rates, or total complications [57–60]. Although these data are compelling, the decision to use an intraoperative intra-abdominal drain should be left at the discretion of the operating surgeon.

Clavien-Dindo Classification of Postoperative Complications

Postoperative complications have historically been reported as either being minor, moderate, or major. Such a reporting can be subjective, which can lead to underestimating the severity of complications. To standardize reporting of surgical complications so that adequate comparisons can be made among different centers, Clavien proposed a 5-scale classification system in 1992 [61] and updated it in 2004 [62]. The Clavien-Dindo classification of surgical complication has been adopted for pancreatic surgery [63] (Table 13.6).

Chemoradiation

In addition to surgical resection, the optimal treatment strategy and the only potential for cure for pancreatic adenocarcinoma includes chemoradiation given either before (neoadjuvant) or after (adjuvant) resection. For patients with localized and resectable cancer, the traditional treatment regimen consists of surgical resection followed by adjuvant chemoradiation. There are approximately eight phase 3 clinical trials that support this approach [64–72] (Table 13.7). Neoadjuvant therapy (NAT) is also an option for localized/clearly resectable disease [73–78], but unlike the adjuvant approach, there are no phase III trials to support this approach (Table 13.8). NAT is more often advocated in the setting of borderline resectable disease.

Table 13.6 Clavien-Dindo classification of surgical complication adopted for pancreatic surgery

Grade	Definition
Grade I	Any deviation from the normal postoperative course without the need for pharmacological treatment or surgical, endoscopic, and radiological interventions
	Allowed therapeutic regimens are drugs as antiemetics, antipyretics, analgesics, diuretics, electrolytes, and physiotherapy. This grade also includes wound infections opened at the bedside
Grade II	Requiring pharmacological treatment with drugs other than such allowed for grade I complications
	Blood transfusions and total parenteral nutrition are also included
Grade III	Requiring surgical, endoscopic, or radiological intervention
Grade IIIa	Intervention not under general anesthesia
Grade IIIb	Intervention under general anesthesia
Grade IV	Life-threatening complication (including CNS complications)[a] requiring IV/ICU management
Grade IVa	Single-organ dysfunction (including dialysis)
Grade IVb	Multiorgan dysfunction
Grade V	Death of a patient
Suffix "d"	If the patient suffers from a complication at the time of discharge, the suffix "d" (for "disability") is added to the respective grade of complication. This label indicates the need for a follow-up to fully evaluate the complication

[a]Brain hemorrhage, ischemic stroke, subarachnoidal bleeding, but excluding transient ischemic attacks. *CNS* central nervous system, *IC* intermediate care, *ICU* intensive care unit

(Reprinted from Dindo et al. [108]. With permission from Lippincott Williams & Wilkins.)

Table 13.7 Randomized phase 3 trials of adjuvant therapy for resectable pancreatic cancer

Trials, year [ref]	# of patients	Treatment regimen	5 years (%)	Median survival (mos) (p-value)
GITSG, 1985 [64]	43	Obs vs ChemoXRT	NA	11 vs 20 (0.03)
Bakkevold, 1993 [65]	61	Obs vs Chemo	8 vs 4	11 vs 23 (0.02)
EORTC, 1999 [66]	114	Obs vs ChemoXRT	10 vs 20	12.6 vs 17.1 (0.099)
ESPAC-1, 2001 [67]	289	No chemo vs Chemo	8 vs 21	15.5 vs 20.1 (0.009)
RTOG-9704, 2008 [68]	538	Gem-5-FU-XRT vs 5-FU-5-FU-XRT	NR	16.9 vs 20.6 (0.03)
CONKO-001, 2007, 2008 [69, 70]	354	Obs vs Chemo	9 vs 21	20.2 vs 22.8 (0.05)
Ueno, 2009 [71]	119	Obs vs Chemo	11 vs 24	5 vs 11.4 (0.01)
			NS	DFS
ESPAC-3, 2010 [72]	1088	5-FU vs Gem	NA	23.0 vs 23.6 (0.39)

DFS disease-free survival, *Obs* observation, *Chemo* chemotherapy, *ChemoXRT* chemoradiotherapy, *GITSG* Gastrointestinal Tumor Study Group, *EORTC* European Organization for Research and Treatment of Cancer, *ESPAC* European Study Group for Pancreatic Cancer, *RTOG* Radiation Therapy Oncology Group, *CONKO* Charité Onkologie, *NA* not available, *NS* not significant

(Courtesy of Quyen D. Chu, MD, MBA, FACS)

Table 13.8 Phase 1 and 2 trials of neoadjuvant therapy for resectable pancreatic cancer

Trials, year [Ref]	# of patients	Treatment regimen	Median survival (mos)
Desai, 2007 [73]	12	Gem/Ox/XRT/Gem/Ox	12.5
Varadhachary, 2008 [74]	79	Gem/Cis/Gem/XRT	17.4
Evans, 2008 [75]	86	Gem/XRT	23
Heinrich, 2008 [76]	28	Gem/Cis	26.5
Le Scodan, 2008 [77]	41	5-FU/Cis/XRT	9.4
Gillen, 2010 [78]	4,394	Meta-analysis of 111 studies	20

5-FU 5-fluorouracil, *Gem* gemcitabine, *Ox* oxalaplatin, *Cis* cisplatin

(Courtesy of Quyen D. Chu, MD, MBA, FACS)

Neoadjuvant Therapy

There are several potential advantages of the neoadjuvant approach. One is that up-front chemotherapy provides the earliest treatment of occult disease. This may be especially important in the treatment of pancreatic cancer as up to 80 % of patients develop distant disease. Furthermore, this approach gives patients the greatest likelihood of receiving the benefits of chemotherapy. Up to 25 % of patients who receive up-front surgery may have surgical complications or prolonged surgical recovery that prevents them from receiving adjuvant treatment or the full course of treatment [79].

Pancreatic tumors may also be downstaged in the course of neoadjuvant treatment, thus increasing the likelihood of the patient having an R0 resection and decreasing the need for concurrent vascular resection/reconstruction. For these reasons, the neoadjuvant approach may be most advantageous in the setting of borderline resectable disease or unresectable locoregional disease (i.e., locally advanced). Locally advanced or unresectable pancreatic cancers are those that are not amenable to surgical resection (i.e., SMA encasement greater than 180°) (Fig. 13.11).

The goal in this setting is to shrink the tumor to become resectable, which can be confirmed by follow-up imaging studies. Among patients with locally advanced disease, approximately 30 % were found to be resectable after such a regimen, and for these patients, the estimated median survival was 20.5 months. This figure is comparable to the survival time of 23.3 months for those with resectable tumors who received adjuvant treatment [78].

The optimal neoadjuvant treatment approach for patients with borderline resectable or locally advanced tumors remains unresolved, although combination chemotherapy regimens appear to yield better response rates [78] (Table 13.9). Options that have been or are currently being investigated include chemoradiation followed by chemotherapy, chemotherapy followed by chemoradiation, or single versus multi-agent

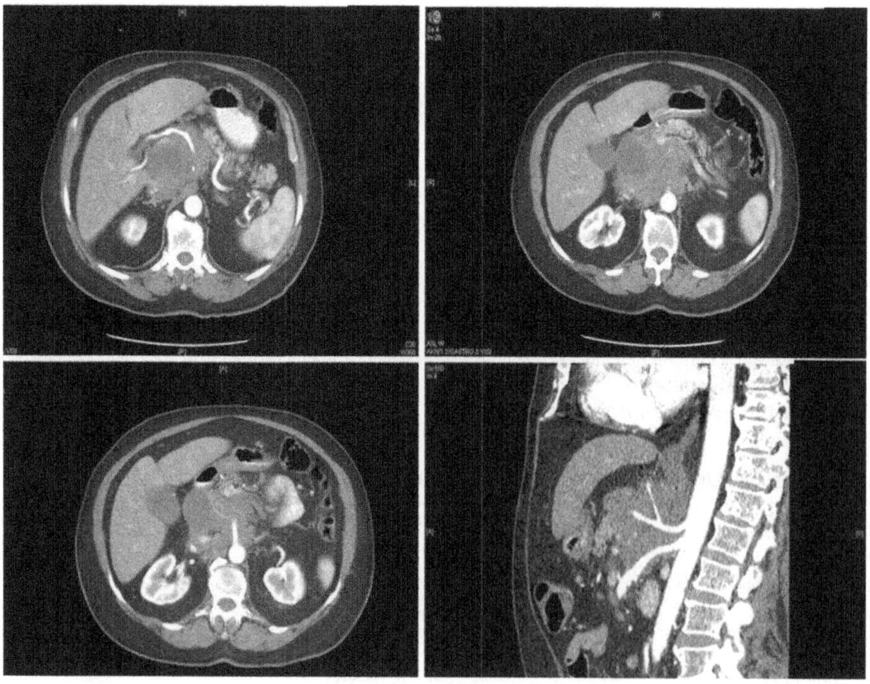

Fig. 13.11 CT scans of a patient with locally advanced or unresectable pancreatic cancer. Note the encasement of major arterial blood vessels (i.e., hepatic artery, celiac artery). This patient remained unresectable despite having completed chemoradiation therapy (Courtesy of Quyen D. Chu, MD, MBA, FACS)

Table 13.9 Selected studies of locally advanced pancreatic cancer

Trial, author, year [Ref]	# of patients	Treatment regimen	Median survival (mos)	p-value	Comments
GITSG, Moertel, 1981 [109]	194	XRT alone vs ChemoXRT (Chemo = 5-FU)	5.7 versus 10.1	<0.01	Favored ChemoXRT
GITSG, 1988 [82]	43	Chemo alone vs ChemoXRT (Chemo = 5-FU, MMC, Strep)	8 vs 10.5	<0.02	Favored ChemoXRT
ECOG, Klaassen, 1985 [110]	91	Chemo alone vs ChemoXRT (Chemo = 5-FU)	8.2 vs 8.3	NS	Retrospective study
ECOG, Cohen, 2005 [84]	114	XRT alone vs ChemoXRT (Chemo = 5-FU, MMC)	7.1 vs 8.4	NS	Toxicity higher in ChemoXRT group
FFCD/SFRO, Chauffert, 2008 [85]	119	Chemo alone vs ChemoXRT (Chemo = 5-FU, GEM, Cis)	13 vs 8.6	0.03	Toxicity higher in ChemoXRT group
ECOG, Loehrer, 2011 [86]	74	Chemo alone vs ChemoXRT (Chemo = GEM)	9.2 vs 11.1	0.017	Acceptable toxicity in ChemoXRT group
GERCOR, Huguet, 2007 [80]	181	Chemo alone vs induction chemo followed by ChemoXRT (Chemo = GEM)	11.7 vs 15	0.0009	Retrospective study
MDACC, Krishnan 2007 [87]	323	ChemoXRT vs induction chemo followed by ChemoXRT (Chemo = GEM)	8.5 vs 11.9	<0.001	Retrospective study

5-FU 5-fluorouracil, *MMC* mitomycin C, *Strep* streptozocin, *GEM* gemcitabine, *Cis* cisplatin, *XRT* radiation therapy, *ChemoXRT* chemoradiotherapy, *Chemo* chemotherapy
(Courtesy of Quyen D. Chu, MD, MBA, FACS)

chemotherapy alone [80–87]. Based on the results of the Oncology Multidisciplinary Research Group (GERCOR), NCCN currently recommends an initial short course of chemotherapy (gemcitabine, up to 4 months) followed by chemoradiation for those with stable disease or with an objective response rather than up-front chemoradiation. This approach allows systemic control of the disease as well as allowing time for the patients to reveal occult metastatic disease [9, 31, 80]. Patients who progress to metastatic disease during the course of up-front chemotherapy may then be spared of radiation therapy. For patients with poorly controlled pain or local obstructive symptoms, up-front chemoradiation is the preferred approach [9].

Lastly, as alluded to above, another potential advantage of the neoadjuvant approach is that it may identify those tumors with more favorable biologic response to chemotherapy. Patients whose disease progresses during the course of neoadjuvant chemotherapy, which can occur in up to 25 % of patients [79], would not have benefitted from up-front surgery, and thus the morbidity of surgical resection can be appropriately avoided.

Opponents of neoadjuvant treatment argue that this approach delays surgery, which is the key component to potential cure. Furthermore, significant side effects of chemotherapy such as myelosuppression may cause clinical deterioration, which may also delay or ultimately preclude surgical resection. Given the ongoing debate, especially among patients with resectable disease, a clinical trial which establishes a head-to-head comparison of neoadjuvant therapy versus adjuvant therapy will provide the most insight. The NEOPAC multicenter phase III trial is currently being conducted and may provide some of these answers. This trial compares adjuvant gemcitabine with neoadjuvant gemcitabine/oxaliplatin plus adjuvant gemcitabine [88].

Until further data is available, adjuvant therapy remains the standard of care for patients with localized/resectable pancreatic cancer. NCCN currently recommends that neoadjuvant therapy should be reserved for special situations such as those who appear to have resectable disease but have poor prognostic features or those who qualify for a clinical trial [9].

Adjuvant Therapy

The first prospective, randomized trial to examine adjuvant chemoradiation following surgical resection for pancreatic adenocarcinoma was conducted by the Gastrointestinal Tumor Study Group (GITSG) [64]. This cooperative group was composed of 14 institutions, with the majority of patients enrolled in the study accrued from Roswell Park Cancer Institute and the University of Miami [89]. The study demonstrated that combined modality treatment doubled median survival time compared to surgery alone (20 vs 11 months; $p=0.03$) [64].

Additional groups studied combined modality treatment regimens, however, with mixed results. The European Organization for Research and Treatment of Cancer (EORTC) trial was a cooperative effort by 29 centers in Europe that assessed the efficacy of adjuvant radiation therapy and 5-FU for pancreatic head and periampullary adenocarcinomas [66, 89]. Although the regimen was well tolerated, there was a lack of demonstrated survival advantage among the adjuvant therapy group compared to the surgery-alone group. The median survival for the treatment and the observation arms was 24 and 19 months, respectively, and the 5-year survival for the treatment and observation arms was 28 % and 22 %, respectively ($p=0.208$). Because the study included periampullary tumors and its possibility of being underpowered, outcomes may have been further obscured.

Another cooperative effort among European institutions, the European Study Group for Pancreatic Cancer Trial (ESPAC-1) was an investigation conducted by 83 clinicians in 61 cancer centers across 11 countries [67]. This study, published in 2001, was the largest randomized trial on adjuvant therapy for pancreatic cancer at the time and found that 5-FU/leucovorin was superior to observation. Additionally, this study determined the addition of radiotherapy had a deleterious effect; however, this study was flawed with complex study design and suboptimal radiotherapy quality control [67].

A subsequent randomized control trial published in 2007, the Charité Onkologie (CONKO-001) trial, was a phase 3 randomized control trial comparing surgery alone versus adjuvant gemcitabine for 24 weeks. This study enrolled 368 patients with at least a macroscopic complete resection (R1 or R0) without any prior chemotherapy or radiation therapy treatment [69]. Findings revealed a median disease-free survival that was significantly higher in the gemcitabine group compared to the observation group (13.4 months vs 6.9 months; $p<0.001$). The final follow-up results published in 2008 demonstrated a significantly higher median overall survival for the gemcitabine group compared to the observation group (22.8 vs 20.2 months; $p=0.005$) [90].

Another phase 3 trial published that year, RTOG 9704, examined the combined modality adjuvant treatment of gemcitabine/fluorouracil (5-FU) and radiation therapy following pancreatic resection [68]. The addition of gemcitabine to 5-FU and radiotherapy did not demonstrate statistically significant improved survival over 5-FU and radiotherapy alone, median survival of 23.6 months (with gemcitabine) versus 23.0 months (p=0.09) [68].

Similar results demonstrating no survival advantage with using adjuvant gemcitabine were published in 2010 with the ESPAC-3 trial [72]. This was a phase 3 trial that randomized patients to receive either a combination of folinic acid and 5-FU or a single agent gemcitabine; neither group was given radiotherapy and both treatment regimens were given over a 24-week period. The median survival times for the 5-FU and gemcitabine groups were 23.0 months and 23.6 months, respectively ($p=0.39$) [72].

There are many ongoing clinical trials to determine an optimal adjuvant treatment regimen for pancreatic adenocarcinoma. The NCCN currently recommends for patients with complete resection and without evidence of recurrent or metastatic disease enrollment into a clinical trial. In the absence of a clinical trial, acceptable options include chemotherapy alone (gemcitabine, 5-FU, or capecitabine) or systemic chemotherapy with gemcitabine or 5-FU given before or after radiation therapy [9].

Radiation therapy as part of the adjuvant treatment regimen remains controversial and is divided between Europe and the United States. As the results of RTOG 9704, ESPAC-1, and ESPAC-3 suggest that adjuvant chemotherapy is beneficial and the addition of radiation is deleterious, most patients in Europe are treated with adjuvant chemotherapy alone, while those in the United States usually receive chemotherapy and radiation.

Treatment for Metastatic Disease

Pancreatic adenocarcinoma is an aggressive disease with no screening protocols and vague presentation, and therefore many cases are diagnosed at late stages when tumors are unresectable and/or metastatic disease is already present. Approximately 50 % of patients diagnosed with pancreatic cancer will present with metastatic disease. Overall survival in patients with metastatic pancreatic cancer is very poor. Untreated, the median survival is approximately 2–3 months [91]. For these cases of metastatic disease, chemotherapy and chemoradiation trials exist, but there are no standard treatment regimens. Furthermore, many of these patients do not have the performance status to tolerate chemoradiation.

According to current National Comprehensive Cancer Network (NCCN) guidelines, treatment of metastatic pancreatic cancer is stratified by ECOG performance status. Good performance status is defined as those with an ECOG score of 0 or 1, having a patent biliary system/stent, good pain control, and adequate nutritional status [11]. For those with a poor performance status, either gemcitabine or supportive care is recommended. For those with good performance status, there are several options available.

Current metastatic therapy recommendations are based on studies of gemcitabine and fluorouracil (5-FU). Results published in 1997 from a randomized trial comparing gemcitabine and 5-FU demonstrated a median survival advantage in the gemcitabine group (5.65 months) versus the 5-FU group (4.41 months; $p=0.0025$). One-year survival rates were 18 % at 1 year for the gemcitabine-treated group versus 2 % for the 5-FU group [92].

Another landmark trial examining gemcitabine combination therapy was the MPACT (Metastatic Pancreatic Adenocarcinoma Clinical Trial) study. This study compared the combination of gemcitabine and Abraxane versus gemcitabine alone in advanced pancreatic cancer and showed an overall survival of 8.5 months versus 6.7 months. Furthermore, 1-year survival increased to 35 % in the combination arm versus 22 % in the single agent arm [93]. Several other studies have also tested combination chemotherapy with gemcitabine, such as gemcitabine/cetuximab [94] and gemcitabine/erlotinib/bevacizumab [95].

Another important study involving the treatment of advanced pancreatic cancer was a multicenter randomized phase 2–3 trial randomizing newly diagnosed patients with metastatic pancreatic cancer to receive either a combination chemotherapy of oxaliplatin, irinotecan, fluorouracil, and leucovorin (FOLFIRINOX) versus gemcitabine [96]. The FOLFIRINOX regimen demonstrated an overall survival advantage with median survival of 11.1 months in the FOLFIRINOX group compared to 6.8 months in the gemcitabine group ($p<0.001$). There were, however, more adverse events in the FOLFIRINOX group. Therefore, because of the intensity of this regimen and concerns regarding tolerability, there have been examinations regarding alternative dosing including dropping the bolus 5-FU given in the regimen [97].

Several combination chemotherapy regimens have been investigated, and additional trials are ongoing. These currently available treatment options demonstrate only modest improvements in survival. The future of pancreatic cancer therapy relies upon the continued advancement of the research and development of more targeted therapy for this aggressive malignancy.

Follow-Up

There are currently no clear guidelines to direct posttreatment surveillance for pancreatic adenocarcinoma. Surveillance methods used to monitor for recurrence or progression of disease include routine physical exam, tumor marker CA19-9 levels, and imaging studies. It is unclear, however, to what degree surveillance improves outcomes for patients who have completed their treatment for pancreatic adenocarcinoma. A national study looking at the use of abdominal imaging among Medicare beneficiaries demonstrated no significant survival benefit among patients who received routine CT scans [98]. Furthermore, studies regarding the use of surveillance imaging reveal that there are no clear patterns, reflecting the lack of established recommendations and the potential need for developing guidelines [98, 99].

Palliative Care

Ultimately, due to the aggressive natural history of pancreatic adenocarcinoma, many patients require palliative treatments. The goal of palliative treatments is to improve the quality of life when cure is not possible. In some circumstances, palliative surgery may be considered to relieve symptoms such as jaundice, nausea/vomiting, or pain.

In patients with advanced or metastatic cancer with poor performance status, unable to tolerate chemotherapy regimens such as those discussed above, palliative care may be the appropriate treatment [100, 101]. Furthermore, it may be of benefit to begin palliative care regimens early. If we can extrapolate the results from other studies of patients with advanced cancers, such as one study of patients with metastatic non-small cell lung cancer, patients receiving palliative care actually also demonstrate a survival benefit in addition to the other comfort benefits of palliative care. In this study, patients were randomized to either early palliative care with standard oncologic care or oncologic care alone. Overall survival was increased 11.6 months versus 8.9 months in the early palliative care group along with improvement in quality of life and less depressive symptoms [102]. It is therefore recommended that involvement of supportive care, especially early, in the setting of metastatic disease should also be done for other solid tumors such as pancreatic cancer.

Depression, pain, and malnutrition are common among patients with advanced pancreatic adenocarcinoma, and palliative medicine care should be initiated early. Pain management is especially important; with identification of the source pain, patients may be able to undergo ablation techniques through endoscopic ultrasound or CT-guided procedures [100]. Directed radiation therapy can also relieve pain from locally advanced disease [100].

In addition to pain, another common complication of locally advanced disease is biliary obstruction; this can be relieved with the placement of an endoscopic biliary stent, preferably a bare metal one as it last longer than plastic [103]. Other options also include percutaneous biliary drainage with subsequent internalization and open biliary-enteric bypass. Gastric outlet obstruction is another possible complication related to locally advanced pancreatic cancer. If a patient has a good performance status, he/she should be considered for an open or laparoscopic gastrojejunostomy with a J-tube, with or without placement of an enteral stent. In patients with poor performance status, an enteral stent placement or placement of percutaneous endoscopic gastrostomy (PEG) tube can be done [102]. Related to feeding, another major impact on quality of end-of-life care involves the use of pancreatic enzyme supplementation, as deficiency is very common in advanced pancreatic cancer. A recent study addressing end-of-life experiences from patients with advanced pancreatic cancer revealed significant distress associated with inadequate dietary management [104]. Finally, support resources are vital for patients dealing with such a devastating malignancy. Several support agencies, websites, and resources are available to patients and families, including the Pancreatic Cancer Action Network (pancan.org) and the American Cancer Society (cancer.org).

Summary

Pancreatic ductal adenocarcinoma is the most common and most aggressive form of pancreatic cancer. This is a solid exocrine tumor arising from the pancreatic ducts and comprises approximately 90 % of all solid tumors of the pancreas. Pancreatic adenocarcinoma develops from precursor lesions (pancreatic intraepithelial neoplasias, or PanINs) in the duct epithelium. Progression is thought to involve telomere shortening and mutations of the oncogene KRAS occurring in early stages, followed by the inactivation of the p16 tumor suppressor gene intermediately and, finally, the inactivation of the p53, SMAD4 (DPC4), and BRCA2 tumor suppressor genes at late stages. Diagnosis of pancreatic adenocarcinoma remains challenging owing to the lack of adequate screening techniques. This leads to the majority of pancreatic adenocarcinoma being diagnosed in late stages. Among the cancers diagnosed in earlier stages, the best chance at cure involves multimodality treatment strategies that include surgical resection as well as chemotherapy and radiation. Chemoradiation may take the form of neoadjuvant (before resection) or adjuvant (after resection) treatment strategies. Neoadjuvant versus adjuvant trials are ongoing, but at this time, neoadjuvant regimens are generally used in cases of borderline resectable disease. Current NCCN guidelines for treatment of resectable disease recommend enrollment in a clinical trial for patients with complete resection and without evidence of recurrent or metastatic disease. In the absence of a clinical trial, acceptable adjuvant treatment options include chemotherapy alone (gemcitabine, 5-FU, or capecitabine) or systemic chemotherapy with gemcitabine or 5-FU given before or after radiation therapy. Current metastatic therapy recommendations include chemotherapy combinations containing gemcitabine or FOLFIRINOX regimens; additional treatments are under investigation. Ultimately, due to the aggressive natural history of the disease, many patients require palliative treatments. Depression, pain, and malnutrition are common among patients with advanced pancreatic adenocarcinoma, and palliative care interventions should be initiated early.

Salient Points

- Pancreatic adenocarcinoma is an aggressive malignancy whose incidence roughly equals its mortality.
- Smoking, chronic pancreatitis, diabetes, high consumption of meat and fat, and obesity are risk factors.
- Pancreatic intraepithelial neoplasias (PanINs) are the most common precursor lesions of invasive pancreatic carcinoma.
- CT scan is the recommended initial imaging studies.
- Endoscopic ultrasound is helpful in detecting small lesions and also allows for biopsy of suspicious lesions.
- CT-guided biopsy should be avoided unless the patient is not a surgical candidate or he/she is being considered for neoadjuvant therapy; a tissue confirmation of malignancy may be required for decision making algorithm.
- Diagnostic laparoscopy to rule out peritoneal and liver metastases is an option and is helpful in those with borderline resectable disease; those with markedly elevated serum CA19-9, large primary tumors, and lymphadenopathy; or those with tumors in the body/tail of the pancreas.
- Patients can be classified as having localized, clearly resectable, borderline resectable, unresectable (locally advanced), or metastatic disease.
- A percutaneous biopsy (i.e., CT-guided biopsy) of a pancreatic mass should be avoided if the patient:
- Is a surgical candidate
- Has resectable, nonmetastatic disease
- Can tolerate surgery (good performance status)

- A percutaneous biopsy can be done if the patient:
- Is not a surgical candidate but a tissue diagnosis is required
- Is considered for neoadjuvant therapy
- For patients with localized, clearly resectable disease, options include surgery followed by adjuvant chemoradiation or neoadjuvant therapy followed by surgery. The adjuvant approach is supported by phase 3 data, while the neoadjuvant approach is supported by phase 2 data.
- NEOPAC is a clinical trial that will compare the adjuvant with the neoadjuvant approach for patients with resectable pancreatic cancer.
- Acceptable options for patients who underwent complete pancreatectomy include:
- Chemotherapy alone (gemcitabine, 5-FU, or capecitabine)
- Systemic chemotherapy with gemcitabine or 5-FU either before or after radiation therapy
- Patients with borderline resectable and locally advanced pancreatic cancer should undergo chemoradiation first.
- There is no difference in outcome between a "classic" Whipple versus the pylorus-sparing Whipple.
- Portal vein resection is a viable option but should be performed by experienced surgeons.
- There is no role for extended lymphadenectomy.
- Preoperative biliary stenting should be avoided unless the patient has cholangitis, severe intractable pruritus, coagulopathy, and will not undergo immediate surgery (i.e., poor nutritional status).
- Self-expanding metallic stents are preferred over plastic stents.
- Somatostatin did not affect reoperation rate, length of hospital stay, incidence of clinically significant fistulas, or mortality.
- The need for routine intraoperative intra-abdominal drain placement is being questioned.
- FOLFIRINOX (oxaliplatin, irinotecan, fluorouracil, leucovorin) or gemcitabine and Abraxane (paclitaxel protein bound) are options for patients with advanced/metastatic pancreatic cancer.

Questions

1. All of the following are true regarding pancreatic ductal adenocarcinoma except:
   A. Most common of all pancreatic cancers
   B. Often diagnosed by screening tests, including serum tests of CA19-9
   C. Exocrine tumor
   D. Incidence rate roughly equals mortality rate
2. Two of the most commonly cited risk factors associated with the development of pancreatic adenocarcinoma include:
   A. Chronic pancreatitis and smoking
   B. Smoking and radiation exposure
   C. Family history and diet rich in fatty foods
   D. Radiation exposure and alcohol intake
3. In the progression of pancreatic cancer from normal epithelium to cancerous lesions, all of the following histopathological changes are noted EXCEPT:
   A. Pancreatic intraepithelial neoplasia (PanIN)-1A flat lesions
   B. Pancreatic intraepithelial neoplasia (PanIN)-1B micropapillary lesions showing minimal cytological and architectural atypia
   C. Pancreatic intraepithelial neoplasia (PanIN)-2 lesions demonstrating severe cytological and architectural atypia
   D. Ductal adenocarcinoma with poorly differentiated tubular structures or cell clusters and dense stromal fibrosis
4. Patients with pancreatic adenocarcinoma may present with the following symptoms:
   A. Painless jaundice
   B. Central abdominal pain radiating to the back
   C. No symptoms
   D. All of the above
5. Diagnostic studies used to evaluate pancreatic cancer may include all of the following EXCEPT:
   A. Serum CA19-9 level
   B. Serum CA-125 level
   C. MRCP
   D. Laparoscopy

6. Borderline resectable pancreatic cancer demonstrates the following features EXCEPT:
   A. No evidence of metastatic disease
   B. Tumor abutment to the hepatic artery without extension to celiac axis
   C. No involvement of SMV
   D. Tumor abutment to the SMA not exceeding 180° of vessel wall
7. Following surgical resection of resectable pancreatic cancer, the following is an option EXCEPT:
   A. Adjuvant chemoradiation
   B. Adjuvant radiation alone
   C. Adjuvant gemcitabine alone
   D. Adjuvant 5-FU alone
8. Goals of neoadjuvant therapy for pancreatic cancer include all of the following EXCEPT:
   A. Provides earliest treatment of occult disease
   B. May downstage more advanced tumors
   C. Allows for identification of tumors with more aggressive biology
   D. May eliminate the need for surgical resection of early stage tumors
9. Palliative treatment for unresectable pancreatic cancer may include:
   A. Surgical intervention
   B. Celiac plexus block
   C. Directed radiation
   D. All of the above

Answers

1. B
2. A
3. C
4. D
5. B
6. C
7. B
8. D
9. D

References

1. Siegel R, Naishadham D, Jemal A. Cancer statistics, 2013. CA Cancer J Clin. 2013;63(1):11–30.
2. Simons JP, Ng SC, McDade TP, Zhou Z, Earle CC, Tseng JF. Progress for resectable pancreatic [corrected] cancer?: a population-based assessment of US practices. Cancer. 2010;116(7):1681–90.
3. Howlader NNA, Krapcho M. SEER cancer statistics review, 1975–2008. Bethesda: National Cancer Institute; 2011.
4. Yadav D, Lowenfels AB. The epidemiology of pancreatitis and pancreatic cancer. Gastroenterology. 2013;144(6):1252–61.
5. Li D, Tang H, Hassan MM, Holly EA, Bracci PM, Silverman DT. Diabetes and risk of pancreatic cancer: a pooled analysis of three large case–control studies. Cancer Causes Control. 2011;22(2):189–97.
6. Rustgi AK. A historical perspective on clinical advances in pancreatic diseases. Gastroenterology. 2013;144(6):1249–51.
7. Zamboni G, Hirabayashi K, Castelli P, Lennon AM. Precancerous lesions of the pancreas. Best Pract Res Clin Gastroenterol. 2013;27(2):299–322.
8. Robbins SL, Kumar V, Cotran RS, editors. Robbins and Cotran pathologic basis of disease. 8th ed. Philadelphia, PA: Saunders/Elsevier; 2010.
9. National Comprehensive Cancer Network (NCCN) guidelines. Available at: www.nccn.org (2013). Accessed 23 May 2013.
10. DiMagno EP. Pancreatic cancer: clinical presentation, pitfalls and early clues. Ann Oncol. 1999;10 Suppl 4:140–2.
11. Porta M, Fabregat X, Malats N, et al. Exocrine pancreatic cancer: symptoms at presentation and their relation to tumour site and stage. Clin Transl Oncol. 2005;7(5):189–97.
12. Ahmed SI, Bochkarev V, Oleynikov D, Sasson AR. Patients with pancreatic adenocarcinoma benefit from staging laparoscopy. J Laparoendosc Adv Surg Tech A. 2006;16(5):458–63.
13. Mayo SC, Austin DF, Sheppard BC, Mori M, Shipley DK, Billingsley KG. Evolving preoperative evaluation of patients with pancreatic cancer: does laparoscopy have a role in the current era? J Am Coll Surg. 2009;208(1):87–95.
14. Karnofsky D, Burchenal J. The clinical evaluation of chemotherapeutic agents in cancer. In: MacLeod C, editor. Evaluation of chemotherapeutic agents. New York: Columbia University Press; 1949. p. 191–205.
15. Oken MM, Creech RH, Tormey DC, et al. Toxicity and response criteria of the Eastern cooperative oncology group. Am J Clin Oncol. 1982;5(6): 649–55.
16. Raut CP, Grau AM, Staerkel GA, et al. Diagnostic accuracy of endoscopic ultrasound-guided fine-needle aspiration in patients with presumed pancreatic cancer. J Gastrointest Surg. 2003;7(1):118–26. discussion 127–118.
17. Callery MP, Chang KJ, Fishman EK, Talamonti MS, William Traverso L, Linehan DC. Pretreatment assessment of resectable and borderline resectable pancreatic cancer: expert consensus statement. Ann Surg Oncol. 2009;16(7):1727–33.
18. Gillen S, Schuster T, Friess H, Kleeff J. Palliative resections versus palliative bypass procedures in pancreatic cancer–a systematic review. Am J Surg. 2012;203(4):496–502.

19. Schnelldorfer T, Adams DB, Warshaw AL, Lillemoe KD, Sarr MG. Forgotten pioneers of pancreatic surgery: beyond the favorite few. Ann Surg. 2008; 247(1):191–202.
20. Whipple AO. Pancreaticoduodenectomy for Islet Carcinoma : a five-year follow-up. Ann Surg. 1945; 121(6):847–52.
21. Rockey EW. Total Pancreatectomy for Carcinoma : case report. Ann Surg. 1943;118(4):603–11.
22. McPhee JT, Hill JS, Whalen GF, et al. Perioperative mortality for pancreatectomy: a national perspective. Ann Surg. 2007;246(2):246–53.
23. Winter JM, Brennan MF, Tang LH, et al. Survival after resection of pancreatic adenocarcinoma: results from a single institution over three decades. Ann Surg Oncol. 2012;19(1):169–75.
24. Simons JP, Shah SA, Ng SC, Whalen GF, Tseng JF. National complication rates after pancreatectomy: beyond mere mortality. J Gastrointest Surg. 2009;13(10):1798–805.
25. Tran KT, Smeenk HG, van Eijck CH, et al. Pylorus preserving pancreaticoduodenectomy versus standard Whipple procedure: a prospective, randomized, multicenter analysis of 170 patients with pancreatic and periampullary tumors. Ann Surg. 2004;240(5): 738–45.
26. Seiler CA, Wagner M, Bachmann T, et al. Randomized clinical trial of pylorus-preserving duodenopancreatectomy versus classical Whipple resection-long term results. Br J Surg. 2005;92(5): 547–56.
27. Kulu Y, Schmied BM, Werner J, Muselli P, Büchler MW, Schmidt J. Total pancreatectomy for pancreatic cancer: indications and operative technique. HPB. 2009;11(6):469–75.
28. Appleby LH. The coeliac axis in the expansion of the operation for gastric carcinoma. Cancer. 1953;6(4):704–7.
29. Evans DB, Farnell MB, Lillemoe KD, Vollmer C, Strasberg SM, Schulick RD. Surgical treatment of resectable and borderline resectable pancreas cancer: expert consensus statement. Ann Surg Oncol. 2009;16(7):1736–44.
30. Yeo CJ, Cameron JL, Lillemoe KD, et al. Pancreaticoduodenectomy with or without distal gastrectomy and extended retroperitoneal lymphadenectomy for periampullary adenocarcinoma, part 2: randomized controlled trial evaluating survival, morbidity, and mortality. Ann Surg. 2002;236(3):355–66. discussion 366–358.
31. Tempero MA, Arnoletti JP, Behrman S, et al. Pancreatic adenocarcinoma. J Natl Compr Canc Netw. 2010;8(9):972–1017.
32. Kloek JJ, Heger M, van der Gaag NA, et al. Effect of preoperative biliary drainage on coagulation and fibrinolysis in severe obstructive cholestasis. J Clin Gastroenterol. 2010;44(9):646–52.
33. Baron TH, Kozarek RA. Preoperative biliary stents in pancreatic cancer–proceed with caution. N Engl J Med. 2010;362(2):170–2.
34. Dixon JM, Armstrong CP, Duffy SW, Davies GC. Factors affecting morbidity and mortality after surgery for obstructive jaundice: a review of 373 patients. Gut. 1983;24(9):845–52.
35. van der Gaag NA, Rauws EA, van Eijck CH, et al. Preoperative biliary drainage for cancer of the head of the pancreas. N Engl J Med. 2010;362(2):129–37.
36. Decker C, Christein JD, Phadnis MA, Wilcox CM, Varadarajulu S. Biliary metal stents are superior to plastic stents for preoperative biliary decompression in pancreatic cancer. Surg Endosc. 2011;25(7):2364–7.
37. Cameron JL, Pitt HA, Yeo CJ, Lillemoe KD, Kaufman HS, Coleman J. One hundred and forty-five consecutive pancreaticoduodenectomies without mortality. Ann Surg. 1993;217(5):430–5. discussion 435–438.
38. Miedema BW, Sarr MG, van Heerden JA, Nagorney DM, McIlrath DC, Ilstrup D. Complications following pancreaticoduodenectomy. Current management. Arch Surg. 1992;127(8):945–9. discussion 949–950.
39. Trede M, Schwall G. The complications of pancreatectomy. Ann Surg. 1988;207(1):39–47.
40. Bassi C, Butturini G, Molinari E, et al. Pancreatic fistula rate after pancreatic resection. The importance of definitions. Dig Surg. 2004;21(1):54–9.
41. Callery MP, Pratt WB, Vollmer CM. Prevention and management of pancreatic fistula. J Gastrointest Surg. 2009;13(1):163–73.
42. Lai EC, Lau SH, Lau WY. Measures to prevent pancreatic fistula after pancreatoduodenectomy: a comprehensive review. Arch Surg. 2009;144(11): 1074–80.
43. Crippa S, Salvia R, Falconi M, Butturini G, Landoni L, Bassi C. Anastomotic leakage in pancreatic surgery. HPB. 2007;9(1):8–15.
44. Bassi C, Dervenis C, Butturini G, et al. Postoperative pancreatic fistula: an international study group (ISGPF) definition. Surgery. 2005;138(1):8–13.
45. van Berge Henegouwen MI, De Wit LT, Van Gulik TM, Obertop H, Gouma DJ. Incidence, risk factors, and treatment of pancreatic leakage after pancreaticoduodenectomy: drainage versus resection of the pancreatic remnant. J Am Coll Surg. 1997;185(1):18–24.
46. Connor S, Alexakis N, Garden OJ, Leandros E, Bramis J, Wigmore SJ. Meta-analysis of the value of somatostatin and its analogues in reducing complications associated with pancreatic surgery. Br J Surg. 2005;92(9):1059–67.
47. Alghamdi AA, Jawas AM, Hart RS. Use of octreotide for the prevention of pancreatic fistula after elective pancreatic surgery: a systematic review and meta-analysis. Can J Surg. 2007;50(6):459–66.
48. Gurusamy KS, Koti R, Fusai G, Davidson BR. Somatostatin analogues for pancreatic surgery. Cochrane Database Syst Rev. 2013;4, CD008370.
49. Lowy AM, Lee JE, Pisters PW, et al. Prospective, randomized trial of octreotide to prevent pancreatic fistula after pancreaticoduodenectomy for malignant disease. Ann Surg. 1997;226(5):632–41.

50. Pessaux P, Sauvanet A, Mariette C, et al. External pancreatic duct stent decreases pancreatic fistula rate after pancreaticoduodenectomy: prospective multicenter randomized trial. Ann Surg. 2011;253(5):879–85.
51. Zhou Y, Zhou Q, Li Z, Lin Q, Gong Y, Chen R. The impact of internal or external transanastomotic pancreatic duct stents following pancreaticojejunostomy. Which one is better? A meta-analysis. J Gastrointest Surg. 2012;16(12):2322–35.
52. Tani M, Kawai M, Hirono S, et al. A prospective randomized controlled trial of internal versus external drainage with pancreaticojejunostomy for pancreaticoduodenectomy. Am J Surg. 2010;199(6):759–64.
53. Kamoda Y, Fujino Y, Matsumoto I, Shinzeki M, Sakai T, Kuroda Y. Usefulness of performing a pancreaticojejunostomy with an internal stent after a pancreatoduodenectomy. Surg Today. 2008;38(6):524–8.
54. Wente MN, Bassi C, Dervenis C, et al. Delayed gastric emptying (DGE) after pancreatic surgery: a suggested definition by the International Study Group of Pancreatic Surgery (ISGPS). Surgery. 2007;142(5):761–8.
55. Malleo G, Crippa S, Butturini G, et al. Delayed gastric emptying after pylorus-preserving pancreaticoduodenectomy: validation of International Study Group of Pancreatic Surgery classification and analysis of risk factors. HPB. 2010;12(9):610–8.
56. Horstmann O, Markus PM, Ghadimi MB, Becker H. Pylorus preservation has no impact on delayed gastric emptying after pancreatic head resection. Pancreas. 2004;28(1):69–74.
57. Conlon KC, Labow D, Leung D, et al. Prospective randomized clinical trial of the value of intraperitoneal drainage after pancreatic resection. Ann Surg. 2001;234(4):487–93. discussion 493–484.
58. Fisher WE, Hodges SE, Silberfein EJ, et al. Pancreatic resection without routine intraperitoneal drainage. HPB. 2011;13(7):503–10.
59. Correa-Gallego C, Brennan MF, D'angelica M, et al. Operative drainage following pancreatic resection: analysis of 1122 patients resected over 5 years at a single institution. Ann Surg. 2013;258(6):1051–8.
60. Mehta VV, Fisher SB, Maithel SK, Sarmiento JM, Staley CA, Kooby DA. Is it time to abandon routine operative drain use? A single institution assessment of 709 consecutive pancreaticoduodenectomies. J Am Coll Surg. 2013;216(4):635–42. discussion 642–634.
61. Clavien PA, Sanabria JR, Strasberg SM. Proposed classification of complications of surgery with examples of utility in cholecystectomy. Surgery. 1992;111(5):518–26.
62. Dindo D, Demartines N, Clavien PA. Classification of surgical complications: a new proposal with evaluation in a cohort of 6336 patients and results of a survey. Ann Surg. 2004;240(2):205–13.
63. DeOliveira ML, Winter JM, Schafer M, et al. Assessment of complications after pancreatic surgery: a novel grading system applied to 633 patients undergoing pancreaticoduodenectomy. Ann Surg. 2006;244(6):931–7. discussion 937–939.
64. Kalser MH, Ellenberg SS. Pancreatic cancer. Adjuvant combined radiation and chemotherapy following curative resection. Arch Surg. 1985;120(8):899–903.
65. Bakkevold KE, Arnesjø B, Dahl O, Kambestad B. Adjuvant combination chemotherapy (AMF) following radical resection of carcinoma of the pancreas and papilla of Vater–results of a controlled, prospective, randomised multicentre study. Eur J Cancer. 1993;29A(5):698–703.
66. Klinkenbijl JH, Jeekel J, Sahmoud T, et al. Adjuvant radiotherapy and 5-fluorouracil after curative resection of cancer of the pancreas and periampullary region: phase III trial of the EORTC gastrointestinal tract cancer cooperative group. Ann Surg. 1999;230(6):776–82. discussion 782–774.
67. Neoptolemos JP, Dunn JA, Stocken DD, et al. Adjuvant chemoradiotherapy and chemotherapy in resectable pancreatic cancer: a randomised controlled trial. Lancet. 2001;358(9293):1576–85.
68. Regine WF, Winter KA, Abrams RA, et al. Fluorouracil vs gemcitabine chemotherapy before and after fluorouracil-based chemoradiation following resection of pancreatic adenocarcinoma: a randomized controlled trial. JAMA. 2008;299(9):1019–26.
69. Oettle H, Post S, Neuhaus P, et al. Adjuvant chemotherapy with gemcitabine vs observation in patients undergoing curative-intent resection of pancreatic cancer: a randomized controlled trial. JAMA. 2007;297(3):267–77.
70. Neuhaus P, Riess H, Post S, et al. CONKO-001: final results of the randomized, prospective, multicenter phase III trial of adjuvant chemotherapy with gemcitabine versus observation in patients with resected pancreatic cancer (PC). J Clin Oncol. 2008; 26 Suppl 1(Abstract LBA 4504).
71. Ueno H, Kosuge T, Matsuyama Y, et al. A randomised phase III trial comparing gemcitabine with surgery-only in patients with resected pancreatic cancer: Japanese Study Group of Adjuvant Therapy for Pancreatic Cancer. Br J Cancer. 2009;101(6):908–15.
72. Neoptolemos JP, Stocken DD, Bassi C, et al. Adjuvant chemotherapy with fluorouracil plus folinic acid vs gemcitabine following pancreatic cancer resection: a randomized controlled trial. JAMA. 2010;304(10):1073–81.
73. Desai SP, Ben-Josef E, Normolle DP, et al. Phase I study of oxaliplatin, full-dose gemcitabine, and concurrent radiation therapy in pancreatic cancer. J Clin Oncol. 2007;25(29):4587–92.
74. Varadhachary GR, Wolff RA, Crane CH, et al. Preoperative gemcitabine and cisplatin followed by gemcitabine-based chemoradiation for resectable adenocarcinoma of the pancreatic head. J Clin Oncol. 2008;26(21):3487–95.

75. Evans DB, Varadhachary GR, Crane CH, et al. Preoperative gemcitabine-based chemoradiation for patients with resectable adenocarcinoma of the pancreatic head. J Clin Oncol. 2008;26(21):3496–502.
76. Heinrich S, Schäfer M, Weber A, et al. Neoadjuvant chemotherapy generates a significant tumor response in resectable pancreatic cancer without increasing morbidity: results of a prospective phase II trial. Ann Surg. 2008;248(6):1014–22.
77. Le Scodan R, Mornex F, Partensky C, et al. Histopathological response to preoperative chemoradiation for resectable pancreatic adenocarcinoma: the French Phase II FFCD 9704-SFRO Trial. Am J Clin Oncol. 2008;31(6):545–52.
78. Gillen S, Schuster T, Meyer Zum Büschenfelde C, Friess C, Kleeff J. Preoperative/neoadjuvant therapy in pancreatic cancer: a systematic review and meta-analysis of response and resection percentages. PLoS Med. 2010;7(4):e1000267.
79. Breslin TM, Hess KR, Harbison DB, et al. Neoadjuvant chemoradiotherapy for adenocarcinoma of the pancreas: treatment variables and survival duration. Ann Surg Oncol. 2001;8(2):123–32.
80. Huguet F, André T, Hammel P, et al. Impact of chemoradiotherapy after disease control with chemotherapy in locally advanced pancreatic adenocarcinoma in GERCOR phase II and III studies. J Clin Oncol. 2007;25(3):326–31.
81. Moertel CGFS, Hahn RG, O'Connell MJ, Reitemeier RJ, Rubin J, Schutt AJ, Weiland LH, Childs DS, Holbrook MA, Lavin PT, Livstone E, Spiro H, Knowlton A, Kalser M, Barkin J, Lessner H, Mann-Kaplan R, Ramming K, Douglas Jr HO, Thomas P, Nave H, Bateman J, Lokich J, Brooks J, Chaffey J, Corson JM, Zamcheck N, Novak JW. Therapy of locally unresectable pancreatic carcinoma: a randomized comparison of high dose (6000 rads) radiation alone, moderate dose radiation (4000 rads + 5-fluorouracil), and high dose radiation + 5-fluorouracil: The Gastrointestinal Tumor Study Group. Cancer. 1981;48(8):1705–10.
82. Treatment of locally unresectable carcinoma of the pancreas: comparison of combined-modality therapy (chemotherapy plus radiotherapy) to chemotherapy alone. Gastrointestinal Tumor Study Group. J Natl Cancer Inst. 1988;80(10):751–755.
83. Klaassen DJMJ, Catton GE, Engstrom PF, Moertel CG. Treatment of locally unresectable cancer of the stomach and pancreas: a randomized comparison of 5-fluorouracil alone with radiation plus concurrent and maintenance 5-fluorouracil–an Eastern Cooperative Oncology Group study. J Clin Oncol. 1985;3(3):373–8.
84. Cohen SJ, Dobelbower R, Lipsitz S, et al. A randomized phase III study of radiotherapy alone or with 5-fluorouracil and mitomycin-C in patients with locally advanced adenocarcinoma of the pancreas: Eastern Cooperative Oncology Group study E8282. Int J Radiat Oncol Biol Phys. 2005;62(5):1345–50.
85. Chauffert B, Mornex F, Bonnetain F, et al. Phase III trial comparing intensive induction chemoradiotherapy (60 Gy, infusional 5-FU and intermittent cisplatin) followed by maintenance gemcitabine with gemcitabine alone for locally advanced unresectable pancreatic cancer. Definitive results of the 2000–01 FFCD/SFRO study. Ann Oncol. 2008;19(9):1592–9.
86. Loehrer PJ, Feng Y, Cardenes H, et al. Gemcitabine alone versus gemcitabine plus radiotherapy in patients with locally advanced pancreatic cancer: an Eastern Cooperative Oncology Group trial. J Clin Oncol. 2011;29(31):4105–12.
87. Krishnan S, Rana V, Janjan NA, et al. Induction chemotherapy selects patients with locally advanced, unresectable pancreatic cancer for optimal benefit from consolidative chemoradiation therapy. Cancer. 2007;110(1):47–55.
88. Heinrich S, Pestalozzi B, Lesurtel M, et al. Adjuvant gemcitabine versus NEOadjuvant gemcitabine/oxaliplatin plus adjuvant gemcitabine in resectable pancreatic cancer: a randomized multicenter phase III study (NEOPAC study). BMC Cancer. 2011;11:346.
89. Chu QD, Khushalani N, Javle MM, Douglass HO, Gibbs JF. Should adjuvant therapy remain the standard of care for patients with resected adenocarcinoma of the pancreas? Ann Surg Oncol. 2003;10(5):539–45.
90. Neuhaus P RH, Post S, Gellert K, Ridwelski K, Schramm H, Zuelke C, Fahlke J, Langrehr J, Oettle Deutsche Krebsgesellschaft H. CONKO-001: final results of the randomized, prospective, multicenter phase III trial of adjuvant chemotherapy with gemcitabine versus observation in patients with resected pancreatic cancer (PC). J Clin Oncol. 2008;26(15S (May 20 Supplement)).
91. Stathis A, Moore MJ. Advanced pancreatic carcinoma: current treatment and future challenges. Nat Rev Clin Oncol. 2010;7(3):163–72.
92. Burris HA, Moore MJ, Andersen J, et al. Improvements in survival and clinical benefit with gemcitabine as first-line therapy for patients with advanced pancreas cancer: a randomized trial. J Clin Oncol. 1997;15(6):2403–13.
93. von Hoff D. Randomized phase 3 study of weekly nab-paclitaxel plus gemcitabine versus gemcitabine alone in patients with metastatic adenocarcinoma of the pancreas (MPACT). Phase 3 metastatic pancreatic cancer (late breaking abstract). San Francisco: American Society of Clinical Oncology (GI); 2013.
94. Philip PA, Benedetti J, Corless CL, et al. Phase III study comparing gemcitabine plus cetuximab versus gemcitabine in patients with advanced pancreatic adenocarcinoma: Southwest Oncology Group-directed intergroup trial S0205. J Clin Oncol. 2010;28(22):3605–10.
95. Van Cutsem E, Vervenne WL, Bennouna J, et al. Phase III trial of bevacizumab in combination with gemcitabine and erlotinib in patients with metastatic pancreatic cancer. J Clin Oncol. 2009;27(13):2231–7.

96. Conroy T, Desseigne F, Ychou M, et al. FOLFIRINOX versus gemcitabine for metastatic pancreatic cancer. N Engl J Med. 2011;364(19):1817–25.
97. Conroy T, Gavoille C, Samalin E, Ychou M, Ducreux M. The role of the FOLFIRINOX regimen for advanced pancreatic cancer. Curr Oncol Rep. 2013;15(2):182–9.
98. Witkowski ER, Smith JK, Ragulin-Coyne E, Ng SC, Shah SA, Tseng JF. Is it worth looking? Abdominal imaging after pancreatic cancer resection: a national study. J Gastrointest Surg. 2012; 16(1):121–8.
99. Sheffield KM, Crowell KT, Lin YL, Djukom C, Goodwin JS, Riall TS. Surveillance of pancreatic cancer patients after surgical resection. Ann Surg Oncol. 2012;19(5):1670–7.
100. Greer JA, Jackson VA, Meier DE, Temel JS. Early integration of palliative care services with standard oncology care for patients with advanced cancer. CA Cancer J Clin. 2013;63(5):349–63.
101. Vincent A, Herman J, Schulick R, Hruban RH, Goggins M. Pancreatic cancer. Lancet. 2011; 378(9791):607–20.
102. Temel JS, Greer JA, Muzikansky A, et al. Early palliative care for patients with metastatic non-small-cell lung cancer. N Engl J Med. 2010;363(8):733–42.
103. Moss A, Morris E, MacMathuna P. Palliative biliary stents for obstructing pancreatic carcinoma. Cochrane Database Syst Rev. 2006; 2(CD004200).
104. Gooden HM, White KJ. Pancreatic cancer and supportive care–pancreatic exocrine insufficiency negatively impacts on quality of life. Support Care Cancer. 2013;21(7):1835–41.
105. Compton C, Byrd D, Garcia-Aguilar J, et al. Exocrine and endocrine pancreas. In: Compton C, Byrd D, Garcia-Aguilar J, Kurtzman S, Olawaiye A, Washington M, editors. AJCC cancer staging atlas. 2nd ed. New York: Springer; 2012. p. 297–308.
106. Bassi C, et al. Postoperative pancreatic fistula: an international study group (ISGPF) definition. Surgery. 2005;138:8–13.
107. Giuseppe M, et al. Delayed gastric emptying after pylorus-preserving pancreaticoduodenectomy: validation of International Study Group of Pancreatic Surgery classification and analysis of risk factors. HPB. 2010;12:610–8.
108. Dindo D, et al. Classification of surgical complications. A new proposal with evaluation in a cohort of 6336 patients and results of a survey. Ann Surg. 2004;240(2):205–13.
109. Moertel CG, Frytak S, Hahn RG, et al. Therapy of locally unresectable pancreatic carcinoma: a randomized comparison of high dose (6000 rads) radiation alone, moderate dose radiation (4000 rads + 5-fluorouracil), and high dose radiation + 5-fluorouracil: The Gastrointestinal Tumor Study Group. Cancer. 1981;48(8):1705–10.
110. Klaassen DJ, MacIntyre JM, Catton GE, Engstrom PF, Moertel CG. Treatment of locally unresectable cancer of the stomach and pancreas: a randomized comparison of 5-fluorouracil alone with radiation plus concurrent and maintenance 5-fluorouracil–an Eastern Cooperative Oncology Group study. J Clin Oncol. 1985;3(3):373–8.

Adrenal Lesions

14

Gazi B. Zibari, Matthew Sanders, and Hosein Shokouh-Amiri

Learning Objectives

After reading this chapter, you should be able to:

- Understand the definition of adrenal incidentalomas (adrenalomas)
- Differentiate between benign, malignant, and hormonally active adrenal lesions
- Learn how to evaluate, manage, and follow-up patients with adrenal masses
- Describe different adrenalectomy techniques
- Discuss different types of adrenal lesion
- Know the indications for adrenalectomy

Background

An adrenal incidentaloma (adrenaloma) is a previously undetected adrenal lesion that is incidentally found on an imaging modality that was performed for an unrelated reason [1–3]. Most investigators agree that the size should measure at least 1 cm to qualify as an adrenal incidentaloma. Autopsy reports found that the average frequency of a clinically silent adrenal nodule is 2.3 %, which is observed for both genders [1–3]. Detection of adrenal incidentaloma is ever escalating because of the skyrocketing number of diagnostic imaging modalities such as computer tomography (CT), magnetic resonance imaging (MRI), abdominal ultrasonography (U/S), and other radiological studies. Although they may be incidental, these lesions warrant proper evaluation and management. It is estimated that up to 5 % of all abdominal and chest CT and MRI exams will identify an adrenal lesion [1–5]. In most cases, these lesions are hormonally inactive adrenal cortical adenomas that require no further treatment. In other cases, they may be malignant or hormonally active. The primary goal of pursuing the work-up of an adrenal incidentaloma is to determine whether it is benign or malignant and whether or not it is functional.

In radiological imaging, adrenalomas were discovered in 2–4 % of middle-aged patients and about 10 % among the elderlies [1–5]. Adrenal incidentaloma can be considered as a disease of modern technology, and it poses a public health concern [6]. Once detected, it is almost obligatory to distinguish adrenalomas, the majority of which are benign, as either benign, malignant, or functionally active tumors. Such diagnostic evaluation might require intervention and, at times, might create considerable anxiety, moderate cost, pain, and risks to the patient, especially if invasive intervention is required. Often, the surgeon is the primary physician, and the onus is put upon her/him to determine whether the neoplasm is

G.B. Zibari, M.D. (✉) • H. Shokouh-Amiri, M.D.
John C. McDonald Regional Transplant Center, Willis Knighton Health System, 2751 Albert Bicknell Dr., Suite 4A, Shreveport, LA 71103, USA
e-mail: gzibari@wkhs.com; hshokouh@wkhs.com

M. Sanders, M.D.
Department of Surgery, LSUHSC-Shreveport, 1501 Kings Hwy, Shreveport, LA 71130, USA
e-mail: msand3@lsuhsc.edu

Q.D. Chu et al. (eds.), *Surgical Oncology: A Practical and Comprehensive Approach*,
DOI 10.1007/978-1-4939-1423-4_14, © Springer Science+Business Media New York 2015

hormonally active and whether it is malignant, and if so, whether it is a primary adrenocortical carcinoma (ACC) or secondary due to metastasis from lung, breast, renal, gastrointestinal malignancies, lymphoma, multiple myeloma, and melanoma. The adrenal gland is the fourth most common site of metastasis and is the second most common cause (up to 20 %) of adrenal incidentalomas. It is extremely important to establish a great working relationship with colleagues who have expertise in the fields of endocrinology and radiology so that they can effectively assist the surgeon with the interpretation of inconclusive work-up as well as render advice regarding additional helpful tests.

Radiologic Evaluation of Adrenal Incidentalomas

Size plays a major role in determining the risk of malignancy. Less than 2 % of theses masses will be ACC if the mass is <4 cm in size. An important step in the evaluation process is to locate previous images of the chest and abdomen that include the adrenal glands. If there have been no significant changes of the adrenal glands over a minimum of 2 years, then the likelihood of malignancy is extremely low, even for lesions greater than 4 cm [7]. On the other hand, if an adrenaloma is detected that was not present on prior radiological images obtained within the past 4–5 years, a high index of suspicion for malignancy should be raised, even for lesions less than 4 cm. Heterogeneous lesions that are large in size have irregular border and invade adjacent tissue and organs are highly suggestive of being malignant. Radiographic characteristics of the lesion beyond size are important in delineating the nature of the mass. On unenhanced CT, low-attenuating lesions with Hounsfield units (HU) ranging between −50 and −150 HU are likely to be benign because of the high lipid content, and the differential diagnosis includes a lipoma or a myelolipoma (Fig. 14.1). For lesions that are more than 10 HU, a contrast-enhanced CT should be performed; benign lesions typically demonstrate more than 40 % washout. Cortisol- and aldosterone-secreting adenoma have Hounsfield values around 30 HU. However, lesions with a high signal intensity and those with architectural heterogeneity are worrisome for malignancy (Fig. 14.2). Most of the pheochromocytomas have single intensity that is similar to that of the spleen on MRI (Fig. 14.3). It should be noted that CT scans cannot determine whether the lesion is a hyperfunctioning or nonfunctioning mass. To summarize, small lesion with low attenuation seen on unenhanced CT can be reassuring, while large lesion with high attenuation can be worrisome. An enhanced CT should be performed for indeterminate lesions, and those that have greater than 40 % washout are less likely to be malignant.

Historically, adrenal scintigraphy with radiocholesterol was used to differentiate benign from malignant adrenal masses. However, a lack of widespread expertise, lack of tracer availability, poor resolution, prolonged time needed to complete the procedure (required over a period of 1 week to complete), and high radiation dose needed are the main limitations of this imaging modality [3, 4]. However, when pheochromocytoma is suspected, scintigraphy with I-123 or I-131 metaiodobenzylguanidine (MIBG) should be performed [3] (Fig. 14.4). Lastly, 18F-fluorodeoxyglucose positron emission tomography (FDG-PET) scan might be very helpful in differentiating malignant (adrenal carcinoma and metastasis) from benign lesions in patients with radiological undetermined adrenal lesion [3, 4] (Fig. 14.5). Adrenal FDG uptake is considered to be malignant when the intensity is higher than hepatic uptake. False positives may be seen in patients with sarcoidosis, tuberculosis, pheochromocytoma, and some adenomas, while false negatives may be seen in patients with necrotic and hemorrhagic cancer lesions as well as in some primary malignant lesions. In a multicenter prospective study of 77 patients who underwent adrenalectomy, preoperative 18F-FDG-PET imaging successfully distinguishes primary adrenal carcinoma from adenomas. An adrenal to liver maximum standardized uptake value (SUV) ratio less than 1.45 was highly predictive of a benign lesion (sensitivity 100 %, specificity 88 %) [8].

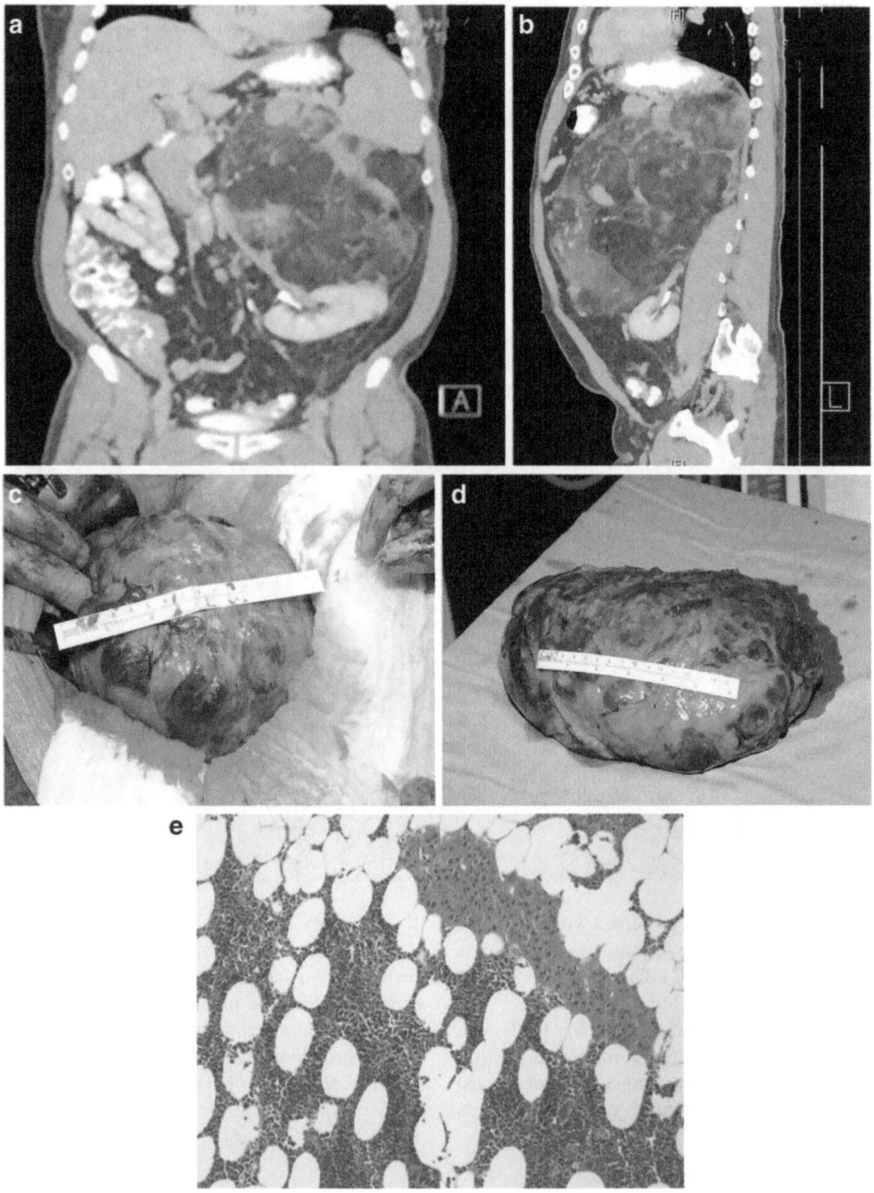

Fig. 14.1 A patient with benign bilateral adrenal lesions. He has a symptomatic left adrenal myelolipoma and underwent a left adrenalectomy. The 5 cm asymptomatic lesion on the *right* side was *left* alone. (**a & b**): CT scan – a large mass occupying most of the left abdomen, pushing the left kidney inferiorly and the gut toward the *right* side of the abdomen. (**c**): Intraoperative photo of a large adrenal lesion that is not amenable to a minimally invasive surgical resection. (**d**): Gross specimen (**e**): Histology slide – adrenal myelolipoma: mature adipocytes are admixed with hematopoietic cells

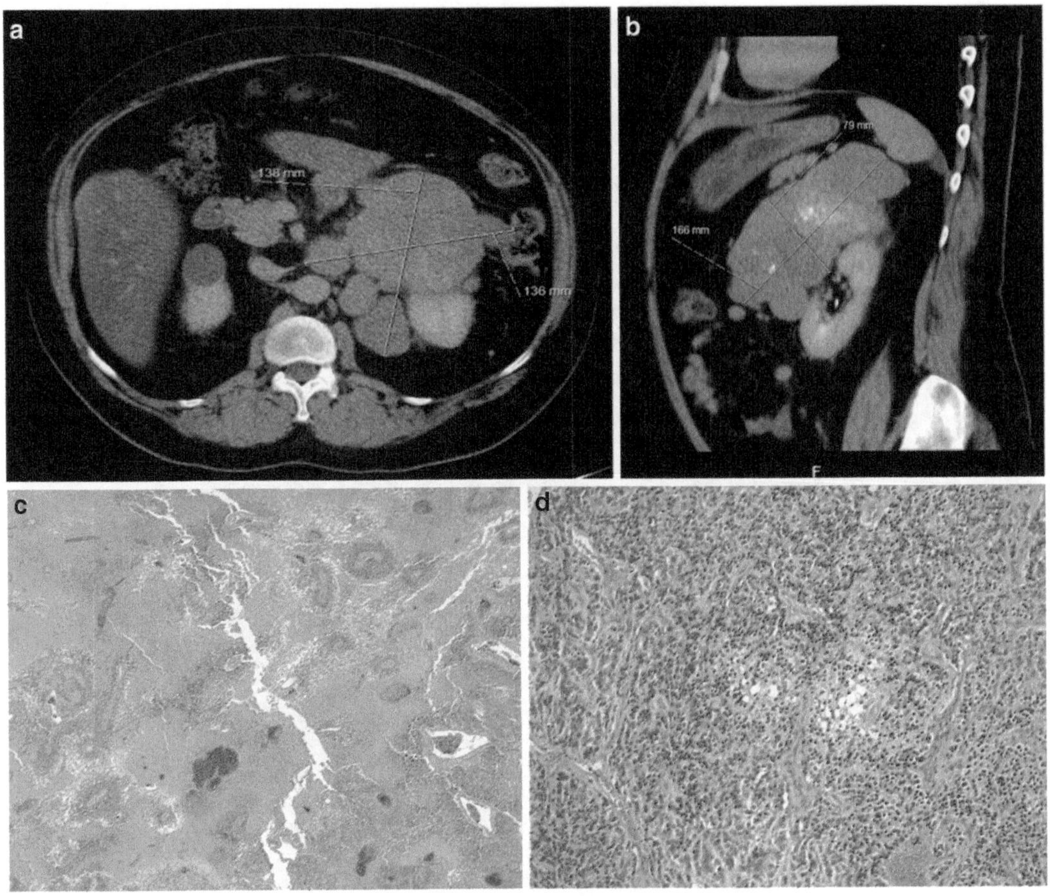

Fig. 14.2 A 33-year-old patient presented with Cushing's disease and was found to have a 17 cm left adrenal mass (adrenocortical carcinoma – ACC). The patient underwent a hand-assisted laparoscopic left adrenalectomy and nephrectomy with clear margins. (**a & b**): CAT scan shows large lobulated left adrenal mass (ACC) (**c**): Histology – low-power photomicrograph (40×) of adrenal cortical carcinoma areas of extensive confluent necrosis (**d**): Histology – medium-power photomicrograph (200X) of an adrenal cortical carcinoma demonstrating cellular pleomorphism and atypia, mitotic activity, and trabecular growth pattern. The tumor also exhibited capsular invasion, and tumor cells showed a typical adrenocortical immunohistochemical profile with positivity for inhibin, melan-A, and synaptophysin, and negativity for EMA and pancytokeratin

Initial Work-Up and Evaluation of Hormonal Function

Majority of adrenal incidentalomas are benign, nonfunctioning adenoma; however, hormonal evaluation can reveal a significant number of patients of having unsuspected adrenal secreting lesions. Adrenalomas ≥1 cm and without prior history of malignancy should undergo hormonal evaluation. All patients with adrenal incidentaloma should be evaluated for possible pheochromocytoma, primary aldosteronism (hypertension, hyperkalemia), and Cushing's syndrome (hypercotisolism) (Table 14.1). Approximately 5–7 % of adrenal incidentalomas are clinically silent pheochromocytoma [1–3, 6, 9, 10]. Primary aldosteronism should be considered in patients with hypertension and/or hypokalemia, although normokalemia can occur in up to 50 % of patients with hyperaldosteronism [11]. However, the diagnosis of primary aldosteronism can virtually be excluded in the absence of hypertension. Thus, laboratory testing should begin not

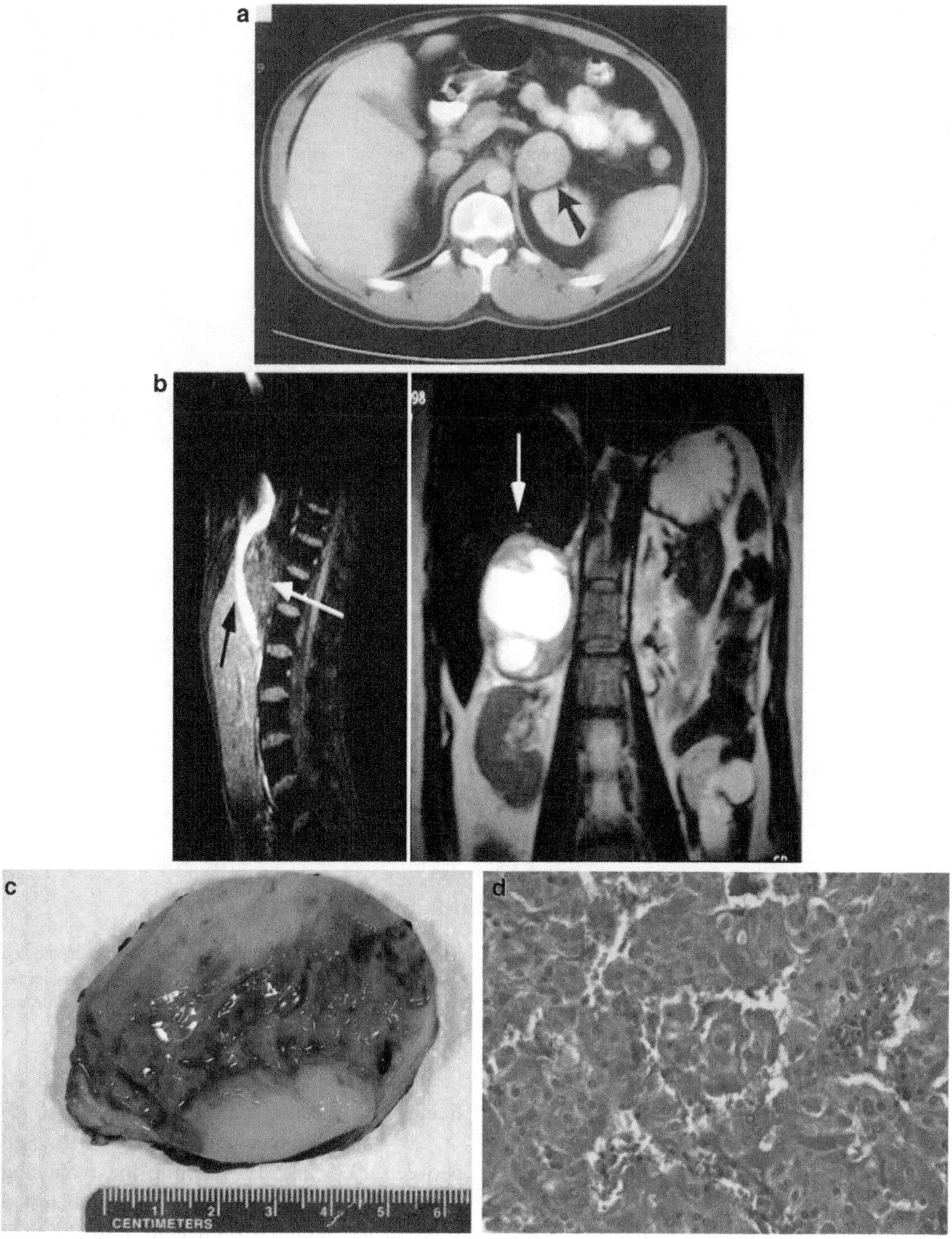

Fig. 14.3 *Patient with a left pheochromocytoma* (**a**): CT scan – *black arrow* is pointing toward the left adrenal mass. (**b**): MRI – *white arrow* pointing toward the left adrenal mass. (**c**): Gross photo (**d**): Histology – this photomicrograph of a pheochromocytoma illustrates the typical "Zellballen" architectural pattern in which balls of tumor cells are supported by a rich vascular framework. The cytoplasm has a finely granular appearance, and nuclei demonstrate a stippled chromatin pattern. Though mitotic activity is typically sparse in these tumors, note the enlarged and hyperchromatic nuclei (hematoxylin and eosin stain, original magnification 200×)

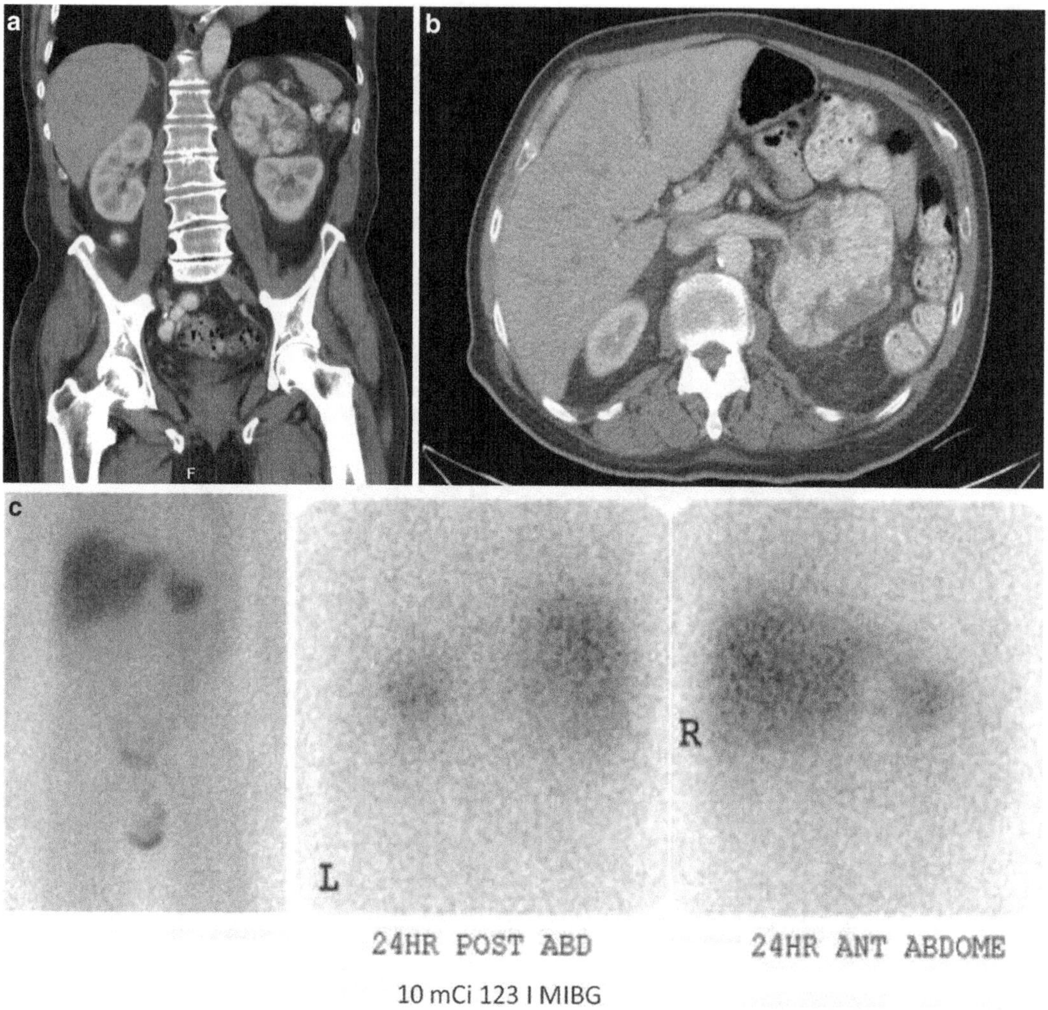

Fig. 14.4 *A patient with a large left adrenal pheochromocytoma* (**a & b**): CT scan reveals a large adrenal mass. (**c**): MIBG scan performed whole-body planar scintigraphic images of I-123 MIBG scan of a patient shows intense uptake in adrenal pheochromocytoma on the *left* side. The scan did not identify any other sites of disease with normal physiologic distribution of the radiotracer elsewhere in the body

only with the most sensitive tests but also with those that are the easiest to perform and the least expensive for the patient [3, 7].

Pheochromocytoma

Approximately 4.7 % of adrenalomas are silent pheochromocytoma, although some studies quote the incidence can be as high as 20 % [12, 13]. Almost 1/3 of all pheochromocytomas are discovered incidentally, and this prevalence increases over the span of time [14–16]. In an Italian retrospective multicenter study, 40 % of 234 pheochromocytomas were diagnosed between 1978 and 1997, while the remaining majority (59 %) were diagnosed in the last 5 years of the study [15]. Of note, prior to 1985 when utilization of ultrasound was limited, less than 10 % of pheochromocytomas were incidentally diagnosed [17]. Thus, the increase prevalence in pheochromocytoma may be a function of earlier detection. Of note, patients with asymptomatic pheochromocytomas tend to be older than those with symptomatic pheochromocytomas [3, 16, 17].

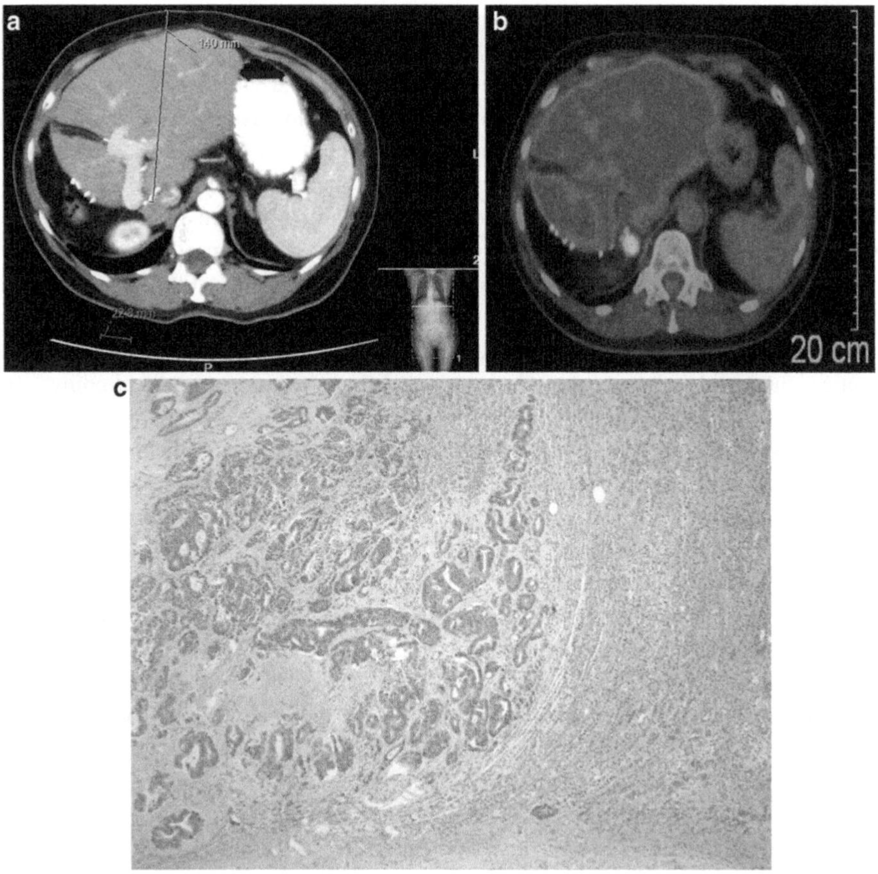

Fig. 14.5 The patient is a 60-year-old with history of a colectomy and right hepatectomy in 2004. She presented with a solitary metastasis to the right adrenal. A biopsy proved to be a metastatic colon cancer. She underwent a successful resection in fall of 2013. (**a**): CT scan shows a mass in the right adrenal gland and a postoperative changes from a right hepatectomy. (**b**): PET scan reveals only uptake in the right adrenal gland. (**c**): Histology – image shows a focus of metastatic colorectal adenocarcinoma involving the adrenal gland. Benign adrenal parenchyma is seen on the right and a metastatic, moderately differentiated adenocarcinoma on the left. The tumor shows obvious glandular formation and areas of "dirty" necrosis, typical of colorectal adenocarcinoma (hematoxylin and eosin stain, original magnification, 100×)

Table 14.1 Evaluation of adrenal masses

Diagnosis	Images	Biochemical listing
Primary aldosteronism (aldosteronoma)	CT/MRI	K^+<3.2; increased plasma aldosterone with decreased renin
Pheochromocytoma	CT/MRI MIBG scan	24-h urine metanephrines; plasma catecholamines
Cushing's syndrome	CT/MRI	1 mg dexamethasone suppression test/
	NP-59 scan	24-h urine cortisol; plasma ACTH
Adrenal cortical carcinoma	CT/MRI	K^+; 1 mg dex-suppression; 24-h urine free cortisol; 17-ketosteroids; and catecholamines
Sex-steroid adenoma	CT/MRI	17-ketosteroids; 24-h urine free cortisol

MIBG metaiodobenzylguanidine, *ACTH* adrenocorticotropic hormone

Some authors found that incidentally found pheochromocytomas tend to be large [3, 16]. By contrast, others found no size differences between incidentally found pheochromocytoma and symptomatic pheochromocytomas; however, they did find that patients with clinically silent pheochromocytoma had lower plasma catecholamine levels than those with symptoms [17].

Pheochromocytomas can be lethal even when they are clinically silent [3, 14]. Clinical presentation can vary, ranging from patients being entirely asymptomatic to those with intermittent headaches, palpitations, and sweating or with a hypertensive crisis. Patients may also be normotensive, which is not uncommon in cases where the pheochromocytoma was incidentally detected. In a multicenter study, Mantero et al. found that about 50 % of patients with incidentally detected pheochromocytoma were normotensive, while the others had mild to moderate hypertension. None of the patients had paroxysmal symptoms of adrenergic excess [9]. Because a significant percentage of patients with pheochromocytoma can be asymptomatic and normotensive, any patient with an incidental adrenaloma should undergo biochemical testing for pheochromocytoma [3]. Outcome for patients with malignant pheochromocytoma is poor; the mean 5-year survival rate is about 40 % [18].

Biochemical Diagnosis of Pheochromocytoma

The diagnosis of pheochromocytoma has evolved over the last six decades. It became apparent in the very early century that the clinical signs and symptoms of pheochromocytoma were due primarily to the excess secretion of catecholamines. In the middle of the last century, a 24-h urinary catecholamines excretion became the test of choice to account for the episodic nature of catecholamines secretion [19–21]. In recent years, metabolites of catecholamine such as normetanephrine and metanephrine, which are respective o-methylated metabolites of norepinephrine and epinephrine, and vanillylmandelic acid (VMA), the final breakdown product of the catecholamines was included as part of the biochemical diagnostic tests [19].

There is no consensus on what the preferred test for pheochromocytoma should be [3, 4, 12, 22]. Recently, Lenders et al. assessed 858 patients with adrenalomas who were at risk for pheochromocytoma [23]. Patients were identified as having a pheochromocytoma based on signs and symptoms suggestive of a pheochromocytoma, or on their genetic predisposition to developing pheochromocytoma. Plasma and urinary catecholamines, urinary fractionated metanephrine and VMA, as well as plasma values of free metanephrine were measured. Findings from this study demonstrated that plasma free metanephrine was the optimal screening test for pheochromocytoma, yielding a 99 % sensitivity and 89 % specificity. The false-negative rate was very low with only 3/214 patients with pheochromocytoma having negative laboratory values [23]. However, plasma metanephrine testing may not be readily available in some centers; therefore, a 24-h urinary metanephrines remains an acceptable initial screening test. The degree of increase in catecholamines and metanephrines can be useful for diagnostic and therapeutic purposes since a mild increase may not necessarily be due to a pheochromocytoma but be due to other causes such as diet and pharmacologic causes [24].

Hereditary Pheochromocytoma and Paraganglioma

Pheochromocytoma and paraganglioma (pheochromocytomas that are outside of the adrenal glands) are neuroendocrine tumors that are derived from sympathetic and parasympathetic paraganglioma. The most common extra-adrenal site of pheochromocytoma is the organ of Zuckerkandl, which comprises of small masses of chromaffin cells along the aorta, with the highest concentration located at the origin of the inferior mesenteric artery and the bifurcation of the aorta.

Most leaders in the field would agree that the rule of 10 applies to pheochromocytoma: 10 % are hereditary (Fig. 14.6), 10 % are bilateral, 10 % are extra-adrenal (Fig. 14.7), 10 % are malignant (Fig. 14.2), and 10 % occur in children. Pheochromocytomas of adrenal and

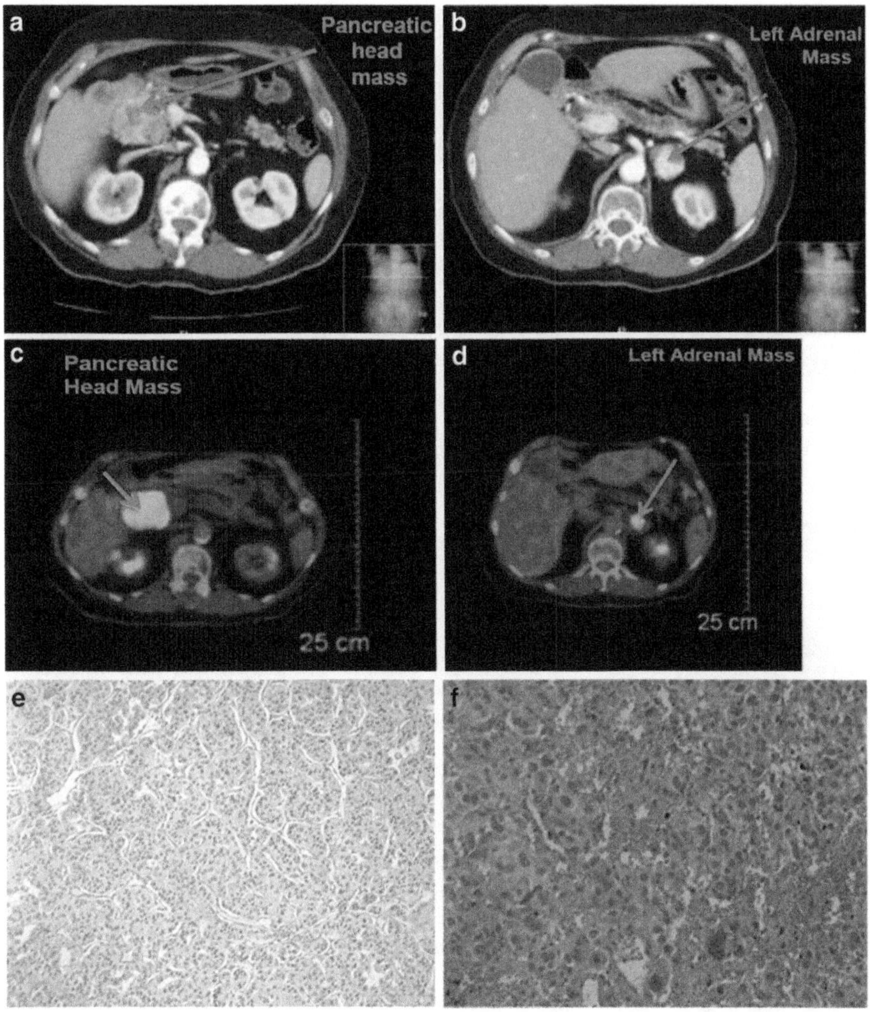

Fig. 14.6 A patient with von Hippel–Lindau disease with a pancreatic head mass and a left adrenal mass. She underwent a left adrenalectomy (pheochromocytoma) and a Whipple procedure (neuroendocrine tumor of the pancreas). (**a**): CT shows a mass in the head of the pancreas (neuroendocrine tumor) (**b**): CT shows a left adrenal mass (pheochromocytoma) (**c**): PET scan shows positive uptake in the head of the pancreas (**d**): PET scan shows positive uptake in the left adrenal gland as well as in the head of the pancreas. (**e**): Histology – this photomicrograph depicts a pancreatic endocrine neoplasm. This tumor manifests a typical trabecular pattern of uniform cells with a granular eosinophilic cytoplasm and round nuclei with finely granular, "salt-and-pepper" chromatin pattern (hematoxylin and eosin stain, original magnification 200×) (**f**): This photomicrograph of a pheochromocytoma illustrates the typical "Zellballen" architectural pattern in which balls of tumor cells are supported by a rich vascular framework. The cytoplasm has a finely granular appearance, and nuclei demonstrate a stippled chromatin pattern. Though mitotic activity is typically sparse in these tumors, note the enlarged and hyperchromatic nuclei (hematoxylin and eosin stain, original magnification 200×)

extra-adrenal sympathetic origin usually secrete catecholamines, whereas lesions of parasympathetic origin (head & neck) usually do not [14]. Roughly one third of pheochromocytomas have germline mutation, and approximately ten tumor susceptibility genes have been identified [25]. These include SDHA/B/C/D (succinate dehydrogenase complex subunits A, B, C, & D), $SDHAF_2$ (succinate dehydrogenase complex assembly factor-2), VHL (von Hippel–Lindau) (Fig. 14.6), RET (REarranged during Transfection), NF1 (neurofibromatosis type 1), and recently reported

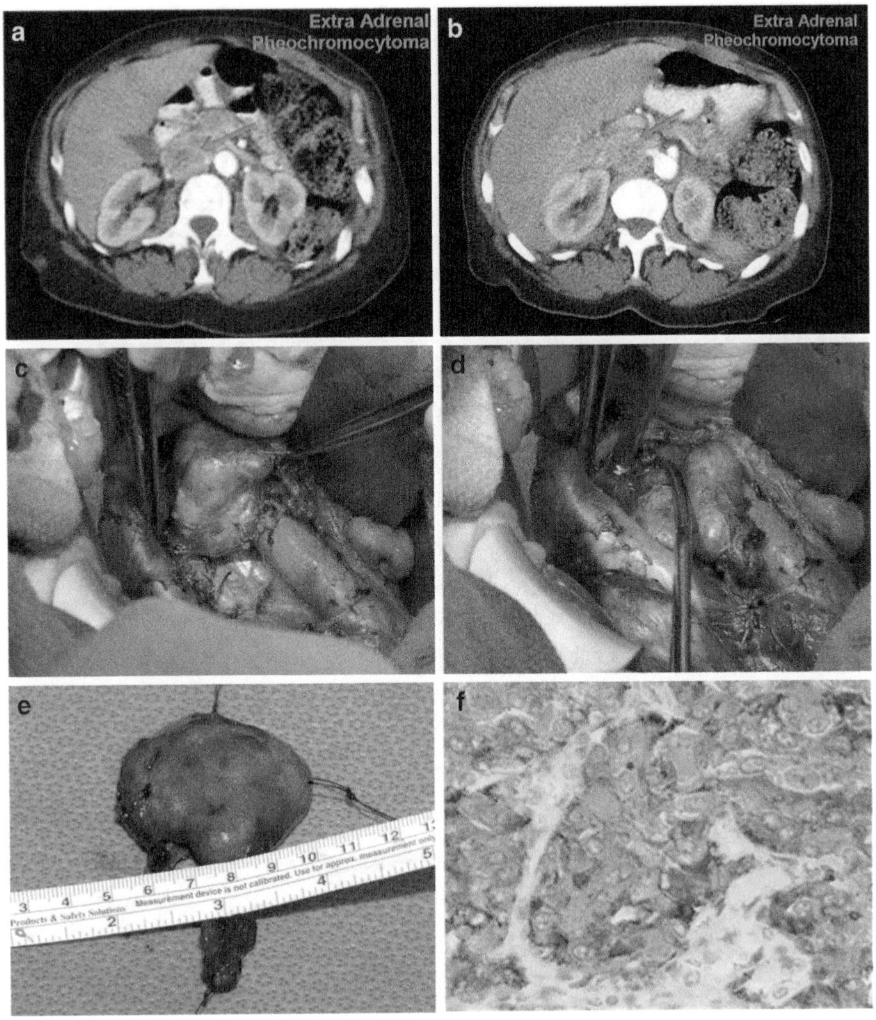

Fig. 14.7 *Extra-adrenal pheochromocytoma (organ of Zuckerkandl)* (**a & b**): CT – *Arrow* points to a retroperitoneal mass, which is inferior to the superior mesenteric artery and between the inferior vena cava, aorta, and left renal vein. (**c & d**): Intraoperative photos of extra-adrenal pheochromocytomas located between the inferior vena cava and aorta and below the left renal vein. (**e**): Gross picture (**f**): Histology – the tumor shows nests and trabecular composed of large polygonal cells with finely granular eosinophilic to somewhat basophilic cytoplasm. There is mild nuclear pleomorphism, and the nucleoli are small and eccentric. The tumor cells reveal positive cytoplasm stain for chromogranin and synaptophysin. Common sites for extra-adrenal pheochromocytomas: between the inferior vena cava and aorta below the left renal vein, and in the organ of Zuckerkandl. Small tumors under the left renal vein may be overlooked unless the area is carefully inspected

TMEM127 (transmembrane protein 127) and MAX (Myc-associated factor X) [25, 26]. Somatic mutations in RET, MAX, VHL, and NF1 have been reported in 17 % of sporadic lesions [26–29]. Succinate dehydrogenase (SDH) is an important part of the mitochondrial electron transport chain, and when it is mutated, the ability of cells to phosphorylate is undermined [30–33].

Preoperative and Intraoperative Management of Pheochromocytoma

The treatment of choice for pheochromocytoma is surgical excision. In the past, poor outcomes following resection of pheochromocytomas were due to uncontrolled hypertensive crisis related to

Table 14.2 Drugs used to treat pheochromocytoma

Drug	Initial dose	Maximum dose	Suggestion
Phenoxybenzamine	10 mg orally twice daily	2 mg/kg/day	Nonselective alpha-blockade may titrate to 3 times per day until postural hypotension is achieved
Prazosin	1 mg orally twice daily	15 mg/day	Selective alpha-blockade, same as above
Labetalol	100 mg orally twice daily	1,200 mg/day	After alpha-blockade, may titrate the dose with target heart rate of 60–70 bpm
Nifedipine	30–90 mg orally once daily	120 mg/day	Calcium channel blocker may increase after 1 week, used for paroxysmal hypertension
Amlodipine	5 mg	10 mg/day	Same as nifedipine
Metyrosine	250–750 mg orally four times daily	4,000 mg/day	Used for refractory hypertension

Modified from Silberfein and Perrier [38]. With permission from Elsevier

excess catecholamine secretion. The first report of surgical excision of a pheochromocytoma in North America was performed by Dr. C. Mayo in 1927 [34]. In the 1950s, the group at the Mayo Clinic reported a decreased operative mortality with successful resection of 61 pheochromocytoma over 11 years by using alpha-blockade with phenoxybenzamine to treat hypertension and epinephrine to treat intraoperative hypotension [35].

However, before surgical intervention, perioperative management requires adequate hydration with isotonic solution and administration of selective alpha 1-adrenergic blocking agents (i.e., doxazosin, prazosin, or terazosin) followed by beta-adrenergic blockade (i.e., propranolol, atenolol) (Table 14.2). It is very important that beta-blockade should never be initiated first because blockade of the vasodilatory peripheral beta-adrenergic receptors with unopposed alpha-adrenergic receptors stimulation can lead to a further elevation of blood pressure.

Calcium channel blockers (i.e., nifedipine) are alternative vasodilator to control blood pressure. These drugs are necessary to normalize heart rate and blood pressure. As mentioned before, it is necessary to replete intravascular volume preoperatively and take precautionary measures to prevent cardiovascular collapse from surgery-induced catecholamine storm [22, 36, 37]. Even with proper and effective preoperative alpha- and beta-adrenergic blockade, hypertensive crisis may occur intraoperatively due to catecholamine surge secondary to manipulation of the adrenal lesion. It is very important for the patient to have an arterial line and a central venous line placed. Additionally, the anesthesiologist must have ready-at-hand premixed intravenous titratable drugs to control blood pressure in the event the blood pressure fluctuates during surgery. Dihydropyridine calcium channel blocker nicardipine (0.5–1.0 mg/ml) and the direct-acting vasodilator sodium nitroprusside (0.5–3 μg/kg/min) are the agents of choice for uncontrolled hypertension. On the other hand, ligation of the adrenal vein can cause an abrupt decrease of catecholamine release, which can lead to unexpected hypotension. Should this occur, epinephrine or norepinephrine should be administered accordingly, along with crystalloid infusion as needed [15, 22, 38].

Operative Management and Technique

Adrenal lesions can be removed by an open technique or by a minimally invasive technique, either via a transabdominal or retroperitoneal approach. Adrenalectomy is effective at treating a number of different diseases and conditions (Table 14.3) including but not limited to pheochromocytoma, aldosteronoma, refractory Cushing's disease,

Table 14.3 Indications for adrenalectomy

Hormonally active
Aldosteronoma
Glucocorticoid adenoma
Pheochromocytoma
Bilateral macronodular adrenal hyperplasia
Selected cases of bilateral adrenal hyperplasia due to Cushing's disease or ectopic ACTH syndrome
Adrenocortical carcinoma
Hormonally inactive
Adrenal carcinoma
Metastatic disease with controlled primary site/otherwise biopsy and systemic treatment
Tumors>5 cm
Tumors that demonstrate growth on serial imaging

adrenal cortical carcinoma, and selected cases of metastatic disease confined to the adrenal gland. Until 1992 when the first laparoscopic adrenalectomy was reported in the literature by Ganger et al., the only operative approach for removal of the adrenal gland was an open adrenalectomy [37]. Laparoscopic and more recently robotic adrenalectomy techniques have been considered by many to be the "gold standard" and the procedure of choice for resecting adrenal lesions. In experienced hands, these techniques are safe and can lead to less postoperative pain, shorter hospital stay, better cosmesis, and less blood loss [37–42]. Open surgery is generally reserved for large lesions, especially those with malignant features and locally advanced. The retroperitoneal approach might be an attractive option for patients who have multiple prior abdominal surgeries. On the other hand, transabdominal approach has the advantage of addressing other intra-abdominal pathology as well as contralateral adrenal lesion. Therefore, most leaders in the field chose the surgical procedure based upon whether the adrenal mass is hereditary or sporadic and whether the lesion is unilateral or bilateral. More importantly, the surgeon should choose the technique for which he or she has the most experience and comfort.

If a patient presents with bilateral hereditary disease, the surgeon may consider performing a unilateral cortex-sparing adrenalectomy on one side and a contralateral total adrenalectomy for pheochromocytoma. For patients with a metachronous contralateral pheochromocytoma after prior unilateral adrenalectomy, a cortex-sparing procedure should be attempted [38, 43].

Adrenal Carcinoma (ACC)

Adrenal cortical carcinoma (ACC) is a very rare cancer that accounts for 1 % of all adrenal lesions. It affects two person per million, worldwide [44]. It is the second most lethal endocrine tumor after anaplastic thyroid malignancy [45]. There is a bimodal age distribution with a peak occurrence in the first decade of childhood and another in the fourth and fifth decades of life. The female to male ratio is approximately 1.5–1.0 [46]. The majority of these cases occur in a sporadic fashion, although ACC can occur in association with several hereditary syndromes including Li–Fraumeni syndrome, Beckwith–Wiedemann syndrome, and multiple endocrine neoplasia syndrome type 1 (MEN-1) [46, 47]. The prognosis of patients with this cancer remains very poor, despite its earlier detection by modern imaging modalities.

The two most important prognostic factors are complete resection and stage of disease [7, 42]. The World Health Organization (WHO) TNM staging system for adrenocortical carcinoma are as follow: (1) stage I, tumor size≤5 cm; (2) stage II, tumor size>5 cm; (3) stage III, tumors with locoregional lymph node involvement or invading peri-adrenal fat; and (4) stage IV, tumors invading adjacent organs or metastatic to remote locations [7, 46, 48]. WHO classification has prognostic significance and predicts overall survival. Additionally, tumor grade is also an important prognostic factor; tumors with mitotic rates >20 mitoses per 50 high-power field (HPF) are associated with a shorter disease-free interval compared to those with lower mitotic rates [3, 46].

Immunohistochemical assessment of high Ki-67 expression is associated with poor clinical outcome as reported by the German ACC Registry. In experienced hands, stages I, II, and most III ACC patients can undergo a successful R0 resection±lymphadenectomy (LND) [7, 46, 49]. The role of LND is not well defined due to the rarity of the disease. However, in select cases, locoregional LND improves tumor staging and possibly leads to a favorable outcome in those with localized ACC [50]. Tumor thrombus in the renal vein or inferior vena cava is not considered a contraindication to surgery. En bloc resection of the kidney is recommended for any patient with renal capsule invasion [44, 51]. Patients with local recurrences after an adrenalectomy can be considered for reoperation if a complete R0 resection can be achieved. Debulking of metastatic cancers should be considered in patients with low-grade tumors, those who are symptomatic because of hormone secretion from the tumor, and those in whom a complete or near-complete resection of the tumor is possible [46]. There is little data on adjuvant radiotherapy following adrenalectomy, although radiating the surgical bed may be considered in patients who are at high risk for developing local recurrence. However, the potential advantage of this therapy is unproven [46].

Occasionally, local recurrences and selected metastatic lesions can be palliated by surgical resection, along with some form of ablative therapy such as radiofrequency ablation and chemoembolization. Overall, 5-year survival depends on the stage of the tumor. One-year survival rate is 40–60 % for stages I and II; 20–30 %, for stage III; and 10 %, for stage IV disease. Early diagnosis and radical resection offers the only chance for long-term cure. Systemic chemotherapy has not proven to be very effective. Mitotane is used to treat metastatic disease, although with only limited success. Further progress in the understanding and treatment of this rare and lethal entity requires novel treatment strategies [46].

Role of Adrenaloma Biopsy

Most experts do not recommend adrenaloma biopsy, despite its frequent recommendation in the radiology literature. These biopsies can often lead to retroperitoneal/adrenal bleed with associated inflammatory changes. Additionally, it can create difficulty with the surgical dissection, resulting in increased surgical complications as well as risk of capsule rupture. Finally, the biopsied tissue is rarely adequate to differentiate malignant from benign adrenal lesions. Needle biopsy of pheochromocytoma is strongly contraindicated due to concerns of tumor seeding and triggering a hypertensive crisis [48, 52]. It is very important that all patients with an adrenaloma who require a work-up should undergo a hormonal evaluation before undergoing a biopsy. An exception to this is when an adrenal metastasis is suspected and a tissue diagnosis is required, especially in patients who are known or suspected to have lung, breast, and renal gastrointestinal malignancies, lymphoma, and melanoma. As a general rule of thumb, metastases to the adrenals tend to be bilateral [7].

Nonfunctioning Incidentaloma Follow-Up

When an adrenal incidentaloma is detected by imaging modalities, the multidisciplinary team must make a decision of whether to treat in the case of symptomatic, malignant, and functioning lesions or to observe in the case of nonfunctioning adrenal lesions. While it is relatively straightforward to determine the functional status of an adrenaloma, it is much more difficult to determine whether it is benign or malignant. Such decision must be based on the clinician's high index of suspicion.

There is a lack of a standardized approach for surveillance of adrenal incidentaloma. As a rule of thumb, most protocols call for biochemical testing and serial CT scans and MRI scans at varying but consistent intervals. In the last decade, a number of expert opinion and consensus statements suggest repeating CT scan or MRI for a suspicious adrenal mass every 3–6 months after the initial diagnostic images. Other lesions of low suspicion can be monitored every 6–12 months and then annually after 3–5 years (Fig. 14.8) [3–5, 7, 53].

Although the threshold for what constitutes as a clinically significant size increase remains controversial, most experts recommend an adrenalectomy if the tumor increases in size by ≥1 cm

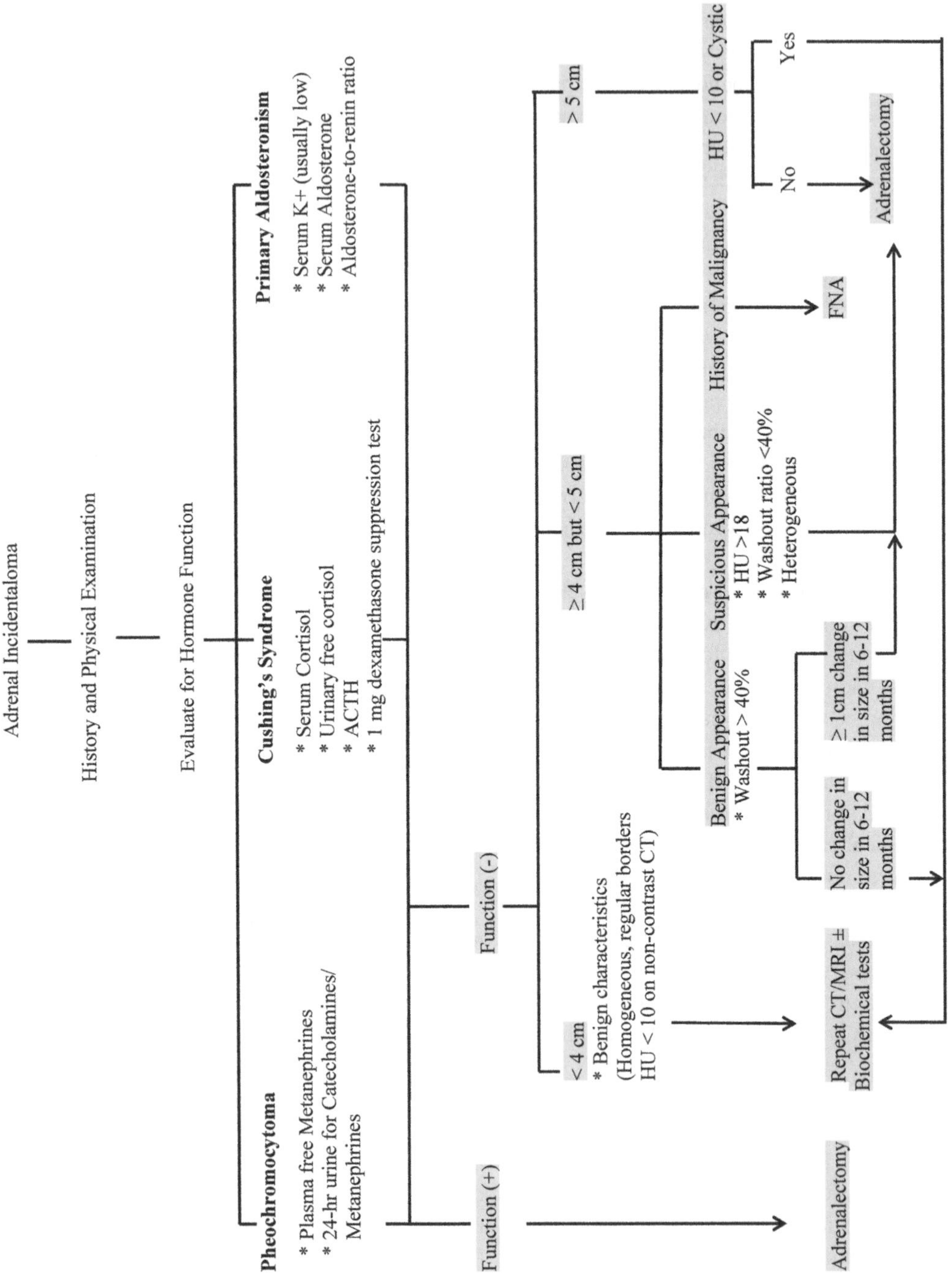

Fig. 14.8 *Algorithm for adrenal incidentaloma* (Courtesy of Quyen D. Chu, MD, MBA, FACS)

and/or has a change in features suggestive of malignancy during the monitoring period [3, 7, 53]. Many authors suggest vigilant clinical monitoring with repeat laboratory screening tests (24-h urinary collection of catecholamine and metanephrine and overnight dexamethasone test) annually for at least 5 years, especially in patients with subclinical hypercortisolism [3]. Others do not recommend routine biochemical testing unless the patient develops symptoms that warrant further investigation [53]. Barry et al. found that none of the follow-up asymptomatic patients developed hyperfunctioning adrenal lesion [53]. Nonfunctioning lesions require repeat biochemical tests for pheochromocytoma and Cushing's syndrome on follow-up, although they are not necessary for primary aldosteronism.

In summary, all nonfunctioning incidentaloma >1 cm but less than 4 cm requires close follow-up with either a CT scan or an MRI every 6–12 months. If the lesion is between 4 and 5 cm, an adrenalectomy is recommended if the mass has the following characteristics: (1) a non-contrast CT with HU density >18, (2) contrast-enhanced CT washout ratio <40 %, and (3) heterogeneous, necrotic, calcified, or evidence of local invasion. Finally, if the lesion is >5 cm, it should be resected unless the HU density is <10, which suggests that it is likely to be a myelolipoma, or if the lesion is entirely cystic (Fig. 14.8) [7].

Summary

The diagnosis of an adrenal incidentaloma (adrenaloma) is skyrocketing secondary to the increase use of abdominal and chest CT and MRI. The clinician's challenging dilemma is to distinguish the majority of benign masses from other malignant or hormone-secreting lesions which will require further intervention and treatment. CT scans and MRI are the best imaging modalities to differentiate malignant from benign masses. In equivocal cases, PET/CT might be a useful adjunct.

It is necessary that all patients with an adrenal incidentaloma be evaluated for a possible pheochromocytoma or hypercortisolism; aldosteronism should be suspected in a hypertensive patient with hypokalemia. The overwhelming majority of adrenalomas are asymptomatic, nonfunctioning adenomas and do not require surgical intervention. Controversy exists in regard to the surgical or medical management of patients with subclinical hypercortisolism. Adrenalectomy is indicated for patients with malignant lesion, pheochromocytoma, aldosteronoma, and adenoma with or without subclinical hypercortisolism that has grown, becomes symptomatic, or is recalcitrant to optimal medical intervention. In these patients, an accurate initial diagnostic assessment is a prerequisite for optimal management. A multidisciplinary approach and tailored strategy is important to differentiate the high-risk patients who might require careful and extensive follow-up from the majority of patients who require only a simplified follow-up.

Salient Points

- Majority of adrenal incidentalomas are hormonally inactive adrenal adenomas requiring no further treatment.
- Clinicians need to determine if incidentalomas are functional or malignant. If yes, they will require intervention.
- All adrenal lesions ≥1 cm require a work-up.
- A work-up for pheochromocytoma and Cushing's syndrome (hypercortisolism) should be pursued, whereas primary aldosteronism should be evaluated in a hypertensive patient only (See Fig. 14.8).
- All functional tumors should be considered for resection (See Fig. 14.8).
- Small nonfunctioning tumors (<4 cm) with benign characteristics (HU <10 on non-contrast CT) can be observed with follow-up CT/MRI and biochemical tests (See Fig. 14.8).
- Tumors ≥4 cm but <5 cm require further work-up which include measurement of HU on non-contrast CT and washout ratio on contrast CT (See Fig. 14.8).
- Tumors >5 cm that are not cystic and HU >10 require resection (See Fig. 14.8).

- Pheochromocytoma can be clinically silent, but nevertheless dangerous. The following applies to pheochromocytomas:
  - When Pheochromocytoma is suspected, MIBG should be performed. PET scan might be helpful in differentiating malignant from benign lesions; however, false positive might be seen in patients with sarcoidosis, tuberculosis, and pheochromocytoma. PET negative scan might be seen in necrotic and hemorrhagic cancer as well as in some primary tumors.
  - Needle biopsy is strongly contraindicated due to concerns regarding tumor seeding and hypertensive crisis.
  - There is no consensus on the test modality for screening pheochromocytoma. Plasma free metanephrine is the best screening test with 99 % sensitivity and 89 % specificity, although a 24-h urine test for catecholamines and their metabolites (metanephrines, normetanephrines, VMA) is acceptable.
  - Preoperative management of pheochromocytoma requires alpha-blockade before beta-blockade and adequate hydration.
  - Hypertension crisis may occur intraoperatively due to catecholamine surge secondary to adrenal lesion manipulation.
  - Anesthesiologist must have premixed intravenous titratable drugs such as nifedipine, Nipride, and nicardipine to control high blood pressure as well as epinephrine and norepinephrine in the event the blood pressure drops during surgery.
  - Laparoscopic and more recently robotic adrenalectomy have become a "gold standard" technique of choice.
  - Retroperitoneal approach is an attractive alternative in a patient who has multiple prior abdominal surgeries.
  - Transabdominal approach has the advantage of addressing other intra-abdominal pathology as well as contralateral adrenal lesion.
  - In a patient with bilateral hereditary disease, the surgeon may attempt a unilateral cortex-sparing adrenalectomy and contralateral total adrenalectomy for pheochromocytoma.
  - For patients with metachronous contralateral pheochromocytoma after prior unilateral adrenalectomy, a cortex-sparing procedure should be attempted.
- Adrenal cortical carcinoma (ACC) is a very rare adrenal cancer and accounts for 1 % of all adrenal lesions. It is the second most lethal endocrine tumor after anaplastic thyroid malignancy. The following are considered for ACC:
  - Prognostic factors include complete resection, stage of disease, and tumor grade.
  - Mitotic rates above 20 mitoses per 50 HPF and high Ki-67 are associated with poor outcome
  - In experienced hands, R0 resection and lymphadenectomy are possible for all stages.
  - Tumor thrombus in the renal vein or inferior cava is not considered a contraindication to surgery.
  - En bloc resection of the kidney is recommended for any patients with renal capsule invasion.
  - Patients with local recurrences after adrenalectomy can still be considered for reoperation, especially if a complete resection can be achieved.
  - Radiation of surgical bed may be considered, although the potential advantage of this therapy is unproven.
  - Local recurrences and selected metastatic lesions can be palliated by surgical resection or by some type of ablation such as radiofrequency ablation and chemoembolization.
  - ACC is an aggressive malignancy with a very poor prognosis. Early diagnosis and radical resection is the only chance for long-term cure.
  - Systemic chemotherapy has not been proven to improve outcome; mitotane is indicated for metastatic disease, which has yielded only limited success.

Questions

1. A patient in her mid-20s is found to have a 3.2 cm solitary left adrenal lesion on a CT scan obtained for right upper abdominal pain. The next step in her treatment should be:
   A. Laparoscopic vs. robotic adrenalectomy
   B. Image-guided biopsy of the mass
   C. Dexamethasone 1 mg test dose
   D. 24-h urine collection for catecholamines
   E. Repeat MRI/CT scan in 2 years
2. Which of the following statements about laparoscopic adrenalectomy for pheochromocytoma is true?
   A. It should not be attempted in any patient with prior abdominal surgery.
   B. During bilateral laparoscopic adrenalectomies, cortical-sparing technique should be considered.
   C. Lesions more than 5 cm should not be attempted with a laparoscopic technique.
   D. Preoperative alpha- and beta-blockade, in contrast to an open adrenalectomy, is not necessary for laparoscopic pheochromocytoma resection.
   E. Laparoscopic adrenal resection should be used only for unilateral lesions.
3. Multiple endocrine neoplasia-2 (MEN-2):
   A. Is an autosomal recessive.
   B. MEN-2 tumors include hyperparathyroidism, pancreatic neuroendocrine tumor, and pituitary adenoma.
   C. MEN-2 is an autosomal dominant transmitted by germline mutation of the RET proto-oncogene.
   D. In MEN-2 syndrome, medullary thyroid cancer should be addressed prior to addressing other associated lesions.
   E. Hyperparathyroidism is a necessary component of MEN-2 syndrome.
4. When a patient presents with an adrenal incidentaloma (adrenaloma), which of the following statements is true?
   A. All patients with adrenal lesions must undergo a biopsy.
   B. When an adrenocortical carcinoma is diagnosed invading the kidney, the lesion should not be resected but rather be treated with chemotherapy.
   C. All functioning adrenal lesions should be resected if the patient is deemed medically suited.
   D. Follow-up images of an incidentaloma should be performed no less than 3 months for a minimum of 5 years.
   E. By definition, an adrenal incidentaloma must be bigger than 3 cm at the time of diagnosis.
5. Which of the following statements about multiple neuroendocrine neoplasia (MEN 1 & 2) syndrome is true?
   A. In MEN-2A, the diagnosis of pheochromocytoma usually precedes the diagnosis of medullary thyroid cancer.
   B. Prophylactic bilateral adrenalectomy should be performed when RET mutations is detected in patients with MEN-2A.
   C. Malignant pheochromocytoma rather than medullary thyroid cancer (MTC) in a patient with MEN-2A is the most common cause of the patient's demise.
   D. The clinical course of MEN-2B is usually aggressive with advanced medullary thyroid cancer (MTC) as the most common cause of death.
   E. In MEN-2A, hyperparathyroidism should be addressed before addressing pheochromocytoma.
6. Which of the following is true about adrenal incidentaloma?
   A. The average frequency of clinically silent adrenal nodule was 10 % in autopsy reports.
   B. All incidentalomas are benign adrenal adenoma and do not require any surgical intervention.
   C. Less than 1 % of abdominal and chest CT scan and MRI exams will identify an adrenal incidentaloma.
   D. Only adrenal adenomas more than 4 cm should be monitored.
   E. In radiological imaging, incidentalomas were found roughly in 2–4 % of middle-aged individuals, and this rate increases to about 10 % in the elderlies.

7. Adrenalectomy might be indicated in all of the following conditions EXCEPT:
   A. Metastatic disease with uncontrolled primary site
   B. Tumors>3.0 cm that demonstrate growth on serial imaging
   C. Adrenal cortical carcinomas without evidence of distant disease
   D. Glucocorticoid adenoma
   E. Asymptomatic pheochromocytoma
8. Which of the following is true about pheochromocytoma?
   A. Scintigraphy with I-123 or I-131 metaiodobenzylguanidine (MIBG) is not recommended for evaluating pheochromocytoma.
   B. Less than 2 % of adrenaloma hide a silent pheochromocytoma.
   C. Patients with a clinically silent pheochromocytoma has higher plasma catecholamine levels than patients with symptoms.
   D. In preparation for surgery, patients with pheochromocytoma should be initiated with a beta-blockade followed by an alpha-blockade.
   E. Rule of "10" applies to pheochromocytoma (10 % are malignant, 10 % occur in pediatrics, 10 % are extra-adrenal, 10 % are bilateral, and 10 % are hereditary).
9. Which is NOT true about adrenal cortical carcinoma (ACC)?
   A. Adrenal cortical carcinoma is relatively common and accounts for 10 % of all adrenal lesions.
   B. It is the second most lethal endocrine tumor after anaplastic thyroid malignancy.
   C. It has a bimodal age distribution with peak occurrence in the first decade and the fourth and fifth decades of life.
   D. The most important prognostic factors are complete resection and stage of disease.
   E. Mitotic rates >20 mitoses per 50 HPF are associated with shorter disease-free interval compared to lower mitotic rates.
10. What statement is NOT true about the role of adrenal mass biopsy?
   A. Adrenal mass biopsy might lead to bleeding.
   B. Needle biopsy of pheochromocytoma is strongly contraindicated due to the risk of initiating a hypertensive crisis and seeding.
   C. Needle biopsy of an adrenal lesion might lead to the rupture of the adrenal capsule.
   D. Needle biopsy should never be attempted when metastasis is suspected.
   E. Tissue obtained by a biopsy is rarely adequate to differentiate malignant from benign adrenal lesion.

Answers

1. D
2. B
3. C
4. C
5. D
6. E
7. A
8. E
9. A
10. D

References

1. Barzon L, Sonino N, Fallo F, Palu G, Boscaro M. Prevalence and natural history of adrenal incidentalomas. Eur J Endocrinol. 2003;149(4):273–85.
2. Kloos RT, Gross MD, Francis IR, Korobkin M, Shapiro B. Incidentally discovered adrenal masses. Endocr Rev. 1995;16(4):460–84.
3. Arnaldi G, Boscaro M. Adrenal incidentaloma. Best Pract Res Clin Endocrinol Metab. 2012;26(4): 405–19.
4. Terzolo M, Stigliano A, Chiodini I, et al. AME position statement on adrenal incidentaloma. Eur J Endocrinol. 2011;164(6):851–70.
5. Grumbach MM, Biller BM, Braunstein GD, et al. Management of the clinically inapparent adrenal mass ("incidentaloma"). Ann Intern Med. 2003;138(5): 424–9.
6. Aron DC. The adrenal incidentaloma: disease of modern technology and public health problem. Rev Endocr Metab Disord. 2001;2(3):335–42.
7. Mazzaglia P, Miner TJ. Adrenal incidentaloma. In: Cameron JLCA, editor. Current surgical therapy. 10th ed. Philadelphia: Elsevier; 2011. p. 565–70.
8. Groussin L, Bonardel G, Silvéra S, et al. 18F-Fluorodeoxyglucose positron emission tomography for the diagnosis of adrenocortical tumors: a

prospective study in 77 operated patients. J Clin Endocrinol Metab. 2009;94(5):1713–22.
9. Mantero F, Terzolo M, Arnaldi G, et al. A survey on adrenal incidentaloma in Italy. Study Group on Adrenal Tumors of the Italian Society of Endocrinology. J Clin Endocrinol Metab. 2000;85(2): 637–44.
10. Cawood TJ, Hunt PJ, O'Shea D, Cole D, Soule S. Recommended evaluation of adrenal incidentalomas is costly, has high false-positive rates and confers a risk of fatal cancer that is similar to the risk of the adrenal lesion becoming malignant; time for a rethink? Eur J Endocrinol. 2009;161(4):513–27.
11. Terzolo M, Bovio S, Pia A, Reimondo G, Angeli A. Management of adrenal incidentaloma. Best Pract Res Clin Endocrinol Metab. 2009;23(2):233–43.
12. Nieman LK. Approach to the patient with an adrenal incidentaloma. J Clin Endocrinol Metab. 2010;95(9): 4106–13.
13. Kim HY, Kim SG, Lee KW, et al. Clinical study of adrenal incidentaloma in Korea. Korean J Intern Med. 2005;20(4):303–9.
14. Lenders JW, Eisenhofer G, Mannelli M, Pacak K. Phaeochromocytoma. Lancet. 2005;366(9486):665–75.
15. Mannelli M, Ianni L, Cilotti A, Conti A. Pheochromocytoma in Italy: a multicentric retrospective study. Eur J Endocrinol. 1999;141(6):619–24.
16. Kopetschke R, Slisko M, Kilisli A, et al. Frequent incidental discovery of phaeochromocytoma: data from a German cohort of 201 phaeochromocytoma. Eur J Endocrinol. 2009;161(2):355–61.
17. Amar L, Servais A, Gimenez-Roqueplo AP, Zinzindohoue F, Chatellier G, Plouin PF. Year of diagnosis, features at presentation, and risk of recurrence in patients with pheochromocytoma or secreting paraganglioma. J Clin Endocrinol Metab. 2005;90(4):2110–6.
18. Loh KC, Fitzgerald PA, Matthay KK, Yeo PP, Price DC. The treatment of malignant pheochromocytoma with iodine-131 metaiodobenzylguanidine (131I-MIBG): a comprehensive review of 116 reported patients. J Endocrinol Invest. 1997;20(11):648–58.
19. Carr JC, Spanheimer PM, Rajput M, et al. Discriminating pheochromocytomas from other adrenal lesions: the dilemma of elevated catecholamines. Ann Surg Oncol. 2013;20(12):3855–61.
20. Engel A, von Euler US. Diagnostic value of increased urinary output of pheochromocytoma. Lancet. 1950; 2(6630):387.
21. Goldenberg M, Serlin I, Edwards T, Rapport MM. Chemical screening methods for the diagnosis of pheochromocytoma. I Nor-epinephrine and epinephrine in human urine. Am J Med. 1954;16(3): 310–27.
22. Zeiger MA, Thompson GB, Duh QY, et al. American Association of Clinical Endocrinologists and American Association of Endocrine Surgeons Medical Guidelines for the Management of Adrenal Incidentalomas: executive summary of recommendations. Endocr Pract. 2009;15(5):450–3.
23. Lenders JW, Pacak K, Eisenhofer G. New advances in the biochemical diagnosis of pheochromocytoma: moving beyond catecholamines. Ann N Y Acad Sci. 2002;970:29–40.
24. Eisenhofer G, Goldstein DS, Walther MM, et al. Biochemical diagnosis of pheochromocytoma: how to distinguish true- from false-positive test results. J Clin Endocrinol Metab. 2003;88(6):2656–66.
25. Welander J, Söderkvist P, Gimm O. Genetics and clinical characteristics of hereditary pheochromocytomas and paragangliomas. Endocr Relat Cancer. 2011;18(6):R253–76.
26. Rao JU, Engelke UF, Rodenburg RJ, et al. Genotype-specific abnormalities in mitochondrial function associate with distinct profiles of energy metabolism and catecholamine content in pheochromocytoma and paraganglioma. Clin Cancer Res. 2013;19(14):3787–95.
27. Burnichon N, Buffet A, Parfait B, et al. Somatic NF1 inactivation is a frequent event in sporadic pheochromocytoma. Hum Mol Genet. 2012;21(26):5397–405.
28. Burnichon N, Vescovo L, Amar L, et al. Integrative genomic analysis reveals somatic mutations in pheochromocytoma and paraganglioma. Hum Mol Genet. 2011;20(20):3974–85.
29. Zhuang Z, Yang C, Lorenzo F, et al. Somatic HIF2A gain-of-function mutations in paraganglioma with polycythemia. N Engl J Med. 2012;367(10):922–30.
30. Favier J, Brière JJ, Burnichon N, et al. The Warburg effect is genetically determined in inherited pheochromocytomas. PLoS One. 2009;4(9):e7094.
31. Gimenez-Roqueplo AP, Favier J, Rustin P, et al. The R22X mutation of the SDHD gene in hereditary paraganglioma abolishes the enzymatic activity of complex II in the mitochondrial respiratory chain and activates the hypoxia pathway. Am J Hum Genet. 2001;69(6):1186–97.
32. Gimenez-Roqueplo AP, Favier J, Rustin P, et al. Functional consequences of a SDHB gene mutation in an apparently sporadic pheochromocytoma. J Clin Endocrinol Metab. 2002;87(10):4771–4.
33. Rapizzi E, Ercolino T, Canu L, et al. Mitochondrial function and content in pheochromocytoma/paraganglioma of succinate dehydrogenase mutation carriers. Endocr Relat Cancer. 2012;19(3):261–9.
34. Mayo C. Paroxysmal hypertension with tumor of retroperitoneal nerve: report of case. JAMA. 1927;89: 1047–50.
35. Kvale WF, Manger WM, Priestley JT, Roth GM. Pheochromocytoma. Circulation. 1956;14(4 (Part 1)): 622–30.
36. Pacak K, Eisenhofer G, Ahlman H, et al. Pheochromocytoma: recommendations for clinical practice from the First International Symposium. October 2005. Nat Clin Pract Endocrinol Metab. 2007;3(2):92–102.
37. Gagner M, Lacroix A, Bolté E. Laparoscopic adrenalectomy in Cushing's syndrome and pheochromocytoma. N Engl J Med. 1992;327(14):1033.
38. Silberfein E, Perrier N. Management of pheochromocytomas. In: Cameron JLCA, editor. Current surgical therapy. 10th ed. Philadelphia: Elsevier; 2011. p. 579–84.

39. Filipponi S, Guerrieri M, Arnaldi G, et al. Laparoscopic adrenalectomy: a report on 50 operations. Eur J Endocrinol. 1998;138(5):548–53.
40. Gagner M, Breton G, Pharand D, Pomp A. Is laparoscopic adrenalectomy indicated for pheochromocytomas? Surgery. 1996;120(6):1076–9. discussion 1079–1080.
41. Janetschek G, Finkenstedt G, Gasser R, et al. Laparoscopic surgery for pheochromocytoma: adrenalectomy, partial resection, excision of paragangliomas. J Urol. 1998;160(2):330–4.
42. Aliyev S, Karabulut K, Agcaoglu O, et al. Robotic versus laparoscopic adrenalectomy for pheochromocytoma. Ann Surg Oncol. 2013;20(13):4190–4.
43. Manny TB, Pompeo AS, Hemal AK. Robotic partial adrenalectomy using indocyanine green dye with near-infrared imaging: the initial clinical experience. Urology. 2013;82(3):738–42.
44. Dackiw AP, Lee JE, Gagel RF, Evans DB. Adrenal cortical carcinoma. World J Surg. 2001;25(7):914–26.
45. Norton J. Adrenal tumors. In: DeVita VTHS, Rosenberg SA, editors. Cancer: principles and practice of oncology. Philadelphia: Lippincott-Raven; 1997. p. 1659–77.
46. Strosberg JR. Update on the management of unusual neuroendocrine tumors: pheochromocytoma and paraganglioma, medullary thyroid cancer and adrenocortical carcinoma. Semin Oncol. 2013;40(1):120–33.
47. Koch CA, Pacak K, Chrousos GP. The molecular pathogenesis of hereditary and sporadic adrenocortical and adrenomedullary tumors. J Clin Endocrinol Metab. 2002;87(12):5367–84.
48. Delellis R, Lloyd R, Heitz P, Eing C, editors. World Health Organization classification of tumors. Pathology and genetics of tumors of endocrine organs. Lyon: Arc Press; 2004.
49. Alaoui OA, Ehirchiou A, Ahallat M, Sabbah F, Mahassini N, Tounsi A. Malignant adrenocortical tumour with inferior vena cava invasion. Ann Chir. 2003;128(4):262–4.
50. Reibetanz J, Jurowich C, Erdogan I, et al. Impact of lymphadenectomy on the oncologic outcome of patients with adrenocortical carcinoma. Ann Surg. 2012;255(2):363–9.
51. Hedican SP, Marshall FF. Adrenocortical carcinoma with intracaval extension. J Urol. 1997;158(6):2056–61.
52. Vanderveen KA, Thompson SM, Callstrom MR, et al. Biopsy of pheochromocytomas and paragangliomas: potential for disaster. Surgery. 2009;146(6):1158–66.
53. Barry MK, van Heerden JA, Farley DR, Grant CS, Thompson GB, Ilstrup DM. Can adrenal incidentalomas be safely observed? World J Surg. 1998;22(6):599–603. discussion 603–594.

Hepatocellular Carcinoma

15

Malcolm H. Squires III and David A. Kooby

Abbreviations

PST	Performance status (ECOG classification)
CLT	Cadaveric liver transplantation
LDLT	Living donor liver transplantation
RF	Radiofrequency ablation
PEI	Percutaneous ethanol injection
TACE	Transarterial chemoembolization
OS	Overall survival

Learning Objectives

After reading this chapter, you should be able to:

- Describe the diagnostic workup for a suspected hepatocellular carcinoma liver lesion
- Understand the multiple staging systems for patients with hepatocellular carcinoma
- Appreciate the treatment paradigm for hepatocellular carcinoma within the context of HCC stage and the severity of underlying liver disease
- Understand the indications for hepatic resection, transplantation, locoregional therapy, and systemic therapy for patients with hepatocellular carcinoma

M.H. Squires III, M.D. • D.A. Kooby, M.D. (✉)
Division of Surgical Oncology, Winship Cancer Institute, Emory University, 1365C Clifton Rd. NE, 2nd Floor, Atlanta 30322, GA, USA
e-mail: msquire@emory.edu; dkooby@emory.edu

Introduction

Hepatocellular carcinoma (HCC) is the most common primary liver malignancy worldwide and ranks as the fifth most common cancer diagnosis overall and the third leading cause of cancer mortality worldwide [1]. In Southeast Asia and sub-Saharan Africa, regions where hepatitis B is endemic and the incidence of HCC is highest, HCC is currently the leading cause of cancer mortality [1, 2]. In the United States, greater than 30,000 new cases of HCC are diagnosed each year, with over 21,000 deaths due to HCC estimated to occur. The annual incidence of both new diagnoses and deaths attributed to HCC continues to increase; in fact, the incidence of HCC in the United States tripled between 1975 and 2005, largely due to the increasing prevalence of hepatitis C-related cirrhosis [1, 3]. Most cases of HCC arise in the setting of chronic liver disease, regardless of the etiology, with viral hepatitis B and C, alcohol abuse, and nonalcoholic steatohepatitis (NASH) constituting the majority of cases. Patients with cirrhosis have a significant risk, estimated at 1–8 % per year and a greater than 30 % lifetime risk, of developing HCC within the cirrhotic liver [4]. Even more concerning are recent data suggesting that the risk of developing HCC may be accentuated in the setting of cirrhosis secondary to nonalcoholic fatty liver disease (NAFLD) or NASH [5].

Despite advances in nonsurgical interventional therapies, the best potential curative treatment

Q.D. Chu et al. (eds.), *Surgical Oncology: A Practical and Comprehensive Approach*,
DOI 10.1007/978-1-4939-1423-4_15, © Springer Science+Business Media New York 2015

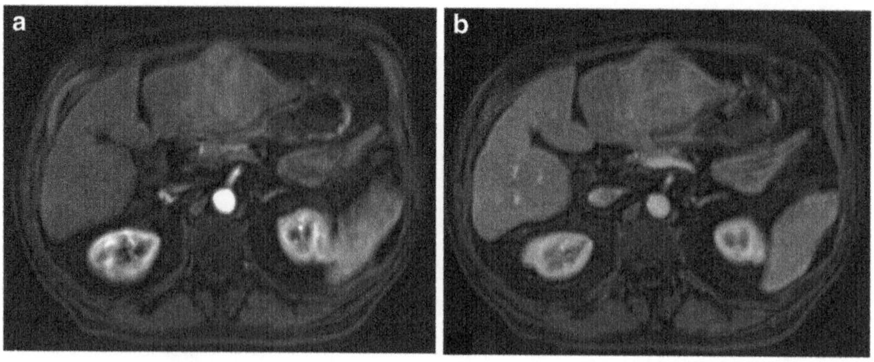

Fig. 15.1 MRI appearance of an HCC lesion in the left liver lobe demonstrating characteristic enhancement in the early arterial phase (**a**), with subsequent contrast washout in the delayed, portal venous phase (**b**)

option for HCC remains resection: either in the form of partial hepatectomy or liver transplantation [6–9]. Optimal surgical management of HCC patients remains a point of debate, due to variability in disease status and degree of liver fibrosis, with practices varying among institutions worldwide.

Diagnostic Workup and Staging

Cross-sectional imaging is a key component of the diagnostic algorithm for patients with suspected HCC. Ultrasound may be valuable in the context of surveillance screening patients at risk for HCC or as an initial imaging modality, but definitive radiologic diagnosis requires contrast-enhanced computed tomography (CT) or magnetic resonance imaging (MRI). Clinical practice guidelines adopted by the American Association for the Study of Liver Diseases (AASLD) and by the European Association for the Study of the Liver/European Organisation for Research and Treatment of Cancer (EASL/EORTC) outline noninvasive diagnostic imaging criteria for HCC [10]. HCC nodules typically have characteristic features of intense arterial enhancement followed by contrast washout during delayed or portal venous phases, as a result of their hypervascularity and dependence on hepatic arterial circulation (Fig. 15.1).

For patients with cirrhosis, lesions greater than 1 cm in size that display these hallmark imaging characteristics are diagnostic of HCC and do not require a confirmatory tissue biopsy. For patients with liver nodules suspicious for HCC but lacking these imaging features on one imaging study, a second modality should be considered. If imaging remains inconclusive, or for patients with liver nodules arising in the absence of underlying cirrhosis, histologic confirmation by core needle biopsy is necessary for pathologic diagnosis. Improved imaging technology and adoption of the diagnostic criteria above have helped limit the need for invasive percutaneous biopsy, which carries risks of potential complications such as tumor rupture or biopsy track seeding, estimated at 0–5.1 % [11, 12]. Serum alpha-fetoprotein (AFP) may play a role as an adjunctive test in patients with suspicious liver lesions, with some degree of AFP elevation observed in the majority of patients, but elevated AFP levels are not a requisite component of the most recent iteration of diagnostic criteria [13]. An initially elevated AFP level, however, can be of benefit to gauge tumor response to therapy and monitor for future recurrence following treatment.

Cross-sectional imaging also provides information regarding morphologic features of the HCC, including tumor focality (uninodular vs. multinodular), macrovascular invasion, presence of main portal or hepatic venous thrombus, and involvement of the biliary tree, as well as potential lymph node involvement or extrahepatic spread of disease (Figs. 15.2 and 15.3). Chest imaging is also appropriate, as HCC commonly

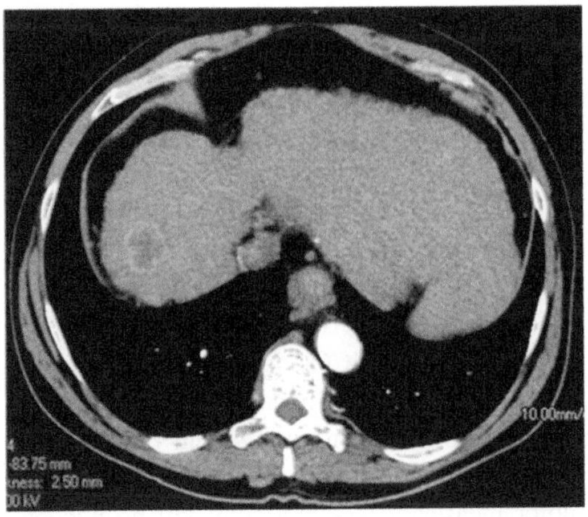

Fig. 15.2 Small HCC lesion arising in the background of a cirrhotic liver. In the absence of any evidence of vascular invasion or distant metastases, this lesion would meet Milan Criteria

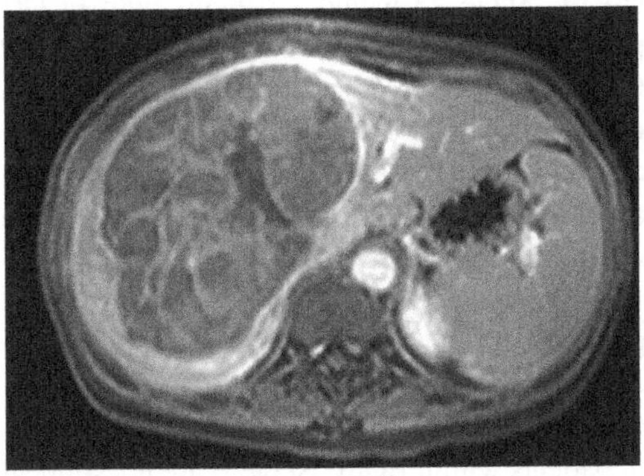

Fig. 15.3 A large HCC lesion arising in the setting of otherwise normal-appearing liver parenchyma

metastasizes to the lungs. Clinical management of patients with HCC requires an understanding of these tumor-specific features as well as the severity of their liver dysfunction and natural history of cirrhosis.

Patients with HCC typically have some degree of underlying liver disease, the severity of which can be quantified on the basis of the Child-Turcotte-Pugh (CTP) score or the Model for End-Stage Liver Disease (MELD) score. The CTP score stratifies patients with underlying cirrhosis on a scale of 5–15 points and incorporates points assigned for quantitative serum values for bilirubin, albumin, and INR (international normalized ratio) as well as the more subjective variables of ascites and encephalopathy (Table 15.1) [14, 15]. Patients with CTP Class A cirrhosis (score of 5–6 points) have a 2-year mortality risk of 10 % versus 20–40 % for those with Class B cirrhosis (score of 7–9 points) or 50–80 % for those with Class C cirrhosis (score 10–15 points) [14].

Table 15.1 Child-Turcotte-Pugh (CTP) classification of hepatic function

Variable	1 Point	2 Points	3 Points
Serum bilirubin (mg/dL)	<2.0	2.0–3.0	>3.0
Serum albumin (g/dL)	>3.5	2.8–3.5	<2.8
INR	<1.7	1.7–2.3	>2.3
Ascites	Absent	Slight	Moderate–severe
Encephalopathy (grade)	None	Mild (I–II)	Severe (III–IV)

CTP Class A = 5–6 points; Class B = 7–9 points; Class C = 10–15 points. Abbreviations: *INR* international normalized ratio

The MELD score, calculated from the patient's serum creatinine, bilirubin, and INR values using a linear regression model, is more objective than the CTP score as it does not incorporate subjective variables such as degree of ascites or encephalopathy [16]. The MELD score ranges from 6 to 40 and has been demonstrated to have prognostic value for survival in patients with underlying chronic liver disease, regardless of the etiology. Importantly, neither of these scoring systems assess tumor involvement.

As compared with other solid tumor types, the TNM staging system is less commonly employed for HCC, as it does not account for liver dysfunction, a crucial variable when examining treatment options for individual patients. The 7th edition American Joint Committee on Cancer (AJCC) staging system defines the stages for HCC as follows (Table 15.2): Stage I as a solitary tumor, any size, without vascular invasion; Stage II as a solitary tumor with vascular invasion or multiple tumors but none >5 cm in size; Stage IIIA as multiple tumors with at least one >5 cm in size; Stage IIIB as one or more tumors of any size involving a major branch of the portal vein or hepatic veins; and Stage IIIC as tumor(s) with perforation of the visceral peritoneum or direct invasion of adjacent organs other than the gallbladder [18].

Table 15.2 American Joint Committee on Cancer (AJCC) TNM Staging for Hepatocellular Carcinoma (7th edition)

Primary tumor (T)	
TX	Primary tumor cannot be assessed
T0	No evidence of primary tumor
T1	Solitary tumor without vascular invasion
T2	Solitary tumor with vascular invasion or multiple tumors, none>5 cm
T3a	Multiple tumors, one or more>5 cm
T3b	Tumor(s), any size, involving major branch of portal vein or hepatic veins
T4	Tumor(s) with perforation of visceral peritoneum or direct invasion of adjacent organs other than the gallbladder

Regional lymph nodes (N)	
NX	Regional lymph nodes cannot be assessed
N0	No regional lymph node metastasis
N1	Regional lymph node metastasis

Distant metastasis (M)	
M0	No distant metastasis
M1	Distant metastasis

Anatomic stage/prognostic groups			
Group	T	N	M
Stage I	T1	N0	M0
Stage II	T2	N0	M0
Stage IIIA	T3a	N0	M0
Stage IIIB	T3b	N0	M0
Stage IIIC	T4	N0	M0
Stage IVA	Any T	N1	M0
Stage IVB	Any T	Any N	M1

Adapted from Compton et al. [17]. With permission from Springer Verlag

Any regional lymph node involvement or distant metastases is classified as Stage IV disease.

Several alternative staging systems have been proposed to better define the prognosis of patients with HCC and appropriately stratify patients for treatment. One of the more established clinical staging systems is the Barcelona Clinic Liver Cancer (BCLC) system [19]. The BCLC classification stratifies patients on the basis of hepatic function as represented by the CTP score, clinical Eastern Cooperative Oncology Group (ECOG) performance status, and tumor stage, which encompasses tumor size, number of lesions, presence of vascular invasion, and extrahepatic spread of disease. Subsequent updates to the BCLC classification scheme have incorporated additional evidence-based treatment recommendations [6, 20]. The widely adopted EASL/EORTC consensus guidelines for management of HCC follow the BCLC staging algorithm (Fig. 15.4).

Very early HCC (BCLC Stage 0) includes patients with an ECOG performance status 0; well-preserved liver function, defined as CTP Class A along with normal serum bilirubin and normal portal pressures; and a solitary HCC tumor, measuring less than 2 cm, with no evidence of vascular invasion. While few patients are typically diagnosed this early in their disease course, resection and transplantation both offer excellent 5-year survival rates of 80–90 % [21]. Early HCC (BCLC Stage A) includes patients with ECOG performance status 0, well-compensated CTP Class A liver disease, and solitary tumors >2 cm or up to three tumors, each <3 cm in diameter. For appropriately selected patients, 5-year survival approaches 50–70 % following hepatic resection or liver transplant [22].

Intermediate HCC (BCLC Stage B) includes patients with ECOG performance status 0, moderate liver dysfunction within CTP Class A or B, and large or multinodular tumors. As the majority of patients within BCLC Stage B are not surgical candidates for resection or transplant, locoregional therapy with chemoembolization generally offers the best chance for improved symptom control and survival within this cohort [19, 23].

Patients with advanced HCC (BCLC Stage C) include patients with diminished ECOG performance status, moderate liver disease within CTP Class A or B, and advanced tumors exhibiting macrovascular invasion and/or extrahepatic spread in the form of nodal disease or distant metastases. Stage C patients have a poor prognosis, and the multi-kinase inhibitor sorafenib (Onyx Pharmaceuticals, San Francisco, CA) is currently the only therapeutic option shown to have a survival benefit, demonstrating a 3-month improvement in overall survival as compared to placebo [24]. For patients without portal

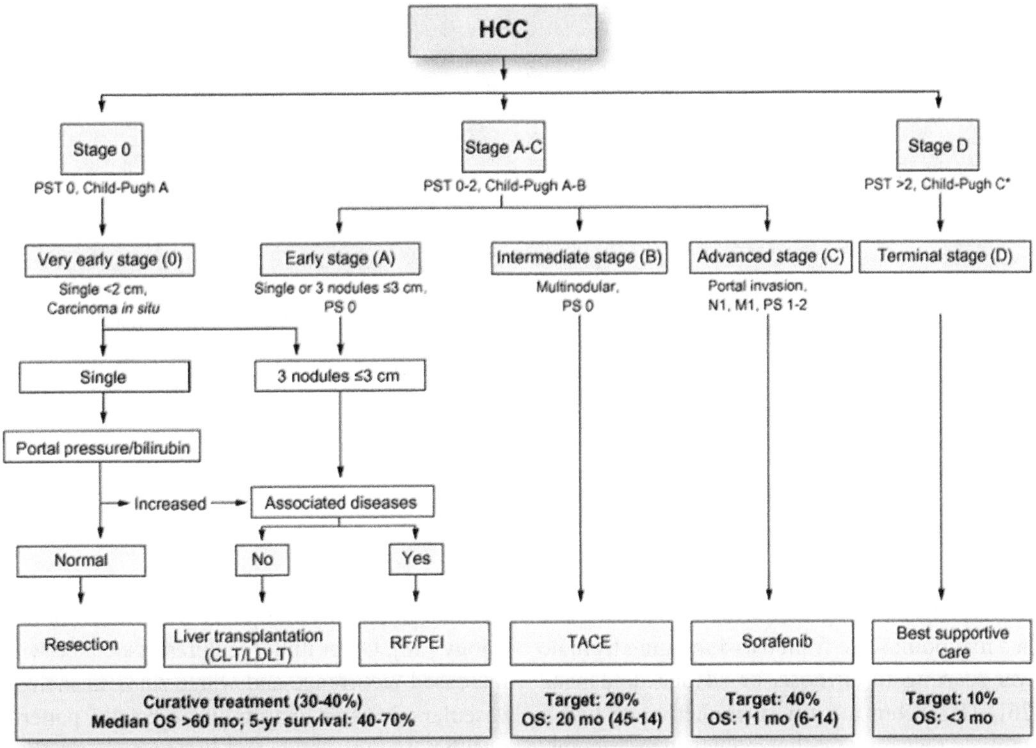

Fig. 15.4 BCLC (Barcelona Clinic Liver Cancer) staging system for management of HCC (Reprinted from European Association for the Study of the Liver, European Organisation for Research and Treatment of Cancer. EASL-EORTC clinical practice guidelines: management of hepatocellular carcinoma. J Hepatol 2012;56(4):908–43. With permission from Elsevier.)

invasion or metastatic disease, locoregional liver-directed therapy with chemoembolization or radioembolization in addition to sorafenib can be considered.

Patients within BCLC Stage D include patients with extremely poor performance status (ECOG 3–4), advanced liver disease within CTP Class C, and advanced HCC. These patients have a terminal prognosis, with median survival of 3–4 months, and are treated with best supportive care and palliation [19].

Hepatic Resection

For patients with normal or minimally diseased underlying liver parenchyma and HCC amenable to surgical resection, liver resection remains the treatment of choice. Most patients, however, develop HCC in the setting of some degree of underlying liver disease or dysfunction, making appropriate patient selection for resection essential. Most patients with well-compensated CTP Class A cirrhosis can typically tolerate hepatic resection, while patients with Class C cirrhosis and nearly all patients with Class B cirrhosis are not candidates for resection. The presence of significant portal hypertension, the sequelae of which are typically detectable on preoperative imaging in the form of parenchymal changes, splenomegaly, and/or varices, is a risk factor for postoperative liver failure following resection. Low preoperative platelet count, another hallmark of portal hypertension, has also been shown to be an important independent risk factor for increased complications, postoperative liver insufficiency, and mortality following hepatic resection for HCC [25]. Pathologically, the

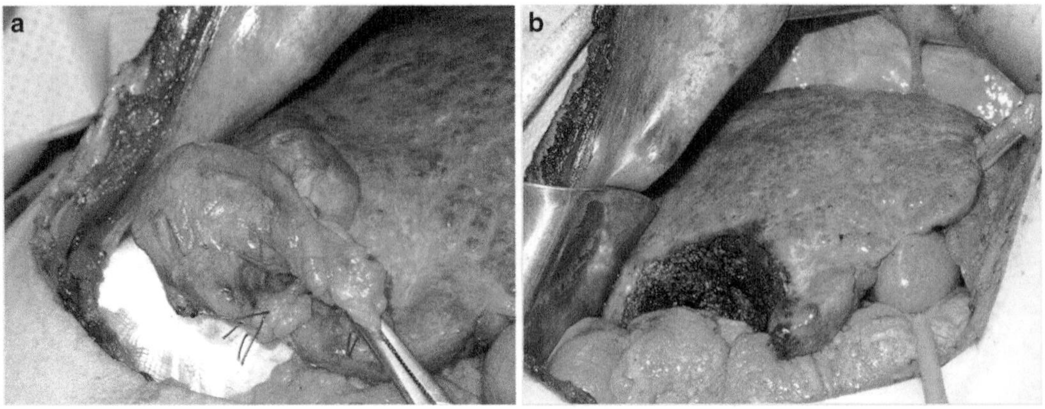

Fig. 15.5 (**a**) Hepatocellular carcinoma arising within a cirrhotic liver (note the fibrotic, nodular appearance of the uninvolved liver). (**b**) Liver remnant following limited hepatic resection of HCC lesion, again demonstrating the characteristic nodular appearance of cirrhosis

degree of hepatic fibrosis can be quantified by the METAVIR scoring system, which assigns a score on a five-point scale from 0 to 4, ranging from no liver scarring to cirrhosis or advanced scarring [26]. This score in turn is predictive of liver's ability to regenerate following hepatic resection.

A key consideration is the extent of the indicated hepatic resection, which must be balanced against the need to preserve an adequate functional liver remnant (FLR) with hepatic portal and arterial inflow, venous outflow, and biliary drainage [27]. The volume of the FLR (ideally >30 % of the total liver volume for patients with normal liver parenchyma or >40 % for well-compensated patients with cirrhotic liver parenchyma) must be taken into account, particularly in the setting of underlying liver disease [27]. Hepatic resection in the setting of fibrosis or cirrhosis carries increased risk of hepatic insufficiency and perioperative complications; this risk increases with the extent of resection (Fig. 15.5a, b). Portal vein embolization is a potential option to induce hypertrophy and increase the size of the FLR in cases where preoperative volumetric calculations suggest an inadequate FLR will remain following partial hepatectomy.

Ideal candidates for resection are patients with minimal or well-compensated liver dysfunction and unifocal, small lesions < 5 cm [7]. While multifocality and larger tumor size are not absolute contraindications for surgical resection, both features are surrogate markers for microscopic vascular invasion and more aggressive tumor histology [28]. Other tumor features associated with increased recurrence and worse survival include vascular invasion, infiltrative growth pattern, positive margin status, and lymph node involvement [29, 30]. In the absence of other adverse features, however, solitary tumors larger than 5 cm can be considered for resection if they involve < 50 % of the liver, as resection may offer 5-year survival rates of 20–25 % (Fig. 15.6a, b) [29, 30]. Resection margins of ≥2 cm are advocated when possible, as long as the adequacy of the FLR size is not compromised, as they are associated with improved recurrence-free and overall survival outcomes versus resection margins of 1 cm [31]. Techniques of resection are beyond the scope of this review, and we refer our readers to the following excellent sources:

- Poon RT. Current techniques of liver transection. HPB. 2007; 9(3): 166–73.
- Cunningham SC, Schulick RD. Management of Primary Malignant Liver Tumors. In: Cameron JL, Cameron AM (eds). Current Surgical Therapy, 10th edition. Philadelphia, PA: Elsevier Saunders; 2010.
- Sicklick JK, D'Angelica M, Fong Y. The Liver. In: Townsend CM, Beauchamp RD, Evers BM, Mattox KL (eds). Sabiston Textbook of Surgery, 19th edition. Philadelphia, PA: Elsevier Saunders; 2012.

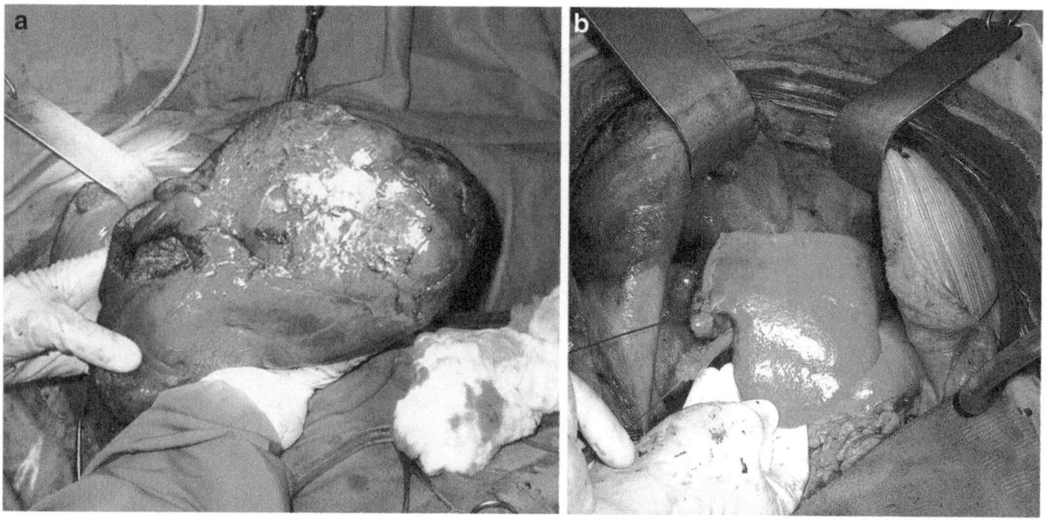

Fig. 15.6 (**a**) Intraoperative photograph of a large HCC lesion. (**b**) Liver remnant after resection of a large HCC lesion

- Fan ST. Major Hepatic Resection for Primary and Metastatic Tumors. In: Fischer JE (ed). Mastery of Surgery, 6th edition. Philadelphia, PA: Lippincott Williams & Wilkins; 2012.
- Maithel SK, Jarnagin WR, Belghiti J. Hepatic Resection for Benign Disease and for Liver and Biliary Tumors. Jarnagin WR (eds). Blumgart's Surgery of the Liver, Biliary Tract, and Pancreas, 5th edition. Philadelphia, PA: Elsevier Saunders; 2012.

Patients with hepatitis B as the etiology of their cirrhosis and HCC often have comparatively well-preserved hepatic function versus patients with underlying hepatitis C, making resection a potentially more viable treatment for these patients. In Asia and Africa, where hepatitis B is endemic and where cadaveric organs are severely limited, resection is commonly employed for most patients with HCC amenable to surgical treatment. HCC arising secondary to NASH presents a new disease paradigm, and results to date suggest that these patients have a greater tendency to develop HCC within noncirrhotic liver parenchyma. These patients may possess a theoretical lower risk of HCC recurrence in the liver remnant as compared with patients with underlying hepatitis B or C, and the benefit of resection may be greater in this patient population [32, 33].

One significant advantage of resection is the potential for immediate treatment, as opposed to the risk of disease progression while on the transplant wait list [34]. A trade-off for more expedited surgical therapy, however, is the significant risk of disease recurrence following partial hepatectomy. Recurrence rates following resection for HCC, whether from true recurrence or de novo tumor development in the cirrhotic liver remnant, have remained extremely high, reaching 50–75 % at 5 years in some series (Table 15.3) [35–47, 48]. Some groups have advocated a strategy of initial resection in patients with HCC within Milan Criteria and with relatively well-preserved liver function, followed by "salvage transplantation" or "secondary transplantation" for those who subsequently develop recurrent disease [49–52]. While primary resection of patients with early HCC and Child-Pugh Class A cirrhosis may be feasible, a significant portion of patients with recurrent disease following resection will not be candidates for transplantation, due to age, comorbidities, or recurrence outside of Milan Criteria [49, 51].

Table 15.3 Representative series of resected hepatocellular carcinoma from Western and Eastern series

						Recurrence-free survival			Overall survival		
Author	Year	Study period	N	% Cirrhosis	Miscellaneous	1 year	3 years	5 years	1 year	3 years	5 years
Llovet [35]	1999	1989–1997	77	100 %	Mean size 3.3 cm	73 %	39 %	25 %	85 %	62 %	51 %
Poon [36]	2001	1989–1994	136	50 %	72 % major resections	42 %	23 %	16 %	68 %	47 %	36 %
		1994–1999	241	43 %	63 % major resections	60 %	38 %	25 %	82 %	62 %	49 %
Belghiti [37]	2002	1990–1999	328	50 %	42 % major resections	NR	NR	NR	61 %	57 %	37 %
Ercolani [38]	2003	1983–1999	224	100 %	Median size 4.1 cm	70 %	43 %	27 %	83 %	63 %	43 %
Cha [39]	2003	1990–2001	164	40 %	85 % major resections	NR	NR	25 %	79 %	51 %	40 %
Ikai [40]	2007	1992–2003	27,062	43 %	27 % multinodular	NR	NR	NR	88 %	69 %	53 %
Shah [41]	2007	1992–2004	193	95 %	Median size 4.5 cm	72 %	48 %	39 %	85 %	68 %	53 %
Park [42]	2009	1994–2007	213	100 %	All within MC	79 %	57 %	44 %	92 %	78 %	69 %
Dahiya [43]	2010	1983–2002	373	100 %	69 % major resections	70 %	43 %	32 %	82 %	63 %	44 %
					31 % minor resections (all tumors < 5 cm)	67 %	43 %	32 %	86 %	65 %	51 %
Lee [44]	2010	1997–2007	130	100 %	63 % within MC	68 %	54 %	50 %	80 %	65 %	52 %
Huang [45]	2011	2000–2005	648	100 %	Mean size 3.6 cm	80 %	57 %	43 %	94 %	83 %	76 %
Arnaoutakis [46]	2013	1992–2011	334	0 %	Median size 6.5 cm	71 %	NR	35 %	87 %	NR	55 %
Sapisochin [47]	2013	1991–2007	95	100 %	All <5 cm in size	81 %	NR	33 %	85 %	NR	62 % (4 years)

Abbreviations: *NR* not reported, *MC* Milan criteria
Adapted from [48]. With permission from Elsevier

Transplantation

Liver transplant offers arguably the most effective cure for HCC, as it removes both the malignancy and the underlying diseased liver parenchyma in which HCC typically arises. Transplantation is limited, however, by access to donor organs and must be balanced against the need for lifelong immunosuppression. Across the globe, the most widely accepted transplant selection criteria are referred to as the Milan Criteria. First reported in 1996 by Mazzaferro et al [53], the Milan Criteria defined transplant criteria for patients as a single HCC lesion < 5 cm in maximum diameter or ≤ 3 lesions each < 3 cm in size, with no evidence of macrovascular invasion or extrahepatic disease on imaging. Numerous studies worldwide, many included in a comprehensive 2011 meta-analysis by the Milan group, have confirmed the favorable outcomes that can be achieved with transplantation for patients meeting these criteria [54]. Others have advocated broader transplantation guidelines, such as the expanded University of California, San Francisco (UCSF) criteria, which include patients with a single lesion < 6.5 cm or up to three tumors, each measuring less than 4.5 cm and a total tumor diameter < 8 cm [55, 56].

As a result of limited organ availability, the drawbacks of transplantation include the risk for disease progression and resulting patient dropout, while patients are on the transplant wait list. Particularly in parts of Asia where HCC is more prevalent, the number of patients with HCC on transplant wait lists far exceeds the supply of deceased donor livers available. In the United States, the UNOS (United Network for Organ Sharing) criteria dictate that patients with HCC meeting Milan Criteria radiographically receive a MELD "exception points" score of 22 when placed on the wait list. If patients remain on the wait list after 3 months, they typically receive an additional three exception points. Within this allocation scheme, wait times vary considerably across UNOS regions and globally, with median times to transplant of 6–12 months in many regions increasing patient dropout and affecting intention-to-treat outcomes [34, 57, 58]. As a result, many centers, particularly those with longer wait times, now offer locoregional neoadjuvant or "bridging" therapy to patients on the transplant wait list to attempt to minimize tumor progression while awaiting a donor organ [59]. Several non-randomized studies to date have reported decreased dropout rates, but none have demonstrated a correlation between pre-transplant bridging therapy with ablation or transarterial chemoembolization and improved posttransplant survival [60–64]. A cost-effective analysis of pretransplantation bridging ablation therapy, however, demonstrated benefit if projected wait time to transplant exceeded 6 months [65].

Downstaging

No randomized controlled trials have evaluated the utility of locoregional therapy for downstaging patients initially outside of Milan Criteria, although several small series have demonstrated comparable 5-year outcomes for such patients successfully treated with radiofrequency ablation or chemoembolization followed by transplantation versus patients who meet Milan Criteria a priori [66–68]. In light of limited donor organ availability, studies are ongoing to better define which patients beyond Milan Criteria are most likely to benefit from downstaging followed by transplantation.

Living Donor Liver Transplantation

Living donor liver transplantation (LDLT) is also an option for patients and avoids the potential limitations of wait times for allocation of deceased donor livers and the restrictions of the Milan Criteria, although LDLT has been slow to be adopted. Some concerns were raised by early studies suggesting patients undergoing LDLT for treatment of HCC had higher rates of recurrence than seen with deceased donor transplantation [69, 70], although overall survival outcomes appear comparable [71, 72]. Because wait times are minimized, patients with more aggressive tumors that would progress and render them ineligible for deceased donor transplant may be undergoing LDLT; thus, an observation period of 2–3 months has been proposed to assess the natural history of a patient's tumor [69, 73]. Markov cost-effectiveness modeling suggests that LDLT is most cost-effective in scenarios where wait list times are projected to exceed 7 months [74].

Locoregional Therapy

Ablation

Local ablation is the treatment of choice for patients with early-stage HCC not amenable to surgical therapies. Modalities include radiofrequency, chemical, and microwave ablation.

Radiofrequency ablation (RFA) involves the delivery of electrical energy to cause coagulative necrosis of tumor tissue and can be performed percutaneously, laparoscopically, or as an adjunct procedure from an open surgical approach. One recent study of early HCC lesions < 2 cm demonstrated sustained complete response in 95 % of patients following ablation, with a local recurrence rate of < 1 % [75]. For tumors >3 cm, the efficacy of ablation diminishes significantly [76]. Only two randomized, controlled comparisons of ablation versus resection for early HCC have been performed to date, with one study demonstrating equivalent recurrence and survival rates for the two treatment modalities and the other study suggesting resection was associated with lower recurrence rates and improved survival compared to RFA [77, 78]. Thus the use of RFA as a first-line definitive therapy in patients with resectable disease is not widely practiced. For patients who are not candidates for resection, however, ablation offers an excellent treatment option for smaller tumors. RFA also can be employed as a bridging therapy for HCC in patients awaiting liver transplantation [79].

Chemical ablation with percutaneous ethanol injection (PEI) was among the earliest ablative therapies tested and also induces coagulative necrosis of the HCC lesion. Effective necrosis rates of nearly 90 % for small tumors <2 cm in size have been demonstrated [80], but local recurrence rates are significant [81]. PEI is currently most often reserved for cases in which RFA is not technically feasible due to tumor location.

Microwave ablation is a newer alternative thermal treatment modality that may be more efficacious than RFA for treatment of lesions in close proximity to large vessels, which can serve as a heat sink for RFA and compromise complete necrosis of tumors. Early results with microwave ablation have been comparable to those with RFA [82, 83], although no prospective controlled head-to-head comparisons have been conducted.

Embolization

Embolization therapies take advantage of the dual blood supply of the liver and the fact that HCC tumors are predominantly supplied by the hepatic artery, whereas the uninvolved liver parenchyma is predominantly supplied by the portal venous circulation, allowing therapeutic agents to be delivered via minimally invasive arterial catheters under image guidance directly to the tumor. Intra-arterial therapeutic options include bland embolization, transarterial chemoembolization (TACE), drug-eluting bead (DEB) chemoembolization, and radioembolization.

Bland embolization, or transarterial embolization (TAE), involves injection of microparticles into the terminal hepatic arterial vessels feeding the tumor, causing occlusion of the vessel and inducing ischemic necrosis of the tumor. Multiple lesions can be treated during the same procedure by super-selective targeting of terminal arterial branches. This procedure can be serially repeated in patients with progressive disease or additional lesions with acceptable safety [84], and multiple studies have demonstrated a survival benefit compared to supportive care [23, 85].

TACE, or conventional chemoembolization, involves injection of hydrophilic cytotoxic chemotherapeutic agents, most commonly doxorubicin, into the arterial branches supplying the tumor(s), followed by occlusion of the feeding vessel with injected embolic particles to prevent washout [86]. This combined cytotoxic and ischemic effect is theorized to induce greater tumor necrosis. Meta-analyses of multiple randomized, controlled trials evaluating TACE have demonstrated minimal procedure-related mortality and significantly improved survival compared to best supportive care, although bland TAE and PEI were also associated with similarly improved survival outcomes [87–90].

Drug-eluting bead chemoembolization (DEB-TACE) takes advantage of embolic microbeads impregnated with doxorubicin and engineered to release the chemotherapeutic agent in a slow, controlled rate over days to weeks within the tumor after being directly injected into the tumor-supplying vessels. This treatment strategy allows for increased, sustained chemotherapy concentrations locally within the tumor without increasing systemic levels [91, 92]. Significantly decreased rates of liver toxicity and systemic side effects compared to conventional TACE and comparable objective response rates of >50 % have been reported, and DEB-TACE has begun replacing TACE at many centers [93, 94].

Arterial catheter-based embolic therapies are recommended for patients with unresectable HCC lesions larger than 4 cm and thus not amenable to RFA or patients with multifocal disease. Per EASL/EORTC guidelines, TACE is the treatment of choice for patients with intermediate, BCLC Stage B, asymptomatic, multifocal HCC in the setting of well-compensated liver dysfunction [10, 95]. The presence of macroscopic vascular invasion or extrahepatic disease is an absolute contraindication to chemoembolization [23, 96]. Chemoembolization is typically limited to patients with Child-Pugh Class A or B cirrhosis, due to the increased risk of liver failure following TACE in patients with more advanced liver disease [97–99]. Other contraindications outlined by Raoul et al [100] include refractory ascites, encephalopathy, extensive bilobar tumor involvement, and renal insufficiency.

Radioembolization

Radioembolization refers to the transarterial catheter-based injection of microspheres loaded with the radioactive isotope yttrium-90 (Y-90). As with chemoembolization, the Y-90 microbeads are selectively injected into the terminal arterial branches supplying the HCC lesion, where they then lodge and deliver a high dose of radiation directly to the tumor, with little penetrance to the surrounding liver parenchyma [101, 102]. Pre-procedure arteriogram mapping of the vasculature and liver-lung shunt studies are required to minimize the risk of radioembolization to the gastrointestinal tract or lungs. The smaller diameter Y-90 microspheres have less embolic effect; therefore portal vein thrombosis is not a contraindication to radioembolization [103]. Trials to date have demonstrated radioembolization is safe and efficacious, with similar objective response rates and overall survival to that seen with chemoembolization [104, 105]. Radioembolization and chemoembolization have yet to be directly compared in a randomized, controlled prospective fashion. Existing retrospective comparisons of these modalities fail to show a survival advantage of one over the other [106, 107].

Among the catheter-based therapies described above, no single therapy has demonstrated a definitive superior survival benefit in a randomized, controlled fashion when compared to the other embolization treatment options. As a result, there is significant heterogeneity among centers as to which liver-directed locoregional therapy is employed.

SBRT

External beam radiation therapy has little role for treatment of HCC due to the risk of radiating the liver in the setting of cirrhosis [108]. Stereotactic body radiation therapy (SBRT) offers a more precise modality for targeting liver lesions with a smaller number of higher doses of radiation, thereby sparing more of the uninvolved liver parenchyma [109, 110]. For unresectable patients with single HCC tumors ≤6 cm in diameter or up to three lesions with a sum diameter ≤6 cm, local control rates of 90 % and overall survival of 60 % at 2 years have been demonstrated with SBRT [111, 112].

Systemic Therapy

Until 2007, no systemic therapeutic agent was approved for the treatment of HCC, and conventional chemotherapy such as doxorubicin, the standard agent for unresectable or metastatic HCC prior to sorafenib, is largely ineffective. Sorafenib, an oral multi-tyrosine kinase inhibitor with activity against vascular endothelial growth factor receptor (VEGFR), platelet-derived growth factor receptor (PDGFR), and other molecular targets, demonstrated a tolerable side effect profile and a nearly 3-month median overall survival improvement in patients with advanced (BCLC Stage C) metastatic HCC versus the placebo arm in phase II and III studies [24, 113, 114]. In a multicenter, phase III trial of 602 patients with HCC who were not eligible for or had disease progression after surgical resection or locoregional therapies, patients who received sorafenib 400 mg twice daily had a median survival of 10.7 months versus 7.9 months in the placebo group [24]. The patients in this study had an ECOG performance status ≤ 2 and CTP Class A liver dysfunction. Based on these trials, sorafenib is currently recommended as standard of care systemic therapy for patients with advanced, BCLC Stage C disease, or disease progression while undergoing locoregional therapies [10]. Treatment guidelines recommend dose maintenance until evidence of disease progression or intolerable side effects [10].

Numerous phase I through III trials are underway to examine the efficacy of additional molecular targeted agents for the treatment of advanced HCC, either alone or in combination with sorafenib.

Conclusion

Management of patients with hepatocellular carcinoma remains a challenge due to the typical combination of malignant disease and organ dysfunction. Resection remains the treatment of choice for patients with early solitary HCC and normal or well-compensated liver dysfunction. Transplantation should be offered to patients with HCC meeting Milan Criteria (a single lesion <5 cm or up to three lesions each <3 cm), although donor organ availability and long wait times pose limitations. For patients with early HCC not amenable to surgical management, radiofrequency ablation is typically indicated for solitary lesions up to 3 cm in size. Patients with multiple HCC lesions and without evidence of macrovascular invasion or extrahepatic disease are candidates for locoregional therapy, typically with TACE, DEB-TACE, or radioembolization. For patients with advanced HCC, sorafenib is currently the only approved therapeutic agent.

Salient Points

- Hepatocellular carcinoma (HCC) most commonly arises in the setting of cirrhosis or chronic liver disease, for which the most common etiologies worldwide include viral hepatitis B and C, alcohol abuse, and nonalcoholic steatohepatitis (NASH).
- HCC lesions characteristically demonstrate intense arterial enhancement followed by delayed contrast washout on portal venous phases of CT or MRI.
- For lesions > 1 cm arising in the background of known cirrhosis and displaying these hallmark imaging characteristics diagnostic of HCC, a tissue biopsy is not necessary, particularly if the patient may be considered for transplant.
- Resection remains the treatment of choice for patients with early solitary HCC and normal or well-compensated liver dysfunction (i.e., CTP Class A).
- Recurrence rates following resection of HCC remain as high as 50–75 % at 5 years in most studies.
- The Milan Criteria define transplant criteria for patients with HCC as a single HCC lesion < 5 cm in size, or ≤ 3 lesions each < 3 cm in size, with no evidence of macrovascular invasion or extrahepatic disease.
- Liver transplantation should be offered to patients with HCC meeting Milan Criteria, although donor organ availability and long wait times pose limitations in many countries and some UNOS regions within the United States.

- For patients with early-stage, small HCC lesions not amenable to surgical therapies, local ablation is the treatment of choice. Modalities include radiofrequency ablation (RFA), percutaneous ethanol injection (PEI), and microwave ablation.
- Patients with multiple HCC lesions and without evidence of macrovascular invasion or extrahepatic disease are candidates for locoregional therapy, typically with transarterial chemoembolization (TACE), drug-eluting bead (DEB)-TACE, or radioembolization.
- The only systemic therapeutic agent approved for advanced or metastatic HCC is sorafenib, an oral multi-kinase inhibitor.

Questions

1. Based on the Milan Criteria, in which of the following scenarios would a patient with HCC NOT be eligible for consideration for transplantation based on these guidelines:
   A. A single 2.5 cm lesion
   B. Three lesions measuring 2.0 cm, 2.5 cm, and 3.0 cm respectively
   C. A single 3.5 cm lesion with evidence of portal vein invasion
   D. Two 2.0 cm lesions involving both the right and left hepatic lobes
2. The characteristic feature of an HCC lesion on cross-sectional imaging with CT or MRI is:
   A. Intense, homogenous contrast enhancement on arterial phase images, with a distinct hypointense central scar
   B. Initial peripheral nodular contrast enhancement with peripheral-to-central progressive infilling of the lesion on delayed phases
   C. Lesion enhancement on arterial phase imaging with contrast washout on delayed phases
   D. Low-attenuation, delayed arterial enhancement
3. The only FDA-approved systemic therapy for a patient with metastatic, Stage IV HCC is:
   A. Everolimus
   B. Sorafenib
   C. Imatinib
   D Herceptin
4. A patient with a serum bilirubin of 2.5, normal serum albumin and INR levels, and no evidence of ascites or encephalopathy would be described as what Child-Turcotte-Pugh (CTP) Class?
   A. CTP Class A
   B. CTP Class B
   C. CTP Class C
   D. CTP Class 3
5. Given a patient with a 7 cm HCC lesion in the setting of cirrhosis and ascites, the most appropriate therapy recommended by BCLC guidelines would be:
   A. Resection
   B. Transplantation
   C. Radiofrequency ablation (RFA)
   D. Transarterial chemoembolization (TACE)
6. Which of the following lab values does NOT factor into the calculation of a patient's MELD (Model for End-Stage Liver Disease) score?
   A. Bilirubin
   B. Albumin
   C. Creatinine
   D. INR
7. In a patient with known cirrhosis and chronic hepatitis C and a large liver lesion suspicious for HCC found on routine surveillance ultrasound, initial workup and staging includes all of the following except:
   A. CT or MRI of abdomen and pelvis
   B. Serum AFP
   C. Percutaneous needle biopsy
   D. Chest imaging
8. All of the following are associated with increased risk of morbidity and mortality following hepatic resection for HCC except:
   A. Splenomegaly
   B. Esophageal varices
   C. Female gender
   D. Low preoperative platelet count
9. All of the following are benefits of transplantation over hepatic resection for the treatment of HCC except:
   A. Clear resection margins
   B. Reduced risk of HCC recurrence
   C. Treatment of the underlying liver disease
   D. Decreased time to surgery

10. Given a patient with CTP Class B cirrhosis, evidence of portal hypertension, and two HCC nodules, each < 3 cm in size, which of the following is the least appropriate therapy by BCLC guidelines?
    A. Transplantation
    B. Radiofrequency ablation (RFA)
    C. Transarterial chemoembolization (TACE)
    D. Hepatic resection

Answers
1. C
2. C
3. B
4. A
5. D
6. B
7. C
8. C
9. D
10. D

References

1. Jemal A, Bray F, Center MM, Ferlay J, Ward E, Forman D. Global cancer statistics. CA Cancer J Clin. 2011;61:69–90.
2. Center MM, Jemal A. International trends in liver cancer incidence rates. Cancer Epidemiol Biomarkers Prev. 2011;20:2362–8.
3. Edwards BK, Ward E, Kohler BA, Eheman C, Zauber AG, Anderson RN, et al. Annual report to the nation on the status of cancer, 1975–2006, featuring colorectal cancer trends and impact of interventions (risk factors, screening, and treatment) to reduce future rates. Cancer. 2010;116:544–73.
4. Bruix J, Sherman M, Llovet JM, Beaugrand M, Lencioni R, Burroughs AK, et al. Clinical management of hepatocellular carcinoma. Conclusions of the Barcelona-2000 EASL conference. European Association for the Study of the Liver. J Hepatol. 2001;35:421–30.
5. Siegel AB, Zhu AX. Metabolic syndrome and hepatocellular carcinoma: two growing epidemics with a potential link. Cancer. 2009;115:5651–61.
6. Llovet JM, Burroughs A, Bruix J. Hepatocellular carcinoma. Lancet. 2003;362:1907–17.
7. Jarnagin WR. Management of small hepatocellular carcinoma: a review of transplantation, resection, and ablation. Ann Surg Oncol. 2010;17:1226–33.
8. Rahbari NN, Mehrabi A, Mollberg NM, Muller SA, Koch M, Buchler MW, et al. Hepatocellular carcinoma: current management and perspectives for the future. Ann Surg. 2011;253:453–69.
9. Kooby DA, Egnatashvili V, Graiser M, Delman KA, Kauh J, Wood WC, et al. Changing management and outcome of hepatocellular carcinoma: evaluation of 501 patients treated at a single comprehensive center. J Surg Oncol. 2008;98:81–8.
10. European Association For The Study Of The L, European Organisation For R, Treatment Of C. EASL-EORTC clinical practice guidelines: management of hepatocellular carcinoma. J Hepatol. 2012;56:908–43.
11. Stigliano R, Marelli L, Yu D, Davies N, Patch D, Burroughs AK. Seeding following percutaneous diagnostic and therapeutic approaches for hepatocellular carcinoma. What is the risk and the outcome? Seeding risk for percutaneous approach of HCC. Cancer Treat Rev. 2007;33:437–47.
12. Silva MA, Hegab B, Hyde C, Guo B, Buckels JA, Mirza DF. Needle track seeding following biopsy of liver lesions in the diagnosis of hepatocellular cancer: a systematic review and meta-analysis. Gut. 2008;57:1592–6.
13. Trevisani F, D'Intino PE, Morselli-Labate AM, Mazzella G, Accogli E, Caraceni P, et al. Serum alpha-fetoprotein for diagnosis of hepatocellular carcinoma in patients with chronic liver disease: influence of HBsAg and anti-HCV status. J Hepatol. 2001;34:570–5.
14. D'Amico G, Garcia-Tsao G, Pagliaro L. Natural history and prognostic indicators of survival in cirrhosis: a systematic review of 118 studies. J Hepatol. 2006;44:217–31.
15. Pugh RN, Murray-Lyon IM, Dawson JL, Pietroni MC, Williams R. Transection of the oesophagus for bleeding oesophageal varices. Br J Surg. 1973;60:646–9.
16. Kamath PS, Wiesner RH, Malinchoc M, Kremers W, Therneau TM, Kosberg CL, et al. A model to predict survival in patients with end-stage liver disease. Hepatology. 2001;33:464–70.
17. Compton CC, Byrd DR, Garcia-Aguilar J. Liver. In: Compton CC, Byrd DR, Garcia-Aguilar J, editors. AJCC cancer staging atlas. New York: Springer; 2012. p. 241–9.
18. Edge SB, Byrd DR, Compton CC, et al., eds.: AJCC Cancer Staging Manual, 7th ed. New York, NY: Springer, 2010, pp 191–9.
19. Llovet JM, Bru C, Bruix J. Prognosis of hepatocellular carcinoma: the BCLC staging classification. Semin Liver Dis. 1999;19:329–38.
20. Llovet JM, Di Bisceglie AM, Bruix J, Kramer BS, Lencioni R, Zhu AX, et al. Design and endpoints of clinical trials in hepatocellular carcinoma. J Natl Cancer Inst. 2008;100:698–711.
21. Takayama T, Makuuchi M, Hirohashi S, Sakamoto M, Yamamoto J, Shimada K, et al. Early hepatocellular carcinoma as an entity with a high rate of surgical cure. Hepatology. 1998;28:1241–6.
22. Llovet JM, Bruix J. Novel advancements in the management of hepatocellular carcinoma in 2008. J Hepatol. 2008;48 Suppl 1:S20–37.
23. Llovet JM, Real MI, Montana X, Planas R, Coll S, Aponte J, et al. Arterial embolisation or chemoem-

bolisation versus symptomatic treatment in patients with unresectable hepatocellular carcinoma: a randomised controlled trial. Lancet. 2002;359:1734–9.
24. Llovet JM, Ricci S, Mazzaferro V, Hilgard P, Gane E, Blanc JF, et al. Sorafenib in advanced hepatocellular carcinoma. N Engl J Med. 2008;359:378–90.
25. Maithel SK, Kneuertz PJ, Kooby DA, Scoggins CR, Weber SM, Martin 2nd RC, et al. Importance of low preoperative platelet count in selecting patients for resection of hepatocellular carcinoma: a multi-institutional analysis. J Am Coll Surg. 2011;212:638–48. discussion 648–50.
26. Poynard T, Bedossa P, Opolon P. Natural history of liver fibrosis progression in patients with chronic hepatitis C. The OBSVIRC, METAVIR, CLINIVIR, and DOSVIRC groups. Lancet. 1997;349:825–32.
27. Melstrom LG, Fong Y. "The management of malignant liver tumors." In: Cameron JL, Cameron AM, eds. Current surgical therapy. 11th ed. Elsevier 2014. p. 328–332.
28. Pawlik TM, Delman KA, Vauthey JN, Nagorney DM, Ng IO, Ikai I, et al. Tumor size predicts vascular invasion and histologic grade: implications for selection of surgical treatment for hepatocellular carcinoma. Liver Transpl. 2005;11:1086–92.
29. Schiffman SC, Woodall CE, Kooby DA, Martin RC, Staley CA, Egnatashvili V, et al. Factors associated with recurrence and survival following hepatectomy for large hepatocellular carcinoma: a multicenter analysis. J Surg Oncol. 2010;101:105–10.
30. Pawlik TM, Poon RT, Abdalla EK, Zorzi D, Ikai I, Curley SA, et al. Critical appraisal of the clinical and pathologic predictors of survival after resection of large hepatocellular carcinoma. Arch Surg. 2005;140:450–7. discussion 457–8.
31. Shi M, Guo RP, Lin XJ, Zhang YQ, Chen MS, Zhang CQ, et al. Partial hepatectomy with wide versus narrow resection margin for solitary hepatocellular carcinoma: a prospective randomized trial. Ann Surg. 2007;245:36–43.
32. Reddy SK, Steel JL, Chen HW, DeMateo DJ, Cardinal J, Behari J, et al. Outcomes of curative treatment for hepatocellular cancer in nonalcoholic steatohepatitis versus hepatitis C and alcoholic liver disease. Hepatology. 2012;55:1809–19.
33. Takuma Y, Nouso K. Nonalcoholic steatohepatitis-associated hepatocellular carcinoma: our case series and literature review. World J Gastroenterol. 2010;16:1436–41.
34. Freeman RB, Edwards EB, Harper AM. Waiting list removal rates among patients with chronic and malignant liver diseases. Am J Transplant. 2006;6:1416–21.
35. Llovet JM, Fuster J, Bruix J. Intention-to-treat analysis of surgical treatment for early hepatocellular carcinoma: resection versus transplantation. Hepatology. 1999;30:1434–40.
36. Poon RT, Fan ST, Lo CM, Ng IO, Liu CL, Lam CM, et al. Improving survival results after resection of hepatocellular carcinoma: a prospective study of 377 patients over 10 years. Ann Surg. 2001;234:63–70.
37. Belghiti J, Regimbeau JM, Durand F, Kianmanesh AR, Dondero F, Terris B, et al. Resection of hepatocellular carcinoma: a European experience on 328 cases. Hepatogastroenterology. 2002;49:41–6.
38. Ercolani G, Grazi GL, Ravaioli M, Del Gaudio M, Gardini A, Cescon M, et al. Liver resection for hepatocellular carcinoma on cirrhosis: univariate and multivariate analysis of risk factors for intrahepatic recurrence. Ann Surg. 2003;237:536–43.
39. Cha C, Fong Y, Jarnagin WR, Blumgart LH, DeMatteo RP. Predictors and patterns of recurrence after resection of hepatocellular carcinoma. J Am Coll Surg. 2003;197:753–8.
40. Ikai I, Arii S, Okazaki M, Okita K, Omata M, Kojiro M, et al. Report of the 17th Nationwide Follow-up Survey of Primary Liver Cancer in Japan. Hepatol Res. 2007;37:676–91.
41. Shah SA, Cleary SP, Wei AC, Yang I, Taylor BR, Hemming AW, et al. Recurrence after liver resection for hepatocellular carcinoma: risk factors, treatment, and outcomes. Surgery. 2007;141:330–9.
42. Park YK, Kim BW, Wang HJ, Kim MW. Hepatic resection for hepatocellular carcinoma meeting Milan criteria in Child-Turcotte-Pugh class a patients with cirrhosis. Transplant Proc. 2009;41:1691–7.
43. Dahiya D, Wu TJ, Lee CF, Chan KM, Lee WC, Chen MF. Minor versus major hepatic resection for small hepatocellular carcinoma (HCC) in cirrhotic patients: a 20-year experience. Surgery. 2010;147: 676–85.
44. Lee KK, Kim DG, Moon IS, Lee MD, Park JH. Liver transplantation versus liver resection for the treatment of hepatocellular carcinoma. J Surg Oncol. 2010;101:47–53.
45. Huang J, Hernandez-Alejandro R, Croome KP, Yan L, Wu H, Chen Z, et al. Radiofrequency ablation versus surgical resection for hepatocellular carcinoma in Childs A cirrhotics-a retrospective study of 1,061 cases. J Gastrointest Surg. 2011;15:311–20.
46. Arnaoutakis DJ, Mavros MN, Shen F, Alexandrescu S, Firoozmand A, Popescu I, et al. Recurrence patterns and prognostic factors in patients with hepatocellular carcinoma in noncirrhotic liver: a multi-institutional analysis. Ann Surg Oncol. 2014; 21(1):147–54.
47. Sapisochin G, Castells L, Dopazo C, Bilbao I, Minguez B, Lazaro JL, et al. Single HCC in cirrhotic patients: liver resection or liver transplantation? Long-term outcome according to an intention-to-treat basis. Ann Surg Oncol. 2013;20:1194–202.
48. Earl TM, Chapman WC. Conventional surgical treatment of hepatocellular carcinoma. Clin Liver Dis. 2011;15:353–70,vii-x.
49. Cherqui D, Laurent A, Mocellin N, Tayar C, Luciani A, Van Nhieu JT, et al. Liver resection for transplantable hepatocellular carcinoma: long-term survival and role of secondary liver transplantation. Ann Surg. 2009;250:738–46.
50. Cucchetti A, Vitale A, Gaudio MD, Ravaioli M, Ercolani G, Cescon M, et al. Harm and benefits of primary liver resection and salvage transplantation

for hepatocellular carcinoma. Am J Transplant. 2010;10:619–27.

51. Fuks D, Dokmak S, Paradis V, Diouf M, Durand F, Belghiti J. Benefit of initial resection of hepatocellular carcinoma followed by transplantation in case of recurrence: an intention-to-treat analysis. Hepatology. 2012;55:132–40.
52. Poon RT, Fan ST, Lo CM, Liu CL, Wong J. Long-term survival and pattern of recurrence after resection of small hepatocellular carcinoma in patients with preserved liver function: implications for a strategy of salvage transplantation. Ann Surg. 2002;235:373–82.
53. Mazzaferro V, Regalia E, Doci R, Andreola S, Pulvirenti A, Bozzetti F, et al. Liver transplantation for the treatment of small hepatocellular carcinomas in patients with cirrhosis. N Engl J Med. 1996;334: 693–9.
54. Mazzaferro V, Bhoori S, Sposito C, Bongini M, Langer M, Miceli R, et al. Milan criteria in liver transplantation for hepatocellular carcinoma: an evidence-based analysis of 15 years of experience. Liver Transpl. 2011;17 Suppl 2:S44–57.
55. Yao FY, Ferrell L, Bass NM, Bacchetti P, Ascher NL, Roberts JP. Liver transplantation for hepatocellular carcinoma: comparison of the proposed UCSF criteria with the Milan criteria and the Pittsburgh modified TNM criteria. Liver Transpl. 2002;8: 765–74.
56. Duffy JP, Vardanian A, Benjamin E, Watson M, Farmer DG, Ghobrial RM, et al. Liver transplantation criteria for hepatocellular carcinoma should be expanded: a 22-year experience with 467 patients at UCLA. Ann Surg. 2007;246:502–9. discussion 509–11.
57. Facciuto ME, Rochon C, Pandey M, Rodriguez-Davalos M, Samaniego S, Wolf DC, et al. Surgical dilemma: liver resection or liver transplantation for hepatocellular carcinoma and cirrhosis. Intention-to-treat analysis in patients within and outwith Milan criteria. HPB (Oxford). 2009;11:398–404.
58. Pelletier SJ, Fu S, Thyagarajan V, Romero-Marrero C, Batheja MJ, Punch JD, et al. An intention-to-treat analysis of liver transplantation for hepatocellular carcinoma using organ procurement transplant network data. Liver Transpl. 2009;15:859–68.
59. Schwartz M, Roayaie S, Uva P. Treatment of HCC in patients awaiting liver transplantation. Am J Transplant. 2007;7:1875–81.
60. Porrett PM, Peterman H, Rosen M, Sonnad S, Soulen M, Markmann JF, et al. Lack of benefit of pre-transplant locoregional hepatic therapy for hepatocellular cancer in the current MELD era. Liver Transpl. 2006;12:665–73.
61. Heckman JT, Devera MB, Marsh JW, Fontes P, Amesur NB, Holloway SE, et al. Bridging locoregional therapy for hepatocellular carcinoma prior to liver transplantation. Ann Surg Oncol. 2008;15: 3169–77.
62. Decaens T, Roudot-Thoraval F, Bresson-Hadni S, Meyer C, Gugenheim J, Durand F, et al. Impact of pretransplantation transarterial chemoembolization on survival and recurrence after liver transplantation for hepatocellular carcinoma. Liver Transpl. 2005; 11:767–75.
63. Mazzaferro V, Battiston C, Perrone S, Pulvirenti A, Regalia E, Romito R, et al. Radiofrequency ablation of small hepatocellular carcinoma in cirrhotic patients awaiting liver transplantation: a prospective study. Ann Surg. 2004;240:900–9.
64. Lu DS, Yu NC, Raman SS, Lassman C, Tong MJ, Britten C, et al. Percutaneous radiofrequency ablation of hepatocellular carcinoma as a bridge to liver transplantation. Hepatology. 2005;41:1130–7.
65. Llovet JM, Mas X, Aponte JJ, Fuster J, Navasa M, Christensen E, et al. Cost effectiveness of adjuvant therapy for hepatocellular carcinoma during the waiting list for liver transplantation. Gut. 2002;50: 123–8.
66. Yao FY, Kerlan Jr RK, Hirose R, Davern 3rd TJ, Bass NM, Feng S, et al. Excellent outcome following down-staging of hepatocellular carcinoma prior to liver transplantation: an intention-to-treat analysis. Hepatology. 2008;48:819–27.
67. Hanje AJ, Yao FY. Current approach to down-staging of hepatocellular carcinoma prior to liver transplantation. Curr Opin Organ Transplant. 2008;13:234–40.
68. Ravaioli M, Grazi GL, Piscaglia F, Trevisani F, Cescon M, Ercolani G, et al. Liver transplantation for hepatocellular carcinoma: results of down-staging in patients initially outside the Milan selection criteria. Am J Transplant. 2008;8:2547–57.
69. Fisher RA, Kulik LM, Freise CE, Lok AS, Shearon TH, Brown Jr RS, et al. Hepatocellular carcinoma recurrence and death following living and deceased donor liver transplantation. Am J Transplant. 2007;7:1601–8.
70. Lo CM, Fan ST, Liu CL, Chan SC, Ng IO, Wong J. Living donor versus deceased donor liver transplantation for early irresectable hepatocellular carcinoma. Br J Surg. 2007;94:78–86.
71. Gondolesi GE, Roayaie S, Munoz L, Kim-Schluger L, Schiano T, Fishbein TM, et al. Adult living donor liver transplantation for patients with hepatocellular carcinoma: extending UNOS priority criteria. Ann Surg. 2004;239:142–9.
72. Todo S, Furukawa H, Japanese Study Group on Organ T. Living donor liver transplantation for adult patients with hepatocellular carcinoma: experience in Japan. Ann Surg. 2004;240:451–9. discussion 459–61.
73. Kulik L, Abecassis M. Living donor liver transplantation for hepatocellular carcinoma. Gastroenterology. 2004;127:S277–82.
74. Sarasin FP, Majno PE, Llovet JM, Bruix J, Mentha G, Hadengue A. Living donor liver transplantation for early hepatocellular carcinoma: a life-expectancy and cost-effectiveness perspective. Hepatology. 2001;33:1073–9.
75. Livraghi T, Meloni F, Di Stasi M, Rolle E, Solbiati L, Tinelli C, et al. Sustained complete response and complications rates after radiofrequency ablation of very early hepatocellular carcinoma in cirrhosis: is

resection still the treatment of choice? Hepatology. 2008;47:82–9.
76. Yan K, Chen MH, Yang W, Wang YB, Gao W, Hao CY, et al. Radiofrequency ablation of hepatocellular carcinoma: long-term outcome and prognostic factors. Eur J Radiol. 2008;67:336–47.
77. Chen MS, Li JQ, Zheng Y, Guo RP, Liang HH, Zhang YQ, et al. A prospective randomized trial comparing percutaneous local ablative therapy and partial hepatectomy for small hepatocellular carcinoma. Ann Surg. 2006;243:321–8.
78. Huang J, Yan L, Cheng Z, Wu H, Du L, Wang J, et al. A randomized trial comparing radiofrequency ablation and surgical resection for HCC conforming to the Milan criteria. Ann Surg. 2010;252:903–12.
79. Martin AP, Goldstein RM, Dempster J, Netto GJ, Katabi N, Derrick HC, et al. Radiofrequency thermal ablation of hepatocellular carcinoma before liver transplantation–a clinical and histological examination. Clin Transplant. 2006;20:695–705.
80. Sala M, Llovet JM, Vilana R, Bianchi L, Sole M, Ayuso C, et al. Initial response to percutaneous ablation predicts survival in patients with hepatocellular carcinoma. Hepatology. 2004;40:1352–60.
81. Livraghi T, Giorgio A, Marin G, Salmi A, de Sio I, Bolondi L, et al. Hepatocellular carcinoma and cirrhosis in 746 patients: long-term results of percutaneous ethanol injection. Radiology. 1995;197: 101–8.
82. Iannitti DA, Martin RC, Simon CJ, Hope WW, Newcomb WL, McMasters KM, et al. Hepatic tumor ablation with clustered microwave antennae: the US Phase II trial. HPB (Oxford). 2007;9:120–4.
83. Swan RZ, Sindram D, Martinie JB, Iannitti DA. Operative microwave ablation for hepatocellular carcinoma: complications, recurrence, and long-term outcomes. J Gastrointest Surg. 2013;17:719–29.
84. Erinjeri JP, Salhab HM, Covey AM, Getrajdman GI, Brown KT. Arterial patency after repeated hepatic artery bland particle embolization. J Vasc Interv Radiol. 2010;21:522–6.
85. Maluccio MA, Covey AM, Porat LB, Schubert J, Brody LA, Sofocleous CT, et al. Transcatheter arterial embolization with only particles for the treatment of unresectable hepatocellular carcinoma. J Vasc Interv Radiol. 2008;19:862–9.
86. Maluccio M, Covey A. Recent progress in understanding, diagnosing, and treating hepatocellular carcinoma. CA Cancer J Clin. 2012;62:394–9.
87. Llovet JM, Bruix J. Systematic review of randomized trials for unresectable hepatocellular carcinoma: Chemoembolization improves survival. Hepatology. 2003;37:429–42.
88. Camma C, Schepis F, Orlando A, Albanese M, Shahied L, Trevisani F, et al. Transarterial chemoembolization for unresectable hepatocellular carcinoma: meta-analysis of randomized controlled trials. Radiology. 2002;224:47–54.
89. Befeler AS. Chemoembolization and bland embolization: a critical appraisal. Clin Liver Dis. 2005;9:287–300, vii.
90. Takayasu K, Arii S, Ikai I, Omata M, Okita K, Ichida T, et al. Prospective cohort study of transarterial chemoembolization for unresectable hepatocellular carcinoma in 8510 patients. Gastroenterology. 2006;131:461–9.
91. Varela M, Real MI, Burrel M, Forner A, Sala M, Brunet M, et al. Chemoembolization of hepatocellular carcinoma with drug eluting beads: efficacy and doxorubicin pharmacokinetics. J Hepatol. 2007;46:474–81.
92. Poon RT, Tso WK, Pang RW, Ng KK, Woo R, Tai KS, et al. A phase I/II trial of chemoembolization for hepatocellular carcinoma using a novel intra-arterial drug-eluting bead. Clin Gastroenterol Hepatol. 2007;5:1100–8.
93. Burrel M, Reig M, Forner A, Barrufet M, de Lope CR, Tremosini S, et al. Survival of patients with hepatocellular carcinoma treated by transarterial chemoembolisation (TACE) using Drug Eluting Beads. Implications for clinical practice and trial design. J Hepatol. 2012;56:1330–5.
94. Lammer J, Malagari K, Vogl T, Pilleul F, Denys A, Watkinson A, et al. Prospective randomized study of doxorubicin-eluting-bead embolization in the treatment of hepatocellular carcinoma: results of the PRECISION V study. Cardiovasc Intervent Radiol. 2010;33:41–52.
95. Bruix J, Sherman M, American Association for the Study of Liver D. Management of hepatocellular carcinoma: an update. Hepatology. 2011;53: 1020–2.
96. Bruix J, Sala M, Llovet JM. Chemoembolization for hepatocellular carcinoma. Gastroenterology. 2004;127:S179–88.
97. Chan AO, Yuen MF, Hui CK, Tso WK, Lai CL. A prospective study regarding the complications of transcatheter intraarterial lipiodol chemoembolization in patients with hepatocellular carcinoma. Cancer. 2002;94:1747–52.
98. Shah SR, Riordan SM, Karani J, Williams R. Tumour ablation and hepatic decompensation rates in multiagent chemoembolization of hepatocellular carcinoma. QJM. 1998;91:821–8.
99. Hwang JI, Chow WK, Hung SW, Li TC, Cheng YP, Ho YJ, et al. Development of a safety index of transarterial chemoembolization for hepatocellular carcinoma to prevent acute liver damage. Anticancer Res. 2005;25:2551–4.
100. Raoul JL, Sangro B, Forner A, Mazzaferro V, Piscaglia F, Bolondi L, et al. Evolving strategies for the management of intermediate-stage hepatocellular carcinoma: available evidence and expert opinion on the use of transarterial chemoembolization. Cancer Treat Rev. 2011;37:212–20.
101. Sangro B, Bilbao JI, Inarrairaegui M, Rodriguez M, Garrastachu P, Martinez-Cuesta A. Treatment of hepatocellular carcinoma by radioembolization using 90Y microspheres. Dig Dis. 2009;27:164–9.
102. Ibrahim SM, Lewandowski RJ, Sato KT, Gates VL, Kulik L, Mulcahy MF, et al. Radioembolization for the treatment of unresectable hepatocellular carci-

noma: a clinical review. World J Gastroenterol. 2008;14:1664–9.
103. Kulik LM, Carr BI, Mulcahy MF, Lewandowski RJ, Atassi B, Ryu RK, et al. Safety and efficacy of 90Y radiotherapy for hepatocellular carcinoma with and without portal vein thrombosis. Hepatology. 2008;47:71–81.
104. Salem R, Lewandowski RJ, Kulik L, Wang E, Riaz A, Ryu RK, et al. Radioembolization results in longer time-to-progression and reduced toxicity compared with chemoembolization in patients with hepatocellular carcinoma. Gastroenterology. 2011; 140:497–507 e2.
105. Salem R, Lewandowski RJ, Mulcahy MF, Riaz A, Ryu RK, Ibrahim S, et al. Radioembolization for hepatocellular carcinoma using Yttrium-90 microspheres: a comprehensive report of long-term outcomes. Gastroenterology. 2010;138:52–64.
106. Carr BI, Kondragunta V, Buch SC, Branch RA. Therapeutic equivalence in survival for hepatic arterial chemoembolization and yttrium 90 microsphere treatments in unresectable hepatocellular carcinoma: a two-cohort study. Cancer. 2010;116: 1305–14.
107. Kooby DA, Egnatashvili V, Srinivasan S, Chamsuddin A, Delman KA, Kauh J, et al. Comparison of yttrium-90 radioembolization and transcatheter arterial chemoembolization for the treatment of unresectable hepatocellular carcinoma. J Vasc Interv Radiol. 2010;21:224–30.
108. Cheng JC, Wu JK, Huang CM, Liu HS, Huang DY, Cheng SH, et al. Radiation-induced liver disease after three-dimensional conformal radiotherapy for patients with hepatocellular carcinoma: dosimetric analysis and implication. Int J Radiat Oncol Biol Phys. 2002;54:156–62.
109. Lo SS, Fakiris AJ, Chang EL, Mayr NA, Wang JZ, Papiez L, et al. Stereotactic body radiation therapy: a novel treatment modality. Nat Rev Clin Oncol. 2010;7:44–54.
110. Tse RV, Hawkins M, Lockwood G, Kim JJ, Cummings B, Knox J, et al. Phase I study of individualized stereotactic body radiotherapy for hepatocellular carcinoma and intrahepatic cholangiocarcinoma. J Clin Oncol. 2008;26:657–64.
111. Price TR, Perkins SM, Sandrasegaran K, Henderson MA, Maluccio MA, Zook JE, et al. Evaluation of response after stereotactic body radiotherapy for hepatocellular carcinoma. Cancer. 2012;118:3191–8.
112. Andolino DL, Johnson CS, Maluccio M, Kwo P, Tector AJ, Zook J, et al. Stereotactic body radiotherapy for primary hepatocellular carcinoma. Int J Radiat Oncol Biol Phys. 2011;81:e447–53.
113. Abou-Alfa GK, Schwartz L, Ricci S, Amadori D, Santoro A, Figer A, et al. Phase II study of sorafenib in patients with advanced hepatocellular carcinoma. J Clin Oncol. 2006;24:4293–300.
114. Cheng AL, Kang YK, Chen Z, Tsao CJ, Qin S, Kim JS, et al. Efficacy and safety of sorafenib in patients in the Asia-Pacific region with advanced hepatocellular carcinoma: a phase III randomised, double-blind, placebo-controlled trial. Lancet Oncol. 2009; 10:25–34.

Colon Cancer

16

Salim Amrani, Michael Polcino, Miguel Rodriguez-Bigas, and Quyen D. Chu

Learning Objectives

After reading this chapter, you should be able to:

- Know screening protocol for colorectal cancer (CRC).
- Understand how to evaluate and manage patients with colon cancer.
- Comprehend the surgical principles of resecting colon cancer.
- Know what circumferential radial margin (CRM) is.
- Identify the high-risk features of stage 2 colon cancer.
- Recognize the indication for adjuvant therapy for colon cancer.
- Appreciate the role of microsatellite instability (MSI) in colon cancer.
- Be cognizant of the data on laparoscopic colectomy for colon cancer.

S. Amrani, M.D.
Department of Surgery, Carlsbad Medical Center, 2111 Calle De Codorniz, Carlsbad, NM 88220, USA
e-mail: samrani75@gmail.com

M. Polcino, M.D.
Department of Surgery, Memorial Sloan Kettering Cancer Center, 1275 York Avenue, C-1067, New York, NY, USA
e-mail: michael.polcino@gmail.com

M. Rodriguez-Bigas, M.D.
Department of Surgical Oncology, UT MD Anderson Cancer Center, 1400 Pressler Street, Unit 1484, Houston, TX, USA
e-mail: mrodbig@mdanderson.org

Q.D. Chu, M.D., MBA, FACS (✉)
Department of Surgery, LSU Health Sciences Center-Shreveport, 1501 Kings Hwy, P.O. Box 33932, Shreveport, LA 71130-3932, USA
e-mail: qchu@lsuhsc.edu

Background

Colon and rectal cancer (CRC) is the 3rd most common cause of cancer and the 2nd most common cause of cancer death in the United States. In women, it ranks 3rd after breast and lung, whereas in men it is preceded by prostate and lung [1]. It is estimated that in 2013 over 50,000 will die from CRC in the United States [2]. The lifetime probability of developing a colon and rectal cancer in the United States is 5.5 % and 5.1 % in men and women, respectively.

The adenocarcinoma sequence in CRC is well described, and it is clear that early detection of CRC and removal of adenomatous polyps have decreased the mortality from the disease [3–9]. Unfortunately, it is estimated that only 50 % of adults over the age of 50 underwent screening for CRC by fecal occult blood test or endoscopy in 2005 [10].

Etiology and Risk Factors

The genesis of CRC is not fully understood; however, it is well established that a combination of genetic predisposition and environmental factors plays a great role [11]. Genomic and epigenetic

Q.D. Chu et al. (eds.), *Surgical Oncology: A Practical and Comprehensive Approach*, DOI 10.1007/978-1-4939-1423-4_16,

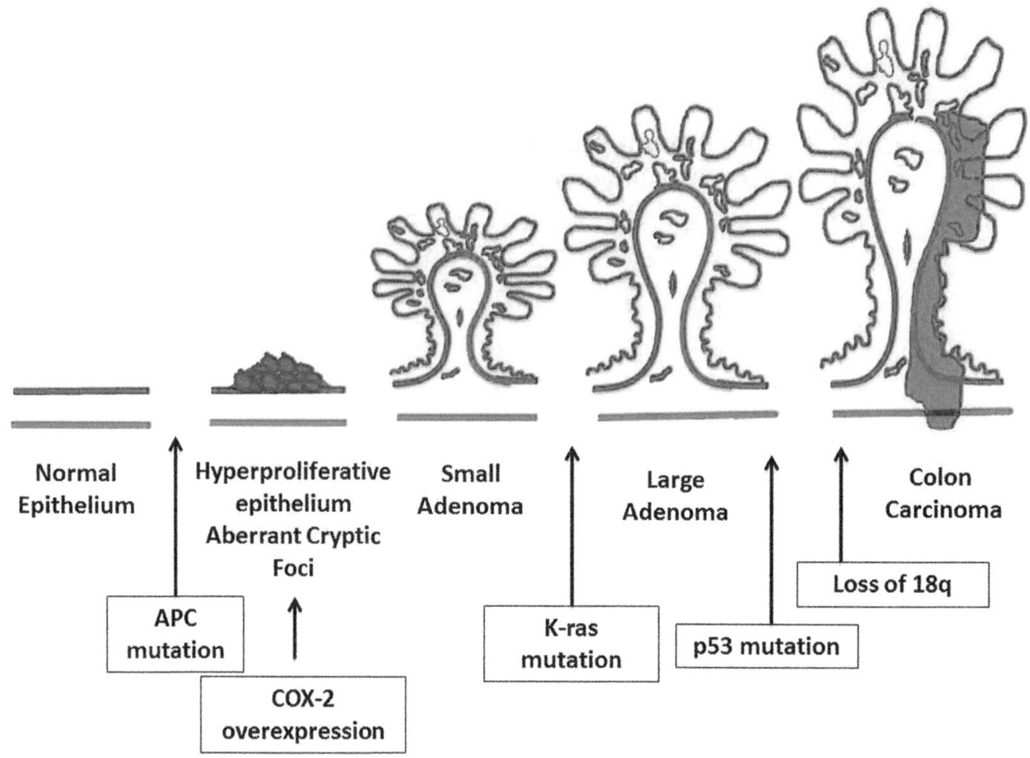

Fig. 16.1 *Fearon and Vogelstein proposed genetic model of colorectal carcinogenesis*. CRC is the result of accumulated mutations of multiple genes that are involved with cell growth and differentiation

alterations are common in CRC, and the two recognized pathways of carcinogenesis are the chromosomal instability pathway (CIN) and the microsatellite instability pathway (MSI). It is thought that colorectal carcinogenesis is a four-step process that begins with the transformation of normal epithelium to an adenoma, proceeding to in situ carcinoma, and ultimately to invasive and metastatic tumor (Fig. 16.1). It was Fearon and Vogelstein who in 1990 proposed specific events that are essential to the development of CRC [12]. These events involved the accumulation of mutations of multiple genes that are involved with cell growth and differentiation [13].

Dietary Fat

Dietary fat and more specifically animal fat have been linked to a higher incidence of CRC [11, 14, 15]. The so-called western diet rich in animal fat has been incriminated due to a higher incidence of CRC in the western world. However, this concept has been challenged by well-conducted case control studies. An association with the total energy consumption rather than animal fat is thought to be responsible for a higher incidence of CRC [16].

Red Meat

The relationship between red meat consumption and an increased incidence of CRC is well established [17]. The proposed hypothesis is that red meat contains high amounts of heme, which in turn damages the colonic mucosa and stimulates epithelial proliferation. Also involved is the role of heme iron that is associated with the increase concentration of fecal N-nitroso compounds, a known carcinogen [18, 19].

Fruits and Vegetables

Due to their significant source of antioxidants, fruits and vegetables have been described in earlier studies as protective against CRC. However, more recent analyses provide conflicting conclusions on their protective/deleterious effect [20].

Dietary Fibers

Because of the low incidence of CRC in high fiber-consuming societies, it was a popular belief that high consumption of dietary fibers was protective against colon cancer. Burkitt has observed the clear differences in the incidence of CRC between the western world and areas of Africa. He concluded that high residue diet was protective by decreasing the transit time of stools and colon carcinogens. These same carcinogens were diluted by the bulk and size of the stools in a high fiber diet [21].

Some authors have challenged this. Studies have attempted to study the relationship between high consumption of fiber and low incidence of recurrent colorectal adenomas [22–26]. A meta-analysis concluded that there was no evidence to suggest that high dietary fiber will reduce the incidence or recurrence of adenomatous polyps within 2–4 years [27].

This being said, these studies were criticized for their weaknesses; compliance to a high fiber diet was not uniform in some of the patients, the duration of the studies was short, the arbitrary amount of daily fiber consumption designated as being sufficient was lower than the amount normally consumed by the high fiber-consuming societies, and patients had a lifelong exposure to a western diet before being enrolled in the studies. In a subsequent subgroup analysis, it was shown that it was possible to decrease the incidence of adenoma recurrence in the highly motivated and compliant patient, thus confirming the protective role of dietary fibers [28].

Insulin Resistance and Obesity

Obesity is linked to insulin resistance, increased levels of insulin, as well as increased activity of insulin-like growth factor type I (IGF-I). This hormone, in turn, is thought to be responsible for increasing cell proliferation, which can lead to an increased risk of developing colon cancer [29]. Weight gain in an adult is associated with an increase in colon cancer risk, thus stressing the importance of weight management as a measure for colon cancer prevention [30].

Folate and Alcohol

Folate is a vitamin commonly found in leafy vegetables, legumes, and some fruits. It plays a role in DNA methylation. A deficiency in folate may interfere with DNA repair and could be associated with certain cancers including CRC. Paradoxically, antifolate chemotherapy agents such as methotrexate and fluorouracil play an essential role in reducing the proliferation of neoplastic cell by inhibiting DNA synthesis. Supplementary folate could have either a beneficial or detrimental effect on CRC development, depending on the timing of the intake.

Recent data suggest that folic acid has a protective role in preventing CRC before its establishment. However, excess intake of folate will increase tumor genesis by providing nucleotide precursors to the multiplying neoplastic cells [31–33].

Alcohol has a role in decreasing the availability of folate in the body by altering its absorption. The consumption of alcohol has an association with CRC and seems to be related to the amount consumed. Compared to nondrinkers, moderate drinkers and heavy drinkers have a 21 % and 52 % increased risk of developing CRC, respectively [34].

Smoking

The link between smoking and adenoma formation as well as the increased incidence of CRC has been demonstrated and seems to be dose dependent [35]. The carcinogens include aromatic amines and nitrosamines, compounds that cause gene mutation by forming aberrant DNA [36].

Bile Acids and Cholecystectomy

High fecal bile acid, mainly deoxycholic acid and lithocholic acid, appears to have a role in the increased incidence of CRC. Similarly, a cholecystectomy increases the quantities of fecal bile acid, resulting in an increase incidence of proximal colonic carcinoma [37].

Inflammatory Bowel Diseases

Crohn's disease and ulcerative colitis (UC) are well-established risk factors for developing CRC. It seems that the duration of the disease, the extent of the colitis, and the severity of the inflammation are related to that increased risk. The age of onset of affected individuals at the time of diagnosis is generally 10–15 years younger than those with sporadic CRC [38].

Family History and Genetic Predisposition

There is a significant risk of developing CRC in individuals with a family history of CRC with a hazard ratio of 2.25 if a patient has a first-degree relative with CRC [39–41]. It is believed that the increased risk is attributed to genetic inheritance and/or exposures to similar environmental factors.

Inheritance of known susceptibility genes such as the APC gene, p53 gene, or the mismatch repair gene also predisposes an individual to developing CRC. Further discussion of the genetics associated with CRC is addressed in Chap. 20, ***Hereditary Colorectal Cancer and Polyposis Syndromes***. It is important to stress that the majority of CRC associated with a family history have no known susceptibility genes.

Screening for Asymptomatic Colon Cancer

The goal of screening is early detection of a surgically resectable and curable cancer in an asymptomatic individual. Multiple tests are available to achieve that goal. For average-risk patients, screening should begin at age 50, whereas high-risk individuals should begin screening at age 40 or ten years prior to the diagnosis of the youngest affected family member.

The digital rectal examination (DRE) should be part of any routine examination in patients over 40 years of age, along with a fecal occult blood testing (FOBT) or a fecal immunochemical testing (FIT). The FOBT is an easy and inexpensive method to identify rectal masses and detect occult fecal blood. It is a proven method of decreasing the mortality from CRC. However, the test has inherent flaws, with approximately 50 % of patients with proven CRC having a negative result, while less than 10 % of test-positive patients will be found to have a CRC. Like all tests, FOBT has to be performed correctly by well-trained healthcare providers to optimize its value. Simply performing an office DRE with a fecal occult blood test or immunochemical testing is inadequate. The correct method is to collect three different stool samples at home. A special diet is recommended and should be free of any type of meat and high in fiber to stimulate bleeding and avoid false negatives. This test should be performed yearly as a screening method.

Colonoscopy is the only test that visualizes the entire colon and should be done every 10 years (Fig. 16.2). It is diagnostic because it can identify small polypoid lesions that would otherwise be missed by other screening modalities. Additionally, it is therapeutic because it can remove existing polyps. In addition to colonoscopy, FOBT should be performed yearly. Flexible sigmoidoscopy every 5 years is another test that

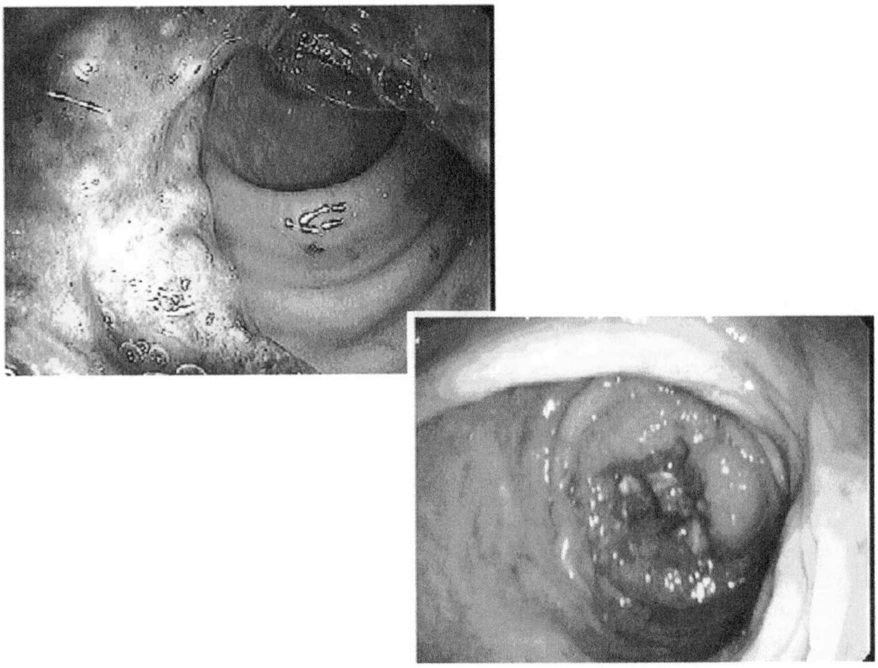

Fig. 16.2 Endoscopic view of colonic cancer (Courtesy of Michael Polcino, MD)

can be used for screening. Double contrast barium enema every 5 years and, more recently, virtual CT colonoscopy every 5 years are offered as alternatives.

CT colonography (CTC) is also a screening option for average-risk individuals and has been endorsed by the American College of Radiology, the United States Multi-Society Task Force on Colorectal Cancer, and the American Cancer Society [8]. CTC has a staging accuracy of 81 %, with a sensitivity of 93 % and a specificity of 97 % for detecting polyps <1 cm. For polyps <1 cm, both sensitivity and specificity fall to 86 % and 86 %, respectively [42, 43]. The advantages with CT colonography include low risk of complications, minimal invasiveness, and high patient tolerance [44]. Although radiation exposure is a concern, the use of newer techniques has decreased the amount of radiation to a level that is close to background level. CT colonography does require colonic cleansing on the day prior to examination, and the patient is also instructed not to eat solids or dairy products a day prior to examination.

Fecal DNA testing is considered an evolving topic. Currently, it is not commercially available in the United States. The FDA molecular and clinical genetics panel of the medical devices advisory committee determined that Cologuard®, the first of its kind stool-based DNA screening test for CRC, has demonstrated safety, effectiveness, and a favorable risk benefit profile. This was based on a recent study that reported a sensitivity for detecting CRC of 92.3 % with DNA testing compared to 73.8 % with FIT ($P=0.002$). The sensitivity for detecting advanced precancerous lesions (adenomas or large sessile serrated polyps) was 42.4 % with DNA testing and 23.8 % with FIT ($P<0.001$) [45]. A positive test should be followed by a direct visualization of the colon by a colonoscopy.

Two categories of patients should be screened according to the American Cancer Society guidelines based on their risk factors (Table 16.1). The screening should begin by determining the individual's level of risk, which could either be average risk or increased risk.

Table 16.1 Screening recommendations for colorectal cancer

Average risk (age > 50 years, without risk factors)
Annual fecal occult blood test (FOBT) or † §
Annual fecal immunochemical test (FIT) or † §
Flexible sigmoidoscopy every 5 years or
Colonoscopy every 10 years or
Double contrast barium enema every 5 years or
CT colonography every 5 years
†Proceed with colonoscopy if test is positive
§Take-home multiple sample should be used
Increased risk
Personal history of polyps removed
Small rectal hyperplastic polyps: treat like average-risk individuals
1–2 small tubular adenomas with low-grade dysplasia: colonoscopy 5–10 years after initial polypectomy
3–10 adenomas or 1 adenoma > 1 cm or any adenoma with villous features or high-grade dysplasia: colonoscopy 3 years after initial polypectomy
>10 adenomas on a single exam: colonoscopy < 3 years after initial polypectomy
Sessile adenomas that are removed piecemeal: colonoscopy 2 to 6 months to confirm complete excision
Personal history of CRC (had curative resection)
Colonoscopy one-year anniversary after initial colon resection; if normal, then
Repeat colonoscopy in 3 years; if normal, then
Repeat colonoscopy in 5 years
Following curative rectal cancer resection
Periodic examination every 3–6 months for the first 2 to 3 years
Family history
First-degree relative (parent, sibling, or child) with CRC or adenomas diagnosed at age ≤60 years or two first-degree relatives at any age
Colonoscopy every 5 years, beginning at age 40 years or 10 years before the age of the youngest affected relative (whichever comes first)
First-degree relative with CRC or adenoma diagnosed at age >60 years, or two second-degree relatives with CRC
Same options as average risk but begin at age 40 years
High risk
Inflammatory bowel disease
Annual or every 2-year screening colonoscopy with biopsies for dysplasia. Significant risk of cancer begins 8 years after onset of pancolitis or 12 to 15 years after onset of left-sided colitis
FAP or suspected to have FAP
Annual screening sigmoidoscopy, beginning at age 10–12 years or refer for genetic testing
HNPCC or suspected to have HNPCC
Colonoscopy every 1–2 years, beginning at age 20–25 years; or 10 years younger than youngest age of CRC diagnosis in family, or refer for genetic testing

Adapted from Levin et al. [8]. With permission from Elsevier

For the average-risk patient, screening should start at age 50; the patient should be offered to choose from each screening method after explaining the advantages and disadvantages of each. The high-risk patient includes those with a personal history of adenomatous colon polyp or colon cancer, a family history of colon cancer, or a personal history of inflammatory bowel disease. A known family history of familial adenomatous polyposis (FAP) or hereditary nonpolyposis colon cancer (HNPCC) also puts the patient at an increased risk of developing CRC. These patients should be offered a screening colonoscopy at a younger age or at more frequent intervals.

An individual with a first-degree relative diagnosed with a CRC before age 60 should undergo a screening colonoscopy at age 40 or 10 years earlier than the affected family member, whichever comes first. A colonoscopy should then be offered every 5 years if no polyps are found.

An individual with proven FAP or at risk of FAP should have an annual sigmoidoscopy beginning at age 10–12. Genetic testing should be considered in these individuals. An individual with a genetic or clinical diagnosis of HNPCC should have a colonoscopy every 1–2 years starting at age 20–25 or 10 years earlier than the youngest age of colon cancer diagnosed in the family.

An individual with inflammatory bowel disease should have a surveillance colonoscopy with systematic random biopsies to rule out dysplasia. This should start 8–10 years after the onset of disease and be performed every 1–2 years.

The surveillance of individuals with a personal history of small hyperplastic polyps should be managed the same as those at average risk. However, those with hyperplastic polyposis syndrome are at an increased risk of developing adenomatous polyps and cancer and should therefore have more intensive follow-up according to the findings of the colonoscopy [46].

Presentation

Most CRC diagnosed are asymptomatic and are detected during a screening examination; moreover the majority of patients who develop CRC have no identifiable risk factor. For those who have symptoms, the location of the cancer usually dictates the symptoms. The most common presenting symptom is abdominal pain, and this can occur regardless of the location of the cancer or whether or not the tumor is obstructive. Change in bowel habits ranks second as the common complaint and varies from being a subtle change to a significant change. Change in frequency, shape, and consistency, usually presenting thinner or looser stools than usual, could be the alerting signs for CRC, especially if these symptoms persist. The location of the tumor can influence the timing of when these symptoms appear; compared to left-sided tumors, right-sided tumors tend to present with symptoms at a later time due to its larger colonic lumen, which can accommodate a larger tumor (Fig. 16.3).

Rectal bleeding could either be dark or bright red, depending on the location of the cancer, with bright red blood being associated with distal cancers. Very often this is a neglected symptom, and its presence should not be taken lightly. Patients with this complaint should be investigated, at the very least, with an endoscopy, even if they are young, to avoid a disastrous outcome stemming from the wrong assumption that such bleeding was due to symptomatic hemorrhoids. Hemorrhoids, if found, should be appropriately treated to avoid them from being blamed for persistent bleeding that may be attributed to cancer. Unexplained weight loss could be associated with advanced CRC, and when present, it usually portends a poor prognosis. Iron deficiency anemia is often due to a digestive disease and therefore deserves an investigation to avoid the risk of missing a malignancy [47].

In up to 15 % of the cases, a colon or rectal cancer will present as an obstructed or perforated cancer with septicemia, the latter of which can be difficult to distinguish from a perforated diverticulitis, thus making the management that much difficult [48].

Evaluation and Staging

When possible, every patient with a presumed or proven CRC diagnosis should undergo a full colonoscopy before initiation of treatment. Although the majority of patients will be diagnosed with a CRC after a full colonoscopy, some will be referred to a surgeon after an alternative method was performed (i.e., rigid sigmoidoscope). A tissue diagnosis must be obtained and synchronous carcinoma should be excluded, as the risk of synchronous carcinoma can be as high as 10 % in the general population [49–51]. In addition, synchronous benign polyps can occur in 13–62 % of cases [49–51], and when identified, they should be removed. In the event that a colonoscopy cannot be completed due to technical problems, a barium

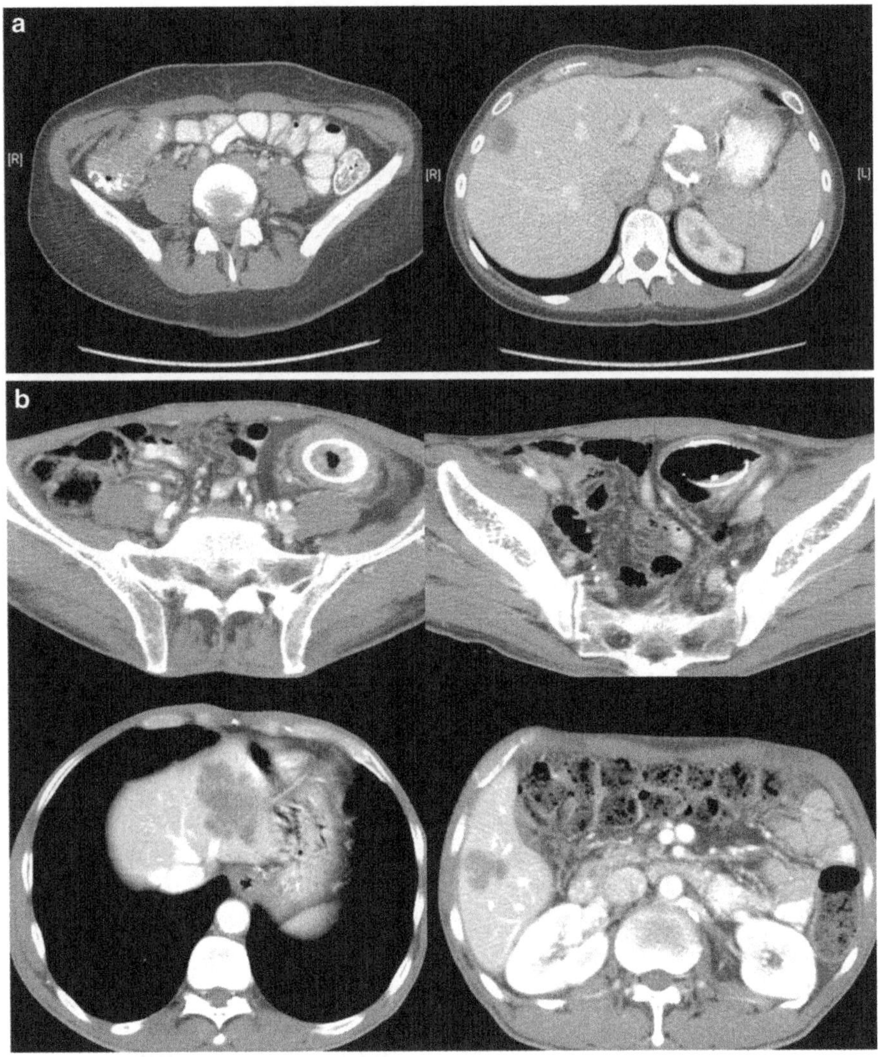

Fig. 16.3 (**a**) CT of a patient with a large cecal mass and metastasis to the liver. (**b**) CT of a patient with synchronous sigmoid mass and bilateral liver metastases. This patient had a colonic stent and underwent chemotherapy. He subsequently underwent a staged operation that included a sigmoidectomy, a left lateral segmentectomy and a right segmentectomy, rendering him disease free (A: Courtesy of Michael Polcino, MD) (B: Courtesy of Quyen D. Chu, MD, MBA, FACS)

enema or a CT colonography and a rigid or flexible sigmoidoscopy should be performed.

Preoperative radiological staging is routinely performed. A CT of the chest abdomen and pelvis will help detect synchronous metastasis (Fig. 16.3); alternatively a PET CT of MRI could be obtained if an allergy to iodine is a concern.

A complete blood count and a carcinoembryonic (CEA) antigen level should be obtained. The latter test establishes a baseline value for which it can be used to compare to subsequent CEA levels during the surveillance phase to detect for possible recurrence.

Colon cancer is staged using the 7th edition of American Joint Committee on Cancer (AJCC)/TNM Staging system (Table 16.2) [53]. While distant disease can be detected prior to treatment, tumor depth (T-stage) and nodal involvement (N-stage) will only be known after surgical resection. The completeness of resection should be

Table 16.2 American Joint Committee on Cancer (AJCC) TNM staging for colorectal carcinoma (7th edition)

Primary tumor (T)*	
TX	Primary tumor cannot be assessed
T0	No evidence of primary tumor
Tis	Carcinoma in situ: intraepithelial or invasion of lamina propria*
T1	Tumor invades submucosa
T2	Tumor invades muscularis propria
T3	Tumor invades through muscularis propria into pericolorectal tissues
T4a	Tumor penetrates to the surface of the visceral peritoneum**
T4b	Tumor directly invades or is adherent to other organs or structures**, ***

*_Note_: Tis includes cancer cells confined within the glandular basement membrane (intraepithelial) or mucosal lamina propria (intramucosal) with no extension through the muscularis mucosae into the submucosa

**_Note_: Direct invasion in T4 includes invasion of other organs or other segments of the colorectum as a result of direct extension through the serosa, as confirmed on microscopic examination (e.g., invasion of the sigmoid colon by a carcinoma of the cecum) or, for cancers in a retroperitoneal or subperitoneal location, direct invasion of other organs or structures by virtue of extension beyond the muscularis propria (i.e., respectively, a tumor on the posterior wall of the descending colon invading the left kidney or lateral abdominal wall, or a mid- or distal rectal cancer with invasion of prostate, seminal vesicles, cervix, or vagina)

***_Note_: Tumor that is adherent to other organs or structures, grossly, is classified cT4b. However, if no tumor is present in the adhesion, microscopically, the classification should be pT1-4a depending on the anatomical depth of wall invasion. The V and L classifications should be used to identify the presence or absence of vascular or lymphatic invasion, whereas the PN site-specific factor should be used for perineural invasion

Regional lymph nodes (N)	
NX	Regional lymph nodes cannot be assessed
N0	No regional lymph node metastasis
N1	Metastasis in 1–3 regional lymph nodes
N1a	Metastasis in 1 regional lymph node
N1b	Metastasis in 2–3 regional lymph nodes
N1c	Tumor deposit(s) in the subserosa, mesentery, or non-peritonealized pericolic or perirectal tissues without regional nodal metastasis
N2	Metastasis in ≥4 regional lymph nodes
N2a	Metastasis in 4–6 regional lymph nodes
N2b	Metastasis in ≥7 regional lymph nodes

(continued)

Table 16.2 (continued)

Regional lymph nodes (N)

Note: A satellite peritumoral nodule in the pericolorectal adipose tissue of a primary carcinoma without histologic evidence of residual lymph node in the nodule may represent discontinuous spread, venous invasion with extravascular spread (V 1/2), or a totally replaced lymph node (N1/2). Replaced nodes should be counted separately as positive nodes in the N category, whereas discontinuous spread or venous invasion should be classified and counted in the site-specific factor category tumor deposits (TD)

Distant metastasis (M)	
M0	No distant metastasis
M1	Distant metastasis
M1a	Metastasis confined to one organ or site (e.g., liver, lung, ovary, nonregional node)
M1b	Metastases > one organ/site or the peritoneum

Anatomic stage/prognostic groups

Stage	T	N	M	Dukes*	MAC*
0	Tis	N0	M0	–	–
I	T1	N0	M0	A	A
	T2	N0	M0	A	B1
IIA	T3	N0	M0	B	B2
IIB	T4a	N0	M0	B	B2
IIC	T4b	N0	M0	B	B3
IIIA	T1-2	N1/N1c	M0	C	C1
	T1	N2a	M0	C	C1
IIIB	T3-T4a	N1/N1c	M0	C	C2
	T2-T3	N2a	M0	C	C1/C2
	T1-T2	N2b	M0	C	C1
IIIC	T4a	N2a	M0	C	C2
	T3-T4a	N2b	M0	C	C2
	T4b	N1-N2	M0	C	C3
IVA	Any T	Any N	M1a	–	–
IVB	Any T	Any N	M1b	–	–

Note: cTNM is the clinical classification, and pTNM is the pathologic classification. The y prefix is used for those cancers that are classified after neoadjuvant pretreatment (e.g., ypTNM). Patients who have a complete pathologic response are ypT0N0cM0 that may be similar to stage group 0 or I. The r prefix is to be used for those cancers that have recurred after a disease-free interval (rTNM)

*Dukes B is a composite of better (T3 N0 M0) and worse (T4 N0 M0) prognostic groups, as is Dukes C (any TN1 M0 and any T N2 M0). MAC is the modified Astler-Coller classification

Adapted from Compton et al. [52]. With permission from Springer Verlag noted and designated by letter R where R0 represents a complete tumor resection, R1 represents an incomplete tumor resection because of involved microscopic surgical margin, and R2 represents an incomplete resection that leaves behind gross residual tumor. Histologic grade should also be noted as it plays a role in the prognosis and treatment consideration [54].

Surgical Management

Surgical resection is the definitive treatment for colon cancer. The depth of bowel wall invasion and lymph node status are the two most important prognostic indicators. A definitive, oncologic resection for colon cancer should include a bowel resection which may require an en bloc resection of adherent structures and removal of the blood supply and lymphatics at the origin of the primary feeding vessel. For colon cancer surgery, 5 cm is an adequate proximal and distal margin so as to decrease the rate of anastomotic recurrence. This distance also allows for adequate nodal clearance. The 2000 National Cancer Institute guidelines for the surgical management of colon cancer recommend that a minimum of 12 lymph nodes should be examined [55]. Additionally, there is improved accuracy in the final pathologic state when there are more lymph nodes examined [56]. Tumor spillage should also be avoided to reduce risk of seeding the cancer into the peritoneum.

The surgeon should be cognizant of the status of the circumferential radial margin (CRM) (Fig. 16.4). CRM pertains to the non-peritonealized (part of the colon that is attached to the retroperitoneum) portion of the colon, and CRM is essentially the retroperitoneal margin. The non-peritonealized colon includes the cecum, ascending colon, descending colon, and upper rectum, areas that are fixed to the retroperitoneum and therefore are "immobile." The fixed portion of the colon limits the surgeon's ability to achieve a wider surgical margin. It is conceivable to appreciate how a bulky, posteriorly located cecal tumor is more likely to have a positive CRM than the same tumor whose bulk is located more anteriorly on the surface of the cecum.

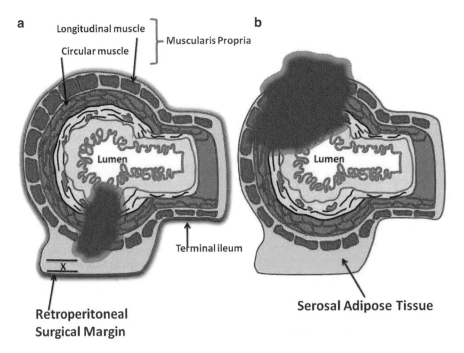

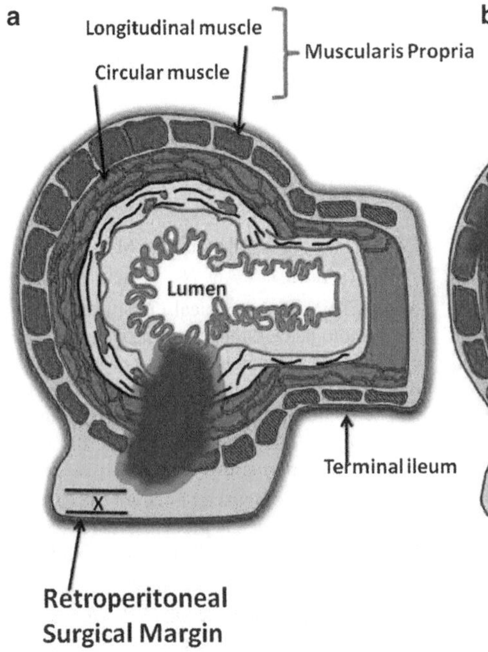

Fig. 16.4 *Circumferential radial margin (CRM) in colon cancer*: The example is a cecal cancer. Note that a tumor that invades posteriorly into the retroperitoneal space runs the risk of having a positive CRM (panel A), whereas an anteriorly located tumor that penetrates into the serosa is not considered to have a positive CRM (panel B) (Redrawn by Quyen D. Chu based on data from Ref. [57])

In contrast, mid-transverse colon and mid-sigmoid colon are mobile and are not likely to result in a positive CRM following resection.

A positive CRM is defined as tumor that is ≤1 mm from the non-peritoneal (i.e., retroperitoneal) surface of the specimen [58]. Although CRM for colon cancer may not be as well recognized as its rectal cancer counterpart, it nevertheless is important because it has prognostic significance. Patients with positive CRM are at risk of developing local recurrence [57, 59, 60]. Note that when the tumor encroaches on the serosal (peritoneal) surface but is not adherent to adjacent structures, it is not considered as having a positive surgical margin. This is an important distinction to make because a T3N0 tumor without CRM involvement does not normally require further treatment following resection, whereas the same tumor with a positive CRM may be treated with adjuvant therapy.

Because there is no anatomic landmark to differentiate the peritonealized and non-peritonealized portion of the colon, the surgeon should work closely with the pathologist to help indicate areas of the tumor that were in close contact with other organs and/or abdominal wall and specify the retroperitoneal margin. Full-thickness tumor with serosal involvement of the peritonealized colon could easily be confused as having a positive CRM when in reality, it represents a T3 lesion. Therefore it is imperative that the surgeon clarifies this subtle difference with the pathologist so as to ensure accurate recording on the final pathology report.

For colon cancer, both the open and minimally invasive techniques have been well described and studied. The discussion of the landmark studies comparing these techniques is done towards the end of this chapter. However, several technical considerations that are common to both surgical approaches shall be highlighted. Of note, safe colorectal oncologic surgery includes the clearance of lateral margins, resection of lymph node-bearing mesentery, and creation of a well-vascularized and tension-free anastomosis.

For a right colectomy, multiple approaches have been described with the two most common being the lateral-medial and the medial-lateral approach (Fig. 16.5). The important surgical tenets for an oncologic right colectomy are elevating the mesentery off of the retroperitoneum

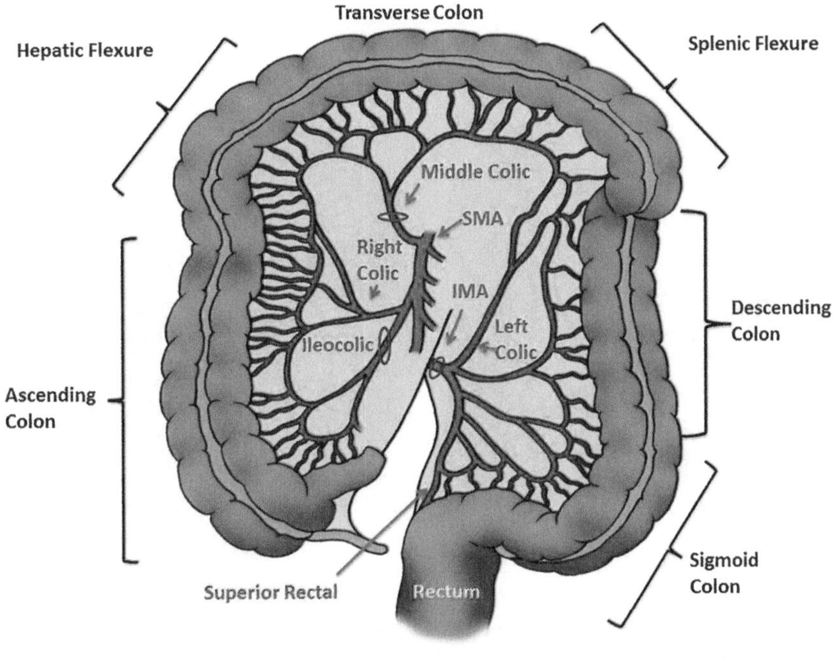

Fig. 16.5 *Anatomy of the colon, its blood supply, and type of operation (A–D).* Note that for cancer involving the cecum, ascending colon, hepatic flexure, and proximal transverse colon (Fig. 16.5B-2), the ileocolic artery, right colic artery, and the right branch of the middle colic artery are ligated. If the middle colic artery is ligated at its origin (Fig. 16.5B-3), then

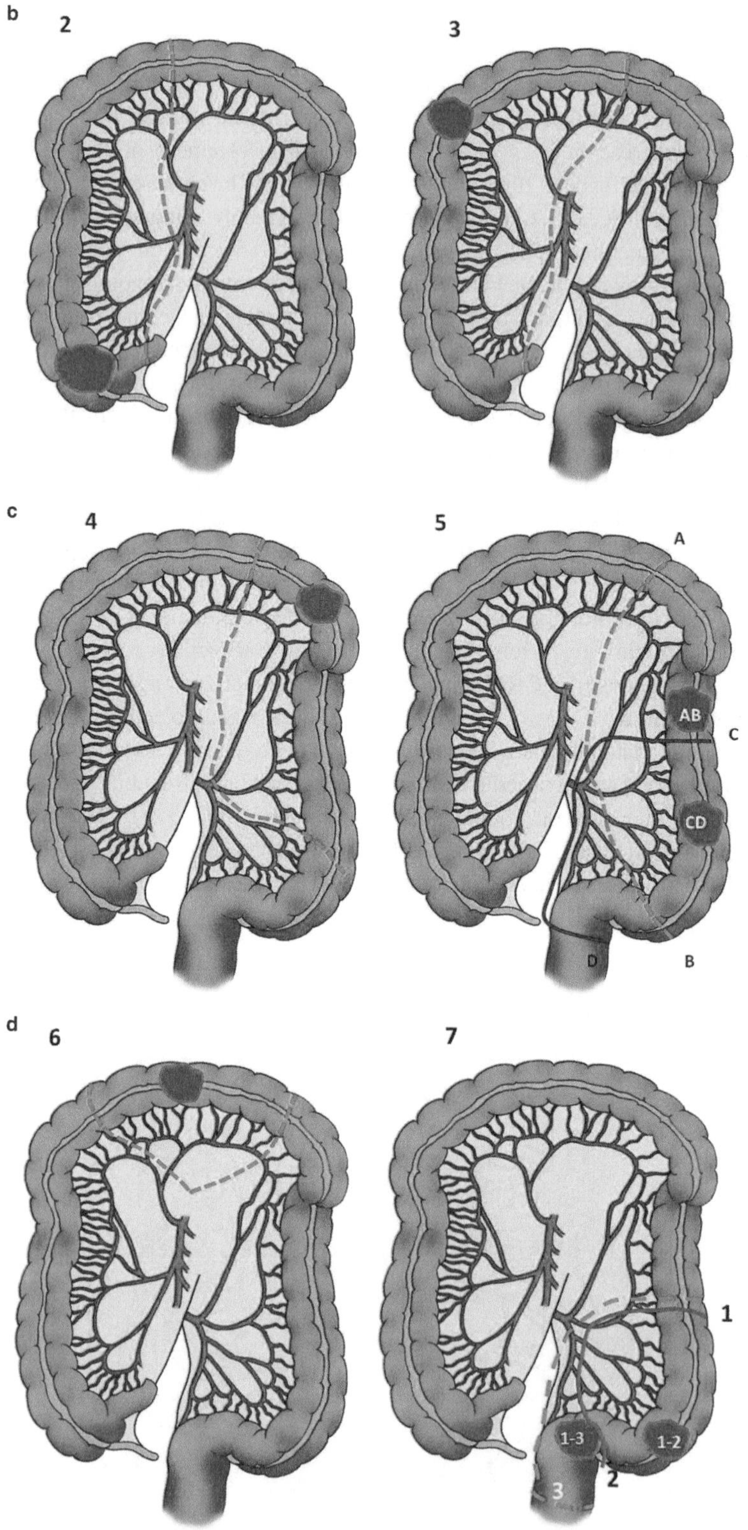

Fig. 16.5 (continued) the distal bowel should be transected just to the distal third of the transverse colon to avoid bowel ischemia. Tumors in the splenic flexure (Fig. 16.5C-4) or descending colon (Fig. 16.5C-5) can be resected by taking the left colic artery without having to ligate the IMA at its origin. Alternatively, if the IMA is ligated at its origin, a sigmoidectomy will be required to ensure bowel viability. Tumors in the transverse colon can be approached with a segmental resection (Fig. 16.5D-6) or an extended right hemicolectomy (Fig. 16.5B-3) (Courtesy of Quyen D. Chu, MD, MBA, FACS)

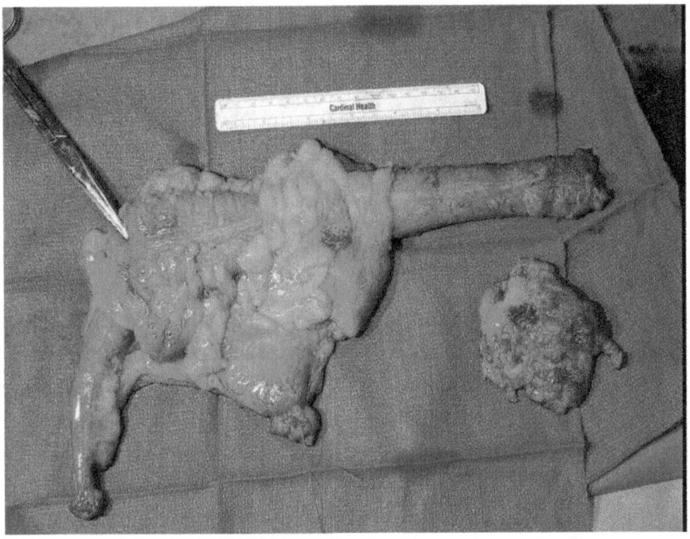

Fig. 16.6 A right colectomy with ligation of its blood supply (Courtesy of Michael Polcino, MD)

and duodenum, identifying and incising the lateral attachments, mobilizing the hepatic flexure, and taking care of not injuring the right ureter. The ileocolic artery, right colic artery, and right branch of the middle colic artery should be ligated at the origin in order to gain an optimal lymph node resection (Fig. 16.6). In the case of proximal transverse colon malignancies, an extended right hemicolectomy should be performed (Fig. 16.5). In the procedure, the entire middle colic artery is ligated at the origin. A well-vascularized and tension-free anastomosis between the ileum and transverse colon should then be created.

For left colectomies, there are similar surgical principles as compared to the right colectomy (Fig. 16.5). The lateral attachments are incised, the mesentery is dissected free from the retroperitoneum, the left ureter is clearly identified, and the splenic flexure is mobilized. The mesentery is ligated at the origin of the main feeding vessel, either at the origin of the IMA or just distal to it at the left colic artery. The main feeding vessel ligated is contingent upon the exact location of the malignancy within the left colon. As mentioned previously, both the medial-lateral and the lateral-medial approach have been described. The medial-lateral approach begins with the identification of both the IMA and IMV. For a true splenic flexure lesion, the left colic artery can be ligated at its origin, thus preserving the remainder of IMA and its branches (Fig. 16.5). The splenic flexure can be approached from posterior as the mesentery is dissected free from the anterior surface of pancreas and Gerota's fascia. Alternatively, the left colon can be dissected in the lateral to medial approach where the white line of Toldt is incised and the dissection is continued proximally until the left colon is completely free from the spleen and retroperitoneal attachments. The IMV is ligated as it enters below the inferior border of the pancreas in order to allow the mobilized proximal bowel to reach the pelvis. The origin of the IMA is ligated, which necessitates a sigmoidectomy to avoid anastomotic dehiscence from an ischemic sigmoid. Both approaches can be utilized as long as the vascular pedicle is ligated at the origin so as to ensure an adequate lymph node harvest.

In the past, it was thought that adhering to the "no touch isolation technique" by early ligation of the regional mesenteric vessels prior to mobilizing the primary tumor would reduce the occurrence of systemic disease. It was believed that such a technique would prevent cancer dissemination into the venous and lymphatic pathways. Unfortunately, this theory has been disproven. A randomized clinical trial of 237 colon cancer patients demonstrated no benefit with this technique [61]. Similarly, a study of over 1800 patients showed that early ligation of regional mesenteric vessels had no impact on the 5- and 10-year disease-free survival (DFS) as compared to late ligation after the tumor was mobilized [62].

Laparoscopic Versus Open Colectomy

Laparoscopic colon surgery has been practiced for the past 15–20 years. Over these past decades, at least 3 major randomized clinical trials and several systemic reviews and meta-analysis have demonstrated the oncologic equivalency of laparoscopic colectomy (LC) with open colectomy (OC) [63–66] (Table 16.3). The COST study (Clinical Outcomes of Surgical Therapy Study Group) was the first landmark study that demonstrated oncologic equivalency between LC and OC [63]. COST was a multicenter, prospective study that randomized 872 patients into two groups, LC and OC. The study demonstrated that not only was overall survival (OS) equivalent in both groups but also that there was no significant difference in cancer recurrence between them. At a median follow-up of 4.4 years, the 3-year OS rate was 86 % in the LC group versus 85 % in the OC group ($P=0.51$), and the recurrence rate was 16 % in the LC group versus 18 % in the OC group ($P=0.32$). Of note, the LC group had a shorter median hospital stay of one day (5 days vs. 6 days; $P<0.001$) and briefer use of parenteral narcotics (3 days vs. 4 days; $P<0.001$) and oral analgesics (1 day vs. 2 days; $P=0.02$) compared to the OC group.

Since the time of the COST study, there have been additional confirmatory trials. The CLASICC (Medical Research Council Conventional versus Laparoscopic-Assisted Surgery in Colorectal Cancer) [64] and the COLOR (Colon Cancer Laparoscopic or Open Resection) Study Group are the two additional prospective randomized studies that produced similar results as the COST study [64, 66].

The CLASICC trial randomized 794 patients with both colon and rectal cancer to either LC or OC. There was no significant difference in the DFS or OS between the two groups. The 3-year DFS was 66.3 % for the LC versus 67.7 % for the OC group ($P=0.70$), and the 3-year OS was 68.4 % for the LC group versus 66.7 % for the OC group ($P=0.55$) [64]. In their long-term follow-up of more than 10 years, they reported the durability of their initial findings. The DFS was 77 months for the LC group versus 89.5 months for the OC group, and the OS was 82.7 months for the LC group versus 78.3 months for the OC group ($P=0.78$) [65]. There were no differences in distant recurrences between OC and LC groups; the 10-year rates were 19.8 % and 22.7 %, respectively ($P=0.588$). Finally, the incidence of wound/port-site recurrences was also not significantly different.

The COLOR trial randomized 1248 patients to either LC or OC. At a median follow-up of 53 months, there was no significant difference in DFS or OS between the two groups. The 3-year DFS for the LC and OC was 74.2 % and 76.2 %, respectively ($P=0.70$), and the 3-year OS for the LC and OC was 81.8 % and 84.2 %, respectively ($P=0.45$). There were no significant differences in the morbidity and mortality rates, positive resection margin rate, local recurrence rate, or distant recurrence rate between LC and OC [66].

Robotic surgery has recently emerged as an alternative minimally invasive technique to laparoscopic colon surgery. The benefit of robotic colon cancer surgery as compared to laparoscopic surgery is currently being evaluated. Specific attention is currently being directed towards intracorporeal anastomoses for right colon cancer surgery [68].

In summary, laparoscopic colectomy yielded similar oncologic outcomes as open colectomy; OS, DFS, local recurrence rate (i.e., port-site recurrence), distant recurrence rate, and long-term quality of life were not significantly different between the LC group and the OC group [65]. Unlike laparoscopic proctectomy for rectal cancer (please see Chap. 18, *Rectal Cancer*), laparoscopic colectomy has been accepted by the healthcare community as a viable option for patients with colon cancer.

Table 16.3 Laparoscopic colon cancer trials

Trial, years	N	Median follow-up (mos)	Median # LNs harvested	DFS	OS	Comments
COST [63], 2004	872	52.8	LC: 12 OC: 12	LC: 16 %[a] OC: 18 % (P=0.32)	LC: 86 %[a] OC: 85 % (P=0.51)	OR time was longer in LC group (150 min vs. 95 min; P<0.001) LC had shorter hospital stay by 1 day, briefer use of narcotics by 1 day Complications were not significantly different between both groups
CLASICC[b] [64], [67] Jayne, 2007, 2013	794[c]	62.9	N/A	LC: 77 mos[d] OC: 89.5 mos (P=0.589)	LC: 82.7 mos[d] OC: 78.3 mos (P=0.78)	No significant differences in Local recurrence rate Distant recurrence rate Wound/port-site recurrences
COLOR [66], Buunen, 2009	1248	53	LC: 10 OP: 10 (P=0.32)	LC: 74.2 %[a] OC: 76.2 % (P=0.70)	LC: 81.8 %[a] OC: 84.2 % (P=0.45)	No significant differences in Morbidity and mortality Positive resection margin rate Local recurrence rate Distant recurrence rate

COST Clinical Outcomes of Surgical Therapy Study Group, *CLASICC* Medical Research Council Conventional versus Laparoscopic-Assisted Surgery in Colorectal Cancer, *COLOR* Colon Cancer Laparoscopic or Open Resection

[a]3-year results

[b]Results are based on latest 10-year follow-up

[c]Included rectal cancer patients (N=381)

[d]Reported as median survival, *N/A* not available, *LC* laparoscopic colectomy, *OC* open colectomy, *OR* operating time

Systemic Therapy: Overview

Stage I colon cancer has an excellent prognosis with a 95 % 5-year survival after resection and therefore does not require adjuvant systemic therapy. Stage II disease also has a favorable prognosis with a 5-year survival rate in the range of 70–80 % after surgical resection. The role of adjuvant systemic therapy is controversial. Stage III disease, on the other hand, has a 40–60 % survival after curative resection. Adjuvant systemic chemotherapy for stage III colon cancer is standard of care. Adjuvant therapy for stage II colon cancer is controversial and will be discussed after the discussion of adjuvant therapy for stage III colon cancer, which is well established.

Adjuvant Therapy for Stage 3 Colon Cancer

The 5-year survival for patients with resected stage 3 colon cancer (positive lymph nodes, irrespective of T-status) is in the range of 75 %. Adjuvant systemic therapy significantly improves this rate to nearly 79 %. In 1990, the Intergroup Trial INT-0035 was the first to report a significant reduction (33 %) in the risk of death with one year of adjuvant 5-FU and levamisole in patients with stage 3 colon cancer [69]. These findings were later confirmed in 1995 [70, 71]. Subsequently, one year of levamisole was replaced with 6 months of leucovorin such that up until 2004, the current standard of care for patients with stage 3 colon cancer was 6 months of 5-FU and leucovorin (5-FU/LV) [72–74]. More recent data established the efficacy of adding oxaliplatin to the fluoropyrimidine-based chemotherapy [75–77] (Table 16.4).

MOSAIC Trial

Over the past decades, multiple newer cytotoxic (irinotecan, oxaliplatin) and targeted therapies (bevacizumab, cetuximab, panitumumab) were successfully combined with 5-FU-based therapy in stage IV colon cancer patients. Naturally, clinicians began testing them in combination with 5-FU-based therapy in the adjuvant setting. Unfortunately, only oxaliplatin, when combined with 5-FU/LV, had any efficacy, and such impact was mainly observed in stage III patients. These findings were reported from two major trials, the MOSAIC (Multicenter International Study of Oxaliplatin/5-Fluorouracil/Leucovorin in the Adjuvant Treatment of Colon Cancer) [75, 76] and the NSABP (National Surgical Adjuvant Breast and Bowel Project) C-07 trials [77, 78].

The MOSAIC investigators were the first to report the efficacy of adding oxaliplatin to ***infusional*** 5-FU/LV regimen in 2004 (Table 16.4). This phase III clinical trial randomized 2,246 patients who had surgically resected stage II ($N=899$) or III ($N=1{,}347$) colon cancer to either traditional 5-FU/LV regimen or ***infusional*** 5-FU/LV plus oxaliplatin (FOLFOX4). The initial study reported a 3-year DFS improvement with FOLFOX4 compared to 5-FU/LV (FOLFOX4 = 78.2 %; 5-FU/LV = 72.9 %; $P=0.002$) [75]. Overall survival was too immature at that time to be reported. In the longer follow-up report with a median follow-up time of 81.9 months, while the DFS benefit remains durable (5-year DFS rates were 73.3 % and 67.4 % in the FOLFOX4 and 5-FU/LV groups, respectively; $P=0.003$), there was an absolute 6-year overall survival benefit of 2.5 % in the FOLFOX4 group (78.5 % vs. 76.0 %; $P=0.046$) [76]. However, OS benefit was observed in the stage III group but not the stage II group. The 6-year OS rates for patients with stage III were 72.9 % and 68.7 % ($P=0.023$) for the FOLFOX4 and 5-FU/LV groups, respectively, while they were 86.9 % and 86.8 % ($P=0.986$) for FOLFOX4 and 5-FU/LV groups, respectively, for stage II disease. Similarly, oxaliplatin resulted in a significant 5-year DFS, which was seen only in stage III disease; the 5-year DFS for stage II disease was 83.7 % for FOLFOX4 and 79.9 % for 5-FU/LV ($P=0.258$), whereas for stage III disease, it was 66.4 % for FOLFOX4 and 58.9 % for 5-FU/LV ($P=0.005$).

Table 16.4 Clinical trials evaluating the role of adding oxaliplatin to fluoropyrimidine-based chemotherapy

Trials, years, authors	N	Median f/u (mos)	5-year DFS	5-year OS	Comments about adjuvant chemotherapy
MOSAIC André 2004 [75], André 2009 [76]	Stage II: 899 Stage III: 1347 (2246)	81.9	Stage II FOLFOX4: 83.7 % FU/LV: 79.9 % ($P=0.258$) Stage III FOLFOX4: 66.4 % FU/LV: 58.9 % ($P=0.005$)	Stage II[a] FOLFOX4:86.9 % FU/LV: 86.8 % ($P=0.986$) Stage III[a] FOLFOX4: 72.9 % FU/LV: 68.7 % ($P=0.023$)	Oxaliplatin benefits were observed only in stage III colon cancer
NSABP C-07 Kuebler 2007 [77],Yothers 2011 [78]	Stage II: 696 Stage III: 1711 (2492)	96	Stage II FLOX: 82.1 % FU/LV: 80.1 % ($P=0.67$) Stage III FLOX: 64.4 % FU/LV: 57.8 % ($P<0.001$)	Stage II FLOX: 89.7 % FU/LV: 89.6 % ($P=0.84$) Stage III FLOX: 76.5 % FU/LV: 73.8 ($P=0.052$)	Oxaliplatin Did not have significant impact on OS for the entire cohort Significantly improved DFS for stage III but not stage II disease OS was borderline significant for stage III disease and insignificant for stage II disease

MOSAIC Multicenter International Study of Oxaliplatin/5-Fluorouracil/Leucovorin in the Adjuvant Treatment of Colon Cancer, *NSABP* National Surgical Adjuvant Breast and Bowel Project, *5-FU* 5-fluorouracil, *LV* leucovorin, *FOLFOX4* infusional 5-FU/LV + oxaliplatin, *FLOX* bolus 5-FU/LV + oxaliplatin

[a]6-year results

NSABP C-07 Trial

Results of the NSABP C-07 are very similar to MOSAIC's, except that OS was not significantly impacted with the addition of oxaliplatin (Table 16.4). NSABP randomized 2,407 patients with stage II ($N=696$) and stage III (1711) disease to either 6 months of 5-FU/LV or ***bolus*** 5-FU/LV + oxaliplatin (FLOX) (*note that infusional 5-FU/LV + oxaliplatin is referred to as FOLFOX4, whereas bolus form is termed FLOX*). At a median follow-up time of 42.5 months, the DFS was 74 % for the FLOX group and 70 % for the 5-FU/LV group ($P=0.005$) [77]. Similar to MOSAIC, OS was too immature at that time to be meaningful. In their follow-up report with a median follow-up time of 96 months, DFS benefit remains durable but OS was not impacted. The 5-year OS was 80.2 % for those who received FLOX and 78.4 % for those treated with 5-FU/LV ($P=0.08$). Similar to MOSAIC, when 5-year OS was analyzed based on the stage of disease, stage III disease was mostly impacted by the addition of oxaliplatin (76.5 % vs. 73.8 %; $P=0.052$), whereas the 5-year OS was nearly identical in stage II disease (89.7 % vs. 89.6 %; $P=0.84$) [78].

Capecitabine Plus Oxaliplatin (CapeOx)

Capecitabine (Xeloda®; Genentech) is an oral prodrug of 5-FU that is commonly used as an oral alternative to intravenous 5-FU in gastrointestinal cancer. Recent clinical trials demonstrated that capecitabine plus oxaliplatin (CapeOx) yielded better DFS compared to 5-FU-based therapy [79, 80]. Because of this, CapeOx is an option for patients with stage III colon cancer.

The above major trials galvanized the role of oxaliplatin as adjuvant therapy for stage III colon cancer. The addition of oxaliplatin to 5-FU/LV increases OS by an absolute value of 3–5 %. Thus, 6 months of FOLFOX4, FLOX, or single agent CapeOx or 5-FU/LV in patients whom oxaliplatin therapy is inappropriate is now the standard of care for patients with resected stage III colon cancer.

Adjuvant Therapy for Stage 2 Colon Cancer

The 5-year survival for patients with resected stage 2 colon cancer (i.e., no evidence of nodal disease) is in the range of 85–89 %. Whether adjuvant systemic therapy can further improve upon this rate remains an area of intense debate (Table 16.5).

NSABP Pooled Analysis

In 1995, Moertel et al., representing the Intergroup Trial INT-0035, reported the results of

Table 16.5 Selected trials evaluating the role of adjuvant chemotherapy for stage II colon cancer

Trials, years, authors	N	Groups	5-year DFS	5-year OS	Comments about adjuvant chemotherapy
IMPACT B2, 1992 [81], [82][a]	1,016	Stage 2	Observation: 73 % FU/LV: 76 % ($P=0.061$)	Observation: 80 % FU/LV: 82 % ($P=0.057$)	No significant DFS, OS benefit with adjuvant therapy
Gill, 2004 (Intergroup analysis) [83][a]	3,302	Stages 2 and 3	Observation: 72 % 5-FU/LV/LM: 76 % ($P=0.49$)	Observation: 80 % 5-FU/LV/LM: 81 % ($P=0.1127$)	Included stage II/III No significant DFS, OS benefit with adjuvant therapy
Gray, 2007 (QUASAR) [84]	3,239	Stage 2	Relative risk of recurrence = 0.78[b] (95 % CI 0.67–0.91; $P=0.001$)	Relative risk of dying = 0.82[b] (95 % CI 0.70–0.95; $P=0.008$)	Only trial that demonstrated OS benefit with adjuvant chemotherapy for stage II disease

IMPACT International Multicenter Pooled Analysis of B2 Colon Cancer Trials, *QUASAR* Quick and Simple and Reliable, *5-FU* 5-fluorouracil, *LV* leucovorin, *LM* levamisole

[a]Pooled or meta-analysis

[b]Calculated as risk of chemotherapy versus observation

318 eligible stage 2 patients and demonstrated no survival benefit with adjuvant 5-FU-based chemotherapy [85]. In 1999, Mamounas et al., representing the National Surgical Adjuvant Breast and Bowel Project (NSABP) group, performed a pooled analysis of four adjuvant studies (C-01 through C-04) and reported that adjuvant chemotherapy improved outcomes for patients with stage 2 colon cancer [86]. A follow-up study reported by Wilkinson et al. in 2010 included an additional trial, the C-05 trial, confirming the advantage of adjuvant chemotherapy in patients with stage 2 colon cancer [87]. Unfortunately, several criticisms were launched against NSABP pooled analysis; only trials C-01 and C-02 had a true control group (surgery alone), different chemotherapy regimens were used, and non-orthodox statistical methods were utilized [88, 89]. Additionally, some of the trials were dated back to the 1970s, and because the quality of lymph node resection was not standardized in many of these older trials, the possibility of incorrectly classifying stage 3 as stage 2 disease (i.e., stage migration) might have had an impact on the results (Table 16.5).

IMPACT B2 Pooled Analysis

In contrast to the results of NSABP pooled analysis, multiple meta-analyses demonstrated that although DFS was significantly improved with adjuvant chemotherapy, there is no overall survival advantage with it [82, 83, 90, 91]. The International Multicenter Pooled Analysis of B2 Colon Cancer Trials (IMPACT B2) pooled analysis of five different trials on 1,016 patients reported no significant advantage with adjuvant chemotherapy for stage II colon cancer; the non-significant absolute risk reduction for treated patients was 2 % for 5-year OS [81, 82].

Intergroup Analysis

Similarly, Gill et al. performed a pooled individual data analysis from 7 intergroup trials of 3302 patients with stage 2 or 3 colon cancer and reported a nonsignificant OS difference of 1 % between the two groups (80 % in surgery alone vs. 81 % in adjuvant arm; $P=0.113$) [83].

Ontario Cochrane Meta-analysis

Figueredo from Ontario performed a Cochrane meta-analysis of over 35 trials and also reported no statistically significant difference in OS with adjuvant chemotherapy, although there was an improved DFS in patients who received adjuvant chemotherapy [90].

SEER-Medicare Analysis

Finally, O'Connor et al. reported no benefit of adjuvant chemotherapy in patients with stage 2 colon cancer [91]. In their 2011 analysis of 43,032 Medicare beneficiaries with stage 2 or 3 colon cancer, O'Connor et al. found that although adjuvant fluorouracil-based chemotherapy improved outcome in stage 3 disease, the same benefit was not seen for stage 2 disease, irrespective of whether the patients had poor prognostic features [91]. Poor prognostic features include elevated preoperative carcinoembryonic antigen (CEA)>5 ng/mL, need for emergent operation, T4 tumors, lymphovascular invasion, poorly differentiated histology, inadequately sampled nodes, and bowel obstruction and perforation. A criticism of this study is that it is based on Surveillance, Epidemiology, and End Results (SEER)-Medicare database, which is an administrative rather than a clinical database. Patients in such a database come from heterogenous populations with major variations in treatment, comorbidities, and follow-up.

QUASAR Results

The recent QUASAR trial (Quick and Simple and Reliable) is the only phase III trial that demonstrated OS benefit with fluoropyrimidine-based adjuvant chemotherapy for patients with resected stage 2 colon cancer [84]. In this trial,

3,239 patients with stage 2 colon cancer were randomly assigned to either adjuvant 5-FU/leucovorin or observation alone. After a median follow-up of 5.5 years, there was an absolute improvement of 3.6 % in the adjuvant group (95 % CI, 1.0 to 6.0; $P=0.04$).

Unfortunately, QUASAR has several limitations. Of the over 3,239 patients with a presumed diagnosis of stage 2 colon cancer, 8.5 % actually had stage I or 3 disease and 29 % had rectal cancer (many of these patients received radiation therapy). Additionally, the median number of lymph nodes examined was only six, which is far less than the recommended 12, suggesting that there is possible contamination by stage 3 patients, a group of patients whose outcome is positively impacted by adjuvant chemotherapy. There were other quality issues associated with the study such as the lack of uniformity in administering chemotherapy and suboptimal method of recording survival (data derived from national mortality records instead of direct communication with the treating physicians), and only 20 % of the pathology was reviewed [92].

One of the challenges facing adjuvant clinical trial is the recruitment of sufficient number of patients to detect a significant difference, if one exists. As such, many of the adjuvant colon cancer trials included both stage 2 and stage 3 colon cancers for which the majority of patients have stage 3 disease. The INT-0035 had 26 % stage 2 and 74 % stage 3 colon cancers [85], and NSABP pooled analysis contained 42 % stage 2 and 58 % stage 3 cancers [87]. Consequently, results tend to be skewed in favor of adjuvant therapy because of the overwhelming majority of stage 3 disease.

ACCENT Studies

To adequately perform an adjuvant clinical trial for stage 2 colon cancer, it would require an enrollment of an astronomical number of patients. To detect a 4 % survival benefit at 5 years with a baseline 5-year survival prognosis of 75 % that includes a nontreatment control arm would require at least 4,700 patients [93]!

Given the large number of patients that are required, a number of investigators evaluated whether disease-free survival (DFS) can be used as a surrogate marker for overall survival (OS). By so doing, the required number of patients needed for a clinical trial would be lower. In 2007, investigators reporting for the ACCENT (Adjuvant Colon Cancer Endpoints) analyzed 18 randomized adjuvant trials in colon cancer and demonstrated a weak correlation between DFS with OS. Whether DFS should be universally accepted as a surrogate marker for OS remains debatable [94, 95].

Impact of Adding Oxaliplatin

As mentioned in the previous section, both the MOSAIC and the NSABP C-07 trials demonstrated that oxaliplatin had no impact on stage II colon cancer. Tournigand et al. recently performed a subgroup analyses of stage II colon cancer and elderly patients who were enrolled in the MOSAIC trial and found that the addition of oxaliplatin yielded no statistically significant benefit (DFS and OS) [96]. Oxaliplatin's long-term side effects include neurotoxicity, which can occur in 10–15 % of patients who receive FOLFOX4 or FLOX [76, 97]. Thus, it could be argued that adding oxaliplatin to 5-FU/LV should not be routinely given for patients with stage 2 colon cancer.

Significance of Microsatellite Instability (MSI)

Prognostic factors and predictive factors are two important concepts that need further emphasis. These concepts were discussed in Chap. 4, ***Early Invasive Breast Cancer***, but will be reiterated here. Prognostic factors are those that are linked to survival but are not affected by treatment, whereas predictive factors are those that predict response to treatment. For example, T-stage is a prognostic factor but not a predictive factor; a T2 lesion has a better prognosis than a T3 or T4 lesion (prognostic factor) but does not necessarily mean that it is less or more responsive to chemotherapy (predictive factor). Of note, it is possible for a factor to be both prognostic and predictive.

There are multiple prognostic as well as predictive molecular markers that have been evaluated for colon cancer. Among these are 18q deletion, thymidylate synthetase (TS) overexpression and/or genotype, K-ras, BRAF, p53 mutations, hypermethylation, multigene assays, and microsatellite instability (MSI)/deficient mismatch repair (MMR). Of all these, only MSI/MMR has proven to be a predictive molecular factor.

The human genome contains at least 500,000 microsatellites [98]. Microsatellites are regions of DNA that contain repeated sequence of either a single nucleotide or units of two or more nucleotides. The actual number of repeated units to be defined as being microsatellites is debatable [98]. During DNA replication, DNA polymerase sometimes makes errors by incorporating the incorrect nucleotides along the long repetitive DNA sequences (i.e., instead of pairing G with C, it might erroneously pair it with T). The DNA mismatch repair (MMR) system is comprised of genes (MLH1, MSH3, PMS1, PMS2) that are involved in identifying and correcting these errors to enhance genomic stability. However, when one of these repair genes is mutated, the fidelity of replication is compromised, resulting in the production of a DNA chain of altered length. This phenomenon is termed microsatellite instability (MSI) [99].

MSI is often considered as the footprint of the DNA mismatch repair (MMR) deficiency. Tumors showing the presence of MSI are classified as being MSI-high (MSI-H) or MSI-low (MSI-L). MMR is classified as either being DNA-repair deficient (dMMR) or DNA-repair proficient (pMMR). MSI/MMR affects not only patients with hereditary nonpolyposis CRC syndrome (HNPPC or Lynch syndrome) but also in about 15–20 % of patients with sporadic colon cancer. Of note, most sporadic CRC have point mutations in tumor suppressor genes and proto-oncogenes including K-ras, p53, and APC, whereas the defect in Lynch syndrome is due to a mutation in the DNA mismatch repair genes [100].

Pathologically, MSI-H tumors are generally located in the proximal colon, poorly differentiated, and mucinous with tumoral lymphocytic infiltration, characteristics that are typical of an aggressive phenotype. However, several large randomized clinical trials [101–106] and a meta-analysis [107] have demonstrated that the presence of MSI-H is associated with a favorable outcome. The mechanism underlying this observation is not clear, but it may be due to the immunogenicity of the mutated or aberrantly expressed proteins that are recognized by the host's immune system as foreign [98]. This is in contrast to sporadic tumors, which are not recognized by the host as being foreign and therefore likely to evade the immune system. A more thorough discourse on MSI/MMR can be found in Chap. 20, Hereditary Colorectal Cancer and Polyposis Syndromes.

Most studies report that patients with MSI-H tumors not only derive no benefit from adjuvant fluoropyrimidine-based chemotherapy but also may be harmed by it. Consequently, it is recommended that poorly differentiated stage II colon tumors that are MSI-H should not be offered adjuvant chemotherapy.

To be complete, BRAF will be briefly mentioned. BRAF mutation in a patient with deficient MMR CRC is a negative prognosticator. Its role in deciding whether or not to give adjuvant chemotherapy for patients with stage II or III colon cancer has not been defined.

Significance of Multigene Assays

In the above discussion, the decision to administer adjuvant chemotherapy for patients with resectable colon cancer has relied mainly on clinical factors. The advent of multigene platforms has ushered a new era of using molecular technology to prognosticate and predict response to chemotherapy. Although there are a number of multigene platforms available, this chapter will only discuss the three more commonly recognized assays: (1) Oncotype DX Colon Cancer Assay, (2) ColDx, and (3) ColoPrint (Table 16.6).

The Oncotype DX Colon Cancer Assay (Genomic Health, Inc) is also referred to as the

Table 16.6 Multigene assays for colon cancer

Authors	Assays	Genetic platforms	Results
O'Connell, 2010 [108]	Oncotype Dx	12-gene RS	Low RS: 12 % Intermediate RS: 18 % High RS: 22 %
Kennedy, 2011 [109]	ColDx	634-probe set signature	HR for high-risk group Recurrence: 2.53 (P<0.001) Death: 2.21 (P=0.0084)
Salazar, 2011 [110]	ColoPrint	18-gene RS	5-year relapse-free survival rate Low RS: 87.6 % High RS: 67.2 %

RS recurrence score

12-gene recurrence score assay [108]. The assay, which uses similar principle to the one developed for breast cancer, quantifies the expression of 7 recurrence-risk genes and 5 reference genes and classifies patients into low, intermediate, or high risk of recurrence groups based on the recurrence score (RS). Data from QUASAR [111], NSABP B-07 [112], and CALGB 9581 [113] validated the utility of Oncotype DX as an independent prognosticator for colon cancer. Based on data from the QUASAR trial, the risk of recurrence at 3 years for patients with stage II colon cancer who have low, intermediate, and high RS was 12 %, 18 %, and 22 %, respectively [111]. These results are similar to data from CALGB 9581; the 5-year recurrence risk in patients with stage II colon cancer who have low and high RS was 13 % and 21 %, respectively [113].

Although Oncotype DX was a useful prognosticator, it did not predict response to chemotherapy. Gray et al. reported that the continuous 12-gene RS was successful at determining the risk of recurrence in stage II colon cancer but not predictive of which patient who will benefit from chemotherapy [111].

The ColDx assay (Almac Diagnostics) is a 634-probe set signature that identifies patients with stage II colon cancer who are at high risk of recurrence [109]. After developing a prognostic signature from their training set, the investigators used the same threshold score to independently validate their findings in a set of 144 patients. The hazard ratio for recurrence and cancer-related death for the high-risk group was 2.53 ($P<0.001$) and 2.21 ($P=0.0084$). ColDx performed independently from known clinical prognostic factors such as tumor stage, grade, histology (mucinous), and number of nodes retrieved.

Finally, ColoPrint (Agendia) uses the expression of 18 genes and classifies tumors as either low or high recurrence risk [110]. From a set of 206 samples from patients with stages I–III CRC, ColoPrint demonstrated that the 5-year relapse-free survival rates were 87.6 % for those with low recurrence risk and 67.2 % for those with high recurrence risk. Among the stage II patients, the HR for recurrence between the high and low groups was 3.34 ($P=0.017$) [110]. Similar to the previous two assays, ColoPrint classifier performs independently from other prognosticators such as T-stage, N-stage, and lymphatic/vascular/perineural invasion.

Despite these encouraging results, current NCCN guidelines and assessment from the US Agency for Healthcare Research and Quality concluded that multigene assays are not yet ready for prime time in the clinical setting [114, 115].

Summary of Adjuvant Chemotherapy for Stage II Colon Cancer

Adjuvant chemotherapy for stage II colon cancer improves DFS but does not necessarily translate to an improved OS. There are multiple divergent viewpoints about this, and it is recommended that clinicians should fully engage their patients with the discussion of the promises and limitations of

Table 16.7 Indications for adjuvant therapy for stage II colon cancer

CEA >5 ng/mL
Poorly differentiated histology (exclusive of those cancers that are MSI-high)
Bowel obstruction
Bowel perforation
T4 lesions
Inadequate nodal resection (<12 nodes)
Peritumoral lymphatic/vascular invasion

adjuvant chemotherapy. It is reasonable to consider adjuvant chemotherapy for the high-risk stage II colon cancer patients who have the following characteristics: elevated preoperative carcinoembryonic antigen (CEA) > 5 ng/mL, T4 tumors, lymphovascular invasion, poorly differentiated histology (except those with MSI-H feature), inadequately sampled nodes, and bowel obstruction and perforation [85, 116] (Table 16.7). It should be stressed that although these features are associated with poor outcomes, they are not predictive of a successful response to adjuvant chemotherapy [117, 118]. NCCN guidelines support adjuvant chemotherapy for high-risk group of patients with stage II colon cancer and even included the addition of oxaliplatin to 5-FU/LV as an option [114].

The Role of Radiotherapy in Colon Cancer

Unlike rectal cancer, the role of postoperative radiation therapy for colon cancer is ill defined. Retrospective data from Massachusetts General Hospital (MGH) of 203 patients demonstrated that postoperative radiation decreased local recurrence for patients with resected colon cancer who had tumor adherence to surrounding structures or tumor penetration through the bowel wall and involvement of regional lymph nodes. The local control rate was 69 % for the group that received postoperative radiation, but 47 % in the group had surgery alone [119]. The largest and only randomized trial of postoperative radiation for colon cancer was conducted by the North Central Cancer Treatment Group. The trial, Intergroup 0130, intended to accrue 700 patients but only accrued 222 patients of whom only 187 patients were evaluable. They reported that the addition of postoperative radiation to conventional chemotherapy had no impact on the outcome of these high-risk patients. High risk was defined as tumor that was adherent or invading into surrounding structures (T4, excluding peritoneal invasion) and T3N + tumor of the ascending and descending colon [120]. The trial did not meet its accrual objective, and because of this, it was thought to lack sufficient statistical power to detect potentially clinically significant differences in outcome. It is unlikely that there will be a randomized trial of adjuvant radiation for patients with colon cancer. As such, the decision to utilize radiation should be tailored on a case-by-case basis. Postoperative radiation may be considered in patients who have CRM < 1 mm. Example of such tumors is the posterior transmural T3 lesion of the right colon or T4 lesions that are adherent or perforated into the abdominal wall for which a wide resection was not achieved.

Metastatic Disease

Unlike rectal cancer which has a dual drainage system (portal venous system and systemic circulation via the inferior and middle rectal veins), colon cancer drains primarily through the portal system. As such its common site of metastasis is the liver (Fig. 16.3). The management of CRC that has metastasized to the liver will be briefly discussed here, but a more thorough discourse on the topic is addressed in Chap. 19, *Management of Liver Metastasis from Colorectal Cancer.* The management of CRC carcinomatosis is discussed in Chap. 21, *Cytoreductive Surgery and Hyperthermic Intraperitoneal Chemotherapy.*

Despite being classified as stage 4 disease, patients with primary colon cancer with resectable metastatic liver disease have an approximately 40 % 5-year survival [121]. Furthermore, metastatic liver lesions that are initially unresectable can be downstaged with chemotherapy and can ultimately be resected. The 5- and 10-year survival in this group is 33 % and 23 %, respectively [122].

There is considerable debate and no clear consensus regarding whether the primary colon cancer and the metastatic liver disease should be resected at the same time. The potential advantage of a single operation is the avoidance of two laparotomies and the operative risk associated with two major operations. In contrast, staged procedures allow for accurate staging of the hepatic metastases and the avoidance of a major liver resection in the setting where disseminated metastatic disease might develop in a short time interval. Furthermore, there is debate as to whether the primary colon cancer should be resected in the setting of unresectable metastatic disease. While local complications from the colon primary tumor will prompt the surgeons to resect the primary tumor, an abdominal operation will delay the initiation and continuation of systemic chemotherapy. Furthermore, patients generally die of uncontrolled metastatic liver disease such that some believe that the liver should be treated before resecting the primary. This is especially true if the patient present with an asymptomatic primary CRC.

Conclusions

Colon cancer is one of the most common cancers diagnosed in developed countries. With the advent of colonoscopic screening, colon cancer continues to be diagnosed at early stages. Surgery offers definitive treatment, and early stage colon cancer has excellent survival after surgical resection. Adjuvant chemotherapy comprising of 6 months of FOLFOX4 (infusional 5-FU/LV + oxaliplatin), FLOX (bolus 5-FU/LV + oxaliplatin), or CapeOx (capecitabine + oxaliplatin) is indicated for patients with stage III colon cancer. However, its role in patients with stage II colon cancer remains controversial. It could be considered in select patients such as those with elevated preoperative carcinoembryonic antigen (CEA) > 5 ng/mL, need for emergent operation, T4 tumors, lymphovascular invasion, poorly differentiated histology (except those with MSI-H feature), inadequately sampled nodes, and bowel obstruction and perforation. Patients with stage II colon cancer that has MSI-H do not benefit from adjuvant chemotherapy. Multigene arrays hold promise to better select which stage II colon cancer patients will benefit from adjuvant chemotherapy, but at this time, they have not been widely accepted to be used in the clinical setting.

Salient Points

- Early detection through screening for CRC and removal of adenomatous polyps decrease the mortality from CRC.
- Fecal occult blood testing (FOBT) or fecal immunochemical testing (FIT) should be done at home rather than in the office to be an effective screening tool.
- Optimal surgical resection requires:
  - Resecting the affected bowel with at least 5 cm proximal and distal margins
  - En bloc resection of adherent structures
  - Ligating primary feeding vessels
  - Harvesting at least 12 lymph nodes
  - Obtaining greater than a 1 mm circumferential radial margin.
- High-risk groups who may need more vigilant CRC screening include:
  - Patients with personal history of adenomatous polyp or colon cancer
  - Family history of colon cancer
  - Personal history of inflammatory bowel disease
  - Family history of FAP or HNPCC
  - Affected first-degree relative with CRC.
- For patients with stage 3 colon cancer, adjuvant chemotherapy for 6 months is the standard. Options include:
  - FOLFOX4 (infusional oxaliplatin + 5-FU/LV) × 6 months
  - FLOX (bolus oxaliplatin + 5-FU/LV) × 6 months
  - CapeOX (capecitabine + oxaliplatin) × 6 months
  - Capecitabine alone or 5-FU/LV alone × 6 months in those who cannot tolerate oxaliplatin
- For patients with stage 2 colon cancer, adjuvant chemotherapy can be considered for patients who are considered to have high-risk features. These are:
  - CEA > 5 ng/mL
  - T4 tumors
  - Lymphovascular invasion

  - Poorly differentiated histology (except for MSI-H)
  - Inadequately sampled nodes (<12 LNs)
  - Bowel obstruction and perforation
- Laparoscopic colectomy yielded oncologic equivalency to open colectomy and is a viable option for patients with colon cancer. However, laparoscopic proctectomy is not widely accepted as an alternative option for patients with rectal cancer (please see Chap. 18, *Rectal Cancer*).
- Microsatellite instability (MSI):
  - Refers to new alleles with small repeated DNA sequences.
  - Considered as footprint of the DNA mismatch repair deficiency (dMMR).
  - MMR is classified as either deficient (dMMR) or proficient (pMMR).
  - MSI/MMR is the only proven molecular predictive marker for colon cancer.
  - Is classified as being high (MSI-H) or low (MSI-L).
  - MSI-H or dMMR tumors have a better prognosis than MSI-L or pMMR.
  - MSI-H/dMMR stage II colon cancer patients will not derive benefit from adjuvant chemotherapy and therefore should not receive it.
- Multigene platforms are attempting to classify colon cancers based on molecular signatures. Their wide clinical use, however, has not been endorsed by NCCN or other organizations.

Questions

1. At what age should a person with a family history of a mother with colon cancer at age 47 begin screening for colon cancer?
   A. 50
   B. 47
   C. 37
   D. 40
2. What is the minimum number of lymph nodes that should be harvested during an oncologic colon resection?
   A. 5
   B. 10
   C. 20
   D. 12
3. A 58-year-old woman who otherwise has no significant comorbidities underwent a successful right hemicolectomy. The final pathology demonstrated a T1N1 disease. Which of the following statement is true?
   A. Because the tumor is small (T1), she will not need further treatment.
   B. Given her small tumor, she is considered to have stage II disease.
   C. Optimal treatment includes adjuvant chemotherapy, which includes 5-FU, leucovorin, and oxaliplatin.
   D. Addition of oxaliplatin to standard 5-FU and leucovorin has not shown to improve outcome.
4. The following statements regarding microsatellite instability (MSI) and DNA mismatch repair gene (MMR) are true EXCEPT
   A. MSI high is a good prognostic factor for patients with stage II colon cancer.
   B. MMR proficient tumors have better prognosis than MMR-deficient tumors.
   C. MSI/MMR is the only proven predictive molecular marker for colon cancer.
   D. Patients with hMSI stage 2 tumors do not need adjuvant chemotherapy.
5. All of the following are considered high-risk features for stage II colon cancer, EXCEPT
   B. T3 tumor
   C. Lymphovascular invasion
   D. Less than 12 lymph nodes harvested
   E. Bowel obstruction/perforation
6. A 60-year-old otherwise healthy man underwent a sigmoidectomy for a cancer and a partial cystectomy due to tumor adherence. The final pathology demonstrated a 5.5 cm adenocarcinoma of the sigmoid colon that has invaded into the bladder. However, margins were all negative. There were 0 out of 10 lymph nodes involved and the tumor is MSI-high. Which of the following statement is true regarding management of this patient?
   A. The patient has stage 3 disease because of the invasion into the bladder.
   B. The patient may benefit from adjuvant chemotherapy because of its involvement into the bladder.

C. Adjuvant therapy is not likely to be helpful because of the tumor being MSI-high.
D. The nodal status is likely to be accurate because he had adequate number of lymph nodes retrieved.

7. ALL of the following statements are true regarding the circumferential radial margin (CRM), EXCEPT:
A. CRM status has prognostic value for both colon and rectal cancer.
B. CRM pertains to the non-peritonealized part of the colon.
C. CRM is more likely to be positive in patients with cecal/ascending colon and descending colon cancer than those with transverse colon cancer.
D. Any tumor that penetrates into the serosal is considered to have positive CRM.

8. The principles of resecting colon cancer include ALL of the following, EXCEPT:
A. Adhere to the "no touch isolation technique" so as to avoid tumor dissemination into the systemic circulation.
B. Achieve at least a 5 cm proximal and distal margin of resection.
C. Retrieve at least 12 lymph nodes so as to accurately stage the patient.
D. Ligate the major feeding vessels at its origin.

Answers

1. C
2. D
3. C
4. B
5. A
6. B
7. D
8. A

Acknowledgment The portion of this work was supported by the Charles D. Knight, Sr. Endowed Professorship.

References

1. Siegel R, Ma J, Zou Z, Jemal A. Cancer statistics, 2014. CA Cancer J Clin. 2014;64(1):9–29.
2. Siegel R, Naishadham D, Jemal A. Cancer statistics, 2013. CA Cancer J Clin. 2013;63(1):11–30.
3. Winawer SJ, Zauber AG, Ho MN, et al. Prevention of colorectal cancer by colonoscopic polypectomy. The National Polyp Study Workgroup. N Engl J Med. 1993;329(27):1977–81.
4. Newcomb PA, Norfleet RG, Storer BE, Surawicz TS, Marcus PM. Screening sigmoidoscopy and colorectal cancer mortality. J Natl Cancer Inst. 1992;84(20):1572–5.
5. Winawer SJ, Flehinger BJ, Schottenfeld D, Miller DG. Screening for colorectal cancer with fecal occult blood testing and sigmoidoscopy. J Natl Cancer Inst. 1993;85(16):1311–8.
6. Müller AD, Sonnenberg A. Protection by endoscopy against death from colorectal cancer. A case–control study among veterans. Arch Intern Med. 1995; 155(16):1741–8.
7. Kronborg O, Fenger C, Olsen J, Jørgensen OD, Søndergaard O. Randomised study of screening for colorectal cancer with faecal-occult-blood test. Lancet. 1996;348(9040):1467–71.
8. Levin B, Lieberman DA, McFarland B, et al. Screening and surveillance for the early detection of colorectal cancer and adenomatous polyps, 2008: a joint guideline from the American Cancer Society, the US Multi-Society Task Force on Colorectal Cancer, and the American College of Radiology. Gastroenterology. 2008;134(5):1570–95.
9. Whitlock EP, Lin JS, Liles E, Beil TL, Fu R. Screening for colorectal cancer: a targeted, updated systematic review for the U.S. Preventive Services Task Force. Ann Intern Med. 2008;149(9): 638–58.
10. Shapiro JA, Seeff LC, Thompson TD, Nadel MR, Klabunde CN, Vernon SW. Colorectal cancer test use from the 2005 National Health Interview Survey. Cancer Epidemiol Biomarkers Prev. 2008;17(7): 1623–30.
11. Potter JD, Slattery ML, Bostick RM, Gapstur SM. Colon cancer: a review of the epidemiology. Epidemiol Rev. 1993;15(2):499–545.
12. Fearon ER, Vogelstein B. A genetic model for colorectal tumorigenesis. Cell. 1990;61(5):759–67.
13. Armaghany T, Wilson JD, Chu Q, Mills G. Genetic alterations in colorectal cancer. Gastrointest Cancer Res. 2012;5(1):19–27.
14. Mathew A, Peters U, Chatterjee N, Kulldorff M, Sinha R. Fat, fiber, fruits, vegetables, and risk of colorectal adenomas. Int J Cancer. 2004;108(2): 287–92.
15. Howell MA. Factor analysis of international cancer mortality data and per capita food consumption. Br J Cancer. 1974;29(4):328–36.
16. Howe GR, Aronson KJ, Benito E, et al. The relationship between dietary fat intake and risk of colorectal cancer: evidence from the combined analysis of 13 case–control studies. Cancer Causes Control. 1997; 8(2):215–28.
17. Larsson SC, Wolk A. Meat consumption and risk of colorectal cancer: a meta-analysis of prospective studies. Int J Cancer. 2006;119(11):2657–64.

18. Sesink AL, Termont DS, Kleibeuker JH, Van der Meer R. Red meat and colon cancer: the cytotoxic and hyperproliferative effects of dietary heme. Cancer Res. 1999;59(22):5704–9.
19. IARC monographs on the evaluation of the carcinogenic risk of chemicals to humans: some N-nitroso compounds. *IARC Monogr Eval Carcinog Risk Chem Man*. 1978;17:1–349.
20. Marques-Vidal P, Ravasco P, Ermelinda Camilo M. Foodstuffs and colorectal cancer risk: a review. Clin Nutr. 2006;25(1):14–36.
21. Burkitt DP. Epidemiology of Burkitt's lymphoma. Proc R Soc Med. 1971;64(9):909–10.
22. Schatzkin A, Lanza E, Corle D, et al. Lack of effect of a low-fat, high-fiber diet on the recurrence of colorectal adenomas. Polyp Prevention Trial Study Group. N Engl J Med. 2000;342(16):1149–55.
23. Alberts DS, Martínez ME, Roe DJ, et al. Lack of effect of a high-fiber cereal supplement on the recurrence of colorectal adenomas. Phoenix Colon Cancer Prevention Physicians' Network. N Engl J Med. 2000;342(16):1156–62.
24. McKeown-Eyssen GE, Bright-See E, Bruce WR, et al. A randomized trial of a low fat high fibre diet in the recurrence of colorectal polyps. Toronto Polyp Prevention Group. J Clin Epidemiol. 1994;47(5): 525–36.
25. MacLennan R, Macrae F, Bain C, et al. Randomized trial of intake of fat, fiber, and beta carotene to prevent colorectal adenomas. J Natl Cancer Inst. 1995;87(23):1760–6.
26. Bonithon-Kopp C, Kronborg O, Giacosa A, Räth U, Faivre J. Calcium and fibre supplementation in prevention of colorectal adenoma recurrence: a randomised intervention trial. European Cancer Prevention Organisation Study Group. Lancet. 2000;356(9238):1300–6.
27. Asano T, McLeod RS. Dietary fibre for the prevention of colorectal adenomas and carcinomas. Cochrane Database Syst Rev. 2002;2, CD003430.
28. Sansbury LB, Wanke K, Albert PS, et al. The effect of strict adherence to a high-fiber, high-fruit and -vegetable, and low-fat eating pattern on adenoma recurrence. Am J Epidemiol. 2009;170(5):576–84.
29. Lin J, Zhang SM, Cook NR, Rexrode KM, Lee IM, Buring JE. Body mass index and risk of colorectal cancer in women (United States). Cancer Causes Control. 2004;15(6):581–9.
30. Aleksandrova K, Pischon T, Buijsse B, et al. Adult weight change and risk of colorectal cancer in the European Prospective Investigation into Cancer and Nutrition. Eur J Cancer. 2013;49(16):3526–36.
31. Logan RF, Grainge MJ, Shepherd VC, Armitage NC, Muir KR, ukCAP Trial Group. Aspirin and folic acid for the prevention of recurrent colorectal adenomas. Gastroenterology. 2008;134(1):29–38.
32. Cole BF, Baron JA, Sandler RS, et al. Folic acid for the prevention of colorectal adenomas: a randomized clinical trial. JAMA. 2007;297(21):2351–9.
33. Ulrich CM, Potter JD. Folate and cancer–timing is everything. JAMA. 2007;297(21):2408–9.
34. Fedirko V, Tramacere I, Bagnardi V, et al. Alcohol drinking and colorectal cancer risk: an overall and dose–response meta-analysis of published studies. Ann Oncol. 2011;22(9):1958–72.
35. Jacobson JS, Neugut AI, Murray T, et al. Cigarette smoking and other behavioral risk factors for recurrence of colorectal adenomatous polyps (New York City, NY, USA). Cancer Causes Control. 1994;5(3): 215–20.
36. Leufkens AM, Van Duijnhoven FJ, Siersema PD, et al. Cigarette smoking and colorectal cancer risk in the European Prospective Investigation into Cancer and Nutrition study. Clin Gastroenterol Hepatol. 2011;9(2):137–44.
37. Schernhammer ES, Leitzmann MF, Michaud DS, et al. Cholecystectomy and the risk for developing colorectal cancer and distal colorectal adenomas. Br J Cancer. 2003;88(1):79–83.
38. Dyson JK, Rutter MD. Colorectal cancer in inflammatory bowel disease: what is the real magnitude of the risk? World J Gastroenterol. 2012;18(29): 3839–48.
39. Baglietto L, Jenkins MA, Severi G, et al. Measures of familial aggregation depend on definition of family history: meta-analysis for colorectal cancer. J Clin Epidemiol. 2006;59(2):114–24.
40. Butterworth AS, Higgins JP, Pharoah P. Relative and absolute risk of colorectal cancer for individuals with a family history: a meta-analysis. Eur J Cancer. 2006;42(2):216–27.
41. Bermejo F, García-López S. A guide to diagnosis of iron deficiency and iron deficiency anemia in digestive diseases. World J Gastroenterol. 2009;15(37): 4638–43.
42. Morrin MM, Farrell RJ, Raptopoulos V, McGee JB, Bleday R, Kruskal JB. Role of virtual computed tomographic colonography in patients with colorectal cancers and obstructing colorectal lesions. Dis Colon Rectum. 2000;43(3):303–11.
43. Halligan S, Altman DG, Taylor SA, et al. CT colonography in the detection of colorectal polyps and cancer: systematic review, meta-analysis, and proposed minimum data set for study level reporting. Radiology. 2005;237(3):893–904.
44. Gluecker TM, Johnson CD, Harmsen WS, et al. Colorectal cancer screening with CT colonography, colonoscopy, and double-contrast barium enema examination: prospective assessment of patient perceptions and preferences. Radiology. 2003;227(2): 378–84.
45. Imperiale TF, Ransohoff DF, Itzkowitz SH, et al. Multitarget stool DNA testing for colorectal-cancer screening. N Engl J Med. 2014;370(14):1287–97.
46. Ko C, Hyman NH. Surgeons SCoTASoCaR. Practice parameter for the detection of colorectal neoplasms: an interim report (revised). Dis Colon Rectum. 2006;49(3):299–301.

47. Johns LE, Houlston RS. A systematic review and meta-analysis of familial colorectal cancer risk. Am J Gastroenterol. 2001;96(10):2992–3003.
48. Finan PJ, Campbell S, Verma R, et al. The management of malignant large bowel obstruction: ACPGBI position statement. Colorectal Dis. 2007;9 Suppl 4:1–17.
49. Langevin JM, Nivatvongs S. The true incidence of synchronous cancer of the large bowel. A prospective study. Am J Surg. 1984;147(3):330–3.
50. Brahme F, Ekelund GR, Nordén JG, Wenckert A. Metachronous colorectal polyps: comparison of development of colorectal polyps and carcinomas in persons with and without histories of polyps. Dis Colon Rectum. 1974;17(2):166–71.
51. Heald RJ, Bussey HJ. Clinical experiences at St. Mark's Hospital with multiple synchronous cancers of the colon and rectum. Dis Colon Rectum. 1975;18(1):6–10.
52. Compton C, Byrd D, Garcia-Aguilar J, et al. Colon and rectum. In: Compton C, Byrd D, Garcia-Aguilar J, Kurtzman S, Olawaiye A, Washington M, editors. AJCC cancer staging atlas. 2nd ed. New York: Springer; 2012. p. 185–201.
53. Edge SB, Compton CC. The American Joint Committee on Cancer: the 7th edition of the AJCC cancer staging manual and the future of TNM. Ann Surg Oncol. 2010;17(6):1471–4.
54. Chang GJ, Kaiser AM, Mills S, Rafferty JF, Buie WD. Surgeons SPTFotASoCaR. Practice parameters for the management of colon cancer. Dis Colon Rectum. 2012;55(8):831–43.
55. Nelson H, Petrelli N, Carlin A, et al. Guidelines 2000 for colon and rectal cancer surgery. J Natl Cancer Inst. 2001;93(8):583–96.
56. Wright FC, Law CH, Last L, et al. Lymph node retrieval and assessment in stage II colorectal cancer: a population-based study. Ann Surg Oncol. 2003;10(8):903–9.
57. Bateman AC, Carr NJ, Warren BF. The retroperitoneal surface in distal caecal and proximal ascending colon carcinoma: the Cinderella surgical margin? J Clin Pathol. 2005;58(4):426–8.
58. Nagtegaal ID, Marijnen CA, Kranenbarg EK, et al. Circumferential margin involvement is still an important predictor of local recurrence in rectal carcinoma: not one millimeter but two millimeters is the limit. Am J Surg Pathol. 2002;26(3):350–7.
59. Stocchi L, Nelson H, Sargent DJ, et al. Impact of surgical and pathologic variables in rectal cancer: a United States community and cooperative group report. J Clin Oncol. 2001;19(18):3895–902.
60. den Dulk M, Marijnen CA, Putter H, et al. Risk factors for adverse outcome in patients with rectal cancer treated with an abdominoperineal resection in the total mesorectal excision trial. Ann Surg. 2007;246(1):83–90.
61. Wiggers T, Jeekel J, Arends JW, et al. No-touch isolation technique in colon cancer: a controlled prospective trial. Br J Surg. 1988;75(5):409–15.
62. Slanetz CA, Grimson R. Effect of high and intermediate ligation on survival and recurrence rates following curative resection of colorectal cancer. Dis Colon Rectum. 1997;40(10):1205–18; discussion 1218–1209.
63. Group COoSTS. A comparison of laparoscopically assisted and open colectomy for colon cancer. N Engl J Med. 2004;350(20):2050–9.
64. Jayne DG, Guillou PJ, Thorpe H, et al. Randomized trial of laparoscopic-assisted resection of colorectal carcinoma: 3-year results of the UK MRC CLASICC Trial Group. J Clin Oncol. 2007;25(21):3061–8.
65. Jayne DG, Thorpe HC, Copeland J, Quirke P, Brown JM, Guillou PJ. Five-year follow-up of the Medical Research Council CLASICC trial of laparoscopically assisted versus open surgery for colorectal cancer. Br J Surg. 2010;97(11):1638–45.
66. Buunen M, Veldkamp R, Hop WC, et al. Survival after laparoscopic surgery versus open surgery for colon cancer: long-term outcome of a randomised clinical trial. Lancet Oncol. 2009;10(1):44–52.
67. Green BL, Marshall HC, Collinson F, et al. Long-term follow-up of the Medical Research Council CLASICC trial of conventional versus laparoscopically assisted resection in colorectal cancer. Br J Surg. 2013;100(1):75–82.
68. Trastulli S, Desiderio J, Farinacci F, et al. Robotic right colectomy for cancer with intracorporeal anastomosis: short-term outcomes from a single institution. Int J Colorectal Dis. 2013;28(6):807–14.
69. Moertel CG, Fleming TR, Macdonald JS, et al. Levamisole and fluorouracil for adjuvant therapy of resected colon carcinoma. N Engl J Med. 1990; 322(6):352–8.
70. Moertel CG, Fleming TR, Macdonald JS, et al. Fluorouracil plus levamisole as effective adjuvant therapy after resection of stage III colon carcinoma: a final report. Ann Intern Med. 1995;122(5):321–6.
71. International Multicentre Pooled Analysis of Colon Cancer Trials (IMPACT) investigators. Efficacy of adjuvant fluorouracil and folinic acid in colon cancer. Lancet. 1995;345(8955):939–44.
72. O'Connell MJ, Mailliard JA, Kahn MJ, et al. Controlled trial of fluorouracil and low-dose leucovorin given for 6 months as postoperative adjuvant therapy for colon cancer. J Clin Oncol. 1997;15(1): 246–50.
73. Wolmark N, Rockette H, Mamounas E, et al. Clinical trial to assess the relative efficacy of fluorouracil and leucovorin, fluorouracil and levamisole, and fluorouracil, leucovorin, and levamisole in patients with Dukes' B and C carcinoma of the colon: results from National Surgical Adjuvant Breast and Bowel Project C-04. J Clin Oncol. 1999;17(11):3553–9.
74. Andre T, Colin P, Louvet C, et al. Semimonthly versus monthly regimen of fluorouracil and leucovorin administered for 24 or 36 weeks as adjuvant therapy in stage II and III colon cancer: results of a randomized trial. J Clin Oncol. 2003;21(15): 2896–903.

75. André T, Boni C, Mounedji-Boudiaf L, et al. Oxaliplatin, fluorouracil, and leucovorin as adjuvant treatment for colon cancer. N Engl J Med. 2004;350(23):2343–51.
76. André T, Boni C, Navarro M, et al. Improved overall survival with oxaliplatin, fluorouracil, and leucovorin as adjuvant treatment in stage II or III colon cancer in the MOSAIC trial. J Clin Oncol. 2009;27(19):3109–16.
77. Kuebler JP, Wieand HS, O'Connell MJ, et al. Oxaliplatin combined with weekly bolus fluorouracil and leucovorin as surgical adjuvant chemotherapy for stage II and III colon cancer: results from NSABP C-07. J Clin Oncol. 2007;25(16):2198–204.
78. Yothers G, O'Connell MJ, Allegra CJ, et al. Oxaliplatin as adjuvant therapy for colon cancer: updated results of NSABP C-07 trial, including survival and subset analyses. J Clin Oncol. 2011;29(28): 3768–74.
79. Haller DG, Tabernero J, Maroun J, et al. Capecitabine plus oxaliplatin compared with fluorouracil and folinic acid as adjuvant therapy for stage III colon cancer. J Clin Oncol. 2011;29(11):1465–71.
80. Schmoll HJ, Cartwright T, Tabernero J, et al. Phase III trial of capecitabine plus oxaliplatin as adjuvant therapy for stage III colon cancer: a planned safety analysis in 1,864 patients. J Clin Oncol. 2007;25(1): 102–9.
81. Marsoni S, Investigators IMPACT. Efficacy of adjuvant fluorouracil and leucovorin in stage B2 and C colon cancer. International Multicenter Pooled Analysis of Colon Cancer Trials Investigators. Semin Oncol. 2001;28 Suppl 1:14–9.
82. International Multicentre Pooled Analysis of B2 Colon Cancer Trials (IMPACT B2) Investigators. Efficacy of adjuvant fluorouracil and folinic acid in B2 colon cancer. J Clin Oncol. 1999;17(5):1356–63.
83. Gill S, Loprinzi CL, Sargent DJ, et al. Pooled analysis of fluorouracil-based adjuvant therapy for stage II and III colon cancer: who benefits and by how much? J Clin Oncol. 2004;22(10):1797–806.
84. Gray R, Barnwell J, McConkey C, et al. Adjuvant chemotherapy versus observation in patients with colorectal cancer: a randomised study. Lancet. 2007;370(9604):2020–9.
85. Moertel CG, Fleming TR, Macdonald JS, et al. Intergroup study of fluorouracil plus levamisole as adjuvant therapy for stage II/Dukes' B2 colon cancer. J Clin Oncol. 1995;13(12):2936–43.
86. Mamounas E, Wieand S, Wolmark N, et al. Comparative efficacy of adjuvant chemotherapy in patients with Dukes' B versus Dukes' C colon cancer: results from four National Surgical Adjuvant Breast and Bowel Project adjuvant studies (C-01, C-02, C-03, and C-04). J Clin Oncol. 1999;17(5): 1349–55.
87. Wilkinson NW, Yothers G, Lopa S, Costantino JP, Petrelli NJ, Wolmark N. Long-term survival results of surgery alone versus surgery plus 5-fluorouracil and leucovorin for stage II and stage III colon cancer: pooled analysis of NSABP C-01 through C-05. A baseline from which to compare modern adjuvant trials. Ann Surg Oncol. 2010;17(4):959–66.
88. Harrington DP. The tea leaves of small trials. J Clin Oncol. 1999;17(5):1336–8.
89. Wein A, Hahn EG, Merkel S, Hohenberger W. Adjuvant chemotherapy for stage II (Dukes' B) colon cancer: too early for routine use. Eur J Surg Oncol. 2000;26(8):730–2.
90. Figueredo A, Coombes ME, Mukherjee S. Adjuvant therapy for completely resected stage II colon cancer. Cochrane Database Syst Rev. 2008;3, CD005390.
91. O'Connor ES, Greenblatt DY, LoConte NK, et al. Adjuvant chemotherapy for stage II colon cancer with poor prognostic features. J Clin Oncol. 2011; 29(25):3381–8.
92. Mayer RJ. Reply to A. Grothey et al and R.S. Midgley et al. J Clin Oncol. 2013;31(12):1612–3.
93. Buyse M, Piedbois P. Should Dukes' B patients receive adjuvant therapy? A statistical perspective. Semin Oncol. 2001;28 Suppl 1:20–4.
94. Mayer RJ. Oxaliplatin as part of adjuvant therapy for colon cancer: more complicated than once thought. J Clin Oncol. 2012;30(27):3325–7.
95. Grothey A, de Gramont A, Sargent DJ. Disease-free survival in colon cancer: still relevant after all these years! J Clin Oncol. 2013;31(12):1609–10.
96. Tournigand C, André T, Bonnetain F, et al. Adjuvant therapy with fluorouracil and oxaliplatin in stage II and elderly patients (between ages 70 and 75 years) with colon cancer: subgroup analyses of the Multicenter International Study of Oxaliplatin, Fluorouracil, and Leucovorin in the Adjuvant Treatment of Colon Cancer trial. J Clin Oncol. 2012;30(27):3353–60.
97. Land SR, Kopec JA, Cecchini RS, et al. Neurotoxicity from oxaliplatin combined with weekly bolus fluorouracil and leucovorin as surgical adjuvant chemotherapy for stage II and III colon cancer: NSABP C-07. J Clin Oncol. 2007;25(16):2205–11.
98. de la Chapelle A, Hampel H. Clinical relevance of microsatellite instability in colorectal cancer. J Clin Oncol. 2010;28(20):3380–7.
99. Boland CR, Goel A. Microsatellite instability in colorectal cancer. Gastroenterology. 2010;138(6): 2073–87.e2073.
100. Drescher KM, Sharma P, Lynch HT. Current hypotheses on how microsatellite instability leads to enhanced survival of Lynch Syndrome patients. Clin Dev Immunol. 2010;2010:170432.
101. Bertagnolli MM, Redston M, Compton CC, et al. Microsatellite instability and loss of heterozygosity at chromosomal location 18q: prospective evaluation of biomarkers for stages II and III colon cancer–a study of CALGB 9581 and 89803. J Clin Oncol. 2011;29(23):3153–62.
102. Roth AD, Tejpar S, Delorenzi M, et al. Prognostic role of KRAS and BRAF in stage II and III resected colon cancer: results of the translational study on the PETACC-3, EORTC 40993, SAKK 60–00 trial. J Clin Oncol. 2010;28(3):466–74.

103. Roth AD, Delorenzi M, Tejpar S, et al. Integrated analysis of molecular and clinical prognostic factors in stage II/III colon cancer. J Natl Cancer Inst. 2012;104(21):1635–46.
104. Halling KC, French AJ, McDonnell SK, et al. Microsatellite instability and 8p allelic imbalance in stage B2 and C colorectal cancers. J Natl Cancer Inst. 1999;91(15):1295–303.
105. Sinicrope FA, Rego RL, Halling KC, et al. Prognostic impact of microsatellite instability and DNA ploidy in human colon carcinoma patients. Gastroenterology. 2006;131(3):729–37.
106. Watanabe T, Wu TT, Catalano PJ, et al. Molecular predictors of survival after adjuvant chemotherapy for colon cancer. N Engl J Med. 2001;344(16):1196–206.
107. Popat S, Hubner R, Houlston RS. Systematic review of microsatellite instability and colorectal cancer prognosis. J Clin Oncol. 2005;23(3):609–18.
108. O'Connell MJ, Lavery I, Yothers G, et al. Relationship between tumor gene expression and recurrence in four independent studies of patients with stage II/III colon cancer treated with surgery alone or surgery plus adjuvant fluorouracil plus leucovorin. J Clin Oncol. 2010;28(25):3937–44.
109. Kennedy RD, Bylesjo M, Kerr P, et al. Development and independent validation of a prognostic assay for stage II colon cancer using formalin-fixed paraffin-embedded tissue. J Clin Oncol. 2011;29(35):4620–6.
110. Salazar R, Roepman P, Capella G, et al. Gene expression signature to improve prognosis prediction of stage II and III colorectal cancer. J Clin Oncol. 2011;29(1):17–24.
111. Gray RG, Quirke P, Handley K, et al. Validation study of a quantitative multigene reverse transcriptase-polymerase chain reaction assay for assessment of recurrence risk in patients with stage II colon cancer. J Clin Oncol. 2011;29(35):4611–9.
112. Yothers G, O'Connell MJ, Lee M, et al. Validation of the 12-gene colon cancer recurrence score in NSABP C-07 as a predictor of recurrence in patients with stage II and III colon cancer treated with fluorouracil and leucovorin (FU/LV) and FU/LV plus oxaliplatin. J Clin Oncol. 2013;31(36):4512–9.
113. Venook AP, Niedzwiecki D, Lopatin M, et al. Biologic determinants of tumor recurrence in stage II colon cancer: validation study of the 12-gene recurrence score in cancer and leukemia group B (CALGB) 9581. J Clin Oncol. 2013;31(14):1775–81.
114. National Comprehensive Cancer Network (NCCN) guidelines. Available at: www.nccn.org (2013). Accessed 23 May 2013.
115. Black E, Falzon L, Aronson N. Gene expression profiling for predicting outcomes in stage II colon cancer. *Agency for Healthcare Research and Quality (US)*. 2012;13 (http://www.ncbi.nlm.nih.gov/books/NBK115808/). Accessed 25 Apr 2014.
116. Le Voyer TE, Sigurdson ER, Hanlon AL, et al. Colon cancer survival is associated with increasing number of lymph nodes analyzed: a secondary survey of intergroup trial INT-0089. J Clin Oncol. 2003;21(15):2912–9.
117. Benson AB, Schrag D, Somerfield MR, et al. American Society of Clinical Oncology recommendations on adjuvant chemotherapy for stage II colon cancer. J Clin Oncol. 2004;22(16):3408–19.
118. Quah HM, Chou JF, Gonen M, et al. Identification of patients with high-risk stage II colon cancer for adjuvant therapy. Dis Colon Rectum. 2008;51(5):503–7.
119. Willett CG, Tepper JE, Skates SJ, Wood WC, Orlow EC, Duttenhaver JR. Adjuvant postoperative radiation therapy for colonic carcinoma. Ann Surg. 1987;206(6):694–8.
120. Martenson JA, Willett CG, Sargent DJ, et al. Phase III study of adjuvant chemotherapy and radiation therapy compared with chemotherapy alone in the surgical adjuvant treatment of colon cancer: results of intergroup protocol 0130. J Clin Oncol. 2004;22(16):3277–83.
121. de Santibañes E, Lassalle FB, McCormack L, et al. Simultaneous colorectal and hepatic resections for colorectal cancer: postoperative and longterm outcomes. J Am Coll Surg. 2002;195(2):196–202.
122. Adam R, Delvart V, Pascal G, et al. Rescue surgery for unresectable colorectal liver metastases downstaged by chemotherapy: a model to predict long-term survival. Ann Surg. 2004;240(4):644–57; discussion 657–648.

Local Excision of Early-Stage Rectal Cancer

17

Matthew Sanders, Benjamin W. Vabi, Phillip A. Cole, and Mahmoud N. Kulaylat

Learning Objectives

After reading this chapter, you should be able to:

- Understand the role of local excision as alternative less radical treatment of early-stage rectal cancer (mainly T1N0 and select T2N0 lesions)
- Recognize selection criteria for local excision of early-stage rectal cancer based on clinical and radiological staging and histopathological features of the primary rectal cancer
- Appreciate the surgical options for local excision of early-stage rectal cancer
- Know the outcome of local excision of early-stage rectal cancer with and without adjuvant therapy

M. Sanders, BA, M.D.
Department of Surgery, LSUHSC-Shreveport, 3806 Richmond Ave., Shreveport, LA, USA
e-mail: msand3@lsuhsc.edu

B.W. Vabi, M.D.
Department of General Surgery, University at Buffalo School of Medicine, 100 High Street, Buffalo, NY, USA
e-mail: bwvabi@buffalo.edu

P.A. Cole, M.D., MHCM, FACS, FASCRS
Department of Surgery, LSUHSC/University Health-Shreveport, 1501 Kings Hwy., Shreveport, LA 71103, USA
e-mail: pcolemd@msn.com

M.N. Kulaylat, M.D. (✉)
Department of Surgery, Buffalo General Medical Center, University at Buffalo-State University of New York, 100 High Street, Buffalo, NY 14203, USA
e-mail: mkulaylat@kaleidahealth.org

Introduction

Colorectal cancer is the fifth most common cancer in adults worldwide and is the most common gastrointestinal (GI) malignancy in the United States. It is the second leading cause of death in the western countries. About 30 % of the colorectal cancers are located in the rectum, and 40,000–42,500 new cases of rectal cancer are diagnosed in the United States annually [1].

Rectal cancer differs from colon cancer in that it is located in the pelvis, in close proximity to the anal sphincter complex, surrounded by major neurovascular structures, and constrained by the bony pelvis. Surgery remains the mainstay treatment modality. The primary goals of treatment are to cure the patient, reduce local recurrence (LR), maximize disease-free survival (DFS), maintain function, and optimize quality of life. Mortality is related to metastatic spread prior to resection and locoregional recurrences after resection, which is related in part to surgical technique.

Evolution of Surgical Treatment of Rectal Cancer

The surgical treatment of rectal cancer continues to evolve, and such evolution is the culmination of our better understanding of the surgical anatomy of the rectum and biologic behavior of the cancer and appreciation of the significance of surgical margins (distal and radial). In addition,

Q.D. Chu et al. (eds.), *Surgical Oncology: A Practical and Comprehensive Approach*,
DOI 10.1007/978-1-4939-1423-4_17, © Springer Science+Business Media New York 2015

the development of new instruments, the introduction of reconstructive surgery, and the advent of effective adjuvant therapy have all contributed to outcome improvement.

Radical resection is standard surgical treatment for cure or palliation. It can be used either as single modality or part of multimodality treatment. For upper, middle, and few distal rectal cancers, the standard surgical treatment is an anterior resection (AR) with or without reconstruction. Abdominoperineal resection (APR) is reserved for very distal rectal cancer (a more in-depth discussion can be found in Chap. 18). Radical resection is associated with low LR and high cure rate and a low 30-day mortality rate (5–7 %). However, radical surgery is associated with a significant morbidity rate of 35 %, a poor or suboptimal bowel and urological functional outcome, a moderate risk of sexual dysfunction, and a high permanent colostomy rate. These disadvantages occur mainly in patients with distal rectal cancers [2–5]. The desire for a less aggressive treatment especially for those with early cancer prompted many to search for an alternative strategy. Such a strategy, coupled with the need to demonstrate oncologic equivalency to radical surgery, prompted many investigators to evaluate the role of local excision.

Local treatment of rectal cancer was described by Lisfranc in 1826 [6]. The anus and distal rectum were removed through an oval perineal incision, leaving the patient with a perineal colostomy. In 1885, Kraske [7] described a transsacral or posterior approach for rectal excision accompanied by the placement of a sacral colostomy or proctotomy and local excision of the cancer. As would be expected, these procedures were associated with suboptimal stoma location, poor healing, and high LR and anastomotic failure, resulting in a poor quality of life for the affected patients.

In the late 1800s, Czerny [8] suggested a more radical resection of rectal cancer that included incorporating the lymphovascular pedicle because it represented the main mode of cancer spread. In 1907, Miles [9] described the APR whereby the entire pelvic colon and mesocolon were removed and a colostomy created. Advances in surgical technique, anesthesia, preoperative and postoperative care, and antibiotic coverage made proctectomy a safer procedure. In the subsequent years, the necessity of obtaining at least a 5 cm margin distal to the tumor was challenged, and the importance of a wide circumferential radial margin (CRM) was recognized [10, 11].

In the 1980s, Heald et al. described the total mesorectal excision (TME) technique whereby the rectum is removed as a package with an intact envelope containing lymph nodes (LN) [12]. With development of newer instruments and the introduction of the concept of multimodality approach to cancer care, other novel approaches were spawned such as sphincter-saving procedures with or without reconstruction, intersphincteric resection, and laparoscopic or robotic surgery.

About 80 % of rectal cancers present with disease beyond the rectal wall (T3) with either direct extension to adjacent organ (T4) or lymphatic spread. The standard treatment is neoadjuvant chemoradiotherapy (neoCRT) followed by radical resection [13]. However, 5–15 % of rectal cancers are T1 or T2 (early stage rectal cancer) that have no or low probability of having LN spread. For these cases, a less radical surgery is a viable option [14]. On occasions, less radical surgery is the only option because of patient's choice (some patients refuse to accept having a permanent colostomy) or because of the biology of the disease (i.e., patients with metastatic disease from a small tumor may prefer local excision followed by palliative chemotherapy for symptomatic relief). Local excision, described by Parks in the 1950s [15], and transanal endoscopic microsurgery (TEM), developed by Buess in 1980s [16], were added to the armamentarium of surgical treatment of rectal cancer as alternative treatment for the 5–15 % of patients with ERC.

Techniques of Local Excision of Early Rectal Cancer

ERC is defined as invasive adenocarcinoma into but not beyond the submucosa (T1) and may present as a small ulcerating or polypoid adenocarcinoma or a focus of adenocarcinoma within

Table 17.1 Criteria for local excision of rectal cancer

T1N0
No evidence of lymphovascular invasion
Well-differentiated to moderately differentiated tumor
Tumor < 3 cm in diameter
Involved < 30 % circumference of rectal wall

an adenoma, i.e., malignant polyp [17]. ERC is stage I, i.e., early-stage rectal cancer (ESRC) [15]. However, stage I cancer also include tumors that have extended to but not through the muscularis propria of the rectum (T2). T3–T4 lesions and/or those that have nodal involvement but without distant metastases are considered as high-risk resectable rectal cancer, a topic that is discussed in Chap. 18, ***Rectal Cancer***.

About 30 % of rectal adenocarcinomas are stage I and historically were treated with radical resection which resulted in excellent local control (local recurrence ranges from 4 % to 16 %) and survival (5-year overall survival (OS) of 90 %) [18, 19]. As mentioned previously, radical resection carries a significant risk of morbidity and mortality and may not be an attractive option for some patients with ESRC. In select cases, local excision is an acceptable alternative for T1 tumors that encompass <30 % of the bowel circumference, are <3 cm in size, are mobile, are well to moderately differentiated, and lack lymphovascular invasion (Table 17.1). These strict criteria are accepted by the National Comprehensive Cancer Network and the American Society of Colon and Rectal Surgeons [20, 21]. For T2 cancer, local excision must be viewed with high reservation since LR after surgery alone is unacceptably high (22 %).

Posterior Approach

The approach to locally resect rectal cancer can be grouped into a posterior approach and the transanal approach (Table 17.2). For the posterior approach, Kraske posterior proctotomy [7] and York-Mason transsphincteric approach [22] are established procedures. However, they are not frequently used nowadays because of the associated

Table 17.2 Approaches for local excision of rectal adenocarcinoma

Posterior approach
Kraske transsacral proctotomy
York-Mason transsphincteric approach
Transanal excision
Park's per anal excision
Transanal endoscopic microsurgery (TEM)
With endoscopic posterior mesorectal excision
With intraperitoneal anastomosis
With two-stage total mesorectal excision
Transanal minimally invasive surgery (TAMIS)
Robotic-TEM

complications (sacral pain after coccygectomy, rectal fistulas, and impairment of sphincter function), the fear of seeding tumor in the retrorectal space, the concern of compromising salvage resection, and the advent of newer and less invasive procedures [23, 24].

Regardless, the approach is briefly mentioned for completeness. The patient is placed in the prone position, an incision is made over the sacrum to the upper border of the sphincter and the coccyx, and the anococcygeal ligament is removed to facilitate exposure. To obtain exposure of the upper rectum, the lower margin of the gluteus maximus muscle and sacrotuberous and sacrospinous ligaments are cut, and the lower most part of the left wing of the sacrum is excised (the classical excision of the lower sacrum is not practiced). The levator muscle is incised in the midline to expose the posterior aspect of the rectum. Proximal dissection is carried along the presacral fascia posteriorly and laterally all the way posterior to the prostate gland. The fascia propria of the rectum is incised, and the mesorectum is divided to the rectal wall that is opened transversely and the lesion is excised. With transsphincteric approach, the sphincter complex is divided, and the cut edges are marked with sutures for precise repair.

Transanal Local Excision (TLE)

Parks' per anal excision [15] [transanal local excision (TLE)] describes excision of tumors under direct visualization through the anal orifice. The

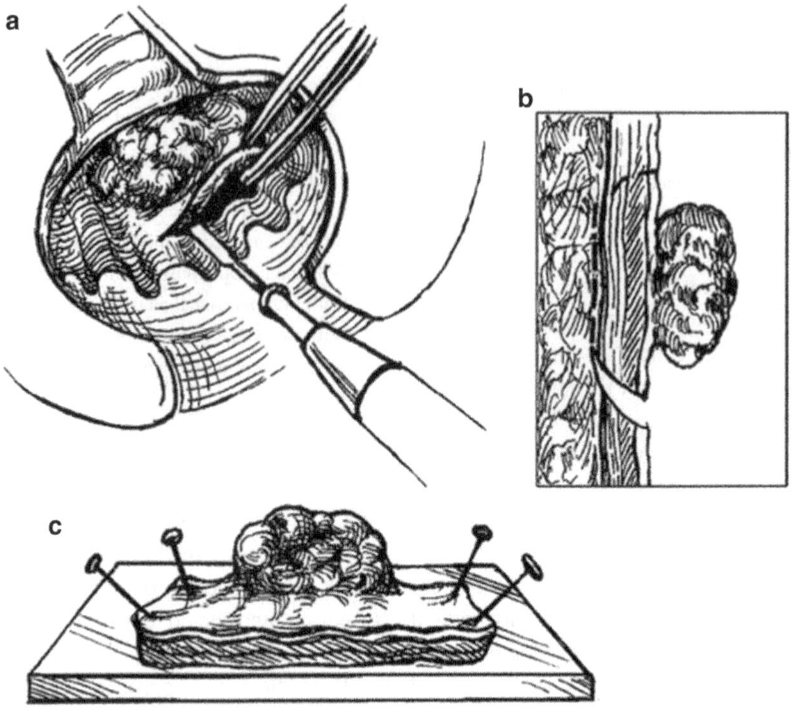

Fig. 17.1 Depiction of transanal local excision (TLE) (Reprinted from Beck et al. [186]. With permission from Springer Verlag)

procedure is limited to small tumors (<3–4 cm or <30 % of the circumference of the rectal lumen) that are not fixed to the levator muscle.

The procedure is performed under general or spinal and local anesthesia (Fig. 17.1). The patient is place in a jackknife position or on stirrups depending on the location of the tumor. Using various retractors, the lesion is assessed, and the tissues surrounding the tumor are infiltrated with epinephrine-containing solution. Traction sutures may be applied at the lateral or superior edge of the tumor to help prolapse the lesion. The lesion is excised with the Bovie cautery to include a 1 cm circumferential mucosal margin and deep into the perirectal fat (full thickness disc excision). The surgical specimen is oriented for the pathologist. The resulting defect is closed transversely with simple interrupted sutures. For anterior lesions, care must be taken not to injure the vagina. Excision using endoscopic linear stapler-cutter does not reliably excise the full thickness of bowel wall. Morbidity of TLE is minimal and usually related to bleeding or urinary retention.

Transanal Endoscopic Microsurgery (TEM)

Transanal endoscopic microsurgery (TEM) describes transanal local excision using specialized equipment that allows for clear and magnified visualization of the rectal lumen and facilitates dissection and removal of larger lesions located higher up in the rectum that are not amenable to be removed by TLE (up to 20 cm from the anal verge) [25, 26] (Fig. 17.2). Compared to TLE, TEM allows exploration of perirectal fat and regional LN basin, provides superior quality of resection, prevents fragmentation of the specimen, and minimizes margin positivity [27]. The tumor is excised, and

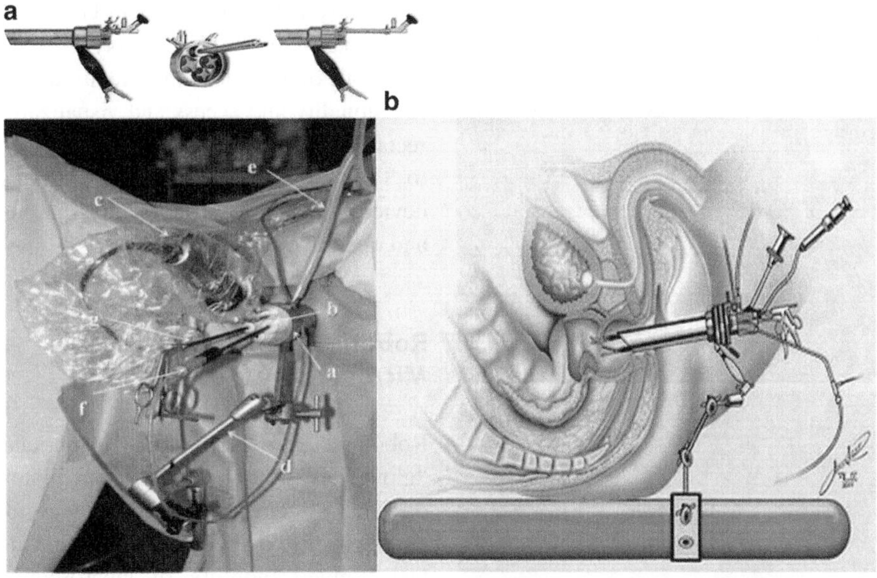

Fig. 17.2 (**a**, **b**) Depiction of surgical equipments and technique of transanal endoscopic microsurgery (TEM) (A: Reprinted from Allaix [185]. With permission from Springer Verlag) (B: Reprinted from Kosinski et al. [184]. With permission from John Wiley & Sons, Inc)

dissection is performed with a spatula, hook, or needle point tip monopolar cautery. A 0.5–1 cm margin with pyramidal volumetric excision of perirectal fat for possible retrieval of regional LN is performed.

Initially, TEM was considered inappropriate for advanced neoplastic lesions and lesions beyond the peritoneal reflection for risk of peritoneal breach and contamination. However, repair of the defect prevents conversion to an open procedure and is not associated with major complication or oncological compromise [28–30]. With larger and more locally advanced lesions, segmental resection with end-to-end anastomosis has been described [31–33].

TEM was developed in early 1980s in Tubingen, Germany, by Dr. Gerald Buess in collaboration with the Richard Wolf Medical Instruments company [25, 26]. The equipment for TEM is prepackaged and includes all that is necessary to perform the surgery: operating proctoscope (4 cm diameter, 12–20 mm long, beveled or straight end, and removable faceplate), angled camera that provides a 3-dimensional stereoscopic vision, and carbon dioxide insufflator. A faceplate with clear window is attached for initial insertion and positioning of the proctoscope over the tumor and then replaced with another faceplate for carrying out the procedure. The faceplate is airtight and has four ports sealed by capped rubber/silastic sleeves and accommodates 3 flexible channels [2 working instruments (5 mm long handle instruments for dissection, excision, and suturing) and one suction irrigation instrument] and one optical stereoscope (binocular eyepiece that provides precise 3-dimentional view of the operative field with up to sixfold magnification). At least 3 mm negative deep and mucosal margins are required. After excision of the lesion, the defect is closed, but for the extraperitoneal rectum, the defect may be left opened.

TEM has been used with other techniques to widen the extent of resection. TEM excision of lower third T1 rectal cancer with mesorectal excision using dorsoposterior extraperitoneal pelviscopy has been described [34, 35]. Also TEM excision of the primary tumor and a two-stage TME have been described as sphincter-saving procedures for locally advanced ultralow rectal cancer after neoCRT [36]. However, long-term

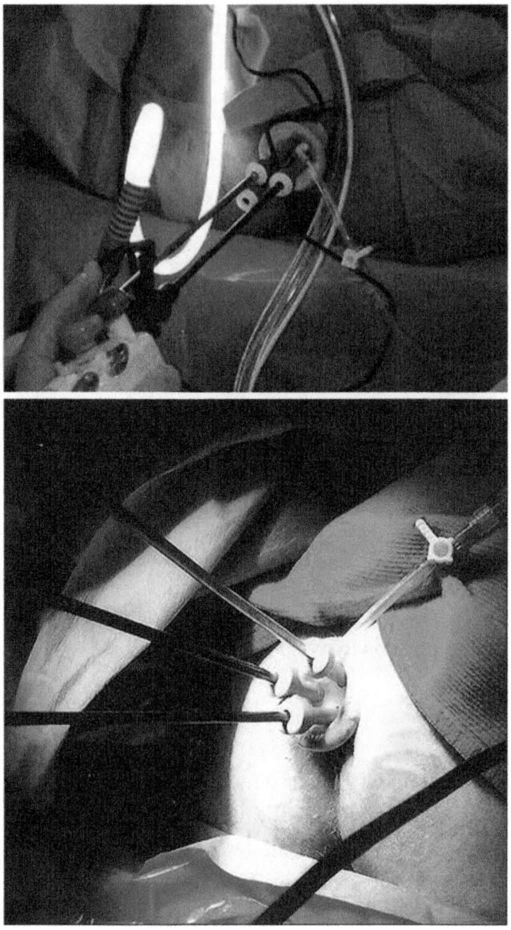

Fig. 17.3 Transanal minimally invasive surgery (TAMIS) (Reprinted from Atallah et al. [39]. With permission from Springer Verlag)

oncologic outcome from such a procedure is not known, and the approach is not widely accepted.

TEM is widely accepted in Europe but is used only in select centers in the United States. The equipment is expensive, and the procedure is technically challenging requiring a long learning curve [37].

Transanal Minimally Invasive Surgery (TAMIS)

Transanal minimally invasive surgery (TMIS) describes transanal excision of rectal tumors using laparoscopic instruments, traditional insufflation device, and a platform adapted from laparoscopic single-port device (Fig. 17.3). It is essentially a hybrid between TEM and single-port laparoscopy. A 5 mm port for the assistant and a flexible endoscope are used to improve functionality and access and visualization of the rectal lumen as high as 15 cm [38–40]. Compared to TEM, the equipment is less expensive, the device is easier to place, setup time is quicker, and operative time is faster [41].

Robotic Transanal Endoscopic Microsurgery (Robotic-TEM)

Robotic-TEM describes TEM using customized "glove port" fitted to circular anal dilator and the da Vinci system that allows maneuverability in deep spaces to overcome some technical difficulties (limited mobility of laparoscopic instruments) with TEM and TAMIS [41–44] (Fig. 17.4). Furthermore, an experienced camera operator is not required. Compared to TEM, the learning curve is shorter [37].

Selection Criteria for Local Excision of Rectal Adenocarcinoma

Surgical treatment of rectal cancer depends on the location of the tumor. Cancers of the upper rectum behave like colon cancer and are treated with anterior resection. Middle and distal third cancers are treated with low anterior resection and mesorectal excision with or without reconstruction or AP resection for lesions too distal to permit an anterior resection. Select cases of rectal cancer, especially distal rectal cancer, may be treated with local excision with or without adjuvant therapy. Thus, the discussion of local treatment of rectal cancer is primarily focused on distal rectal tumors.

Selecting patients for local excision is based on patient factors, location, and clinical stage of the tumor as determined by a digital rectal examination (DRE) and endoscopy, staging radiological studies, and endoscopic biopsies and at the time of excisional biopsy results. The ideal candidates for "curative" local excision are those whose tumors are confined to the rectal wall, more likely to be free of LN involvement and less likely to locally

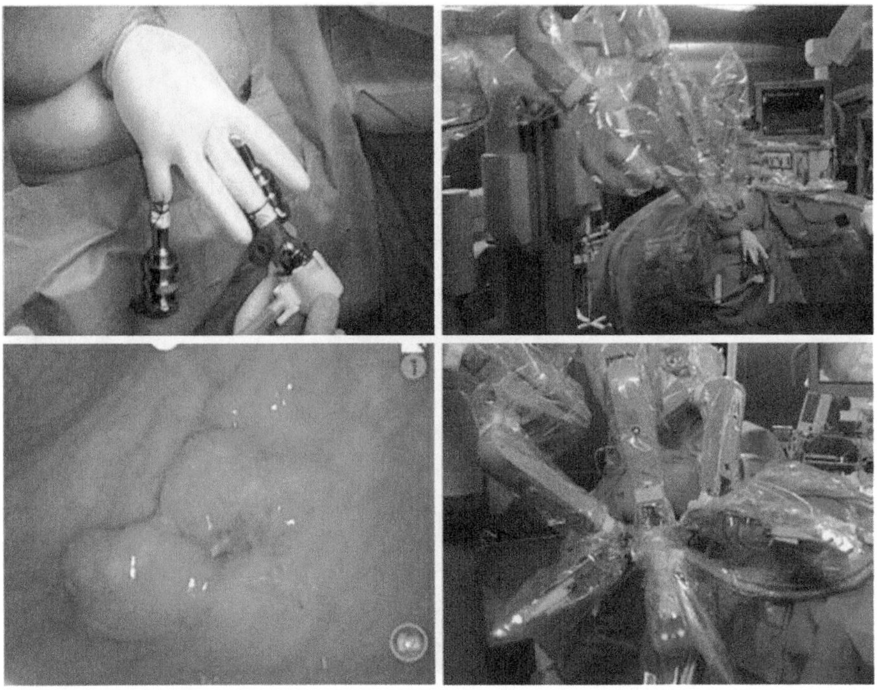

Fig. 17.4 Robotic transanal endoscopic microsurgery (Robotic-TEM) (Reprinted from Valls [183]. With permission from Springer Verlag)

recur. These strict clinical criteria, however, remain imperfect, and surgeons therefore must be vigilant in their follow-up of these patients.

Examination

The initial assessment of the patient includes a history and physical examination, a DRE, and a proctoscopic examination. The patient's medical conditions (comorbidities), physical limitations, and anal control are assessed. On DRE, the size, morphology, location, and mobility of the tumor and its distance from the anal verge are assessed. On proctoscopy, characteristics of the tumor such as its gross appearance, whether it is ulcerated or polypoid; its dimensions; its distance from the anal verge or dentate line; and its relationship to anatomical luminal landmarks are determined as well as a tissue biopsy for diagnosis is obtained.

Tumor size predicts LR and LN involvement. The risk of LN involvement is 29 % for lesions <2 cm, 17–31 % for lesions <3 cm, and 43–50 % for lesions <4 cm [45–47]. In a recent study, tumor size with a threshold of 34 mm has been suggested to complement clinical staging of patients with rectal cancer [48]

Ulcerated lesions are associated with a greater failure rate and increased risk for LN involvement when compared to polypoid lesions, 49 % versus 11 % [45, 48, 49] (Fig. 17.5). It is advisable that patients with such a characteristic and without contraindication are best considered for radical surgery.

Radiological Studies

Endorectal Ultrasound (ERUS)

ERUS has the ability to delineate the layers of rectal wall and identifies enlarged regional LN. Based on the depth of invasion and LN involvement, the tumor is classified into uT0 to uT4 and uN0 or uN1 (Table 17.3) [50].

The accuracy of ERUS is operator dependent and varies with pathological stage of the primary tumor and quality of the scanner used (length of the probe, 7 vs. 10 MHz, and resolution). It is superior

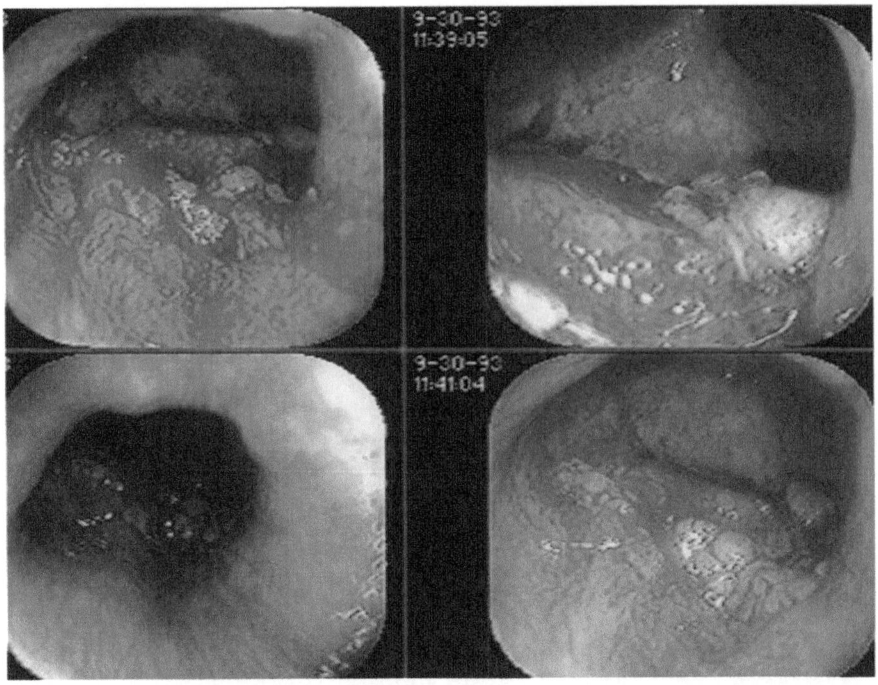

Fig. 17.5 *Small distal rectal lesions not amenable to local rectal excision*. Ulcerated, bleeding small distal rectal cancer should undergo radical surgery due to a greater failure rate and risk of lymph node involvement

Table 17.3 Ultrasound staging of rectal adenocarcinoma

uT0 – tumor confined to the mucosa
uT1 – tumor confined to the mucosa and submucosa
uT2 – tumor penetrates into but not through the muscularis propria
uT3 – tumor extends into the perirectal fat
uT4 – tumor extends into the adjacent structure
uN0-N1 – absence or presence of suspicious metastatic LN

to conventional CT scan and MRI in detecting LN. ERUS does not determine whether the enlarged LN is inflammatory or neoplastic and does not assess the involvement of the mesorectum or the mesorectal envelope. Unlike the 2-D ERUS, 3-D ERUS has the ability to demonstrate spatial relationship of the tumor in the transverse, sagittal, and coronal planes and determine distance to anal sphincter and is better at differentiating LN from blood vessels [51, 52]. Compared to 2-D ERUS, the accuracy of 3-D ERUS for T stage is 85–91 % versus 83–90 % and for N stage is 76–88 % versus 67–83 % respectively [51–55].

Magnetic Resonance Imaging (MRI)

MRI is more accurate than CT scan at assessing the circumferential radial margin (CRM). With the use of the endorectal coil (EMRI), the accuracy of MRI approaches that of ERUS. The accuracy of EMRI for T and N staging is 85 % and 82 %, respectively, compared to 87 % and 74 %, respectively for ERUS. When compared to CT scans, the accuracy of EMRI for T and N staging is 82 % and 74 %, respectively, and 73 % and 66 % for CT scan [56–60]. However, the wide use of MRI is prohibitive in many centers because of its high cost.

Since up to 50 % of positive LNs in the mesorectum are <1 cm in size, LN staging by size criterion alone is inaccurate and understages the cancer. Spiculated or indistinct border and a mottled heterogeneous appearance are new criteria used to increase the accuracy of predicting LN involvement [61]. The 3 tesla MRI accurately predicts tumor depth and CRM involvement as well as reliably stages the LNs by morphologically evaluating it and the blood vessels within the mesorectum [62–64]. Regardless of the imaging modality being used, accurate staging remains imperfect. This may partly explain the sobering recurrence rate of 10–29 % for T1 and 26–47 % for T2 cancers following local excision [65–67].

Computerized Tomography Scan (CT Scan)

CT scan is useful in detecting distant metastasis and tumor extension into adjacent organs, but it is inadequate for T staging of ESRC since it does not delineate the layers of the rectal wall. Additionally, CT scan is limited in its ability to detect regional LN. The accuracy for T staging is 46–75 % and for LN staging is 56–72 % [58, 68].

Positron Emission Tomography Scan (PET Scan)

PET scan can help detect locoregional and distant spread and has been used to determine response to chemoradiation therapy (CRT) in patients with advanced rectal cancer. Its role in staging the cancer preoperatively is yet to be determined, although some studies have shown that PET scan alters management in up to a third of patients.

Histopathological Features of the Primary Tumor

The histopathological features of the primary tumor are helpful in selecting patients who may be candidates for local excision. Such features are determined from endoscopic biopsies or after complete removal of the tumor (Table 17.4). These features are discussed in details in the following section, and recommendations assumed that the patient is a surgical candidate for cure. Of note, the decision for definitive operation is easily made when many or all of the histological features are available from the initial biopsy. However, in situations where some or all of the features are known only after a definitive local rectal excision has been performed, the surgeon must consider counseling the patient to undergo a definitive operation within a thirty-day window period [69].

Table 17.4 Histopathological features important in selecting patients for local excision of rectal adenocarcinoma

Histological type
Grade
Depth of invasion
Presence or absence of
Blood vessel invasion
Perineural invasion
Angiolymphatic invasion
Lymphocytic infiltration
Increased tumor infiltration with lymphocytes
Extramural lymphocytosis
Infiltration in the stroma in the region of tumor and lymphoid nodules often in the region of the tumor edge
Infiltration at the edge of the muscularis propria analogous to Crohn's Disease
Budding at edge of tumor
Surgery-related factors:
Completeness of excision
Fragmentation

Table 17.5 Histologic classification of rectal cancer

Adenocarcinoma
Mucinous adenocarcinoma (>50 % mucinous)
Signet cell adenocarcinoma (>50 % signet cell)
Small cell (oat cell) carcinoma
Squamous cell carcinoma (epidermoid)
Adenosquamous carcinoma
Medullary carcinoma
Undifferentiated carcinoma
Others (e.g., papillary carcinoma)

Tumor Type

The World Health Organization (WHO) classification of rectal cancer is depicted in Table 17.5 with the most common carcinoma being adenocarcinoma [70].

Tumor type is not an independent prognostic factor, except for signet cell and small cell carcinomas. Small cell carcinoma is a high-grade carcinoma with neuroendocrine differentiation that presents with higher stage and has dismal prognosis even with early lesions than non-signet cell carcinomas [71–73]. Local rectal excision must not be performed with these histologies.

Grade

The College of American Pathologists recommends a two-tier classification scheme of rectal cancer: low-grade (well-differentiated and moderately differentiated) and high-grade (poorly differentiated and undifferentiated) carcinomas [74]. Grade of the tumor is a stage-independent prognostic factor with high-grade predicting LN metastasis and adverse outcome [74–77].

Lymph node involvement in well-differentiated to moderately differentiated adenocarcinomas is 0–30 % compared to 50–69 % for poorly differentiated carcinomas [74, 78]. Lymph node involvement is <10 % for T2 well-differentiated adenocarcinoma without adverse histological features compared to 70 % for poorly differentiated with lymphovascular invasion [79]. Thus, patients with high-grade histology are not candidates for local excision.

Depth of Tumor Invasion

The primary tumor in rectal cancer is classified into Tx to T4 depending on the depth of invasion into the rectal wall (Table 17.6) [71]. On occasion, a malignant polyp is found following a routine lower endoscopic examination. T1 malignant polyps are further classified into substages depending on the extent of invasion into the polyp (Haggitt classification) [80] (Fig. 17.6) or into the submucosa (Kikuchi classification) [81] (Fig. 17.7). The Haggitt classification applies mainly for pedunculated polyps with levels of invasion ranging from 0 to 4. The Haggitt classification is as follows: level 0, carcinoma in situ; level 1, invasion of the submucosa but limited to the head of the polyp; level 2, invasion extending into the neck of the polyp; level 3, invasion into any part of the stalk; and level 4, invasion beyond the stalk but above the muscularis propria. By definition, sessile polyps are classified as Haggitt level 4. However, not all sessile polyps behave the same. Because Haggitt classification does not take this into account, the Kikuchi classification of sessile polyp becomes a useful tool to further identify patients who are candidate for local excision. Essentially, Kikuchi classification divides the submucosa layer into thirds, Sm1 through Sm3.

Table 17.6 T staging of colorectal adenocarcinoma

Tx = primary tumor cannot be assessed
T0 = no evidence of primary
Tis = carcinoma in situ (intraepithelial invasion of the lamina propria or muscularis mucosae)
High-grade dysplasia = no stromal invasion
Intramucosal carcinoma = stromal invasion identified
T1 = tumor invades into the submucosa
T2 = tumor invades into the muscularis propria
T3 = tumor invades through the muscularis propria into the subserosa or into nonperitonealized pericolic or perirectal fat (pT3a-3d)
T4 = tumor directly invading other organs or structure T4a or perforates the visceral peritoneum T4b

The risk of LN involvement is related to T stage. Carcinoma in situ is not a "true carcinoma" and has no risk of LN metastasis; patients with carcinoma in situ only require wide excision with a negative margin. The risk of LN involvement based on T stage is as follows: T1 = 5–25 %, T2 = 20–28 %, T3 = 36–67 %, and T4 = 53 % [78, 82–89]. The risk of LN metastasis is <1 % for Haggitt levels 1–3 and 12–25 % for level 4 [80, 86, 87, 90]. The depth of the submucosal invasion is related to LN metastasis with none found if invasion is less than 1,075 μm [91, 92]. For pedunculated polyps, LN metastasis is zero for invasive cancer confined to the head and neck and for those where the stalk invasion is less than 3,000 μm without evidence of lymphatic invasion [92, 93]. Lymph node metastasis increases with Kikuchi level: 1–3 % for Sm1, 8 % for Sm2, and 23 % for Sm3 [81, 87, 94].

Angiolymphatic Invasion

Lymphatic invasion is associated with increased regional LN metastasis particularly with pT1 and superficial pT2 lesions [39, 80, 95–100]. Invasion of extramural large vessel in the perirectal fat and outside the muscularis propria is associated with a predisposition for hepatic metastasis. Angiolymphatic invasion is a stage-independent prognostic factor and identifies patients at increased risk for LN metastasis and diverse outcome [76, 101, 102]. Patients with angiolymphatic invasion are not candidates or local excision.

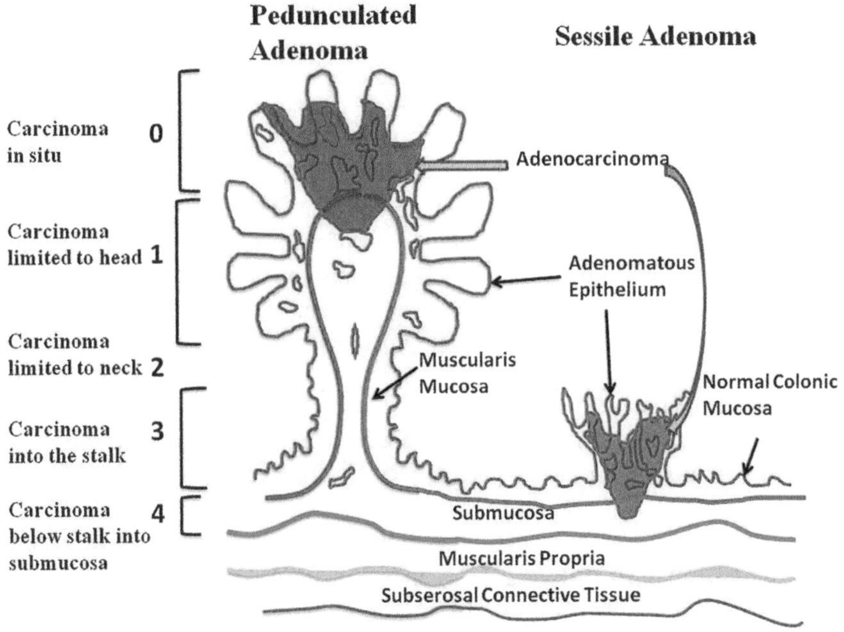

Fig. 17.6 *Haggitt classification*. Level 0, carcinoma in situ; level 1, invasion of the submucosa but limited to the head of the polyp; level 2, invasion extending into the neck of the polyp; level 3, invasion into any part of the stalk; and level 4, invasion beyond the stalk but above the muscularis propria (Courtesy of Quyen D. Chu, MD, MBA, FACS)

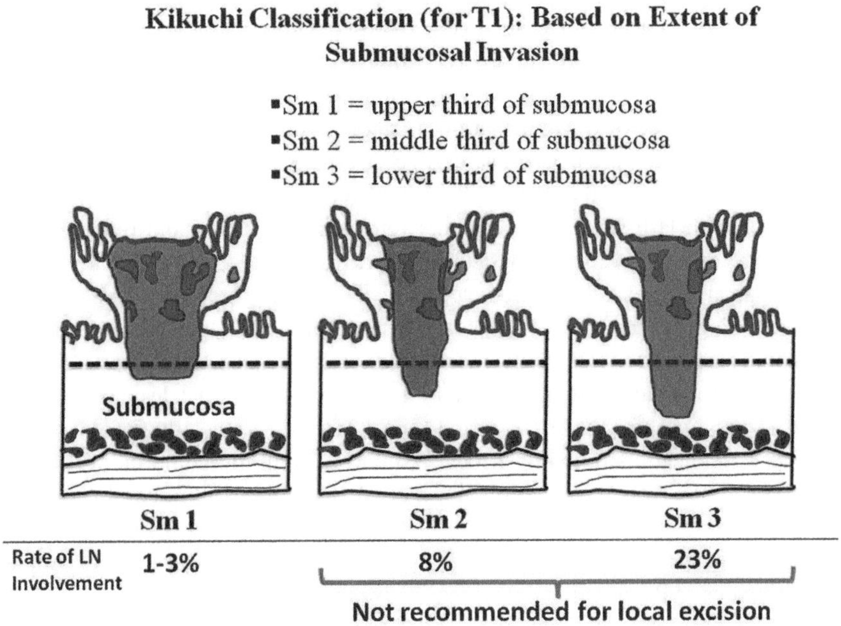

Fig. 17.7 *Kikuchi levels*. Sm1, invasion of superficial third of the submucosa; Sm2, invasion of middle third of the submucosa; and Sm3, invasion of deep third of the submucosa (Courtesy of Quyen D. Chu, MD, MBA, FACS)

Neural Invasion

Perineural invasion identifies rectal carcinomas that are at increased risk for LN metastasis and worse prognosis [97, 101–103]. Local excision is contraindicated for those with neural invasion.

Tumor Budding

This refers to microscopic clusters of undifferentiated cancer cells located ahead of the invasive front of a well-differentiated to moderately differentiated tumor. It has greater prognostic value than overall grade and predicts regional LN metastasis in APR specimens of T1 and superficial T2 rectal cancers [97, 104]. Patients with this feature are not considered for local rectal excision.

Host Lymphoid Response to Tumor

Lymphoid infiltration of tumor or peritumoral tissue is indicative of host immunologic response to invasive malignancy and is associated with microsatellite instability and favorable prognosis [105, 106]. This favorable feature is not a contraindication for local rectal excision.

LN Involvement

Perirectal LNs include mesorectal, lateral sacral, presacral, sacral promontory, and superior, middle, and inferior rectal LNs. None of these LNs are included in TLE but may be included in the TEM or TAMIS. The absence of LN in the surgical specimen limits their predictive value. Perhaps this partly explains [107] the higher recurrence rate seen with TLE when compared to TEM. The presence of LN metastasis is determined on radiological studies and is predicted based on histopathological features of the primary tumor. A high suspicion of LN involvement as determined on preoperative imaging (i.e., ERUS, MRI, CT) must prompt the surgeon and patient to consider a radical operation over local rectal excision.

Surgery-Related Factors

Following anterior or AP resection, margins assessed are proximal, distal, transverse, and circumferential. After local excision, margins assessed are lateral (circumferential around the tumor) and deep. Surgical margins involved by tumor, either microscopically or grossly, are indicative of residual tumor within the operative field, which predispose the patient to having LR. Piecemeal excision (fragmented excision) is an adverse prognostic factor resulting in a higher proportion of local failures [108]. Thus, patients with positive margins after local rectal excision or those whose tumors underwent piecemeal excision must be considered for definitive radical operation.

Candidates (Patient/Tumor) for Local Excision

Local excision is an attractive treatment option since it preserves rectal function, is associated with rapid recovery, low morbidity, and mortality, and does not result in the need for a colostomy. The operation, however, is controversial since there is lack of level I/level II evidence supporting its oncologic equivalency with standard radical surgery [18, 109]. As an aside, prospective clinical trials are classified as being phase I, II, or III. Phase III trials compare new treatments with the best currently available treatment (i.e., the standard treatment) and are considered the highest level of evidence to guide treatment decision. In the literature on local excision of rectal cancer, although there are a number of phase II trials, there are no phase III trials.

Breen et al. [110] summarized the results of retrospective studies and reported a local recurrence (LR) rate of 0–33 % for ERC following local excision. Yet, local excision has been on the rise despite poor locoregional control with and without adjuvant CRT therapy [18, 66, 111, 112]. Local excision of T2 lesions has tripled in the past 25 years, especially for elderly patients who often have multiple comorbidites [18]. Stitzenberg et al. recently confirmed this trend using the National Cancer Data Base [111]. There is also an increasing rate of local excision in patients with advanced rectal cancer who develop complete response after neoCRT where the risk of occult LN is reportedly to be as low as 3–6 % [113–116]. Surgeons must be aware of the limitations of the current available data and be cautious when selecting patients for local rectal excision. When selecting local excision, patient and tumor factors must be considered, and clinical and radiological staging of local tumor is the most important aspect of the selection.

Patient Factors

Patients with anal incontinence and poor mobility are not candidates for a sphincter-saving procedure. On the other hand, those who are unfit or refuse to undergo major abdominal surgery, even with advance disease such as those with ≥T3 or ≥N1, may be considered for local excision for symptomatic relief (bleeding and discharge) [117]. Local excision is also an attractive alternative to radical surgery in patients with recurrent cancer for whom a major operation is prohibitive. This is especially applicable to elderly patients with multiple comorbidities [118].

Tumor Factors

Local excision is restricted to tumors that are confined to but do not involve full thickness rectal wall (T2 or less) or regional LN and have favorable histopathological features. Classically, tumors that are polypoid and not ulcerated, located with proximal margin <10 cm from the anal verge, appeared <3–4 cm in size, encompassed <30 % of luminal circumference of the rectum, and not fixed to the sphincter or puborectalis muscle may be considered for local excision. Conversely, local excision is not appropriate for:

- Large lesions encompassing >40 % of rectal circumference, since local excision can lead to a loss of rectal volume and/or stricture formation resulting in poor function
- Proximal anterior or lateral lesions since excision is associated with a risk of peritoneal contamination and potential tumor dissemination
- Stage III cancer since local excision does not adequately address the LN and nodal involvement is substantial high in this population

However, there is no conclusive evidence that size is a limiting factor in the selection criteria for local excision. A more suitable criterion is the ability to achieve an adequate tumor-free margin. It is thought that adjuvant therapy may improve LR rates after local excision, although these highly selected results are based on uncontrolled studies (i.e., retrospective studies). Reduction in tumor size after neoadjuvant therapy is found to be a reliable prognostic factor of success of local excision [109, 119]. Again, such data are limited due to their retrospective nature. TEM, TAMIS, and Robotic-TEM do not only facilitate the resection of more proximal, larger, and locally advanced lesions but allow for more complex excision/resection. With the advent of effective neoCRT that results in significant or complete response of locally advanced rectal cancer, the use of such modality along with local excision has been on the rise [113, 115, 116, 120, 121]. Whether such a practice yields oncologic equivalence with standard radical resection remains a controversial topic.

As mentioned in the previous section, factors that affect recurrence rate and outcome after local excision of rectal adenocarcinoma include T stage, degree of differentiation, lymphovascular invasion, and positivity of resection margins [67, 78, 94, 109, 122–126]. Local recurrence for ERC, especially those with adverse histopathological features, i.e., high-risk early ERC [poorly differentiated and mucinous adenocarcinoma, signet ring and undifferentiated adenocarcinomas, lymphovascular invasion (absence of lymphoid infiltration and tumor budding are relative factors)], is higher than previously reported [66, 127]. More importantly, the risk of leaving behind nodal disease after local excision of a T2 lesion with adverse histopathological features is 70 % compared to 10 % for T2 with no adverse histopathological features [101, 128].

Hence, local excision alone is ideal for incidental adenocarcinoma following polypectomy, especially for sessile polyp that was incidentally removed and found to have involved margins. It is ideal for Haggitt 1–3 or Kikuchi Sm1 T1 with favorable histological features and T1 lesions that have no adverse features and clear margin.

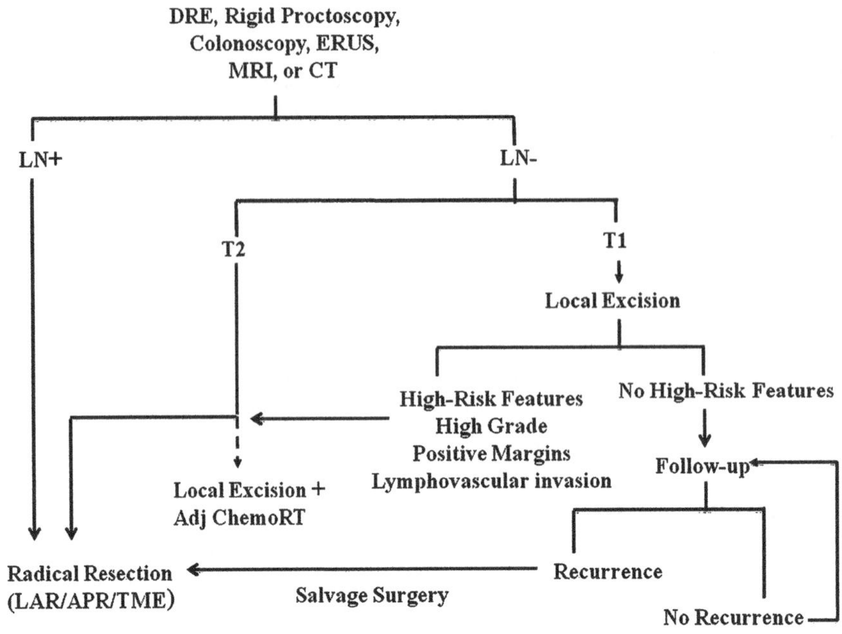

Fig. 17.8 Algorithm for evaluating small distal rectal cancer

Local excision alone is controversial for Kikuchi Sm2 T1N0 and T2N0.

The following situations require further treatment after local excision:

- Positive margins or inadequate tissue for accurate pathological staging histological: patient can be considered for re-excision or proceed with radical surgery.
- Radical resection for:
  - T1 with unfavorable histological features
  - For T1 Kikuchi Sm3 where risk of LN metastasis mirrors T2
  - T2
  - T3 lesions because of high LR rate
- Adjuvant therapy has been considered for the following patient population, although radical surgery should seriously be considered:
  - T1 with unfavorable histopathological features
  - T2
  - Higher-risk patient not amenable to more radical surgery

An algorithm for evaluating patients with distal rectal cancer is depicted in Fig. 17.8.

Outcome of Local Excision of Rectal Adenocarcinoma

Transanal Local Excision (TLE)

There is great variation in the oncological results following TLE that is mostly related to the number of patients included in the study, patient selection for TLE, and follow-up period after TLE [109]. With short-term follow-up, local excision is associated with a favorable outcome, 10–13 % LR [18, 66, 77, 82, 83, 110, 112, 129]. With long-term follow-up, however, the risk of LR is higher 15–30 %, 12–18 % for T1 and 28–47 % for T2, and recent studies have shown even higher recurrence rate [65–67, 130–135]. The pattern of first recurrence is predominantly local, 50 % LR only, 18 % local and distant, and 32 % distant [66, 130]. Local recurrence after local excision develops quickly, whereas distal recurrence is delayed [67]. The overall recurrence (local + systemic) is higher with TLE compared to radical resection, 21 % versus 0% for T1 and 47 % versus 16 % for

T2 [65, 131, 132]. With radical resection, failure is mostly distal with LR occurring in 6–10 % [136, 137].

Bhangu et al. [138] reported the survival outcome of TLE (n=7,378) versus radical resection (n=36,116) of colon and rectal cancer in a Surveillance, Epidemiology, and End Results (SEER)-based study in 2013. Cancer survival rates for carcinoma in situ and T1 rectal cancer were not significantly different but reduced for T2 rectal cancer. In a nationwide cohort study from the National Cancer Data Base, 2124 patients with T1 and T2 diagnosed with rectal cancer between 1994 and 1996 were treated with TLE (n=765) and standard surgery (n=1,359) [18]. The 5-year LR rate in the TLE group was 12.5 % for T1 and 22.1 % for T2 compared to 6.9 % for T1 and 15.1 % for T2 in the standard surgery group. The 5-year OS rate in the TLE group was 77.4 % for T1 and 67.6 % for T2 compared to 69 % for T1 and 76.5 % for T2 in the standard surgery group. For ERC with favorable histology, low LR and high 5-year OS rate approaching 100 % are possible [18, 133, 139]. Since about half of the recurrences are locoregional, radical resection may be curative. However, there is limited data on salvage surgery [65, 133]. Few patients can be treated successfully, at the first clinical recurrence, but the actuarial survival after salvage surgery for LR is low (30–50 %% at 5 years) [65, 66]. In a retrospective study of 155 patients, Baron et al. reported definite survival advantage with immediate radical surgery. The 5-year DFS was 94 % compared to 55 % for delayed salvage [140].

Transanal Local Excision and Adjuvant Therapy

Since LR in patients with T2 cancers treated with TLE is high, it is thought that adjuvant therapy may reduce the risk of recurrence. Minsky [141] noted that with local excision and postoperative RT, local failure was 3 % for T1, 10 % for T2, and 24 % for T3. Fortunato et al. [142] reported less favorable outcome in 21 patients (mostly T2 lesions) with 19 % LR that occurred up to 48 months following resection and 19 % of patients developing distant metastasis; the 5-year DFS was 59 %. Paty et al. [66] noted that RT delayed LR (median 2.1 years vs. 1.1 years for LE only), but overall rates of local and overall recurrence and survival rates were similar to patients not receiving RT. Thus, postoperative RT had no impact on recurrences.

In a phase II multi-institutional trial of TLE or TLE + adjuvant CRT, the overall recurrence rate at 3 years for T1 or T2 was 4 % [143]. In another prospective study of patients with T1 treated with TLE and T2 with TLE and adjuvant CRT, no T2 patient recurred [144]. In an initial prospective phase II study by the Radiation Therapy Oncology Group, low-grade T1 tumors with negative margins were observed, and CRT or RT was administered based on post-excision results. Local recurrence rates were 7 %, 8 %, and 23 % for T1, T2, and T3 tumors, respectively [145]. Recent data suggest that the recurrence rate for T1, especially those with unfavorable histopathological features, was high and that neoCRT may be administered to sterilize the regional LN, especially when further surgery is not contemplated [128, 139, 146]. The results of other studies are depicted in Table 17.7.

TEM and TAMIS

There is a paucity of well-designed studies comparing TLE to TEM, but TEM is superior in terms of visualizing and resecting more proximal lesions and may have better oncologic outcome [147]. Moore et al., in a systematic review of all TEM over 22 years (including 55 case series and 3 comparative studies), noted that TEM is superior to Park's per anal excision with a 6 % local recurrence rate for TME versus 22 % for Park's; TEM was more likely to yield negative margins (90 % vs. 71 %) and non-fragmented specimen (94 % vs. 65 %) [148]. Compared to radical surgery, TEM has significantly shorter operating time, lower blood loss, shorter hospital stay, and lower perioperative analgesia requirement [26, 27, 149]. Early and late complications of TEM patients are similar or lower than those undergoing

Table 17.7 Studies evaluating outcome of transanal local excision with and without adjuvant therapy

Study	Treatment	Local recurrence
CALBG [182]	T1 = TLE (n = 59)	T1 = 7 %
	T2 = TLE (n = 51)	T2 = 14 %
	T1 and T2	6-year OS = 85 %
		6-year DFS = 78 %
MEDLINE database		
Retrospective review, 41 studies [109]	TLE	T1 = 9.7 % (0–24 %)
		T2 = 25 % (0–67 %)
		T3 = 38 % (0–100 %)
	TLE + adjuvant CRT	T1 = 9.5 % (0–50 %)
		T2 = 16.6 % (0–24 %)
		T3 = 18.8 % (0–50 %)
National Cancer Data Base [18]	TLE:	
	T1 (*n* = 601)	12.5 %
	T2 (*n* = 164)	22.1 %
	Standard surgery:	
	T1 (*n* = 493)	6.9 %
	T2 (*n* = 866)	15.1 %

CALGB Cancer and Leukemia Group B, *CRT* chemoradiation therapy, *DFS* disease-free survival, *OS* overall survival, *TLE* transanal local excision

open radical surgery [149–151]. Complication rate is low <10 % (ranges from 6 % to 31 %) and complications are minor [26, 27, 152–156]. Perioperative complications that require converting to laparotomy are hemorrhage and peritoneal entry. However, primary repair of the peritoneal entry can prevent the need to convert to open procedure and is not associated with major complications or oncological compromise [28, 29].

It should be noted that evidence to support TEM is based on case series and retrospective studies, which mostly focused on the technical aspect of the procedure, individual selection criteria, and its value in comparison with TLE and radical resection rather than on its oncologic impact.

T1N0

For T1 cancer, local failure of 0–13 % has been reported with TEM [99, 100, 153, 154, 157]. However, Doornebosch and colleagues, in a systematic review of T1 lesions treated with TEM, noted LR varied between 4 % and 33 % [156]. In a series of 88 patients who underwent TEM for T1 rectal cancer, 18 patients (20.5 %) had LR [158]. Local recurrence rates depend on margin positivity, tumor grade, status of lymphovascular invasion, and muscle penetration (T2) [122–126]. The recurrence rate for low-risk T1 is 6 % and for high-risk T1 is 39 %, and immediate operation for high-risk T1 lesions results in a reduction of LR to 6 % [126].

Carefully selected patients have excellent survival, low recurrence rate, and outcomes comparable to radical resection [149, 159–162]. Lee and colleagues retrospectively compared the outcomes of 74 patients with TEM to 100 patients with radical surgery [162]. For T1 cancer, there was no difference in 5-year recurrence or survival between the two groups, but for T2 lesions, there was a higher recurrence rate for the TEM group, although OS was similar for both. In a systematic review of 55 case series, one randomized study and two nonrandomized comparative studies, Middleton et al. noted there was no difference in the recurrence or survival rates or complication rates between TEM and radical resection [27]. In a meta-analysis of 5 studies (one prospective and 4 retrospective, nonrandomized; total of 397; T1 rectal cancer), Wu et al. [163] noted that patients with T1 cancer who received TEM ($n=216$) had higher rates of local or distant metastasis at 40 months' follow-up but with no significant difference in the 5-year OS rate compared to patients receiving radical surgery ($n=181$). In another meta-analysis of 11 studies (three randomized controlled, one prospective, 7 retrospective; total of 1,191 patients; T1 and T2) in which 514 patients received TEM, 386 TAE, and 291 standard resection, Sgourakis et al. found that for T1 tumors, local and overall recurrence rates were significantly higher for TEMS versus standard surgery, but there was no significant difference in the distant metastasis rate or OS rate between the groups [164].

The outcome of salvage surgery depends on the timing of surgery. Baatrup et al. reported the outcome of 143 consecutive individuals (multicenter study) treated with TEM for rectal cancer, curative in 43 % and palliative in 5 % [165]. Immediate reoperation was performed in 15 % of cases. Cancer-specific survival for T1 was 94 % [165]. In a series of 88 patients who underwent TEM for T1 rectal cancer, 18 patients developed local recurrence, and of those, 16 underwent salvage surgery with a 3-year OS rate of 31 % and cancer-related survival of 58 % [156].

T2N0

The LR rate of T2 with TEM alone is unacceptably high at ≥17 % [162, 166, 167]. However, compared to radical resection, OS is similar (80.5 % vs. 83.3 %). The addition of neoCRT to downstage T2 lesion may improve results. However, several studies have shown that overall recurrence after TEM for T2 lesions with or without neoCRT or adjuvant therapy was 6–18 % [122, 128, 150, 154, 155, 157, 168].

On the other hand, in one study of 21 patients, recurrence with TEM followed by RT was 0 % compared to 50 % in those without RT [169]. In another study where 196 patients with rectal cancer with T1, T2, or T3 underwent TEM (T2 and T3 patients received neoadjuvant therapy), the overall LR rate was 4.1 % [154]. Other studies suggested equivalent results to radical resection when neoCRT was used [113, 151, 170]. Lezoche et al. recruited 70 patients with T2N0 and treated them with neoCRT and then randomized them to receive either TEM or laparoscopic surgery with total mesorectal excision. At a median follow-up of 56 months, the local failure rate and distant metastasis rate were similar (5 %), and the probability of survival was 95 % for TEM and 83 % for laparoscopic group [151]. In another prospective randomized trial, patients with clinical stage T2N0, histological grade 1–2, and tumors less than 3 cm and within 6 cm from anal verge received neoadjuvant therapy followed by TEM or laparoscopic TME [170]. Downstaging and downsizing were similar in both groups and all had R0 resection. Long-term follow-up showed that LR developed in 8 % in the TEM group and 6 % in the laparoscopic TME group and distant recurrence was 4 % in both groups. There was no difference in DFS or OS; OS rate was 75 % for TEM and 80 % for laparoscopic TME. Other data also suggest equivalent results with TEM after CRT.

The American College of Surgeons Oncology Group (ACOSG) Z6041 trial is a prospective, multicenter, single-arm, phase II trial that assesses the efficacy and safety of neoCRT and local excision for T2N0 rectal cancer [113]. A recent preliminary publication on 90 patients reports a high complete pathological response rate (44 %), a high rate of tumor downstaging (64 %), and a high negative resection margin rate (99 %). However, the complication rate was substantially high; 39 % of patients developed CRT-related grade ≥3 complications.

It should be stressed that given the current data on multimodality therapy for locally excised rectal cancer, such an approach should be considered as investigational and not standard of care.

Local Excision of Local Tumor After Major Response to CRT

It is well accepted that neoCRT improves local control of more advanced rectal cancers (T3/T4, N0/N+) and that some patients achieve complete pathological response, i.e., no residual tumor, following neoCRT. Complete pathological response after neoCRT is associated with improved outcome. In some patients, neoCRT may be curative [171]. The standard-of-care treatment for patients with T2 lesion or more advanced rectal cancer who have had a major response after CRT is radical resection. Local excision may be offered not only to patients who are unfit for surgery or refuse surgery but as an organ-preserving alternative procedure to radical resection for select patients with T2 lesion. The selected patients are those with luminal but no rectal wall or LN disease (no risk of leaving tumor behind after excision). Since there is 20–30 % discordance between clinical and pathological complete response (pCR), patient selection is based on imaging and excisional biopsy results [172, 173].

Restaging with CT or MRI has a negative predictive value for LN metastasis of 88–100 % [120]. PET/CT scan can predict early and sustained clinical response after CRT [174–176]. Endoscopic biopsies will exclude only luminal disease but not rectal wall disease [177, 178]. On the other hand, complete local excision will exclude rectal wall involvement [120]. A 0.5–1 cm margin is considered adequate, but in irradiated tumors, a wide circumferential excision is required since microscopic tumor can be found outside the ulcer boundary overlying normal mucosa in 50 % of the cases [121]. Defect closure may be performed, but dehiscence occurs in 70 % of the times, and significant symptoms (pain, tenesmus, discharge, and bleeding) are common after surgery [113, 171, 179]. The complication rate with this approach is high, 27–56 % [120].

There has been an increase in the use of local excision in patients with T2 lesion who had a major response after neoadjuvant therapy where the risk of occult LN is low (3–6 %) [113–116]. In a review of 8 studies (237 patients underwent LE after CRT), Borscht et al. [179] reported LR ranging from 6 % to 20 % for ypT2. In a prospective multicenter phase II clinical trial, Pucciarelli et al. [120] reported the results of 63 patients with clinically T3 or low-lying T2 rectal adenocarcinoma treated with neoCRT followed by local excision. Patients ($n=43$) with ypT0 or ypT1 (all with negative margins after LE) were observed, and none developed LR. Patients ($n=11$) with ypT$\geq$2 or positive margins after LE underwent TME, and none developed LR. The estimated cumulative 3-year OS rate was 91.5 %, 3-year DFS was 91 %, and local DFS was 96.9 %. Again, it should be reiterated that these modalities are investigational and have not been embraced as standard of care.

Outcomes After Salvage Surgery for Recurrence of Locally Excised Rectal Cancer

There is no prospective data reporting the outcomes of patients who had salvage surgery for recurrence of locally excised rectal cancer. Retrospective data, however, revealed that salvage surgery is not very promising. Most recurrent cancers present at a more advanced stage than the original tumor, and the salvage rate is approximately 50–59 % at best. This implies that 40–50 % of patients who otherwise would have been cured by conventional radical surgery had they undergone this at the onset will die [65, 119, 180]. These grim statistics should be put in context with the realization that radical surgery for stage I disease carries a local control rate of approximately 95 % and 5-year OS rate in excess of 90 % [181]. Additionally, the morbidity rate of salvage operation following failed local excision is also substantial at 34 %, and the surgery generally requires multivisceral organ resection that frequently leaves the patient with a permanent stoma. Finally, patients are generally treated with chemoradiation prior to salvage surgery, a treatment regimen that is unnecessary in patients with stage I disease for whom a definitive radical surgery was all that is needed.

Whether immediate salvage surgery within 30 days of the local excision could make a difference was reported by Hahnloser et al. [69]. In a review of 52 patients who underwent an APR (24 patients) or LAR (28 patients) for a cancerous polyp, positive margins, lymphovascular invasion, or T3 cancer, there was no significant difference in LR in this patient population (3 %) versus matched patients who had primary radical surgery (5 %) or those who had local excision alone (8 %). Additionally, there was no difference in the 5-year OS rate among these groups. Although encouraging, the study was small and retrospective in nature.

Summary

Patients with early distal rectal cancer are faced with difficult choices. On the one hand, standard radical operation is highly curative but potentially leaves the patient with less than quality of life (i.e., permanent stoma, urologic/sexual dysfunction). On the other hand, local excision avoids many of the quality of life issue associated with radical surgery, but the trade-off is recurrent disease and chance of a cure. There are multiple studies, none of which are phase III trials, examining the impact of adjuvant or neoadjuvant therapy to reduce recurrences in patients who undergo local excision of their rectal cancer. However, such strategies are considered investigational at this time. Accepted indications for local excision include T1N0, no evidence of lymphovascular invasion, well-differentiated to moderately differentiated tumor, size <3 cm in diameter, and tumor encompassing less than 30 % of the circumference of the rectal wall. ACOSOG Z6041 is a phase II trial that is evaluating the role of neoCRT for T2N0 rectal cancer. Although response rate is promising, toxicity is high and long-term oncologic implication is unknown.

Salient Points

- Early-stage rectal cancer includes stage I, which encompasses TINOMO and T2NOMO.
- Preoperative risk stratification in addition to the patient's desire for sphincter preservation, colostomy, and maintaining sexual and genitourinary function must be considered in choosing the best therapy.
- Radical resection such as low anterior resection or APR is the mainstay therapy for stage I rectal cancer. It offers excellent oncologic outcomes, albeit limited by significant morbidity, compromised bowel, sexual and urological function, and permanent colostomy, especially with distal rectal cancer.
- Local excision is a rectum-preserving, function-maintaining limited surgery that is associated with low morbidity and mortality, rapid recovery, and no colostomy. The oncological adequacy of this treatment is controversial.
- Recurrence rates for T1N0 and T20 range from 8 % to 30 %.
- There are no randomized trials comparing local excision with radical surgery for stage T1N0 and T2N0 cancers.
- The indications for local excision based on recommendations by the National Comprehensive Cancer Network (NCCN) and the American Society of Colorectal Surgeons are:
  - T1N0
  - No evidence of lymphovascular invasion
  - Well-differentiated to moderately differentiated tumor
  - Tumor <3 cm in diameter
  - Involved <30 % circumference of rectal wall
- The Haggitt classification classifies polyp into level 0–4. It is useful for pedunculated polyps but not for sessile polyps (all sessile polyps are classified as Haggitt level 4).
- Kikuchi classification divides T1 sessile polyps into thirds, based on the extent of the submucosal invasion.
- Local excision is ideal for Haggitt 1–3 or Kikuchi Sm1.
- Multimodality treatment (chemoradiation) along with local excision has been proposed to reduce local recurrence. However, this is considered investigational and has not been accepted as standard of care.
- Selection of patients for local excision is based on patient factors, location, and clinical stage of the tumor that are determined by digital rectal examination (DRE) and endoscopy, staging radiological studies, and histopathological features of the primary tumor.
- Recurrence rates after local excision are higher than after radical resection. Patients must be informed about the compromise between lower surgical morbidity and higher disease recurrence. For the frail and high-risk patients, recurrence rate may not be an issue.

- The risk of LR after local excision of ERC is related to T stage (and substage of T1) and adverse histopathological features of the primary tumor [poorly differentiated and mucinous adenocarcinoma, signet ring and undifferentiated adenocarcinomas, lymphovascular invasion (absence of lymphoid infiltration and tumor budding are relative factors)] and positivity of excision margins.
- Compared to radical resection, the first recurrence is predominantly local, and the overall recurrence (local + systemic) is higher.
- Survival after local excision of in situ and T1 rectal cancer is not significantly different but reduced for T2 rectal cancer.
- The outcome of salvage surgery depends on the timing of surgery with more favorable outcome with immediate reoperation.
- There has been an increase in the use of local excision in patients with advance rectal cancer who have major response after neoadjuvant therapy. Short-term follow-up has shown favorable outcome. However, long-term data are needed.
- Salvage multimodality therapy with radical resection and adjuvant or neoadjuvant chemoradiation remains a viable option for patients with recurrent disease, although outcome is suboptimal.
- ACOSOG Z6041 is evaluating the role of neoCRT in T2N0 rectal cancers. Preliminary results demonstrate:
  - High complete pathological response rate (44 %).
  - High rate of tumor being downstaged (64 %).
  - High negative margin rate (99 %).
  - High toxicity rate of almost 40 %.
  - Long-term oncologic outcome is not known.

Questions

A 65-year-old man complains of a 2-month history of rectal bleeding on defecation. Other than constipation, he denied other associated symptoms including abdominal pain, nausea, vomiting, tenesmus, or unintentional weight loss. He takes hydrochlorothiazide and aspirin 81 mg prescribed by his primary care physician and has never had any surgeries in the past. Physical exam including a digital rectal exam was pertinent for an anterior 4 cm mobile mass located approximately 5 cm from the anal verge. Fecal occult blood testing was positive.

The following series of questions pertains to the above case scenario.

1. What is the next best approach in the management of this patient?
   A. Reassure him that his clinical presentation is classic for grade I internal hemorrhoids and reschedule a repeat physical exam in one year.
   B. Schedule the patient for examination under anesthesia (EUA) and excision of the mass.
   C. Perform proctoscopy and biopsy of the mass.
   D. Refer the patient to gastroenterology associates for a screening colonoscopy as he likely has inflammatory bowel disease.
2. Upon further evaluation, the patient is found to be anemic, and the rectal lesion reveals a 3 cm polypoid, fungating mobile lesion occupying one-third of the rectal mucosal circumference at about 2 cm above the sphincter complex. Multiple biopsies are obtained. What should be the next step in managing this patient?
   A. Nothing can be done at this point until pathology results are available.
   B. Obtain CT scan of the abdomen and pelvis.
   C. Consent for abdominoperineal resection.
   D. Counsel and proceed with a completion diagnostic colonoscopy to further evaluate for synchronous rectal and colonic lesions.
3. What is the role of CT scan in the evaluation of a patient with a suspected rectal cancer?
   A. It is the gold standard diagnostic tool in the evaluation of patients with rectal lesions.

B. It provides morphologic details that can exclusively help differentiate benign versus malignant lesions.
C. It is useful in the detection of distant metastases and local tumor extension into adjacent structures.
D. It can clearly identify nodal invasion into the mesorectal space and therefore be helpful in the N staging of rectal cancer.

4. Endorectal rectal ultrasound (ERUS) revealed a lesion that had extended into the second hypoechoic line corresponding to the submucosal layer. There was no ultrasonographic evidence of perirectal lymph node invasion. Based on this information alone, what is the ultrasound stage of this lesion?
   A. uT0N0
   B. uT1N0M0
   C. uT1N1
   D. uT1N0
5. Had the tumor extended through the muscularis propria and into the perirectal tissue (mesorectum) and only two lymph nodes were identified sonographically, what would be the new stage for this rectal lesion?
   A. uT1N0
   B. uT1N0M0
   C. uT2N2
   D. uT2N0
   E. uT3N1
6. What is the most predictive factor determining the risk of nodal invasion and distant metastases in patients with rectal cancer?
   A. Depth of rectal wall invasion
   B. Presence of tumor ulceration
   C. Tumor size
   D. Distance from anal verge and sphincter complex
   E. Presence of synchronous lesions
7. The tumor was staged as T1N0, what is the best treatment option for this patient with the least morbidity and potential for cure?
   A. Transanal local excision
   B. Neoadjuvant chemoradiation therapy followed by low anterior resection, TME, and primary anastomosis
   C. Neoadjuvant chemoradiation therapy (CRT) to downstage the tumor and then subsequent local excision under local anesthesia
   D. Observation with frequent surveillance and only offer surgery if tumor is >4 cm
8. What characteristics would potentially prohibit transanal local resection of rectal cancer and may require further treatment? *SELECT ALL THAT APPLIES.*
   A. Tumor size >4 cm.
   B. Well-differentiated to moderately differentiated tumor.
   C. Presence of ulceration on rigid proctoscopy.
   D. Tumor occupies LESS than one-third of the rectal mucosal circumference.
   E. Tumor shows evidence of active bleeding at time of rigid proctoscopy.
   F. Evidence of perirectal lymphatic invasion.
   G. Negative margins after transanal excision.

Answer Key
1: C
2: D
3: C
4: D
5: E
6: A
7: A
8: A,C,E,F

References

1. Siegel R, Desantis C, Jemal A. Colorectal cancer statistics, 2014. CA Cancer J Clin. 2014;64 (2):104–17.
2. Merchant NB, Guillem JG, Paty PB, et al. T3N0 rectal cancer: results following sharp mesorectal excision and no adjuvant therapy. J Gastrointest Surg. 1999;3(6):642–7.
3. Chessin DB, Guillem JG. Abdominoperineal resection for rectal cancer: historic perspective and current issues. Surg Oncol Clin N Am. 2005;14(3):569–86, vii.
4. Hallböök O, Sjödahl R. Anastomotic leakage and functional outcome after anterior resection of the rectum. Br J Surg. 1996;83(1):60–2.
5. Kingham TP, Pachter HL. Colonic anastomotic leak: risk factors, diagnosis, and treatment. J Am Coll Surg. 2009;208(2):269–78.
6. Lisfranc J. Observation sur une affection cancereuse du rectume guire par l'excision. Red Med Franc Etrang. 1826;2:380–2.
7. Kraske P. Zur exstirpation hoch sitzender mastdarmkrebse. Verh Dtsch Ges Chir. 1885;14:464.
8. Czerny V. Casuistische mittheilugan aus der Chirurg Klin zu Heidelberg. Munch Med Wchnschr. 1894;12:11–4.
9. Miles E. A method of performing abdominoperineal excision for carcinoma of the rectum and the terminal portion of pelvic colon. Lancet. 1908;2:1812–3.
10. Quirke P, Durdey P, Dixon MF, Williams NS. Local recurrence of rectal adenocarcinoma due to inadequate surgical resection. Histopathological study of lateral tumour spread and surgical excision. Lancet. 1986;2(8514):996–9.
11. Pollet W, Nicholls R. The relationship between the extent of distal clearance and survival and local recurrence rates after curative resection for carcinoma of the rectum. Ann Surg. 1983;198:1059–63.
12. Heald RJ, Husband EM, Ryall RD. The mesorectum in rectal cancer surgery–the clue to pelvic recurrence? Br J Surg. 1982;69(10):613–6.
13. Jemal A, Bray F, Center MM, Ferlay J, Ward E, Forman D. Global cancer statistics. CA Cancer J Clin. 2011;61(2):69–90.
14. Bailey AA, Debinski HS, Appleyard MN, et al. Diagnosis and outcome of small bowel tumors found by capsule endoscopy: a three-center Australian experience. Am J Gastroenterol. 2006;101(10): 2237–43.
15. Parks AG. A technique for excising extensive villous papillomatous change in the lower rectum. Proc R Soc Med. 1968;61(5):441–2.
16. Buess G, Theiss R, Günther M, Hutterer F, Pichlmaier H. Transanal endoscopic microsurgery. Leber Magen Darm. 1985;15(6):271–9.
17. Day D, Jass J, Price A, et al. Epithelial tumors of the large intestine. In: Morson and Dawson's gastrointestinal pathology. 4th ed. Oxford: Blackwell Science; 2003. p. 551–609.
18. You YN, Baxter NN, Stewart A, Nelson H. Is the increasing rate of local excision for stage I rectal cancer in the United States justified?: a nationwide cohort study from the National Cancer Database. Ann Surg. 2007;245(5):726–33.
19. Blumberg D, Paty PB, Picon AI, et al. Stage I rectal cancer: identification of high-risk patients. J Am Coll Surg. 1998;186(5):574–9; discussion 579–580.
20. Tjandra JJ, Kilkenny JW, Buie WD, et al. Practice parameters for the management of rectal cancer (revised). Dis Colon Rectum. 2005;48(3):411–23.
21. National Comprehensive Cancer Network (NCCN) guidelines. Available at: www.nccn.org (2013). Accessed 23 May 2013.
22. Mason AY. Transsphincteric approach to rectal lesions. Surg Annu. 1977;9:171–94.
23. Huber PJ, Reiss G. Rectal tumors: treatment with a posterior approach. Am J Surg. 1993;166(6):760–3.
24. Stearns MW, Sternberg SS, DeCosse JJ. Treatment alternatives. Localized rectal cancer. Cancer. 1984;54(11 Suppl):2691–4.
25. Buess G, Hutterer F, Theiss J, Böbel M, Isselhard W, Pichlmaier H. A system for a transanal endoscopic rectum operation. Chirurg. 1984;55(10):677–80.
26. Buess G, Kipfmüller K, Hack D, Grüssner R, Heintz A, Junginger T. Technique of transanal endoscopic microsurgery. Surg Endosc. 1988;2(2):71–5.
27. Middleton PF, Sutherland LM, Maddern GJ. Transanal endoscopic microsurgery: a systematic review. Dis Colon Rectum. 2005;48(2):270–84.
28. Ganai S, Kanumuri P, Rao RS, Alexander AI. Local recurrence after transanal endoscopic microsurgery for rectal polyps and early cancers. Ann Surg Oncol. 2006;13(4):547–56.
29. Baatrup G, Borschitz T, Cunningham C, Qvist N. Perforation into the peritoneal cavity during transanal endoscopic microsurgery for rectal cancer is not associated with major complications or oncological compromise. Surg Endosc. 2009;23(12): 2680–3.
30. Morino M, Allaix ME, Famiglietti F, Caldart M, Arezzo A. Does peritoneal perforation affect short- and long-term outcomes after transanal endoscopic microsurgery? Surg Endosc. 2013;27(1):181–8.
31. Bhattacharjee HK, Buess GF, Becerra Garcia FC, et al. A novel single-port technique for transanal rectosigmoid resection and colorectal anastomosis on an ex vivo experimental model. Surg Endosc. 2011;25(6):1844–57.
32. Whiteford MH, Denk PM, Swanström LL. Feasibility of radical sigmoid colectomy performed as natural orifice translumenal endoscopic surgery (NOTES) using transanal endoscopic microsurgery. Surg Endosc. 2007;21(10):1870–4.
33. Eyvazzadeh DJ, Lee JT, Madoff RD, Mellgren AF, Finne CO. Outcomes after transanal endoscopic microsurgery with intraperitoneal anastomosis. Dis Colon Rectum. 2014;57(4):438–41.
34. Zerz A, Müller-Stich BP, Beck J, Linke GR, Tarantino I, Lange J. Endoscopic posterior mesorectal resection

after transanal local excision of T1 carcinomas of the lower third of the rectum. Dis Colon Rectum. 2006;49(6):919–24.
35. Walega P, Kenig J, Richter P, Nowak W. Functional and clinical results of transanal endoscopic microsurgery combined with endoscopic posterior mesorectum resection for the treatment of patients with t1 rectal cancer. World J Surg. 2010;34(7):1604–8.
36. Wang T, Wang J, Deng Y, Wu X, Wang L. Neoadjuvant therapy followed by local excision and two-stage total mesorectal excision: a new strategy for sphincter preservation in locally advanced ultra-low rectal cancer. Gastroenterol Rep (Oxf). 2014;2(1):37–43.
37. Koebrugge B, Bosscha K, Ernst MF. Transanal endoscopic microsurgery for local excision of rectal lesions: is there a learning curve? Dig Surg. 2009;26(5):372–7.
38. Hompes R, Lindsey I, Jones OM, et al. Step-wise integration of single-port laparoscopic surgery into routine colorectal surgical practice by use of a surgical glove port. Tech Coloproctol. 2011;15(2): 165–71.
39. Atallah S, Albert M, Larach S. Transanal minimally invasive surgery: a giant leap forward. Surg Endosc. 2010;24(9):2200–5.
40. Lezoche E, Guerrieri M, Paganini AM, et al. Transanal endoscopic versus total mesorectal laparoscopic resections of T2-N0 low rectal cancers after neoadjuvant treatment: a prospective randomized trial with a 3-years minimum follow-up period. Surg Endosc. 2005;19(6):751–6.
41. Lorenz C, Nimmesgern T, Back M, Langwieler TE. Transanal single port microsurgery (TSPM) as a modified technique of transanal endoscopic microsurgery (TEM). Surg Innov. 2010;17(2):160–3.
42. Hompes R, Rauh SM, Hagen ME, Mortensen NJ. Preclinical cadaveric study of transanal endoscopic da Vinci® surgery. Br J Surg. 2012;99(8): 1144–8.
43. Buchs NC, Pugin F, Volonte F, Hagen ME, Morel P, Ris F. Robotic transanal endoscopic microsurgery: technical details for the lateral approach. Dis Colon Rectum. 2013;56(10):1194–8.
44. Bardakcioglu O. Robotic transanal access surgery. Surg Endosc. 2013;27(4):1407–9.
45. Graham RA, Garnsey L, Jessup JM. Local excision of rectal carcinoma. Am J Surg. 1990;160(3): 306–12.
46. Jessup J, Bothe A, Stone M, et al. Preservation of sphincter function in rectal carcinoma by a multimodality treatment approach. Surg Oncol Clin N Am. 1992;1:137–45.
47. Zlobec I, Minoo P, Karamitopoulou E, et al. Role of tumor size in the pre-operative management of rectal cancer patients. BMC Gastroenterol. 2010;10:61.
48. Greaney MG, Irvin TT. Criteria for the selection of rectal cancers for local treatment: a clinicopathologic study of low rectal tumors. Dis Colon Rectum. 1977;20(6):463–6.
49. Patel SA, Chen YH, Hornick JL, et al. Early-stage rectal cancer: clinical and pathologic prognostic markers of time to local recurrence and overall survival after resection. Dis Colon Rectum. 2014;57(4): 449–59.
50. Hildebrandt U, Feifel G. Preoperative staging of rectal cancer by intrarectal ultrasound. Dis Colon Rectum. 1985;28(1):42–6.
51. Kim JC, Cho YK, Kim SY, Park SK, Lee MG. Comparative study of three-dimensional and conventional endorectal ultrasonography used in rectal cancer staging. Surg Endosc. 2002;16(9): 1280–5.
52. Kim JC, Kim HC, Yu CS, et al. Efficacy of 3-dimensional endorectal ultrasonography compared with conventional ultrasonography and computed tomography in preoperative rectal cancer staging. Am J Surg. 2006;192(1):89–97.
53. Hünerbein M, Pegios W, Rau B, Vogl TJ, Felix R, Schlag PM. Prospective comparison of endorectal ultrasound, three-dimensional endorectal ultrasound, and endorectal MRI in the preoperative evaluation of rectal tumors. Preliminary results. Surg Endosc. 2000;14(11):1005–9.
54. Harewood GC. Assessment of publication bias in the reporting of EUS performance in staging rectal cancer. Am J Gastroenterol. 2005;100(4):808–16.
55. Hildebrandt U, Klein T, Feifel G, Schwarz HP, Koch B, Schmitt RM. Endosonography of pararectal lymph nodes. In vitro and in vivo evaluation. Dis Colon Rectum. 1990;33(10):863–8.
56. Kim NK, Kim MJ, Yun SH, Sohn SK, Min JS. Comparative study of transrectal ultrasonography, pelvic computerized tomography, and magnetic resonance imaging in preoperative staging of rectal cancer. Dis Colon Rectum. 1999;42(6):770–5.
57. Gualdi GF, Casciani E, Guadalaxara A, d'Orta C, Polettini E. Pappalardo G Local staging of rectal cancer with transrectal ultrasound and endorectal magnetic resonance imaging: comparison with histologic findings. Dis Colon Rectum. 2000;43(3): 338–45.
58. Kwok H, Bissett IP, Hill GL. Preoperative staging of rectal cancer. Int J Colorectal Dis. 2000;15(1):9–20.
59. Brown G, Davies S, Williams GT, et al. Effectiveness of preoperative staging in rectal cancer: digital rectal examination, endoluminal ultrasound or magnetic resonance imaging? Br J Cancer. 2004;91(1):23–9.
60. Bipat S, Glas AS, Slors FJ, Zwinderman AH, Bossuyt PM, Stoker J. Rectal cancer: local staging and assessment of lymph node involvement with endoluminal US, CT, and MR imaging–a meta-analysis. Radiology. 2004;232(3):773–83.
61. Kim JH, Beets GL, Kim MJ, Kessels AG, Beets-Tan RG. High-resolution MR imaging for nodal staging in rectal cancer: are there any criteria in addition to the size? Eur J Radiol. 2004;52(1):78–83.
62. Klessen C, Rogalla P, Taupitz M. Local staging of rectal cancer: the current role of MRI. Eur Radiol. 2007;17(2):379–89.

63. Torricelli P, Lo Russo S, Pecchi A, Luppi G, Cesinaro AM, Romagnoli R. Endorectal coil MRI in local staging of rectal cancer. Radiol Med. 2002;103(1–2):74–83.
64. Brown G, Richards CJ, Bourne MW, et al. Morphologic predictors of lymph node status in rectal cancer with use of high-spatial-resolution MR imaging with histopathologic comparison. Radiology. 2003;227(2):371–7.
65. Mellgren A, Sirivongs P, Rothenberger DA, Madoff RD, García-Aguilar J. Is local excision adequate therapy for early rectal cancer? Dis Colon Rectum. 2000;43(8):1064–71; discussion 1071–1064.
66. Paty PB, Nash GM, Baron P, et al. Long-term results of local excision for rectal cancer. Ann Surg. 2002;236(4):522–9; discussion 529–530.
67. Madbouly KM, Remzi FH, Erkek BA, et al. Recurrence after transanal excision of T1 rectal cancer: should we be concerned? Dis Colon Rectum. 2005;48(4):711–9; discussion 719–721.
68. Rifkin MD, Ehrlich SM, Marks G. Staging of rectal carcinoma: prospective comparison of endorectal US and CT. Radiology. 1989;170(2):319–22.
69. Hahnloser D, Wolff BG, Larson DW, Ping J, Nivatvongs S. Immediate radical resection after local excision of rectal cancer: an oncologic compromise? Dis Colon Rectum. 2005;48(3):429–37.
70. Hamilton S, Rubio C, Vogelstein B, et al. Carcinoma of the colon and rectum. In: Hamilton A, Aaltonen L, editors. World Health Organization classification of tumors. Tumors of the digestive system. Lyon: IARC Press; 2000. p. 101–19.
71. Compton CC, Fielding LP, Burgart LJ, et al. Prognostic factors in colorectal cancer. College of American Pathologists Consensus Statement 1999. Arch Pathol Lab Med. 2000;124(7):979–94.
72. Crucitti F, Sofo L, Doglietto GB, et al. Prognostic factors in colorectal cancer: current status and new trends. J Surg Oncol Suppl. 1991;2:76–82.
73. Staren ED, Gould VE, Warren WH, et al. Neuroendocrine carcinomas of the colon and rectum: a clinicopathologic evaluation. Surgery. 1988; 104(6):1080–9.
74. Cohen AM, Wood WC, Gunderson LL, Shinnar M. Pathological studies in rectal cancer. Cancer. 1980;45(12):2965–8.
75. Gospodarowicz M, Mackillop W, O'Sullivan B, et al. Prognostic factors in clinical decision making: the future. Cancer. 2001;91(8 Suppl):1688–95.
76. Wiggers T, Arends JW, Volovics A. Regression analysis of prognostic factors in colorectal cancer after curative resections. Dis Colon Rectum. 1988;31(1):33–41.
77. Killingback M. Local excision of carcinoma of the rectum: indications. World J Surg. 1992;16(3):437–46.
78. Minsky BD, Rich T, Recht A, Harvey W, Mies C. Selection criteria for local excision with or without adjuvant radiation therapy for rectal cancer. Cancer. 1989;63(7):1421–9.
79. Saclarides TJ, Bhattacharyya AK, Britton-Kuzel C, Szeluga D, Economou SG. Predicting lymph node metastases in rectal cancer. Dis Colon Rectum. 1994;37(1):52–7.
80. Haggitt RC, Glotzbach RE, Soffer EE, Wruble LD. Prognostic factors in colorectal carcinomas arising in adenomas: implications for lesions removed by endoscopic polypectomy. Gastroenterology. 1985;89(2):328–36.
81. Kikuchi R, Takano M, Takagi K, et al. Management of early invasive colorectal cancer. Risk of recurrence and clinical guidelines. Dis Colon Rectum. 1995;38(12):1286–95.
82. Bailey HR, Huval WV, Max E, Smith KW, Butts DR, Zamora LF. Local excision of carcinoma of the rectum for cure. Surgery. 1992;111(5):555–61.
83. Morson BC, Bussey HJ, Samoorian S. Policy of local excision for early cancer of the colorectum. Gut. 1977;18(12):1045–50.
84. Huddy SP, Husband EM, Cook MG, Gibbs NM, Marks CG, Heald RJ. Lymph node metastases in early rectal cancer. Br J Surg. 1993;80(11):1457–8.
85. Baron PL, Sigurdson ER. Local surgical treatment of rectal cancer. Cancer Invest. 1995;13(6):612–6.
86. Nivatvongs S, Rojanasakul A, Reiman HM, et al. The risk of lymph node metastasis in colorectal polyps with invasive adenocarcinoma. Dis Colon Rectum. 1991;34(4):323–8.
87. Nascimbeni R, Burgart LJ, Nivatvongs S, Larson DR. Risk of lymph node metastasis in T1 carcinoma of the colon and rectum. Dis Colon Rectum. 2002;45(2):200–6.
88. Chok KS, Law WL. Prognostic factors affecting survival and recurrence of patients with pT1 and pT2 colorectal cancer. World J Surg. 2007;31(7):1485–90.
89. Sitzler PJ, Seow-Choen F, Ho YH, Leong AP. Lymph node involvement and tumor depth in rectal cancers: an analysis of 805 patients. Dis Colon Rectum. 1997;40(12):1472–6.
90. Cooper HS, Deppisch LM, Gourley WK, et al. Endoscopically removed malignant colorectal polyps: clinicopathologic correlations. Gastroenterology. 1995;108(6):1657–65.
91. Shimomura T, Ishiguro S, Konishi H, et al. New indication for endoscopic treatment of colorectal carcinoma with submucosal invasion. J Gastroenterol Hepatol. 2004;19(1):48–55.
92. Kitajima K, Fujimori T, Fujii S, et al. Correlations between lymph node metastasis and depth of submucosal invasion in submucosal invasive colorectal carcinoma: a Japanese collaborative study. J Gastroenterol. 2004;39(6):534–43.
93. Kyzer S, Bégin LR, Gordon PH, Mitmaker B. The care of patients with colorectal polyps that contain invasive adenocarcinoma. Endoscopic polypectomy or colectomy? Cancer. 1992;70(8):2044–50.
94. Tytherleigh MG, Warren BF, Mortensen NJ. Management of early rectal cancer. Br J Surg. 2008;95(4):409–23.

95. Cooper HS, Deppisch LM, Kahn EI, et al. Pathology of the malignant colorectal polyp. Hum Pathol. 1998;29(1):15–26.
96. Lipper S, Kahn LB, Ackerman LV. The significance of microscopic invasive cancer in endoscopically removed polyps of the large bowel. A clinicopathologic study of 51 cases. Cancer. 1983;52(9):1691–9.
97. Goldstein NS, Hart J. Histologic features associated with lymph node metastasis in stage T1 and superficial T2 rectal adenocarcinomas in abdominoperineal resection specimens. Identifying a subset of patients for whom treatment with adjuvant therapy or completion abdominoperineal resection should be considered after local excision. Am J Clin Pathol. 1999;111(1):51–8.
98. Volk EE, Goldblum JR, Petras RE, Carey WD, Fazio VW. Management and outcome of patients with invasive carcinoma arising in colorectal polyps. Gastroenterology. 1995;109(6):1801–7.
99. Lezoche G, Guerrieri M, Baldarelli M, et al. Transanal endoscopic microsurgery for 135 patients with small nonadvanced low rectal cancer (iT1-iT2, iN0): short- and long-term results. Surg Endosc. 2011;25(4):1222–9.
100. Floyd ND, Saclarides TJ. Transanal endoscopic microsurgical resection of pT1 rectal tumors. Dis Colon Rectum. 2006;49(2):164–8.
101. Chapuis PH, Dent OF, Fisher R, et al. A multivariate analysis of clinical and pathological variables in prognosis after resection of large bowel cancer. Br J Surg. 1985;72(9):698–702.
102. Mulcahy HE, Skelly MM, Husain A, O'Donoghue DP. Long-term outcome following curative surgery for malignant large bowel obstruction. Br J Surg. 1996;83(1):46–50.
103. Hermanek P, Guggenmoos-Holzmann I, Gall FP. Prognostic factors in rectal carcinoma. A contribution to the further development of tumor classification. Dis Colon Rectum. 1989;32(7):593–9.
104. Hase K, Shatney C, Johnson D, Trollope M, Vierra M. Prognostic value of tumor "budding" in patients with colorectal cancer. Dis Colon Rectum. 1993;36(7):627–35.
105. Harrison JC, Dean PJ, el-Zeky F, Vander Zwaag R. From Dukes through Jass: pathological prognostic indicators in rectal cancer. Hum Pathol. 1994;25(5):498–505.
106. Jass JR, Do KA, Simms LA, et al. Morphology of sporadic colorectal cancer with DNA replication errors. Gut. 1998;42(5):673–9.
107. Halvorsen TB, Seim E. Association between invasiveness, inflammatory reaction, desmoplasia and survival in colorectal cancer. J Clin Pathol. 1989;42(2):162–6.
108. Willett CG, Tepper JE, Donnelly S, et al. Patterns of failure following local excision and local excision and postoperative radiation therapy for invasive rectal adenocarcinoma. J Clin Oncol. 1989;7(8):1003–8.
109. Sengupta S, Tjandra JJ. Local excision of rectal cancer: what is the evidence? Dis Colon Rectum. 2001;44(9):1345–61.
110. Breen E, Bleday R. Preservation of the anus in the therapy of distal rectal cancers. Surg Clin N Am. 1997;77(1):71–83.
111. Stitzenberg KB, Sanoff HK, Penn DC, Meyers MO, Tepper JE. Practice patterns and long-term survival for early-stage rectal cancer. J Clin Oncol. 2013;31(34):4276–82.
112. Endreseth BH, Myrvold HE, Romundstad P, et al. Transanal excision vs. major surgery for T1 rectal cancer. Dis Colon Rectum. 2005;48(7):1380–8.
113. Garcia-Aguilar J, Shi Q, Thomas CR, et al. A phase II trial of neoadjuvant chemoradiation and local excision for T2N0 rectal cancer: preliminary results of the ACOSOG Z6041 trial. Ann Surg Oncol. 2012;19(2):384–91.
114. Kundel Y, Brenner R, Purim O, et al. Is local excision after complete pathological response to neoadjuvant chemoradiation for rectal cancer an acceptable treatment option? Dis Colon Rectum. 2010;53(12): 1624–31.
115. Bedrosian I, Rodriguez-Bigas MA, Feig B, et al. Predicting the node-negative mesorectum after preoperative chemoradiation for locally advanced rectal carcinoma. J Gastrointest Surg. 2004;8(1):56–62; discussion 62–53.
116. Bujko K, Nowacki MP, Nasierowska-Guttmejer A, et al. Prediction of mesorectal nodal metastases after chemoradiation for rectal cancer: results of a randomised trial: implication for subsequent local excision. Radiother Oncol. 2005;76(3):234–40.
117. Türler A, Schäfer H, Pichlmaier H. Role of transanal endoscopic microsurgery in the palliative treatment of rectal cancer. Scand J Gastroenterol. 1997;32(1):58–61.
118. Perrotta S, Quarto G, Desiato V, Benassai G, Amato B. TEM in the treatment of recurrent rectal cancer in elderly. BMC Surg. 2013;13 Suppl 2:S56.
119. Friel CM, Cromwell JW, Marra C, Madoff RD, Rothenberger DA, Garcia-Aguílar J. Salvage radical surgery after failed local excision for early rectal cancer. Dis Colon Rectum. 2002;45(7):875–9.
120. Pucciarelli S, De Paoli A, Guerrieri M, et al. Local excision after preoperative chemoradiotherapy for rectal cancer: results of a multicenter phase II clinical trial. Dis Colon Rectum. 2013;56(12):1349–56.
121. Hayden DM, Jakate S, Pinzon MC, et al. Tumor scatter after neoadjuvant therapy for rectal cancer: are we dealing with an invisible margin? Dis Colon Rectum. 2012;55(12):1206–12.
122. Park YJ, Kim WH, Paeng SS, Park JG. Histoclinical analysis of early colorectal cancer. World J Surg. 2000;24(9):1029–35.
123. Choi PW, Yu CS, Jang SJ, Jung SH, Kim HC, Kim JC. Risk factors for lymph node metastasis in submucosal invasive colorectal cancer. World J Surg. 2008;32(9):2089–94.
124. Tominaga K, Nakanishi Y, Nimura S, Yoshimura K, Sakai Y, Shimoda T. Predictive histopathologic factors for lymph node metastasis in patients with nonpedunculated submucosal invasive colorectal carcinoma. Dis Colon Rectum. 2005;48(1):92–100.

125. Sakuragi M, Togashi K, Konishi F, et al. Predictive factors for lymph node metastasis in T1 stage colorectal carcinomas. Dis Colon Rectum. 2003; 46(12):1626–32.
126. Borschitz T, Heintz A, Junginger T. The influence of histopathologic criteria on the long-term prognosis of locally excised pT1 rectal carcinomas: results of local excision (transanal endoscopic microsurgery) and immediate reoperation. Dis Colon Rectum. 2006;49(10):1492–506; discussion 1500–1495.
127. García-Aguilar J, Hernandez de Anda E, Sirivongs P, Lee SH, Madoff RD, Rothenberger DA. A pathologic complete response to preoperative chemoradiation is associated with lower local recurrence and improved survival in rectal cancer patients treated by mesorectal excision. Dis Colon Rectum. 2003;46(3): 298–304.
128. Le Voyer TE, Hoffman JP, Cooper H, Ross E, Sigurdson E, Eisenberg B. Local excision and chemoradiation for low rectal T1 and T2 cancers is an effective treatment. Am Surg. 1999;65(7):625–30; discussion 630–621.
129. Willett CG, Compton CC, Shellito PC, Efird JT. Selection factors for local excision or abdominoperineal resection of early stage rectal cancer. Cancer. 1994;73(11):2716–20.
130. Rothenberger DA, Garcia-Aguilar J. Role of local excision in the treatment of rectal cancer. Semin Surg Oncol. 2000;19(4):367–75.
131. Garcia-Aguilar J, Mellgren A, Sirivongs P, Buie D, Madoff RD, Rothenberger DA. Local excision of rectal cancer without adjuvant therapy: a word of caution. Ann Surg. 2000;231(3):345–51.
132. Taylor RH, Hay JH, Larsson SN. Transanal local excision of selected low rectal cancers. Am J Surg. 1998;175(5):360–3.
133. Chakravarti A, Compton CC, Shellito PC, et al. Long-term follow-up of patients with rectal cancer managed by local excision with and without adjuvant irradiation. Ann Surg. 1999;230(1):49–54.
134. Nash GM, Weiser MR, Guillem JG, et al. Long-term survival after transanal excision of T1 rectal cancer. Dis Colon Rectum. 2009;52(4):577–82.
135. Greenberg JA, Shibata D, Herndon JE, Steele GD, Mayer R, Bleday R. Local excision of distal rectal cancer: an update of cancer and leukemia group B 8984. Dis Colon Rectum. 2008;51(8):1185–91; discussion 1191–1184.
136. Enker WE, Merchant N, Cohen AM, et al. Safety and efficacy of low anterior resection for rectal cancer: 681 consecutive cases from a specialty service. Ann Surg. 1999;230(4):544–52; discussion 552–544.
137. Paty PB, Enker WE, Cohen AM, Lauwers GY. Treatment of rectal cancer by low anterior resection with coloanal anastomosis. Ann Surg. 1994;219(4):365–73.
138. Bhangu A, Brown G, Nicholls RJ, Wong J, Darzi A, Tekkis P. Survival outcome of local excision versus radical resection of colon or rectal carcinoma: a Surveillance, Epidemiology, and End Results (SEER) population-based study. Ann Surg. 2013;258(4):563–9; discussion 569–571.
139. Bouvet M, Milas M, Giacco GG, Cleary KR, Janjan NA, Skibber JM. Predictors of recurrence after local excision and postoperative chemoradiation therapy of adenocarcinoma of the rectum. Ann Surg Oncol. 1999;6(1):26–32.
140. Baron PL, Enker WE, Zakowski MF, Urmacher C. Immediate vs salvage resection after local treatment for early rectal cancer. Dis Colon Rectum. 1995;38(2):177–81.
141. Minsky BD. Clinical experience with local excision and postoperative radiation therapy for rectal cancer. Dis Colon Rectum. 1993;36(4):405–9.
142. Fortunato L, Ahmad NR, Yeung RS, et al. Long-term follow-up of local excision and radiation therapy for invasive rectal cancer. Dis Colon Rectum. 1995;38(11):1193–9.
143. Ota DM, Skibber J, Rich R, Anderson MD. Cancer Center experience with local excision and multimodality therapy for rectal cancer. Surg Oncol Clin N Am. 1992;1:147–52.
144. Bleday R, Breen E, Jessup JM, Burgess A, Sentovich SM, Steele G. Prospective evaluation of local excision for small rectal cancers. Dis Colon Rectum. 1997;40(4):388–92.
145. Russell AH, Harris J, Rosenberg PJ, et al. Anal sphincter conservation for patients with adenocarcinoma of the distal rectum: long-term results of radiation therapy oncology group protocol 89–02. Int J Radiat Oncol Biol Phys. 2000;46(2):313–22.
146. Wagman RT, Minsky BD. Conservative management of rectal cancer with local excision and adjuvant therapy. Oncology (Williston Park). 2001;15(4):513–9, 524;discussion 524–518.
147. Christoforidis D, Cho HM, Dixon MR, Mellgren AF, Madoff RD, Finne CO. Transanal endoscopic microsurgery versus conventional transanal excision for patients with early rectal cancer. Ann Surg. 2009;249(5):776–82.
148. Moore JS, Cataldo PA, Osler T, Hyman NH. Transanal endoscopic microsurgery is more effective than traditional transanal excision for resection of rectal masses. Dis Colon Rectum. 2008;51(7):1026–30; discussion 1030–1021.
149. Winde G, Nottberg H, Keller R, Schmid KW, Bünte H. Surgical cure for early rectal carcinomas (T1). Transanal endoscopic microsurgery vs anterior resection. Dis Colon Rectum. 1996;39(9):969–76.
150. Lezoche E, Guerrieri M, Paganini AM, Baldarelli M, De Sanctis A, Lezoche G. Long-term results in patients with T2-3 N0 distal rectal cancer undergoing radiotherapy before transanal endoscopic microsurgery. Br J Surg. 2005;92(12):1546–52.
151. Lezoche G, Baldarelli M, Guerrieri M, et al. A prospective randomized study with a 5-year minimum follow-up evaluation of transanal endoscopic microsurgery versus laparoscopic total mesorectal excision after neoadjuvant therapy. Surg Endosc. 2008;22(2):352–8.

152. Buess G, Mentges B, Manncke K, Starlinger M, Becker HD. Technique and results of transanal endoscopic microsurgery in early rectal cancer. Am J Surg. 1992;163(1):63–9; discussion 69–70.
153. Saclarides TJ, Smith L, Ko ST, Orkin B, Buess G. Transanal endoscopic microsurgery. Dis Colon Rectum. 1992;35(12):1183–91.
154. Guerrieri M, Baldarelli M, Organetti L, et al. Transanal endoscopic microsurgery for the treatment of selected patients with distal rectal cancer: 15 years experience. Surg Endosc. 2008;22(9):2030–5.
155. Stipa F, Burza A, Lucandri G, et al. Outcomes for early rectal cancer managed with transanal endoscopic microsurgery: a 5-year follow-up study. Surg Endosc. 2006;20(4):541–5.
156. Doornebosch PG, Tollenaar RA, De Graaf EJ. Is the increasing role of Transanal Endoscopic Microsurgery in curation for T1 rectal cancer justified? A systematic review. Acta Oncol. 2009;48(3): 343–53.
157. Maslekar S, Pillinger SH, Monson JR. Transanal endoscopic microsurgery for carcinoma of the rectum. Surg Endosc. 2007;21(1):97–102.
158. Doornebosch PG, Ferenschild FT, de Wilt JH, Dawson I, Tetteroo GW, de Graaf EJ. Treatment of recurrence after transanal endoscopic microsurgery (TEM) for T1 rectal cancer. Dis Colon Rectum. 2010;53(9):1234–9.
159. Palma P, Horisberger K, Joos A, Rothenhoefer S, Willeke F, Post S. Local excision of early rectal cancer: is transanal endoscopic microsurgery an alternative to radical surgery? Rev Esp Enferm Dig. 2009;101(3):172–8.
160. Heintz A, Mörschel M, Junginger T. Comparison of results after transanal endoscopic microsurgery and radical resection for T1 carcinoma of the rectum. Surg Endosc. 1998;12(9):1145–8.
161. Lee SH, Jeon SW, Jung MK, Kim SK, Choi GS. A comparison of transanal excision and endoscopic resection for early rectal cancer. World J Gastrointest Endosc. 2009;1(1):56–60.
162. Lee W, Lee D, Choi S, Chun H. Transanal endoscopic microsurgery and radical surgery for T1 and T2 rectal cancer. Surg Endosc. 2003;17(8):1283–7.
163. Wu Y, Wu YY, Li S, et al. TEM and conventional rectal surgery for T1 rectal cancer: a meta-analysis. Hepato-gastroenterol. 2011;58(106):364–8.
164. Sgourakis G, Lanitis S, Gockel I, et al. Transanal endoscopic microsurgery for T1 and T2 rectal cancers: a meta-analysis and meta-regression analysis of outcomes. Am Surg. 2011;77(6):761–72.
165. Baatrup G, Breum B, Qvist N, et al. Transanal endoscopic microsurgery in 143 consecutive patients with rectal adenocarcinoma: results from a Danish multicenter study. Colorectal Dis. 2009;11(3): 270–5.
166. Allaix ME, Arezzo A, Giraudo G, Morino M. Transanal endoscopic microsurgery vs. laparoscopic total mesorectal excision for T2N0 rectal cancer. J Gastrointest Surg. 2012;16(12):2280–7.
167. Stipa F, Lucandri G, Ferri M, Casula G, Ziparo V. Local excision of rectal cancer with transanal endoscopic microsurgery (TEM). Anticancer Res. 2004;24(2C):1167–72.
168. Steele RJ, Hershman MJ, Mortensen NJ, Armitage NC, Scholefield JH. Transanal endoscopic microsurgery–initial experience from three centres in the United Kingdom. Br J Surg. 1996;83(2):207–10.
169. Duek SD, Issa N, Hershko DD, Krausz MM. Outcome of transanal endoscopic microsurgery and adjuvant radiotherapy in patients with T2 rectal cancer. Dis Colon Rectum. 2008;51(4):379–84; discussion 384.
170. Lezoche E, Baldarelli M, Lezoche G, Paganini AM, Gesuita R, Guerrieri M. Randomized clinical trial of endoluminal locoregional resection versus laparoscopic total mesorectal excision for T2 rectal cancer after neoadjuvant therapy. Br J Surg. 2012;99(9):1211–8.
171. Perez RO, Habr-Gama A, São Julião GP, Proscurshim I, Scanavini Neto A, Gama-Rodrigues J. Transanal endoscopic microsurgery for residual rectal cancer after neoadjuvant chemoradiation therapy is associated with significant immediate pain and hospital readmission rates. Dis Colon Rectum. 2011;54(5):545–51.
172. Hiotis SP, Weber SM, Cohen AM, et al. Assessing the predictive value of clinical complete response to neoadjuvant therapy for rectal cancer: an analysis of 488 patients. J Am Coll Surg. 2002;194(2):131–5; discussion 135–136.
173. Glynne-Jones R, Wallace M, Livingstone JI, Meyrick-Thomas J. Complete clinical response after preoperative chemoradiation in rectal cancer: is a "wait and see" policy justified? Dis Colon Rectum. 2008;51(1):10–9; discussion 19–20.
174. Perez RO, Habr-Gama A, Gama-Rodrigues J, et al. Accuracy of positron emission tomography/computed tomography and clinical assessment in the detection of complete rectal tumor regression after neoadjuvant chemoradiation: long-term results of a prospective trial (National Clinical Trial 00254683). Cancer. 2012;118(14):3501–11.
175. Lambregts DM, Maas M, Bakers FC, et al. Long-term follow-up features on rectal MRI during a wait-and-see approach after a clinical complete response in patients with rectal cancer treated with chemoradiotherapy. Dis Colon Rectum. 2011;54(12):1521–8.
176. van Stiphout RG, Lammering G, Buijsen J, et al. Development and external validation of a predictive model for pathological complete response of rectal cancer patients including sequential PET-CT imaging. Radiother Oncol. 2011;98(1):126–33.
177. Maretto I, Pomerri F, Pucciarelli S, et al. The potential of restaging in the prediction of pathologic response after preoperative chemoradiotherapy for rectal cancer. Ann Surg Oncol. 2007;14(2):455–61.
178. Perez RO, Habr-Gama A, Pereira GV, et al. Role of biopsies in patients with residual rectal cancer following neoadjuvant chemoradiation after downsizing: can they rule out persisting cancer? Colorectal Dis. 2012;14(6):714–20.

179. Borschitz T, Wachtlin D, Möhler M, Schmidberger H, Junginger T. Neoadjuvant chemoradiation and local excision for T2-3 rectal cancer. Ann Surg Oncol. 2008;15(3):712–20.
180. Weiser MR, Landmann RG, Wong WD, et al. Surgical salvage of recurrent rectal cancer after transanal excision. Dis Colon Rectum. 2005;48(6):1169–75.
181. Lange MM, Martz JE, Ramdeen B, et al. Long-term results of rectal cancer surgery with a systematical operative approach. Ann Surg Oncol. 2013;20(6): 1806–15.
182. Steele GD, Herndon JE, Bleday R, et al. Sphincter-sparing treatment for distal rectal adenocarcinoma. Ann Surg Oncol. 1999;6(5):433–41.
183. Beck DE, Roberts PL, Rombeau JL, et al. Surgical treatment of rectal cancer. In: The ASCRS manual of colon and rectal surgery. New York: Springer; 2009. p. 571–604.
184. Allaix ME. Transanal endoscopic microsurgery for rectal neoplasms. How I do it. J Gastrointest Surg. 2013;17(3):586–92.
185. Kosinski L, et al. Shifting concepts in rectal cancer management. A review of contemporary primary rectal cancer treatment strategies. CA Can J Clin. 2012;62:173–202.
186. Valls F. Robotic transanal endoscopic microsurgery in benign rectal tumour. J Robot Surg. 2013. doi:10.1007/s11701-013-0429-9.

Rectal Cancer

18

Quyen D. Chu, Guillermo Pablo Sangster, and Mahmoud N. Kulaylat

Learning Objectives

After reading this chapter, you should be able to:

- Recognize what constitutes operable rectal cancer
- Understand how to evaluate and manage patients with rectal cancer
- Appreciate the treatment paradigm of rectal cancer
- Understand the role of neoadjuvant chemoradiation and total mesorectal excision (TME) in controlling rectal cancer
- Select options for local, regional, and systemic control of the disease

Q.D. Chu, M.D., M.B.A., FACS (✉)
Department of Surgery, Louisiana State University Health Sciences Center – Shreveport, 1501 Kings Highway, P.O. Box 33932, Shreveport, LA 71130-3392, USA
e-mail: qchu@lsuhsc.edu

G.P. Sangster, M.D.
Department of Radiology, Louisiana State University Health Sciences Center – Shreveport, 1501 Kings Highway, P.O. Box 33932, Shreveport, LA 71130-3392, USA
e-mail: gsangs@lsuhsc.edu

M.N. Kulaylat, M.D.
Department of Surgery, Buffalo General Medical Center, University at Buffalo-State University of New York, 100 High Street, Buffalo, NY 14203, USA
e-mail: mkulaylat@kaleidahealth.org

Introduction, Incidence, and Epidemiology

Colorectal cancer (CRC) is currently the third most common cancer and the third leading cause of cancer death for women and men in the United States [1]. It is estimated that 136,830 new cases of CRC will be diagnosed in 2014, of which 40,000 will be rectal cancer (29 %) [1, 2]. The overall incidence rate of CRC has decreased by an average of 3.4 % per year during 2001–2010 [1]. Outcomes for patients with rectal cancer have significantly improved over the decades; the relative 5-year survival rate for rectal cancer for the years from 1975 to 1977 was 48 % and has risen to 68 % for the years between 2003 and 2009 ($P<0.05$) [2]. The 5-year survival rates for patients with localized disease, regional disease, and distant disease are 88 %, 70 %, and 13 %, respectively [1, 2]. Such progress is a testament to our advances in the treating, introduction and dissemination of early detection tests, and addressing the risks factors associated with CRC (i.e., smoking cessation, reduction in red meat consumption, and increased use of aspirin) [1, 3]. This chapter addresses the evaluation and management of patients with stage II/III rectal adenocarcinoma, while the other chapters address related topics: *Chapter 17- Local Excision of Early-Stage Rectal Cancer, Chap. 19- Management of Liver Metastases from Colorectal Cancer, and Chap. 21- Cytoreductive Surgery and Hyperthermic Intraperitoneal Chemotherapy.*

Q.D. Chu et al. (eds.), *Surgical Oncology: A Practical and Comprehensive Approach*,
DOI 10.1007/978-1-4939-1423-4_18,

Risk factors for CRC include advancing age, obesity, personal behavioral (lack of physical activity, cigarette smoking, and excessive alcohol consumption) and dietary habits (high-fat diet, high red or processed meat consumption), and personal history of adenomatous polyps, CRC, inflammatory bowel disease, and prior treatment for Hodgkin's lymphoma. More details regarding these factors are discussed in *Chap. 16, Colon Cancer*. Also inherited genetic risk (FAP and HNPCC) and family history of CRC and adenomatous polyps are also risk factors. By and large, the majority of CRC is sporadic for which the underlying etiology is unknown. HNPCC accounts for 2–6 % of CRC and FAP <1 % of all CRC. Further elucidation of their natural history and treatment can be found in *Chap. 20, Hereditary Colorectal Cancer and Polyposis Syndromes*.

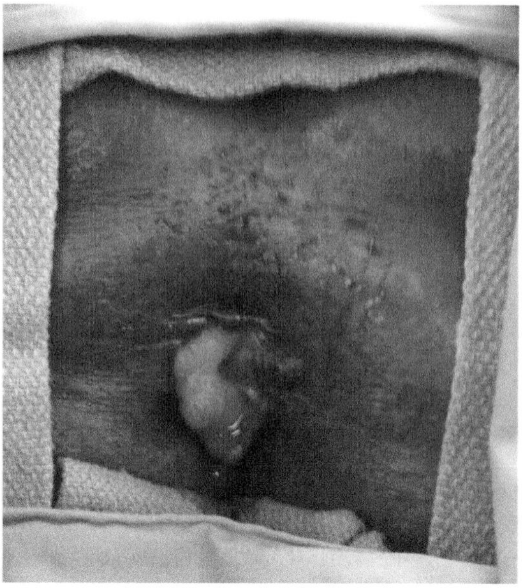

Fig. 18.1 A 62-year-old woman who presents with a rectal adenocarcinoma involving the sphincter complex. She is not a candidate for sphincter-preserving operation. The patient underwent neoadjuvant chemoradiation therapy followed by a successful abdominoperineal resection (Courtesy of Quyen D. Chu, MD, MBA, FACS)

Clinical Presentation

While rectal cancer may not be associated with symptoms in a minority of patients, most generally present with complaints of change in bowel habits, rectal pressure, a constant urge to move their bowels (tenesmus), and/or rectal bleeding that is often mistaken for hemorrhoids. Complaints of constant anal pain, pain upon defecation, and fecal incontinence suggest advanced disease such as cancer invading into the sphincter complex or pelvic floor (Fig. 18.1). Straining at defecation, constipation with periods of diarrhea, and increased abdominal girth are suggestive of partial large bowel obstruction from the cancer.

Evaluation

The initial evaluation of a patient who presents with the above complaints includes a complete physical examination, digital rectal examination (DRE), and proctoscopy. The patient's nutritional status should also be recorded, although unlike patients with upper gastrointestinal cancers (i.e., esophageal cancer, pancreatic cancer, gastric cancer), poor nutrition is often not observed in patients with CRC. If present, this would suggest advanced disease.

Abdominal examination may reveal enlarged liver suggestive of liver metastasis, ascites indicative of intra-abdominal carcinomatosis, and nodules in the umbilicus or abdominal wall that may represent Sister Mary Joseph nodule. The presence of inguinal adenopathy may be suggestive of metastatic disease. On DRE, if a rectal mass is palpated, location, size, mobility, and distance of the distal edge from the anal verge or anorectal ring are assessed. The integrity and adequacy of the anal sphincter complex are evaluated. Knowing the length of one's own examining digit is helpful in estimating the distance of the cancer from the anal verge. Information on DRE is helpful in ordering appropriate imaging studies and designing treatment plan. A small tumor within 8 cm from the anal verge may be considered for a transanal excision, while a large fixed tumor is best treated with neoadjuvant chemoradiation (neoCRT) and radical resection. In a male, a large anterior tumor that appears to involve the prostate may require a concomitant prostatectomy at the time of a definitive operation, especially if the tumor has not regressed significantly following neoadjuvant therapy. Similarly, in a female, anterior involvement of the posterior vagina might necessitate a partial vaginectomy with reconstruction. Patients with fecal incontinence and compromised anal sphincter function or integrity are not candidates for sphincter-sparing operation (Fig. 18.1). Patients presenting with obstructive symptoms may be candidates for an endoluminal stent or a diverting colostomy, the latter of which can be performed laparoscopically.

Proctoscopy is important not only to accurately visualize and localize the lesion but also to help determine its gross appearance, size, and distance from the anal verge and obtain biopsies. Morphologic features help in prognosticating patients with small rectal cancers who may be candidate for local excision. Ulcerated or flat raised tumors (nonexophytic) tend to have a worse prognosis than those that are polypoid or sessile (exophytic) lesions [4, 5]. Biopsies determine the type of tumor (adenocarcinoma, squamous cell carcinoma, small cell carcinoma, undifferentiated carcinoma, etc.) and histopathological features that are essential in the selection of small tumors for local versus local + adjuvant versus radical resection.

As part of the complete work-up, a colonoscopy is warranted to exclude synchronous lesions in the colon and determine the proximal extent of the tumor. Synchronous benign polyps occur in 13–62 % of cases, while synchronous cancers occur in 2–8 % of cases [6–8]. The rectum can be divided into thirds: upper, middle, and lower thirds. Such division can be based on the valves of Houston or by dividing the rectum into thirds using either the 12 cm or 15 cm as the cutoff point (Fig. 18.2). The National Cancer Institute Guidelines for Colon and Rectal Cancer defined the most proximal boundary of the rectum as no more than 12 cm from the anal verge [9], while the European Society for Medical Oncology (ESMO) defined rectal tumors as those with distal extension < 15 cm from the anal verge [10] . Establishing which thirds of the rectum to which the tumor belongs is essential in determining the treatment modality and type of operation the patient will ultimately require.

Unlike colon cancer which drains mainly into the portal venous system (route that leads to metastasis to the liver), rectal cancer drains into both the portal venous system and the systemic circulation, the latter via the inferior and middle rectal veins to the iliac veins and finally to the inferior vena cava. Consequently, rectal cancer can bypass the portal venous system to reside in the lungs, which explains why the incidence of isolated lung metastases is higher in rectal cancer (12 % vs. 6 %) than it is in colon cancer [11, 12]. Given rectal cancer's affinity to metastasize to the lungs, it is reasonable to obtain CT scans of the chest as part of the work-up of patients with rectal cancer.

Imaging Modalities

Computed tomography (CT) scanning, magnetic resonance imaging (MRI), and transrectal ultrasound (TRUS) have all been extensively evaluated in the initial staging of rectal carcinoma [13–15]. Pretreatment imaging to accurately stage the patient is extremely important because it can potentially alter treatment and affect patients' outcome. For a patient with a low-lying T1 lesion who is concerned about having a permanent colostomy and/or sexual dysfunction, a local rectal excision may be an option. However, the same patient with a T2 lesion will likely be treated with radical surgery, which may result in a permanent colostomy and/or sexual dysfunction. Thus, these decisions cannot be made without accurate presurgical staging. Although reports suggest that MRI and TRUS are better at staging rectal cancer than CT, to date, they have not been reliable enough to be used routinely as the sole imaging modality [16, 17]. Furthermore, because of the prohibitive cost associated with MRI, such modality may not be widely available in many centers.

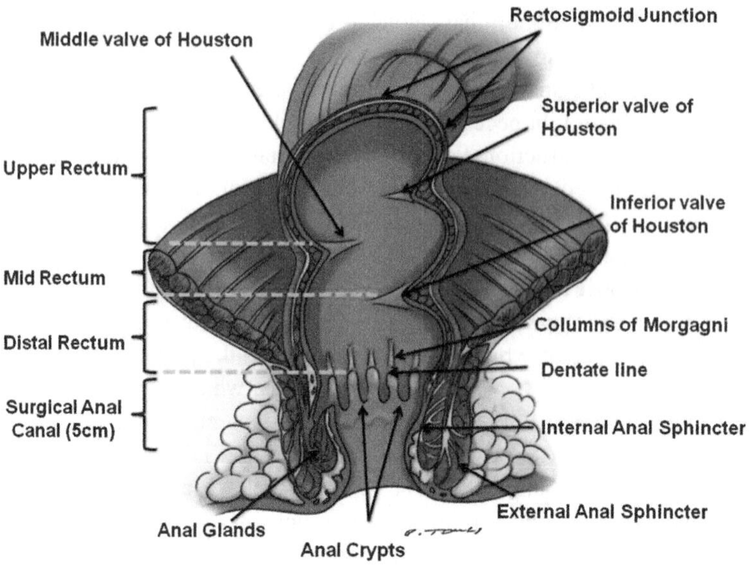

Fig. 18.2 **Anatomy of the rectum**: the rectum can be divided into thirds: upper, middle, and lower thirds. Such division can be based on the valves of Houston or by dividing the rectum into thirds using either the 12 cm or 15 cm as the cutoff point (Illustrated by Paul Tomljanovich, MD and modified by Karen Howard and Lory Tubbs. Courtesy of Quyen D. Chu, MD, MBA, FACS)

Computed Tomography

CT was the first "staging" modality used to evaluate rectal cancer (Figs. 18.3 and 18.6a). Early enthusiasms reported its accuracy to range between 85 % and 90 % [18], and it was championed to be an excellent preoperative staging modality for characterizing both tumor and metastases. CT is still recommended in the initial evaluation of all patients scheduled for colorectal carcinoma surgery because of its ability to obtain a rapid global evaluation of the extent of disease and helpful in revealing complications (perforation, obstruction) that may not be clinically apparent. Larger, more carefully controlled studies, however, have shown that the overall accuracy of CT is in the 50–70 % range, varying directly with the stage of the lesion (i.e., T4 lesions are more accurately assessed than T2 or T3 lesions) [13, 15, 19]. Overstaging is a far more common problem as it is difficult to accurately determine T-stage (depth of bowel wall penetration) on CT [20]. Another complicating factor, particularly in rectal cancer, is that perirectal spiculation can be confused with desmoplastic peritumoral inflammation, which can lead to overstaging.

There is little agreement on the critical cutoff diameter to determine if lymph nodes are involved. One study suggests that the cutoff value should be 4.5 mm; however, nodal size does not correlate with nodal status [21, 22]. The specificity for detecting lymph nodes involved with tumor is only 45 % [23].

Liver metastases are detected by CT with an 85 % accuracy rate and a 97 % specificity rate [15]. Detection of liver metastases by CT improves with increasing stage of disease. Among a group of 100 patients who underwent CT, CT arterioportography (CTAP), and MRI, the sensitivity and specificity for liver metastases were 73 % and 96.5 % for CT, 87.1 % and 89.3 % for CTAP, and 81.9 % and 93.2 % for MRI [19]. In addition, abdominal/pelvic CT has a high negative predictive value of 90 % [21].

As mentioned previously, rectal cancer can spread to the lungs via the systemic portal circulation route. Among patients with potentially

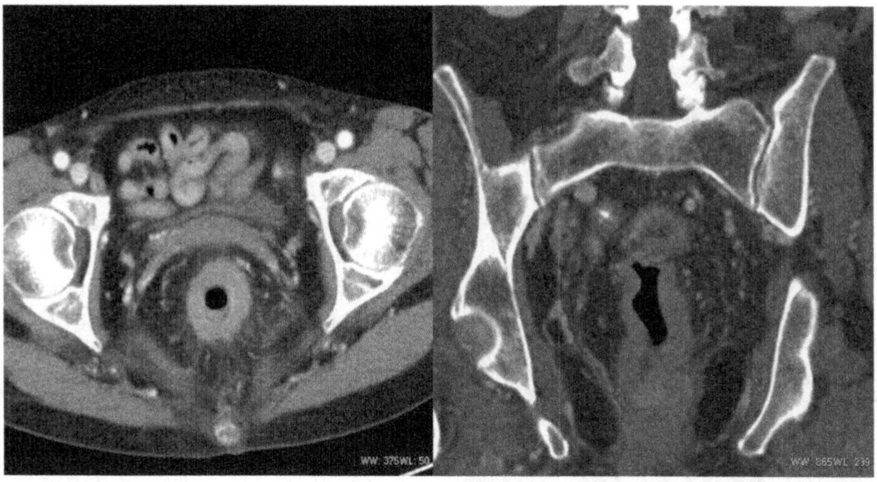

Fig. 18.3 A 64-year-old woman with an advanced rectal cancer. She underwent neoadjuvant chemoradiation therapy and a laparoscopic abdominoperineal resection (Courtesy of Quyen D. Chu, MD, MBA, FACS)

resectable liver metastases and a negative initial chest radiograph, additional imaging with a chest CT revealed pulmonary metastases in only 5 % of patients [24]. However, one study showed that rectal cancer is more likely than colon cancer to present with lung metastases without liver metastases and that this risk increases with advancing T-stage. Although this study advised CT imaging of the chest in all rectal cancer patients, it was limited by the lack of pathologic correlation [25].

Magnetic Resonance Imaging

The Radiology Diagnostic Oncology Group (RDOG) study showed that MRI had an accuracy rate of 58 % for detecting local staging of rectal cancer [15] (Fig. 18.4). Accuracy in identifying lymph node metastases was similar to CT with a sensitivity of 85 %, but MRI was slightly superior for detecting liver metastases. Endorectal MR coils and 3.0 T magnets [27] have shown impressive results in depicting the layers of the rectal wall with resultant improvement in the accuracy of assessing the depth of bowel wall penetration [17]. There is no consensus in the literature as to whether endorectal coils should be used routinely in practice. Some studies contend that endorectal coils provide improved diagnostic accuracy as compared to phased-array coils alone for T-stage, with sensitivity reaching 100 % and specificity of 86 %. Endorectal coils have limitations in assessing upper rectal tumors and lateral pelvic and inferior mesenteric lymph nodes. Although phased-array coils are far superior in detecting lymph node metastases, they are limited in the imaging of obese patients and in the evaluation of lower rectal tumors [28, 29]. With the advent of 3.0 T imaging, most imaging can be performed with a pelvic phased-array coil only.

MRI is accurate at identifying high-risk features such as extramural venous invasion, extramural spread beyond 5 mm, and potentially positive circumferential resection margin (CRM). CRM, which is the distance of the leading edge of the tumor to the mesorectal fascia, is an important prognostic factor for determining risk of local recurrence. The accuracy, sensitivity, and specificity of MRI to predict CRM involvement are 86 %, 94–100 %, and 85–88 %, respectively [30]. From a surgical perspective, assessment of the mesorectal fascia involvement and tumor-free CRM is crucial for surgical planning [31].

Diffusion-weighted imaging (DWI) has shown to be more sensitive and specific than standard contrast-enhanced MRI with gadolinium-enhanced MRI, with values of 82 % and 94 %, respectively [32]. It is believed to be superior for

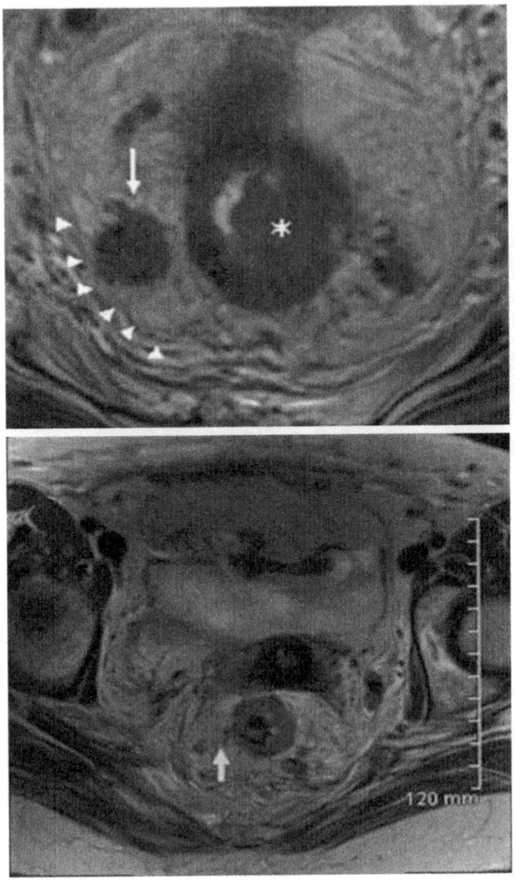

Fig. 18.4 **MRI of the rectum**, high-resolution magnetic resonance imaging of rectal cancer used for staging. (*Top*) An axial, T2-weighted, nonfat-saturated image demonstrating a rectal tumor identified invading the muscularis propria (*). There is an adjacent enlarged heterogenous lymph node (*arrow*) in contact with the mesorectal fascia (*arrow heads*). Incidental note is made of another heterogenous lymph node to the left of the rectum. (*Bottom*) Vascular invasion in the linear area of an abnormal T2 signal extending from the tumor margin (*arrow*) (Reprinted from Ref. [26]. With permission from John Wiley & Sons, Inc.)

tumor detection and characterization and for monitoring tumor response. Adding DWI to conventional MRI yields better diagnostic accuracy than conventional MRI alone [32]. DWI does not use contrast and is more sensitive than contrast-enhanced CT in detecting metastases [33]. It also has the potential to be clinically effective for the evaluation of preoperative TNM staging and the postoperative follow-up of colorectal cancer.

Transrectal Ultrasound

TRUS has become the standard imaging procedure for staging rectal carcinoma [34]. Because TRUS enables one to distinguish the layers within the rectal wall, it is an accurate method for detecting depth of tumor penetration and perirectal spread. Reported sensitivities range between 83 % and 97 %. The T-stage accuracy for TRUS (84.6 %) is far superior to that of CT (70.5 %) [22]. TRUS is of value in assessing apparently superficial rectal carcinomas that are potentially suitable for treatment by transanal or local excision or endocavitary radiation [23]. Detection of lymph node involvement with TRUS is difficult; the sensitivity rate is 50–57 % [29] and the overall accuracy is between 62 % and 83 % [35]. Although TRUS is frequently used to assess regional lymph nodes, it is not very reliable in predicting actual nodal involvement. Many lymph nodes measuring <5 mm in diameter have associated micrometastases, while some early stage T1 and T2 tumors that have lymph node micrometastases were missed by TRUS. Such limitations partly explain the high pelvic recurrence rate observed within this patient population who underwent local rectal excision.

Nuclear Medicine

Positron emission tomography (PET) and PET/CT have been shown to alter therapy in almost a third of patients with advanced primary rectal cancer. In a study comparing PET/CT with TRUS, MRI, and helical CT in imaging patients with low rectal carcinoma, PET/CT identified discordant findings and was far superior in 38 % of patients. The result was an upstaging in half the patients while downstaging in almost a quarter of patients (21 %) [36]. A relatively new concept of using PET/CT has been reported to be significantly more accurate in defining TNM stage than CT alone [36]. However, it is not used routinely in most centers. The accuracy of PET/CT is similar to that of CT in terms of T-stage but is far superior in detecting hepatic and peritoneal metastases (sensitivity, 89 %, and specificity, 64 %) [37]. The sensitivity of detecting nodal metastases is only 43 % with a specificity of 80 %, and again, size is not a helpful characteristic. There is also a potential role for PET in restaging colorectal cancer after chemoradiotherapy by measuring the pretreatment and posttreatment standard uptake volume (SUV) and assessing response by the amount of decreasing SUV [38]. Limitations of PET include decreased sensitivity in detecting small colonic lesions (5–10 mm in diameter) and decreased 18F-fluorodeoxyglucose (FDG) uptake by mucinous tumors.

The 2012 European Society for Medical Oncology consensus guidelines recommend pelvic MRI for staging of primary rectal cancer [39], while NCCN guidelines (version 4.2013) recommend either a pelvic MRI or endorectal ultrasound [40].

Staging

Clinical stage of rectal cancer is determined by preoperative DRE and imaging studies (CT scan, ERUS, endorectal coil MRI, and/or PET scan). Pathologic staging is determined after excision of the cancer. Rectal cancer is staged using the seventh edition of the American Joint Committee on Cancer (AJCC)/TNM staging system (Table 18.1) [42]. By definition, stage II has uninvolved nodes, whereas stage III has involved lymph nodes. There are several important changes made to the sixth edition. T4 lesions are subdivided into T4a (tumor penetrates to the surface of the visceral peritoneum) and T4b (tumor directly invades or is adherent to other organs or structures). The number of involved lymph nodes also has an impact on outcomes; thus, N1 is subdivided into N1a (metastasis in 1 regional lymph node), N1b (metastasis in 2–3 lymph nodes), and N1c (no nodal disease, but tumor deposits in the subserosa, mesentery, or non-personalized pericolic or perirectal tissues); N2 is subdivided into N2a (metastasis in 4–6 nodes) and N2b (metastasis in ≥ 7 nodes) [40].

In the seventh edition, stage group II was subdivided into three subdivisions instead of two: stage IIA (T3N0), IIB (T4aN0), and IIC (T4bN0).

Table 18.1 American Joint Committee on Cancer (AJCC) TNM staging for colorectal carcinoma (7th edition)

Primary tumor (T)*	
TX	Primary tumor cannot be assessed
T0	No evidence of primary tumor
Tis	Carcinoma in situ: intraepithelial or invasion of lamina propria*
T1	Tumor invades submucosa
T2	Tumor invades muscularis propria
T3	Tumor invades through muscularis propria into pericolorectal tissues
T4a	Tumor penetrates to the surface of the visceral peritoneum**
T4b	Tumor directly invades or is adherent to other organs or structures**, ***

**Note*: Tis includes cancer cells confined within the glandular basement membrane (intraepithelial) or mucosal lamina propria (intramucosal) with no extension through the muscularis mucosae into the submucosa

***Note*: Direct invasion in T4 includes invasion of other organs or other segments of the colorectum as a result of direct extension through the serosa, as confirmed on microscopic examination (e.g., invasion of the sigmoid colon by a carcinoma of the cecum) or, for cancers in a retroperitoneal or subperitoneal location, direct invasion of other organs or structures by virtue of extension beyond the muscularis propria (i.e., respectively, a tumor on the posterior wall of the descending colon invading the left kidney or lateral abdominal wall or a mid or distal rectal cancer with invasion of prostate, seminal vesicles, cervix, or vagina)

****Note*: Tumor that is adherent to other organs or structures, grossly, is classified cT4b. However, if no tumor is present in the adhesion, microscopically, the classification should be pT1–4a depending on the anatomical depth of wall invasion. The V and L classifications should be used to identify the presence or absence of vascular or lymphatic invasion, whereas the PN site-specific factor should be used for perineural invasion

Regional lymph nodes (N)	
NX	Regional lymph nodes cannot be assessed
N0	No regional lymph node metastasis
N1	Metastasis in 1–3 regional lymph nodes
N1a	Metastasis in 1 regional lymph node
N1b	Metastasis in 2–3 regional lymph nodes
N1c	Tumor deposit(s) in the subserosa, mesentery, or nonperitonealized pericolic or perirectal tissues without regional nodal metastasis
N2	Metastasis in ≥4 regional lymph nodes
N2a	Metastasis in 4–6 regional lymph nodes
N2b	Metastasis in ≥7 regional lymph nodes

(continued)

Table 18.1 (continued)

Regional lymph nodes (N)
Note: A satellite peritumoral nodule in the pericolorectal adipose tissue of a primary carcinoma without histologic evidence of residual lymph node in the nodule may represent discontinuous spread, venous invasion with extravascular spread (V 1/2), or a totally replaced lymph node (N1/2). Replaced nodes should be counted separately as positive nodes in the N category, whereas discontinuous spread or venous invasion should be classified and counted in the site-specific factor category tumor deposits (TD)

Distant metastasis (M)	
M0	No distant metastasis
M1	Distant metastasis
M1a	Metastasis confined to one organ or site (e.g., the liver, lung, ovary, nonregional node)
M1b	Metastases>one organ/site or the peritoneum

Anatomical stage/prognostic groups

Stage	T	N	M	Dukes*	MAC*
0	Tis	N0	M0	–	–
I	T1	N0	M0	A	A
	T2	N0	M0	A	B1
IIA	T3	N0	M0	B	B2
IIB	T4a	N0	M0	B	B2
IIC	T4b	N0	M0	B	B3
IIIA	T1–2	N1/N1c	M0	C	C1
	T1	N2a	M0	C	C1
IIIB	T3–T4a	N1/N1c	M0	C	C2
	T2–T3	N2a	M0	C	C1/C2
	T1–T2	N2b	M0	C	C1
IIIC	T4a	N2a	M0	C	C2
	T3–T4a	N2b	M0	C	C2
	T4b	N1–N2	M0	C	C3
IVA	Any T	Any N	M1a	–	–
IVB	Any T	Any N	M1b	–	–

Note: cTNM is the clinical classification; pTNM is the pathologic classification. The y prefix is used for those cancers that are classified after neoadjuvant pretreatment (e.g., ypTNM). Patients who have a complete pathologic response are ypT0N0cM0 that may be similar to stage group 0 or I. The r prefix is to be used for those cancers that have recurred after a disease-free interval (rTNM)

*Dukes B is a composite of better (T3N0M0) and worse (T4N0M0) prognostic groups, as is Dukes C (any TN1M0 and any TN2M0). MAC is the modified Astler-Coller classification

Adapted from Ref. [41]. With permission from Springer Verlag

Additionally, several stage group III were reclassified (i.e., T4bN1 is reclassified as IIIC instead of IIIB, T1N2a is IIIA instead of IIIC, T1N2b, T2N2a–b, and T3N2a are IIIB instead of IIIC). Finally, M1 is subdivided into M1a (single metastatic site) and M1b (multiple metastatic sites).

Treatment

Management of rectal cancer requires a multidisciplinary approach. However, surgery remains the mainstay treatment modality of rectal cancer. The primary goals are to cure the patient, maintain function, reduce local recurrence, maximize disease-free survival (DFS), and optimize quality of life. Locoregional recurrence after surgery is related in part to surgical technique. Treatment of rectal cancer depends on location of the tumor and staging information. Selected cases of rectal cancer can be treated with local excision (discussed in *Chap. 17, Local Excision of Early-Stage Rectal Cancer*); however, the majority of rectal cancers are treated with radical resection with or without adjuvant therapy.

Upper Rectal Cancer

The rectosigmoid junction is identified at the level of the promontory of the sacrum and where the teniae coli coalesce to form the continuous longitudinal muscle layer around the rectum. The anterior and lateral wall of the upper rectum is covered with peritoneum, and unlike the middle and distal rectum, it is not confined within the bony pelvis. The concern of sphincter preservation is therefore not relevant.

While it is widely accepted that combination therapy comprising of chemoradiation therapy (CRT) and surgery is the treatment of choice for patients with stage II and III rectal cancer in the mid and distal rectum, the benefit of CRT does not extend to patients with upper rectal or rectosigmoid cancers. Lopez-Kostner et al found that local recurrence and survival for upper rectal cancer were similar to those of sigmoid cancer and because of this, the upper rectum is treated more like colon cancer than rectal cancer [43]. In other words, chemoradiation and possibly total mesorectal excision (TME) may be spared in patients with upper rectal/rectosigmoid cancer, especially those that are T3N0 (Stage II). Both the Swedish Rectal Trial and Dutch Rectal Trial found that, compared to surgery alone, preoperative radiation followed by surgery had no significant impact on local recurrence rate for upper rectal tumors [44].

For upper rectal cancer, anterior resection with tumor specific rather than TME is required. The mesorectum is divided 3–5 cm below the lesion [45]. Alternatively, anterior resection without TME for upper rectosigmoid cancer is also an acceptable option.

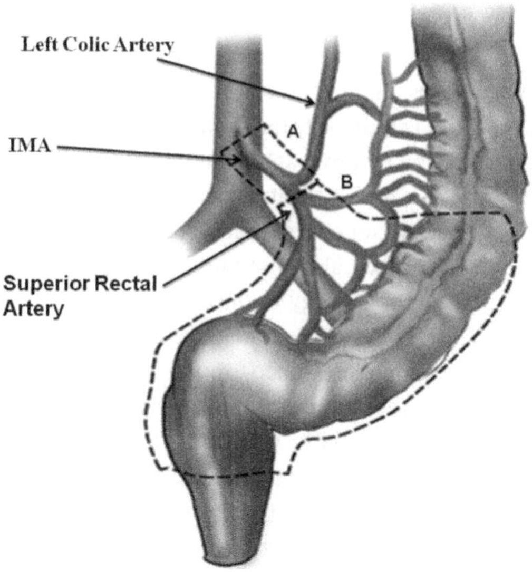

Fig. 18.5 Surgical approaches to rectal cancer. In addition to resecting sufficient segment of bowel proximal and distal to the tumor and mesorectal excision, the major feeding vessel accompanied by lymphatics and LN are ligated at the level of their origin from the aorta. The inferior mesenteric artery (IMA) close to the aorta is taken (high ligation, Fig. 18.5A), but ligation above the bifurcation of the aorta distal to the left colic artery is sufficient (low ligation at the level of the superior rectal artery, Fig. 18.5B) (Reprinted from Ref. [46]. Available from http://www.intechopen.com/books/cancer-treatment-conventional-and-innovative-approaches/current-strategies-in-the-management-of-adenocarcinoma-of-the-rectum with permission from InTech)

Mid and Distal Rectal Cancer

Unlike the colon, the mid and distal rectum are confined in the pelvis, constrained by the bony pelvis, surrounded by major neurovascular structures, and in close proximity to urogenital organs which makes it difficult to achieve a wide resection around the tumor. Consequently, the risk of local recurrence is higher than with colon cancer. Also, unlike colon cancer, adjuvant radiation is required with stage II rectal cancer.

For the majority of rectal cancers, radical or major surgical resection is optimal, sphincter-sparing operation such as a low or ultralow anterior resection (LAR or ULAR) with or without reconstruction for mid to low rectal cancer, and an abdominoperineal resection (APR) for some mid rectal cancers and all low rectal cancer (Fig. 18.5). Better stapling devices have increased the success of low anastomoses, thus allowing more liberal use of sphincter-sparing surgeries. The decision to perform an LAR versus an APR depends mainly on whether an adequate distal margin can be achieved and whether the sphincter complex is compromised. With LAR, the colorectal anastomosis is performed hand sewn or stapled. To perform ULAR without reconstruction, a straight low rectal or coloanal anastomosis is performed either with hand sewn at the dentate line after excision of the columnar to the level of the anorectal ring or stapled at or just above the level of the anorectal ring. For ULAR with construction, the neorectum is fashioned (transverse coloplasty or colonic J-pouch) and anastomosed to the low rectum or just above the anorectal ring. With reconstruction, the functional outcome is superior to straight coloanal or low colorectal anastomosis [47, 48]. Other procedures that involve posterior or intersphincteric resection are not widely used and will not be further discussed. Kraske transsacral and York-Mason transphincteric resections are of historic interest. Transabdominal coloanal anastomosis after removal part of or the entire internal sphincter (intersphincteric resection) is associated with high positive circumferential margin.

Mortality of rectal cancer is related to metastatic disease present prior to surgery and recurrence after surgery. Local recurrence is related to technique and adequacy of resection. Pelvic recurrence poses a management dilemma because the morbidity is quite substantial and the majority of patients who recurred are not amenable to a reoperation. The high LR rate observed in the past is likely due to suboptimal surgical techniques as well as the medical community's lack of knowledge about the biology of the disease.

The goal of radical or major resection is to (1) obtain adequate clearance around the tumor and tumor-free resection margins (proximal, distal, and circumferential), (2) remove LN-bearing mesorectum with an intact envelope, (3) ligate the IMA at its origin, (4) harvest at least ≥12 regional LN, (5) minimize the risk of tumor perforation or rupture, and (6) en bloc resection of any adherent structure.

Margins

Surgery requires resection of a sufficient segment of bowel proximal and distal to the tumor. Generally, proximal margin ≥ 5 cm is sufficient and 2 cm for distal margins is ideal. However, for distal rectal cancers a 1–2 cm is acceptable. Appreciable distal intramural spread of rectal adenocarcinoma is noted in only 25 % of cases and is almost always within 1.5 cm of the primary tumor. Tumor spread > 1.5 cm is found in poorly differentiated or widely metastatic cancer. In the era of neoCRT, the required 2 cm distal margin can be reduced to 1 cm [49]. To reiterate, patients whose tumors that cannot be safely resected with a clear distal margin or have evidence of sphincter involvement or dysfunction should undergo an APR. Inadequate number of lymph nodes retrieved is associated with increased mortality in both node-negative and node-positive rectal cancer [50, 51].

Circumferential margin is the nonperitonealized surface of the rectal specimen created by mesorectal dissection at surgery (Fig. 18.6c). Circumferential margin is considered positive if the distance between the deepest extent of the tumor and closed surgical clearance around the tumor, i.e., circumferential resection margin (CRM), is 0 to 1 mm. In radical resection, a > 1 mm circumferential resection margin (CRM) is optimal. CRM has been found to be an independent predictor of outcome in patients with rectal cancer. An involved CRM is defined as tumor within or equal to 1 mm or less from the CRM [52]. When CRM is < 1 mm, local recurrence rate was 22 %, but when it was more than 1 mm, this rate drops to 5 % [53]. Furthermore, CRM < 1 mm was predictive of an increased risk of distant metastases (37 % vs. 15 % for those with CRM > 1 mm) and shorter survival (70 % vs. 90 % at 2 years for those with CRM > 1 mm) [54]. However, other investigators have considered 2 mm as the cutoff point [55]. Nagtegaal reported that the local recurrence was 16 % for CRM <2 mm versus 6 % for patients with radial margins > 2 mm [55]. Although the ideal CRM has not been universally accepted, the general principle is that the operating surgeon should strive for as wide of a CRM margin as possible.

Mesorectal Excision

Radical surgery also requires resection of the mesorectum that contains fat, LN (regional LN), and the lymphatics. Heald et al described total mesorectal excision (TME) that involves complete removal of the LN-bearing mesorectum along with its intact enveloping fascia [56]. TME requires sharp dissection, instead of the conventional blunt dissection, in the extrafascial plane between the presacral fascia and the fascia propria of the rectum. TME requires the complete excision of the visceral mesorectal tissue not only the proximal mesorectum but also the distal mesorectum down to the level of the levators [57, 58] (Figs. 18.6b, c and 18.7a–c). TME does require intense training, but when done properly, it can result in substantial locoregional control in long-term outcomes for patients with rectal cancer. Proper identification and preserving branches of the hypogastric nerves innervating the pelvic organ can spare the patient the sequelae of urinary retention and sexual dysfunction (retrograde ejaculation). TME results in a higher number of lymph nodes retrieved because the lymph node

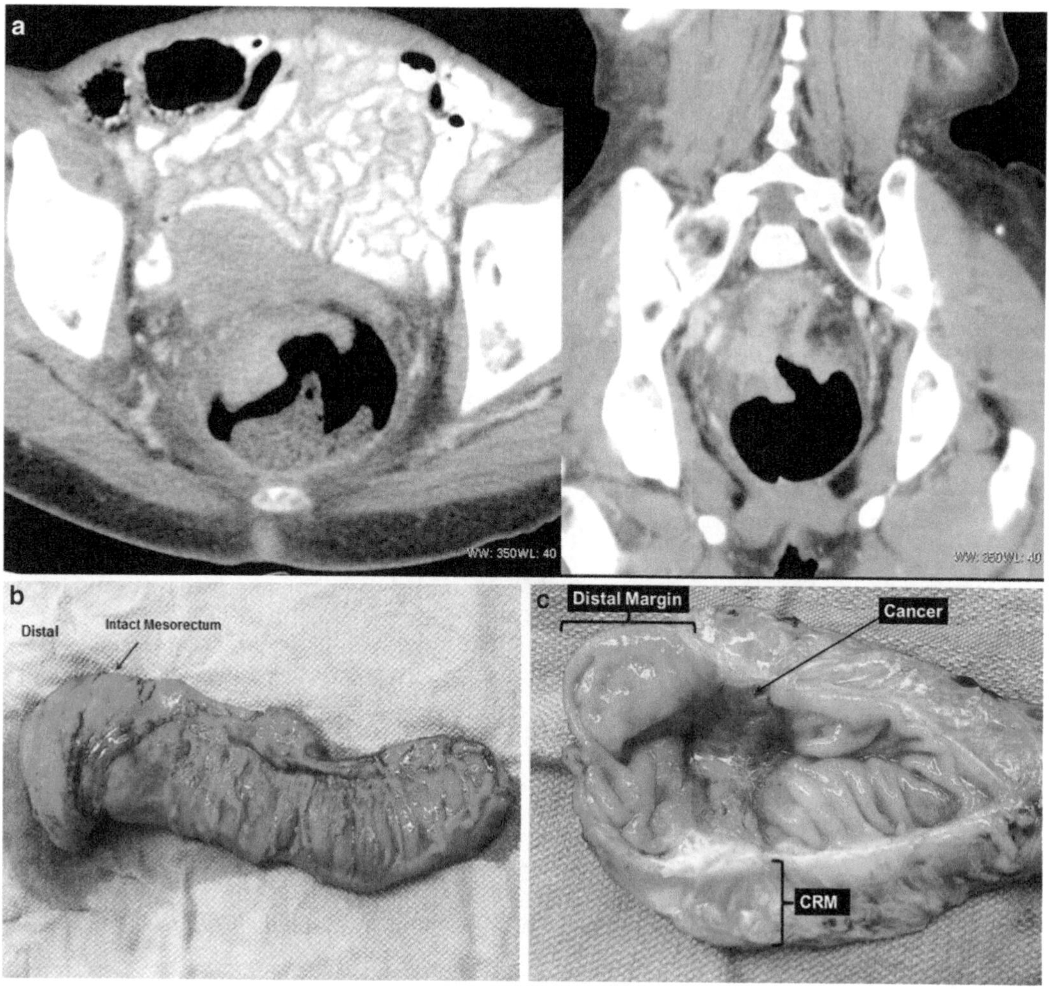

Fig. 18.6 A 67-year-old woman with a rectal cancer located approximately 5 cm from the anal verge. CT demonstrated an advanced rectal cancer (**a**). She underwent preoperative chemoradiotherapy, followed by a low anterior resection, total mesorectal excision, and a diverting loop ileostomy (**b**). The final pathology demonstrated a T3N0M0 disease. None of the 16 lymph nodes were involved; the distal margin was 3 cm from the tumor and the circumferential margin was 8 mm (**c**) (Courtesy of Quyen D. Chu, MD, MBA, FACS)

bearing the mesorectum is resected. Finally, TME accomplishes adequate circumferential radial margin (CRM) (Fig. 18.6b, c.)

Vascular Pedicle

In addition to resecting sufficient segment of bowel proximal and distal to the tumor and mesorectal excision, the major feeding vessel accompanied by the lymphatics and LN are ligated at the level of their origin from the aorta. The inferior mesenteric artery (IMA) close to the aorta is taken, but ligation above the bifurcation of the aorta distal to the left colic artery is sufficient (Figs. 18.5 and 18.8). Along with mobilization of the splenic flexure, the inferior mesenteric vein (IMV) may be ligated at the lower edge of the pancreas to allow the colon to reach the pelvis so as to construct a tension-free anastomosis. The IMV can be identified after taking down the ligament of Treitz; it is located just to the left of the ligament.

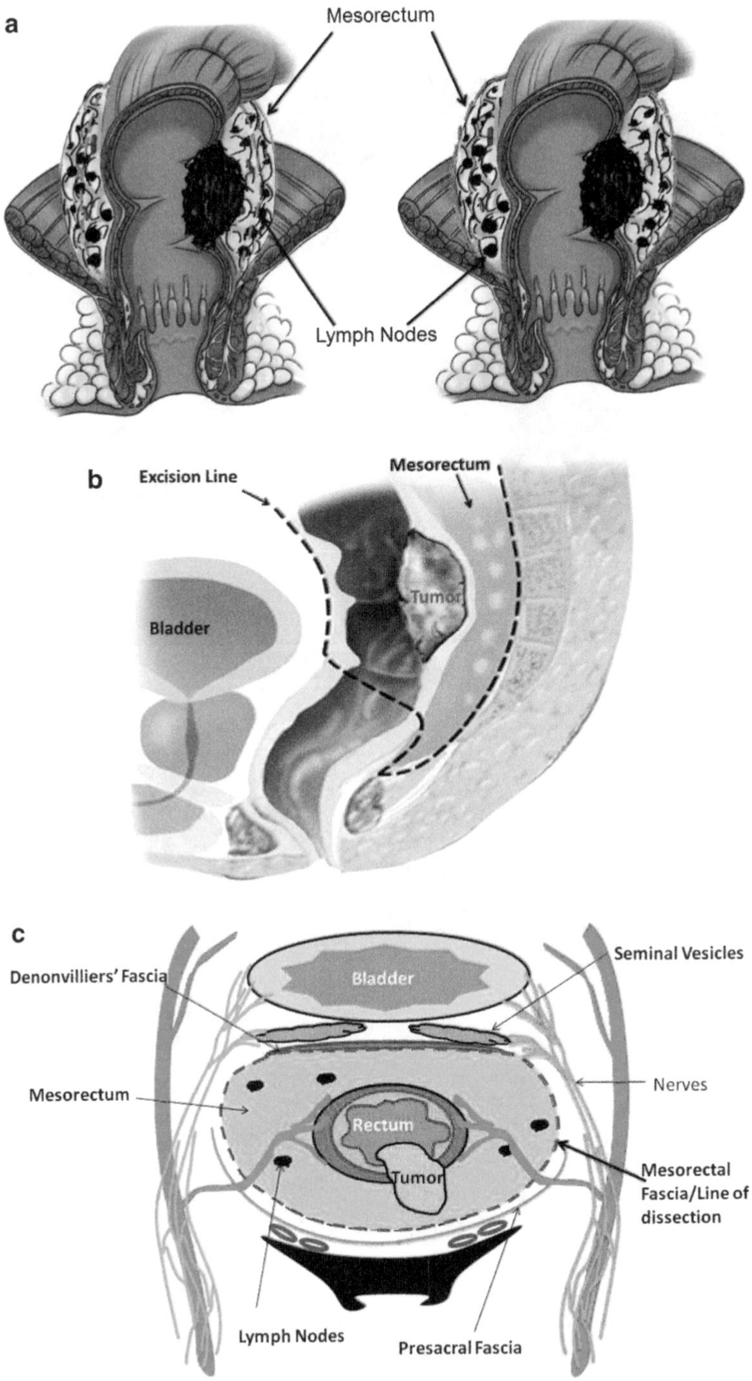

Fig. 18.7 (**a**) Total mesorectal excision (TME): TME requires resection of the mesorectum that contains fat, LN (regional LN), and the lymphatics, along with its intact enveloping fascia. *Panel A* of Fig. 18.7a demonstrates inadequate TME when the line of resection (*red dotted lines*) does not incorporate the mesorectum. *Panel B* of Fig. 18.7a depicts an adequate TME that incorporates the lymph node-bearing mesorectum. (**b**) Sagittal view of a male pelvis: the mesorectum is resected at least 5 cm below the tumor. *Dotted lines* depict extent or resection to achieve sufficient TME. (**c**) Cross section showing TME and the relationship with other pelvic structures: care should be taken to avoid injury to the hypogastric nerve. (**a**: Illustrator-Paul Tomljanovich, MD, modified by Karen Howard and Quyen D. Chu, MD; Courtesy of Quyen D. Chu, MD, MBA, FACS) (**b**: Reprinted from Ref. [46]. Available from http://www.intechopen.com/books/cancer-treatment-conventional-and-innovative-approaches/current-strategies-in-the-management-of-adenocarcinoma-of-the-rectum with permission from InTech.) (**c**: Courtesy of Quyen D. Chu, MD, MBA, FACS)

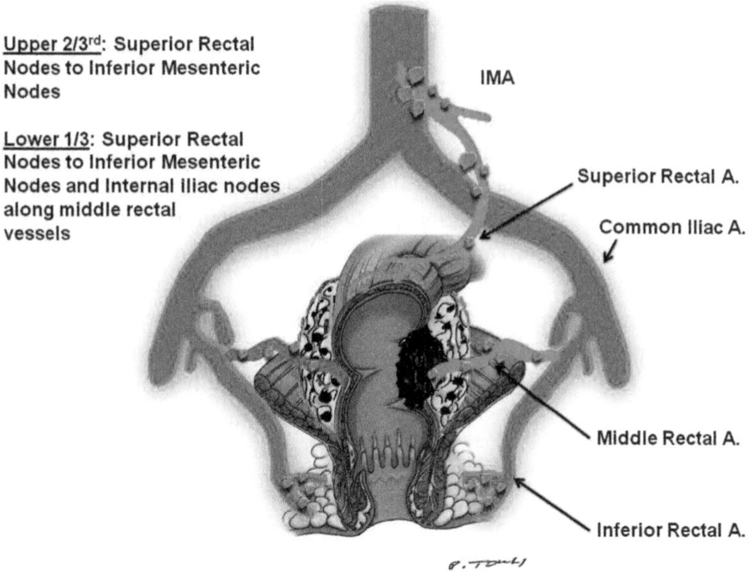

Fig. 18.8 Lymph nodes of the rectum. Note that the upper 2/3 of the rectum is drained by lymph nodes along the superior rectal artery to the lymph nodes along the inferior mesenteric artery (IMA). The lower 1/3 of the rectum is drained by lymph nodes along the superior rectal artery to the lymph nodes along the IMA. It also drains into the lymph nodes along the middle rectal artery, which drains into the nodes along the internal iliac artery and then to the nodes along the para-aortic LN. (Illustrator-Paul Tomljanovich, MD, modified by Karen Howard and Quyen D. Chu, MD; Courtesy of Quyen D. Chu, MD, MBA, FACS)

Lymph Node Dissection

For adequate staging of rectal cancer, at least ≥12 regional lymph nodes, as recommended by the American College of Surgeons, the American College of Pathology, the National Comprehensive Cancer Network (NCCN), and the American Association of Clinical Oncology (ASCO) for colorectal cancers [40, 59–61], must be harvested.

The lymphatics from the rectum drain to the mesorectal LN then upward along the superior rectal artery (or superior hemorrhoidal artery, SHA) toward the mesenteric LN along the IMA to the lateral aortic and para-aortocaval LN (Figs. 18.5 and 18.8). Drainage into paracolic LN is unusual. From the middle and lower rectum, there are two pathways for lymphatic drainage: upward along SHA and laterally to lateral pelvic LN. Downward spread is uncommon. Lateral drainage occurs to intermediate lateral LN (LN along the middle hemorrhoidal artery outside fascia propria) and lateral main LN (along internal iliac artery and obturator artery) to para-aortic LN. The lower rectum however has a cloacal origin and its lymphatic channels are part of the pedicles draining to lateral LN. The number of LN found in the mesorectum ranges from 14 to 28 depending on the method of preparation of specimens. The majority of the mesorectal LNs are located posteriorly with few on each side. There are relatively few LNs in the mesorectum of the lower rectum. Most of the LNs (70 %) are found around the branches of the SHA proximal to the peritoneal reflection, and 30 % are found distal to the peritoneal reflection. In surgical terms, the lymphatic spread of cancer occurs to perirectal (mesorectal LN) and upward along the IMA. With mesorectal excision and ligation of the IMA close to its origin, enough LN will be harvested. Lateral spread to lateral LN is more clinically important in tumors with lower margin below 5 cm from the dentate line, and the incidence becomes significantly higher with lower margin below 3 cm above the dentate line. Spread from the lower rectum laterally to the iliac LN occurs in about 15 % of cases. Lateral spread occurs to LN along the middle rectal artery that lies outside the fascia propria. More extensive nodal dissection such as lateral LN dissection that removes nodal tissue along the common and internal iliac artery demonstrated no survival benefits but increased morbidity (18 % urinary dysfunction, 50 % sexual dysfunction) and therefore should not be performed [62–64]. To reiterate, a TME should be a part of the surgical operation, especially for tumors in the middle and lower rectum.

Tumor Rupture and En Bloc Resection

Inadvertent rupture of the tumor during dissection is associated with increase in LR and decrease in 5-year survival. Separation of structure adherent to the tumor is considered incomplete resection and associated with adverse outcome [9].

Adjuvant and Neoadjuvant Therapy

Patients with early stage rectal cancer (T1-2, N0, M0, or stage I disease) enjoy a 5-year survival rates greater than 90 % after radical surgery alone, and therefore, adjuvant or neoadjuvant therapy is not necessary. For patients with clinical stage II (cT3–4, N0, M0) and III (any T, N+, M0) diseases according to the AJCC/TNM and International Union Against Cancer (IUCC), multimodality therapy (chemotherapy, radiotherapy, surgery) is the treatment of choice. However, this has not always been the case. Historically, surgery alone in this high-risk group resulted in an unacceptably high rate of local recurrence (LR); pelvic recurrence occurs in approximately 30–65 % when surgery alone was performed [65–69].

Pelvic recurrence poses a management dilemma because the morbidity is quite substantial and the majority of patients who recurred are not amenable to a reoperation. The high LR rate observed in the past was likely due to suboptimal surgical techniques (the use of blunt dissection rather than sharp dissection) as well as the paucity of knowledge about the natural history of the disease.

In 1985, the Gastrointestinal Tumor Study Group (GITSG), spearheaded by members of Roswell Park Cancer Institute, Buffalo, New York, conducted a randomized trial to assess the efficacy of postoperative chemoradiation (postCRT) in a group of high-risk patients who underwent "curative" rectal resection [70, 71] (Table 18.2). This landmark study altered the landscape of the management of rectal cancer because it established that adjuvant therapy was better than surgery alone; combination of postoperative chemotherapy (5-fluorouracil or 5-FU based) and radiation therapy significantly reduced recurrence rate from 55 % in the surgery alone group to 33 % in the postCRT group ($P<0.04$). A subsequent study comparing postoperative radiation alone with postCRT confirmed the superiority of postCRT [73]. In this study, postCRT not only significantly reduced rectal recurrence by 34 % ($P=0.0016$) but also reduced cancer-related deaths by 36 % ($P=0.0071$) and overall deaths by 29 % ($P=0.025$).

The National Surgical Adjuvant Breast and Bowel Project (NSABP) R01 trial reported that adjuvant 5-FU after rectal surgery was associated with improved survival compared with either surgery alone or surgery with adjuvant radiation [72]. Based on these studies, the National Institute of Health (NIH) consensus conference in circa 1990 recommended ***postCRT*** as standard treatment for patients with stage II and III rectal cancer [79]. These recommendations, however, have changed with the advent of subsequent clinical trials.

Role of Preoperative Radiation Therapy

In 1997, the Swedish Rectal Cancer Trial group reported a large phase III trial of over 1100 patients comparing a short course of preoperative radiation therapy followed by surgery (*please see section on short-course versus long-course radiation therapy below*) versus surgery alone and found that the preoperative radiation group not only had a significantly lower local recurrence rate (11 % vs. 27 %; $P<0.001$) but also an improved 5-year overall survival (OS) rate

Table 18.2 Summary of selected trials on adjuvant and neoadjuvant treatment of rectal adenocarcinoma

Authors, year	N	Median follow-up (mos)	Treatment groups	TME performed?	Outcome
GITSG 1985 [70, 71]	202	80	1. Adjuvant chemoXRT 2. Observation	No	Adjuvant chemoXRT significantly reduces LR rate from 55 % to 33 % ($P<0.04$)
NSABP R-01, 1988 [72] (Fisher)	555	64	1. Adjuvant chemo 2. Adjuvant XRT 3. Observation	No	Adjuvant chemo significantly reduced DFS and OS compared to observation
Krook 1991 [73]	204	84	1. Adjuvant chemoXRT 2. Adjuvant XRT	No	Adjuvant chemoXRT reduces Recurrence by 34 % ($P=0.0016$) Cancer-related deaths by 36 % ($P=0.0071$) Overall deaths by 29 % ($P=0.025$)
Frykholm 1993 [74]	471	60	1. Preoperative SC XRT 2. Postoperative LC XRT	No	LR lower in preoperative group (13 % vs. 22 %; $P=0.02$) Overall survival: no difference Morbidity: no difference
Swedish Trial, 1997 [75], Folkesson, 2005 [76]	1168	156	1. Preoperative SC XRT 2. Observation	No	**Only trial that demonstrated survival benefit with preoperative XRT**
Colorectal Cancer Collaborative Group 2001 [77]*	8507	NA	1. Preoperative XRT 2. Postoperative XRT 3. Observation	NA	Overall survival: no differences 5-year LR rates Preop XRT, 12.5 % Observation, 22.2 % ($P<0.00001$)
Dutch Trial, 2001 [44] (Kapiteijn), 2011 [78] (van Gijn)	1861	144	1. Preoperative SC XRT + TME 2. TME	Yes	Preop XRT significantly reduces LR rates by > 50 % relative to surgery alone Overall survival: no differences 10-year LR rates Preop XRT/TME, 5 % TME, 11 % ($P<0.0001$)

GITSG Gastrointestinal Tumor Study Group, *NSABP* National Surgical Adjuvant Breast and Bowel Project, *SC* short course, *LC* long course, *OS* overall survival, *DFS* disease-free survival, *LR* local recurrence, *meta-analysis of 22 randomized, controlled trial, *NA* not available, *CRT* chemoradiotherapy, *XRT* radiation therapy, *TME* total mesorectal excision, *chemo* chemotherapy

(58 % vs. 48 %; $P=0.004$) [75]. These results were demonstrated to be durable in their follow-up report (median follow-up time = 13 years [76]). In 2001, the Colorectal Cancer Collaborative Group performed a systematic review of over 8,500 patients from 22 randomized trials and found that both preoperative XRT (neoRT) and postoperative XRT (postRT) were effective at decreasing local recurrence rate when compared to surgery alone [77]. Of note, while multiple subsequent rectal cancer trials by other investigators demonstrated an improved local control rate, the Swedish trial is the only one thus far that had demonstrated an additional OS benefit with combination therapy (Table 18.2).

Total Mesorectal Excision (TME) Era

Almost all of the above earlier studies did not emphasize the importance of surgical techniques in reducing locoregional recurrences. The Dutch Colorectal Cancer Group was the first to assess the role of TME in controlling LR [44]. Over 1800 patients with resectable rectal cancer were randomized to either a short course of neoRT followed by TME or TME alone. Although 2-year OS was not significantly different between the groups (82 % vs. 81.8 %; $P=0.84$), the rate of local recurrence at 2 years was significantly reduced in the neoRT/TME group (2.4 % vs. 8.2 %; $P<0.001$) [44]. The 12-year follow-up results confirmed a 10-year cumulative incidence of local recurrence of 5 % in the neoRT/TME group versus 11 % in the TME alone group ($P<0.0001$) [78] (Table 18.2). The Dutch study galvanized the importance of TME in the management of patients with rectal cancer, which became standard procedure in subsequent clinical trials.

Preoperative Chemoradiotherapy Versus Preoperative Radiotherapy Alone

Although neoRT was effective at controlling local disease, significant tumor downsizing rarely occurred, especially when short-course radiation regimen is used. To improve tumor response, several investigators evaluated the efficacy of adding chemotherapy to neoadjuvant radiation (neoCRT) [80–85] (Table 18.3).

A large phase III trial conducted by the European Organisation for Research and Treatment of Cancer (EORTC) found that neoCRT was better at controlling local disease than neoRT [86, 88]. EORTC 22921 randomized over 1000 patients into four groups, neoRT alone, neoCRT alone, neoRT + adjuvant chemotherapy, and neoCRT + adjuvant chemotherapy. The initial results were reported in 2006 [88] and the latest long-term results were reported in 2014 [86]. With a median follow-up of 10.4 years, the 10-year cumulative risk of local relapse was significantly higher in the preRT alone arm than in any of the three chemotherapy groups ($P=0.0017$). This confirms the efficacy of neoCRT over neoRT in controlling local disease. OS, disease-free survival (DFS), rate of distant metastases, and long-term side effects were not significantly different among the different groups.

A 2013 Cochrane meta-analysis of five major clinical trials reported that although 5-year OS (63.9 % in neoCRT vs. 65.2 % in neoRT; $P=0.58$) and DFS (57.5 % in neoCRT vs. 54.9 % in neoRT; $P=0.27$) were not statistically different between the two groups, the incidence of LR was significantly lower in the neoCRT group compared to neoRT group (9.4 % vs. 16.5 %; $P<0.001$). Although moderate acute toxicity and postoperative complications ($P=0.05$) were higher when chemotherapy was added, there was no increase in the postoperative mortality (2.8 % in neoCRT vs. 1.9 % in neoRT; $P=0.17$) or anastomotic leak rate ($P=0.81$). Finally, neoCRT increased the rate of pathologic complete response (pCR; 11.8 % in neoCRT vs. 3.5 % in neoRT group; $P<0.00001$) but did not result in a higher sphincter preservation rate (50.4 % in neoCRT vs. 48.3 % in neoRT; $P=0.32$). *Based on these results, one can surmise that the major advantage of adding chemotherapy to neoRT is the significant reduction of local recurrence in patients with stage II/III resectable rectal cancer* (Table 18.3).

Table 18.3 Selected randomized trials comparing preoperative chemoradiotherapy with preoperative radiotherapy alone in resectable rectal cancer

Authors/year	N	Median follow-up (mos)	Outcome	Summary
Boulis-Wassif 1984 [80]	247	84	5-year OS NeoCRT, 59 % PreRT, 46 % (P=0.06) 5-year LR rates NeoCRT, 85 % PreRT, 85 %	NeoCRT had borderline significance in OS
Bosset 2014 [86] (EORTC 22921)	1011	125	10-year OS NeoCRT, 50.7 % PreRT, 49.9 % (P=0.91) 10-year DFS NeoCRT, 46.4 % PreRT, 44.2 % (P=0.38) 10-year LR rate NeoCRT, 11.8 % PreRT, 22.4 % (P=0.0017)	LR significantly higher in preRT No differences in OS, DFS, distant metastases rate Long-term side effects
Bujko 2004, 2006 [82, 87] (Polish Trial)	316	48	4-year OS NeoCRT, 66.2 % PreRT, 67.2 % (P=0.96) 4-year DFS NeoCRT, 55.6 % PreRT, 58.4 % (P=0.82) LR rate NeoCRT, 14.2 % PreRT, 9 % (P=0.17)	No differences in OS, DFS, LR rate Incidence of distant metastases Late toxicity
Gerard 2006 [83] (FFCD 9203)	742	81	5-year OS NeoCRT, 67.4 % PreRT, 67.9 % (P=0.684) 5-year PFS NeoCRT, 59.4 % PreRT, 55.5 % (P=0.82) 5-year LR rate NeoCRT, 8.1 % PreRT, 16.5 % (P=0.004)	Grade 3 and 4 toxicity higher in neoCRT No differences in Sphincter preservation rate OS LR was lower in neoCRT
Latkauskas 2012 [85]	83	N/A	N/A	NeoCRT significantly downsizes and downstages tumor No difference in R0 resection rate Sphincter preservation rate Postoperative morbidity rate

(continued)

Table 18.3 (continued)

Authors/year	N	Median follow-up (mos)	Outcome	Summary
De Caluwé, 2013 [84] (Cochrane meta-analysis)	2399	N/A	5-year OS	NeoCRT
			NeoCRT, 63.9 %	Higher toxicity with neoCRT
			PreRT, 65.2 % ($P=0.58$)	Lower LR rate
			5-year DFS	No differences in
			NeoCRT, 57.5 %	OS, DFS
			PreRT, 54.9 % ($P=0.27$)	Sphincter preservation rate
			5-year LR rate,	Postoperative mortality
			NeoCRT, 9.4 %	Anastomotic leak rate
			PreRT, 16.5 % ($P<0.001$)	

neoCRT neoadjuvant chemoradiation therapy, *preRT* preoperative radiotherapy, *LR* local recurrence, *N/A* not available, *EORTC* European Organisation for Research and Treatment of Cancer, *FFCD* Fédération Francophone de Cancérologie Digestive, *PFS* progression-free survival, *DFS* disease-free-survival, *OS* overall survival

Preoperative Chemoradiotherapy Versus Postoperative Chemoradiotherapy

Whether preoperative chemoradiotherapy (neoCRT) is better than postoperative chemoradiotherapy (postCRT) was the focus of three randomized trials, the Intergroup (INT) 0147, the National Surgical Adjuvant Breast and Bowel Project (NSABP) R-03 [89], and the German Rectal Cancer Study Group (Working Group of Surgical Oncology/Working Group of Radiation Oncology/Working Group of Medical Oncology of the Germany Cancer Society or CAO/ARO/AIO) [90] (Table 18.4). Unfortunately, INT 0147 had to close prematurely because it accrued only 53 patients, while NSABP R-03 accrued 267 patients instead of the intended 900 patients [93]. The latter trial, with a median follow-up of 8.4 years, demonstrated a significantly improved DFS and a trend toward improved OS in favor of the preoperative arm, although there was no improvement in the rate of local control [89].

It was the German group that in 2004 successfully defined the ideal sequence of therapy for patients with stage II/III rectal cancer [90]. Over 800 patients with clinical stage T3/T4 or node-positive disease were randomized to receive either neoCRT or postCRT. TME was performed in all patients. At a median follow-up of 46 months, OS was not statistically significant between the groups (76 % in neoCRT group vs. 74 % in the postCRT group; $P=0.80$). However, the 5-year cumulative incidence of local relapse was 6 % in the neoCRT group versus 13 % in the postCRT group ($P=0.006$). In addition, the preoperative group had lower incidence of grade 3 or 4 acute toxicities (27 % vs. 40 %; $P=0.001$), lower long-term toxic effects (14 % vs. 24 %; $P=0.01$), and higher sphincter preservation rate in patients for whom an APR would have been required as deemed by the surgeon (39 % vs. 19 %; $P=0.004$) [90]. Additionally, postoperative complications were similar, assuaging the fear that preoperative chemoradiation might lead to an increased rate of wound breakdown.

An update of this study with a median follow-up of 11 years confirmed the durability of these results; the 10-year cumulative incidence of local relapse was 7.1 % and 10.1 % in the neoCRT and postCRT groups, respectively, ($P=0.048$) [91]; for low-lying tumors that required up-front APR, the rates of local recurrences increased to 20.7 % at 10 years with the postoperative approach, which could have been reduced to 12.3 % had the tumors been treated with the preoperative approach. Both DFS and OS were not significantly different between the two groups (10-year OS was 59.6 % in the preoperative arm and 59.9 % in the postoperative arm; $P=0.85$). In fact, the rate of distant recurrences was 30 % at 10 years in both arms ($P=0.9$). This, alone, allays

Table 18.4 Selected trials comparing neoadjuvant chemoradiotherapy versus adjuvant chemoradiotherapy

Authors, year	*N*	Median follow-up (mos)	Treatment groups	TME performed?	Outcome
German Trial, 2004 2012 (Sauer) [90, 91]	800	134	1. NeoCRT/TME 2. PostCRT/TME (5-FU-based chemotherapy)	Yes	10-year OS, 59.6 % vs. 59.9 % (*P*=0.85) 10-year DFS, 68.1 % vs. 67.8 % (*P*=0.65) 10-year local relapse, 7.1 % vs. 10.1 % (*P*=0.048) 10-year distant relapse, 29.8 % vs. 29.6 % (*P*=0.9) NeoCRT/TME has better local control than postCRT/TME NeoCRT regimen doubled sphincter preservation rate from 19 % to 39 %
NSABP R-03, 2009 [89] (Roh)	267	100	1. NeoCRT 2. PostCRT (5-FU-based chemotherapy)	No/yes	Low accrual rate (only 267 instead of 900 patients). Trial closed early Included patients who had local excision Not all patients had TME 5-year DFS NeoCRT, 64.7 % PostCRT, 53.4 % (*P*=0.011) 5-year OS NeoCRT, 74.5 % PostCRT, 65.6 % (*P*=0.065) 5-year LR control rates (10.7 % vs. 10.7 %; *P*=0.693)
Korean Trial, 2011 [92] (Park)	240	52	1. NeoCRT/TME 2. PostCRT/TME (Capecitabine chemotherapy)	Yes	No significant differences in 5-year DFS (74 % vs. 74 %; *P*=0.86) 5-year OS (90 % vs. 85 %; *P*=0.62) LR rate (6 % vs. 6 %; *P*=0.39) Distant metastasis rate (24 % vs. 24 %; *P*=0.73) Acute or late complication rates Sphincter preservation is higher in neoCRT group for low-lying tumors (68 % vs. 42 %; *P*=0.008)

NSABP National Surgical Adjuvant Breast and Bowel Project, *neoCRT* neoadjuvant chemoradiation therapy, *postCRT* postoperative chemoradiation therapy, *TME* total mesorectal excision, *DFS* disease-free survival, *OS* overall survival

the theoretical concern that delaying surgery might lead to a loss opportunity of a cure for patients undergoing neoadjuvant therapy. Thus, the German trial cemented the role of neoCRT in treating patients with stage II/III rectal cancer because it demonstrated that neoCRT had better local control, sphincter-sparing rate, and treatment-related toxicities compared to neoCRT, although DFS or OS was not affected.

Some investigators questioned whether neoCRT actually leads to a higher rate of sphincter-sparing surgery. Although the German trial reported a doubling of sphincter preservation rate in patients undergoing neoCRT for whom an APR would have been required as deemed by the surgeon (39 % vs. 19 %; *P*=0.004), the absolute rate of APR was not statistically different when compared to the postCRT group.

Additionally, a review of 17 randomized trials found that compared to postCRT, neoCRT did not necessarily increase the rate of sphincter-sparing surgery [94].

One of the concerns of the preoperative approach is overtreatment. Up to 18 % of patients in the German trial who were thought to have had cT3N0 disease based on endorectal ultrasound (ERUS) underwent up-front surgery and were found to actually have pT1–2 N0 disease (stage I disease). Obviously, surgery alone in these patients is all that is required. However, preoperative staging using MRI/TRUS is imperfect and can also understage patients. In a review of 188 patients who underwent neoCRT and were deemed to have T3N0 disease by MRI/TRUS, 22 % actually had nodal involvement (i.e., stage III disease) [95]. This rate may actually be higher given that preoperative treatment can sterilize involved LNs.

One is tempted to argue that cT3N0 patients should undergo surgery first while waiting for the final pathology. CRT can then be spared in those who were downstaged, while postCRT can be given to those who had stage II or III disease. While this is a legitimate argument, it should be recalled that compared to neoCRT, postCRT is associated with increased toxicity and local recurrence rates (German trial), as well as decreased compliance to adjuvant chemotherapy following surgery, and abnormal bowel function due to radiation of low pelvic anastomosis [77, 95].

Given these reasons, neoCRT is the preferred approach for patients with stage II/III cancer.

Of note, guidelines on the minimal number of lymph nodes retrieved (≥12 LNs) are extrapolated from data for colon cancer, and the number of lymph nodes retrieved may be influenced by neoadjuvant therapy. In a study of over 700 patients by Govindarajan et al at Memorial Sloan Kettering Cancer Center, there was a significantly fewer number of lymph nodes retrieved in the neoadjuvant group compared to surgery alone (10.8 vs. 15.5; $P<0.001$). The investigators concluded that in a major tertiary cancer center such as theirs, the 12 LN threshold may not be relevant and may not be an accurate quality indicator since lower LN count following neoadjuvant therapy was not associated with understaging or inferior survival [96]. Like many things in clinical practice, guidelines should be used in a context of clinical judgment. Surgeons caring for patients with rectal cancer should be aware of these guidelines, but also be cognizant of their own outcomes.

Short-Course Versus Long-Course Radiation Therapy

Preoperative external beam radiation therapy (RT) for rectal cancer is given either as short-course (SC) regimen or long-course (LC) therapy. The SC regimen delivers 25 Gy over a 5-day period (5 × 5 Gy regimen) followed by immediate surgery within 1–2 weeks of completing RT, while the LC regimen delivers smaller fraction of radiation (1.8–2 Gy) over a period of 25–28 days, giving a higher total dose of radiation (45–54 Gy); chemotherapy can be given concurrently with the LC regimen but not with the SC because of potential toxicity. Unlike the SC regimen, surgery is delayed for 6 weeks to 8 weeks after RT in the LC regimen. The LC regimen is used mainly in the United States as well as some part of Europe, whereas the SC schedule is used mainly in Europe; in fact, a number of rectal cancer clinical trials stemming from Europe use the SC regimen.

Compared to LC regimen, the benefits of SC schedule include lower rate of early toxicity, less expense, and more convenience to the patients [82]. However, SC does not allow enough time for the tumor to shrink (i.e., downsizing) and thus has no effect on sphincter preservation rate. Proponents of the LC argue that chemotherapy can be given concomitantly with RT and that the 6–8-week interval before surgery allows time for the tumor to shrink, thus increasing the rate of sphincters being spared. Whether this is true is controversial because recent data would suggest otherwise [87, 97].

Several randomized trials comparing SC with LC regimen found that the two are equivalent. There are no statistically significant differences in survival, local recurrence rate, incidence of

Table 18.5 Selected randomized trials comparing preoperative short-course with long-course radiation therapy in resectable rectal cancer

Authors/year	N	Stage	Median follow-up (mos)	Survival	Local recurrence rate	Late toxicity rate	Summary
Bujko 2004, 2006 [82, 87] (Polish Trial)	312	cT3–4	48	4-year OS SC, 67.2 % LC, 66.2 % $P=0.96$ 4-year DFS SC, 58.4 % LC, 55.6 % $P=0.82$	SC, 9 % LC, 14.2 % $P=0.17$	SC, 10.1 % LC, 7.1 % $P=0.36$	No differences in Survival LR rate Incidence of distant metastases Late toxicity
Ngan 2012 [97] TROG	326	T3N0–2M0	70.8	5-year OS SC, 74 % LC, 70 % $P=0.62$	3-years SC, 7.5 % LC, 4.4 % $P=0.24$	SC, 5.8 % LC, 8.2 % $P=0.53$	No differences in Survival LR rate Incidence of distant metastases Late toxicity

TROG Trans Tasman Radiation Oncology Group, *SC* short-course radiation therapy, *LC* long-course radiation therapy, *LR* local recurrence, *OS* overall survival, *DFS* disease-free survival

distant metastases, or late toxicity rates between the two (Table 18.5). Although some investigators have found a difference in the degree of downstaging, rate of complete tumor response, or rate of R0 surgery in one regimen over another, the lack of a difference in the more important metrics such as local control and OS has prompted some to abandon the other metrics used to assess efficacy [82].

For patients who had TME and SC preoperative radiotherapy, the late side effects can be substantial when compared to those who just had TME. At a median follow-up of 5 years, the Dutch Colorectal Cancer Group Study reported a significantly higher rates of fecal incontinence (62 % vs. 38 %; $p<0.001$), pad wearing as a result of incontinence (56 % vs. 33 %, $P<0.001$), anal blood loss (11 % vs. 3 %, $P=0.004$), and mucus loss (27 % vs. 15 %, $P=0.005$) in those who had SC radiotherapy [98].

Choice of Chemotherapy for Neoadjuvant Chemoradiotherapy

The fluoropyrimidine 5-fluorouracil (5-FU) is the widely used chemotherapeutic agents in the management of patients with advanced colorectal cancer. 5-FU is given intravenously and can be delivered either as a bolus or continuous infusions. Infusional chemotherapy during RT is preferred over bolus because it increases the likelihood of a pCR [99]. Unfortunately, administration of 5-FU requires central venous access via a Port-a-Cath, Hickman catheter, or Groshong, which can be an inconvenience to patients. These catheters can be infected or thrombosed and compliance can also be a problem. In the EORTC 22921 study, less than 43 % of patients who were randomized to receive postoperative chemotherapy received the planned dose within the scheduled time interval [88]. Thus, the need for an oral agent such as capecitabine would potentially address many of these concerns.

Capecitabine (Xeloda®) is an oral fluoropyrimidine that has been used as an oral alternative to continuous infusion 5-FU in gastrointestinal cancer. It has been tested in several phase III trials in patients with rectal cancer and was found to be comparable to concurrent intravenous 5-FU with radiotherapy in the neoadjuvant setting [100, 101].

Five phase III trials reported that adding oxaliplatin to preoperative 5-FU or capecitabine chemoradiation regimen added no benefit to the patients, but instead, resulted in high toxicity and noncompliance rate [102–107]. Grade 3/4 toxicity such as diarrhea was significantly higher in patients receiving oxaliplatin compared to controls. At this time, NCCN guidelines recommend infusional 5-FU or daily capecitabine for patients with T3/T4 rectal cancer, but advised against adding oxaliplatin [40].

Is Postoperative Chemotherapy Necessary After Neoadjuvant Chemoradiotherapy?

Although current multimodality therapy is excellent at controlling local disease, distant disease remains a problem; approximately 20–25 % of patients who underwent curative treatment for apparently localized disease will succumb to the disease. The rationale for adding adjuvant chemotherapy following neoCRT and surgery is to eliminate micrometastatic disease. However, the value of such an approach remains an area of intense controversy. There are four randomized trials that demonstrated that adjuvant chemotherapy following neoCRT had no impact on outcome or incidence of metastasis when compared to observation [86, 108–110] (Table 18.6). The Italian study compared observation versus adjuvant chemotherapy (5-FU/LV) in 634 patients with clinical T3/T4 rectal cancer, all of whom had neoCRT and TME surgery, and found that adding adjuvant chemotherapy had no impact on OS [108]. Similar results were also reported by the Dutch Colorectal Cancer Group (PROCTOR/SCRIPT) (PROCTOR, Preoperative Radiotherapy and/or Adjuvant Chemotherapy Combined with TME Surgery in Operable Rectal Cancer; SCRIPT, Simply Capecitabine in Rectal Cancer after Irradiation Plus TME Surgery) [109]. The European Organisation for Research and Treatment of Cancer (EORTC) 22921 recently reported their long-term results of a phase III study that evaluated 5-FU-based adjuvant chemotherapy after neoCRT in rectal cancer [86]. EORTC 22921 randomized 1,011 patients with clinical stage T3 or T4 resectable rectal cancer to receive neoCRT followed by either adjuvant chemotherapy or surveillance. At a median follow-up of 10.4 years, postoperative chemotherapy provided no improved DFS or OS (Table 18.6). Possible reasons for the lack of benefit might be poor compliance to the postoperative chemotherapy regimen; more than a quarter of patients were not able to start the adjuvant regimen due to postoperative complications.

Besides the large EORTC 22921 trial, the other three trials accrued small number of patients and were published in abstract form only. The UK Chronicle trial originally intended to accrue 800 patients but had to terminate the study prematurely due to poor accrual (only accrued 113 patients). In addition, compliance was poor [110]. The lack of sufficient power might be the reason why the smaller studies were unable to demonstrate a significant difference with adjuvant chemotherapy. A meta-analysis that will combine data from the 470 patients of the PROCTOR/SCRIPT, 113 patients from Chronicle (who are receiving capecitabine/oxaliplatin), and 634 from the Italian study is currently in progress to evaluate the role of adjuvant chemotherapy.

Members of the European Registration of Cancer Care (EURECCA) consensus conference could not arrive at a consensus on recommending adjuvant chemotherapy following neoCRT [111], while NCCN guidelines recommend 6 months of postoperative chemotherapy, irrespective of whether or not pCR was achieved following neoCRT [40]. The European Society for Medical Oncology (ESMO) recommends adjuvant chemotherapy for pT3–4 or N+tumors, but questioned its routine use in pT3N0 tumors [10]. A 2012 Cochrane meta-analysis of randomized controlled trials supports the use of 5-FU-based adjuvant chemotherapy for patients who had resectable rectal cancer [112]

It is not known what the preferred adjuvant chemotherapy regimen should be for patients with rectal cancer. 5-FU and leucovorin have traditionally been used in the past, and in more recent years, oxaliplatin has been added to the 5-FU/leucovorin (FOLFOX) regimen. The rationale for adding oxaliplatin was based on the

Table 18.6 Role of postoperative chemotherapy following neoadjuvant chemoradiotherapy for resectable rectal cancer

Authors, year	N	Study group	Treatment group	Median follow-up	Outcome	Conclusions
Cionini 2010 [108]	634	cT3–T4	1. Postop 5-FU/LV 2. Observation	25 mos	**5-year OS** Postop chemo 68 % Observation, 69.8 % *P*=NS **LR** Postop chemo, 7.4 % Observation, 8.7 %	Postoperative chemotherapy had no impact on OS and did not have an impact on the incidence of distant metastasis
Breugom 2013 [109] PROCTOR/ SCRIPT	470	Stage II Stage III	1. Postop 5-FU/LV or capecitabine 2. Observation	4 years	**5-year OS** Postop chemo, 74.4 % Observation, 75.9 % *P*=0.527 **5-year DFS** Postop chemo, 62.0 % Observation, 58.4 % *P*=0.247	Postoperative chemotherapy had no impact on OS and DFS
Glynne-Jones 2013 [110] CHRONICLE	113	N/A	1. Postop capecitabine + oxaliplatin 2. Observation	44.8 mos	**3-year OS** Postop chemo, 89.0 % Observation 88.0 % *P*=0.75 **3-year DFS** Postop chemo, 78.0 % Observation 71.0 % *P*=0.56	Postoperative chemotherapy had no impact on OS and DFS Poor accrual and poor compliance
Bosset 2014 [86] EORTC 22921	1011	cT3–T4	1. Preop XRT alone 2. Preo chemoX RT alone 3. Preoperative XRT and postop chemo 4. Preop chemo XRT and postop chemo (Chemo: 5-FU/LV)	10.4 years	**10-year OS** Postop chemo, 51.8 % Observation, 48.4 % *P*=0.32 **10-year DFS,** Postop chemo, 47 % Observation, 43.7 % *P*=0.29	Postoperative chemotherapy had no impact on OS and DFS. No difference in incidence of distant metastasis

PROCTOR, Preoperative Radiotherapy and/or Adjuvant Chemotherapy Combined with TME Surgery in Operable Rectal Cancer, *SCRIP*, Simply Capecitabine in Rectal Cancer After Irradiation Plus TME Surgery, *EORTC* European Organisation for Research and Treatment of Cancer, *LR* local recurrence, *OS* overall survival, *DFS* disease-free survival, *5-FU/LV* 5-fluorouracil and leucovorin

MOSAIC trial, an adjuvant trial that demonstrated a 40–50 % reduction in recurrence when oxaliplatin was added to the fluorouracil regimen versus a 30–50 % reduction with fluorouracil alone for patients with stage III colon cancer [113]. Capecitabine, with or without oxaliplatin, is also an acceptable option as adjuvant therapy [40]. Of note, oxaliplatin is acceptable as *adjuvant therapy*, but not as *neoadjuvant therapy* along with 5-FU.

Induction Chemotherapy Before Standard Neoadjuvant Chemoradiation Therapy

As mentioned above, postoperative chemotherapy following neoCRT and TME surgery is optional. However, one of the concerns with postoperative chemotherapy is the low adherence rate; up to one third of patients are not able to start adjuvant chemotherapy due to postoperative complications, absence of tumor resection, disease progression, clinician discretion, or patient refusal [86, 88]. Therefore, instead of giving chemotherapy postoperatively, several investigators have thought about giving the entire intended chemotherapy preoperatively with the standard neoCRT [114–118]. Such a strategy is called induction chemotherapy. The advantage with this strategy is that the patient benefits from having received the full scheduled dose and intensity of the planned chemotherapy without the worries associated with postoperative chemotherapy. While this strategy does sound attractive in principle, however in practice, induction chemotherapy has not been demonstrated to improve OS. Thus, induction chemotherapy should be considered investigational at this time.

Other Considerations

Is a Diverting Ostomy Necessary?

A temporary diverting stoma (colostomy or ileostomy) to reduce the risk of symptomatic anastomotic leaks and urgent reoperation is highly recommended. This is especially applicable in patients who had very low anastomosis. A multi-institutional study found that patients who had a stoma had significantly less symptomatic leaks (10.3 % vs. 18.0 %; $P<0.001$) and three times less likely to require an urgent abdominal reoperation compared to those who did not have a stoma [119]. A 2010 Cochrane review and a meta-analysis also confirmed the role of a defunctionalized stoma to reduce the rate of clinically relevant anastomotic leakages and urgent abdominal reoperation [120, 121]. The stoma, however, does not prevent an anastomotic separation but limits the extent of dehiscence that can lead to pelvic sepsis from fecal contamination. Patients at high risk for an anastomotic leak include obese patients, those who had preoperative radiation therapy or on steroids, and those whose anastomosis is 5 cm or less from the anal verge.

T3N0M0 Mid to Distal Rectal Cancer

Chemoradiotherapy does come with a price, despite all of its advantages. This price comes in a form of radiation enteritis, diarrhea, ileus, bowel obstruction, hematologic toxicities, and treatment-related deaths. In the era before TME and neoCRT, retrospective data suggest that adjuvant therapy can be avoided in a subset of patients with pT3N0M0 rectal cancer, mainly patients who had adequate node dissection and whose tumors (1) have well-differentiated to moderately differentiated histology, (2) extend ≤ 2 mm into the perirectal fat, (3) possess no evidence of lymphovascular invasion, and (4) located in the upper rectum [43, 122–125]. However, with the widespread preference of the neoCRT approach, it becomes difficult to identify preoperatively those patients who are truly pT3N0M0. As mentioned previously, the German Rectal Cancer Study Group trial reported an 18 % of overtreatment of patients who were thought to have had cT3N0 but actually had T1–2N0 disease [90]. This study reveals the limitations of being able to accurately predict T-stage in the preoperative setting.

Guillem et al performed a retrospective analysis of 188 patients from six institutions who were deemed to have cT3N0 mid to distal rectal cancer by preoperative ERUS/MRI [95]. All patients had neoCRT followed by surgery. The investigators found that 22 % of patients were upstaged because they had mesorectal lymph node involvement (N+), suggesting that ERUS/MRI had ***understaged*** a significant proportion of patients who were thought to have had N0 disease. Although 18 % of patients may be overstaged, a larger percentage of patients were understaged (22 %). Thus, Guillem et al concluded that because of the limited accuracy of preoperative ERUS/MRI in staging mid to distal cT3N0 rectal cancer, neoCRT should be given to all patients with cT3N0M0 disease [95]. As mentioned previously, one might argue in favor of up-front surgery, reserving postCRT to those with more advanced disease. To reiterate, compared to neoCRT, postCRT was associated with inferior local control, higher toxicity, and worse functional outcome [90, 91].

Given the limitations of current pretreatment imaging modality to accurately predict T3N0 disease, it is recommended that all mid to distal cT3N0 rectal cancer should be treated using the neoCRT approach [126].

Optimal Timing of Surgery After NeoCRT

The optimal time between neoCRT and surgery is debatable. The Lyon R90-01 is the only randomize trial that compared short-interval (within 2 weeks) and long (6–8 weeks)-interval groups following preoperative radiotherapy and reported that the long interval group resulted in better clinical response, pathologic downstaging, and a nonsignificant trend toward increased sphincter preservation [127]. Following this report, the 6–8-week interval following completion of RT became the accepted time frame for treating mid to low rectal cancer [128].

Radiation-induced necrosis is a time-dependent event, and over the recent years, several investigators have advocated extending this time interval up to 12 weeks so as to increase the rates of pCR and downstage the tumor [128, 129]. However, most surgeons are more comfortable using the 6–8-week interval because of the concern of radiation-induced pelvic fibrosis, which can make the surgery more technically challenging, which can result in a higher risk of surgical complications and locoregional recurrence [130].

Laparoscopic Proctectomy

Laparoscopic colectomy has proven to be oncologically equivalent to open colectomy in at least 4 large, prospective, randomized trials [131–134] and is considered an acceptable option to open colectomy. Laparoscopic proctectomy (LP), however, has not received such universal endorsement due to a lack of long-term follow-up data from randomized trials. LP is demanding in that TME and autonomic nerve preservation are required for acceptable functional and oncologic outcomes. Several prospective clinical trials have demonstrated that LP had similar short-term oncologic outcomes as well as perioperative advantages when compared with open rectal surgery [135–138] (Table 18.7). LP resulted in a significantly lower amount of blood loss, quicker recovery of bowel function, and less analgesic requirement, although the operative time was significantly longer than the open technique. Surgical quality indicators such as the number of lymph nodes retrieved, involvement of CRM, quality of TME, length of hospital stay, morbidity, mortality, and OS and DFS were similar between LP and open rectal surgery [135–138].

The COLOR II (Colorectal Cancer Laparoscopic or Open Resection) trial is an ongoing clinical trial that compares laparoscopic with open surgery for rectal cancer [138]. Short-term results on 1044 patients found no differences in circumferential or distal margin, anastomotic leak rate (13 % vs. 10 % after LP vs. open surgery, respectively; $P=0.46$), or number of nodes retrieved. However, LP had less blood loss and analgesic use, earlier return of GI function, and shorter hospital stay. Approximately 17 % of patients required conversion from laparoscopic to open approach [138].

The American College of Surgeons Oncology Group (ACOSOG) Z6051 trial is a phase III randomized trial that will test the hypothesis that LP is not inferior to open resection in patients with stage IIA–IIIB rectal cancer. The expected enrollment is 650 patients and the primary objectives will compare the incidence of circumferential and radial margin involvement and completeness of TME. Secondary objectives will compare amount of blood loss, length of hospital stay, pain medication requirements, sexual function, bowel and stoma function, quality of life, and disease-free survival and local pelvic recurrence at 2 years (NCT00726622).

Another ongoing phase 3 trial is the Japan Clinical Oncology Group Study (JCOG 0404), which began in 2004 and intended to recruit 818

Table 18.7 Selected randomized trials comparing laparoscopic rectal surgery with open rectal surgery

Authors, year	N	# LNs retrieved	EBL	Operative time (min)	Time to flatus	Time to normal diet	Analgesic used (mg)	Additional comments
Ng, 2008 [135]	99	L, 12.4	L, 322 cc	L, 214	L, 3.1 d	L, 4.3 d	L, 6 inj	No differences in
		O, 13.0	O, 556 cc	O, 164	O, 4.6 d	O, 5.1 d	O, 11 in	LOS
		P=0.72	*P*=0.09	*P*<0.001	*P*<0.001	*P*=0.001	*P*=0.007	Morbidity and mortality
								OS, DFS
Lujan, 2009 [136]	204	L, 13.6	L, 128 cc	L, 194	N/A	L, 2.8 d	N/A	No differences in
		O, 11.6	O, 234 cc	O, 173		O, 3.6 d		Circumferential margin involvement
		P=0.026	*P*<0.001	*P*=0.02		*P*=0.198		Morbidity
								LOS
								Local recurrence
								OS, DFS
Kang, 2010 [137] (COREAN)	340	NS	L, 200 cc	L, 245	L, 38.5 hr	L, 85 hr	L, 107	No differences in
			O, 217 cc	O, 197	O, 60 hr	O, 93 hr	O, 157	Circumferential margin involvement
			P=0.006	*P*<0.001	*P*<0.001	*P*<0.001	*P*<0.0001	Quality of TME
								Morbidity
van der Pas, 2013 [138] (COLOR II)	1044	L, 13	L, 200 cc	L, 240	L, 2 d	N/A	NS	No differences in
		O, 14	O, 400 cc	O, 188	O, 3 d			Circumferential margin involvement
		P=0.085	*P*<0.0001	*P*<0.001	*P*<0.0001			Morbidity and mortality
								L group had shorter LOS

L laparoscopic, *O* open, *NS* not significant, *hr* hours, *d* days, *LOS* length of hospital stay, *OS* overall survival, *DFS* disease-free survival, *N/A* no available or missing data, *inj* injections, *COREAN* Comparison of Open Versus Laparoscopic Surgery for Mid and Low Rectal Cancer After Neoadjuvant Chemoradiotherapy, *COLOR* Colorectal Cancer Laparoscopic or Open Resection, *TME* total mesorectal excision patients with T3/T4 colorectal cancer. Its plan is to evaluate the benefits of laparoscopic surgery with open surgery [139]. Finally, the ROLARR (Robotic versus Laparoscopic Resection for Rectal Cancer) trial is an international, multicenter, randomized trial that will compare robotic-assisted versus laparoscopic surgery for rectal cancer [140]. As of 2014, laparoscopic proctectomy is still considered investigational in the United States. NCCN prefers that laparoscopic surgery for rectal cancer be done in a clinical trial [40].

Is There a Role to "Watch and Wait" and Not Operate After Chemoradiotherapy?

Similar to other malignancies (breast, esophageal), there is a subset of patients with resectable rectal cancer who achieve a complete clinical response (cCR) and pathologic complete response (pCR) following neoCRT. cCR means no evidence of disease on clinical exam, although there may be residual cancer on the final pathologic specimen. pCR means no evidence of residual cancer in the primary and draining lymphatic nodal basin on final pathologic specimen. pCR occurs in about 10–40 % of patients and obviously can only be known after surgical resection [88, 90, 107]. Patients who achieve pCR have excellent 5-year survival rates of 95 % and local recurrence rates close to 0 % [141, 142].

Given the excellent outcomes when pCR is achieved and the significant postoperative morbidity associated with radical TME, Habr-Gama from Brazil questioned the paradigm of subjecting every patient with rectal cancer to immediate surgery [143]. Using cCR as a surrogate marker of pCR, Habr-Gama reported a series of patients who had cCR following neoCRT who did not undergo immediate radical surgery. Such a strategy is referred to as the "watch and wait" approach and is a topic of intense debate.

In their seminal 2004 studies, Habr-Gama reported 5-year OS, DFS, and LR of 100 %, 92 %, and 3 %, respectively, in a series of 71 patients who were observed after achieving cCR 8–10 weeks after neoCRT and sustained such a status at 1 year after neoCRT. An updated report of 99 patients demonstrated the 5-year OS and DFS rates to be 93 % and 85 %, respectively [144]. Maas et al from the Netherlands also reported similar findings as Habr-Gama's. Using high-resolution MRI, Maas identified 21 patients who underwent the watch and wait strategy and found only one LR and no DRs at a median follow-up of 25 months [145].

The Memorial Sloan Kettering also reported a cohort of 32 patients who were managed nonoperatively after being deemed to have pCR following neoCRT. At a median follow-up of 28 months, there were six cases (19 %) that had recurred locally, of which three had concomitant distant disease [146].

Although provocative, the watch and wait strategy should be approached with extreme caution. A recent systematic review of 30 published articles on this subject concluded that patients who were observed but failed to sustain cCR had worse outcome than those who had undergone immediate surgical resection [147]. Furthermore, there are no randomized trials comparing surgery versus the "watch and wait" approach. Therefore, prospective randomized trials and long-term follow-up are needed to determine the safety of the watch and wait strategy. Therefore, the standard of care for patients with rectal cancer remains neoCRT followed by TME surgical resection, even in those who appear to have a complete clinical response to neoCRT.

Management of Local Recurrences

Recurrent rectal cancer, although not as common as it once was, remains a challenge. Factors associated with local recurrence include tumor depth of invasion (T-stage), number of lymph nodes involved (N-stage), status of CRM and radial margin, evidence of lymphovascular invasion, and poor differentiation [148, 149].

The work-up of patients suspected to have recurrent rectal cancer should include CT scans

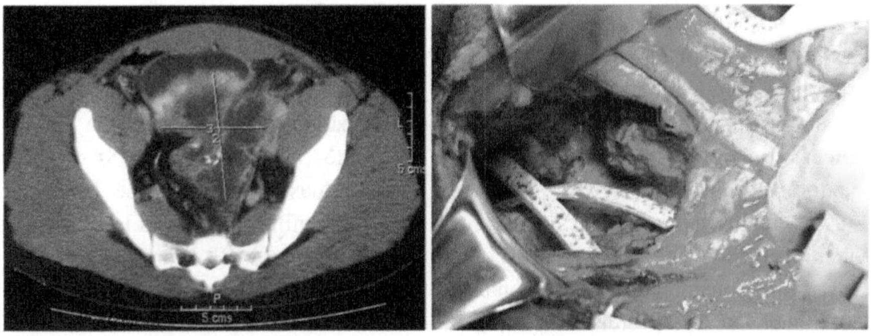

Fig. 18.9 A 43-year-old gentleman who presented with a recurrent rectal cancer that necessitated a pelvic exenteration (total proctectomy, bladder resection, and prostatectomy) (Courtesy of Quyen D. Chu, MD, MBA, FACS)

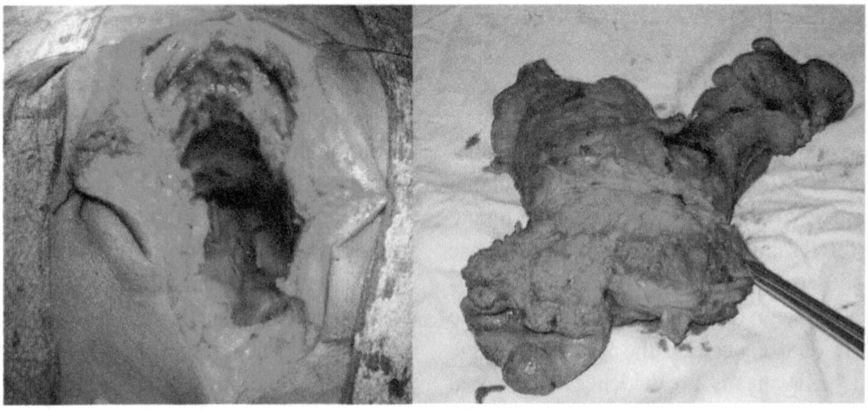

Fig. 18.10 A 56-year-old woman who presented with a recurrent rectal cancer that involved the sacrum. She underwent a successful abdominosacral resection (Courtesy of Quyen D. Chu, MD, MBA, FACS)

of the chest, abdomen, and pelvis and a PET scan to rule out for possible distant disease. A colonoscopy may be warranted to assess for possible anastomotic recurrence. Patients who have no evidence of distant disease but recurrent local disease can be considered for salvage re-resection. Almost 50 % of recurrences occurred in the low pelvic or presacral areas with an additional 14 % occurring in the high to mid pelvis [150].

For patients who do not have metastatic disease, preoperative chemoradiotherapy can be given if the patient is radiotherapy naïve, followed by re-resection. Alternatively, adjuvant chemoradiotherapy is also an option. Some studies have reported acceptable toxicity with re-irradiation [151, 152]. To prepare the patient for surgery, the surgeon should counsel her/him that an extensive resection, which may include a sacral resection and/or pelvic exenteration (resection of bladder, prostate, or a hysterectomy), may be required to achieve an R0/R1 resection (Figs. 18.9 and 18.10). Such extensive operations may require the assistance of urologic or neurosurgical colleagues. Debulking that leaves gross disease behind is not recommended.

Surveillance

Surveillance recommendations for rectal cancer are similar to those for colon cancer, except that a proctoscopy is recommended every 6 months for

3–5 years for those who had an LAR or transanal excision. The purpose of surveillance following curative intent surgery is to detect recurrent diseases that are amenable for further surgical intervention. CRC metastases to the liver and local recurrences are examples of recurrent diseases that can potentially extend survival following re-resection.

Approximately 80 % of CRC recurrences occur within the first 3 years after surgical resection of the primary tumor [125]. This is the basis for an intensive surveillance program within the first 3 years following curative intent surgery. The optimal strategy of surveillance is controversial and based on consensus rather than high level of evidence. In general, following surgery, the patient should be seen every 3–6 months for the first 2 years and then every 6 months thereafter up to year 5. The patient can be seen annually after reaching the 5-year anniversary. A complete history and physical examination should be performed as well as a CEA level obtained during these visits. A colonoscopy and a proctoscopy for those with a low anastomosis should be performed at the 1-year anniversary of the surgery. If negative, a repeat colonoscopy is recommended to be done at 3 years and then every 5 years thereafter. If there is evidence of advanced adenoma(s) (villous polyp, polyp >1 cm, or high-grade dysplasia), then a colonoscopy should be repeated in 1 year. The choice of proctoscopy (i.e., rigid vs. flexible) and ERUS is left at the discretion of the clinician.

It is recommended that an annual chest, abdomen, and pelvic CT should be done up to 5 years. Routine PET scans are not recommended and CEA monitoring and CT scans beyond 5 years are also not recommended.

On occasions, a patient may present with a rising CEA level, and despite all investigative efforts, the source remains elusive. In such a situation, it is recommended to practice the wait and see approach, which entails a repeat CT scan every 3 months until the source is found or CEA level stabilizes or declines, rather than performing a blind or CEA-directed laparotomy.

Future Prospects

It has become apparent that perhaps not all patients with rectal cancer will require neoCRT. How to identify such a group is an area of investigation. Perhaps using a high-resolution MRI to stage and identify high-risk features such as positive CRM, extramural venous invasion, and extramural spread beyond 5 mm might help with predicting the risk of local or systemic relapse and thereby spare those who do not have these features.

A preliminary study from Memorial Sloan Kettering Cancer Center found that preoperative FOLFOX or FOLFOX plus bevacizumab without XRT followed by TME had resulted in no local recurrences in a small group of select patients with 4 years of follow-up [153]. This study prompted a validation study, the PROSPECT (Preoperative Radiation or Selective Preoperative Radiation and Evaluation Before Chemotherapy and TME; NCT01515787) study, which intends to recruit 1,000 patients to determine whether a subgroup of patients with low-risk rectal cancer can be treated with neoadjuvant chemotherapy alone. High-risk tumors such as T4 tumors, tumors with bulky nodal disease (defined as 4LNs>1 cm), and those that are adjacent to (defined as within 3 mm of) the mesorectal fascia on preoperative MRI or ERUS/pelvic CT scan are excluded from the study. Final results will not be available until the foreseeable future.

Summary

In summary, for patients with stage II or III rectal cancer, multimodality therapy is the standard of care. Although surgery followed by adjuvant chemoradiotherapy (postCRT) is an acceptable option, neoadjuvant chemoradiotherapy (neoCRT) is the preferred approach for patients with T3/T4, N+disease, and/or mesorectal fascia involvement as seen on pretherapy imaging. Even though neoCRT overtreats 18 % and undertreats

22 % of patients, it is still preferred over postCRT. NeoCRT results in tumor regression, tumor downstaging, improved respectability rate, improved local control, and increased in pathologic complete response rates. There is no overall survival advantage with the neoCRT approach compared to the postCRT approach. Patients who achieved pCR tend to have better long-term outcomes compared to those who only have a partial response or no response at all [154]. Regardless, besides the Swedish trial, none of the clinical trials demonstrated a survival advantage of using one multimodal therapy over another.

Salient Points

- Unlike colon cancer, which drains into the portal system, rectal cancer drains through 2 systems: the portal venous system and systemic circulation through the inferior and middle rectal veins (bypassing the portal venous system). This explains why rectal cancer can metastasize to the lungs without liver involvement.
- TRUS is good for assessing tumor stage but not very good at assessing nodal involvement.
- MRI is good at assessing tumor stage, nodal involvement, and involvement of the circumferential radial margin (CRM).
- PET scan is important because it can alter the management in almost a third of patients with advanced rectal cancer.
- PET scan is not useful in mucinous tumors.
- Important principles to keep in mind when operating on patients with rectal cancer:
  - Strive to obtain > 1 mm circumferential radial margin (employ total mesorectal excision or TME).
  - Obtain ≥ 12 lymph nodes.
  - 5 cm proximal margin and 2 cm distal margin (1 cm distal margin for those who had neoadjuvant chemoradiation therapy.
- Preoperative chemoradiotherapy (neoCRT) and optimal surgery with TME are standard of care for patients with stage II/III rectal cancer.
- NeoCRT + TME results in:
  - Reduced local recurrence rate
  - Increased tumor downstaging
  - Possibly greater rates of sphincter preservation
- Preoperative and postoperative chemoradiotherapy resulted in similar 10-year OS (60 %) and DFS (68 %), but preoperative CRT resulted in:
  - Lower local recurrence rate
  - Lower incidence of acute toxicities
  - Lower incidence of long-term morbidity
- Although neoCRT overstages 18 % and understages 22 % of patients, it is still preferred over adjuvant CRT because of the above advantages.
- NeoCRT may not necessarily increase the rate of sphincter-sparing surgery compared to postCRT.
- Indications for neoCRT:
  - T3/T4.
  - N + disease.
  - CRM is “threatened”; the tumor is within 1–2 mm of the mesorectal fascia as deemed by preoperative imaging.
- Both short-course preoperative radiotherapy and long-course preoperative radiotherapy are acceptable radiation techniques. Short-course XRT is more common in Europe and select centers in the United States, while long-course XRT is more common in the United States.
- Short-course radiation therapy:
  - Does not include chemotherapy
  - Is given over a 5-day period followed by immediate surgery within 1–2 weeks
  - Has lower rate of early toxicity compared to long-course therapy
  - More convenient to patient than long-course therapy
- Capecitabine is an oral a fluoropyrimidine, which is similar to 5-FU. It is an alternative to infusional 5-FU.
- Adding oxaliplatin to conventional neoCRT regimen should not be used because it increases toxicity without any additional benefits.
- Postoperative chemotherapy is recommended by NCCN following neoCRT and surgery. However, recent phase 3 trials found no benefit.
- Induction chemotherapy (giving chemotherapy along with standard neoCRT instead of adjuvant chemotherapy) is considered investigational at this time.

- T3N0 upper rectal cancer can be treated like colon cancer:
  - Combination chemoXRT might not be necessary.
  - TME might not be necessary.
- T3N0 mid to distal rectal cancer should receive neoCRT.
- Laparoscopic proctectomy:
  - Appears to be similar to open in oncologic outcome, although long-term follow-up from phase 3 trials is needed.
  - Has many advantages over open, although the operative time is longer than the open technique.
  - Is considered investigational in the United States. NCCN prefers that it be done in a clinical trial.
- Diverting ostomy should be considered in:
  - Obese patients
  - Those who had neoCRT or on steroids
  - Those whose anastomosis is ≤ 5 cm from anal verge
- Watch and wait approach has been suggested by some for patients with complete clinical response. However, such an approach is considered investigational at this time. Current standard of care requires surgical resection following neoCRT, irrespective of tumor's response.

Questions

1. A 65-year-old man presented with a rectal mass located approximately 8 cm from the anal verge. A biopsy confirmed a poorly differentiated adenocarcinoma and an endoscopic ultrasound demonstrated a T3 lesion. Which of the following is the most appropriate treatment option?
   A. Surgery alone
   B. Chemoradiation therapy followed by surgery
   C. Radiation therapy followed by surgery followed by chemotherapy
   D. Surgery followed by chemotherapy
   E. Chemotherapy followed by surgery
2. Which of the following statement is true regarding laparoscopic proctectomy (LP)?
   A. LP is a standard option for patients with rectal cancer.
   B. LP retrieves a lower number of lymph nodes than open proctectomy.
   C. LP is considered investigational at this time.
   D. LP requires less operative time than open proctectomy.
   E. LP results in a better overall survival than open proctectomy.
3. Compared to adjuvant chemoradiation therapy, neoadjuvant chemoradiation has:
   A. Lower recurrence rate
   B. Better overall survival
   C. No impact on tumor downstaging
   D. Lower rate of sphincter preservation
   E. Higher acute toxicities
4. Which statement is correct regarding neoadjuvant chemoradiation therapy (neoCRT) for patients with rectal cancer?
   A. NeoCRT results in better overall survival than adjuvant therapy.
   B. Adding oxaliplatin to neoCRT regimen resulted in improved outcome.
   C. NeoCRT is not necessary in patients with T3 mid rectal tumor.
   D. Capecitabine or 5-FU is acceptable chemotherapy regimen.
   E. Induction chemotherapy to neoCRT is the current standard of care.
5. Which of the following is true regarding the "watch and wait" approach to rectal cancer?
   A. It is the preferred approach to most patients who had a complete clinical response to neoCRT.
   B. Randomized clinical trials confirmed its role in patients with mid to distal rectal cancer.
   C. Retrospective data demonstrated it to yield a higher survival rate in elderly patients.
   D. It is preferred in patients with upper rectal cancer.
   E. It is considered investigational at this time.
6. Which of the following is a correct statement regarding surgical management of rectal cancer?
   A. The behavior of upper rectal cancer is similar to mid rectal cancer than it is to colon cancer.

B. Total mesorectal excision (TME) should be performed for patients with mid and distal rectal cancer
C. Lateral lymph node dissection results in better outcome since more lymph nodes are retrieved.
D. A distal margin of 5 cm is needed for mid rectal cancer.
E. The minimum number of lymph nodes recommended is 15.

7. Which of the following is true regarding short-course radiation therapy for rectal cancer?
 A. Short-course therapy yields equivalent outcome as long-course therapy.
 B. Short-course therapy has a higher rate of early toxicity.
 C. Short-course therapy allows more tumor downsizing due to the intensity of therapy given.
 D. Short-course therapy can be administered along with chemotherapy.
 E. Short-course therapy has lower compliance rate than long-course therapy.
8. All of the following statements are correct EXCEPT:
 A. NeoCRT overstaged approximately 18 % of patients with rectal cancer.
 B. NeoCRT understaged approximately 22 % of patients with rectal cancer.
 C. To avoid overstaging and understaging, surgery followed by adjuvant therapy is recommended.
 D. NeoCRT results in lower local recurrence rate compared to adjuvant therapy.
 E. Circumferential radial margin (CRM) of greater than 1 mm results in a local recurrence rate of 5 %.

Answers

1. B
2. C
3. A
4. D
5. E
6. B
7. A
8. C

References

1. Siegel R, Desantis C, Jemal A. Colorectal cancer statistics, 2014. CA Cancer J Clin. 2014;64:104–17.
2. Siegel R, Ma J, Zou Z, Jemal A. Cancer statistics, 2014. CA Cancer J Clin. 2014;64(1):9–29.
3. Vogelaar I, van Ballegooijen M, Schrag D, et al. How much can current interventions reduce colorectal cancer mortality in the U.S.? Mortality projections for scenarios of risk-factor modification, screening, and treatment. Cancer. 2006;107(7):1624–33.
4. Leong AF, Seow-Choen F, Tang CL. Diminutive cancers of the colon and rectum: comparison between flat and polypoid cancers. Int J Colorectal Dis. 1998;13(4):151–3.
5. Chambers WM, Khan U, Gagliano A, Smith RD, Sheffield J, Nicholls RJ. Tumour morphology as a predictor of outcome after local excision of rectal cancer. Br J Surg. 2004;91(4):457–9.
6. Langevin JM, Nivatvongs S. The true incidence of synchronous cancer of the large bowel. A prospective study. Am J Surg. 1984;147(3):330–3.
7. Brahme F, Ekelund GR, Nordén JG, Wenckert A. Metachronous colorectal polyps: comparison of development of colorectal polyps and carcinomas in persons with and without histories of polyps. Dis Colon Rectum. 1974;17(2):166–71.
8. Heald RJ, Bussey HJ. Clinical experiences at St. Mark's Hospital with multiple synchronous cancers of the colon and rectum. Dis Colon Rectum. 1975;18(1):6–10.
9. Nelson H, Petrelli N, Carlin A, et al. Guidelines 2000 for colon and rectal cancer surgery. J Natl Cancer Inst. 2001;93(8):583–96.
10. Glimelius B, Tiret E, Cervantes A, Arnold D, Group EGW. Rectal cancer: ESMO clinical practice guidelines for diagnosis, treatment and follow-up. Ann Oncol. 2013;24 Suppl 6:vi81–8.
11. Scheele J, Altendorf-Hofmann A, Stangl R, Gall FP. Pulmonary resection for metastatic colon and upper rectum cancer. Is it useful? Dis Colon Rectum. 1990;33(9):745–52.
12. Tan KK, Lopes GL, Sim R. How uncommon are isolated lung metastases in colorectal cancer? A review from database of 754 patients over 4 years. J Gastrointest Surg. 2009;13(4):642–8.
13. Balthazar EJ, Megibow AJ, Hulnick D, Naidich DP. Carcinoma of the colon: detection and preoperative staging by CT. AJR Am J Roentgenol. 1988;150(2):301–6.
14. Thoeni RF. Colorectal cancer. Radiologic staging. Radiol Clin North Am. 1997;35(2):457–85.
15. Zerhouni EA, Rutter C, Hamilton SR, et al. CT and MR imaging in the staging of colorectal carcinoma: report of the Radiology Diagnostic Oncology Group II. Radiology. 1996;200(2):443–51.
16. Vogl TJ, Pegios W, Mack MG, et al. Radiological modalities in the staging of colorectal tumors: new

perspectives for increasing accuracy. Recent Results Cancer Res. 1996;142:103–20.
17. Zagoria RJ, Schlarb CA, Ott DJ, et al. Assessment of rectal tumor infiltration utilizing endorectal MR imaging and comparison with endoscopic rectal sonography. J Surg Oncol. 1997;64(4):312–7.
18. Bernini A, Deen KI, Madoff RD, Wong WD. Preoperative adjuvant radiation with chemotherapy for rectal cancer: its impact on stage of disease and the role of endorectal ultrasound. Ann Surg Oncol. 1996;3(2):131–5.
19. Bhattacharjya S, Bhattacharjya T, Baber S, Tibballs JM, Watkinson AF, Davidson BR. Prospective study of contrast-enhanced computed tomography, computed tomography during arterioportography, and magnetic resonance imaging for staging colorectal liver metastases for liver resection. Br J Surg. 2004;91(10):1361–9.
20. Rotte KH, Klühs L, Kleinau H, Kriedemann E. Computed tomography and endosonography in the preoperative staging of rectal carcinoma. Eur J Radiol. 1989;9(3):187–90.
21. Perez RO, Pereira DD, Proscurshim I, et al. Lymph node size in rectal cancer following neoadjuvant chemoradiation–can we rely on radiologic nodal staging after chemoradiation? Dis Colon Rectum. 2009;52(7):1278–84.
22. Ju H, Xu D, Li D, Chen G, Shao G. Comparison between endoluminal ultrasonography and spiral computerized tomography for the preoperative local staging of rectal carcinoma. Biosci Trends. 2009;3(2):73–6.
23. Caseiro-Alves F, Gonçalo M, Cruz L, et al. Water enema computed tomography (WE-CT) in the local staging of low colorectal neoplasms: comparison with transrectal ultrasound. Abdom Imaging. 1998;23(4):370–4.
24. Kronawitter U, Kemeny NE, Heelan R, Fata F, Fong Y. Evaluation of chest computed tomography in the staging of patients with potentially resectable liver metastases from colorectal carcinoma. Cancer. 1999;86(2):229–35.
25. Kirke R, Rajesh A, Verma R, Bankart MJ. Rectal cancer: incidence of pulmonary metastases on thoracic CT and correlation with T staging. J Comput Assist Tomogr. 2007;31(4):569–71.
26. Kosinski L, et al. Shifting concepts in rectal cancer management. A review of contemporary primary rectal cancer treatment strategies. CA: Cancer J Clin. 2012;62:173–202.
27. Kim SH, Lee JM, Lee MW, Kim GH, Han JK, Choi BI. Diagnostic accuracy of 3.0-Tesla rectal magnetic resonance imaging in preoperative local staging of primary rectal cancer. Invest Radiol. 2008;43(8):587–93.
28. Tatli S, Mortele KJ, Breen EL, Bleday R, Silverman SG. Local staging of rectal cancer using combined pelvic phased-array and endorectal coil MRI. J Magn Reson Imaging. 2006;23(4):534–40.
29. Wong EM, Leung JL, Cheng CS, Lee JC, Li MK, Chung CC. Effect of endorectal coils on staging of rectal cancers by magnetic resonance imaging. Hong Kong Med J. 2010;16(6):421–6.
30. Videhult P, Smedh K, Lundin P, Kraaz W. Magnetic resonance imaging for preoperative staging of rectal cancer in clinical practice: high accuracy in predicting circumferential margin with clinical benefit. Colorectal Dis. 2007;9(5):412–9.
31. Kim SH, Lee JM, Park HS, Eun HW, Han JK, Choi BI. Accuracy of MRI for predicting the circumferential resection margin, mesorectal fascia invasion, and tumor response to neoadjuvant chemoradiotherapy for locally advanced rectal cancer. J Magn Reson Imaging. 2009;29(5):1093–101.
32. Kim SH, Lee JM, Hong SH, et al. Locally advanced rectal cancer: added value of diffusion-weighted MR imaging in the evaluation of tumor response to neoadjuvant chemo- and radiation therapy. Radiology. 2009;253(1):116–25.
33. Sugita R, Ito K, Fujita N, Takahashi S. Diffusion-weighted MRI in abdominal oncology: clinical applications. World J Gastroenterol. 2010;16(7):832–6.
34. Snady H, Merrick MA. Improving the treatment of colorectal cancer: the role of EUS. Cancer Invest. 1998;16(8):572–81.
35. Low G, Tho LM, Leen E, et al. The role of imaging in the pre-operative staging and post-operative follow-up of rectal cancer. Surgeon. 2008;6(4):222–31.
36. Kinner S, Antoch G, Bockisch A, Veit-Haibach P. Whole-body PET/CT-colonography: a possible new concept for colorectal cancer staging. Abdom Imaging. 2007;32(5):606–12.
37. Shin SS, Jeong YY, Min JJ, Kim HR, Chung TW, Kang HK. Preoperative staging of colorectal cancer: CT vs integrated FDG PET/CT. Abdom Imaging. 2008;33(3):270–7.
38. Capirci C, Rubello D, Pasini F, et al. The role of dual-time combined 18-fluorodeoxyglucose positron emission tomography and computed tomography in the staging and restaging workup of locally advanced rectal cancer, treated with preoperative chemoradiation therapy and radical surgery. Int J Radiat Oncol Biol Phys. 2009;74(5):1461–9.
39. Schmoll HJ, Van Cutsem E, Stein A, et al. ESMO consensus guidelines for management of patients with colon and rectal cancer a personalized approach to clinical decision making. Ann Oncol. 2012;23(10):2479–516.
40. National Comprehensive Cancer Network (NCCN) guidelines. 2013. Available at: www.nccn.org. Accessed 23 May 2013.
41. Compton C, Byrd D, Garcia-Aguilar J, et al. Colon and rectum. In: Compton C, Byrd D, Garcia-Aguilar J, Kurtzman S, Olawaiye A, Washington M, editors. AJCC cancer staging atlas. 2nd ed. New York: Springer; 2012. p. 185–201.

42. Edge SB, Compton CC. The American Joint Committee on Cancer: the 7th edition of the AJCC cancer staging manual and the future of TNM. Ann Surg Oncol. 2010;17(6):1471–4.
43. Lopez-Kostner F, Lavery IC, Hool GR, Rybicki LA, Fazio VW. Total mesorectal excision is not necessary for cancers of the upper rectum. Surgery. 1998;124(4):612–7; discussion 617–618.
44. Kapiteijn E, Marijnen CA, Nagtegaal ID, et al. Preoperative radiotherapy combined with total mesorectal excision for resectable rectal cancer. N Engl J Med. 2001;345(9):638–46.
45. Law WL, Chu KW. Anterior resection for rectal cancer with mesorectal excision: a prospective evaluation of 622 patients. Ann Surg. 2004;240(2):260–8.
46. Huerta S, Dineen SP. Current strategies in the management of adenocarcinoma of the rectum. In: Rangel L, editor. Cancer treatment-conventional and innovative approaches. Rijeka: Intech; 2013.
47. Ortiz H, De Miguel M, Armendáriz P, Rodriguez J, Chocarro C. Coloanal anastomosis: are functional results better with a pouch? Dis Colon Rectum. 1995;38(4):375–7.
48. Ho YH, Seow-Choen F, Tan M. Colonic J-pouch function at six months versus straight coloanal anastomosis at two years: randomized controlled trial. World J Surg. 2001;25(7):876–81.
49. Moore HG, Riedel E, Minsky BD, et al. Adequacy of 1-cm distal margin after restorative rectal cancer resection with sharp mesorectal excision and preoperative combined-modality therapy. Ann Surg Oncol. 2003;10(1):80–5.
50. Swanson RS, Compton CC, Stewart AK, Bland KI. The prognosis of T3N0 colon cancer is dependent on the number of lymph nodes examined. Ann Surg Oncol. 2003;10(1):65–71.
51. Stocchi L, Nelson H, Sargent DJ, et al. Impact of surgical and pathologic variables in rectal cancer: a United States community and cooperative group report. J Clin Oncol. 2001;19(18):3895–902.
52. Adam IJ, Mohamdee MO, Martin IG, et al. Role of circumferential margin involvement in the local recurrence of rectal cancer. Lancet. 1994; 344(8924):707–11.
53. Wibe A, Rendedal PR, Svensson E, et al. Prognostic significance of the circumferential resection margin following total mesorectal excision for rectal cancer. Br J Surg. 2002;89(3):327–34.
54. Nagtegaal ID, van Krieken JH. The role of pathologists in the quality control of diagnosis and treatment of rectal cancer-an overview. Eur J Cancer. 2002;38(7):964–72.
55. Nagtegaal ID, Quirke P. What is the role for the circumferential margin in the modern treatment of rectal cancer? J Clin Oncol. 2008;26(2):303–12.
56. Heald RJ, Husband EM, Ryall RD. The mesorectum in rectal cancer surgery–the clue to pelvic recurrence? Br J Surg. 1982;69(10):613–6.
57. Lowry AC, Simmang CL, Boulos P, et al. Consensus statement of definitions for anorectal physiology and rectal cancer: report of the Tripartite Consensus Conference on Definitions for Anorectal Physiology and Rectal Cancer, Washington, D.C., May 1, 1999. Dis Colon Rectum. 2001;44(7):915–9.
58. Lowry AC, Simmang CL, Boulos P, et al. Consensus statement of definitions for anorectal physiology and rectal cancer. Colorectal Dis. 2001;3(4):272–5.
59. Compton CC, Fielding LP, Burgart LJ, et al. Prognostic factors in colorectal cancer. College of American Pathologists Consensus Statement 1999. Arch Pathol Lab Med. 2000;124(7):979–94.
60. Marks JH, Valsdottir EB, Rather AA, Nweze IC, Newman DA, Chernick MR. Fewer than 12 lymph nodes can be expected in a surgical specimen after high-dose chemoradiation therapy for rectal cancer. Dis Colon Rectum. 2010;53(7):1023–9.
61. Tepper JE, O'Connell MJ, Niedzwiecki D, et al. Impact of number of nodes retrieved on outcome in patients with rectal cancer. J Clin Oncol. 2001; 19(1):157–63.
62. Nagawa H, Muto T, Sunouchi K, et al. Randomized, controlled trial of lateral node dissection vs. nerve-preserving resection in patients with rectal cancer after preoperative radiotherapy. Dis Colon Rectum. 2001;44(9):1274–80.
63. Michelassi F, Block GE. Morbidity and mortality of wide pelvic lymphadenectomy for rectal adenocarcinoma. Dis Colon Rectum. 1992;35(12):1143–7.
64. Kyo K, Sameshima S, Takahashi M, Furugori T, Sawada T. Impact of autonomic nerve preservation and lateral node dissection on male urogenital function after total mesorectal excision for lower rectal cancer. World J Surg. 2006;30(6):1014–9.
65. Berge T, Ekelund G, Mellner C, Pihl B, Wenckert A. Carcinoma of the colon and rectum in a defined population. An epidemiological, clinical and post-mortem investigation of colorectal carcinoma and coexisting benign polyps in Malmö, Sweden. Acta Chir Scand Suppl. 1973;438:1–86.
66. Gilbertsen VA. Adenocarcinoma of the rectum: incidence and locations of recurrent tumor following present-day operations performed for cure. Ann Surg. 1960;151(3):340–8.
67. Gunderson LL, Sosin H. Areas of failure found at reoperation (second or symptomatic look) following "curative surgery" for adenocarcinoma of the rectum. Clinicopathologic correlation and implications for adjuvant therapy. Cancer. 1974;34(4):1278–92.
68. Påhlman L, Glimelius B. Local recurrences after surgical treatment for rectal carcinoma. Acta Chir Scand. 1984;150(4):331–5.
69. Rao AR, Kagan AR, Chan PM, Gilbert HA, Nussbaum H, Hintz BL. Patterns of recurrence following curative resection alone for adenocarcinoma of the rectum and sigmoid colon. Cancer. 1981; 48(6):1492–5.
70. Group GTS. Prolongation of the disease-free interval in surgically treated rectal carcinoma. N Engl J Med. 1985;312(23):1465–72.
71. Douglass HO, Moertel CG, Mayer RJ, et al. Survival after postoperative combination treatment of rectal cancer. N Engl J Med. 1986;315(20):1294–5.

72. Fisher B, Wolmark N, Rockette H, et al. Postoperative adjuvant chemotherapy or radiation therapy for rectal cancer: results from NSABP protocol R-01. J Natl Cancer Inst. 1988;80(1):21–9.
73. Krook JE, Moertel CG, Gunderson LL, et al. Effective surgical adjuvant therapy for high-risk rectal carcinoma. N Engl J Med. 1991;324(11):709–15.
74. Frykholm GJ, Glimelius B, Påhlman L. Preoperative or postoperative irradiation in adenocarcinoma of the rectum: final treatment results of a randomized trial and an evaluation of late secondary effects. Dis Colon Rectum. 1993;36(6):564–72.
75. Trial SRC. Improved survival with preoperative radiotherapy in resectable rectal cancer. N Engl J Med. 1997;336(14):980–7.
76. Folkesson J, Birgisson H, Pahlman L, Cedermark B, Glimelius B, Gunnarsson U. Swedish Rectal Cancer Trial: long lasting benefits from radiotherapy on survival and local recurrence rate. J Clin Oncol. 2005;23(24):5644–50.
77. Group CCC. Adjuvant radiotherapy for rectal cancer: a systematic overview of 8507 patients from 22 randomized trials. Lancet. 2001;358:1291–304.
78. van Gijn W, Marijnen CA, Nagtegaal ID, et al. Preoperative radiotherapy combined with total mesorectal excision for resectable rectal cancer: 12-year follow-up of the multicentre, randomised controlled TME trial. Lancet Oncol. 2011;12(6):575–82.
79. NIH consensus conference. Adjuvant therapy for patients with colon and rectal cancer. JAMA. 1990;264(11):1444–50.
80. Boulis-Wassif S, Gerard A, Loygue J, Camelot D, Buyse M, Duez N. Final results of a randomized trial on the treatment of rectal cancer with preoperative radiotherapy alone or in combination with 5-fluorouracil, followed by radical surgery. Trial of the European Organization on Research and Treatment of Cancer Gastrointestinal Tract Cancer Cooperative Group. Cancer. 1984;53(9):1811–8.
81. Bosset JF, Calais G, Mineur L, et al. Enhanced tumorocidal effect of chemotherapy with preoperative radiotherapy for rectal cancer: preliminary results–EORTC 22921. J Clin Oncol. 2005;23(24): 5620–7.
82. Bujko K, Nowacki MP, Nasierowska-Guttmejer A, Michalski W, Bebenek M, Kryj M. Long-term results of a randomized trial comparing preoperative short-course radiotherapy with preoperative conventionally fractionated chemoradiation for rectal cancer. Br J Surg. 2006;93(10):1215–23.
83. Gérard JP, Conroy T, Bonnetain F, et al. Preoperative radiotherapy with or without concurrent fluorouracil and leucovorin in T3-4 rectal cancers: results of FFCD 9203. J Clin Oncol. 2006;24(28):4620–5.
84. De Caluwé L, Van Nieuwenhove Y, Ceelen WP. Preoperative chemoradiation versus radiation alone for stage II and III resectable rectal cancer. Cochrane Database Syst Rev. 2013;2, CD006041.
85. Latkauskas T, Pauzas H, Gineikiene I, et al. Initial results of a randomized controlled trial comparing clinical and pathological downstaging of rectal cancer after preoperative short-course radiotherapy or long-term chemoradiotherapy, both with delayed surgery. Colorectal Dis. 2012;14(3):294–8.
86. Bosset JF, Calais G, Mineur L, et al. Fluorouracil-based adjuvant chemotherapy after preoperative chemoradiotherapy in rectal cancer: long-term results of the EORTC 22921 randomised study. Lancet Oncol. 2014;15(2):184–90.
87. Bujko K, Nowacki MP, Nasierowska-Guttmejer A, et al. Sphincter preservation following preoperative radiotherapy for rectal cancer: report of a randomised trial comparing short-term radiotherapy vs conventionally fractionated radiochemotherapy. Radiother Oncol. 2004;72(1):15–24.
88. Bosset JF, Collette L, Calais G, et al. Chemotherapy with preoperative radiotherapy in rectal cancer. N Engl J Med. 2006;355(11):1114–23.
89. Roh MS, Colangelo LH, O"Connell MJ, et al. Preoperative multimodality therapy improves disease-free survival in patients with carcinoma of the rectum: NSABP R-03. J Clin Oncol. 2009; 27(31):5124–30.
90. Sauer R, Becker H, Hohenberger W, et al. Preoperative versus postoperative chemoradiotherapy for rectal cancer. N Engl J Med. 2004;351(17):1731–40.
91. Sauer R, Liersch T, Merkel S, et al. Preoperative versus postoperative chemoradiotherapy for locally advanced rectal cancer: results of the German CAO/ARO/AIO-94 randomized phase III trial after a median follow-up of 11 years. J Clin Oncol. 2012;30(16):1926–33.
92. Park JH, Yoon SM, Yu CS, Kim JH, Kim TW, Kim JC. Randomized phase 3 trial comparing preoperative and postoperative chemoradiotherapy with capecitabine for locally advanced rectal cancer. Cancer. 2011;117(16):3703–12.
93. Minsky BD. Is preoperative chemoradiotherapy still the treatment of choice for rectal cancer? J Clin Oncol. 2009;27(31):5115–6.
94. Gerard JP, Rostom Y, Gal J, et al. Can we increase the chance of sphincter saving surgery in rectal cancer with neoadjuvant treatments: lessons from a systematic review of recent randomized trials. Crit Rev Oncol Hematol. 2012;81(1):21–8.
95. Guillem JG, Díaz-González JA, Minsky BD, et al. cT3N0 rectal cancer: potential overtreatment with preoperative chemoradiotherapy is warranted. J Clin Oncol. 2008;26(3):368–73.
96. Govindarajan A, Gönen M, Weiser MR, et al. Challenging the feasibility and clinical significance of current guidelines on lymph node examination in rectal cancer in the era of neoadjuvant therapy. J Clin Oncol. 2011;29(34):4568–73.
97. Ngan SY, Burmeister B, Fisher RJ, et al. Randomized trial of short-course radiotherapy versus long-course chemoradiation comparing rates of local recurrence in patients with T3 rectal cancer: Trans-Tasman Radiation Oncology Group trial 01.04. J Clin Oncol. 2012;30(31):3827–33.
98. Peeters KC, van de Velde CJ, Leer JW, et al. Late side effects of short-course preoperative radiotherapy

combined with total mesorectal excision for rectal cancer: increased bowel dysfunction in irradiated patients–a Dutch colorectal cancer group study. J Clin Oncol. 2005;23(25):6199–206.

99. Mohiuddin M, Regine WF, John WJ, et al. Preoperative chemoradiation in fixed distal rectal cancer: dose time factors for pathological complete response. Int J Radiat Oncol Biol Phys. 2000;46(4): 883–8.
100. Hofheinz RD, Wenz F, Post S, et al. Chemoradiotherapy with capecitabine versus fluorouracil for locally advanced rectal cancer: a randomised, multicentre, non-inferiority, phase 3 trial. Lancet Oncol. 2012;13(6):579–88.
101. Allegra C, Yothers G, O'Connell M, et al. Neoadjuvant therapy for rectal cancer. Mature results from NSABP R-04. J Clin Oncol. 2014;32(Suppl 3):Abstract 390.
102. Aschele C, Cionini L, Lonardi S, et al. Primary tumor response to preoperative chemoradiation with or without oxaliplatin in locally advanced rectal cancer: pathologic results of the STAR-01 randomized phase III trial. J Clin Oncol. 2011;29(20):2773–80.
103. Gérard JP, Azria D, Gourgou-Bourgade S, et al. Comparison of two neoadjuvant chemoradiotherapy regimens for locally advanced rectal cancer: results of the phase III trial ACCORD 12/0405-Prodige 2. J Clin Oncol. 2010;28(10):1638–44.
104. Gérard JP, Azria D, Gourgou-Bourgade S, et al. Clinical outcome of the ACCORD 12/0405 PRODIGE 2 randomized trial in rectal cancer. J Clin Oncol. 2012;30(36):4558–65.
105. Rödel C, Liersch T, Becker H, et al. Preoperative chemoradiotherapy and postoperative chemotherapy with fluorouracil and oxaliplatin versus fluorouracil alone in locally advanced rectal cancer: initial results of the German CAO/ARO/AIO-04 randomised phase 3 trial. Lancet Oncol. 2012;13(7):679–87.
106. Schmoll H, Haustermans K, Price T, et al. Preoperative chemoradiotherapy and postoperative chemotherapy with capecitabine and oxaliplatin versus capecitabine alone in locally advanced rectal cancer: first results of the PETACC-6 randomized trial. J Clin Oncol. 2013;31:Abstract 3531.
107. Roh M, Yothers G, O'Connell M, et al. The impact of capecitabine and oxaliplatin in the preoperative multimodality treatment in patients with carcinoma of the rectum: NSABP R-04. J Clin Oncol. 2011;29(15 (Suppl)):Abstract 3503.
108. Cionini L, Sainato A, De Paoli A, et al. Final results of randomized trial on adjuvant chemotherapy after preoperative chemoradiation in rectal cancer. Radiother Oncol. 2010;96(Suppl 1):Abstract S113–4.
109. Breugom A, van den Broek C, van Gijn W, et al. The value of adjuvant chemotherapy in rectal cancer patients after preoperative radiotherapy or chemoradiation followed by TME-surgery: the PROCTOR/SCRIPT study. Eur Cancer Congr. 2013;Abstract 1.
110. Glynne-Jones R, Counsell N, Meadows H, Ledermann J, Sebag-Montefiore D. Chronicle: a phase III trial in locally advanced rectal cancer after neoadjuvant chemoradiation randomising postoperative adjuvant capecitabine/oxaliplatin versus control. Ann Oncol. 2013;24(4):iv11–24.
111. van de Velde CJ, Boelens PG, Borras JM, et al. EURECCA colorectal: multidisciplinary management: European consensus conference colon & rectum. Eur J Cancer. 2014;50(1):1.e1–34.
112. Petersen SH, Harling H, Kirkeby LT, Wille-Jørgensen P, Mocellin S. Postoperative adjuvant chemotherapy in rectal cancer operated for cure. Cochrane Database Syst Rev. 2012;3, CD004078.
113. André T, Boni C, Navarro M, et al. Improved overall survival with oxaliplatin, fluorouracil, and leucovorin as adjuvant treatment in stage II or III colon cancer in the MOSAIC trial. J Clin Oncol. 2009;27(19):3109–16.
114. Chua YJ, Barbachano Y, Cunningham D, et al. Neoadjuvant capecitabine and oxaliplatin before chemoradiotherapy and total mesorectal excision in MRI-defined poor-risk rectal cancer: a phase 2 trial. Lancet Oncol. 2010;11(3):241–8.
115. Rödel C, Arnold D, Becker H, et al. Induction chemotherapy before chemoradiotherapy and surgery for locally advanced rectal cancer : is it time for a randomized phase III trial? Strahlenther Onkol. 2010;186(12):658–64.
116. Dewdney A, Cunningham D, Tabernero J, et al. Multicenter randomized phase II clinical trial comparing neoadjuvant oxaliplatin, capecitabine, and preoperative radiotherapy with or without cetuximab followed by total mesorectal excision in patients with high-risk rectal cancer (EXPERT-C). J Clin Oncol. 2012;30(14):1620–7.
117. Fernández-Martos C, Pericay C, Aparicio J, et al. Phase II, randomized study of concomitant chemoradiotherapy followed by surgery and adjuvant capecitabine plus oxaliplatin (CAPOX) compared with induction CAPOX followed by concomitant chemoradiotherapy and surgery in magnetic resonance imaging-defined, locally advanced rectal cancer: Grupo cancer de recto 3 study. J Clin Oncol. 2010;28(5):859–65.
118. Maréchal R, Vos B, Polus M, et al. Short course chemotherapy followed by concomitant chemoradiotherapy and surgery in locally advanced rectal cancer: a randomized multicentric phase II study. Ann Oncol. 2012;23(6):1525–30.
119. Matthiessen P, Hallböök O, Rutegård J, Simert G, Sjödahl R. Defunctioning stoma reduces symptomatic anastomotic leakage after low anterior resection of the rectum for cancer: a randomized multicenter trial. Ann Surg. 2007;246(2):207–14.
120. Montedori A, Cirocchi R, Farinella E, Sciannameo F, Abraha I. Covering ileo- or colostomy in anterior resection for rectal carcinoma. Cochrane Database Syst Rev. 2010;5, CD006878.

121. Hüser N, Michalski CW, Erkan M, et al. Systematic review and meta-analysis of the role of defunctioning stoma in low rectal cancer surgery. Ann Surg. 2008;248(1):52–60.
122. Willett CG, Badizadegan K, Ancukiewicz M, Shellito PC. Prognostic factors in stage T3N0 rectal cancer: do all patients require postoperative pelvic irradiation and chemotherapy? Dis Colon Rectum. 1999;42(2):167–73.
123. Merchant NB, Guillem JG, Paty PB, et al. T3N0 rectal cancer: results following sharp mesorectal excision and no adjuvant therapy. J Gastrointest Surg. 1999;3(6):642–7.
124. Faerden AE, Naimy N, Wiik P, et al. Total mesorectal excision for rectal cancer: difference in outcome for low and high rectal cancer. Dis Colon Rectum. 2005;48(12):2224–31.
125. Tepper JE, O'Connell M, Niedzwiecki D, et al. Adjuvant therapy in rectal cancer: analysis of stage, sex, and local control–final report of intergroup 0114. J Clin Oncol. 2002;20(7):1744–50.
126. Lombardi R, Cuicchi D, Pinto C, et al. Clinically-staged T3N0 rectal cancer: is preoperative chemoradiotherapy the optimal treatment? Ann Surg Oncol. 2010;17(3):838–45.
127. Francois Y, Nemoz CJ, Baulieux J, et al. Influence of the interval between preoperative radiation therapy and surgery on downstaging and on the rate of sphincter-sparing surgery for rectal cancer: the Lyon R90-01 randomized trial. J Clin Oncol. 1999; 17(8):2396.
128. de Campos-Lobato LF, Geisler DP, da Luz MA, Stocchi L, Dietz D, Kalady MF. Neoadjuvant therapy for rectal cancer: the impact of longer interval between chemoradiation and surgery. J Gastrointest Surg. 2011;15(3):444–50.
129. Habr-Gama A, Perez RO, Proscurshim I, et al. Interval between surgery and neoadjuvant chemoradiation therapy for distal rectal cancer: does delayed surgery have an impact on outcome? Int J Radiat Oncol Biol Phys. 2008;71(4):1181–8.
130. Garcia-Aguilar J, Smith DD, Avila K, et al. Optimal timing of surgery after chemoradiation for advanced rectal cancer: preliminary results of a multicenter, nonrandomized phase II prospective trial. Ann Surg. 2011;254(1):97–102.
131. Group COoSTS. A comparison of laparoscopically assisted and open colectomy for colon cancer. N Engl J Med. 2004;350(20):2050–9.
132. Buunen M, Veldkamp R, Hop WC, et al. Survival after laparoscopic surgery versus open surgery for colon cancer: long-term outcome of a randomised clinical trial. Lancet Oncol. 2009;10(1):44–52.
133. Jayne DG, Thorpe HC, Copeland J, Quirke P, Brown JM, Guillou PJ. Five-year follow-up of the Medical Research Council CLASICC trial of laparoscopically assisted versus open surgery for colorectal cancer. Br J Surg. 2010;97(11):1638–45.
134. Leung KL, Kwok SP, Lam SC, et al. Laparoscopic resection of rectosigmoid carcinoma: prospective randomised trial. Lancet. 2004;363(9416):1187–92.
135. Ng SS, Leung KL, Lee JF, et al. Laparoscopic-assisted versus open abdominoperineal resection for low rectal cancer: a prospective randomized trial. Ann Surg Oncol. 2008;15(9):2418–25.
136. Lujan J, Valero G, Hernandez Q, Sanchez A, Frutos MD, Parrilla P. Randomized clinical trial comparing laparoscopic and open surgery in patients with rectal cancer. Br J Surg. 2009;96(9):982–9.
137. Kang SB, Park JW, Jeong SY, et al. Open versus laparoscopic surgery for mid or low rectal cancer after neoadjuvant chemoradiotherapy (COREAN trial): short-term outcomes of an open-label randomised controlled trial. Lancet Oncol. 2010;11(7): 637–45.
138. van der Pas MH, Haglind E, Cuesta MA, et al. Laparoscopic versus open surgery for rectal cancer (COLOR II): short-term outcomes of a randomised, phase 3 trial. Lancet Oncol. 2013;14(3):210–8.
139. Kitano S, Inomata M, Sato A, Yoshimura K, Moriya Y, Study JCOG. Randomized controlled trial to evaluate laparoscopic surgery for colorectal cancer: Japan Clinical Oncology Group Study JCOG 0404. Jpn J Clin Oncol. 2005;35(8):475–7.
140. Collinson FJ, Jayne DG, Pigazzi A, et al. An international, multicentre, prospective, randomised, controlled, unblinded, parallel-group trial of robotic-assisted versus standard laparoscopic surgery for the curative treatment of rectal cancer. Int J Colorectal Dis. 2012;27(2):233–41.
141. Martin ST, Heneghan HM, Winter DC. Systematic review and meta-analysis of outcomes following pathological complete response to neoadjuvant chemoradiotherapy for rectal cancer. Br J Surg. 2012;99(7):918–28.
142. Stipa F, Chessin DB, Shia J, et al. A pathologic complete response of rectal cancer to preoperative combined-modality therapy results in improved oncological outcome compared with those who achieve no downstaging on the basis of preoperative endorectal ultrasonography. Ann Surg Oncol. 2006;13(8):1047–53.
143. Habr-Gama A, Perez RO, Nadalin W, et al. Operative versus nonoperative treatment for stage 0 distal rectal cancer following chemoradiation therapy: long-term results. Ann Surg. 2004;240(4):711–7; discussion 717–718.
144. Habr-Gama A, Perez RO, Proscurshim I, et al. Patterns of failure and survival for nonoperative treatment of stage c0 distal rectal cancer following neoadjuvant chemoradiation therapy. J Gastrointest Surg. 2006;10(10):1319–28; discussion 1328–1319.
145. Maas M, Beets-Tan RG, Lambregts DM, et al. Wait-and-see policy for clinical complete responders after chemoradiation for rectal cancer. J Clin Oncol. 2011;29(35):4633–40.
146. Smith JD, Ruby JA, Goodman KA, et al. Nonoperative management of rectal cancer with complete clinical response after neoadjuvant therapy. Ann Surg. 2012;256(6):965–72.
147. Glynne-Jones R, Hughes R. Critical appraisal of the "wait and see" approach in rectal cancer for clinical

complete responders after chemoradiation. Br J Surg. 2012;99(7):897–909.
148. Kim YW, Kim NK, Min BS, et al. Factors associated with anastomotic recurrence after total mesorectal excision in rectal cancer patients. J Surg Oncol. 2009;99(1):58–64.
149. Quirke P, Durdey P, Dixon MF, Williams NS. Local recurrence of rectal adenocarcinoma due to inadequate surgical resection. Histopathological study of lateral tumour spread and surgical excision. Lancet. 1986;2(8514):996–9.
150. Yu TK, Bhosale PR, Crane CH, et al. Patterns of locoregional recurrence after surgery and radiotherapy or chemoradiation for rectal cancer. Int J Radiat Oncol Biol Phys. 2008;71(4):1175–80.
151. Valentini V, Morganti AG, Gambacorta MA, et al. Preoperative hyperfractionated chemoradiation for locally recurrent rectal cancer in patients previously irradiated to the pelvis: A multicentric phase II study. Int J Radiat Oncol Biol Phys. 2006;64(4):1129–39.
152. Das P, Delclos ME, Skibber JM, et al. Hyperfractionated accelerated radiotherapy for rectal cancer in patients with prior pelvic irradiation. Int J Radiat Oncol Biol Phys. 2010;77(1):60–5.
153. Schrag D. Evolving role of neoadjuvant therapy in rectal cancer. Curr Treat Options Oncol. 2013;14(3):350–64.
154. Maas M, Nelemans PJ, Valentini V, et al. Long-term outcome in patients with a pathological complete response after chemoradiation for rectal cancer: a pooled analysis of individual patient data. Lancet Oncol. 2010;11(9):835–44.

Management of Liver Metastases from Colorectal Cancer

19

Junichi Shindoh, Giuseppe Zimmitti, and Jean-Nicolas Vauthey

Learning Objectives

After reading this chapter, you should be able to:

- Recognize how to determine surgical indication for patients with colorectal liver metastases.
- Understand how to expand surgical indication and improve safety of major hepatectomy.
- Appreciate new prognostic predictors in patients undergoing preoperative chemotherapy.

Background

Colorectal cancer (CRC) is the second leading cause of cancer mortality in the United States. Approximately 20–25 % of patients are found to have synchronous colorectal liver metastases (CLM) [1, 2], and 35–55 % of patients develop CLM during the course of the disease [3]. However, the 5-year survival after curative resection of CLM has been reported to be as high as 58 % [4–6], while the median survival of CLM without any treatment is approximately 6 months [2]. Therefore, adequate assessment and preoperative management are important in selecting patients with resectable or potentially resectable CLM who are candidates for liver resection.

J. Shindoh, M.D., Ph.D. • G. Zimmitti, M.D.
J.-N. Vauthey, M.D. (✉)
Department of Surgical Oncology, MD Anderson Cancer Center, 1515 Holcombe Boulevard, Unit 1484, Houston 77030-4009, TX, USA
e-mail: jvauthey@mdanderson.org

With recent advancements in chemotherapy and surgical management, resectability of CLM has dramatically increased, and long-term survival after resection of CLM has also significantly improved [7]. The practical points in the initial clinical evaluation and management of patients with CLM include (1) precise assessment of extension of disease and (2) proper selection of the initial therapeutic options. Surgical resection is potentially the most curative therapeutic strategy for liver metastases. However, to select the patients who would benefit the most from surgery, a multidisciplinary approach by surgeons, medical oncologist, radiologist, and pathologist is essential (Fig. 19.1) [8].

Pre-therapeutic Imaging Evaluation

Adequate imaging is essential for patients with suspected CLM for diagnosis, staging, treatment planning, and evaluation of response to chemotherapy. The choice of imaging technique for pretreatment assessment of CLM depends on the local expertise and availability of imaging modalities. However, computed tomography (CT) and magnetic resonance imaging (MRI) are the most common modalities utilized for diagnosing and evaluating patients with CLM.

Niekel et al. [9] reviewed 39 articles (3,391 patients) and showed that the estimated sensitivities on a per-lesion basis for CT, MRI, and

Q.D. Chu et al. (eds.), *Surgical Oncology: A Practical and Comprehensive Approach*,
DOI 10.1007/978-1-4939-1423-4_19,

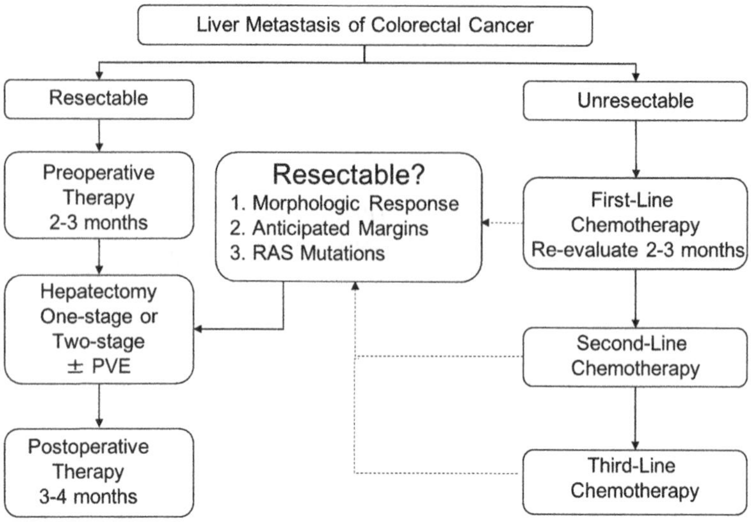

Fig. 19.1 Multidisciplinary approach for CLM (Adapted from Ref. [8]. With permission from Elsevier)

18F-fluorodeoxyglucose positron emission topography (^{18}F-FDG-PET) were 74.4 %, 80.3 %, and 81.4 %, respectively. Per-patient sensitivities were 83.6 %, 88.2 %, and 94.1 %, respectively. MRI combining gadolinium ethoxybenzyl diethylenetriamine pentaacetic acid (Gd-EOB-DTPA) delayed images and diffusion-weighted imaging has the best performance characteristics for detecting and characterizing liver lesions, particularly those smaller than 10 mm in size [10]. In addition, the usefulness of ^{18}F-FDG-PET has been reported especially for detecting extrahepatic metastases or local recurrence [11, 12]. However, increased sensitivity is usually associated with reduced specificity. Also, limitations of these new imaging modalities include limited availability, high cost, limited access to specialized techniques, and lack of expertise to interpret the results. Therefore, from a practical clinical perspective, CT still plays a central role in characterizing CLM because of its accessibility, practicality, low cost, and acceptable sensitivity/specificity to characterize CLM. At MD Anderson Cancer Center, a CT of chest, abdomen, and pelvis is routinely performed for evaluating patients with CLM [13]. PET and MRI are selectively used.

Evaluation of Resectability

After confirming the patient's physical status to tolerate surgery and determining his/her tumor distributions, the eligibility for resection in patients with CLM is determined by two factors: oncological benefit and technical feasibility.

Oncological Resectability

From an oncological standpoint, complete resection of all viable disease in patients with CLM is crucial if the patient is to derive the most benefit from surgery. Selection of surgical candidate depends on the presence or absence of extrahepatic disease and tumor response to chemotherapy.

Because lack of extrahepatic disease is associated with the ability to perform curative surgery, careful preoperative screening is important to make this determination. Lung, abdominal lymph nodes, and peritoneum represent the most common sites of extrahepatic disease. However, location of extrahepatic disease plays less of a role in determining outcome so long as complete resection is feasible [14]. In appropriately selected patients, the presence of extrahepatic disease does not necessarily represent an absolute contraindication for surgery, since there are reports of relatively favorable long-term survivals in those who had extrahepatic metastasectomy [15]. Isolated lung metastases or periportal adenopathy has reportedly been associated with a high 5-year survival rate (30–40 %) when complete resection is feasible [16]. Localized peritoneal disease correlates with intermediate 5-year survival rates (15–30 %), whereas para-aortic adenopathy or evidence of multiple sites of extrahepatic disease is rarely associated with good survival after resection of CLM (5-year survivals <15 %) [17]. These data suggest that patients harboring limited extrahepatic disease are amenable to surgical resection with a reasonable expectation for long-term control with adjuvant therapies [18]. When the extrahepatic disease burden is unresectable or uncontrollable, hepatic resection for CLM is contraindicated.

Another important factor in determining resectability is response to chemotherapy. When patients are treated with preoperative systemic therapy, biologic behavior of the tumor can be assessed during treatment. With modern effective chemotherapy, disease progression during preoperative systemic therapy is relatively rare. However, there are patients who occasionally (5–15 %) do have disease progression during receipt of systemic therapy, and development of new lesions is associated with a poor prognosis after CLM resection [19]. In contrast, growth of preexisting intrahepatic lesion itself does not seem to be associated with poor outcomes as long as new lesions do not develop during treatment. Therefore, patients who show this pattern of progression who have resectable lesions should remain candidates for a hepatectomy.

A recent study reviewing LiverMetSurvey international registry reported that although tumor progression during chemotherapy is a negative prognostic factor, surgical resection might still be a viable option with acceptable long-term outcomes. Exceptions include patients with >3 liver metastases, liver tumor size ≥50 mm, and/or serum carcinoembryonic antigen (CEA) level ≥200 ng/mL; in such situations, further chemotherapy is recommended [20].

Technical Resectability

Technical resectability is based on adequate knowledge of liver anatomy, histopathology, and hepatic function, all of which are best evaluated in a multidisciplinary setting with inputs from hepatobiliary surgeons, radiologists, hepatologists, and pathologists. Conventionally, technical resectability has been defined as removal of all viable tumors with a negative margin, leaving behind a minimum of two contiguous segments of hepatic parenchyma that have adequate vascular inflow and outflow and adequate biliary drainage [21]. More recently, the selection of patients with resectable CLM has greatly improved from the enhanced ability to predict future liver remnant (FLR) volume and liver function.

Currently, functional reserve of the liver is estimated by both static and dynamic measurements. The most reliable static variable is the FLR volume. Because absolute volume of FLR against standardized liver volume (SLV) (i.e., sFLR: standardized FLR) has strong correlation with the rates of postoperative morbidity and mortality (Fig. 19.2) [22, 23], minimal requirements of sFLR have currently been set at >20 % in normal liver, >30 % in damaged liver after extensive treatment, and >40 % in cirrhotic liver (Fig. 19.3) [22, 24–27]. In a recent analysis on the clinical impact of duration of systemic therapy and the minimal requirement of sFLR in patients undergoing preoperative chemotherapy, those who underwent more than 3 months of systemic therapy required at least 30 % of sFLR to prevent postoperative hepatic insufficiency [27]. These cutoff values offer a good practical decision making metric in patients requiring major hepatectomy.

In addition to the FLR volume, dynamic measurements such as degree of hypertrophy [23] and kinetic growth rate (KGR) [28] after portal vein embolization (PVE) have also been reported to be sensitive predictors of functional liver reserve

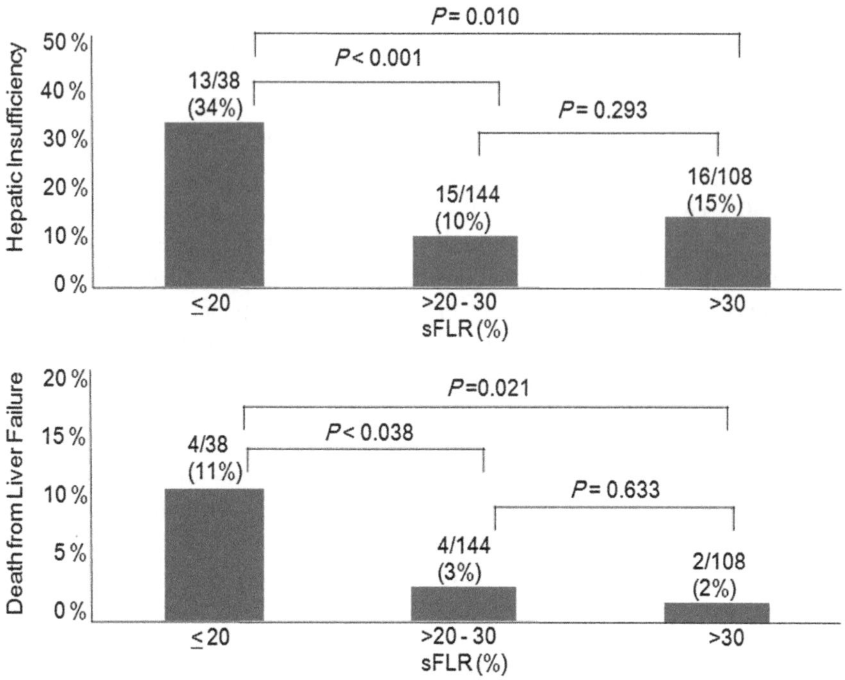

Fig. 19.2 FLR volume and surgical outcomes (Adapted from Ref. [22]. With permission from Wolters Kluwer Health)

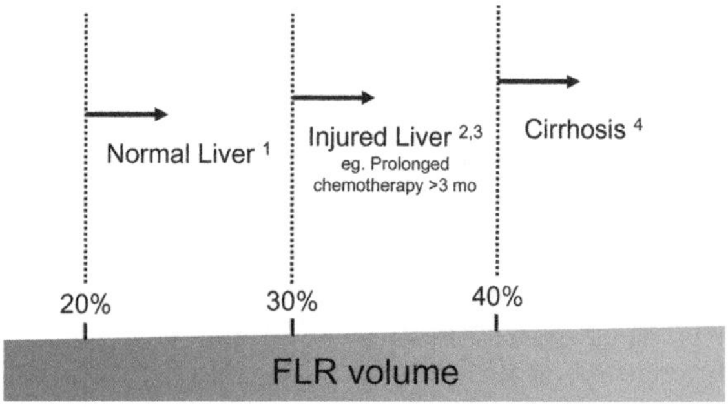

Fig. 19.3 Minimal requirement of FLR volume

1. **Kishi Y, et al. Ann Surg 2009 [22]**
2. **Shindoh J, et al. Ann Surg Oncol 2013 [27]**
3. **Azoulay D, et al., Ann Surg 2000 [25]**
4. **Kubota K, et al. Hepatology 1997 [26]**

in patients undergoing extended hepatectomy. The KGR, defined as the degree of hypertrophy divided by the number of weeks elapsed after portal vein embolization, well predicts underlying liver function and short-term surgical outcomes independent of sFLR or the timing of initial volume assessment. KGR of at least 2 % per week reduces hepatic complications and liver failure-related deaths [28].

Furthermore, indocyanine green clearance test [29] or hepatic scintigraphy [30] has also been reported to be a good indicator of hepatic functional reserve with regard to metabolic function. Because FLR volume itself is not correlated with functional reserve, dynamic measurements should be integrated to estimate the total functional reserve of FLR in individual patients.

Strategies to Increase Resectability

Portal Vein Embolization (PVE)

PVE is a safe, minimally invasive procedure that leads to atrophy of the liver to be resected and compensatory hypertrophy of FLR [31–33]. Based on the baseline status of liver parenchyma, PVE should be considered if a patient is found to have

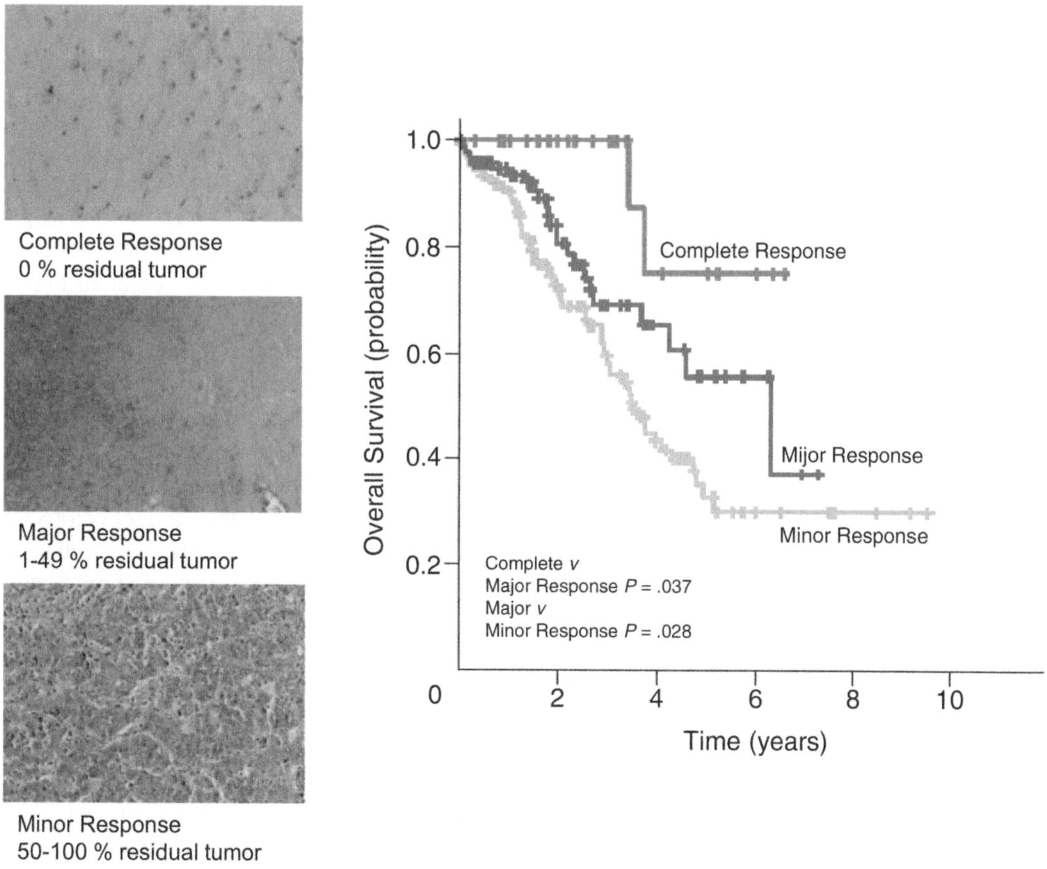

Fig. 19.4 Pathologic response to preoperative chemotherapy (Adapted from Ref. [54]. With permission from American Society of Clinical Oncology)

insufficient volume in the pretreatment measurement of FLR. To maximize the regeneration of FLR in PVE, optimal selection of embolic materials [34] and concurrent embolization of segment IV portal vein [35, 36] have been recommended, the latter often has evidence of disease. Our previous work comparing right PVE with and without segment IV embolization revealed significant difference in volume increase rates in segment II+III (median, 26 % vs. 54 %; $p=0.021$).

Two-Stage Liver Resection

With limited liver tumor burden including small tumors and anatomically favorably positioned bilateral metastases, a one-stage strategy involving one or more simultaneous partial to lobar hepatic resection is safe and effective [37–42]. In contrast, when extensive bilobar metastases are present (i.e., extensive right lobe disease including disease in segment 4 and one or more lesions in the left lateral segment and/caudate lobe), different surgical strategies are required.

Two-stage liver resection (TSR) is indicated in patients with advanced bilateral CLM who responded to chemotherapy and in whom limited resection can clear the less affected side of the liver before a planned extended contralateral liver resection. In the majority of cases, patients undergo first-stage limited resection of metastases of the left lobe, followed by right PVE with segment IV embolization to allow hypertrophy of the FLR (i.e., left lateral segment and segment 1), and extended right hepatectomy is completed after sFLR meets the volume criteria. A previous study from MD Anderson Cancer Center reported that 72.3 % (47/65) of the patients among planned TSR completed TSR, and the 5-year survival in these patients was 51 % compared to 15 % in the cases treated with chemotherapy only [44].

Associating Liver Partition and Portal Vein Ligation for Staged Hepatectomy (ALPPS) Procedure

Recently, a European group reported safety and efficacy data for a short-interval (median waiting period of 9 days) two-stage liver surgery technique consisting of an initial open right portal vein ligation with in situ splitting of the liver parenchyma followed by re-exploration for right trisectionectomy, named Associating Liver Partition and Portal Vein Ligation for Staged hepatectomy or "ALPPS" [45]. Wedge resection of the left lobe is generally performed at the initial operation so as to render the left lobe disease-free. The combination of portal vein ligation and in situ splitting of the liver to prevent cross-portal circulation between the lobes of the liver was believed to lead to a profound hypertrophy of the FLR. However, preliminary data suggested a high incidence of major morbidity (40 %) and inpatient mortality (12 %) associated with this new procedure.

In our recent study comparing the ALPPS and PVE for patients with very small FLR volume, we demonstrated that right PVE with segment IV embolization may offer equivalent hypertrophy of FLR (62 % vs. 74 %) but with less perioperative bile leak (5.8 % vs. 24 %) and sepsis (0 % vs. 20 %) compared to the ALPPS procedure [46]. Although the time duration from the hemodynamic modulation to surgery was significantly longer in the PVE group (34 days vs. 9 days), this waiting period is oncologically meaningful because it allows selection of patients who would truly benefit from surgical resection while avoiding unnecessary resection of those with disease progression.

Strategies for Synchronous Metastases

Nearly 25 % of patients with colorectal cancer have CLM at the same time the primary tumor is diagnosed (synchronous presentation). The major problem in these patients is that both colectomy and hepatectomy are needed to resect all tumor burdens, either by a simultaneous or in a stepwise fashion. The traditional surgical strategy for patients with resectable synchronous CLM includes resection of the primary tumor followed by chemotherapy and then liver resection (classic strategy). A combined strategy that includes simultaneous resection of the primary colorectal lesion and the liver metastases has also been used to avoid delaying surgical resection of metastatic lesions. However, the limitation with the combined strategy is the associated increased risk of postoperative complications.

With recent advancements in effective chemotherapy, a reverse strategy, in which preoperative chemotherapy is followed by resection of the CLM and then by resection of the colorectal primary at a second operation, has been proposed especially for patients with advanced synchronous CLM. A study comparing these three approaches (classic, combined, and reverse approaches) demonstrated similar surgical outcomes among the three approaches despite patients undergoing the reverse strategy having more extensive disease. Therefore, a reverse strategy should be considered as an alternative approach for treating advanced CLM in patients with synchronous liver metastases and an asymptomatic primary tumor (i.e., no evidence of obstruction, bleeding, intractable pain, or perforation) [47].

Surgical Outcomes

Short-Term Outcomes

A systematic review of short-term results of liver resection reported a mortality rate of 0 % to 6.6 % (median 2.8 %) [48]. The main cause of mortality related to liver resection was hepatic failure (18.4 %), followed by hemorrhage (17.5 %) and sepsis (16.5 %). However, the definition of liver failure varied among institutions, making it difficult to compare surgical risk according to individual criteria for FLR volumes.

Mullen et al. have reviewed 1,059 noncirrhotic patients who underwent major hepatectomy at 3 hepatobiliary centers and found that peak serum bilirubin level of > 7.0 mg/dL was a potent predictor of any (odds ratio [OR] 83.3) or major complication (OR 10.0), 90-day mortality (OR 10.8), and 90-day liver-related mortality (OR 250). Importantly, combining INR with bilirubin did not improve the high sensitivity (93 %) and high specificity (94 %) of bilirubin alone in the predicting liver failure. Therefore, peak bilirubin level of >7.0 mg/dL is defined as "postoperative hepatic insufficiency" and is a potent predictor of "death from liver failure" [49].

Based on the clear definition of hepatic insufficiency, minimal requirement of FLR volume could be analyzed and determined according to the histopathologic status of underlying liver [22, 27], This has also contributed to develop further advance the concept of dynamic measurement of liver volumes such as degree of hypertrophy [23] or kinetic growth rate [28] after PVE as mentioned in the previous section.

The reported overall complication rates after hepatectomy range from 16 % to 44 %. Factors associated with the risk for postoperative complications include complexity of liver resection (number of liver segments to be resected, whether or not a biliary-enteric anastomosis is performed, the need for vascular resection, etc.), intraoperative blood loss and blood transfusion, concomitant major extrahepatic procedure, and patient medical conditions [50]. In a recent study, we compared short-term outcomes of 2,628 liver resections at MD Anderson Cancer Center in two different periods (before and after 2006) and found that overall morbidity rates, hepatic insufficiency, and 90-day mortality have not changed over time, even though the complexity of surgery such as extended hepatectomy, repeated resection, two-stage surgery, or use of preoperative PVE has increased. However, the rate of bile leak has increased over time (3.7 vs. 5.9 % before and after 2006, respectively) which is likely related to the increasing complexity of liver resection. With the systematic use of a new air leak test to detect bile leak, the rate of biliary fistula has significantly decreased over the recent years [51, 52].

Long-Term Outcomes and Prognostic Factors

With the development of effective chemotherapy and strategies for surgical management as mentioned previously, recent series reported the 5-year survival rate after curative resection of CLM to be as high as 58 % [4–6]. However, there is considerable heterogeneity in oncological feature of the tumor and patients and variable degree of aggressiveness of CLM among patients, which lead to a variable 5-year survival rates reported in the literature

Traditionally, large liver tumor size and number of tumor, evidence of bilobar distribution, short disease-free interval, and high serum CEA level before hepatectomy have been regarded as important poor prognostic factors following resection of CLM [38, 39, 53]. However, increasing evidence has suggested that these traditional prognostic factors are losing their clinical significance in the era of effective chemotherapy and increasing use of biologic agents. In the era of effective preoperative chemotherapy, several new criteria have been proposed that appeared to be sensitive in predicting patient survival.

Pathologic Response

Pathologic response to preoperative chemotherapy is a strong predictor of survival outcomes in patients undergoing hepatic resection after preoperative chemotherapy (Fig. 19.4) [54, 55]. Pathologic response is excellent in stratifying both overall and recurrence-free survival of patients who undergo hepatic resection of CLM. However, the limitation in the clinical setting is that pathologic response is difficult to assess prior to surgery.

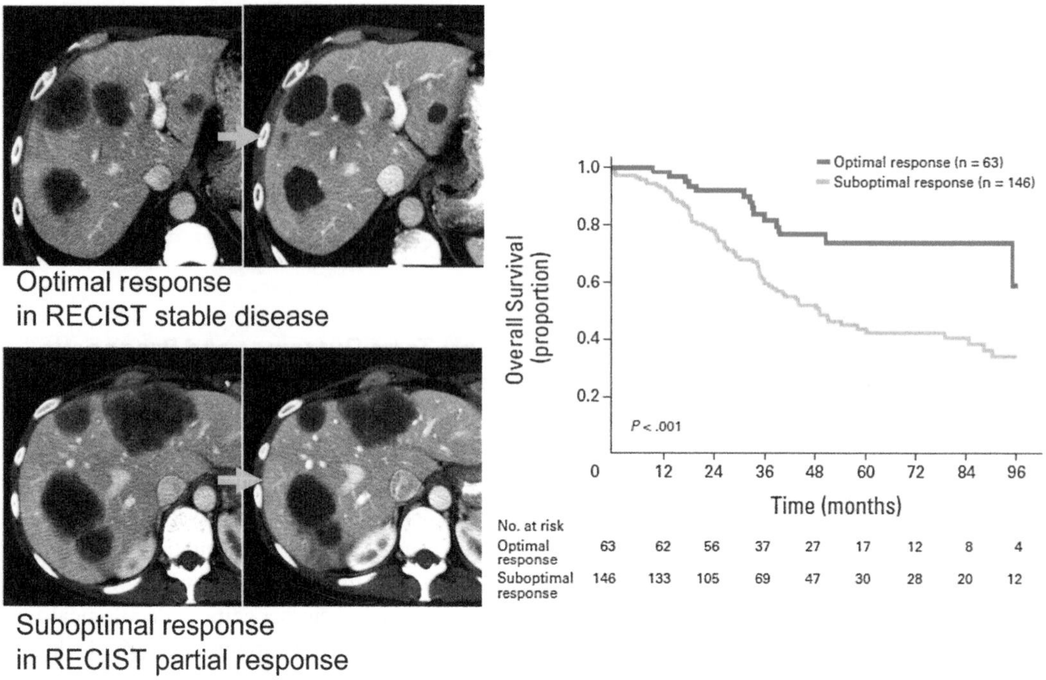

Fig. 19.5 Morphological response to preoperative chemotherapy (Adapted from Ref. [64]. With permission from American Society of Clinical Oncology)

Table 19.1 Definition of CT morphologic groups

Group	Overall attenuation	Tumor-liver interface	Peripheral rim of enhancement
3	Heterogeneous	Ill defined	May be present
2	Mixed	Variable	If initially present, partially resolved
1	Homogeneous and hypoattenuating	Sharp	If initially present, completely resolved

Reprinted from Ref. [63]. With permission from the Journal of the American Medical Association
Optimal response, from group 3 or 2 to group 1; *incomplete response*, group 3 to group 2; *no response*, no change in group 2 or 3, or progression

Radiologic Response

Radiologic response to chemotherapy was conventionally assessed by changes in tumor size according to the Response Evaluation Criteria in Solid Tumors (RECIST) [56–58]. However, recent studies have reported that the RECIST criteria may underestimate the response to chemotherapy since the traditional size-based response criteria can be unreliable [59–62]. To overcome this issue, our group first reported that changes consisting of a "cystic-like" alteration in the texture of tumor seen on CT image (morphologic response) is a better alternative criterion for evaluating response to preoperative therapy in patients with CLM (Table 19.1 and Fig. 19.5) [63, 64]. In a recent validation study with 209 patients, we confirmed that these non-size-based observations were also applicable for patients who were not given bevacizumab. Morphologic response was well correlated with pathologic response, and suboptimal morphologic response was a strong "preoperative" prognostic factors for both overall survival (Hazard ratio [HR] 2.1, 95 % CI 1.2–3.8) and recurrence-free survival (HR 1.8, 95 % CI 1.2–2.8) [64].

Fig. 19.6 RAS mutations and pathologic response (Adapted from Ref. [69]. With permission from Annals of Surgical Oncology)

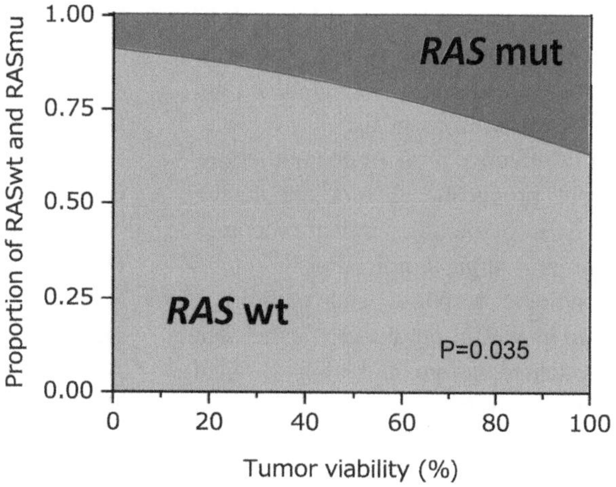

Estimated RAS mutation rate according to the degree of pathologic response in 165 patients with >5% viable tumor cells

Somatic Mutational Status

The variability of the individual CLM in clinical presentation, degree of aggressiveness, and patterns of treatment failure suggests the presence of variability in genotypes and phenotypes among the individual patients. Over the past decades, numerous biomarkers and molecular pathways have been investigated to explain such biologic heterogeneity. Among the molecular candidates, *RAS* mutation is the most important marker that predicts efficacy of anti-EGFR (epidermal growth factor receptor) biologic agents. Recent studies have clarified that *RAS* mutation status in clinical practice is likely to expand beyond its current role just as a predictor of response to anti-EGFR agents.

First, *RAS* mutations independently predict worse overall and disease-free survival after resection of CLM [65–67]. Second, *RAS* mutation status is also predictive of patterns of recurrence or metastases to other organs. Tie et al. reported higher *KRAS* mutation rates in lung (62 %), and brain (56 %) colorectal metastases than in primary colorectal cancer (35 %) [68]. Our group also confirmed that patients with *RAS* mutation undergoing resection of CLM had a worse lung recurrence-free survival than patients with *RAS* wild type [67]. In another study, RAS mutational status also predicted radiologic and pathologic response in patients treated with preoperative chemotherapy for CLM (Fig. 19.6) [69]. Though the clinical significance of mutation in *RAS* has not been fully understood, it may offer clinicians the ability to predict outcome at presentation before response to chemotherapy and can serve as a basis for personalized medicine in the near future.

Salient Points

- Prior to considering resection of colorectal liver metastases (CLM), pretreatment radiologic staging is required to assess for the presence and extent of intra- and extrahepatic disease.
- Resectability includes the expectation that a margin-negative resection (i.e., R0) can be achieved leaving sufficient volume of future liver remnant (FLR) with adequate blood flow and biliary drainage.
- Patients harboring limited extrahepatic disease amenable to surgical resection or with reasonable expectations for long-term control with adjuvant therapies may be considered for hepatic resection.
- Patients with significant progression of metastatic disease during preoperative systemic therapy should have surgical resection deferred until achieving disease control with second-line systemic or regional therapies.
- Portal vein embolization (PVE) is indicated when FLR volume is expected to be insufficient according to the status of the underlying liver. At least 20 % of standardized FLR volume is

required for patients with normal liver, 30 % for patients heavily pretreated with prolonged chemotherapy greater than 3 months, and 40 % for patients with cirrhosis.

- In the era of effective modern chemotherapy, conventional prognostic factors are losing their priority in predicting surgical outcomes and determining surgical indication.
- CT morphologic response and pathologic response are powerful prognostic factors that can be evaluated before and after surgical resection, respectively.
- RAS mutations predict patterns of recurrence and long-term outcomes of patients undergoing resection of CLM.

Questions

1. Regarding two-stage resection of advanced bilateral colorectal liver metastases, which of the following statements is true?
   A. The procedure is associated with an intent to treat 5-year overall survival of > 50 %.
   B. The procedure is associated with a 90-day perioperative mortality of more than 10 %.
   C. The results are not better than those of a match cohort of medical patients with best response to chemotherapy alive after 1 year of chemotherapy.
   D. Is contraindicated in patients with more than 10 metastases.
2. Methods to improve resectability include:
   A. Two-stage hepatectomy
   B. The "reverse approach" (resection of liver metastases before primary in patients with synchronous liver metastases)
   C. Portal vein embolization extended to segment IV
   D. All of the above
3. Regeneration after portal vein embolization can be compromised
   A. By the use of spherical microspheres in addition to coils
   B. If right portal vein embolization is extended to segment IV prior to extended right hepatectomy
   C. If performed while chemotherapy with bevacizumab is administered
   D. If performed in patients with splenomegaly
4. Major pathologic response to chemotherapy (<50 % viable cancer cells):
   A. Is easy to assess preoperatively
   B. Is associated with improved overall survival after resection
   C. Has no association with morphologic response on computed tomography
   D. Has no impact on outcome
5. Which of the following is the strongest predictor of postoperative liver-related death?
   A. Postoperative peak INR >1.6
   B. Ascites drained >500 ml/day postoperatively
   C. Postoperative total bilirubin level of > 7.0 mg/dL
   D. Postoperative alanine aminotransferase level of >300 mg/dL
6. All of the following statements are true regarding the ALPPS procedure (associated liver partition and portal vein ligation for staged hepatectomy) <u>EXCEPT</u>:
   A. The long-term results of the procedure are unknown.
   B. It is the only effective approach to resect liver tumors in patients with a very small future liver remnant (liver to patient weight ratio of less than .5).
   C. The reported perioperative mortality is more than 10 %.
   D. It induces hypertrophy of the liver remnant without the need for portal vein embolization.
7. Major resection for CLM can be performed safely in patients with:
   A. Standardized future liver remnant (sFLR) >20 % and a normal liver
   B. A kinetic growth rate (KGR) > 2 % per week following portal vein embolization
   C. Standardized future liver remnant (sFLR) >30 % after prolonged preoperative chemotherapy (>3 months)
   D. All of the above
8. Optimal morphologic radiologic response to chemotherapy is:
   A. Defined by a "cystic-like" appearance of colorectal liver metastases on computed tomography (CT)
   B. Associated with a two-fold (HR2.0) decrease in overall survival after resection of CLM

C. More commonly observed in liver metastases with a *RAS* mutation
D. All of the above

Answers

1. A
2. D
3. D
4. B
5. C
6. B
7. D
8. A

References

1. Almersjo O, Bengmark S, Hafstrom L. Liver metastases found by follow-up of patients operated on for colorectal cancer. Cancer. 1976;37(3):1454–7.
2. Bengmark S, Hafstrom L. The natural history of primary and secondary malignant tumors of the liver. I. The prognosis for patients with hepatic metastases from colonic and rectal carcinoma by laparotomy. Cancer. 1969;23(1):198–202.
3. Pawlik TM, Choti MA. Surgical therapy for colorectal metastases to the liver. J Gastrointest Surg. 2007;11(8):1057–77.
4. Fong Y, Cohen AM, Fortner JG, et al. Liver resection for colorectal metastases. J Clin Oncol. 1997;15(3): 938–46.
5. Ito H, Are C, Gonen M, et al. Effect of postoperative morbidity on long-term survival after hepatic resection for metastatic colorectal cancer. Ann Surg. 2008;247(6):994–1002.
6. Pawlik TM, Scoggins CR, Zorzi D, et al. Effect of surgical margin status on survival and site of recurrence after hepatic resection for colorectal metastases. Ann Surg. 2005;241(5):715–22; discussion 722–4.
7. Kopetz S, Chang GJ, Overman MJ, et al. Improved survival in metastatic colorectal cancer is associated with adoption of hepatic resection and improved chemotherapy. J Clin Oncol. 2009;27(22):3677–83.
8. Kopetz S, Vauthey JN. Perioperative chemotherapy for resectable hepatic metastases. Lancet. 2008;371(9617):963–5.
9. Niekel MC, Bipat S, Stoker J. Diagnostic imaging of colorectal liver metastases with CT, MR imaging, FDG PET, and/or FDG PET/CT: a meta-analysis of prospective studies including patients who have not previously undergone treatment. Radiology. 2010;257(3):674–84.
10. Koh DM, Collins DJ, Wallace T, et al. Combining diffusion-weighted MRI with Gd-EOB-DTPA-enhanced MRI improves the detection of colorectal liver metastases. Br J Radiol. 2012;85(1015):980–9.
11. Chen LB, Tong JL, Song HZ. (18)F-DG PET/CT in detection of recurrence and metastasis of colorectal cancer. World J Gastroenterol. 2007;13(37): 5025–9.
12. Truant S, Huglo D, Hebbar M, et al. Prospective evaluation of the impact of [18F]fluoro-2-deoxy-D-glucose positron emission tomography of resectable colorectal liver metastases. Br J Surg. 2005;92(3):362–9.
13. Vauthey JN, Rousseau Jr DL. Liver imaging. A surgeon's perspective. Clin Liver Dis. 2002;6(1): 271–95.
14. Elias D, Liberale G, Vernerey D, et al. Hepatic and extrahepatic colorectal metastases: when resectable, their localization does not matter, but their total number has a prognostic effect. Ann Surg Oncol. 2005;12(11):900–9.
15. Carpizo DR, Are C, Jarnagin W, et al. Liver resection for metastatic colorectal cancer in patients with concurrent extrahepatic disease: results in 127 patients treated at a single center. Ann Surg Oncol. 2009;16(8):2138–46.
16. Brouquet A, Vauthey JN, Contreras CM, et al. Improved survival after resection of liver and lung colorectal metastases compared with liver-only metastases: a study of 112 patients with limited lung metastatic disease. J Am Coll Surg. 2011;213(1):62–9; discussion 69–71.
17. Chua TC, Saxena A, Liauw W, et al. Hepatectomy and resection of concomitant extrahepatic disease for colorectal liver metastases–a systematic review. Eur J Cancer. 2012;48(12):1757–65.
18. Adams RB, Aloia TA, Loyer E, et al. Selection for hepatic resection of colorectal liver metastases: expert consensus statement. HPB (Oxford). 2013;15(2):91–103.
19. Nordlinger B, Sorbye H, Glimelius B, et al. Perioperative chemotherapy with FOLFOX4 and surgery versus surgery alone for resectable liver metastases from colorectal cancer (EORTC Intergroup trial 40983): a randomised controlled trial. Lancet. 2008;371(9617):1007–16.
20. Vigano L, Capusotti L, Barroso E, et al. Progression while receiving preoperative chemotherapy should not be an absolute contraindication to liver resection for colorectal metastases. Ann Surg Oncol. 2012;19(9):2786–96.
21. Charnsangavej C, Clary B, Fong Y, et al. Selection of patients for resection of hepatic colorectal metastases: expert consensus statement. Ann Surg Oncol. 2006;13(10):1261–8.
22. Kishi Y, Abdalla EK, Chun YS, et al. Three hundred and one consecutive extended right hepatectomies: evaluation of outcome based on systematic liver volumetry. Ann Surg. 2009;250(4):540–8.
23. Ribero D, Abdalla EK, Madoff DC, et al. Portal vein embolization before major hepatectomy and its effects on regeneration, resectability and outcome. Br J Surg. 2007;94(11):1386–94.
24. Zorzi D, Laurent A, Pawlik TM, et al. Chemotherapy-associated hepatotoxicity and surgery for colorectal liver metastases. Br J Surg. 2007;94(3):274–86.

25. Azoulay D, Castaing D, Krissat J, et al. Percutaneous portal vein embolization increases the feasibility and safety of major liver resection for hepatocellular carcinoma in injured liver. Ann Surg. 2000; 232(5):665–72.
26. Kubota K, Makuuchi M, Kusaka K, et al. Measurement of liver volume and hepatic functional reserve as a guide to decision-making in resectional surgery for hepatic tumors. Hepatology. 1997;26(5):1176–81.
27. Shindoh J, Tzeng CW, Aloia TA, et al. Optimal future liver remnant in patients treated with extensive preoperative chemotherapy for colorectal liver metastases. Ann Surg Oncol. 2013;20(8):2493–500.
28. Shindoh J, Truty MJ, Aloia TA, et al. Kinetic growth rate after portal vein embolization predicts posthepatectomy outcomes: toward zero liver-related mortality in patients with colorectal liver metastases and small future liver remnant. J Am Coll Surg. 2013; 216(2):201–9.
29. Takamoto T, Hashimoto T, Sano K, et al. Recovery of liver function after the cessation of preoperative chemotherapy for colorectal liver metastasis. Ann Surg Oncol. 2010;17(10):2747–55.
30. Dinant S, de Graaf W, Verwer BJ, et al. Risk assessment of posthepatectomy liver failure using hepatobiliary scintigraphy and CT volumetry. J Nucl Med. 2007;48(5):685–92.
31. Abulkhir A, Limongelli P, Healey AJ, et al. Preoperative portal vein embolization for major liver resection: a meta-analysis. Ann Surg. 2008;247(1): 49–57.
32. Giraudo G, Greget M, Oussoultzoglou E, et al. Preoperative contralateral portal vein embolization before major hepatic resection is a safe and efficient procedure: a large single institution experience. Surgery. 2008;143(4):476–82.
33. Mueller L, Hillert C, Moller L, et al. Major hepatectomy for colorectal metastases: is preoperative portal occlusion an oncological risk factor? Ann Surg Oncol. 2008;15(7):1908–17.
34. Madoff DC, Abdalla EK, Gupta S, et al. Transhepatic ipsilateral right portal vein embolization extended to segment IV: improving hypertrophy and resection outcomes with spherical particles and coils. J Vasc Interv Radiol. 2005;16(2 Pt 1):215–25.
35. Kishi Y, Madoff DC, Abdalla EK, et al. Is embolization of segment 4 portal veins before extended right hepatectomy justified? Surgery. 2008;144(5):744–51.
36. Nagino M, Kamiya J, Kanai M, et al. Right trisegment portal vein embolization for biliary tract carcinoma: technique and clinical utility. Surgery. 2000;127(2): 155–60.
37. Rees M, Tekkis PP, Welsh FK, et al. Evaluation of long-term survival after hepatic resection for metastatic colorectal cancer: a multifactorial model of 929 patients. Ann Surg. 2008;247(1):125–35.
38. Nordlinger B, Guiguet M, Vaillant JC, et al. Surgical resection of colorectal carcinoma metastases to the liver. A prognostic scoring system to improve case selection, based on 1568 patients. Association Francaise de Chirurgie. Cancer. 1996;77(7):1254–62.
39. Fong Y, Fortner J, Sun RL, et al. Clinical score for predicting recurrence after hepatic resection for metastatic colorectal cancer: analysis of 1001 consecutive cases. Ann Surg. 1999;230(3):309–18; discussion 318–21.
40. Wei AC, Greig PD, Grant D, et al. Survival after hepatic resection for colorectal metastases: a 10-year experience. Ann Surg Oncol. 2006;13(5):668–76.
41. Kato T, Yasui K, Hirai T, et al. Therapeutic results for hepatic metastasis of colorectal cancer with special reference to effectiveness of hepatectomy: analysis of prognostic factors for 763 cases recorded at 18 institutions. Dis Colon Rectum. 2003;46(10 Suppl):S22–31.
42. Scheele J, Altendorf-Hofmann A, Grube T, et al. Resection of colorectal liver metastases. What prognostic factors determine patient selection? Chirurg. 2001;72(5):547–60.
43. Jaeck D, Oussoultzoglou E, Rosso E, et al. A two-stage hepatectomy procedure combined with portal vein embolization to achieve curative resection for initially unresectable multiple and bilobar colorectal liver metastases. Ann Surg. 2004;240(6):1037–51.
44. Brouquet A, Abdalla EK, Kopetz S, et al. High survival rate after two-stage resection of advanced colorectal liver metastases: response-based selection and complete resection define outcome. J Clin Oncol. 2011;29(8):1083–90.
45. Schnitzbauer AA, Lang SA, Goessmann H, et al. Right portal vein ligation combined with in situ splitting induces rapid left lateral liver lobe hypertrophy enabling 2-staged extended right hepatic resection in small-for-size settings. Ann Surg. 2012;255(3): 405–14.
46. Shindoh J, Vauthey JN, Zimmitti G, et al. Analysis of the efficacy of portal vein embolization for patients with extensive liver malignancy and very low future liver remnant volume, including a comparison with the associating liver partition with portal vein ligation for staged hepatectomy approach. J Am Coll Surg. 2013;217(1):126–33; discussion 133–4.
47. Brouquet A, Mortenson MM, Vauthey JN, et al. Surgical strategies for synchronous colorectal liver metastases in 156 consecutive patients: classic, combined or reverse strategy? J Am Coll Surg. 2010; 210(6):934–41.
48. Simmonds PC, Primrose JN, Colquitt JL, et al. Surgical resection of hepatic metastases from colorectal cancer: a systematic review of published studies. Br J Cancer. 2006;94(7):982–99.
49. Mullen JT, Ribero D, Reddy SK, et al. Hepatic insufficiency and mortality in 1,059 noncirrhotic patients undergoing major hepatectomy. J Am Coll Surg. 2007;204(5):854–62; discussion 862–4.
50. Jarnagin WR, Gonen M, Fong Y, et al. Improvement in perioperative outcome after hepatic resection: analysis of 1,803 consecutive cases over the past decade. Ann Surg. 2002;236(4):397–406; discussion 406–7.
51. Zimmitti G, Vauthey JN, Shindoh J, et al. Systematic use of an intraoperative air leak test at the time of major liver resection reduces the rate of postoperative

biliary complications. J Am Coll Surg [In press, 2013].

52. Zimmitti G, Roses RE, Andreou A, et al. Greater complexity of liver surgery is not associated with an increased incidence of liver-related complications except for bile leak: an experience with 2,628 consecutive resections. J Gastrointest Surg. 2013;17(1):57–64; discussion p 64–5.
53. Minagawa M, Makuuchi M, Torzilli G, et al. Extension of the frontiers of surgical indications in the treatment of liver metastases from colorectal cancer: long-term results. Ann Surg. 2000; 231(4):487–99.
54. Blazer 3rd DG, Kishi Y, Maru DM, et al. Pathologic response to preoperative chemotherapy: a new outcome end point after resection of hepatic colorectal metastases. J Clin Oncol. 2008;26(33):5344–51.
55. Maru DM, Kopetz S, Boonsirikamchai P, et al. Tumor thickness at the tumor-normal interface: a novel pathologic indicator of chemotherapy response in hepatic colorectal metastases. Am J Surg Pathol. 2010;34(9):1287–94.
56. Eisenhauer EA, Therasse P, Bogaerts J, et al. New response evaluation criteria in solid tumours: revised RECIST guideline (version 1.1). Eur J Cancer. 2009;45(2):228–47.
57. Jaffe CC. Measures of response: RECIST, WHO, and new alternatives. J Clin Oncol. 2006;24(20): 3245–51.
58. Therasse P, Arbuck SG, Eisenhauer EA, et al. New guidelines to evaluate the response to treatment in solid tumors. European Organization for Research and Treatment of Cancer, National Cancer Institute of the United States, National Cancer Institute of Canada. J Natl Cancer Inst. 2000;92(3):205–16.
59. Antoch G, Kanja J, Bauer S, et al. Comparison of PET, CT, and dual-modality PET/CT imaging for monitoring of imatinib (STI571) therapy in patients with gastrointestinal stromal tumors. J Nucl Med. 2004;45(3):357–65.
60. Choi H, Charnsangavej C, de Castro FS, et al. CT evaluation of the response of gastrointestinal stromal tumors after imatinib mesylate treatment: a quantitative analysis correlated with FDG PET findings. AJR Am J Roentgenol. 2004;183(6):1619–28.
61. Stroobants S, Goeminne J, Seegers M, et al. 18FDG-Positron emission tomography for the early prediction of response in advanced soft tissue sarcoma treated with imatinib mesylate (Glivec). Eur J Cancer. 2003;39(14):2012–20.
62. Thiam R, Fournier LS, Trinquart L, et al. Optimizing the size variation threshold for the CT evaluation of response in metastatic renal cell carcinoma treated with sunitinib. Ann Oncol. 2010;21(5):936–41.
63. Chun YS, Vauthey JN, Boonsirikamchai P, et al. Association of computed tomography morphologic criteria with pathologic response and survival in patients treated with bevacizumab for colorectal liver metastases. JAMA. 2009;302(21):2338–44.
64. Shindoh J, Loyer EM, Kopetz S, et al. Optimal morphologic response to preoperative chemotherapy: an alternate outcome end point before resection of hepatic colorectal metastases. J Clin Oncol. 2012;30(36):4566–72.
65. Nash GM, Gimbel M, NShia J, et al. KRAS mutation correlates with accelerated metastatic progression in patients with colorectal liver metastases. Ann Surg Oncol. 2010;17(2):572–8.
66. Stremitzer S, Stift J, Gruenberger B, et al. KRAS status and outcome of liver resection after neoadjuvant chemotherapy including bevacizumab. Br J Surg. 2012;99(1):1575–82.
67. Vauthey JN, Zimmitti G, Kopetz S, et al. RAS mutation status predicts survival and patterns of recurrence in patients undergoing hepatectomy for colorectal liver metastases. Ann Surg. 2013;258(4):619–27.
68. Tie J, Lipton L, Desai J, et al. KRAS mutation is associated with lung metastasis in patients with curatively resected colorectal cancer. Clin Cancer Res. 2011; 17(5):1122–30.
69. Mise Y, Zimmitt G, Shindo J, et al. RAS mutations predict radiologic and pathologic response in patients treated with chemotherapy prior to resection of colorectal liver metastases. Ann Surg Oncol. [In press].

Hereditary Colorectal Cancer and Polyposis Syndromes

20

Edward Eun Cho, John F. Gibbs, Miguel Rodriguez-Bigas, and Luz Maria Rodriguez

Learning Objectives

After reading this chapter, you should be able to:

- Describe the epidemiology, genetic mutation, clinical presentation, surveillance recommendations, and treatment options for Lynch syndrome and familial adenomatous polyposis (FAP) and attenuated FAP (aFAP)
- Describe the various extracolonic manifestations associated with Lynch syndrome and FAP
- Understand the various medical and surgical treatment options for FAP and its various extracolonic manifestations especially duodenal polyps and periampullary neoplasm
- Understand the difference between FAP and aFAP
- Describe the epidemiology, genetic mutation, clinical presentation, surveillance recommendations, and treatment options for MYH-associated polyposis, Peutz–Jeghers syndrome, and juvenile polyposis syndrome

E.E. Cho, M.D., Sc.M.
Department of Surgery, Kaleida Health/Buffalo General Med Center, State University of New York at Buffalo, 100 High St. Buffalo, 14203 NY, USA
e-mail: eecho@buffalo.edu

J.F. Gibbs, M.D.
Department of Surgery, Jersey Shore University Medical Center/Meridian Health, 1945 State Highway 33, 4 floor Ackerman, Neptune, 07753 NJ, USA
e-mail: jgibbs@meridianhealth.com

M. Rodriguez-Bigas, M.D.
Department of Surgical Oncology, UT MD Anderson Cancer Center, 1400 Pressler Street, Unit 1484, Houston 77044, TX, USA
e-mail: mrodbig@mdanderson.org

L.M. Rodriguez, M.D. (✉)
Department of Surgery, Walter Reed National Military Medical Center/National Cancer Institute, 9609 Medical Center Drive, Rm 5E- 228, MSC 9782, Bethesda 20892-9782, MD, USA
e-mail: rodrigul@mail.nih.gov

Background

Colorectal cancer (CRC) is the leading cause of death in the United States, with an estimated diagnosis of approximately 140,000 cases per year [1]. Approximately 10–30 % of patients with CRC have a positive family history [2]. The majority of these inherited CRC are accounted by two syndromes, Lynch syndrome and familial adenomatous polyposis (FAP). Lynch syndrome accounts for approximately 2–3 % of all CRC cases. Next most common is FAP, which accounts for 1 % of CRC cases [3] (Fig. 20.1). In addition, attenuated FAP (aFAP) and MUTYH-associated polyposis (MAP) are being seen with more frequency. This chapter will also focus on two additional less common polyposis syndromes, Peutz–Jeghers syndrome (PJS) and juvenile polyposis syndrome (JPS).

Lynch Syndrome

The most common form of heritable CRC is Lynch syndrome, which accounts for 1–3 % of all cases of CRC [4, 5]. It is inherited in an

Q.D. Chu et al. (eds.), *Surgical Oncology: A Practical and Comprehensive Approach*,
DOI 10.1007/978-1-4939-1423-4_20, © Springer Science+Business Media New York 2015

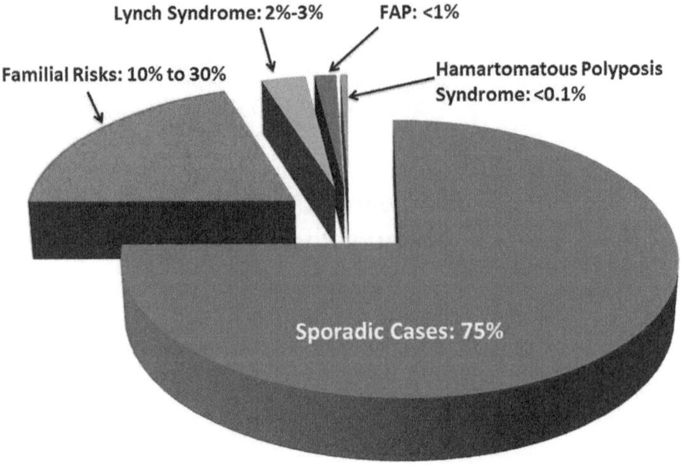

Fig. 20.1 Distribution of colorectal cancer cases (Courtesy of Quyen D. Chu, MD, MBA, FACS)

autosomal-dominant fashion. Lifetime risk of CRC in Lynch syndrome is approximately 10–69 % depending on gender and mismatch repair gene mutations [6–8]. Lynch syndrome is used in preference to hereditary nonpolyposis colorectal cancer (HNPCC) given that polyps can occur, and it involves a group of extracolonic cancer types.

Genetics

Lynch syndrome is characterized by a mutation in one of the DNA mismatch repair (MMR) genes – MLH1, MSH2, MSH6, and PMS2 (Fig. 20.2). These genetic mutations lead to errors in the number of repetitive sequences replicated, causing microsatellite instability (MSI). The errors that occur during DNA replication are not efficiently repaired, causing mutant changes and subsequent unrestrained growth that leads to adenoma and then to carcinoma. MSI occur in approximately 90–95 % of cancers in Lynch syndrome due to uncorrected errors in DNA replication [3].

In a report published by the International Collaborative Group on HNPCC, 63 % of total mutations reported in Lynch patients were MLH1 mutations, 25 % were MSH2 mutations, 6 % were MSH6 mutations, and 0.4 % were PMS2 mutations [3]. No clear genotype–phenotype relationship has been established except in Lynch patients that present with endometrial cancer, which is most commonly associated with MSH6 mutations [3]. However, patients with mutations in the other MMR genes can develop endometrial cancer.

Sometimes, patients will display mutations in mismatch repair proteins or high microsatellite instability (MSI-H) without evidence of germline mutations. This can be due to current technology that cannot identify the mutations. Also, deletions in epithelial cell adhesion molecule gene (*EpCAM*), also known as TACSTD1, located just upstream of MSH2 can account for Lynch syndrome [9]. This mutation leads to hypermethylation of MSH2 that can ultimately lead to an *EpCAM–MSH2* fusion protein that can cause aberrant protein transcription. This is responsible for the Lynch phenotype in 6–19 % of families without MMR gene mutation [10].

Clinical Evaluation

A detailed family history of at least three generations should be obtained in all patients being evaluated for Lynch syndrome. Clinical criteria such as the Amsterdam I and II were developed to identify high-risk families to aid in the discovery of the MMR genes. These criteria are useful and are still being used to identify Lynch syndrome kindreds. Lynch syndrome is suspected in those that fit the Amsterdam II criteria [11]. This criteria requires that at least three relatives, of which

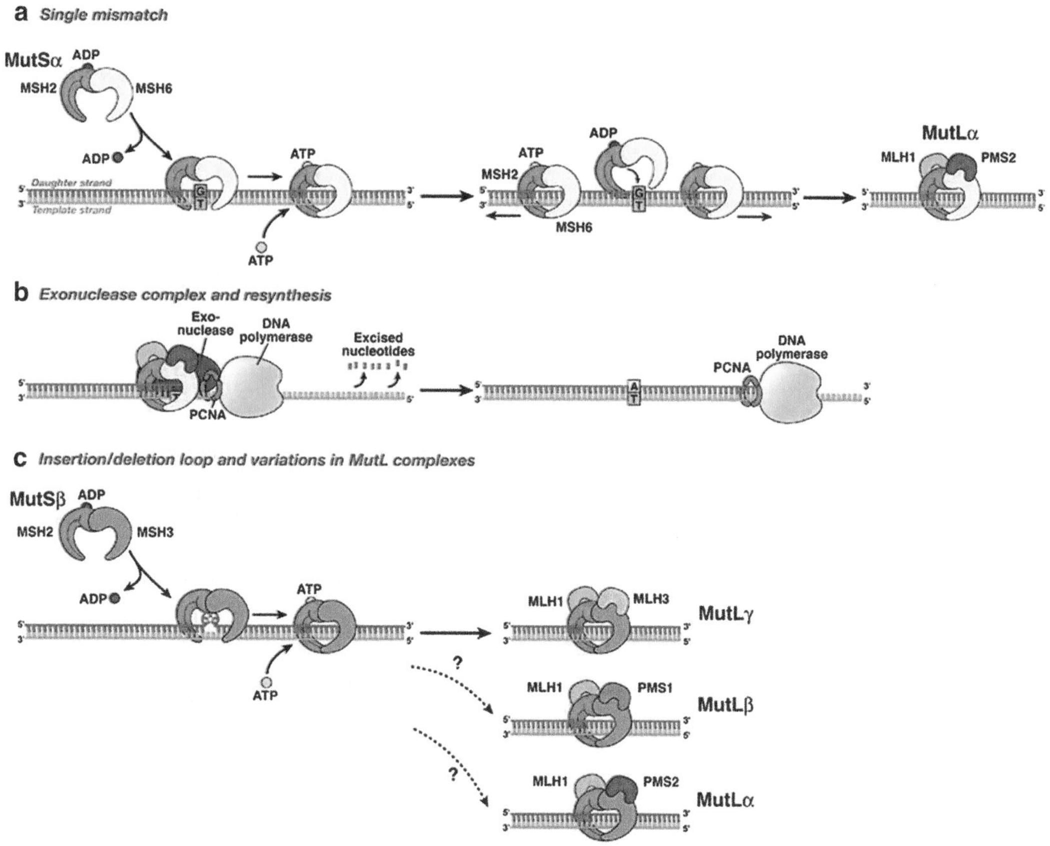

Fig. 20.2 The DNA MMR system functions through a series of steps. (**a**) MSH2–MSH6 (MutSα) recognizes single base-pair mismatches, in which the DNA polymerase has matched the wrong base (G) with the T on the template (shown on *left*), and creates a sliding clamp around the DNA. This step that requires the exchange of adenosine triphosphate (ATP) for adenosine diphosphate (ADP) (by MSH2, but not MSH6 or MSH3). The complex diffuses away from the mismatch site, which is then bound by the MLH1–PMS2 (MutLα) complex (*right*). This "matchmaker" complex moves along the new DNA chain until it encounters the DNA polymerase complex. (**b**) The DNA MMR protein sliding clamp interacts with exonuclease-1, proliferating cell nuclear antigen (PCNA), and DNA polymerase. This complex excises the daughter strand back to the site of the mismatch (shown on *left*). Eventually, the complex falls off the DNA and resynthesis occurs, correcting the error. (**c**) Variations on the DNA MMR theme. Whereas MSH2–MSH6 recognizes single-pair mismatches and small IDLs, MSH2–MSH3 (MutSα) complements this by also recognizing larger IDLs (shown on *left*). The right side shows the possible interactions with different MutL dimers, as MLH1 can dimerize with PMS2, PMS1, or MLH3. The preferred interaction with MSH2–MSH3 is MLH1–MLH3 (MutLα), but the precise roles of the other MutL heterodimers in this reaction are not entirely understood (Reprinted from Ref. [128]. With permission from W.B. Saunders Co.)

one must be a first-degree relative of the other two, have a diagnosis of some cancers associated with Lynch syndrome (CRC, endometrial, ureter/renal pelvis, small bowel), that at least two successive generations be affected, that at least one relative had a diagnosis of cancer associated with Lynch syndrome before the age of 50, and where FAP has been excluded. The Bethesda guidelines [12] linked the diagnostic criteria of Lynch syndrome to the presence of microsatellite instability (Table 20.1). However, with the advent of molecular technologies such as polymerase chain reaction (PCR) and immunohistochemistry for MMR gene protein expression in colorectal tumors (and in some cases extracolonic tumors), neoplasms can be screened for mismatch repair deficiency (and proficiency) thus identifying individuals that would be missed if only clinical

Table 20.1 Amsterdam II criteria/Bethesda guidelines

Greater than 3 relatives with Lynch/HNPCC-associated cancer and
1. One should be a first-degree relative of the other two
2. At least two successive generations should be affected
3. At least one diagnosed before the age of 50
4. FAP should be ruled out
5. Tumors verified by pathological examination
Tumors should be tested for microsatellite instability in following situations:
1. Colorectal cancer under age of 50
2. Presence of synchronous, metachronous colorectal, or other HNPCC-related cancers
3. Colorectal cancer with high microsatellite instability histology diagnosed in patients below age of 60
4. Colorectal cancer diagnosed in patient with one or more first-degree relatives with an HNPCC-related tumor confirmed under age of 50
5. Colorectal cancer diagnosed in patient with two or more first-degree relatives with an HNPCC-related tumor confirmed at any age

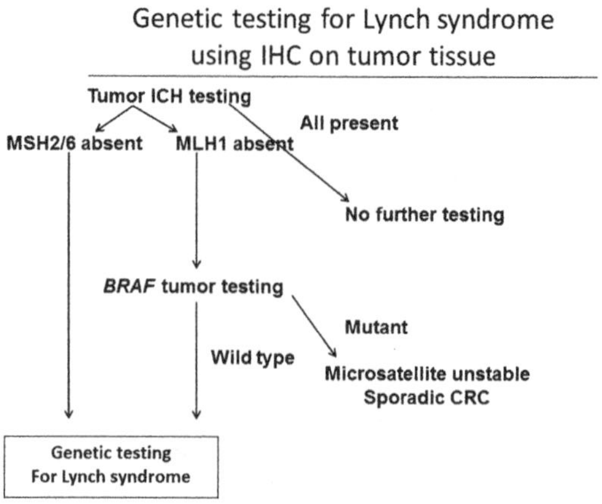

Fig. 20.3 Algorithm for genetic testing for Lynch syndrome. CRCs are tested via immunohistochemistry first for presence or absence of DNA mismatch repair proteins. If all proteins are present, then Lynch syndrome is ruled out. If MLH1 is absent, then the tumor is analyzed for BRAF mutations. If BRAF protein is present in its original state or if MSH 2 or 6 is absent, then the patient is tested genetically for Lynch syndrome. If BRAF protein is present as a mutant state, then CRC is likely a sporadic tumor due to microsatellite instability (Reprinted from Ref. [129]. With permission from Nature Publishing Group)

criteria were used for guidance in identifying Lynch syndrome patients.

Extracolonic cancers include endometrial, gastric, urinary tract, pancreas, biliary tract, brain, sebaceous gland adenomas, keratoacanthomas in Muir–Torre syndrome, carcinoma of the small bowel, and ovarian neoplasias [13, 14].

Muir–Torre variant of Lynch syndrome is associated with dermatologic manifestations such as sebaceous adenomas and carcinomas, keratoacanthomas, and basal carcinomas with sebaceous differentiation in addition to the other Lynch-associated tumors [15].

Surveillance

Those patients that meet the Bethesda guidelines should be offered screening by MSI testing or by immunohistochemistry to look for loss of MMR protein expression. However, the Bethesda guidelines were sensitive but not specific enough. There has been a move toward universal testing of colorectal tumors because it will help identify patients with Lynch syndrome as well as the status of the mismatch repair (either proficient or deficient) [16]. A more selective approach for testing colorectal cancers has been recommended by Moreira et al. and the Epicolon consortium [17]. These authors recommend testing all CRC diagnosed at age 70 or less and in older patients who fulfill the revised Bethesda guidelines. Using this approach, 4.9 % of Lynch syndrome cases were missed, but 34.8 % fewer cases required tumor MMR testing and 28.6 % fewer patients underwent germline mutation testing compared to a universal approach to all colorectal tumors [17]. It must be emphasized that tumors that show loss of protein expression of MLH 1 should undergo BRAF mutation and/or methylation testing of the promoter of MLH1. BRAF mutations are demonstrated in high levels in sporadic MSI CRC and rarely in Lynch syndrome CRC [18] (Fig. 20.3). Those patients whose tumors display loss of MSH2 protein are considered to have Lynch syndrome either secondary to the mutation in MSH2 or less commonly a mutation in EpCAM causing epigenetic silencing of MSH2. Less commonly isolated loss of either PMS2 and MSH6 will be noted directing the clinician to test for germline mutations in these genes. Most commonly loss of MSH6 is accompanied by loss of MSH2 and loss of PMS2 by loss of MLH1.

Annual full colonoscopy starting at age 20–25 is recommended for those with diagnosis of Lynch syndrome[3]. Strong clinical evidence suggests more rapid transition from adenoma to carcinoma in those with Lynch syndrome, thus a more frequent endoscopic surveillance than for the general population is warranted. Colonoscopic surveillance in Lynch syndrome has been shown to decrease CRC incidence and decrease mortality from CRC [19].

Some literature advocates for annual transvaginal ultrasonography, measurement of CA 125 levels and annual endometrial aspiration for affected females starting at age 25–35 [20]. In those patients with Lynch syndrome and family history of gastric cancer, annual EGD is recommended. Ultrasonography and urine cytology can be considered annually or every other year to screen for urinary tract malignancy. Data for these screening tools to decrease mortality is limited at best.

Surgical Treatment

Due to a high lifetime risk of CRC, prophylactic surgical options should be presented to patients diagnosed with Lynch syndrome. However, if the colon is normal in appearance on colonoscopic exam, surgery is not recommended unless there are extenuating circumstances. The options of treatment in Lynch syndrome include total abdominal colectomy with ileorectal anastomosis (IRA) with yearly flexible sigmoidoscopy in those with normal rectal and anal sphincter function or segmental colectomy with yearly colonoscopy. To date, there have been no prospective or retrospective studies demonstrating a survival improvement in patients undergoing a total abdominal colectomy versus a segmental colectomy. What has been demonstrated is a decrease in metachronous colorectal cancer and abdominal procedures related to CRC in patients undergoing more extensive procedures [21, 22]. In the study by Parry et al., the risk of metachronous CTC after a segmental colectomy was 16 %, 41 %, and 62 % at 10, 20, and 30 years after segmental resection in MMR mutation carriers, respectively. Careful surveillance should also be advocated for those that opt for IRA, since the risk of metachronous rectal cancer after total colectomy was reported to be approximately 12 % at 10–12 years [23]. Because of the risk of metachronous CRC, most recommend a total abdominal colectomy at the time of diagnosis of colon cancer in Lynch syndrome. If the index cancer is in the rectum, the alternatives include segmental resection versus restorative proctocolectomy with ileal pouch-anal anastomosis (IPAA) if the sphincters are not involved. Similar to the colon, there is an increased incidence of metachronous colon cancer in patients undergoing segmental rectal resection. These have been reported to be 19%, 47% and 69% at 10, 20, and 30 years post-segmental rectal resection in mutation carriers [24].

Extracolonic Manifestations

Endometrial cancer risk has been reported to be from 15 % to 71 % in MMR gene carriers [6–9, 25]. Endometrial cancer can be the index cancer in a Lynch syndrome patient. Similar to CRC, the age of presentation is younger than the general populations. There is retrospective data reported where females who underwent prophylactic hysterectomy and salpingo-oophorectomy did not develop endometrial or ovarian cancer. In those that did not have the prophylactic procedure, 61 out of 315 females developed cancer [26]. In patients who have completed their families or are postmenopausal, discussion about prophylactic hysterectomy and salpingo-oophorectomy should be entertained, especially at the time of colectomy for CRC.

Other extracolonic manifestations associated with Lynch syndrome include gastric, urinary tract, pancreatic, biliary, brain cancers, sebaceous glands, and keratoacanthomas. There has been a suggestion that both prostate and breast cancer are part of the tumor spectrum of Lynch syndrome, but because these tumors are so common in the general population, there is still controversy about their link to Lynch syndrome [24].

Familial Adenomatous Polyposis

Familial adenomatous polyposis (FAP) is the second most common inherited colon cancer, affecting approximately 1 in 10,000 individuals and accounting for approximately 1 % of all colon cancers [27]. It is inherited in an autosomal-dominant fashion with nearly 100 % penetrance. Those affected are at nearly 100 % risk of CRC by the age of 60 [3].

Genetics

Adenomatous polyposis coli (APC) gene is a tumor suppressor gene that spans 108 kb of DNA on chromosome 5q21. The gene encodes a protein that negatively regulates the β-catenin oncoprotein. In the absence of the APC gene, the β-catenin protein interacts with various transcription factors as it accumulates in the nucleus to upregulate genes that propagate the cell cycle progression [28]. Germline mutations include deletions, insertions, nonsense, and missense mutations. Overall, it is predicted that a mutant truncated APC protein is produced as a consequence of these mutations in as much as 92 % of the cases [29] (Fig. 20.4).

Majority of the germline mutations are clustered in the 5′ portion of exon 15. Miyoshi and colleagues reported that 40 % of all mutations occurred in five specific codons (302, 625, 1061, 1309, and 1546), and 65 % of somatic mutations and 23 % of germline mutations in FAP patients occurred between codons 1286 and 1513 in exon 15 [30]. Genotype–phenotype correlation studies have demonstrated that severe polyposis in FAP patients usually have mutations between codons 1250 and 1464. Correlation between severe FAP and earlier age of onset (defined as symptoms in teen years, cancer before 30), higher number of polyps, and higher mean of diagnosis and death were seen in those with codon 1309 mutations and those more downstream [31–33]. However, subsequent studies have shown more heterogeneity and variability between and within family members with FAP and codon 1309 mutations, showing that a specific APC mutation was not the only determinant of phenotype [34].

Clinical Evaluation

Classically, FAP is diagnosed in those with greater than 100 adenomatous colorectal polyps. Polyp development is usually evident around puberty.

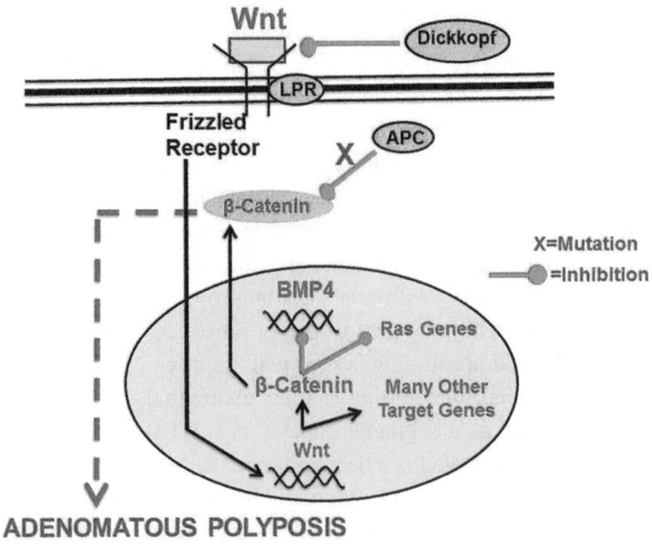

Fig. 20.4 Wnt/β-catenin pathway and adenomatous polyposis. APC (adenomatous polyposis coli) normally targets β-catenin for degradation. In familial adenomatous polyposis and in sporadic adenomatous polyps, mutations in APC are associated with an increase in β-catenin (Reprinted from Ref. [130]. With permission from Springer Verlag)

In a review of a national polyposis registry, median age for development of colorectal adenomatous polyps was 16 years (range 5–38 years), first symptoms from lower GI tract developed by median age of 29 years (range 2–73 years), and development of colorectal carcinoma occurred at a median age of 36 years (range 17–67 years) [3]. Earliest symptoms and signs of lower GI involvement in patients with FAP are blood per rectum, vague abdominal pain, tenesmus, diarrhea and/or constipation, or obstipation.

Polyps develop by age 20 in 75 % of cases and are usually less than 1 cm in size [3]. They may be pedunculated or sessile and may have tubular, villous, or tubulovillous histology. In severe polyposis, thousands may carpet the colorectal epithelium. The risk of invasive cancer is proportional to the severity of polyposis. CRC in the setting of FAP tends to be more commonly located on the left side, unlike CRC in the setting of Lynch syndrome [4].

A number of extracolonic manifestations have been reported in patients with FAP. Those include desmoid tumors, periampullary neoplasms, osteomas, odontomas, supernumerary teeth, fused teeth roots, sebaceous and epidermoid cysts, hepatoblastomas, thyroid tumors, and congenital hypertrophy of the retinal pigmented epithelium (CHRPE).

Surveillance

Patients in whom the diagnosis of FAP is suspected should undergo a complete history, paying particular attention to family history and physical examination with emphasis in areas affected by extracolonic manifestations, including neurologic, ophthalmic, dental, dermatologic, thyroid, abdominal, and digital rectal examinations.

If a mutation is known in the family, then the at-risk individual(s) should be tested for that mutation. In general, genetic testing is not recommended before age 10–12 years. Patients with normal gene study can be dismissed from further screening with a nearly 100 % certainty that any known mutation is absent. These patients should still be counseled to undergo CRC screening starting at age of 50, which is the recommendation for the general population. Surveillance for at-risk family members should begin at 10–12 years of age with a flexible sigmoidoscopy, repeated at 1–2 year intervals. Those that present with adenomatous polyps should undergo a full colonoscopy to determine the extent of polyposis. It is understood that if there are any symptoms prior to the recommended age of surveillance, at-risk individuals should be immediately evaluated at the onset of symptoms.

About 25 % of patients with FAP have no family history of polyposis; therefore, the mutation is de novo [35]. Grover et al. reported the prevalence of germline mutations in the APC gene according to the number of adenomas [36]. The prevalence of APC germline mutation in patients with 10–19 adenomas was 5 %, whereas if there are greater than 1,000 adenomas, it was 80 %.

Treatment

Surgical

Due to the nearly 100 % risk of colorectal cancer, prophylactic surgery has become the standard of care in patients with FAP. The timing of surgical treatment partially depends on the age of the patient, extent of polyposis, symptoms, family history of desmoids, genetic test results (if available), experience of the surgeon, and patient's input. The risk of CRC in FAP patients less than 20 years of age is less than 1 % [37]. If a prophylactic colectomy is to be performed due to severe polyposis, then ideally it should be performed between high school and college. Patients with severe polyposis, severe dysplasia, adenomas greater than 5 mm, and those with severe symptoms that impair quality of life should undergo surgery as soon as possible [38]. Prophylactic colectomy may also be delayed in those with a family history of aggressive desmoids tumors because the risk of desmoids-related complications may outweigh the risk of developing CRC. In females, Ileal pouch anal anastomosis (IPAA) has been associated with decreased fecundity. Therefore, it is also reasonable to delay surgery if deemed safe [39].

The three basic surgical options are: (1) total proctocolectomy (TPC) with permanent ileostomy, (2) total abdominal colectomy with ileorectal anastomosis (IRA), or (3) restorative proctocolectomy (with or without mucosectomy) with ileal pouch-anal anastomosis (IPAA).

TPC with permanent ileostomy is rarely chosen as the first-line option for prophylactic surgery. More commonly, it is considered when sphincter sparing surgery is not feasible due to rectal cancer presenting in the lower third of the rectum, if the patient has poor sphincter function or in the extremely rare situation of a patient presenting with desmoid disease that shortens the small bowel mesentery and not enough length can be technically achieved for an IRA or IPAA. Additionally, the patient's lifestyle has to be taken into consideration.

The choice between IRA and IPAA is more challenging, and considerations for the risk of rectal cancer development and/or differences in functional outcome and quality of life must be taken into account. One of the advantages of an IRA is that it is a one-stage procedure, whereas IPAA, due to the creation of a diverting loop ileostomy to protect the distal anastomosis, is a two-stage procedure (although in expert hands, it can be a one-stage procedure). Besides the increased risk in morbidity that comes from an ileostomy takedown, IPAA has been cited by several studies to have increased rate of complications. Nyam et al. reported a complication rate of 24 % in 187 patients that underwent IPAA for FAP [39]. The most common complication reported was intestinal obstruction in 13 % of the patients. Other complications included wound infection, pelvic infection, urinary tract infection or retention, and sexual dysfunction. Later study by Kartheuser and colleagues reported similar findings, with a complication rate of 27 %. Approximately 15 % experienced small bowel obstruction, and approximately 14 % experienced other complications including pelvic sepsis, fistula formation, necrotizing enterocolitis, and anastomotic stricture (4 %). Impotence and retrograde ejaculation reported after IPAA has only been 1–3 %. More commonly seen is dyspareunia in females and stool leakage during intercourse [40].

A disadvantage with IRA is its association with rectal cancer risk. According to various studies, the risk of developing rectal cancer following IRA in patients with FAP is between 4 and 14 % after 10 years and 9 to 32 % after 20 years [41–45]. It is important to note that in some of these studies, figures were derived when only IRA was available even in the setting of more extensive rectal disease. Also clear documentation of the length of the rectal stump in some series was not provided. Therefore, rectal cancer occurrence after IRA may be overestimated. Iwama et al. noted that 3 % of patients with rectal stump shorter than or equal to 7 cm developed rectal cancer after IRA as opposed to 17 % in those with rectal stump longer than 7 cm [44].

The risk of developing rectal cancer after primary prophylactic surgery may be estimated on the basis of a specific location on the APC mutation. Those that had mutations downstream of codon 1250 had threefold higher incidence of rectal cancer than those with a mutation upstream of 1250 [46]. In another study, those that had an APC mutation between codons 1250 and 1464 were 6.2 times more likely to develop rectal cancer than those with mutations upstream of 1250 or downstream of 1464 [47]. Nevertheless, having APC mutations at other sites will not preclude potential rectal cancer after an IRA.

Furthermore, in a genotype–phenotype study, the cumulative risk of needing a secondary proctectomy within 20 years after IRA and the cumulative risk of developing rectal cancer were compared based on the location of the APC mutation. In the attenuated phenotype (discussed in separate section below) group, which correlated with codons 1–157, 312–412, and 1596–2843, the risks were 10 % and 3.7 %, respectively. In the intermediate phenotype group, correlating with codons 158–311, 413–1249, and 1465–1595, the risks were 39 % and 9.3 %, respectively. In the severe phenotype group, correlating with codons 1250–1464, the risks were 61 % and 8.3 %, respectively [48]. Church et al. correlated the number of rectal polyps at the time of prophylactic IRA with subsequent need for secondary proctectomy [49]. None of the patients with less than five rectal adenomas and less than 1,000 adenomas in the colon had to undergo proctectomy. Patients who had 5–20 rectal adenomas had a 13 % chance of subsequent proctectomy. Those with greater than 20 adenomas had a 54 % chance of subsequent proctectomy.

Patients that develop rectal cancer after IRA may undergo completion proctectomy. The rate of this procedure ranges from 36.6 % to 74 %. The 5-year survival rate following metachronous rectal cancer in FAP patients who had undergone IRA originally ranges from 60 % to 78 % [3]. Other factors that also influenced this rate were stage of the tumor, comorbidities, and performance status of the patient.

The risk of developing polyps and subsequent cancer is not limited to IRA. One report found the risk of developing polyps in the ileal pouch in patients who had undergone IPAA to be 7 % at 5 years, 35 % at 10 years, and 75 % at 15 years [50]. Another study reported a higher incidence of neoplasia occurring at the site of anastomosis in FAP patients who had undergone IPAA after staple use (31 %) versus those that received a hand-sewn anastomosis with anal mucosectomy (10 %).

In terms of bowel function and quality of life, stool frequency ranged from 4.5 to 5 after IPAA compared to 3–4 after IRA. Normal continence was reported in 60–87 % in patients after IPAA compared to 72–83 % after IRA [51, 52]. Night defecation was significantly less in the IRA group, although fecal urgency was reduced in the IPAA patients. Reoperation rate is higher in the IPAA group. No significant difference was shown in terms of sexual dysfunction, dietary restriction, or postoperative complications [53].

Regardless of the procedure, endoscopic surveillance is recommended at intervals of 6 months to 1 year, either to examine the rectal stump (in the case of IRA) or the ileal pouch (in the case of IPAA). After IRA, small adenomas less than 5 mm can be safely observed with biopsies taken. If adenomas increase in number, endoscopic surveillance should occur more frequently. Any polyps larger than 5 mm should be removed and examined by histology. Any development of dysplasia or a villous adenoma larger than 1 cm may be an indication for proctectomy if it cannot be addressed endoscopically. Chemoprevention is discussed in a separate section below.

Extracolonic Manifestations

Desmoid tumors are histologically collagen abundant, spindle cell populated benign tumors arising from fibroaponeurotic tissues. They are usually referred to as benign without metastatic potential but can be locally invasive with ill-defined margins[3]. The prevalence of desmoid tumors in FAP has been estimated to be as high as 38 % [54]. Desmoid tumors occur in approximately 10 % of FAP patients. One study estimated the cumulative risk of 21 % for patients with FAP to develop a desmoid tumor by age 60 [55]. Desmoid tumors are associated with high morbidity and can be the cause of death in 10–23 % of FAP patients [54]. A high proportion of desmoid tumors develop after colonic resection in FAP patients [46]. Patients that have had total colectomy with IRA more frequently developed intra-abdominal desmoids compared to those that of IPAA [56], and due to mesenteric shortening, IPAA may be technically impossible for patients needing a completion proctectomy after an initial IRA [37]. Females of reproductive age seem to be more prone to developing intra-abdominal desmoids [29], possibly due to the expression of estrogen receptors that have been shown in some desmoid tumors [57].

Pharmacological intervention has been used to treat desmoid diseases. NSAID therapy such as sulindac and indomethacin has shown to show partial to complete regression in small, non-randomized studies [58]. However, it is associated with significant side effects and delayed response. Hormonal agents such as tamoxifen have also shown variable partial or complete regression of desmoid tumors [59]. Either NSAIDs or hormonal agents are viable first-line options to treat clinically inert desmoid tumors. For fast-growing tumors or those unresponsive to NSAID or hormonal agents, cytotoxic agents such as doxorubicin and dacarbazine can achieve some degree of response [58–60]. There is no definite effective

Table 20.2 Desmoid tumor staging system

Stages	
I	Asymptomatic, less than 10 cm maximum diameter and not growing
II	Mildly symptomatic, less than 10 cm maximum diameter and not growing
III	Moderately symptomatic or bowel/ureteric obstruction or 10–20 cm or slowly growing
IV	Severely symptomatic or greater than 20 cm or rapidly growing

treatment for desmoid tumors. Church et al. proposed a classification system for desmoids in FAP patients that can serve as a guide for management of these difficult problems [61] (Table 20.2).

Surgical resection is limited to those that are symptomatic (e.g., from intestinal obstruction) (Fig. 20.5). Unfortunately, resection is associated with a high rate of and more aggressive recurrence.

Duodenal cancer has become the leading cause of death in patients with FAP who have already undergone prophylactic colectomy [60]. Nearly 90 % of patients with FAP will develop duodenal polyps, and 4.5 % will develop duodenal adenocarcinoma in their lifetime [62].

Surveillance by EGD with biopsy of suspicious polyps should begin at age 20 or at the time of prophylactic colectomy, whichever is earlier [57]. Staging for duodenal polyposis can be staged using the Spigelman classification [63] (Table 20.3).

Having no polyps is designated as stage 0. One to four points is classified as stage 1. For these stages, the surveillance should be every 5 years. Five to six points is stage 2, with surveillance recommended every 3 years. Seven to eight points is stage 3 with surveillance recommended every 1–2 years. Nine to twelve points is stage 4, which warrants surgical intervention.

Surgical options include endoscopic ablation and transduodenal excision. Duodenal surgery, specifically pancreas-preserving duodenectomy or pancreaticoduodenectomy, is currently indicated for patients with severe duodenal polyposis (Spigelman IV) or duodenal carcinoma.

Several small-powered studies have investigated the role of sulindac in stabilizing or regressing duodenal polyposis [64, 65]. So far, no significant benefits have been seen. A randomized placebo study using celecoxib showed that there was no significant difference among the groups in number of polyps, although there was significant qualitative improvement in polyposis among those on high-dose celecoxib when the patients' endoscopies were reviewed independently by other physicians [66]. Overall, chemoprevention studies of duodenal polyposis with NSAIDs have been disappointing. One plausible explanation is that because the duodenum expresses higher levels of COX-2 than colon in FAP patients [67], higher dosage of NSAIDS may be needed to suppress polyp burden in the duodenum. However, higher dosages of NSAIDs, especially COX-2 inhibitors, may be limited by the potentially serious cardiovascular side effects.

Other extracolonic manifestations include gastric cancer, osteomas, odontomas, sebaceous and epidermoid cysts, and CHRPE (congenital hypertrophy of the retinal pigment epithelium).

Attenuated Familial Adenomatous Polyposis

A milder form of FAP known as attenuated familial adenomatous polyposis (aFAP) has been defined as less than 100 adenomatous polyps in the colon. Similar to FAP, aFAP is passed onto progeny by autosomal-dominant pattern and is associated with APC gene mutations and upper GI lesions [3]. Historically, aFAP has been reported to be predominantly right sided with rectal sparing, unlike FAP. However, recent studies indicate that adenoma location be uniform throughout the colon, although rectal adenomas are considerably less common than in FAP [68]. Mean age of cancer diagnosis has been reported in the early 50's [69, 70]. Cumulative risk of CRC in patients with aFAP is estimated to be 69 % by the age of 80 [71].

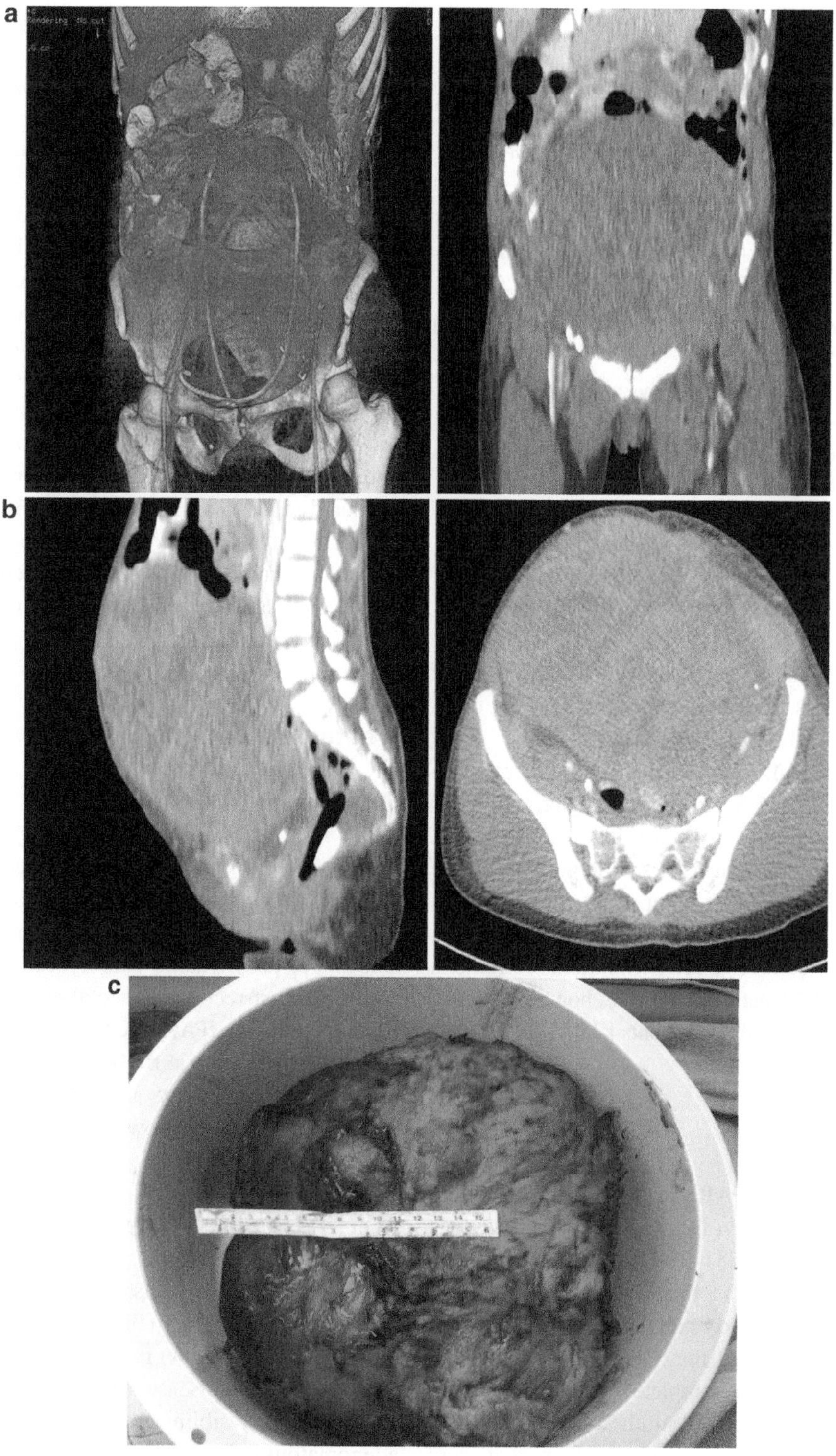

Fig. 20.5 A 24-year old woman with familial adenomatous polyposis presented with small bowel obstruction because of a large abdominal desmoids. She underwent a palliative debulking of her desmoids tumor (Courtesy of Quyen D. Chu, MD, MBA, FACS)

Table 20.3 Spigelman classification

	Points		
	1	2	3
Polyp number	1–4	5–20	Greater than 20
Polyp size (mm)	1–4	5–10	Greater than 10
Histology	Tubular	Tubulovillous	Villous
Dysplasia	Mild	Moderate	Severe

Table 20.4 Clinical diagnostic criteria for attenuated FAP (aFAP)

1. No family members with > 100 adenomas diagnosed before the age of 30 and one of two below
(a) ≥2 patients with 10–99 adenomas at age >30 years
(b) One patient with 10–99 adenomas at age ≥30 years and a first-degree relative with CRC

Clinical Evaluation

The aFAP phenotype occurs in less than 10 % of FAP patients. The clinical criteria [72] for diagnosis is listed in the table (Table 20.4).

Pathologically, adenomas may be either pedunculated or sessile and may have tubular, villous, or tubulovillous histology, much like FAP. However, there is a higher chance of sessile polyps that are seen in aFAP patients compared to FAP patients [71]. Extracolonic manifestation, such as desmoids, osteomas, and periampullary tumors, occurs in aFAP patients. CHRPE, however, has not been reported in aFAP patients [73].

Genetics

Mutations in the aFAP patients tend to be at either the 5′ end or 3′ end of APC gene, usually codons 78–167, codons 1581–2843, and in exon 9 [74]. It is hypothesized that the mutations seen in aFAP may result in a weakly functional protein, whereas other APC mutations may cause more severe phenotypes through a complete dysfunctionality of the transcribed protein. Smith et al. reported that 5′ mutations led to unstable proteins that were ultimately degraded, while 3′ mutations resulted in proteins that formed heterodimers which inhibited tumor suppressor function [75].

Surveillance

In patients with a known APC mutation and a family history of AAPC, initial colonoscopy should begin at age 15. If the study shows findings consistent with FAP, then surgery is warranted. If the polyposis is not severe, endoscopic control with regular polypectomies may be feasible and repeated annually. If no polyps are found and the patient is APC mutation positive, colonoscopy annually starting at 20 is recommended. If the APC mutation status is unknown, colonoscopy every 2 years is sufficient. If no polyps are found and the patient tests negative for the APC mutation, routine colorectal cancer screening can be applied. Individuals with a positive family history but negative APC mutation should have a screening colonoscopy at age 15. If no adenomas are found, they can be followed with a colonoscopy every 2 years starting at age 20 [3].

Treatment

Surgical

In patients with mild adenomas, repeated endoscopic polypectomies may be preferable to surgery. In those where the colonic polyps cannot be controlled, prophylactic surgery can be recommended. Most recommend total colectomy with IRA as oppose to IPAA due to rectal sparing [3]. One study reported a 10 % cumulative risk of secondary proctectomy and 3.7 % cumulative risk of rectal cancer following IRA [48].

MYH-Associated Polyposis

MYH-associated polyposis (MAP) is an autosomal recessive disorder due to biallelic mutations (pertaining to both alleles) in *MYH*, a base excision repair gene. This disease came into light in 2002 when 3 out of 7 siblings presented with multiple adenomatous colorectal polyps and cancer without germline APC mutations [76]. Subsequent APC mutation analysis revealed a result that was characteristic for a defective base excision repair.

Unaffected relatives were heterozygous for MYH mutations or wild type, confirming the autosomal recessive pattern of disease inheritance.

The mean age of diagnosis is late 40's and 50's, similar to aFAP. Approximately 60 % of MAP patients with polyposis have colorectal cancer initially [77]. Synchronous cancers occur in up to 24 % of patients [78]. The estimated cumulative risk of CRC by age 70 in biallelic MYH mutation carriers has been reported to be as high as 80 % [79]. Penetrance of CRC in MAP patients has been shown to be approximately 19 % at age 50 and 43 % by age 60 [80]. Additionally, there is a twofold increase in risk of CRC for heterozygous carriers of MYH mutations compared to the general population [81].

Genetics

The MUTYH gene, located on chromosome locus 1p34.3–p32.1, is a base excision repair gene that codes for a glycosylase protein [82]. This protein is involved in repairing guanine residues that have undergone oxidative damage. Over 105 mutations have been identified for the MUTYH gene, majority of them being missense mutations. In the western population and in the northern European descent, the most common mutations within the MUTYH gene are the Y179C and the G396D mutations, with reports of approximately 90 % of the MAP patients carrying at least one of these mutations. Different mutations in patients of Indian (E480X), Pakistani (Y90X), southern European (1395 del GGA), and Portuguese (1186–1187 insertion GG) descent have been reported.

Clinical Evaluation

Most patients with biallelic MUTYH mutations present with between 10 and a few hundred polyps. There is a slight propensity for CRC to arise proximal to the splenic flexure [83]. Phenotypic presentation for MAP patients with biallelic G396D mutations was less severe than for Y179C mutation patients [77].

Extracolonic lesions associated with MUTYH mutations include small bowel polyposis, specifically duodenal polyposis, gastric cancer, endometrial cancer, breast cancer, and low to moderate risks in skin, ovarian, and bladder cancers [82]. Very rarely, MAP patients have developed sebaceous gland tumors [84].

Surveillance

Current recommendation [85] is to begin colonoscopic surveillance for MAP patients by age 18–20 to be repeated every 2 years. If polyposis is mild, patients can be followed with polypectomy. When the polyposis becomes severe, surgery is indicated.

Upper gastrointestinal tract screening is advised to begin at the age of 25–30. Recommended screening interval is determined by the Spigelman classification (see FAP section).

Treatment

Polyposis can be controlled with endoscopic polypectomies. Surgical intervention depends on rectum involvement. If rectum is not involved, TAC/IRA is recommended. If rectum is involved, total proctocolectomy with IPAA is recommended. Postsurgically, yearly surveillance with endoscopy is warranted.

Peutz–Jeghers Syndrome

Peutz–Jeghers syndrome (PJS) is an autosomal-dominant disorder with variable penetrance characterized by mucocutaneous melanotic macules and intestinal hamartomatous polyps. Although dysplastic and carcinomatous changes in hamartomas are low (approximately 1 %), malignant transformations are found in PJS patients due to their high polyp burden, especially in the intestines. Incidence of disease varies, ranging from 1 in 8,500 to 1 in 200,000 depending on various reports in the literature [86], showing that the true incidence remains unclear.

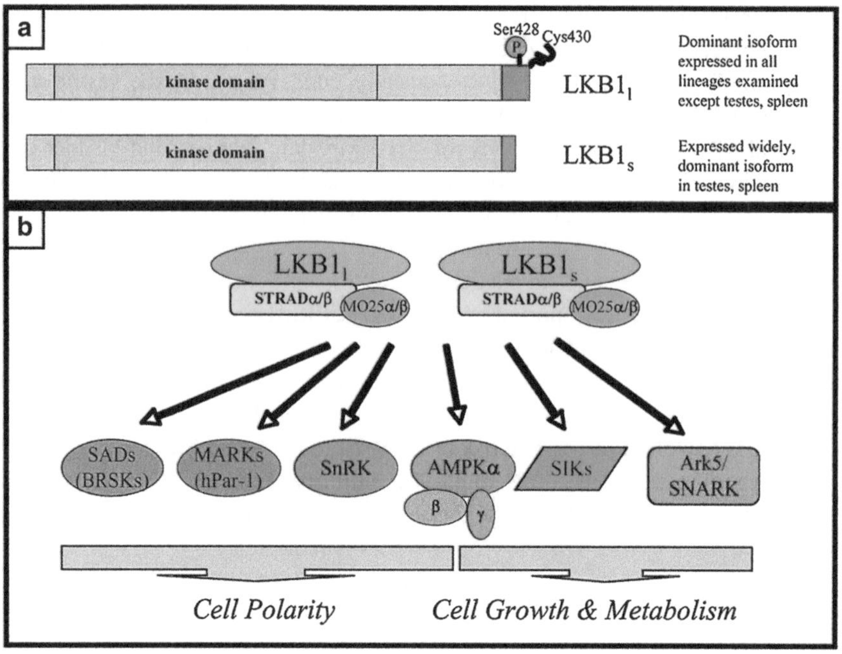

Fig. 20.6 LKB1 is a serine/threonine kinase which complexes with STRAD to phosphorylate downstream kinases in the AMP-activated protein kinase family (AMPK) (Reprinted from Ref. [131]. With permission from Portland Press Limited)

Lifetime risk of small bowel cancer risk for patients with PJS has been estimated to be approximately 57 % [87]. Cumulative risk of colonic or extracolonic cancer is 85–93 % by age 70 in PJS patients [87, 88].

Genetics

PJS is caused by a mutation in the LKB1 gene, located on the telomeric region of chromosome 19p13.3. LKB1 is a serine/threonine kinase which complexes with STE-20-related adaptor (STRAD) and mouse protein 25 (MO25) to phosphorylate and mediate downstream cell signaling cascade [89]. It is the only known tumor suppressor kinase. The Human Genome Organization designated the name serine/threonine kinase 11 (STK11) for LKB1. It is the only gene whose mutation is associated with PJS. It can be found in approximately 75 % of PJS patients [86] (Fig. 20.6).

For those without detectable LKB1 mutation, possibilities include large rearrangements of the LKB1 gene due to deletions, duplications or inversions, mutations to the LKB1 promoter, or the existence of additional PJS loci that is yet to be discovered. Thus far, no additional mutations have been found [86].

Gene sequencing is used for genetic screening. Those that come back with a negative result may opt for a multiplex ligation-dependent probe amplification (MLPA). Reported accuracy for genetic testing in at-risk individuals with established family mutations is 95 % [90]. Due to the high false-negative rate, a clinical diagnosis of PJS stands even when the genetic testing is negative. Genetic testing can also be difficult to coordinate due to a limited number of laboratories offering the test and the cost.

Clinical Evaluation

Mucocutaneous melanin pigmentation on or around the lips generally appear by the end of the first year of life and are almost always present by the age of 5 [91]. They can also be seen in the buccal mucosa, periorbital or periaural area, dorsal surface of fingers or toes, and around the anus and genitalia. By puberty and adulthood, these skin pigmentations can disappear so the absence of these lesions in adults does not rule out PJS. They are usually macules 1–5 mm in diameter and vary in color from light brown to black.

Gastrointestinal polyps can occur anywhere in the GI tract, with jejunum being the most common location. Other common locations include the ileum, colon, rectum, stomach, duodenum, appendix, and esophagus [92]. Polyp numbers can vary, from only a handful to thousands.

The majority of PJS patients initially present with small bowel obstruction secondary to intussusception of hamartomas. Most present between the ages of 6 and 18 [93]. Symptoms include abdominal pain, nausea, vomiting, and bloody stool. CT scan is the imaging choice for diagnosis.

According to the guidelines from Mayo Clinic [86], in patients without a family history of PJS, if either of the following two is present, a diagnosis of PJS can be made:

1. Characteristic mucocutaneous melanotic macules and one or more intestinal polyps with PJS-type histology
2. Two intestinal polyps with PJS-type histology

In patients with a family history of PJS in a parent or sibling, if any of the following are present, a diagnosis of PJS can be made:

1. Characteristic melanotic macules
2. One intestinal polyp with PJS-type histology
3. An *LKB1* mutation

Histologically, the polyps seen in PJS are disorganized hamartomas characterized by hypertrophy or hyperplasia of smooth muscle in the muscularis mucosa. Unique to PJS-type polyps, smooth muscle cells arborize into the superficial epithelial layer. Sometimes the epithelium can invade and be entrapped in the smooth muscle layer, termed pseudo-invasion [86]. This can be mistaken for malignant invasion and can be misdiagnosed as cancer. Therefore, to diagnose a malignancy in PJS polyps, cellular atypia or increased mitotic rate must be seen [94]. In a past review, 10 % of PJS-type polyp specimen examined under microscopy had pseudo-invasion.

Patients with PJS are at increased risk of developing both intestinal and extraintestinal malignancies. One study reported a 15.2 relative risk for PJS patients for all cancers, with statistically increased risk for developing cancer in the esophagus, stomach, small intestines, colon, pancreas, lung, breast, uterus, and ovary [88]. Another study reported an association of PJS and nasal polyposis [91]. Nasopharyngeal carcinoma has also been reported in PJS patients [95]. Gallbladder polyps, gallbladder cancer, and bile duct cancer have also manifested in PJS patients [96–98]. Rarely, hamartomatous polyps have been reported in the ureter [99] and respiratory tract [100] in PJS patients. Finally, several rare cancers have a special association with PJS. In female PJS patients, a highly differentiated adenocarcinoma of the cervix can develop called adenoma malignum (ADM). Special sex cord tumor with annular tubules (SCTAT) can also develop in the ovaries. In males, the corresponding sex cord tumor is the Sertoli cell testicular tumors[83].

Surveillance

Riegert-Johnson et al. outlined the surveillance protocol from two institutions, Johns Hopkins Hospital and Mayo Clinic [86]. Both institutions recommend breast self-examination at age 18 with clinical semiannual examination and optional annual mammography annually starting at age 25, endoscopy surveys for stomach and small intestines every 1–8 years starting at age 8, and colonic endoscopic examination every 2–3 years starting at age 18. Johns Hopkins recommends surveillance of pancreas (with endoscopic ultrasound, CT or MR, and/or CA 19–9 as options) and female reproductive organs (ultrasound, serum CA-125, Pap smear) at age 25 and repeated annually, whereas Mayo Clinic recommends these examinations to start at age 18. Clinical examination with ultrasound adjunct for testicular screening should begin at birth and offered annually until age 12.

Treatment

Surgical

Polyps greater than 1–1.5 cm in size should be removed [86]. The polyps should be removed by extended upper endoscopy if accessible. If not, double-balloon endoscopy (DBE) can be considered. If the polyps cannot be removed by DBE, then surgical intervention should be considered. Options are laparoscopic-assisted endoscopic polypectomy versus an open procedure with intraoperative endoscopy and polypectomy. In patients where polyps are too large to remove endoscopically, polyps are incompletely removed, or polyp-associated complications arise such as intussusception, surgery can be warranted.

If a patient presents with intussusception, the treatment is surgical, not endoscopic management. The approach depends on location, timing of extend of intussusception, and associated inflammation, bowel edema, and any degree of ischemia. Most common intussusception in PJS patients are jejunum telescoping into another segment of jejunum, and the recommended surgical technique is reduction, enterotomy, and polyp resection. In the rare case where the polyp is suspected to be malignant, enterotomy should be made first prior to reduction to prevent dissemination of cancer. Intraoperative endoscopy is an option after to inspect and remove other polyps. Another option is to prolapse the small intestine through the enterotomy incision so that the mucosa near the incision can be inspected for the presence of polyps [86].

Prophylactic colectomy in patients at risk is unclear at this time. Due to the unclear risk of CRC in PJS patients and the limited availability of genetic testing, no consensus exists at this time for prophylactic surgery.

Juvenile Polyposis Syndrome

Juvenile polyposis syndrome (JPS) is a rare autosomal-dominant syndrome. It is characterized by multiple distinct juvenile polyps throughout the GI tract as well as multiple extracolonic manifestations. The cumulative lifetime risk of colorectal cancer is 39 % [101]. This syndrome is defined by the presence of greater than 5 juvenile polyps in the colorectum, juvenile polyps throughout the GI tract, or any number of juvenile polyps plus a positive family history.

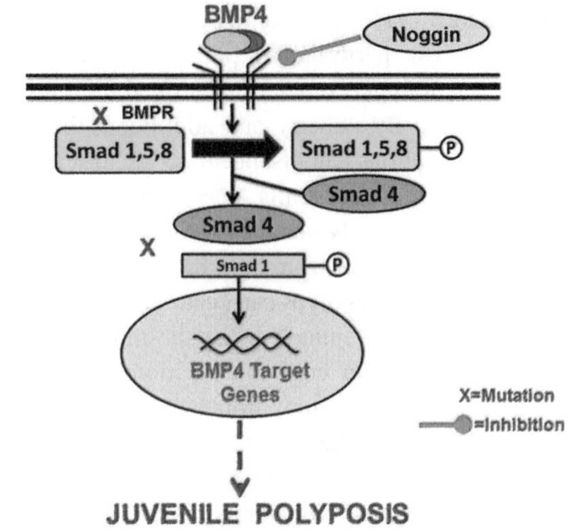

Fig. 20.7 BMP4–BMPR–Smad pathway and juvenile polyposis. Mutation of the BMP receptor 1A, introduction of Noggin, which inhibits BMP4 receptor binding, and mutation of Smad4 can suppress expression of BMP4 target genes. These interruptions of BMP4 signaling are associated with development of juvenile polyposis syndrome and related predisposition to juvenile polyps (Reprinted from Ref. [130]. With permission from Springer Verlag)

Genetics

JPS is associated with a germline mutation, usually a point mutation or small base-pair deletion, in the SMAD4 gene in chromosome 18q21.1 or BMPR1A gene on chromosome 10q22–q23 [91]. These mutations are found in about 50–60 % of JPS patients [102]. Both of these genes are involved in the bone morphogenetic protein (BMP)/transforming growth factor (TGF)-beta signaling pathway (Fig. 20.7). About 15 % of these defects are large deletions, necessitating the use of techniques such as multiplex ligation-dependent probe amplification (MLPA) for identification [103]. Upper GI polyposis and gastric cancer have been associated with SMAD4 germline mutation [104].

Clinical Evaluation

The clinical presentation of JPS can be divided into two main variants [101]. The first is called juvenile polyposis of infancy. This is a nonsex-linked recessive condition characterized by failure to thrive, diarrhea, protein-losing enteropathy, bleeding, intussusception, rectal prolapse, and congenital abnormalities including macrocephaly and generalized hypotonia. Polyps generally are 1 mm–3 cm, sessile or pedunculated, and occur in stomach, small bowel, or colon. Death usually occurs before the age of 2. The second form, termed generalized juvenile polyposis or juvenile polyposis coli, seems to be different expressions of the same disease. GI juvenile polyps are usually present in the first decade of life or in adulthood, which are at increased risk of cancer. A number of other extraintestinal manifestations may arise. In approximately 50 % of cases, a heterozygous germline mutation in the SMAD4 or BMPR1A gene has been identified [105].

Diagnosis of JPS is made by ruling out other hamartomatous GI polyps and having:

1. Greater than 5 juvenile polyps in the colorectum
2. Juvenile polyps throughout the GI tract
3. Any number of juvenile polyps plus a family history for JPS [106]

Polyps in JPS predominantly occur in the colon and rectum, although they can be found in the stomach and small bowel. Their numbers vary from tens to hundreds. Their size can vary from 5 mm to 5 cm and typically have a spherical, lobulated, and pedunculated appearance with surface erosion. Histology shows an abundance of edematous lamina propria infiltrated with inflammatory cells and cystically dilated mucous-filled glands lined with cuboidal or columnar epithelium with reactive changes.

Extracolonic manifestations of JPS include malrotation of midgut and mesenteric lymphangiomas. Extraintestinal manifestations include hypertrophic pulmonary osteoarthropathy, cleft lip and palate abnormalities, porphyria, congenital cardiac and AV malformation, vitellointestinal duct abnormalities, and renal, uterus, and vaginal abnormalities. Cowden disease, associated with PTEN mutation and characterized by hamartomatous polyposis and is associated with other cancers including thyroid and breast, may be a phenotypic variant of JPS [4].

Surveillance

Patients with JPS or at risk should have endoscopic screening beginning at age 15 or at the time of first symptom. At diagnosis, the entire GI tract should be examined for the presence of polyps. Endoscopic examination of colon and upper GI is recommended every 2–3 years. If the patient has polyps, endoscopic exam should occur yearly until the patient is polyp free [101].

Treatment

Surgery

Patients with mild polyposis can be managed with frequent endoscopy and polypectomy. Prophylactic surgery can be considered in patients with severe polyposis that is unmanageable by endoscopy or with those with unmanageable symptoms. Surgical options include total colectomy with ileorectal anastomosis or proctocolectomy with ileal pouch-anal anastomosis [101]. Due to recurrence of rectal polyps in half of the individuals who require subsequent proctectomy [101], the initial surgery of choice is the IPAA. Patients need frequent yearly surveillance of the rectum or the ileal pouch regardless of the surgery for polyp recurrence [101].

POLE- and POLD1-Associated Polyposis

Recently, germline mutation in POLE and POLD1 has been associated with oligopolyposis inherited in an autosomal-dominant fashion [107, 108].

POLE and POLD1 are DNA polymerases ε and δ which are involved in DNA replication. The syndrome has been referred to as polymerase proofreading-associated polyposis (PPAP). In addition to oligopolyposis, colorectal cancer has been described in affected individuals, and in those with POLD1 mutations, endometrial cancer has also been described. The syndrome is relatively new and still needs to be elucidated.

A summary of all polyposis syndromes discussed above is discussed in Table 20.5.

Chemoprevention

The development of chemopreventive agents follow a standard algorithm for drug development, starting with mechanically based drug screens, preclinical, efficacy tests, toxicology assessments, and an orderly sequence of carefully designed clinical trials. Before proceeding to clinical trials, promising agents are identified and then prioritized on the basis of complementary lines of evidence. The prioritization criteria include efficacy data obtained from in vitro and in vivo animal models and observational studies.

Today, many of these agents fall short, but choosing the correct population to do the trials is crucial, and thus individuals falling into the high-risk category include the FAP and HNPCC. Table 20.6 shows some of the studies and the agents that have been utilized in hereditary colorectal cancer syndrome patients.

This section will focus on studies providing the most compelling evidence for their use in these cohorts.

Efficacy of NSAIDs such as sulindac and its metabolites (sulfide and sulfone), as well as aspirin, has been studied in patients with FAP. NSAIDs inhibit cyclooxygenase (COX), the key enzyme in the formation of prostaglandins and other eicosanoids from arachidonic acid. Prostaglandins have been postulated in having a role in altering cell adhesion, inhibiting apoptosis and promoting angiogenesis [109, 110], all important components that are implicated in transforming tumors from benign to malignant lesions. Subsequent studies have suggested that NSAIDS exert most of their antineoplastic effects via the inhibition of the COX-2 enzyme and inhibition of other biochemical pathways independent of COX suppression [111].

One of the earlier reports of chemopreventive agents in FAP came from Waddell and Loughry who in 1983 reported regression of adenomas in three patients on sulindac after ileorectal anastomosis and on one patient with an intact colon [112]. Others subsequently confirmed the efficacy of sulindac in decreasing the number and size of polyps in patients with FAP. One such study was a randomized, double-blind placebo-controlled study of 22 patients with FAP including 18 who had not undergone colectomy [113]. In this study, sulindac 150 mg twice daily was shown to reduce the size and number of polyps in patients treated compared to placebo. The effect disappeared once the study drug was discontinued. None of the patients had complete disappearance of the polyps. It must be noted that there are reports in the literature where FAP patients who were on sulindac after colectomy went on to develop colorectal adenocarcinoma [114, 115]. If sulindac is to be used, it should be used in conjunction with strict endoscopic surveillance regimen [111].

Giardello et al. also evaluated the effect of sulindac in 41 patients aged 8–25 years with APC germline mutations but not yet phenotypically affected [116]. In this double-blind placebo-controlled trial over a 48-month period, sulindac did not prevent the development of adenomas in individuals with FAP.

Combination therapy has also been looked at using sulindac. In a randomized, double-blind study reported by Meyskens Jr. et al., 375 patients with a history of adenomas greater than 3 mm that were resected were assigned to receive either oral difluoromethylornithine (DFMO) and low-dose sulindac versus placebo (DFMO and sulindac trial) [117]. Follow-up colonoscopy was performed at 3 years looking for colorectal adenoma recurrence. They reported a significant decrease in recurrence of one or more adenomas and a decrease in advanced adenomas in the DFMO plus sulindac group. They reported no statistically significant increase in gastrointestinal,

Table 20.5 Summary table of hereditary polyposis syndromes

Syndrome	Genetic basis	GI manifestation	Surveillance	Extracolonic manifestation	Surgical management
Lynch	DNA mismatch genes MLH1, MSH2, MSH6, PMS2	Right-sided tumor in 60–70 % MSI high tumor	Colonoscopy starting at age 25 or 10 years younger than youngest family history affected Consider transvaginal U/S, CA 125 levels, EGD, and urine cytology	Endometrial, gastric, urinary tract, pancreas, biliary tract, brain, sebaceous gland, keratoacanthomas	TAC/IRA with annual rectal surveillance or segmental colectomy with annual colonoscopy
FAP	APC gene 5q21 in >90 %	>100 adenomatous polyps of colorectum or polyps positive for APC mutation	Sigmoidoscopy at age 10–12 years Consider protein truncation test Upper GI surveillance with EGD at age 20 or time of prophylactic colectomy	Desmoids, periampullary neoplasms, osteomas, odontomas, sebaceous and epidermoid cysts, and CHRPE	Options include TAC with ileostomy, TAC/IRA, or TPC with IPAA
aFAP	APC gene Usually codons 78–167 or 1581–2843	10–99 adenomatous polyps of colorectum or polyps positive for APC mutation	Initial colonoscopy at age 15. If no adenomas, colonoscopy every 2 years starting at age 20	Desmoids, periampullary neoplasms, and osteomas	Options include TAC with ileostomy, TAC/IRA, or TPC with IPAA
MYH-associated polyposis	Biallelic mutation of MYH	MYH mutation in polyp	Colonoscopy at age 18–20. Repeat every 2 years if negative or polyposis mild Upper GI screening at age 25–30	Desmoids, periampullary neoplasms, osteomas, odontomas, sebaceous and epidermoid cysts, and CHRPE	Options include TAC with ileostomy, TAC/IRA, or TPC with IPAA
PJS	LKB1	Hamartomas of GI tract and at least two of the following: Small bowel disease, mucocutaneous melanin pigmentation, or positive family history	Colonoscopy at age 18, then every 2–3 years	Mucocutaneous melanin pigmentation of perioral and buccal areas	Polypectomy If not amenable, segmental bowel resection with intraoperative endoscopy Prophylactic colectomy not recommended at this time
JPS	SMAD4 in gene 18q2 or BMPR1A gene 10q22–23	Greater than 3 juvenile colonic polyps and juvenile polyps anywhere in GI tract or any number of polyps with positive family history	Colonoscopy at age 15 with EGD and SBS. If negative, repeat every 2–3 years	Stomach, pancreas, and duodenum	Polypectomy If disease diffuse, TAC/IRA with rectal surveillance every 1–3 years
POLE- and POLD1-associated polyposis	POLE and POLD1 DNA polymerase mutations	Confirmed germline mutation in POLE and POLD1 in unexplained adenomatous polyposis	Colonoscopy at age 30	Endometrial	Polypectomy. No consensus on prophylactic colectomy

CHRPE Congenital Hypertrophy of the Retinal Pigmented Epithelium, *TAC/IRA* Total Abdominal Colectomy/Ileorectal Anastomosis, *TPC* Total Proctectomy, *IPAA* Ileal Pouch-Anal Anastomosis.

Table 20.6 Hereditary colorectal chemoprevention in colorectal neoplasia: antioxidant micronutrients and NSAIDs

Study	Sample size[a]	Design/cohort[b]	Intervention[c]	Primary results
Labayle et al. [132]	9	DBRCT/phenotypic FAP	Sulindac 100 mg po TID × 4 months	Adenoma number and size reduced*
Giardiello et al. [133, 134]	22	DBRCT/phenotypic FAP	Sulindac 150 mg po BID × 9 months	Adenoma number and size reduced* mucosal prostanoids reduced*d
Nugent et al. [135]	14	DBRCT/phenotypic FAP	Sulindac 200 mg po BID × 6 months	Adenoma burden reduced* proliferative index reduced*
Winde et al. [136]	38	CCTRL/phenotypic FAP	Sulindac 25–150 mg BID × 3–48 months	Adenoma number and size reduced*; proliferative index reduced*; prostonoids reduced
Steinbach et al. [137]	77	DBRCT/phenotypic FAP	Celecoxib 100, 400 mg po BID × 6 months	Focal and global adenoma number and burden reduced* (400 mg BID vs. placebo)
Bussey et al. [138]	49	DBRCT/phenotypic FAP	Vitamin C 3 g/d followed for up to 24 months	Rectal adenoma number reduced(NS)
DeCosse et al. [139]	58	DBRCT/phenotypic FAP	Placebo wheat bran fiber 2.2 g/d versus Vitamin C (4 g/d), Vitamin E (400 mg/d) +/- Wheat bran fiber (22.5 g/d) over a 4 year period	Rectal adenoma number reduced in high fiber supplement group (NS)
Burn et al. [140]	861	DBRCT/HNPCC	HNPCC versus placebo 600 mg ASA qd	44 % reduction of CRC in HNPCC at 5 years. At 2 years, 63 %. No difference in the polyps burden
Ishikawa et al. [141]	34	DBRCT/FAP	ASA 100 mg qd 6–10 months	Reduction in the number and size of polyps
Glebov et al. [142]	**	HNPCC carriers	Celecoxib 200 mg BID versus 400 mg BID for 6 months	Biomarker modulation Pattern of gene expression

*Statistically significant result ($P<0.05$). *NS* nonsignificant
**Not disclosed
[a]Number of subjects evaluated at study completion
[b]*DBRCT* double-blind, randomized, controlled trial, *DBRXT* double-blind, randomized, crossover trial, *CCTRL* case-control, *PBRCT* partially blind, randomized, controlled trial
[c]Duration of agent administration until described effect
[d]One subject with adenocarcinoma on extended follow-up

hematologic, cardiovascular, or cerebrovascular toxicity with sulindac use, although the study was not adequately powered to identify the differences in the two treatment groups. Currently, an NIH-funded randomized double-blind study is in recruitment to determine if the combination of DFMO plus sulindac is superior to sulindac or DFMO alone in delaying the first time occurrence of any FAP pathology.

A metabolite of sulindac, sulindac sulfone (exisulind), has also been investigated in FAP. Burke et al. reported a 25 % decrease in rectal adenomas in patients receiving exisulind compared to placebo [118]. In an open-label extension of the study by Burke et al., Phillips reported that patients who continued treatment with exisulind had a 58 % polyp reduction [119]. Side effects of exisulind include increase in liver enzymes and abdominal pain [120].

COX-2 inhibitors such as rofecoxib and celecoxib have been shown to reduce polyp number and polyp burden in the short term [121, 122]. However, significant side effects, especially cardiovascular adverse effects including myocardial infarction, stroke, and heart failure, limit rofecoxib and to a lesser extent celecoxib use. In the celecoxib study, a double-blinded study by Steinbach et al., 77 patients were randomized to receive celecoxib or placebo for 6 months. Individuals receiving celecoxib at 400 mg twice daily showed a 28 % reduction in colorectal polyp numbers and a 30.7 % reduction in polyp burden (as calculated by the sum of polyp diameter) compared to a lesser dose of celecoxib or to placebo.

Aspirin has also been studied in the FAP as well as Lynch syndrome patients. In the Colorectal Adenoma/Carcinoma Prevention Program 1 (CAPP1) study, aspirin was studied alone or in combination with dietary nonabsorbable starch (resistant starch) and compared to resistant starch alone or to placebo in patients with FAP [123]. After median treatment duration of 17 months, no significant reduction in polyp size or count was noted, but the study did show a trend toward a decrease in both the polyp size and count in the aspirin 600 mg daily group with no effect noted on the resistant starch. Aspirin's role in FAP remains under investigation.

The combination of curcumin, an antioxidant and free radical scavenger, and quercetin, an antiflavonoid and antiinflammatory, both which are widely available as diet-derived nonprescription supplements, has been shown to reduce the size and number of ileal and rectal adenomas in five FAP patients with much toxicity [124]. Further studies are being planned to evaluate this combination.

In Lynch syndrome, only one prospective randomized study has been published with both short- and long-term results [125, 126]. In the CAPP2 study, Lynch syndrome patients defined as those with mismatch repair gene mutation or those whose family met the Amsterdam criteria and had a personal history of a cured Lynch syndrome neoplasm with an intact colon were randomized in a two by two design to either aspirin at 600 mg daily with or without resistant starch, placebo, and/or resistant starch alone [125]. At the 4-year follow-up, neither aspirin nor resistant starch alone or in combination had any effect on the incidence of adenoma or carcinoma [125]. However, at a mean follow-up of 55.7 months, 600 mg of aspirin daily for a mean of 25 months reduced cancer (overall) incidence [126].

CAPP3 trial is a double-blind randomized dose inferiority trial designed to compare the degree of cancer prevention in Lynch syndrome patients after administering three different doses of aspirin – 600 mg, 300 mg, and 100 mg [127]. The results are still pending.

Conclusion

Hereditary colon cancer represents a minority of colorectal cancer but with severe and life-threatening consequences. Lynch syndrome and familial adenomatous polyposis represent the majority of hereditary colon cancers. Due to their high risk of polyp formation and transformation, aggressive surveillance and prophylactic surgical intervention are indicated. Extracolonic manifestations and their increased malignant potential also necessitate frequent surveillance and possible surgical resection. Chemoprevention trials are ongoing, with NSAIDs such as aspirin showing promise in reducing polyp burden in individuals with FAP. However, at this time, chemopreventive agents are not a substitute for surgery and should be used as an adjunct to surgery. In Lynch syndrome, it appears that after about 2 years of aspirin intake, cancer incidence is reduced. The optimal dosage is yet to be determined.

Salient Points

- Approximately 10–30 % of colorectal cancer (CRC) patients have a positive family history. Of these inherited CRCs, majority are accounted by Lynch syndrome and familial adenomatous polyposis (FAP).
- Lynch syndrome is characterized by a mutation in one of the DNA mismatch repair genes that cause microsatellite instability and replication of repetitive sequences.
- Diagnosis of Lynch syndrome should follow the Amsterdam criteria and the Bethesda guidelines. If positive, screening should start with immunohistochemistry to look for loss of MMR protein expression.

- Those diagnosed with Lynch syndrome should start annual colonoscopy at age 25.
- The preferred surgical treatment in those with Lynch syndrome is subtotal colectomy with ileorectal anastomosis.
- Extracolonic manifestations occur with great frequency in those with Lynch syndrome, with a reported incidence as high as 43 % of those developing endometrial cancer.
- Majority of patients with FAP have a genetic mutation to the adenomatous polyposis coli (APC) gene, a tumor suppressor gene.
- FAP is diagnosed in those with greater than 100 adenomatous colorectal polyps, with these polyps developing by age 20 in 75 % of cases.
- Screening should begin at age 10–12 years of age.
- Three surgical options for FAP are total proctocolectomy with permanent ileostomy, total abdominal colectomy with ileorectal anastomosis, or proctocolectomy with ileal pouch-anal anastomosis. Each option has its advantages and disadvantages. Typically, the ideal time to have prophylactic surgery is the summer between high school and college.
- FAP is associated with many extracolonic manifestations. Desmoid tumors and duodenal cancers occur with high frequency. Patients with FAP should be screened routinely for these pathologies.
- Attenuated familial adenomatous polyposis (aFAP) is diagnosed in patients with APC mutations with less than 100 adenomatous polyps and is mainly located in the right side of the colon.
- In those whose colonic polyps cannot be controlled endoscopically, total abdominal colectomy with ileorectal anastomosis is the procedure of choice.
- MYH-associated polyposis (MAP) is an autosomal recessive disorder due to biallelic mutation in MYH, a base excision repair gene.
- In MAP, polyposis is controlled with endoscopic polypectomies. If surgical intervention is warranted, in patients without involvement of the rectum, total abdominal colectomy with ileorectal anastomosis is recommended. If rectum is involved, then total proctocolectomy with ileal pouch-anal anastomosis is indicated.
- Peutz–Jeghers syndrome (PJS) is an autosomal-dominant disorder caused by a mutation in the LKB1 gene, the only known tumor suppressor kinase.
- Hamartomatous polyps in PJS can occur anywhere in the GI tract, with the jejunum being the most common location.
- Dysplastic hamartomatous polyps must be distinguished from pseudo-invasion by histology.
- Patients often present with intussusceptions and/or bowel obstructive symptoms.
- Prophylactic colectomy in PJS is unclear.
- Juvenile polyposis syndrome (JPS) is a rare autosomal-dominant syndrome. Cumulative lifetime risk of colorectal cancer is 39 %.
- In JPS, polyposis is controlled with endoscopic polypectomies. If surgical intervention is warranted, the surgical procedure of choice has to be individualized.
- Polyps seen in PJS are disorganized hamartomas characterized by hypertrophy or hyperplasia of smooth muscle in the muscularis mucosa. Polyps in JPS are typically spherical, lobulated, or pedunculated in appearance with histology showing abundance of edematous lamina propria infiltrated with inflammatory cells and cystically dilated mucous-filled glands.
- There are differing reports on the efficacy of sulindac on colorectal recurrence and reducing polyp number and size. Currently, it is not recommended as a first-line treatment for polyp reduction.
- In CAPP1 study, aspirin was studied alone or in combination with dietary nonabsorbable starch (resistant starch) and compared to resistant starch alone or to placebo in patients with FAP. The study did show a trend toward a decrease in both the polyp size and count in the aspirin 600 mg daily group with no effect noted on the resistant starch. Aspirin's role in FAP remains under investigation.
- CAPP2 trial showed a reduction in all cancers in Lynch syndrome patients with when they were treated with 600 mg of aspirin daily for a

mean of 25 months and at a mean follow-up of 55.7 months.

- CAPP3 trial is investigating the effects of different doses of aspirin on cancer prevention in Lynch syndrome patients.
- NSAID such as sulindac decreases the number and size of polyps in FAP patients; however, they are not a substitute for surgical management.

Questions

1. What genetic mutations are linked with Lynch syndrome?
   A. SMAD4
   B. MMR genes
   C. APC
   D. LKB1
2. What is the next step in the algorithm for genetic testing in Lynch syndrome patients if MLH1 is found to be absent?
   A. Test for MSH2
   B. Test for PMS2
   C. Test for BRAF
   D. No more testing necessary
3. Which of the following is not an extracolonic manifestations linked with Lynch syndrome?
   A. Endometrial cancer
   B. Gastric cancer
   C. Intestinal hamartomas
   D. Keratoacanthomas
4. At what age does the colonic surveillance schedule for FAP patients recommended to start?
   A. At birth
   B. 10–12 years of age
   C. 16–18 years of age
   D. 28–30 years of age
5. Which of the following is not a surgical treatment options for FAP?
   A. Total colectomy with ileostomy
   B. Segmental colectomy with primary anastomosis
   C. Total colectomy with ileorectal anastomosis
   D. Total proctocolectomy with ileal pouch-anal anastomosis
6. Which of the following is not an extracolonic manifestation associated with FAP?
   A. Desmoid cancer
   B. Gastric cancer
   C. CHRPE
   D. Urogenital cancer
7. How is aFAP distinguished from FAP?
   A. Less than 100 adenomatous polyps in the colon
   B. Less than 150 adenomatous polyps in the colon
   C. Less than 500 adenomatous polyps in the colon
   D. Less than 1,000 adenomatous polyps in the colon
8. Which of the following studies looked at the role of aspirin in reducing cancer recurrence in FAP patients?
   A. DFMO trial
   B. CAPP2 trial
   C. CAPP1 trial
   D. CAPP3 trial

Answers

1. B
2. C
3. C
4. B
5. B
6. A
7. A
8. C

References

1. Siegel R, Ma J, Zou Z, Jemal A. Cancer statistics, 2014. CA Cancer J Clin. 2014;64(1):9–29.
2. Lynch HT, de la Chapelle A. Hereditary colorectal cancer. N Engl J Med. 2003;348:919–32.
3. Merg A, Lynch HT, Lynch JF, et al. Hereditary colon cancer part I. Curr Probl Surg. 2005;42(4):195–256.
4. Hampel H, Frankel W, Martin E, et al. Feasibility of screening for Lynch syndrome among patients with colorectal cancer. J Clin Oncol. 2008;26:5783–8.
5. Vasen HFA, et al. Revised guidelines for the clinical management of Lynch syndrome (HNPCC): recommendations by a group of European experts. Gut. 2013;62(6):812–23.
6. Hampel H, Stephens J, Pukkala E, et al. Cancer risk in hereditary nonpolyposis colorectal cancer syndrome: later age of onset. Gastroenterol. 2005; 129:415–21.

7. Quehenberger F, Vasen H, van Houwelingen H. Risk of colorectal and endometrial cancer for carriers of mutations of the hMLH1 and hMSH2 gene: correction for ascertainment. J Med Genet. 2006;42: 491–6.
8. Bonadonna V, Bonaiti B, Olschwang S, et al. Cancer risks associated with germline mutations in MLH1, MSH2, and MSH8 genes in Lynch syndrome. JAMA. 2011;305:2304–10.
9. Kovacs M, Papp J, Szentirmay Z, et al. Deletions removing the last exon of TACSTD1 constitute a distinct class of mutations predisposing to Lynch syndrome. Hum Mutat. 2009;30:197–203.
10. Niessen R, Hofstra R, Westers H, et al. Germline hypermethylation of MLH1 and EPCAM deletions are a frequent cause of Lynch syndrome. Genes Chromosomes Cancer. 2009;48:737–44.
11. Vasen H, Mecklin J, Khan P, et al. New clinical criteria for hereditary nonpolyposis colorectal cancer (HNPCC) proposed by the International Collaborative Group on HNPCC. Gastroenterology. 1999;116:1453–6.
12. Rodriguez-Bigas M, Boland C, Hamilton S, et al. A National Cancer Institute workshop on Hereditary Nonpolyposis Colorectal Cancer Syndrome: meeting highlights and Bethesda guidelines. J Natl Cancer Inst. 1997;89:1758–62.
13. Baglietto L, Lindor N, Dowty J, et al. Risks of Lynch syndrome cancers for MSH6 mutation carriers. J Nat Cancer Inst. 2010;102:193–201.
14. Lynch HT, Fitzgibbons Jr R. Surgery, desmoid tumors, and familial adenomatous polyposis: case report and literature review. Am J Gastroenterol. 1996;91:2598–601.
15. Ponti G, de Ponz Loen M. Muir-Torre syndrome. Lancet Oncol. 2005;6:980–7.
16. Sargent D, Marsoni S, Monges G, et al. Defective mismatch repair as a predictive marker for lack of efficacy of fluorouracil based adjuvant therapy in colon cancer. J Clin Oncol. 2010;28(20):3219–26.
17. Moreira L, et al. Identification of Lynch syndrome among patients with colorectal cancer. JAMA. 2012;308:1555–65.
18. Nakagawa H, Nagasaka T, Cullings H, et al. Efficient molecular screening of Lynch syndrome by specific 3′ promoter methylation of MLH1 or BRAF mutation in colorectal cancer with high frequency microsatellite instability. Oncol Rep. 2009;21:1577–83.
19. Heiskanen I, Luostarinen T, Jarvinen H. Impact of screening examinations on survival in familial adenomatous polyposis. Scand J Gastroenterol. 2000; 35(12):1284–7.
20. Lynch H, Riley B, Weissman S, et al. Hereditary nonpolyposis colorectal carcinoma and HNPCC-like families: problems in diagnosis, surveillance and management. Cancer. 2004;100:53–64.
21. Natarajan N, Watson P, Silva-Lopez E, et al. Comparison of extended colectomy and limited resection in patients with Lynch syndrome. Dis Colon Rectum. 2010;53(1):77–82.
22. Parry S, Win A, Parry B, et al. Metachronous colorectal cancer risk for mismatch repair gene mutation carriers: the advantage of more extensive colon surgery. Gut. 2011;60(7):950–7.
23. Rodriguez-Bigas M, Vasen H, Pekka-Mecklin J, et al. Rectal cancer risk in hereditary nonpolyposis colorectal cancer after abdominal colectomy. International Collaborative Group on HNPCC. Ann Surg. 1997;225:202–7.
24. Win A, Lindor N, Young J, et al. Risks of primary extracolonic cancers following colorectal cancer in Lynch syndrome. J Nat Cancer Inst. 2012;104(18):1363–72.
25. Chen S, Wang W, Lee S, et al. Prediction of germline mutations and cancer risk in the Lynch syndrome. JAMA. 2006;296:1479–87.
26. Schmeler K, Lynch H, Chen L, et al. Prophylactic surgery to reduce the risk of gynecologic cancers in the Lynch syndrome. N Engl J Med. 2006;354:261–9.
27. Bisgaard M, Fenger K, Bulow S, et al. Familial adenomatous polyposis (FAP): frequency, penetrance and mutation rate. Hum Mutat. 1994;3:121–5.
28. Kerr S, Thomas C, Thibodeau S, et al. APC germline mutations in individuals being evaluated for familial adenomatous polyposis. A review of the Mayo experience with 1591 consecutive tests. J Mol Diagn. 2013;15(1):31–43.
29. Miyoshi Y, Ando H, Nagase H, et al. Germ-line mutations of the APC gene in 53 familial adenomatous polyposis patients. Proc Natl Acad Sci U S A. 1992;89:4452–6.
30. Miyoshi Y, Nagase H, Ando H, et al. Somatic mutations of the APC gene in colorectal tumors: mutation cluster in the APC gene. Hum Mol Genet. 1992;1:229–33.
31. Gayther SA, Wells D, Sengupta SB, et al. Regionally clustered APC mutations are associated with a severe phenotype and occur at a high frequency in new mutation cases of adenomatous polyposis coli. Hum Mol Genet. 1994;3:53–6.
32. Nugent KP, Phillips RKS, Hodgson SV, et al. Phenotypic expression in familial adenomatous polyposis: partial prediction by mutation analysis. Gut. 1994;35:1622–3.
33. Caspari R, Friedl F, Mandl M, et al. Familial adenomatous polyposis: mutation at codon 1309 and early onset of colon cancer. Lancet. 1994;343:629–32.
34. Giardiello FM, Krush AJ, Petersen GM, et al. Phenotypic variability of familial adenomatous polyposis in 11 unrelated families with identical APC gene mutation. Gastroenterology. 1994;106: 1542–7.
35. Giardiello FM. The use and interpretation of commercial APC gene testing for familial adenomatous polyposis. N Engl J Med. 1997;336:823–7.
36. Grover S, Kastrinos F, Steyerberg E, et al. Prevalence and phenotypes of APC and MUTYH mutations in patients with multiple colorectal adenomas. JAMA. 2012;308(5):485–92.

37. Church J, Simmang C. Practice parameters for the treatment of patients with dominantly inherited colorectal cancer (familial adenomatous polyposis and hereditary nonpolyposis colorectal cancer). Dis Colon Rectum. 2003;46(8):1001–12.
38. Olsen K, Juul S, Bulow S, et al. Female fecundity before and after operation for familial adenomatous polyposis. Br J Surg. 2003;90(2):227–31.
39. Nyam DC, Brillant PT, Dozois RR, et al. Ileal pouch-anal canal anastomosis for familial adenomatous polyposis: early and late results. Ann Surg. 1997; 226:514–9.
40. Metcalf AM, Dozois RR, Kelly KA. Sexual function in women after proctocolectomy. Ann Surg. 1986; 204:624–7.
41. Bussey HJ, Eyers AA, Ritchie SM, et al. The rectum in adenomatous polyposis: the St Mark's policy. Br J Surg. 1985;72:S29–31.
42. De Cosse JJ, Bulow S, Neale K, et al. Rectal cancer risk in patients treated for familial adenomatous polyposis. Br J Surg. 1992;79:1372–5.
43. Bulow C, Vasen H, Jarvinen H, et al. Ileorectal anastomosis is appropriate for a subset of patients with familial adenomatous polyposis. Gastroenterology. 2000;119:1454–60.
44. Iwama T, Mishima Y. Factors affecting the risk of rectal cancer following rectum-preserving surgery in patients with familial adenomatous polyposis. Dis Colon Rectum. 1994;37:1024–6.
45. Bess MA, Adson MA, Elveback LR, et al. Rectal cancer following colectomy for polyposis. Arch Surg. 1980;115:460–7.
46. Vasen H, van der Luijt R, Slors J, et al. Molecular genetic tests as a guide to surgical management of familial adenomatous polyposis. Lancet. 1996;348: 433/435.
47. Bertario L, Russo A, Radice P, et al. Genotype and phenotype factors as determinants for rectal stump cancer in patients with familial adenomatous polyposis. Ann Surg. 2000;231:538–43.
48. Nieuwenhuis M, Bulow S, Bjork J, et al. Genotype predicting phenotype in familial adenomatous polyposis: a practical application to the choice of surgery. Dis Colon Rectum. 2009;52:1259–63.
49. Church J, Burke C, McGannon E, et al. Predicting polyposis severity by proctoscopy: how reliable is it? Dis Colon Rectum. 2001;44(9):1249–54.
50. Parc YR, Moslein G, Dozois RR, et al. Familial adenomatous polyposis: results after ileal pouch-anal anastomosis in teenagers. Dis Colon Rectum. 2000;43:893–8.
51. Jagelman DG. Choice of operation in familial adenomatous polyposis. World J Surg. 1991;15:47–9.
52. Madden MV, Neale KF, Nicholls RJ, et al. Comparison of morbidity and function after colectomy with ileorectal anastomosis or restorative proctocolectomy for familial adenomatous polyposis. Br J Surg. 1991;78:789–92.
53. Aziz O, Athanasiou T, Fazio V, et al. Meta-analysis of observational studies of ileorectal versus ileal pouch anal anastomosis for familial adenomatous polyposis. Br J Surg. 2006;93(4):407–17.
54. Rodriguez-Bigas MA, Mahoney MC, Karakousis CP, et al. Desmoid tumors in patients with familial adenomatous polyposis. Cancer. 1994;74:1270–4.
55. Heiskanen I, Jarvinen HJ. Occurrence of desmoid tumours in familial adenomatous polyposis and results of treatment. Int J Colorectal Dis. 1996;11: 157–62.
56. Heiskanen I, Jarvinen H. Occurrence of desmoid tumors in familial adenomatous polyposis and results of treatment. Int J Colorectal Dis. 1996;11:1157–62.
57. Lim CL, Walker MJ, Mehta RR, et al. Estrogen and antiestrogen binding sites in desmoid tumors. Eur J Cancer Clin Oncol. 1986;22:583–7.
58. Tsukada K, Church JM, Jagelman DG, et al. Noncytotoxic drug therapy for intra-abdominal desmoid tumor in patients with familial adenomatous polyposis. Dis Colon Rectum. 1992;35:29–33.
59. Lynch HT, Fitzgibbons Jr R, Chong S, et al. Use of doxorubicin and dacarbazine for the management of unresectable intra-abdominal desmoid tumors in Gardner's syndrome. Dis Colon Rectum. 1994; 37:260–7.
60. Nugent KP, Spigelman AD, Phillips RK. Life expectancy after colectomy and ileorectal anastomosis for familial adenomatous polyposis. Dis Colon Rectum. 1993;36:1059–62.
61. Church J, Berk T, Boman B, et al. Staging intra-abdominal desmoid tumors in familial adenomatous polyposis: a search for a uniform approach to a troubling disease. Dis Colon Rectum. 2005;48(8): 1528–34.
62. Wallace MH, Phillips RKS. Upper gastrointestinal disease in patients with familial adenomatous polyposis. Br J Surg. 1998;85:742–50.
63. Spigelman A, Williams C, Napoleaon B, et al. Upper gastrointestinal cancer in patients with familial adenomatous polyposis. Lancet. 1989;2:783–5.
64. Debinski HS, Trojan J, Nugent KP, et al. Effect of sulindac on small polyps in familial adenomatous polyposis. Lancet. 1995;345:855–6.
65. Richard CS, Berk T, Bapat BV, et al. Sulindac for periampullary polyps in FAP patients. Int J Colorectal Dis. 1997;12:14–8.
66. Phillips RKS, Wallace MH, Lynch PM, et al. A randomised, double blind, placebo controlled study of celecoxib, a selective cyclooxygenase 2 inhibitor, on duodenal polyposis in familial adenomatous polyposis. Gut. 2002;50:857–60.
67. Brosens LAA, Iacobuzio-Donahue CA, Keller JJ, et al. Increased cyclooxygenase-2 expression in duodenal compared with colonic tissues in familial adenomatous polyposis and relationship to the $-765G \rightarrow C$ COX-2 polymorphism. Clin Cancer Res. 2005;11:4090–6.
68. Knudsen A, Bulow S, Tomlinson I, et al. Attenuated familial adenomatous polyposis: results from an international collaborative study. Colorectal Dis. 2010;12:243–9.

69. Lynch HT, Smyrk T, McGinn T, et al. Attenuated familial adenomatous polyposis (AFAP): a phenotypically and genotypically distinctive variant of FAP. Cancer. 1995;76:2427–33.
70. Brensinger JD, Laken SJ, Luce MC, et al. Variable phenotype of familial adenomatous polyposis in pedigrees with 3 mutation in the APC gene. Gut. 1998;43:548–52.
71. Burt RW, Leppert MF, Slattery ML, et al. Genetic testing and phenotype in a large kindred with attenuated familial adenomatous polyposis. Gastroenterology. 2004;127:444–51.
72. Nielsen M, Hes F, Nagengast F, et al. Germline mutations in APC and MUTYH are responsible for the majority of families with attenuated familial adenomatous polyposis. Clin Genet. 2007;71:427–33.
73. Anaya D, Chang G, Rodriguez-Bigas M. Extracolonic manifestations of hereditary colorectal cancer syndromes. Clin Colon Rectal Surg. 2008;21:263–72.
74. Lipton L, Tomlinson I. The genetics of FAP and FAP-like syndromes. Fam Cancer. 2006;5:221–6.
75. Smith KJ, Johnson KA, Bryan TM, et al. The APC gene product in normal and tumor cells. Proc Natl Acad Sci U S A. 1993;90:2846–50.
76. Al-Tassan N, Chmiel N, Maynard J, et al. Inherited variants of MYH associated with somatic G:C to T:A mutations in colorectal tumors. Nat Genet. 2002;30:227–32.
77. Nielsen M, van de Joerink-Beld MC, Jones N, et al. Analysis of MUTYH genotypes and colorectal phenotypes in patients with MUTYH-associated polyposis. Gastroenterology. 2009;136:471–6.
78. Olschwang S, Blanhe H, de Moncuit C, et al. Similar colorectal cancer risk in patients with monoallelic and biallelic mutations in the MYH gene identified in a population with adenomatous polyposis. Genet Test. 2007;11:315–20.
79. Jenkins M, Croitoru M, Monga N, et al. Risk of colorectal cancer in monoallelic and biallelic carriers of MYH mutations: a population based case family study. Cancer Epidemiol Biomarkers Prev. 2006;15:312–4.
80. Lubbe SJ, Di Bernardo MC, Chandler IP, et al. Clinical implications of the colorectal cancer risk associated with MUTYH mutation. J Clin Oncol. 2009;27:3975–80.
81. Jones N, Vogt S, Nielsen M, et al. Increased colorectal cancer incidence in obligate carriers of heterozygous mutations in MUTYH. Gastroenterology. 2009;137:489–94.
82. Nielsen M, Morreau H, Hans F, et al. MUTYH-associated polyposis (MAP). Crit Rev Oncol Hematol. 2011;79(1):1–16.
83. Nielsen M, Franken P, Reinards T, et al. Multiplicity in polyp count and extracolonic manifestations in 40 Dutch patients with MYH associated polyposis coli. J Med Genet. 2005;42:e54.
84. Jith Kumar VK, Gold JA, Mallon E, et al. Sebaceous adenomas in an MYH associated polyposis patient of Indian (Gujarati) origin. Fam Cancer. 2008; 7:187–9.
85. Vasen HF, Moslein G, Alonso A, et al. Guidelines for the clinical management of familial adenomatous polyposis (FAP). Gut. 2008;57:704–13.
86. Riegert-Johnson D, Gleeson F, Westra W, et al. Peutz Jeghers syndrome. Cancer Syndr. 2008 Jul.
87. Hearle N, Schumacher V, Menko F, et al. Frequency and spectrum of cancers in the Peutz-Jeghers syndrome. Clin Cancer Res. 2006;12(10):3209–15.
88. Giardiello F, Brensinger J, Tersmette A. Very high risk of cancer in familial Peutz-Jeghers syndrome. Gastroenterology. 2000;119(6):1447–53.
89. Boudeau J, Baas A, Deak M, et al. MO25alpha/beta interact with STRADalpha/beta enhancing their ability to bind, activate and localize LKB1 in the cytoplasm. Embo J. 2003;22(19):5102–14.
90. Burt R. Colon cancer screening. Gastroenterology. 2000;119(3):837–53.
91. Westerman A, Entius M, de Baar E, et al. Peutz-Jeghers syndrome: 78-year follow-up of the original family. Lancet. 1999;353(9160):1211–5.
92. Bartholomew L, Dahlin D, Waugh J. Intestinal polyposis associated with mucocutaneous melanin pigmentation Peutz-Jeghers syndrome; review of literature and report of six cases with special reference to pathologic findings. Gastroenterology. 1957;32:434–51.
93. Sarlos P, Kiraly A, Nagy L. Family study in Peutz-Jeghers syndrome. Orv Hetil. 2007;148(6):255–8.
94. Westerman A, van Velthuysen M, Bac D, et al. Malignancy in Peutz-Jeghers syndrome? The pitfall of pseudo-invasion. J Clin Gastroenterol. 1997;25: 387–90.
95. Mehenni H, Resta N, Park J, et al. Cancer risks in LKB1 germline mutation carriers. Gut. 2006; 55(7):984–90.
96. Parker M, Knight M. Peutz-Jeghers syndrome causing obstructive jaundice due to polyp in common bile duct. J R Soc Med. 1983;76(8):701–3.
97. Wada K, Tanaka M, Yamaguchi K. Carcinoma and polyps of the gallbladder associated with Peutz-Jeghers syndrome. Dig Dis Sci. 1987;32(8):943–6.
98. Olschwang S, Boisson C, Thomas G. Peutz-Jeghers families unlinked to STK11/LKB1 gene mutations are highly predisposed to primitive biliary adenocarcinoma. J Med Genet. 2001;38(6):356–60.
99. Sommerhaug RG, Mason T. Peutz-Jeghers syndrome and ureteral polyposis. Jama. 1970;211(1):120–2.
100. Jancu J. Peutz-Jeghers syndrome. Involvement of the gastrointestinal and upper respiratory tracts. Am J Gastroenterol. 1971;56(6):545–9.
101. Brosens L, Langeveld D, van Hattem W, et al. Juvenile polyposis syndrome. World J Gastroenterol. 2011;17(44):439–4844.
102. Van Hattem W, Brosens L, de Leng W, et al. Large genomic deletions of SMAD4, BMPR1A and PTEN in juvenile polyposis. Gut. 2008;57:623–7.
103. Aretz S, Stieven D, Uhlhaas S, et al. High proportions of large genomic deletions and a genotype phenotype

update in 80 unrelated families with juvenile polyposis syndrome. J Med Genet. 2007;44:702–9.
104. Friedl W, Uhlhaas S, Schulmann K, et al. Juvenile polyposis: massive gastric polyposis is more common in MADH4 mutation carriers than in BMPR1A mutation carriers. Hum Genet. 2002;111:108–11.
105. Delnatte C, Sanlaville D, Mougenot J, et al. Contiguous gene deletion within chromosome arm 10q is associated with juvenile polyposis of infancy, reflecting cooperation between the BMPR1A and PTEN tumor suppressor gene. Am J Hum Genet. 2006;78:1066/1074.
106. Aaltonen L. Hereditary intestinal cancer. Semin Cancer Biol. 2000;10(4):289–98.
107. Church D, Briggs S, Palles C. DNA polymerase ε and δ exonuclease domain mutations in endometrial cancer. Hum Mol Genet. 2013;22:2820–8.
108. Briggs S, Tomlinson I. Germline and somatic polymerase ε and δ mutations define a new class of hypermutated colorectal and endometrial cancers. J Pathol. 2013;230(2):148–53.
109. Tsujii M, Kawano S, Tsuji S, et al. Cyclooxygenase regulates angiogenesis induced by colon cancer cells. Cell. 1998;93:705–16.
110. Giardiello FM, Offerhaus GJA, DuBois RN. The role of nonsteroidal anti-inflammatory drugs in colorectal cancer prevention. Eur J Cancer. 1995; 31A:1071–6.
111. Kim B, Giardiello FM. Chemoprevention in familial adenomatous polyposis. Best Pract Res Clin Gastroenterol. 2011;25:607–22.
112. Waddell W, Loughry R. Sulindac for polyposis of the colon. J Surg Oncol. 1983;24(1):83–7.
113. Giardello F, Hamilton S, Krush A, et al. Treatment of colonic and rectal adenomas with sulindac in familial adenomatous polyposis. N Engl J Med. 1993;328(18):1313–6.
114. Thorson A, Lynch H, Smyrk T. Rectal cancer in FAP patients after sulindac. Lancet. 1994;343:417–8.
115. Niv Y, Fraser GM. Adenocarcinoma in the rectal segment in familial polyposis coli is not prevented by sulindac therapy. Gastroenterology. 1994;107:854–7.
116. Giardiello FM, Yang VW, Hylind LM, et al. Primary chemoprevention of familial adenomatous polyposis with sulindac. N Engl J Med. 2002;346:1054–9.
117. Meyskens Jr F, McLaren C, Pelot D, et al. Difluoromethylornithine plus sulindac for the prevention of sporadic colorectal adenomas: a randomized placebo-controlled double-blind trial. Cancer Prev Res. 2008;1:32–8.
118. Burke CA, et al. Exisulind prevents adenoma formation in familial adenomatous polyposis (FAP). Gastroenterology. 2000;118:A657.
119. Philips R, et al. Exisulind, a pro-apoptotic drug prevents new polyp formation in patients with familial adenomatous polyposis. Gut. 2000;47 suppl 3:A2–3.
120. Arber N, Kuwada S, Leshno M, et al. Sporadic adenomatous polyp regression with exisulind is effective but toxic: a randomised, double blind, placebo controlled, dose–response study. Gut. 2006; 55:367–73.
121. Higuchi T, Iwama T, Yoshinaga K, et al. A randomized double blind placebo controlled trial of the effects of rofecoxib, a selective cyclooxygenase 2 inhibitor, on rectal polyps in familial adenomatous polyposis patients. Clin Cancer Res. 2003;9: 4756–60.
122. Steinbach G, Lynch PM, Phillips RK, et al. The effect of celecoxib, a cyclooxygenase-2 inhibitor, in familial adenomatous polyposis. N Engl J Med. 2000;342:1946–52.
123. Burn J, Bishop D, Chapman P, et al. A randomized placebo controlled prevention trial of aspirin and/or resistant starch in young people with familial adenomatous polyposis. Cancer Prev Res. 2011;4(5):655–65.
124. Cruz-Correa M, Shoskes D, Sanchez P, et al. Combination treatment with curcumin and quercetin of adenomas in familial adenomatous polyposis. Clin Gastroenterol Hepatol. 2006;4(8):1035–8.
125. Burn J, Bishop D, Mecklin J, et al. Effects of aspirin or resistant starch on colorectal neoplasia in the Lynch Syndrome. N Engl J Med. 2008;359:2567–78.
126. Burn J, Gerdes A, Macrae F, et al. Long term effect of aspirin on cancer risk in carriers of hereditary colorectal cancer: an analysis from the CAPP2 randomized controlled trial. Lancet. 2011;378(9809): 2081–7.
127. Burn et al. A randomised double blind dose non-inferiority trial of a daily dose of 600 mg versus 300 mg versus 100 mg of enteric coated aspirin as a cancer preventive in carriers of a germline pathological mismatch repair gene defect, Lynch syndrome. Project 3 in the Cancer Prevention Programme. Published May 2013. Retrieved April 2014. http://www.mallorca-group.eu/pdf/CaPP3_version_0.96_May_2013.pdf.
128. Boland C, Goel A. Microsatellite instability in colorectal cancer. Gastroenterology. 2010;138(6): 2073–87.
129. Ahnen DJ. The American College of gastroenterology Emily Couric Lecture [mdash]. The adenoma-carcinoma sequence revisited. Has the era of genetic tailoring finally arrived? Am J Gastroenterol. 2011;106:190–8.
130. Bhattacharyya S, et al. Carrageenan reduces bone morphogenetic protein-4 (BMP4) and activates the Wnt/β-Catenin pathway in normal human colonocytes. Dig Dis Sci. 2007;52(10):2766–74.
131. Shaw R. LKB1: cancer, polarity, metabolism and now fertility. Biochem J. 2008;416:e1–3. doi:10.1042/BJ20082023.
132. Labayle D, Fischer D, Vielh P, et al. Sulindac causes regression of rectal polyps in familial adenomatous polyposis. Gastroenterology. 1991;101(3):635–9.
133. Giardiello FM, Hamilton SR, Krush AJ, et al. Treatment of colonic and rectal adenomas with sulindac in familial adenomatous polyposis. N Engl J Med. 1993;328(18):1313–6.
134. Giardiello FM, Spannhake EW, DuBois RN, et al. Prostaglandin levels in human colorectal mucosa:

effects of sulindac in patients with Familial adenomatous polyposis. Dig Dis Sci. 1998;43(2):311–6.
135. Nugent KP, Farmer KC, Spigelman AD, et al. Randomized controlled trial of the effect of sulindac on duodenal and rectal polyposis and cell proliferation in patients with familial adenomatous polyposis. Br J Surg. 1993;80(12):1618–9.
136. Winde G, Schmid KW, Brandt B, et al. Clinical and genomic influence of sulindac on rectal mucosa in familial adenomatous polyposis. Dis Colon Rectum. 1997;40(10):1156–68. Discussion 1168–69
137. Steinbach G, Lynch PM, Phillips RK, et al. The effects of celecoxib, a cyclooxygenase 2 inhibitor, in familial adenomatous polyposis. N Engl J Med. 2000;342(26):1946–52.
138. Bussey HJ, DeCosse JJ, Deschner EE, et al. A randomized trial of ascorbic acid in polyposis coli. Cancer. 1982;50(7):1434–9.
139. DeCosse J, Miller H, Lesser M. Effects of wheat fiber and vitamins C and E on rectal polyps in patients with familial adenomatous polyposis. J Natl Cancer Inst. 1989;81(17):1290–7.
140. Burn J, Gerdes AM, Macrae F, et al. Long term effect of aspirin on cancer risk in carriers of hereditary colorectal cancer: an analysis from the CAPP2 randomized controlled trial. Lancet. 2011;378(9809):2081–7.
141. Ishikawa H, Wakabayashi K, Suzuki S, et al. Preventive effects of low dose aspirin on colorectal adenoma growth in patients with familial adenomatous polyposis: double blind randomized clinical trial. Cancer Med. 2013;2(1):50–6.
142. Glebov OK, Rodriguez LM, Soballe P, et al. Celecoxib treatment alters the gene expression profile of normal colonic mucosa. Cancer Epidemiol Biomarkers Prev. 2006;15(7):1382–91.

21 Cytoreductive Surgery and Hyperthermic Intraperitoneal Chemotherapy

Reese W. Randle, Konstantinos I. Votanopoulos, Perry Shen, Edward A. Levine, and John H. Stewart IV

Abbreviations

CC	Completeness of cytoreduction
CDDP	Cisplatin
CRC	Colorectal cancer
CRS	Cytoreductive surgery
CT	Computed tomography
DPAM	Disseminated peritoneal adenomucinosis
ECOG	Eastern Cooperative Oncology Group
GIST	Gastrointestinal stromal tumor
HIPEC	Hyperthermic intraperitoneal chemotherapy
MMC	Mitomycin C
MRI	Magnetic resonance imaging
OS	Overall survival
PCI	Peritoneal carcinomatosis index
PET	Positron-emission tomography
PFS	Progression-free survival
PMCA	Peritoneal mucinous carcinomatosis
PMP	Pseudomyxoma peritonei
PSD	Peritoneal surface disease
ULS	Uterine leiomyosarcoma

R.W. Randle, M.D. • K.I. Votanopoulos, M.D., Ph.D.
P. Shen, M.D. • E.A. Levine, M.D.
Department of Surgery, Wake Forest School of Medicine, Medical Center Boulevard, Winston-Salem 27157, NC, USA

J.H. Stewart, IV, M.D., M.B.A. (✉)
Department of General Surgery, Wake Forest Baptist Health, Medical Center Boulevard, Winston-Salem 27157, NC, USA
e-mail: jhstewar@wakehealth.edu

Learning Objectives

After reading this chapter, you should be able to:

- Define peritoneal surface disease and cytoreductive surgery (CRS) with hyperthermic intraperitoneal chemotherapy (HIPEC)
- Recognize indications for CRS-HIPEC
- Describe an appropriate candidate for CRS-HIPEC
- Understand the primary goal and basic components of cytoreduction
- Appreciate the limitations of HIPEC and identify factors influencing its efficacy
- Convey realistic expectations to patients regarding the clinical outcomes of CRS-HIPEC

Background

Peritoneal surface disease (PSD) involves the intra-abdominal dissemination of neoplasms to peritoneal surfaces and encompasses disseminated mucinous adenomas, peritoneal carcinomatosis, and abdominal sarcomatosis (Fig. 21.1). It is thought to spread from the primary tumor by rupture either spontaneously or during the initial resection and is a lethal condition regardless of its primary origin [1, 2]. Intraperitoneal free cancer cells preferentially deposit on peritoneal surfaces, the diaphragms, and the small bowel

Q.D. Chu et al. (eds.), *Surgical Oncology: A Practical and Comprehensive Approach*,
DOI 10.1007/978-1-4939-1423-4_21, © Springer Science+Business Media New York 2015

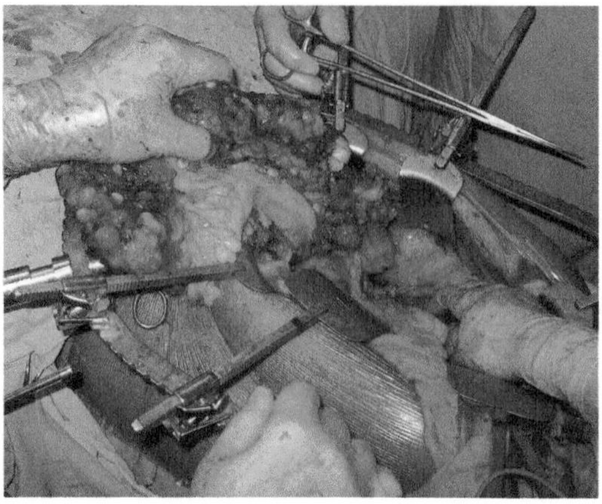

Fig. 21.1 Photograph depicting tumor implants from pseudomyxoma peritonei nearly replacing the omentum, a finding referred to as "omental cake," from a ruptured appendiceal neoplasm

mesentery [3]. The number, size, and distribution of the individual tumor deposits on peritoneal surfaces vary greatly. In most cases PSD is diagnosed incidentally during surgical exploration, during evaluation of abdominal pain, or on radiographic imaging for other indications [4]. These patients have a dismal prognosis with median survival reported between 3 and 7 months [3, 5–7]. Due to the extent, location, or microscopic nature of tumor implants in the peritoneal cavity, surgery alone is infrequently sufficient. Furthermore, systemic chemotherapy is largely ineffective for these patients; thus, a combination of modalities has been developed over the past three decades [3].

Regional approaches to peritoneal surface disease have included cytoreduction via peritonectomy procedures [8, 9], intraperitoneal injection of a streptococcal preparation OK432 [10], debulking with photodynamic therapy [11–13], intracavitary immunotherapy [14], and early postoperative intraperitoneal chemotherapy [2, 15–17]. In fact, intraperitoneal chemotherapy has also been studied preceding and following cytoreduction [18]. Delivery at the time of cytoreduction has been thought to have a more complete distribution throughout the peritoneal cavity given that adhesions may be present before and after surgery. Intraperitoneal chemotherapy has achieved higher concentrations at the level of the peritoneal surfaces than systemic chemotherapy before reaching toxic endpoints, and the addition of heat has been thought to have a synergistic effect with the chemotherapy [19]. Thus, the advantage of CRS-HIPEC is that it addresses macroscopic diseases surgically and microscopic diseases chemically and is now routinely performed in specialized centers across America, Europe, Asia, and Australia [3]. Although hyperthermic chemotherapy has carried many names during its development including continuous hyperthermic peritoneal perfusion (CHPP), hyperthermic antiblastic peritoneal perfusion (HAPP), heated intraoperative intraperitoneal chemotherapy (HIIC), intraperitoneal hyperthermic chemotherapy (IPHC), and intraperitoneal hyperthermic perfusion (IPHP), "HIPEC" is now the preferred acronym by international consensus [2, 20].

Decision Process

Once a diagnosis of peritoneal surface disease has been made and the patient wishes to pursue treatment, the clinician should ask the following important question: is this patient an appropriate candidate for CRS-HIPEC? The answer to the above question requires a thorough assessment of the disease process, the patient's performance status, and an in depth understanding of the clinical utility of CRS-HIPEC.

Goal of CRS-HIPEC

Complete cytoreduction of all gross diseases is the primary objective of CRS-HIPEC as complete cytoreduction is a strong predictor of improved survival [14, 21, 22]. To this end, many guidelines for selecting appropriate situations for CRS-HIPEC are aimed at identifying cases in which complete cytoreduction is feasible. While cure can be achieved in a minority of cases, it is important to realize that most patients will recur despite a complete resection. Attempts are made to reduce as much of the tumor burden as possible without compromising the safety of the patient for cases in which complete cytoreduction is not feasible [14].

Evaluation of Patients with PSD for Possible CRS-HIPEC

Indications

The classic indication for CRS-HIPEC is PSD from low-grade appendiceal neoplasms otherwise known as pseudomyxoma peritonei (PMP) [14]. Other generally accepted indications include PSD arising from appendiceal adenocarcinoma, colorectal cancer, gastric cancer, ovarian cancer, and peritoneal mesothelioma [19]. This therapy has also been applied to small bowel adenocarcinoma [23, 24], appendiceal adenocarcinoid [19], sarcomatosis [25–30], endometrial cancer [31], and urachal cancer [32]. Although CRS-HIPEC has been offered to patients with PSD from biliary or pancreatic primary tumors, these are generally avoided due to difficulty in controlling the primary tumor [14].

In general, lower-grade primary tumors have better outcomes with CRS-HIPEC than higher-grade lesions given the lower rate of locoregional recurrence. The rate of recurrence in high-grade tumors is attributable to the early invasion of peritoneal surfaces and subsequent smaller margins of excision obtained with peritonectomy procedures [19].

Patient Selection

It is imperative that appropriate candidates be selected for CRS-HIPEC due to the considerable morbidity associated with this therapy. A determination of the appropriateness of CRS-HIPEC in a given patient is based upon a thorough clinical assessment and extensive imaging [33, 34]. Preoperative evaluation generally includes complete history, physical examination, pathologic review, contrast-enhanced computed tomography (CT), and laboratory examination including blood counts, electrolytes, and liver function panel. Previously published selection criteria include:

1. The patient is sufficiently medically fit to undergo CRS-HIPEC.
2. There is no extra-abdominal disease.
3. Peritoneal disease burden is potentially completely resectable or at least significantly reducible.
4. There are no parenchymal hepatic metastasis.
5. There is no bulky retroperitoneal disease [35].

Besides being largely subjective, selection criteria are quite variable. A patient may be considered medically unfit for CRS-HIPEC if they display signs of organ dysfunction evidenced by elevations in serum creatinine or liver enzymes or abnormally low white blood cell or platelet counts [14]. Although not an absolute contraindication, poor performance status has predicted worse outcomes for patients presenting for consideration for CRS-HIPEC. Patients with Eastern Cooperative Oncology Group (ECOG) performance status scores of 2 or greater have significantly worse survival outcomes than those with better scores [36].

The extent of previous surgery has been shown to correlate with the extent of tumor implants throughout the peritoneal cavity. Sugarbaker and Chang created a prior surgical score (Table 21.1) and found that patients with scores of 3 had significantly worse survival when compared with patients with lesser scores [37].

Other clinical factors are able to predict outcome and can be used to identify the most appropriate candidates for CRS-HIPEC. The presence of a bowel obstruction with subsequent malnutrition has also predicted worse survival in this population of patients [35]. Data from our own

Table 21.1 Prior surgical score

Prior surgical score	Description
0	PSD diagnosed via biopsy or laparoscopy
1	Previous laparotomy without resection
2	Previous laparotomy with resection
3	Previous attempt at complete cytoreduction

Reprinted from Sugarbaker and Chang [37]. With permission from Springer Verlag
PSD peritoneal surface disease

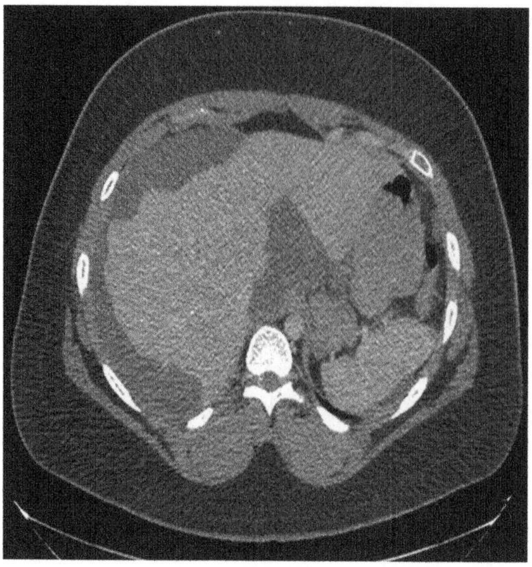

Fig. 21.2 Contrast-enhanced computed tomography of a patient with large-volume pseudomyxoma peritonei. Tumor encases the lateral liver and porta hepatis. A smaller amount of disease is deposited on the spleen

institution indicates that malignant ascites is a strong predictor of incomplete resection, and as such also predicts worse survival [38].

Preoperative imaging plays an important role in determining the location and extent of disease. Specifically, radiographic studies are used to exclude extra-abdominal disease, parenchymal hepatic metastases, extensive small bowel involvement, and obstruction of the small bowel, ureters, or biliary tree [14]. Contrast-enhanced CT of the chest, abdomen, and pelvis is the standard preoperative imaging modality (Fig. 21.2). Sensitivity for detecting peritoneal lesions ranges from 25 to 37 % and improves with increasing lesion size [32, 37]. For example, lesions less than 5 mm in thickness were only detected in 28 % of cases [39]. Although the sensitivity for detecting peritoneal lesions is low, this imaging modality is good for determining retroperitoneal solid organ involvement and overall operability [35]. Furthermore, patients without mesenteric tumors greater than 5 mm and small bowel obstruction have more than a 90 % chance of having a complete resection [34, 40]. Magnetic resonance imaging (MRI) with both oral and intravenous contrast is able to detect PSD with 84–100 % sensitivity [41, 42]. Unfortunately, MRI is also associated with a significant rate of false positives as it is incapable of distinguishing between postoperative scar formation and PSD [19]. Positron-emission tomography (PET) is good both for high-volume disease and for ruling out extra-abdominal disease, yet sensitivity and specificity decrease to 10 % and 42 %, respectively, in patients with low-volume disease [35, 43, 44].

Despite the shortcomings for PSD, modern imaging is able to provide valuable information during the preoperative patient evaluation. Some centers will offer CRS-HIPEC to patients with parenchymal hepatic metastasis if they are amenable to resection at the time of surgery [43]. Others have specific criteria for offering CRS-HIPEC to patients with PSD from different primary tumors based on estimations of disease volume [21]. In the case of PSD from ovarian cancer, no contraindications regarding tumor metastases have been agreed upon [45]. Extensive disease in the lesser sac has been shown to decrease the likelihood of complete cytoreduction and can be identified on cross-sectional imaging when this potential space is distended in the setting of known carcinomatosis [46].

Beyond radiographic imaging, other components of a thorough preoperative evaluation may be case specific. Endoscopy with or without endoscopic ultrasonography can provide valuable information for patients with gastric or colorectal primary tumors [21]. Diagnostic laparoscopy has also been employed to determine the resectability of PSD prior to CRS-HIPEC [47, 48].

Staging Peritoneal Surface Disease

Although the majority of staging will occur at cytoreduction, the use of diagnostic laparoscopy makes it possible to stage patients prior to CRS-HIPEC. The two most commonly used staging systems for PSD are the Gilly carcinomatosis index [49] and the peritoneal carcinomatosis index (PCI) [50]. Both are based upon lesion size and extent of distribution throughout the abdomen. The Gilly carcinomatosis index is the simpler of the two with a designation of Stage 0 to Stage 4 as follows: Stage 0 for no macroscopic disease, Stage 1 for localized tumor implants less

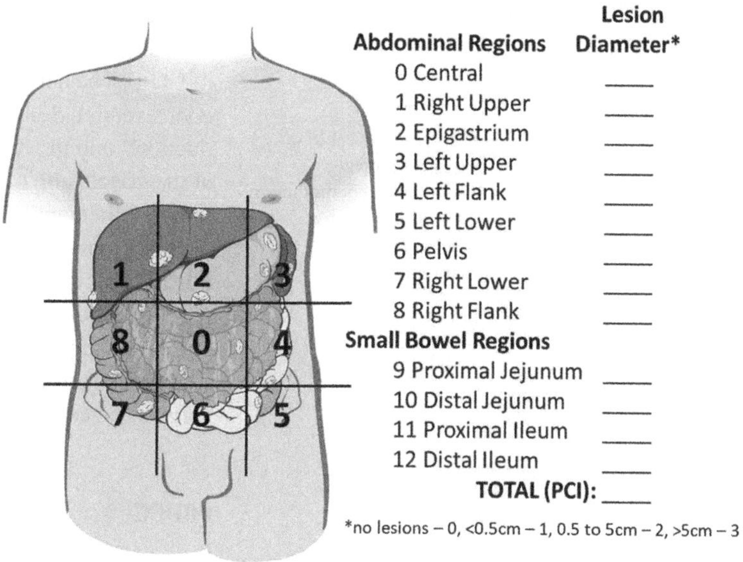

Fig. 21.3 Schematic for calculating the peritoneal carcinomatosis index (PCI) staging system. Scores based on lesion size for each of nine abdominal regions plus 4 small bowel regions are added together to reach the PCI

than 0.5 cm in diameter, Stage 2 for non-localized tumor implants less than 0.5 cm in diameter, Stage 3 for localized or non-localized implants 0.5–2 cm in diameter, and Stage 4 for any implants greater than 2 cm in diameter. As expected, higher stage correlates with worse prognosis [15, 49, 51, 52]. Despite being more complex, the PCI is the most widely used PSD staging system largely due its prognostic value [35, 41, 53–55]. Furthermore, it has provided a way to standardize volume and extent of disease and is even used as a gauge of when HIPEC is warranted [43]. Calculating the PCI involves dividing the abdomen into nine regions and the small bowel into four regions. For each region, a score of 0 (no tumor), 1 (tumor up to 0.5 cm), 2 (tumor up to 5 cm), or 3 (tumor > 5 cm) is applied. Scores for each of the 12 regions are tabulated to derive the PCI score (Fig. 21.3) [35, 54].

Management of PSD with CRS-HIPEC

Preoperative Preparation

Once it has been decided that a patient has an acceptable indication for CRS-HIPEC and is an appropriate candidate, he or she is scheduled for surgery. Patients are generally admitted the day prior to surgery for final assessment and preparation. Final assessment includes an interval history, physical examination, and laboratory evaluation consisting of blood counts, comprehensive chemistry panel, appropriate tumor markers, and a blood type with crossmatch of 4 units of packed red blood cells. For patients felt to have a higher likelihood of ureteral involvement based on disease volume or prior surgery, a urology consultation may be obtained for the placement of externalized ureteral stents. A bowel preparation is routine for all patients and may be accomplished with the use of enemas in cases where a bowel obstruction is present.

Cytoreduction

Patients may be placed in a supine or in a modified lithotomy position for CRS-HIPEC. If a modified lithotomy position is used, the surgeon must be cautious about positioning the legs to prevent myonecrosis of the posterior compartment of the legs [8]. After a thorough prep, an incision is made from the xiphoid to the pubis for generous exposure of the peritoneal cavity. If the falciform ligament is present, it is resected prior to placing a fixed retractor. All adhesions from the disease process or previous operations are

Table 21.2 Grading resection

Size of residual disease (cm)	R status	CC score [19]
0	– R0 – negative margins on final pathology R1 – positive margins on final pathology	CC-0N – no visible disease following neoadjuvant chemotherapy CC-0S – no visible disease following cytoreduction
0.25	R2a	CC-1
0.5		CC-2
>0.5–2	R2b	
>2–2.5	R2c	
>2.5		CC-3

CC Completeness of cytoreduction

lysed to facilitate penetration of HIPEC to all areas of the peritoneal cavity. Cytoreductive surgery is then undertaken to remove all gross disease if technically feasible. Peritoneal surfaces with tumor deposits are stripped from the abdominal wall and diaphragm using electrocautery [8, 9, 19]. The greater omentum is routinely removed along with any involved tissue or organ not vital to the patient. If at any time during the procedure, complete cytoreduction is believed to be either not feasible or unsafe for the patient, the remaining tumor is debulked as much as possible. If a bowel resection is required, an anastomosis may be created prior to or following HIPEC. Ostomies are created following HIPEC to allow exposure of the chemotherapy to any potential microscopic disease remaining on the serosal surfaces.

Grading Resection

The degree of resection is judged by the surgeon at the conclusion of the cytoreduction. Residual disease is evaluated by measuring the diameter of the largest remaining tumor deposits. The two predominating classification systems are the R status of resection and the completeness of cytoreduction (CC) score (Table 21.2). Complete cytoreduction of all gross disease is designated with an R status of R0 or R1 or a CC designation of CC-0. The definition of a complete resection is controversial. Some consider a "complete cytoreduction" one in which there is no visible disease at the conclusion of the cytoreductive procedure. Other authors tailor the definition based upon the primary tumor and the expected response to HIPEC. For example, complete cytoreduction for gastric cancer is limited to CC-0, while complete cytoreduction for low-grade appendiceal primary tumors includes CC-0 to CC-1 and CC-0 to CC-2 for ovarian cancer [1, 19].

HIPEC

The decision to perfuse the patient with HIPEC is based primarily on the degree of resection achieved but is also influenced by the institution and primary tumor. Sugarbaker [19] has described 11 well-defined factors influencing the success rates of HIPEC:

1. Dose of chemotherapeutic agent
2. Timing of delivery in relation to surgery
3. Distribution within the peritoneal cavity
4. Temperature of the tumor implants during perfusion
5. Size of the tumor implant
6. Mucinous versus solid tumor morphology
7. Tumor response to chemotherapy
8. Number of cycles of chemotherapy
9. Peritoneal to plasma drug concentration ratio
10. Synergistic effect with systemic chemotherapy
11. Extent of previous surgery

While HIPEC is ideal for patients following a complete cytoreduction, it may be beneficial in selected patients following incomplete cytoreduction [19]. Perfusion following R2a or CC-1 resection is routine given that locally administered chemotherapy is expected to penetrate tumors at depths ranging from 0.1 cm up to 0.25 cm [19, 33]. Thus, tumor deposits up to 0.5 cm in diameter can be effectively treated with chemotherapy penetration of 0.25 cm from either side.

The advantage of administering chemotherapy directly into the peritoneal cavity is that higher drug concentrations can be achieved at the tumor

Table 21.3 Comparison of chemotherapeutic agents used in HIPEC

Agent	Molecular weight (Da)	Peritoneal fluid to plasma concentration ratio	Applications
5-Fluorouracil	130	300:1 [63]	PMP, gastric
Cisplatin	300	20:1 [57]	PMP, ovarian, mesothelioma, sarcoma
Doxorubicin	544	975:1 [62]	Ovarian, sarcoma
Floxuridine	246	2,000:1 [59]	PMP, CRC, gastric
Mitomycin C	334	75:1 [60]	PMP, CRC, gastric
Oxaliplatin	397	25:1 [58]	CRC, gastric
Paclitaxel	808	1,000:1 [61]	ovarian

PMP pseudomyxoma peritonei, *CRC* colorectal cancer

interface with decreased systemic absorption and toxicity [21]. Peritoneal to plasma drug concentration ratios vary depending on the molecular weight and water solubility of the agent used and may vary between 20:1 and 2,000:1 (Table 21.3) [19, 35, 56–63]. Selection of a particular agent is largely determined by the primary tumor or response to previous systemic chemotherapy.

Although one randomized-controlled trial was unable to demonstrate improved response rate with the addition of hyperthermia [64], heating the chemotherapy is believed to both increase the penetration of agents into tissue and enhance their cytotoxic effects [19, 65, 66]. In vitro studies have also shown that hyperthermia can lead to blunted angiogenesis, increased enzyme denaturation, and apoptosis [67]. The desired temperature of the perfusate in the abdomen ranges from 40 to 42 °C [14, 21], as temperatures greater than 42 °C have been associated with increased morbidity [68].

If perfusion with HIPEC is anticipated, the patient's core body temperature is cooled using a variety of passive means including lowering room temperature and ceasing to warm intravenous fluids and airway gases [2, 14, 69]. These maneuvers prevent systemic hyperthermia during hyperthermic peritoneal perfusion. The delivery of HIPEC to the patient has evolved into several different modalities (Table 21.4) [2, 70–73]. Each technique utilizes a closed continuous circuit to maintain consistent hyperthermia and temperature probes located at different points throughout the circuit to monitor the temperature. This circuit involves the use of inflow and outflow catheters carrying the perfusate to and from the abdominal cavity respectively, a pump, and a heat exchanger (Fig. 21.4). Once sufficient flow is established, the chemotherapeutic agent is added to the circuit. Although much debate exists regarding the optimal perfusion modality, the majority of experts agree that there is a lack of evidence favoring one modality over another [2].

One of the most common modalities is the closed abdominal technique (Fig. 21.5). This involves the placement of inflow and outflow catheters through the skin prior to suturing the skin closed in a watertight manner. Temporarily closing at the skin level and leaving the fascia opened allow contact of the perfusate to the abdominal wall. Once flow is established and chemotherapy is added, the abdomen is massaged by the operating room personnel to help distribute the perfusate throughout the abdomen. The increased pressure in the closed technique can facilitate deeper penetration of chemotherapeutic agents into tumor deposits [74, 75].

The open, or coliseum, technique involves suturing a plastic sheet to either side of the patient's skin incision and to the fixed retractor in effect extending the peritoneal cavity with a "coliseum-like" device. This allows the abdominal contents to float beyond the abdominal wall in a greater volume of perfusate theoretically increasing exposure of all surfaces to the chemotherapy. It also allows the surgeon to manipulate the intra-abdominal contents further facilitating equal distribution of heat and drug throughout the peritoneal cavity. Due to concern regarding exposure of operating room personnel to the chemotherapeutic agent, certain precautions are made

Table 21.4 Comparison of HIPEC modalities

Perfusion modality	Advantages	Disadvantages
Open abdomen (coliseum)	Equal exposure of all surfaces to perfusate Equal temperature distribution Easy access to abdominal cavity	Difficult to maintain high temperature Risk of contamination Risk of exposure to operating room personnel
Closed abdomen	Hyperthermia easily maintained Better tissue penetration Minimal risk of exposure to operating room personnel	Unequal exposure of all surfaces to perfusate Unequal temperature distribution
Peritoneal cavity expander [71]	Equal exposure of intra-abdominal contents to perfusate Equal temperature distribution	Separates abdominal wall from perfusate Risk of exposure to operating room personnel Complex
Abdominal cavity expander [72]	Equal exposure of all surfaces to perfusate Equal temperature distribution Minimal risk of exposure to operating room personnel	Complex
Containment instrument [73]	Equal exposure of all surfaces to perfusate Equal temperature distribution Easy access to abdominal cavity Minimal risk of exposure to operating room personnel	Complex

Based on data from Refs. [2, 70–73]

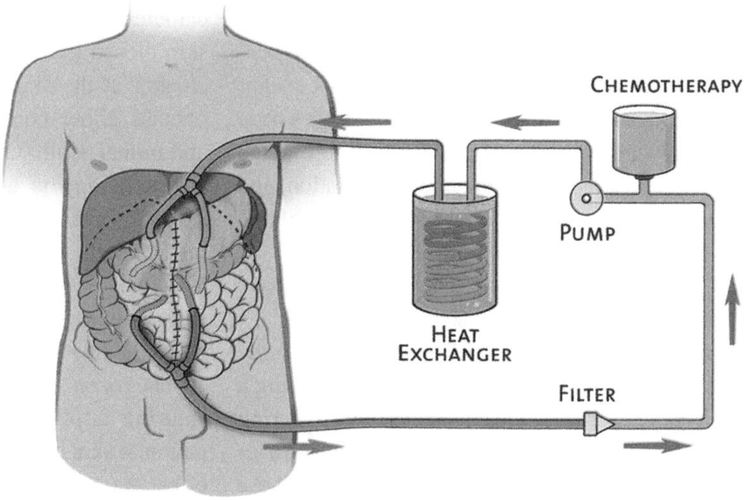

Fig. 21.4 Schematic of hyperthermic intraperitoneal chemotherapy perfusion circuit. (closed technique) (Reprinted from Shen et al. [154]. With permission from Springer Verlag)

including smoke evacuators, education and training of involved personnel, restriction of operating room traffic, filtration masks, and waterproof gowns [76].

Other modalities of perfusion have been developed in an attempt to combine the advantages of both the open and closed techniques. These attempts include the development of a peritoneal cavity expander by a Japanese group [71], an abdominal cavity expander by a French group [72], and an instrument to provide containment of the perfusate by Sugarbaker [73]. While these techniques generally provide equal drug and temperature distribution, they are generally complex and may not eliminate the risk of drug exposure to operating room personnel.

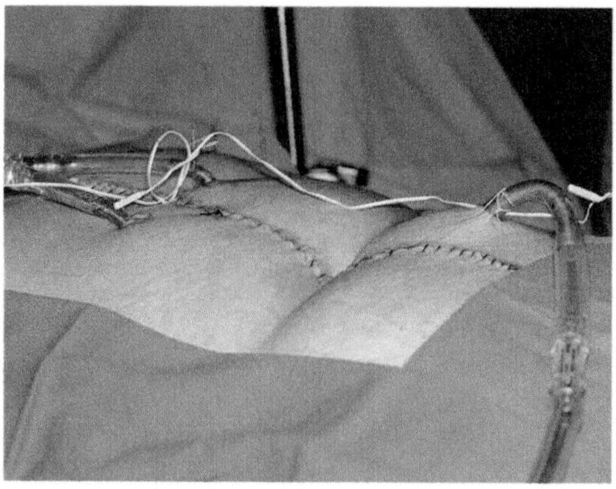

Fig. 21.5 Inflow and outflow catheters in the closed abdominal perfusion technique for hyperthermic intraperitoneal chemotherapy (Reprinted from Stewart et al. [35]. With permission from Springer Verlag)

Perfusion is generally maintained for 30–120 min depending on the primary and desired effect. Perfusion times may be decreased to avoid systemic absorption in patients deemed to be particularly susceptible. Factors that may make a patient more susceptible to drug toxicity include extensive peritonectomy, poor performance status, and old age [14]. Once perfusion is completed, the perfusate is drained, and the abdomen re-explored. Ostomies and anastomoses may be made at this time, and drains may be inserted. The abdomen is closed and the procedure is concluded.

Follow-Up

Patients are initially seen for a postoperative checkup 2–4 weeks following discharge from the hospital. Follow-up thereafter includes an examination, tumor markers, and CT imaging and ranges from 0- to 12-month intervals as recommended by a majority of clinicians [14, 33, 77–80].

Clinical Outcomes for CRS-HIPEC

Complete Cytoreduction

Much effort is devoted to selecting candidates whom will tolerate a complete cytoreduction and thus derive the maximal benefit of CRS-HIPEC [3]. Regardless of the primary tumor, resection status has been shown to be an important independent predictor of survival [14, 81–84]. Although the definition of a complete cytoreduction differs among institutions and primary tumors, the average rate of cytoreduction among high-volume centers is about 75 % [4]. Predictors of complete cytoreduction include good performance status, disease limited to the peritoneal cavity, no more than three resectable hepatic metastases, absence of biliary or ureteral obstruction, absence of more than one intestinal obstruction, absence of small bowel mesenteric implants, and limited disease in the gastrohepatic ligament [43].

Morbidity

Given the extent of the surgical resection required to achieve adequate cytoreduction morbidity is significant. Overall major morbidity following CRS-HIPEC ranges from 12 to 68 % though comparison between studies is difficult due to the lack of a universally accepted grading system [85]. Complications are frequently divided into two groups based on whether they are believed to have arisen from the operation itself or represent toxicity from the chemotherapeutic agent. A multi-institutional review examining the results of over 1,200 procedures found that common complications include reoperation (14 %), neutropenia (13 %), fistula (10 %), pneumonia (9 %), bleeding (8 %), abscess (7 %), sepsis (2 %), bowel obstruction (2 %), and renal insufficiency (1 %) [4]. In addition to bone marrow suppression and renal insufficiency, other observed toxicities attributed to the chemotherapeutic component include transient hepatic toxicity and ileus [27]. More than half of the patients are likely to require a blood transfusion at some point during their operation or hospitalization [36]. Predictors of morbidity include older age, higher PCI, greater number of visceral resections, poorer performance status, and higher drug dose [85, 86]. It is also important to note that morbidity is related to the experience of the center performing CRS-HIPEC as many large centers have displayed a substantial learning curve [85, 87].

Table 21.5 Survival following CRS-HIPEC for pseudomyxoma peritonei

First author	Year	*n*	Drug	5-year progression-free survival (%)	5-year survival (%)	10-year survival (%)
Deraco [93]	2004	33	MMC+CDDP	43	97	–
Stewart [97]	2006	110	MMC	–	53	–
Yan [99]	2006	50	MMC	–	69	–
Murphy [96]	2007	83	MMC	75	–	–
Smeenk [78]	2007	103	MMC	37	60	–
Cioppa [92]	2008	53	MMC+CDDP	80	94	85
Elias [94]	2008	105	Oxaliplatin	67	80	–
Baratti [91]	2009	102	MMC+CDDP	48	84	79
Vaira [98]	2009	60	MMC±CDDP	80	94	85
Elias [95]	2010	255	MMC or oxaliplatin	–	79	–
Arjona-Sanchez [90]	2013	38	MMC	49 (3 years)	59	–

CDDP cisplatin, *MMC* mitomycin C

Mortality

Operative mortality has been reported as high as 11 % following CRS-HIPEC but is generally about 4 % [35, 85]. Common causes of death are bowel perforation, respiratory failure, bone marrow suppression, thromboembolic events, and various infections. Preoperatively, the presence of ascites, bowel obstruction, and poor performance status predict mortality [35, 36].

Survival by Primary Tumor

Despite the significant rates of morbidity and mortality, CRS-HIPEC remains the only hope many of these patients have for long-term survival. Therefore, any legitimate evaluation of the complications following CRS-HIPEC must be compared to the inherent complications of PSD and its natural history without such treatment. In order to accurately represent expected outcomes, survival is discussed within the context of PSD arising from specific primary tumors.

Pseudomyxoma Peritonei

PMP most commonly results from the peritoneal seeding of ruptured mucinous appendiceal neoplasms and is the classic indication for CRS-HIPEC. PMP has been subdivided based on the relative proportions of mucin and epithelial cells. Disseminated peritoneal adenomucinosis (DPAM) consists primarily of mucin and rare, generally benign-appearing epithelial cells, while peritoneal mucinous carcinomatosis (PMCA) consists of less or no mucin and abundant epithelial cells with cytologic findings consistent with typical carcinomas. PSD with features of both DPAM (abundant mucin) and PMCA (malignant appearing cells) are grouped into a third category [52]. Recent work by our group demonstrated that PMP can be classified as either low grade or high grade with the intermediate cohort being considered low grade except for cases with a signet-ring cell component [88]. Patients with lower-grade lesions or a higher mucin to cell ratio experience better survival [52, 88].

Prior to CRS-HIPEC, patients were subjected to repeated debulking procedures with little hope for long-term survival [22, 33, 89]. Long-term survival following CRS-HIPEC is now common [78, 90–99], but direct comparisons between studies should be made with caution as each contains a different proportion of low- and high-grade lesions, all of which are considered PMP (Table 21.5). A recent multi-institutional review of outcomes following CRS and intraperitoneal chemotherapy (including 2,050 cases where HIPEC was used) reported a median progression-free survival of 98 months and a 10-year overall

Table 21.6 Survival following CRS-HIPEC for colorectal cancer

First author	Year	*n*	Drug	Median OS (months)	5-year survival (%)
Witkamp [100]	2001	29	MMC	–	23 (3 years)
Pilati [101]	2003	34	MMC + CDDP	18	–
Glehen [103]	2004	506	Multiple regimens	19	19
Glehen [104]	2004	53	MMC	13	11
da Silva [105]	2006	70	MMC	33	32
Zanon [106]	2006	25	MMC	30	40 (2 years)
Verwaal [102, 107]	2008	105	MMC	22	28 (3 years)
Shen [110]	2009	197	MMC	16	–
Elias [108]	2009	48	Oxaliplatin	63	51
Franko [109]	2010	67	MMC	35	25

OS Overall survival, *CDDP* cisplatin, *MMC* mitomycin C

survival rate of 63 % [84]. Thus, CRS-HIPEC has become the treatment of choice for patients with PMP due to the fact that it has a poor response to systemic chemotherapy and is universally fatal if left untreated [35]. Patients with the lowest-grade lesions amenable to complete resection may expect to do particularly well [33].

Colorectal Cancer

A consensus statement on the locoregional treatment of colorectal PSD recommends CRS-HIPEC as the treatment of choice for patients without distant metastatic disease and in whom complete cytoreduction is feasible [43]. This combined therapy has achieved 5-year survival rates in terminally ill patients ranging from 11 to 51 % (Table 21.6) [100–110]. Verwaal and colleagues [102, 107] have undertaken a phase III trial randomizing patients to standard chemotherapy and palliative surgery in cases of obstruction or CRS-HIPEC with a goal of complete cytoreduction prior to HIPEC. They found that disease-specific survival was better in the patients receiving CRS-HIPEC (22.2 months vs. 12.6 months, $p = 0.028$). Furthermore, 45 % of patients were alive at 5 years following complete macroscopic cytoreductions [102, 107]. Despite these results, HIPEC for this cohort has not been universally accepted in the oncology community, and controversy remains [43, 111].

Gastric Cancer

CRS-HIPEC for peritoneal carcinomatosis arising from gastric cancer has been heavily evaluated and has shown benefits over cytoreduction alone. A randomized control study comparing cytoreduction with HIPEC with cytoreduction without HIPEC observed a median overall survival of 6.5 months for the CRS arm and 11 months for the CRS-HIPEC arm [112]. A systematic review of the literature found that overall median survival for PSD from gastric cancer was 7.9 months, but complete CRS extended survival to 15 months [113]. Typical median survival for these patients following CRS-HIPEC ranges from 6 to 12 months (Table 21.7) [110, 112, 114–120]. Interestingly, HIPEC has also been evaluated in the adjuvant setting in high-risk patients at the time of their initial resection. In one randomized control study, HIPEC delayed recurrence and conferred a survival benefit in patients with either serosal invasion or lymph node metastasis [121].

Ovarian Cancer

Five-year survival rates for women diagnosed with advanced (stage III/IV) ovarian cancer remain low at less than 50 % for women younger than 65 and less than 30 % for women older than 65 [122]. Although ovarian cancer is often confined to the peritoneal cavity, many women

Table 21.7 Survival following CRS-HIPEC for gastric cancer

First author	Year	*n*	Drug	Median OS (months)	5-year survival (%)
Glehen [114]	2004	49	MMC	10	16
Hall [115]	2004	34	MMC	8	6
Yonemura [116]	2005	107	MMC + CDDP + etoposide	12	–
Scaringi [117]	2008	26	MMC + CDDP	7	–
Shen [110]	2009	43	MMC	6	–
Glehen [118]	2010	159	Multiple regimens	9	13
Yang [120]	2011	34	MMC + CDDP	11	6 (3 years)
Strohlein [112]	2011	34	MMC + CDDP	11	–

OS Overall survival, *CDDP* cisplatin, *MMC* mitomycin C

Table 21.8 Survival following CRS-HIPEC for ovarian cancer

First author	Year	*n*	Drug	Median PFS (months)	Median OS (months)	3-year survival (%)
Deraco [128]	2001	27	CDDP + MMC	16	22	55 (2 years)
de Bree [129]	2003	19	Docetaxel	–	–	63
Zanon [131]	2004	30	CDDP	17	28	60 (2 years)
Piso [130]	2004	19	CDDP or mitoxantrone	18	–	15 (5 years)
Reichman [132]	2005	13	CDDP	15	–	55
Armstrong [126]	2006	205	CDDP and paclitaxel[a]	24	66	–
Helm [133]	2007	18	CDDP or MMC	10	31	60
Carrabin [134]	2010	18	Oxaliplatin	10–17	–	83
Frenel [136]	2011	31	Oxaliplatin	13–14	–	–
Deraco [135]	2011	26	CDDP + doxorubicin	30	–	61
Parson [137]	2011	51	MMC, carboplatin, or paclitaxel	–	29	48
Spiliotis [83]	2011	24	–	–	19.4	50
Ansaloni [138]	2012	39	Multiple regimens	~12	–	~60
Fagotti [139]	2012	30	Oxaliplatin	26	–	68 (5 years)

[a]Early postoperative intraperitoneal chemotherapy instead of HIPEC
PFS Progression-free survival, *OS* Overall survival, *CDDP* cisplatin, *MMC* mitomycin C

present late with advanced-stage disease making these patients difficult to treat [123, 124].

A meta-analysis of over 6,000 patients with ovarian cancer showed that maximal cytoreduction was an independent predictor of better survival [125]. Armstrong and colleagues [126] performed a phase III randomized controlled trial of 415 patients with peritoneal spread of ovarian cancer and reported that following cytoreduction, the addition of early postoperative intraperitoneal cisplatin and paclitaxel to the routine management of patients conferred a significant progression-free and overall survival benefit [126]. Taken together, these results provide substantial evidence in favor of using CRS with some form of intraperitoneal chemotherapy for the treatment of ovarian carcinomatosis. Currently, three additional large-scale trials are underway evaluating carboplatin-based intraperitoneal chemotherapy for a broad range of patients with ovarian cancer [127]. Previously published reviews of the combination of CRS and HIPEC have reported a progression-free interval ranging from 10 to 30 months and a 5-year survival rate as high as 68 % (Table 21.8) [83, 128–139].

Peritoneal Mesothelioma

Peritoneal mesothelioma is rare with only two cases per million people in the United States, but given the origination of this malignancy from the

Table 21.9 Survival following CRS-HIPEC for peritoneal mesothelioma

First author	Year	*n*	Drug	Median OS (months)	5-year survival (%)
Costamagna [141]	2003	19	CDDP+MMC, CDDP+doxorubicin, or doxorubicin	40	–
Sugarbaker [142]	2003	68	Multiple regimens	67	–
Brigand [143]	2006	14	CDDP+MMC	36	–
Yan [144]	2009	405	Multiple regimens	53	47
Blackham [145]	2010	34	CDDP or MMC	41	17
Deraco [147]	2013	116	CDDP+MMC or CDDP+doxorubicin	40	49
Alexander [81]	2013	211	CDDP or MMC	38	41

OS Overall survival, *CDDP* cisplatin, *MMC* mitomycin C

Table 21.10 Survival following CRS-HIPEC for sarcomatosis

First author	Year	*n*	Excluded histologies	Drug	Median OS (months)	5-year survival (%)
Rossi [28]	2004	60	None	CDDP+doxorubicin	36	38
Lim [27]	2007	19	None	CDDP	17	–
Gusani [26]	2008	6	None	MMC	40	–
Baratti [25]	2010	37	None	CDDP+MMC or CDDP+doxorubicin	26	24
Salti [29]	2012	13	GIST, ULS	CDDP+doxorubicin	12	–
Randle [30]	2013	7	GIST, ULS	MMC±mitoxantrone	22	43

OS Overall survival, *CDDP* cisplatin, *MMC* mitomycin C, *GIST* gastrointestinal stromal tumor, *ULS* uterine leiomyosarcoma

peritoneal surface, all patients have an indication for CRS-HIPEC [35, 140]. Current median survival ranges between 36 and 41 months following CRS-HIPEC (Table 21.9) [141–146]. Although many regimens are used, some evidence suggests better outcomes with cisplatin than with mitomycin C [81, 145].

Sarcomatosis

CRS-HIPEC for patients with sarcomatosis is somewhat controversial given the tendency for sarcomas to spread hematogenously and resist chemotherapy. Median overall survival following CRS-HIPEC ranges from 3 to 40 months (Table 21.10) [25–30]. However, direct comparisons between studies are difficult given the varying proportions of complete resections and the differences in specific histologies included. A randomized control study revealed similar survival in patients randomized to CRS alone and those randomized to CRS with early postoperative intraperitoneal chemotherapy [17]. Furthermore, current studies achieve survival similar to historical controls of CRS alone prior to the induction of HIPEC [30, 147].

Quality of Life

Patient quality of life is another key outcome following CRS-HIPEC. Most reviews indicate that patients return to their baseline quality of life between 3 and 12 months postoperatively [27, 148–150]. One review reported a longer but meaningful recovery with emotional quality of life returning to baseline at 1 year, physical quality of life at 2 years, and social and cognitive quality of life at 3 years [151]. In fact, more than 90 % of patients surviving at least 3 years report minimal or no limitations in activity despite the fact that many of these patients will have recurrent disease [152]. Although depressive symptoms are common in patients with PSD, slight improvement is observed following CRS-HIPEC; yet, most patients will continue to experience significant sleep disturbances [150, 153]. Overall, reasonably good quality of life can be anticipated for patients recovering from CRS-HIPEC. The expected decrease in quality of life immediately following such therapy and its likelihood of persisting up to a year should be communicated openly to potential candidates of CRS-HIPEC, but not used as a justification for denying therapy [151].

Salient Points

- Peritoneal surface disease refers to the intra-abdominal dissemination of malignancy. CRS-HIPEC is a regional treatment modality combining surgical resection with locally administered chemotherapy.
- Current indications for CRS-HIPEC include PSD arising from appendiceal, colorectal, ovarian, gastric, or peritoneal mesothelioma primary tumors.
- Appropriate candidates for CRS-HIPEC should be fit for surgery and have a disease burden that is limited to the peritoneal cavity and amenable to complete or near-complete cytoreduction.
- Complete cytoreduction remains the goal of CRS. CRS consists of peritonectomy procedures and the removal of all involved tissue and organs not vital to the patients.
- HIPEC is most efficacious against microscopic diseases following a complete macroscopic cytoreduction. Other variables affecting its utility include tumor sensitivity, disease distribution, perfusate temperature, and drug concentration.
- Phase III trials support the application of cytoreduction and some form of intraperitoneal chemotherapy for colorectal and ovarian carcinomatosis.
- Although surgical morbidity is high and operative mortality is less than negligible, CRS-HIPEC is the treatment that is most likely to prolong survival in patients with peritoneal surface disease.

Questions

1. A 54-year-old woman is being evaluated for cytoreductive surgery with HIPEC for ovarian carcinomatosis. Her work-up should include all of the following EXCEPT:
   A. Thorough history and physical examination
   B. Laboratory evaluation of blood counts, electrolytes, and liver function
   C. Contrast-enhanced CT of the chest, abdomen, and pelvis
   D. Esophagogastroduodenoscopy
   E. Additional tests as determined by past medical history
2. A young, healthy man is referred to you for evaluation for cytoreductive surgery (CRS) and HIPEC. He was diagnosed by his local surgeon during a diagnostic laparoscopy and pathologic confirmation. His disease is limited and appears to originate from a high-grade appendiceal primary tumor. You determine that he is medically fit to undergo CRS-HIPEC. The next step in evaluation and management includes:
   A. Imaging to rule out extra-abdominal disease
   B. Repeat laparoscopy to estimate a peritoneal carcinomatosis index
   C. Diagnostic paracentesis
   D. Nutritional supplementation with parenteral nutrition
   E. Scheduling for CRS-HIPEC
3. A 47-year-old man is being evaluated for cytoreductive surgery with HIPEC for peritoneal surface disease originating from an appendiceal primary tumor. Which of the following scenarios would be associated with the most favorable outcomes?
   A. Low-grade disease with diffuse involvement of small bowel mesentery
   B. Low-grade disease involving the right-lower-quadrant peritoneal surfaces
   C. Low-grade disease with massive malignant ascites
   D. High-grade disease limited to the pelvis
   E. High-grade disease with a 1 cm focus in the right lung parenchyma
4. Several patients with peritoneal surface disease are presenting for evaluation for possible cytoreductive surgery with HIPEC. Which of the following patients represents the best candidate for such therapy?
   A. A 72-year-old man with clearly resectable disease, emphysema, and renal insufficiency

B. A 35-year-old man with a tumor invading his retroperitoneum
C. A 58-year-old woman with a negative CT scan but pathology confirmed peritoneal surface disease from a diagnostic laparoscopy
D. A 45-year-old woman with an albumin of 2.7 and two areas of partial small bowel obstruction
E. A 66-year-old woman with a parenchymal hepatic metastasis and an Eastern Cooperative Oncology Group performance status of 3.

5. Upon initial exploration of a patient with peritoneal surface disease, you note sparing of the entire small bowel and mesentery, but the central, right-lower, and pelvic regions all have tumor deposits greater than 5 cm in diameter. What is the peritoneal carcinomatosis index (PCI) score?
   A. 3
   B. 6
   C. 9
   D. 12
   E. 15
6. A 62-year-old man is being admitted in preparation of his cytoreductive surgery with HIPEC tomorrow. Although his primary tumor was resected 1 year ago, he had extensive disease in his pelvis visible on a CT scan performed in clinic 2 weeks ago. His preoperative preparation should include all of the following EXCEPT:
   A. Interval history and physical
   B. Blood typing and crossmatch
   C. Bowel preparation
   D. Urology consult for possible ureteral stent placement
   E. Repeat CT scan to evaluate for tumor progression
7. You are performing cytoreductive surgery with HIPEC on a 52-year-old man for a low-grade appendiceal neoplasm with peritoneal dissemination. You have lysed all adhesions and have resected all visible disease. The next step in management is to:
   A. Conclude the procedure because HIPEC is no longer necessary
   B. Conclude the procedure and await final pathology to determine if HIPEC is necessary
   C. Perform HIPEC only if frozen sections return with microscopic positive margins
   D. Prepare for HIPEC only if the tumor ruptured during resection
   E. Begin passively cooling the patient while you prepare to administer HIPEC
8. A 47-year-old woman is undergoing HIPEC for peritoneal carcinomatosis from a colonic primary tumor. All of the following are thought to influence the efficacy of HIPEC EXCEPT:
   A. Size of the tumor implant
   B. Temperature of the tumor implant
   C. Distribution of HIPEC within the peritoneal cavity
   D. Ratio of mucin to tumor
   E. Location of the primary tumor along the colon

Answers

1. D
2. A
3. B
4. C
5. C
6. E
7. E
8. E

References

1. Sugarbaker PH. Cytoreductive surgery and perioperative intraperitoneal chemotherapy as a curative approach to pseudomyxoma peritonei syndrome. Eur J Surg Oncol. 2001;27(3):239–43.
2. Glehen O, Cotte E, Kusamura S, Deraco M, Baratti D, Passot G, et al. Hyperthermic intraperitoneal chemotherapy: nomenclature and modalities of perfusion. J Surg Oncol. 2008;98(4):242–6.
3. Al-Shammaa HA, Li Y, Yonemura Y. Current status and future strategies of cytoreductive surgery plus intraperitoneal hyperthermic chemotherapy for peritoneal carcinomatosis. World J Gastroenterol. 2008; 14(8):1159–66.
4. Glehen O, Gilly FN, Boutitie F, Bereder JM, Quenet F, Sideris L, et al. Toward curative treatment of peritoneal carcinomatosis from nonovarian origin by

cytoreductive surgery combined with perioperative intraperitoneal chemotherapy: a multi-institutional study of 1,290 patients. Cancer. 2010;116(24):5608–18.
5. Blair SL, Chu DZ, Schwarz RE. Outcome of palliative operations for malignant bowel obstruction in patients with peritoneal carcinomatosis from nongynecological cancer. Ann Surg Oncol. 2001;8(8):632–7.
6. Jayne DG, Fook S, Loi C, Seow-Choen F. Peritoneal carcinomatosis from colorectal cancer. Br J Surg. 2002;89(12):1545–50.
7. Sadeghi B, Arvieux C, Glehen O, Beaujard AC, Rivoire M, Baulieux J, et al. Peritoneal carcinomatosis from non-gynecologic malignancies: results of the EVOCAPE 1 multicentric prospective study. Cancer. 2000;88(2):358–63.
8. Sugarbaker PH. Peritonectomy procedures. Ann Surg. 1995;221(1):29–42.
9. Sugarbaker PH. Parietal peritonectomy. Ann Surg Oncol. 2012;19(4):1250.
10. Torisu M, Katano M, Kimura Y, Itoh H, Takesue M. New approach to management of malignant ascites with a streptococcal preparation, OK-432. I. Improvement of host immunity and prolongation of survival. Surgery. 1983;93(3):357–64.
11. Hendren SK, Hahn SM, Spitz FR, Bauer TW, Rubin SC, Zhu T, et al. Phase II trial of debulking surgery and photodynamic therapy for disseminated intraperitoneal tumors. Ann Surg Oncol. 2001;8(1):65–71.
12. Sindelar WF, DeLaney TF, Tochner Z, Thomas GF, Dachoswki LJ, Smith PD, et al. Technique of photodynamic therapy for disseminated intraperitoneal malignant neoplasms. Phase I study. Arch Surg. 1991;126(3):318–24.
13. Bauer TW, Hahn SM, Spitz FR, Kachur A, Glatstein E, Fraker DL. Preliminary report of photodynamic therapy for intraperitoneal sarcomatosis. Ann Surg Oncol. 2001;8(3):254–9.
14. Levine EA, Stewart JH, Russell GB, Geisinger KR, Loggie BL, Shen P. Cytoreductive surgery and intraperitoneal hyperthermic chemotherapy for peritoneal surface malignancy: experience with 501 procedures. J Am Coll Surg. 2007;204(5):943–53.
15. Beaujard AC, Glehen O, Caillot JL, Francois Y, Bienvenu J, Panteix G, et al. Intraperitoneal chemohyperthermia with mitomycin C for digestive tract cancer patients with peritoneal carcinomatosis. Cancer. 2000;88(11):2512–9.
16. Sugarbaker PH, Jablonski KA. Prognostic features of 51 colorectal and 130 appendiceal cancer patients with peritoneal carcinomatosis treated by cytoreductive surgery and intraperitoneal chemotherapy. Ann Surg. 1995;221(2):124–32.
17. Bonvalot S, Cavalcanti A, Le Péchoux C, Terrier P, Vanel D, Blay JY, et al. Randomized trial of cytoreduction followed by intraperitoneal chemotherapy versus cytoreduction alone in patients with peritoneal sarcomatosis. Eur J Surg Oncol. 2005;31(8):917–23.
18. Averbach AM, Sugarbaker PH. Methodologic considerations in treatment using intraperitoneal chemotherapy. Cancer Treat Res. 1996;82:289–309.
19. Sugarbaker PH. Intraperitoneal chemotherapy and cytoreductive surgery for the prevention and treatment of peritoneal carcinomatosis and sarcomatosis. Semin Surg Oncol. 1998;14(3):254–61.
20. Gonzalez-Moreno S. Peritoneal surface oncology: a progress report. Eur J Surg Oncol. 2006;32(6):593–6.
21. Glockzin G, Schlitt HJ, Piso P. Peritoneal carcinomatosis: patients selection, perioperative complications and quality of life related to cytoreductive surgery and hyperthermic intraperitoneal chemotherapy. World J Surg Oncol. 2009;7:5.
22. Sugarbaker PH. New standard of care for appendiceal epithelial neoplasms and pseudomyxoma peritonei syndrome? Lancet Oncol. 2006;7(1):69–76.
23. Chua TC, Koh JL, Yan TD, Liauw W, Morris DL. Cytoreductive surgery and perioperative intraperitoneal chemotherapy for peritoneal carcinomatosis from small bowel adenocarcinoma. J Surg Oncol. 2009;100(2):139–43.
24. Jacks SP, Hundley JC, Shen P, Russell GB, Levine EA. Cytoreductive surgery and intraperitoneal hyperthermic chemotherapy for peritoneal carcinomatosis from small bowel adenocarcinoma. J Surg Oncol. 2005;91(2):112–7.
25. Baratti D, Pennacchioli E, Kusamura S, Fiore M, Balestra MR, Colombo C, et al. Peritoneal sarcomatosis: is there a subset of patients who may benefit from cytoreductive surgery and hyperthermic intraperitoneal chemotherapy? Ann Surg Oncol. 2010;17(12):3220–8.
26. Gusani NJ, Cho SW, Colovos C, Seo S, Franko J, Richard SD, et al. Aggressive surgical management of peritoneal carcinomatosis with low mortality in a high-volume tertiary cancer center. Ann Surg Oncol. 2008;15(3):754–63.
27. Lim SJ, Cormier JN, Feig BW, Mansfield PF, Benjamin RS, Griffin JR, et al. Toxicity and outcomes associated with surgical cytoreduction and hyperthermic intraperitoneal chemotherapy (HIPEC) for patients with sarcomatosis. Ann Surg Oncol. 2007;14(8):2309–18.
28. Rossi CR, Deraco M, De Simone M, Mocellin S, Pilati P, Foletto M, et al. Hyperthermic intraperitoneal intraoperative chemotherapy after cytoreductive surgery for the treatment of abdominal sarcomatosis: clinical outcome and prognostic factors in 60 consecutive patients. Cancer. 2004;100(9):1943–50.
29. Salti GI, Ailabouni L, Undevia S. Cytoreductive surgery and hyperthermic intraperitoneal chemotherapy for the treatment of peritoneal sarcomatosis. Ann Surg Oncol. 2012;19(5):1410–5.
30. Randle RW, Swett KR, Shen P, Stewart JH, Levine EA, Votanopoulos KI. Cytoreductive surgery with hyperthermic intraperitoneal chemotherapy in peritoneal sarcomatosis. Am Surg. 2013;79(6):620–4.

31. Bakrin N, Cotte E, Sayag-Beaujard A, Raudrant D, Isaac S, Mohamed F, et al. Cytoreductive surgery with hyperthermic intraperitoneal chemotherapy for the treatment of recurrent endometrial carcinoma confined to the peritoneal cavity. Int J Gynecol Cancer. 2010;20(5):809–14.
32. Krane LS, Kader AK, Levine EA. Cytoreductive surgery with hyperthermic intraperitoneal chemotherapy for patients with peritoneal carcinomatosis secondary to urachal adenocarcinoma. J Surg Oncol. 2012;105(3):258–60.
33. Moran B, Baratti D, Yan TD, Kusamura S, Deraco M. Consensus statement on the loco-regional treatment of appendiceal mucinous neoplasms with peritoneal dissemination (pseudomyxoma peritonei). J Surg Oncol. 2008;98(4):277–82.
34. Sulkin TV, O'Neill H, Amin AI, Moran B. CT in pseudomyxoma peritonei: a review of 17 cases. Clin Radiol. 2002;57(7):608–13.
35. Stewart JH, Shen P, Levine EA. Intraperitoneal hyperthermic chemotherapy for peritoneal surface malignancy: current status and future directions. Ann Surg Oncol. 2005;12(10):765–77.
36. Shen P, Levine EA, Hall J, Case D, Russell G, Fleming R, et al. Factors predicting survival after intraperitoneal hyperthermic chemotherapy with mitomycin C after cytoreductive surgery for patients with peritoneal carcinomatosis. Arch Surg. 2003;138(1):26–33.
37. Sugarbaker PH, Chang D. Results of treatment of 385 patients with peritoneal surface spread of appendiceal malignancy. Ann Surg Oncol. 1999;6(8):727–31.
38. Randle RW, Swett KR, Swords DS, Shen P, Stewart JH, Levine EA, Votanopoulos KI. Efficacy of cytoreductive surgery with hyperthermic intraperitoneal chemotherapy in the management of malignant ascites. Ann Surg Oncol. 2014;21(5):1474-9.
39. Jacquet P, Jelinek JS, Steves MA, Sugarbaker PH. Evaluation of computed tomography in patients with peritoneal carcinomatosis. Cancer. 1993;72(5):1631–6.
40. Jacquet P, Jelinek JS, Chang D, Koslowe P, Sugarbaker PH. Abdominal computed tomographic scan in the selection of patients with mucinous peritoneal carcinomatosis for cytoreductive surgery. J Am Coll Surg. 1995;181(6):530–8.
41. Kubik-Huch RA, Dorffler W, von Schulthess GK, Marincek B, Kochli OR, Seifert B, et al. Value of (18F)-FDG positron emission tomography, computed tomography, and magnetic resonance imaging in diagnosing primary and recurrent ovarian carcinoma. Eur Radiol. 2000;10(5):761–7.
42. Low RN, Barone RM, Lacey C, Sigeti JS, Alzate GD, Sebrechts CP. Peritoneal tumor: MR imaging with dilute oral barium and intravenous gadolinium-containing contrast agents compared with unenhanced MR imaging and CT. Radiology. 1997;204(2):513–20.
43. Esquivel J, Elias D, Baratti D, Kusamura S, Deraco M. Consensus statement on the loco regional treatment of colorectal cancer with peritoneal dissemination. J Surg Oncol. 2008;98(4):263–7.
44. Rose PG, Faulhaber P, Miraldi F, Abdul-Karim FW. Positive emission tomography for evaluating a complete clinical response in patients with ovarian or peritoneal carcinoma: correlation with second-look laparotomy. Gynecol Oncol. 2001;82(1):17–21.
45. Helm CW, Bristow RE, Kusamura S, Baratti D, Deraco M. Hyperthermic intraperitoneal chemotherapy with and without cytoreductive surgery for epithelial ovarian cancer. J Surg Oncol. 2008;98(4):283–90.
46. Nougaret S, Addley HC, Colombo PE, Fujii S, Al Sharif SS, Tirumani SH, et al. Ovarian carcinomatosis: how the radiologist can help plan the surgical approach. Radiographics. 2012;32(6):1775–800.
47. Garofalo A, Valle M. Staging videolaparoscopy of peritoneal carcinomatosis. Tumori. 2003;89(4 Suppl):70–7.
48. Pomel C, Appleyard TL, Gouy S, Rouzier R, Elias D. The role of laparoscopy to evaluate candidates for complete cytoreduction of peritoneal carcinomatosis and hyperthermic intraperitoneal chemotherapy. Eur J Surg Oncol. 2005;31(5):540–3.
49. Gilly FN, Carry PY, Sayag AC, Brachet A, Panteix G, Salle B, et al. Regional chemotherapy (with mitomycin C) and intra-operative hyperthermia for digestive cancers with peritoneal carcinomatosis. Hepatogastroenterology. 1994;41(2):124–9.
50. Portilla AG, Sugarbaker PH, Chang D. Second-look surgery after cytoreduction and intraperitoneal chemotherapy for peritoneal carcinomatosis from colorectal cancer: analysis of prognostic features. World J Surg. 1999;23(1):23–9.
51. Rey Y, Porcheron J, Talabard JN, Szafnicki K, Balique JG. Peritoneal carcinomatosis treated by cytoreductive surgery and intraperitoneal chemohyperthermia. Ann Chir. 2000;125(7):631–42.
52. Ronnett BM, Zahn CM, Kurman RJ, Kass ME, Sugarbaker PH, Shmookler BM. Disseminated peritoneal adenomucinosis and peritoneal mucinous carcinomatosis. A clinicopathologic analysis of 109 cases with emphasis on distinguishing pathologic features, site of origin, prognosis, and relationship to "pseudomyxoma peritonei". Am J Surg Pathol. 1995;19(12):1390–408.
53. Berthet B, Sugarbaker TA, Chang D, Sugarbaker PH. Quantitative methodologies for selection of patients with recurrent abdominopelvic sarcoma for treatment. Eur J Cancer. 1999;35(3):413–9.
54. Sebbag G, Sugarbaker PH. Peritoneal mesothelioma proposal for a staging system. Eur J Surg Oncol. 2001;27(3):223–4.
55. Tentes AA, Tripsiannis G, Markakidis SK, Karanikiotis CN, Tzegas G, Georgiadis G, et al. Peritoneal cancer index: a prognostic indicator of survival in advanced ovarian cancer. Eur J Surg Oncol. 2003;29(1):69–73.

56. Jacquet P, Sugarbaker PH. Peritoneal-plasma barrier. Cancer Treat Res. 1996;82:53–63.
57. Bartlett DL, Buell JF, Libutti SK, Reed E, Lee KB, Figg WD, et al. A phase I trial of continuous hyperthermic peritoneal perfusion with tumor necrosis factor and cisplatin in the treatment of peritoneal carcinomatosis. Cancer. 1998;83(6):1251–61.
58. Elias D, Bonnay M, Puizillou JM, Antoun S, Demirdjian S, El OA, et al. Heated intra-operative intraperitoneal oxaliplatin after complete resection of peritoneal carcinomatosis: pharmacokinetics and tissue distribution. Ann Oncol. 2002;13(2):267–72.
59. Israel VK, Jiang C, Muggia FM, Tulpule A, Jeffers S, Leichman L, et al. Intraperitoneal 5-fluoro-2′-deoxyuridine (FUDR) and (S)-leucovorin for disease predominantly confined to the peritoneal cavity: a pharmacokinetic and toxicity study. Cancer Chemother Pharmacol. 1995;37(1–2):32–8.
60. Kuzuya T, Yamauchi M, Ito A, Hasegawa M, Hasegawa T, Nabeshima T. Pharmacokinetic characteristics of 5-fluorouracil and mitomycin C in intraperitoneal chemotherapy. J Pharm Pharmacol. 1994;46(8):685–9.
61. Markman M, Brady MF, Spirtos NM, Hanjani P, Rubin SC. Phase II trial of intraperitoneal paclitaxel in carcinoma of the ovary, tube, and peritoneum: a Gynecologic Oncology Group Study. J Clin Oncol. 1998;16(8):2620–4.
62. Ozols RF, Young RC, Speyer JL, Sugarbaker PH, Greene R, Jenkins J, et al. Phase I and pharmacological studies of adriamycin administered intraperitoneally to patients with ovarian cancer. Cancer Res. 1982;42(10):4265–9.
63. Speyer JL, Collins JM, Dedrick RL, Brennan MF, Buckpitt AR, Londer H, et al. Phase I and pharmacological studies of 5-fluorouracil administered intraperitoneally. Cancer Res. 1980;40(3): 567–72.
64. Fujimura T, Yonemura Y, Muraoka K, Takamura H, Hirono Y, Sahara H, et al. Continuous hyperthermic peritoneal perfusion for the prevention of peritoneal recurrence of gastric cancer: randomized controlled study. World J Surg. 1994;18(1):150–5.
65. Elias DM, Ouellet JF. Intraperitoneal chemohyperthermia: rationale, technique, indications, and results. Surg Oncol Clin N Am. 2001;10(4):915–33, xi.
66. Glehen O, Mohamed F, Gilly FN. Peritoneal carcinomatosis from digestive tract cancer: new management by cytoreductive surgery and intraperitoneal chemohyperthermia. Lancet Oncol. 2004; 5(4):219–28.
67. Sugarbaker PH. Laboratory and clinical basis for hyperthermia as a component of intracavitary chemotherapy. Int J Hyperthermia. 2007;23(5):431–42.
68. Jacquet P, Stephens AD, Averbach AM, Chang D, Ettinghausen SE, Dalton RR, et al. Analysis of morbidity and mortality in 60 patients with peritoneal carcinomatosis treated by cytoreductive surgery and heated intraoperative intraperitoneal chemotherapy. Cancer. 1996;77(12):2622–9.
69. Sarnaik AA, Sussman JJ, Ahmad SA, Lowy AM. Technology of intraperitoneal chemotherapy administration: a survey of techniques with a review of morbidity and mortality. Surg Oncol Clin N Am. 2003;12(3):849–63.
70. Sarnaik AA, Sussman JJ, Ahmad SA, McIntyre BC, Lowy AM. Technology for the delivery of hyperthermic intraoperative intraperitoneal chemotherapy: a survey of techniques. Recent Results Cancer Res. 2007;169:75–82.
71. Fujimura T, Yonemura Y, Fushida S, Urade M, Takegawa S, Kamata T, et al. Continuous hyperthermic peritoneal perfusion for the treatment of peritoneal dissemination in gastric cancers and subsequent second-look operation. Cancer. 1990;65(1):65–71.
72. Rat P, Benoit L, Cheynel N, Osmak L, Favoulet P, Peschaud F, et al. Intraperitoneal chemohyperthermia with “overflow” open abdomen. Ann Chir. 2001;126(7):669–71.
73. Sugarbaker PH. An instrument to provide containment of intraoperative intraperitoneal chemotherapy with optimized distribution. J Surg Oncol. 2005; 92(2):142–6.
74. Esquis P, Consolo D, Magnin G, Pointaire P, Moretto P, Ynsa MD, et al. High intra-abdominal pressure enhances the penetration and antitumor effect of intraperitoneal cisplatin on experimental peritoneal carcinomatosis. Ann Surg. 2006;244(1):106–12.
75. Jacquet P, Stuart OA, Chang D, Sugarbaker PH. Effects of intra-abdominal pressure on pharmacokinetics and tissue distribution of doxorubicin after intraperitoneal administration. Anticancer Drugs. 1996;7(5):596–603.
76. Gonzalez-Bayon L, Gonzalez-Moreno S, Ortega-Perez G. Safety considerations for operating room personnel during hyperthermic intraoperative intraperitoneal chemotherapy perfusion. Eur J Surg Oncol. 2006;32(6):619–24.
77. Yan TD, Bijelic L, Sugarbaker PH. Critical analysis of treatment failure after complete cytoreductive surgery and perioperative intraperitoneal chemotherapy for peritoneal dissemination from appendiceal mucinous neoplasms. Ann Surg Oncol. 2007; 14(8):2289–99.
78. Smeenk RM, Verwaal VJ, Antonini N, Zoetmulder FA. Survival analysis of pseudomyxoma peritonei patients treated by cytoreductive surgery and hyperthermic intraperitoneal chemotherapy. Ann Surg. 2007;245(1):104–9.
79. Bijelic L, Yan TD, Sugarbaker PH. Treatment failure following complete cytoreductive surgery and perioperative intraperitoneal chemotherapy for peritoneal dissemination from colorectal or appendiceal mucinous neoplasms. J Surg Oncol. 2008;98(4):295–9.
80. Deraco M, Bartlett D, Kusamura S, Baratti D. Consensus statement on peritoneal mesothelioma. J Surg Oncol. 2008;98(4):268–72.
81. Alexander Jr HR, Bartlett DL, Pingpank JF, Libutti SK, Royal R, Hughes MS, et al. Treatment factors associated with long-term survival after cytoreductive

surgery and regional chemotherapy for patients with malignant peritoneal mesothelioma. Surgery. 2013;153(6):779–86.
82. Van Sweringen HL, Hanseman DJ, Ahmad SA, Edwards MJ, Sussman JJ. Predictors of survival in patients with high-grade peritoneal metastases undergoing cytoreductive surgery and hyperthermic intraperitoneal chemotherapy. Surgery. 2012; 152(4):617–24.
83. Spiliotis J, Vaxevanidou A, Sergouniotis F, Lambropoulou E, Datsis A, Christopoulou A. The role of cytoreductive surgery and hyperthermic intraperitoneal chemotherapy in the management of recurrent advanced ovarian cancer: a prospective study. J BUON. 2011;16(1):74–9.
84. Chua TC, Moran BJ, Sugarbaker PH, Levine EA, Glehen O, Gilly FN, et al. Early- and long-term outcome data of patients with pseudomyxoma peritonei from appendiceal origin treated by a strategy of cytoreductive surgery and hyperthermic intraperitoneal chemotherapy. J Clin Oncol. 2012;30(20):2449–56.
85. Mohamed F, Moran BJ. Morbidity and mortality with cytoreductive surgery and intraperitoneal chemotherapy: the importance of a learning curve. Cancer J. 2009;15(3):196–9.
86. Baratti D, Kusamura S, Mingrone E, Balestra MR, Laterza B, Deraco M. Identification of a subgroup of patients at highest risk for complications after surgical cytoreduction and hyperthermic intraperitoneal chemotherapy. Ann Surg. 2012;256(2):334–41.
87. Kusamura S, Baratti D, Deraco M. Multidimensional analysis of the learning curve for cytoreductive surgery and hyperthermic intraperitoneal chemotherapy in peritoneal surface malignancies. Ann Surg. 2012;255(2):348–56.
88. Bradley RF, Stewart JH, Russell GB, Levine EA, Geisinger KR. Pseudomyxoma peritonei of appendiceal origin: a clinicopathologic analysis of 101 patients uniformly treated at a single institution, with literature review. Am J Surg Pathol. 2006;30(5):551–9.
89. Moran BJ, Cecil TD. The etiology, clinical presentation, and management of pseudomyxoma peritonei. Surg Oncol Clin N Am. 2003;12(3):585–603.
90. Arjona-Sanchez A, Munoz-Casares FC, Casado-Adam A, Sanchez-Hidalgo JM, Ayllon Teran MD, Orti-Rodriguez R, et al. Outcome of patients with aggressive pseudomyxoma peritonei treated by cytoreductive surgery and intraperitoneal chemotherapy. World J Surg. 2013;37(6):1263–70.
91. Baratti D, Kusamura S, Nonaka D, Cabras AD, Laterza B, Deraco M. Pseudomyxoma peritonei: biological features are the dominant prognostic determinants after complete cytoreduction and hyperthermic intraperitoneal chemotherapy. Ann Surg. 2009;249(2):243–9.
92. Cioppa T, Vaira M, Bing C, D'Amico S, Bruscino A, De Simone M. Cytoreduction and hyperthermic intraperitoneal chemotherapy in the treatment of peritoneal carcinomatosis from pseudomyxoma peritonei. World J Gastroenterol. 2008;14(44):6817–23.
93. Deraco M, Baratti D, Inglese MG, Allaria B, Andreola S, Gavazzi C, et al. Peritonectomy and intraperitoneal hyperthermic perfusion (IPHP): a strategy that has confirmed its efficacy in patients with pseudomyxoma peritonei. Ann Surg Oncol. 2004;11(4):393–8.
94. Elias D, Honore C, Ciuchendea R, Billard V, Raynard B, Lo DR, et al. Peritoneal pseudomyxoma: results of a systematic policy of complete cytoreductive surgery and hyperthermic intraperitoneal chemotherapy. Br J Surg. 2008;95(9):1164–71.
95. Elias D, Gilly F, Quenet F, Bereder JM, Sideris L, Mansvelt B, et al. Pseudomyxoma peritonei: a French multicentric study of 301 patients treated with cytoreductive surgery and intraperitoneal chemotherapy. Eur J Surg Oncol. 2010;36(5):456–62.
96. Murphy EM, Sexton R, Moran BJ. Early results of surgery in 123 patients with pseudomyxoma peritonei from a perforated appendiceal neoplasm. Dis Colon Rectum. 2007;50(1):37–42.
97. Stewart JH, Shen P, Russell GB, Bradley RF, Hundley JC, Loggie BL, et al. Appendiceal neoplasms with peritoneal dissemination: outcomes after cytoreductive surgery and intraperitoneal hyperthermic chemotherapy. Ann Surg Oncol. 2006;13(5):624–34.
98. Vaira M, Cioppa T, DE Marco G, Bing C, D'Amico S, D'Alessandro M, et al. Management of pseudomyxoma peritonei by cytoreduction+HIPEC (hyperthermic intraperitoneal chemotherapy): results analysis of a twelve-year experience. In Vivo. 2009;23(4):639–44.
99. Yan TD, Links M, Xu ZY, Kam PC, Glenn D, Morris DL. Cytoreductive surgery and perioperative intraperitoneal chemotherapy for pseudomyxoma peritonei from appendiceal mucinous neoplasms. Br J Surg. 2006;93(10):1270–6.
100. Witkamp AJ, de Bree E, Kaag MM, van Slooten GW, van Coevorden F, Zoetmulder FA. Extensive surgical cytoreduction and intraoperative hyperthermic intraperitoneal chemotherapy in patients with pseudomyxoma peritonei. Br J Surg. 2001;88(3): 458–63.
101. Pilati P, Mocellin S, Rossi CR, Foletto M, Campana L, Nitti D, et al. Cytoreductive surgery combined with hyperthermic intraperitoneal intraoperative chemotherapy for peritoneal carcinomatosis arising from colon adenocarcinoma. Ann Surg Oncol. 2003;10(5):508–13.
102. Verwaal VJ, van Ruth S, de Bree E, van Slothen GW, van Tinteren H, Boot H, et al. Randomized trial of cytoreduction and hyperthermic intraperitoneal chemotherapy versus systemic chemotherapy and palliative surgery in patients with peritoneal carcinomatosis of colorectal cancer. J Clin Oncol. 2003;21(20):3737–43.
103. Glehen O, Kwiatkowski F, Sugarbaker PH, Elias D, Levine EA, De Simone M, et al. Cytoreductive surgery combined with perioperative intraperitoneal chemotherapy for the management of peritoneal

carcinomatosis from colorectal cancer: a multi-institutional study. J Clin Oncol. 2004;22(16): 3284–92.
104. Glehen O, Cotte E, Schreiber V, Sayag-Beaujard AC, Vignal J, Gilly FN. Intraperitoneal chemohyperthermia and attempted cytoreductive surgery in patients with peritoneal carcinomatosis of colorectal origin. Br J Surg. 2004;91(6):747–54.
105. da Silva RG, Sugarbaker PH. Analysis of prognostic factors in seventy patients having a complete cytoreduction plus perioperative intraperitoneal chemotherapy for carcinomatosis from colorectal cancer. J Am Coll Surg. 2006;203(6):878–86.
106. Zanon C, Bortolini M, Chiappino I, Simone P, Bruno F, Gaglia P, et al. Cytoreductive surgery combined with intraperitoneal chemohyperthermia for the treatment of advanced colon cancer. World J Surg. 2006;30(11):2025–32.
107. Verwaal VJ, Bruin S, Boot H, van Slooten G, van Tinteren H. 8-year follow-up of randomized trial: cytoreduction and hyperthermic intraperitoneal chemotherapy versus systemic chemotherapy in patients with peritoneal carcinomatosis of colorectal cancer. Ann Surg Oncol. 2008;15(9):2426–32.
108. Elias D, Lefevre JH, Chevalier J, Brouquet A, Marchal F, Classe JM, et al. Complete cytoreductive surgery plus intraperitoneal chemohyperthermia with oxaliplatin for peritoneal carcinomatosis of colorectal origin. J Clin Oncol. 2009;27(5):681–5.
109. Franko J, Ibrahim Z, Gusani NJ, Holtzman MP, Bartlett DL, Zeh III HJ. Cytoreductive surgery and hyperthermic intraperitoneal chemoperfusion versus systemic chemotherapy alone for colorectal peritoneal carcinomatosis. Cancer. 2010;116(16):3756–62.
110. Shen P, Stewart JH, Levine EA. Cytoreductive surgery and intraperitoneal hyperthermic chemotherapy for peritoneal surface malignancy: non-colorectal indications. Curr Probl Cancer. 2009;33(3):168–93.
111. Newman NA, Votanopoulos KL, Stewart JH, Shen P, Levine EA. Cytoreductive surgery and hyperthermic intraperitoneal chemotherapy for colorectal cancer. Minerva Chir. 2012;67(4):309–18.
112. Strohlein MA, Bulian DR, Heiss MM. Clinical efficacy of cytoreductive surgery and hyperthermic chemotherapy in peritoneal carcinomatosis from gastric cancer. Expert Rev Anticancer Ther. 2011;11(10):1505–8.
113. Gill RS, Al-Adra DP, Nagendran J, Campbell S, Shi X, Haase E, et al. Treatment of gastric cancer with peritoneal carcinomatosis by cytoreductive surgery and HIPEC: a systematic review of survival, mortality, and morbidity. J Surg Oncol. 2011;104(6):692–8.
114. Glehen O, Schreiber V, Cotte E, Sayag-Beaujard AC, Osinsky D, Freyer G, et al. Cytoreductive surgery and intraperitoneal chemohyperthermia for peritoneal carcinomatosis arising from gastric cancer. Arch Surg. 2004;139(1):20–6.
115. Hall JJ, Loggie BW, Shen P, Beamer S, Douglas CL, McQuellon R, et al. Cytoreductive surgery with intraperitoneal hyperthermic chemotherapy for advanced gastric cancer. J Gastrointest Surg. 2004;8(4):454–63.
116. Yonemura Y, Kawamura T, Bandou E, Takahashi S, Sawa T, Matsuki N. Treatment of peritoneal dissemination from gastric cancer by peritonectomy and chemohyperthermic peritoneal perfusion. Br J Surg. 2005;92(3):370–5.
117. Scaringi S, Kianmanesh R, Sabate JM, Facchiano E, Jouet P, Coffin B, et al. Advanced gastric cancer with or without peritoneal carcinomatosis treated with hyperthermic intraperitoneal chemotherapy: a single western center experience. Eur J Surg Oncol. 2008;34(11):1246–52.
118. Glehen O, Gilly FN, Arvieux C, Cotte E, Boutitie F, Mansvelt B, et al. Peritoneal carcinomatosis from gastric cancer: a multi-institutional study of 159 patients treated by cytoreductive surgery combined with perioperative intraperitoneal chemotherapy. Ann Surg Oncol. 2010;17(9):2370–7.
119. Yang XJ, Li Y, Yonemura Y. Cytoreductive surgery plus hyperthermic intraperitoneal chemotherapy to treat gastric cancer with ascites and/or peritoneal carcinomatosis: results from a Chinese center. J Surg Oncol. 2010;101(6):457–64.
120. Yang XJ, Huang CQ, Suo T, Mei LJ, Yang GL, Cheng FL, et al. Cytoreductive surgery and hyperthermic intraperitoneal chemotherapy improves survival of patients with peritoneal carcinomatosis from gastric cancer: final results of a phase III randomized clinical trial. Ann Surg Oncol. 2011;18(6):1575–81.
121. Yonemura Y, de Aretxabala X, Fujimura T, Fushida S, Katayama K, Bandou E, et al. Intraoperative chemohyperthermic peritoneal perfusion as an adjuvant to gastric cancer: final results of a randomized controlled study. Hepatogastroenterology. 2001;48(42): 1776–82.
122. Lowe KA, Chia VM, Taylor A, O'Malley C, Kelsh M, Mohamed M, et al. An international assessment of ovarian cancer incidence and mortality. Gynecol Oncol. 2013;130(1):107–14.
123. Cannistra SA. Cancer of the ovary. N Engl J Med. 2004;351(24):2519–29.
124. Thigpen T. The if and when of surgical debulking for ovarian carcinoma. N Engl J Med. 2004; 351(24):2544–6.
125. Bristow RE, Tomacruz RS, Armstrong DK, Trimble EL, Montz FJ. Survival effect of maximal cytoreductive surgery for advanced ovarian carcinoma during the platinum era: a meta-analysis. J Clin Oncol. 2002;20(5):1248–59.
126. Armstrong DK, Bundy B, Wenzel L, Huang HQ, Baergen R, Lele S, et al. Intraperitoneal cisplatin and paclitaxel in ovarian cancer. N Engl J Med. 2006;354(1):34–43.
127. Fujiwara K. Three ongoing intraperitoneal chemotherapy trials in ovarian cancer. J Gynecol Oncol. 2012;23(2):75–7.
128. Deraco M, Rossi CR, Pennacchioli E, Guadagni S, Somers DC, Santoro N, et al. Cytoreductive surgery followed by intraperitoneal hyperthermic perfusion

in the treatment of recurrent epithelial ovarian cancer: a phase II clinical study. Tumori. 2001; 87(3):120–6.
129. de Bree E, Romanos J, Michalakis J, Relakis K, Georgoulias V, Melissas J, et al. Intraoperative hyperthermic intraperitoneal chemotherapy with docetaxel as second-line treatment for peritoneal carcinomatosis of gynaecological origin. Anticancer Res. 2003;23(3C):3019–27.
130. Piso P, Dahlke MH, Loss M, Schlitt HJ. Cytoreductive surgery and hyperthermic intraperitoneal chemotherapy in peritoneal carcinomatosis from ovarian cancer. World J Surg Oncol. 2004;2:21.
131. Zanon C, Clara R, Chiappino I, Bortolini M, Cornaglia S, Simone P, et al. Cytoreductive surgery and intraperitoneal chemohyperthermia for recurrent peritoneal carcinomatosis from ovarian cancer. World J Surg. 2004;28(10):1040–5.
132. Reichman TW, Cracchiolo B, Sama J, Bryan M, Harrison J, Pliner L, et al. Cytoreductive surgery and intraoperative hyperthermic chemoperfusion for advanced ovarian carcinoma. J Surg Oncol. 2005;90(2):51–6.
133. Helm CW, Randall-Whitis L, Martin III RS, Metzinger DS, Gordinier ME, Parker LP, et al. Hyperthermic intraperitoneal chemotherapy in conjunction with surgery for the treatment of recurrent ovarian carcinoma. Gynecol Oncol. 2007;105(1): 90–6.
134. Carrabin N, Mithieux F, Meeus P, Tredan O, Guastalla JP, Bachelot T, et al. Hyperthermic intraperitoneal chemotherapy with oxaliplatin and without adjuvant chemotherapy in stage IIIC ovarian cancer. Bull Cancer. 2010;97(4):E23–32.
135. Deraco M, Kusamura S, Virzi S, Puccio F, Macri A, Famulari C, et al. Cytoreductive surgery and hyperthermic intraperitoneal chemotherapy as upfront therapy for advanced epithelial ovarian cancer: multi-institutional phase-II trial. Gynecol Oncol. 2011;122(2):215–20.
136. Frenel JS, Leux C, Pouplin L, Ferron G, Berton RD, Bourbouloux E, et al. Oxaliplatin-based hyperthermic intraperitoneal chemotherapy in primary or recurrent epithelial ovarian cancer: a pilot study of 31 patients. J Surg Oncol. 2011;103(1):10–6.
137. Parson EN, Lentz S, Russell G, Shen P, Levine EA, Stewart JH. Outcomes after cytoreductive surgery and hyperthermic intraperitoneal chemotherapy for peritoneal surface dissemination from ovarian neoplasms. Am J Surg. 2011;202(4):481–6.
138. Ansaloni L, Agnoletti V, Amadori A, Catena F, Cavaliere D, Coccolini F, et al. Evaluation of extensive cytoreductive surgery and hyperthermic intraperitoneal chemotherapy (HIPEC) in patients with advanced epithelial ovarian cancer. Int J Gynecol Cancer. 2012;22(5):778–85.
139. Fagotti A, Costantini B, Petrillo M, Vizzielli G, Fanfani F, Margariti PA, et al. Cytoreductive surgery plus HIPEC in platinum-sensitive recurrent ovarian cancer patients: a case-control study on survival in patients with two year follow-up. Gynecol Oncol. 2012;127(3):502–5.
140. Loggie BW. Malignant peritoneal mesothelioma. Curr Treat Options Oncol. 2001;2(5):395–9.
141. Costamagna D, Scuderi S, Vaira M, Barone R, De Simone M. Treatment of peritoneal mesothelioma using cytoreduction and intraperitoneal hyperthermic chemotherapy. Tumori. 2003;89(4 Suppl):40–2.
142. Sugarbaker PH, Welch LS, Mohamed F, Glehen O. A review of peritoneal mesothelioma at the Washington Cancer Institute. Surg Oncol Clin N Am. 2003;12(3):605–21, xi.
143. Brigand C, Monneuse O, Mohamed F, Sayag-Beaujard AC, Isaac S, Gilly FN, et al. Peritoneal mesothelioma treated by cytoreductive surgery and intraperitoneal hyperthermic chemotherapy: results of a prospective study. Ann Surg Oncol. 2006; 13(3):405–12.
144. Yan TD, Deraco M, Baratti D, Kusamura S, Elias D, Glehen O, et al. Cytoreductive surgery and hyperthermic intraperitoneal chemotherapy for malignant peritoneal mesothelioma: multi-institutional experience. J Clin Oncol. 2009;27(36):6237–42.
145. Blackham AU, Shen P, Stewart JH, Russell GB, Levine EA. Cytoreductive surgery with intraperitoneal hyperthermic chemotherapy for malignant peritoneal mesothelioma: mitomycin versus cisplatin. Ann Surg Oncol. 2010;17(10):2720–7.
146. Deraco M, Baratti D, Hutanu I, Bertuli R, Kusamura S. The role of perioperative systemic chemotherapy in diffuse malignant peritoneal mesothelioma patients treated with cytoreductive surgery and hyperthermic intraperitoneal chemotherapy. Ann Surg Oncol. 2013;20(4):1093–100.
147. Karakousis CP, Blumenson LE, Canavese G, Rao U. Surgery for disseminated abdominal sarcoma. Am J Surg. 1992;163(6):560–4.
148. Hill AR, McQuellon RP, Russell GB, Shen P, Stewart JH, Levine EA. Survival and quality of life following cytoreductive surgery plus hyperthermic intraperitoneal chemotherapy for peritoneal carcinomatosis of colonic origin. Ann Surg Oncol. 2011;18(13):3673–9.
149. McQuellon RP, Danhauer SC, Russell GB, Shen P, Fenstermaker J, Stewart JH, et al. Monitoring health outcomes following cytoreductive surgery plus intraperitoneal hyperthermic chemotherapy for peritoneal carcinomatosis. Ann Surg Oncol. 2007; 14(3):1105–13.
150. Alves S, Mohamed F, Yadegarfar G, Youssef H, Moran BJ. Prospective longitudinal study of quality of life following cytoreductive surgery and intraperitoneal chemotherapy for pseudomyxoma peritonei. Eur J Surg Oncol. 2010;36(12):1156–61.
151. Tsilimparis N, Bockelmann C, Raue W, Menenakos C, Perez S, Rau B, et al. Quality of life in patients after cytoreductive surgery and hyperthermic intraperitoneal chemotherapy: is it worth the risk? Ann Surg Oncol. 2013;20(1):226–32.
152. McQuellon RP, Loggie BW, Lehman AB, Russell GB, Fleming RA, Shen P, et al. Long-term survivorship

and quality of life after cytoreductive surgery plus intraperitoneal hyperthermic chemotherapy for peritoneal carcinomatosis. Ann Surg Oncol. 2003;10(2):155–62.

153. Duckworth KE, McQuellon RP, Russell GB, Cashwell CS, Shen P, Stewart JH, et al. Patient rated outcomes and survivorship following cytoreductive surgery plus hyperthermic intraperitoneal chemotherapy (CS+HIPEC). J Surg Oncol. 2012;106(4):376–80.

154. Shen P, Thai K, Stewart JH, Howerton R, Loggie BW, Russell GB, Levine EA. Peritoneal surface disease from colorectal cancer: comparison with the hepatic metastases surgical paradigm in optimally resected patients. Ann Surg Oncol. 2008;15(12):3422–32.

Squamous Cell Carcinoma of the Anal Canal

22

Mahmoud N. Kulaylat

Learning Objectives

After reading this chapter, you should be able to:

- Understand the importance of HPV and HIV in the etiogenesis of anal canal SCC and the similarities between genital and anal cancer
- Understand the natural history of anal canal SCC
- Understand the evolution of the treatment of anal canal SCC

Introduction

Anal neoplasms comprise tumors of the anal canal and anal margin. Squamous cell carcinoma (SCC) is the most common carcinoma of the anal canal and constitutes 80–90 % of all malignant anal tumors and is the focus of this review. Anal carcinoma is a rare tumor and accounts for 1.5–2 % of all gastrointestinal (GI) tract malignancies, 2–4 % of lower GI tract cancers, nearly 4 % of anorectal tumors, and less than 0.3 % of all cancers (excluding skin BCC and SCC) [1–4].

The incidence of anal cancer is estimated to be between 0.2 and 1.4 persons/100,000 persons with a slight female predominance [5–7]. There is a trend towards younger patients in both gender, largely in part due to the increased prevalence of immunosuppressed conditions such as transplantation and human immunodeficiency virus (HIV), along with transmission of the human papillomavirus (HPV) [8, 9].

The incidence of anal cancer in the United States and worldwide has been rising in men and women. According to Surveillance, Epidemiology, and End Results (SEER) data collected between 1973 and 2000, the incidence has increased from 10 patients/100,000 to 20 patients/100,000 [10]. The incidence has been steadily increasing: in the year 2000, 3,400 cases were reported and in 2012 approximately 6,230 new cases were diagnosed [2, 4, 11]. The annual incidence of anal cancer among men climbed 5.7-fold, from 1.9/100,000 to 10.8/100,000 between 1973 and 2000 [3, 4]. African-American (AA) men had the sharpest increase followed by Caucasian men, Caucasian women, and AA women [3, 4]. The risk is higher among homosexual men [men having sex with men (MSM)], patients on chronic immunosuppression, HIV-positive or AIDS patients, and women with history of cervical precancer or cancer [12, 13]. In HIV-negative MSM, the incidence is 35/100,000; it is higher in HIV-positive MSM (70/100,000) [3, 13–16].

Anatomy

The anal canal represents the caudal part of the large intestine (Fig. 22.1). The exact definition of the anal canal is not generally agreed upon

M.N. Kulaylat, M.D. (✉)
Department of Surgery, Buffalo General Medical Center, University at Buffalo-State University of New York, 100 High Street, Buffalo 14203, NY, USA
e-mail: mkulaylat@kaleidahealth.org

Q.D. Chu et al. (eds.), *Surgical Oncology: A Practical and Comprehensive Approach*,
DOI 10.1007/978-1-4939-1423-4_22, © Springer Science+Business Media New York 2015

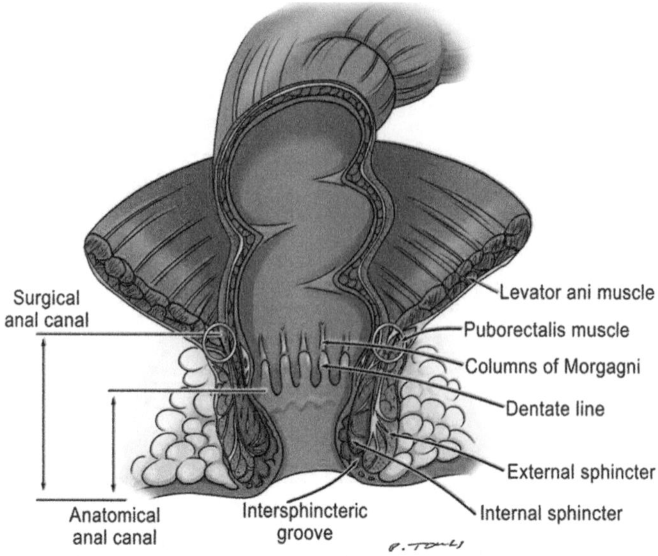

Fig. 22.1 *Anatomy of the anorectal region*: The anatomic anal canal is between the anal verge below and the dentate line above. The surgical anal canal is approximately 4 cm, with one-third below the dentate line and two-thirds above it (Illustrated by Paul Tomljanovich, MD and modified by Karen Howard, Medical Student. Courtesy of Quyen D. Chu, MD, MBA, FACS)

among mists, the anal canal extends from the dentate line to the top of anorectal ring, while the anal margin extends from the dentate line to within 5 cm of the verge. Anatomical definition is based on studies showing lymphatic drainage and histology relative to the dentate line [16]. Lymphatic drainage above the dentate line is to the mesorectal, pararectal, inferior mesenteric, and retroperitoneal lymph nodes (LN) [16]. The lymphatics from the area of the puborectalis drain into the internal iliac LN. Drainage below the dentate line is to inguinal and femoral LN [17]. External and common iliac and para-aortic LN are not considered regional [18]. There are, however, numerous connections between the lymphatics and their drainage patterns are variable [19]. The dentate line lies 1–2 cm above the anal verge and is at the termination of the anal columns [4]. The anal margin extends distal to the anal verge to a 5 cm circumferential area, which is referred to as the perianal skin [6].

There are three histologic zones, the proximal glandular (rectal columnar), distal squamous (keratinizing, modified skin devoid of appendages), and squamocolumnar or transitional (nonkeratinizing) zone, which span about 0–1.2 cm above the dentate line. Squamous metaplastic tissue occurs above the dentate line and represents a transformation of the epithelium from fully developed columnar epithelium to relatively immature or incompletely developed squamous epithelium overlying columnar epithelium (6–10 cm).

According to surgeons, the anal canal extends from the rectum to the perianal skin that does not include the hair-bearing skin [4, 17]. Outside the verge is the perianal skin and encompasses a radius of 5 cm. The anal canal is 3–5 cm in men and shorter in women. It begins where the rectum enters the puborectalis sling at the apex of the anal sphincter complex and ends at the anal verge that roughly coincides with the palpable intersphincteric groove.

Pathology

The lining of the anal canal and perianal area represents progressive transition from the digestive system to the skin, with many different types of cells and tissue. Anal cancers can arise from any of these cells and include adenocarcinoma, mucinous adenocarcinoma, undifferentiated carcinoma, small cell carcinoma, melanoma, and SCC. SCC may be keratinizing or nonkeratinizing depending on its relation to the dentate line. The majority of cancers are SCC with adenocarcinoma and melanoma making up the rest. Keratinzing SCC is rare in the anal canal above the dentate line. Variants of nonkeratinizing SCC include basaloid, large cell nonkeratinzing (transitional) and mucoepidermoid cancer. These cancers contain a mixture of squamous cells, mucin-secreting cells and cells of intermediate type [20]. Variants of SCC have similar natural history, patterns of spread, and prognosis as SCC. The other non-SCC anal cancers have distinct clinical features, natural history, and radiation sensitivity and will not be discussed.

Etiology

It was recognized in 1984 that genital and anal cancer have similar epidemiology: both are associated with the human papillomavirus (HPV) and represent sexually transmitted diseases (STD) [21]. In recent years, it became well established that the most important risk or causative factor for anal cancer is HPV [9, 22, 23]. The epithelium that is particularly susceptible to HPV infection and cancers is the transitional zone and transformational epithelium situated at variable height above dentate line [4]. Like genital cancer, HPV causes anal intraepithelial neoplasia (AIN) [squamous intraepithelial lesion (SIL)], and like cervical and vulvar intraepithelial neoplasia (CIN and VIN), AIN progresses from low-grade AIN (LG-AIN) to high-grade AIN (HG-AIN) to cancer [24]. Anal LG-AIN may not progress to HG-AIN and may regress but does not go directly to cancer without going through HG-AIN. Once established, HG-AIN rarely regresses to LG-AIN and it progresses to cancer without treatment. Although data on progression to invasive cancer is not available, it is reported in two studies with follow-up spanning nearly 20 years that about 5 % of LG-AIN undergo malignant change [25, 26]. In a recent study, malignant progression of HG-AIN occurs in 11 % of patients who were immunosuppressed for over 8 years [27].

Several risk factors are associated with anal cancer and include genetic, environmental, female gender, sexual orientation and activity, associated anogenital disease, immunosuppression (due to solid organ transplantation or HIV infection), and persistent high-risk infection with multiple HPV types (Table 22.1).

Table 22.1 Risk factors for anal cancer

Human papillomavirus (HPV 16 and 18)
Human immunodeficiency virus infection
Sexual behavior:
Homosexuality
History of anal receptive intercourse
History of more than 10 lifetime sexual partners among heterosexual men and women
History of anal receptive intercourse before age 30 in women
History of genital disease:
Cervical, vulvar, or vaginal cancer
Sexually transmitted diseases among heterosexual men and women
History of anogenital warts
Immunosuppression after sold organ transplantation
Cigarette smoking
Inflammatory bowel disease

Human Papillomavirus (HPV)

Infection with HPV is the first step in the pathogenesis of anal cancer. There are about 30,000 cases of anal cancer per year worldwide and 90 % are associated with HPV [28]. It is estimated that 75–80 % of sexually active Americans will likely acquire genital HPV at some point of their life, and the most common mode of transmission is sexual contact [9, 28] At times, HPV does not require direct sexual intercourse since "normal tissue trauma" and repair in the transformational zone can facilitate HPV infection. The infection causes field change throughout the perineum and may cause latent subclinical (10–40 %) or clinically apparent (1 %) disease. The virus becomes established as a result of blunted cell-mediated immune response [13, 29].

HPV subtypes 16 and 18 are strongly linked to premalignant and malignant lesions of the anus, uterus, cervix, and vulva [9, 30–33]. The prevalence of the high-risk HPV serotypes in patients with anal cancer is about 85 %, with HPV 16 and 18 occurring in the majority of the cases; HPV 16 is the most common serotype (70 %), and 80 % of affected patients have at least two HPV types [22, 34–36].

HIV

HIV represents a marker for coinfection with other STD such as HPV. HIV-positive men infected with HPV tend to carry multiple serotypes compared with HIV-negative men infected with HPV, 73 % vs. 23 %, respectively [37]. This is also true for both MSM and heterosexual men and women who do not report anoreceptive intercourse [38]. The prevalence of anal HPV infection is greater than cervical HPV infection in women who are HIV positive or have a high risk of having HIV infection [39].

SCC is the third common neoplasm observed in patients with HIV with a substantially higher incidence in MSM and in long-standing infection [40, 41]. MSM who are HIV positive have doubled the risk of developing anal cancer compared with MSM who are HIV negative [8, 14]. The risk of cancer increases with total time elapsed with CD 4+ count below 200 cells/μl and viral load >100,000 copies/ml [40, 42]. There is a 60-fold increase in relative risk of anal cancer in HIV-positive compared to HIV-negative patients [12].

With the introduction of highly active antiretroviral treatment (HAART), HIV/AIDS patients have gained improved life expectancy, but at a price of being at an increased risk for developing tumors and dying from neoplasia including AIDS-defining cancers. There is increased incidence of anal cancer in HIV-infected individuals (120-fold higher than in age- and gender-matched controls) treated with HAART as a result of increased longevity with their altered immune status [43]. SCC of the anal canal is third (8.2 %) among neoplasms in that population with higher incidence in MSM and long-standing infected people [40, 41].

Sexual Behavior

The risk of developing AIN and anal SCC is associated with sexual behavior, and the most important risk factors are lifetime number of sexual partners in homosexual and heterosexual men, engagement in anal intercourse, and presence of HIV [9]. HPV infection and high-risk sexual behavior are associated with marked increase of AIN in HIV-positive patients [44].

About 28 % of patients with anal cancer give history of genital warts as a result of HPV infection compared to 1–2 % control, and a history of receptive anal intercourse in men increases the relative risk of developing anal cancer by 33x compared with control who have colon cancer [14].

In unmarried women, history of partners with STD, 10 or more lifetime sexual partners, having at least two anal intercourse sexual partners, history of anal intercourse at young age (before the age 30), homosexuality, history of anogenital disease (warts, syphilis, gonorrhea, genital dysplasia, or cancer), and HIV infection are associated with increased risk for anal cancer [9, 29]. History of cervical or vulvar HPV infection and VIN increases the risk of anal cancer with an incidence rate ratio of 3.97–31.09 depending on age at diagnosis compared to control [32, 45].

Solid Organ Transplantation

Cell-mediated immunity is important in the host response that prohibits HPV from establishing a prolonged existence. All immunosuppression regimens used in renal transplantation are cyclosporin-based with direct suppressive effect on cellular (T cell) immunity. Among the side effects of immunosuppression is the increased incidence of neoplasms and viral infections (HPV, Epstein-Barr, and CMV) [13, 23, 46].

Kidney transplant patients, as a result of chronic immunosuppression, have a 100-fold increase risk of anogenital cancer [13]. Anogenital carcinoma, as a result of HPV infection, may be 20x more frequent in renal transplant recipient receiving immunosuppression than in the general population [46].

Smoking

Smoking is an independent factor for increasing the risk of anal cancer [14, 47, 48]. There is a 5x increased risk compared to control and the relative risks are 9.4 and 7.7 compared to nonsmoking controls [14, 47, 48]. The mechanism behind smoking and anal cancer development is unknown but may be related to interference with apoptosis and/or suppression of the immune system.

IBD

In patients with Crohn's disease (anorectal disease), the incidence of SCC is ten times higher than in the general population [49].

Presentation

The median age of diagnosis of anal canal cancer in the United States is 60–65 years. There is a trend from older to younger patients of both genders as sexually transmitted diseases such as HIV and HPV become more prevalent. The diagnosis of SCC is often delayed because the clinical presentation is nonspecific and the coexistence of benign anorectal conditions is not uncommon. About 70–80 % of patients are initially diagnosed with benign anorectal condition, and 20 % have no symptoms [1, 5]. Invasive cancer is occasionally an unexpected finding after excision of hemorrhoids or skin tag in up to 20 % of cases [1]. AIN is present in 28–35 % of excised condylomas [50].

Patients may present with anorectal bleeding, pruritus, pain, and soiling. Bleeding is described in 45 % of patients, with pain and a progressive growth of an anal mass as among the presenting complaints in one of three cases (Fig. 22.2). Bleeding and presence of a mass are the complaints in 80 % of cases. Locally advanced cancers may present with incontinence (due to infiltration of the anal sphincter), perianal infection, and fistula. The average tumor size measures approximately 3–4 cm at the time of diagnosis.

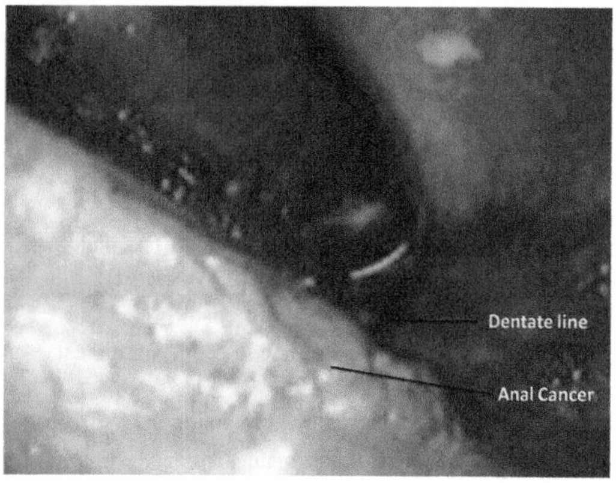

Fig. 22.2 Endoscopic view of a squamous cell carcinoma of the anal canal

Diagnostic Procedures and Staging

The widely used staging system for anal cancer is endorsed by the American Joint Committee on Cancer, 7th ed, 2010 [6] (Table 22.2). Pathologic staging was based on historical data when surgery was the gold standard and in few tumors that were locally excised. Nowadays, staging is based on clinical assessment of the primary tumor and inguinal LN, supplemented by radiologic studies such as transanal ultrasound (US) or MRI, abdominal and pelvic CT scan or MRI, PET scan, and sentinel LN biopsy (SLNBx).

Clinical Assessment

Location, size, and mobility of the primary lesion are carefully assessed on examination. The anal verge remains closed when the buttocks are gently spread. Unlike perianal cancers that can be visualized by gentle traction on the buttocks, cancers of the anal canal cannot be seen in their entirety with this method alone [5]; about 50 % are <3 cm, 24 % are superficial or in situ, and 71 % invade into the muscle or fat [51].

Clinical examination for inguinal LN involvement is carefully performed since their involvement with cancer is a major independent poor prognostic factor and their presence helps gauge therapy. About 10–20 % of patients present with synchronous inguinal LN metastasis [51–53]. Tumors located laterally drain to homolateral side and those in the midline drain to bilateral groin LN [54]. Most (70–90 %) tumors are located laterally in the anal canal and have clinically negative inguinal LN at initial presentation [13, 55, 56].

Table 22.2 American Joint Committee on Cancer (AJCC) TNM staging for anal cancer (7th edition)

Primary tumor (T)	
TX	Primary tumor cannot be assessed
T0	No evidence of primary tumor
Tis	Carcinoma in situ, Bowen disease, high-grade squamous intraepithelial lesion (HSIL), anal intraepithelial neoplasia II–III (AIN II–III)
T1	Tumor ≤2 cm in greatest dimension
T2	Tumor more than >2 cm and <5 cm in greatest dimension
T3	Tumor >5 cm in greatest dimension
T4	Tumor of any size that invades adjacent organ(s), e.g., vagina, urethra, bladder*

*Note: Direct invasion of the rectal wall, perirectal skin, subcutaneous tissue, or the sphincter muscle(s) is not classified as T4

Regional lymph nodes (N)	
NX	Regional lymph nodes cannot be assessed
N0	No regional lymph nodes metastasis
N1	Metastasis in perirectal lymph node(s)
N2	Metastasis in unilateral internal iliac and/or unilateral inguinal lymph node(s)
N3	Metastasis in perirectal and inguinal lymph nodes and/or bilateral internal iliac and/or bilateral inguinal lymph nodes

Distant metastasis (M)	
M0	No distant metastasis
M1	Distant metastasis

Anatomic stage/prognostic groups			
Group	T	N	M
Stage 0	Tis	N0	M0
Stage I	T1	N0	M0
Stage II	T2, T3	N0	M0
Stage IIIA	T1-T3	N1	M0
	T4	N0	M0
Stage IIIB	T4	N1	M0
	Any T	N2-N3	M0
Stage IV	Any T	Any N	M1

Adapted from Compton et al. [179]. With permission from Springer Verlag

Synchronous groin LN metastasis increases with tumor size and extent of the primary tumor [53]. Half of the clinically positive LNs are <5 mm in size, and of all patients presenting with palpable inguinal LN, only 50 % will turn out to be metastatic. HIV-positive patients, however, commonly present with palpable enlarged LN that are histologically positive in 50 % of cases. Needle biopsy is indicated when LNs are enlarged or are >10 mm on CT or MRI [57]. Some, however, do not advocate biopsy and recommend RT boost to the affected groin if there is palpable or radiologically suspicious LN [58].

Examination under anesthesia may be necessary to relax the sphincter and allow adequate examination. Biopsy is recommended for patients who present with pruritus or anal discharge with a suspicious raised, scaly, white plaques, erythematous, pigmented, fissured, or eczematous lesions.

Transanal US and MRI

Transanal US and MRI allow accurate determination of depth of invasion by the tumor, sphincter involvement, and local LN metastasis [18, 59]. Three-dimensional US has improved accuracy in detecting perirectal LN and tumor invasion compared to two-dimensional US [60, 61]. Proper positioning of the US probe or MRI coil may be hampered by pain and stricture. Transanal US has been mostly used in follow-up of patients treated with chemoradiation therapy (CRT) [18, 62]. Its ability to differentiate residual tumor from posttreatment fibrosis is, however, limited.

CT Scan and MRI

CT scan and MRI can delineate tumor dimension, invasion to adjacent structures, and LN involvement. MRI is more sensitive as it delineates soft tissue planes more clearly. The efficacy of CT scan and MRI to detect inguinal LN is suboptimal [49, 63]. After CRT, MRI is used with clinical evaluation to assess for therapeutic response [49].

PET Scan

PET scan has become the standard of care in staging anal canal cancer in many centers and is used as an adjunct to CT scan. It evaluates the status of LN and identifies distant metastasis. The sensitivity of PET scan for nodal disease is 89 % in comparison to 62 % for CT scan and or MRI [39]. PET identifies sites of metastasis not observed in CT scan in about 20 % of cases [39, 63–65]. It is also used in posttreatment evaluation since clinical assessment is subjective and confounded by radiation-related skin toxicity and nonmalignant residual masses [66, 67]. Furthermore, PET scan is used to assess response to treatment as it correlates with the end point of progression-free survival (PFS), overall survival (OS), and cause-specific survival [63, 68].

PET-CT is useful in the initial staging of perirectal/pelvic LN or inguinal LN, more so in high-risk advanced tumors. It also alters the RT fields in 16–35 % of patients and identifies synchronous cancer [69–72].

Sentinel LN

Management of nonpalpable inguinal LN (clinically negative) at presentation is controversial. Elective LN dissection is not widely applied since metastasis is found only in 50 % of cases and 44 % of pathologically positive LN are smaller than 5 mm [51]. Inclusion of inguinal LN in the radiation field is not standard and is empirically made according to institutional practice. Some suggest prophylactic RT whereby radiotherapy is delivered to the primary tumor, pelvic LN, and the groin with the intent to reduce the risk of late nodal metastasis [73]. Others recommend the "watch and see" policy and treating the nodal basin only when LN metastasis becomes evident after the completion of treatment of the primary tumor [61]. Others adopt a more selective approach and deliver RT based on the size of the primary tumor [74]. Sentinel LN biopsy (SLNBx) is yet another tool that can be used to improve detection of metastatic disease in clinically unsuspicious nodes. It may upstage patients with small primary anal cancer who may otherwise be excluded from radiotherapy and avoid overtreating patients who have no nodal involvement [53, 54, 71, 75–79].

SLNBx must not be performed for clearly clinically positive or suspicious LN. Some advocate its routine use in patients with nonpalpable LN, while others suggest exclusion of T4 patients and patients with prior anal manipulation [54, 80].

Markers

Lampejo et al. in a systemic review of biomarkers found that tumor suppressor genes p53 and p21 were the only markers of prognostic value in more than one study [81].

Treatment

Management of keratinizing and nonkeratinizing anal canal carcinomas is similar. In the past, treatment included single-modality therapy, either abdominoperineal resection (APR) or RT. The treatment paradigm has changed to concurrent CRT as primary treatment and APR as salvage treatment. Below is an in-depth description of the evolution of the treatment for anal SCC.

Surgery

APR was the gold standard and treatment of choice for advanced anal cancer before 1974 [26]. The treatment was associated with an over-all survival (OS) of 40–70 %, morbidity up to 72 %, and local recurrence as high as 40 % [1, 51, 82]. With pelvic nodal involvement and tumor size larger than 5 cm, prognosis was worsened by 50 % and survival reduced to below 20 % [1, 82]. The paradigm shifted to primary CRT after Nigro published the results of neoadjuvant CRT [83]. APR became a salvage procedure offered to patients with persistent and progressive disease, and those with local recurrence and CRT-related complications such as anal stenosis and incontinence [84–90].

Local excision is suitable for in situ lesions, those that are confined to the epithelial and subepithelial connective tissue, and for small (<2 cm) well-differentiated lesions occupying <50 % of the anal circumference [51, 87]. Local excision of selected lesions is associated with a 5-year OS of 87 % and cancer-specific survival of 100 %.

Colostomy is indicated for patients who are incontinent, those who cope poorly with RT-related acute toxicity, or those who are at risk of developing a rectovaginal fistula.

Sphincter Preservation Treatments

Radiation Therapy (RT) Alone

In 1984, Cummings et al. demonstrated that survival rates with RT alone were equivalent to CRT (70 %), but primary tumor control was better with the combined therapy (60 % vs. 93 %) [91]. In a later study, they demonstrated that the 4-year actuarial cause-specific rates were better with CRT compared to RT alone (80 % vs. 68 %) [92]. Radiotherapy alone is highly effective for selected patients with small tumors (T1, T2, N0, M0) but not for those with larger tumors or those with positive LNs [93, 94]. It is also an acceptable modality for the frail and elderlies [95].

Concurrent Chemoradiation Therapy (CRT)

The Nigro protocol originally used CT as a precursor (neoadjuvant) to APR to improve survival [83]. Low-dose RT (3,000 cGy full pelvis radiation) and continuous 5-fluorouracil (5-FU infusion) and a single bolus of mitomycin C (MMC) were given during RT. Overall, 86 % of patients had at least a clinical complete response (CR), 79 % were alive and disease-free at time of analysis, and the majority had no residual tumor after APR [83]. The treatment was later modified to decrease toxicity [96]. The presence of CR subsequently led most centers to adopt CRT as primary curative treatment to avoid the morbidity and mortality associated with an APR.

Concurrent CRT evolved from a precursor to an alternative to surgery as an organ preserving, sphincter-saving, and colostomy-sparing treatment that is associated with a good outcome. It became the standard of care supported by retrospective and prospective studies, although there is no head-to-head prospective randomized trial comparing CRT to surgery. Subsequent studies focused on the selection of the chemotherapeutic agent and RT to improve the efficacy of and reduce toxicity of the treatment.

5-FU + MMC

Randomized trials conducted by the United Kingdom Coordinating Committee on cancer Research (UKCCCR) [55] and the European Organisation for Research and Treatment of cancer (EORTC) [52] demonstrated that the addition of CT yielded higher local control, colostomy-free survival (CFS), and complete remission rates than RT alone.

In the British trial (ACT I), 585 patients with T1–T4 epidermoid SCC of the anal canal or margin were randomized to RT alone ($n=290$) or RT with concurrent 5-FU and MMC ($n=295$) [55]. There was no significant difference in OS between the two therapies at 36 months, but CRT resulted in less local failure and decreased cancer-related risk of death (Table 22.3). With CRT, CR rate was obtained in 70 % of patients (range, 64–86 %). The long-term follow-up data (median 13 years) was recently reported and demonstrated that the full benefit with CRT can be seen at about 5 years after start of treatment and sustained at least 7 years after [97]. There was a 9.1 % increase in non-anal cancer death in the first 5 years of CRT that disappeared by 10 years. The benefits of CRT outweighed an early excess risk of non-anal cancer death.

In all, 84 % of recurrences were detected within the first 2 years, and most anal cancer deaths occurred in the first few years (53 % in the first 2 years). Patients who survived to 5 years were considered cured since the cause of deaths thereafter were due to other causes. Only 7 % of patients developed metastatic disease without earlier locoregional recurrence. For every 100 patients, there was an expected 25.3 fewer patients with locoregional relapse and 12.5 fewer anal cancer deaths compared with 100 patients given RT alone.

The EORTC randomized 110 patients (T3–T4 or N1–N3) to RT alone or RT + concurrent 5-FU and MMC [52]. The study demonstrated no difference in the OS (58 % vs. 54 %). However, CR and colostomy-free survival (CFS) were higher in the CRT compared to RT group (Table 22.3). The locoregional control rate improved by 18 % at 5 years, and the event-free and progression-free survival rates were higher in the CRT. Unlike the

Table 22.3 Randomized clinical trials of chemoradiation therapy for anal SCC

Clinical trial	*N*	Treatment	Results
UKCCCR (ACT I) [55]	577/585	RT vs. 5-FU/MMC/RT (*RT=45 Gy; boost RT to responders*)	*At 3 years*:
			Survival = 58 % vs. 65 %
			Local failure = 61 % vs. 39 %
			Cancer mortality = 28 % vs. 39 %
			Complete response rate = 70 %
			Early toxicity = 48 % vs. 39 %
			Late toxicity = no difference
EORTC [52]	110	RT vs. 5-FU/MMC/RT	Overall survival = 58 % vs. 54 %
			Locoregional control rate = 68 % vs. 50 %
			Complete response rate = 54 % vs. 80 %
RTOG and ECOG [58]	310	5-FU/RT vs. 5-FU/MMC/RT (*RT=45–54.4 Gy*)	*At 4 years*:
			Colostomy rate = 23 vs. 9 %
			Colostomy-free survival = 59 % vs. 71 %
			Tumor regression rate = 87 % vs. 92 %
			Disease-free survival = 68 % vs. 75 %
			High-grade toxicity = 7 % vs. 23 %
RTOG 98-11 [102, 103]	644/682	5-FU/MMC/RT vs. 5-FU/cisplatin/RT + induction 5-FU/cisplatin (*RT=55–59 Gy*)	*At 5 years*:
			Overall survival = 73 % vs. 70 %
			Disease-free survival = 60 % vs. 54 %
			Local failure rate = 25 % vs. 33 %
			Colostomy rate = 10 % vs. 19 %
			Locoregional failure = 25 % vs. 33 %
			Distant metastasis = 15 % vs. 19 %
			Time to relapse = 60 % vs. 42 %
			Hematologic toxicity = 60 % vs. 42 %
			Nonhematologic toxicity = no difference (74 %)
ECOG E4292 [164]	32	5-FU/cisplatin/RT	Overall response rate = 92 %
			5-year OS = 69 %
			5-year progression-free survival = 55 %
			Overall high-grade toxicity = 31 %
			Severe hematologic toxicity = 16 %
EXTRA [108]	31	Xeloda/MMC/RT (*RT 50.4 Gy*)	Complete response rate = 77 %
			No related deaths

5-FU 5-fluorouracil, *MMC* mitomycin C, *RT* radiotherapy

UKCCCR study, the morbidity and mortality were not significantly different.

5-FU + MMC vs. 5-FU (Is MMC Necessary?)

A phase III randomized joint trial, the Radiation Therapy Oncology Group (RTOG 87-04) and Eastern Cooperative Oncology Group (ECOG 1289), was designed to determine the importance of MMC [58]. In the study, 310 patients with stages I to IIIa were randomized to 5-FU/RT or 5-FU/MMC/RT (Nigro regimen). Patients in the MMC arm compared to the 5-FU arm had significantly higher-grade 4–5 toxicity rates (23 % vs. 7 %). However, at 4 years, patients in the 5-FU/MMC arm had lower colostomy rate, higher CFS, and improved disease-free survival (DFS) than the 5-FU arm (Table 22.3). There was also higher tumor regression response in the MMC arm (92 % vs. 87 %) but no significant difference in survival (75 % vs. 68 %). Elimination of MMC resulted in almost doubling of 5-year local recurrence (from 17 % in FU/MMC to 36 % in 5-FU alone) and 17 % decrease in 5-year DFS (from 64 % in FU-MMC to 50 % in FU alone). Although 5-FU-MMC was associated with increased hematologic toxicity, this did not compromise OS. The study confirmed the superiority of MMC+5-FU as it improved sphincter preservation and disease control, despite greater associated toxicity.

5-FU+Cisplatin (Can Platinum-Based Therapy Replace MMC?)

MMC was associated with 60 % incidence of serious (grade 3–4) toxicity, life-threatening hematologic, lung, renal toxicities, as well as an increased incidence in hemolytic-uremic syndrome [19, 65]. Cisplatinum was introduced as a possible alternative regimen given its proven efficacy in other SCC. Initial studies demonstrated high local control rates (up to 85 %) at 2 years [98–101].

The Radiation Therapy Oncology Group and the US Gastrointestinal Intergroup Randomized Trial (RTOG 98-11) conducted a randomized trial to compare RT+5-FU/MMC and RT+5-FU/cisplatin and to determine whether induction 5-FU/cisplatin CT followed by concurrent CRT would be more effective than standard concurrent CRT [102]. 644 of 682 patients (T2-T4, M0) received either standard CRT (5-FU/MMC) or two cycles of induction 5-FU/cisplatin followed by RT with concurrent 5-FU/cisplatin. The mean follow-up was 2.51 years. There was no difference in nonhematologic toxicity, 3- and 5-year OS, and 5-year DFS or time to relapse between the groups (Table 22.3). However, the 5-year locoregional recurrence (LRF), distant metastasis, and cumulative colostomy-free survival (CFS) rates were significantly better with the MMC-based therapy. 5-FU/MMC/RT has better DSF and lower colostomy failure (CF) rate than with induction 5-FU/cisplatin and 5-FU/cisplatin/RT. In a multivariate analysis of patients with tumor >5 cm and or node-positive disease, significant relapses occurred locoregionally (40–64 %) compared to 20 % in T2N0 or T3N0 disease [102]. In an updated long-term follow-up, it was found that RT+5-FU/MMC had a statistically better DFS and OS than RT+5-FU/CCDP (5-year DFS, 67.8 % vs. 57.8 %; $P=0.008$; 5-year OS, 78.3 % vs. 70.7 %; $P=0.026$). Additionally, the 5-FU/MMC group trended towards statistical significance for CFS ($P=0.05$), LRF ($P=0.087$), and CF ($P=0.074$) [103].

Other studies questioned whether cisplatin could replace MMC and whether maintenance (consolidation; adjuvant) 5-FU/cisplatin would improve on those results [104, 105]. The second UK Anal Cancer Trial II (ACT II) evaluated the role of adjuvant 5-FU/cisplatin after concurrent 5-FU/cisplatin/RT or 5-FU/MMC/RT [104]. In this study, 940 non-HIV patients with SCC T1–T4 were randomized to 5-FU/cisplatin ($n=469$) with RT or 5-FU/MMC ($n=471$) with RT. Both groups were further randomized to receive two courses of consolidation (adjuvant) therapy, either 5-FU/cisplatin ($n=448$) after CRT or no consolidation ($n=446$). At 26 weeks, there was no difference in CR rate in patients receiving adjuvant CT vs. observation alone (85 % vs. 82 %). The results of the recently completed study, phase III ACT II, which showed no differences in CR, DFS, and OS in both groups, are depicted in Table 22.3 [106]. Unlike the RTOG 98-11, the colostomy rate was lower in the cisplatin arm (11 % vs. 14 % with MMC). As in RTOG 98-11, grade 3–4 acute hematologic toxicity occurred significantly more often in the MMC arm (25 % vs. 13 %), whereas nonhematologic toxicity did not differ between the two arms (60 % vs. 65 %) [106].

The European Action Clinique Coordonnees en Cancerologie Digestive (ACCORD-03) phase III trial evaluated the benefit of cisplatin-based neoadjuvant CT prior to concurrent 5-FU/cisplatin/RT and assessed the impact of higher RT boost to responding patients [high-dose boost (25 Gy vs. standard dose boost (15 Gy)] on CFS in patients with advanced anal cancer [107]. The study showed no benefit for the addition of cisplatin-based neoadjuvant CT prior to CRT or from increase in RT boost (Table 22.4).

Table 22.4 Neoadjuvant vs. adjuvant chemotherapy

Study	*N*	Treatment	Outcome
ACT II [104, 106]	940	*Cisplatin group*	CR: similar (94 %)
		5-FU/cisplatin/RT	OS: similar (85 %)
		± adjuvant 5-FU/cisplatin	3 year RFS: similar
			T1–T2 = 75 %
		MMC group	T3–T4 = 68 %
		5-FU/MMC/RT	Toxicity:
		± adjuvant 5-FU/cisplatin	Nonhematologic: similar 60 % vs. 65 %
			Hematologic: MMC > cis 13 % vs. 25 %
ACCORD 03 [107]	307	*NACT + 5-FU/cisplatin/RT*	*5-year CFS*:
		Standard boost RT (group A)	Group A and B = 76.5 %
		High-dose boost RT (group B)	Group A and C = 73.7 %
		No NACT + 5-FU/cisplatin/RT	
		Standard boost RT (group C)	Group C and D = 75 %
		High-dose boost RT (group D)	Group B and D = 77.8 %
		Standard boost RT = 15 Gy	
		High-dose boost RT = 25 Gy	

5-FU 5-fluorouracil, *CFS* colostomy-free survival, *CR* complete response, *NACT* neoadjuvant chemotherapy, *OS* overall survival, *RFS* relapse-free survival

Capecitabine and MMC

In gastrointestinal cancer, oral capecitabine (Xeloda®) is at least as effective with similar toxicity profile as intravenous 5-FU. The efficacy and toxicity of capecitabine in the treatment of anal SCC was explored in a multicenter phase II study (EXTRA) that replicated ACT II treatment but substituted capecitebine for 5-FU [108]. Thirty one patients were treated with CRT using intravenous MMC on day 1 and oral capecitabine on each RT treatment day in two divided doses (825 mg/m^2 BID). The combination of MMC/capecitabine was well tolerated. Complete CR occurred in 77 % of patients and partial response occurred in 16 %, and there were no treatment-related deaths (Table 22.3).

In another phase I study of 18 patients with locally advanced anal cancer who were treated with intensity-modulated RT (IMRT) and concomitant capecitabine and MMC, 83 % of patients achieved CR. At a follow-up of 28 months, none of the patients with CR relapsed [109]. The predominant acute toxicity (grade ≥3) was radiation dermatitis (50 %) [109].

Cetuximab and Cisplatin

Early results of treatment with EGFR inhibitor (Cetuximab) in metastatic anal SCC are promising [110–113]. Patients with KRAS wild-type showed partial response or at least stabilization of the tumor, whereas patients harboring KRAS mutation had progressive disease [112, 113]. A phase I study of cetuximab with cisplatin and RT for locally advanced anal cancer showed 78 % of patients (7/9) achieved CR [114].

HIV Status and CRT

HIV-negative patients with anal cancer treated with concurrent CRT often required a break from RT and dose reduction of at least one CT agent and have a local failure rate of 30 % and a 5-year OS near 70 %; more than 50 % succumb to death for which the causes are unrelated to anal cancer [52, 55, 58, 102, 115]. HIV-negative patients with anal cancer differ from HIV-positive patients by age (60–65 years vs. 40–45 years), male gender

(35–40 % vs. 90–95 %), and homosexuality [116–118]. Currently in the Western world, up to 50 % of patients with anal SCC are relatively young (40–60 years) male homosexuals under highly active antiretroviral therapy (HAART) [119].

In the pre-HAART era, HIV-positive patients were excluded from major studies. Small studies, however, have shown that HIV-positive patients had poor tolerance to MMC-based CRT protocol, experienced frequent local recurrence, but had satisfactory local control and survival rates [40, 41, 117, 120–123]. Despite poor tolerance, standard CRT was given whenever possible, especially when the CD 4+ count was >200/mm^3 [123]. Many of these young patients eventually died of AIDS with or without evidence of residual anal cancer since the median survival with the diagnosis of AIDS was 17 months. In one study where many patients did not receive standard CT because of fear of significant hematologic toxicity, after 38 months follow-up, 40–50 % had local recurrence, 50 % were alive and disease-free, and 50 % died from complications of AIDS [115]. Acute toxicity was frequent (>50 %). In another study, the median time to cancer-related death was 1.4 years (vs. 5.3 years in HIV-negative patient) [117].

In the HAART era, HIV-positive patients were able to tolerate CRT if CD 4+ count >200 [123]. In a multicenter cohort study and retrospective analysis of 40 HIV-positive patients (on HAART) and 81 HIV-negative patients treated with either CRT or RT alone, the CR rate was high in both groups (92 % vs. 96 %), although HIV-positive patients were more likely to experience grade 3–4 skin and hematologic toxicity [120]. The 5-year OS was similar in both groups (61 % vs. 65 %), but the locoregional recurrence was higher in the HIV-positive patients (61 % vs. 13 %), and the majority of HIV-positive patients died of anal cancer [120]. In the Veterans Affairs study, the authors noted that survival was equivalent between HIV-positive and HIV-negative patients (overall 4-year survival 66 % vs. 62 %) [118]. Overall, HIV-positive individuals with anal SCC in the HAART era carry a 50 % risk of local recurrence and 33 % risk of dying from the cancer [40].

Radiotherapy: Standard RT vs. Intensity-Modulated RT (IMRT)

Standard Radiotherapy [Conventional 3D-Conformal Radiotherapy (3D CRT)]

The RT that has been used is 3D conformal radiation therapy (3D CRT). It delivered RT using opposed anteroposterior and posteroanterior fields during a 6-week period with a therapeutic break between sequences [94, 124–126]. The delivery covered gross disease and elective pelvic and inguinal LN including extensive portions of the bowel, bladder, and perineum. The total dose of RT continues to be evaluated. Nigro initially utilized low-dose RT, 30 Gy [83]. However, escalating or higher doses has been shown to improve locoregional recurrence [127, 128]. Dose 50–55 Gy is effective in obtaining local control and eradication of the tumor, resulting in a cure in 70–90 % of patients [1, 124, 127–129]. Local recurrence dropped to less than 10 % and 5-year survival improved to 60–90 %. Escalating the dose up to 60 Gy is associated with 90 % locoregional control at 5 years and improves survival in patients with T3 and T4 tumors [129, 130]. The benefit of a dose >60 Gy is doubtful and is associated with complications [88, 89, 131–133].

Extensive portions of the bowel, urinary bladder, and perineum and large volume of bone marrow are included within each RT field arrangement, leading to increase in acute toxicity and chronic sequelae that can pose life-threatening complications and adversely affect quality of life [53, 88, 134–136]. Death from RT toxicity is reported in 2–2.7 % of cases [53]. Hematologic and nonhematologic toxicities are observed in 42–74 % of the patients, and the incidence of grade ≥3 GI and skin toxicity ranged from 34 to 48 % [52, 55, 58, 102–104, 106, 137]. Irradiation to groin LN cancer results in significant early and late toxicity: external genitalia edema, epidermolysis with super infection of the skin, inguinal fibrosis, osteonecrosis of femoral head, femoral head fracture, small bowel injury, lymphedema of lower extremities, edema of genitalia, and stenosis of iliac artery that occur in 33 % of irradiated patients [89, 134–136]. There is a threefold increase in the risk of pelvic fractures in elderly women [138]. High-dose radiation is associated with anal stenosis, ulcers, and necrosis that may require a colostomy in up to 6–12 % of patients [88, 89, 124]. With increasing doses of RT, the need for a diverting colostomy increases, and with a dose >65 Gy, necrosis of the anal canal occurs [132]. Potential toxicity of 3D CRT results in significant dose reduction of CT and increases incidence of treatment breaks (gap) and overall treatment time. Prolonged treatment with frequent treatment interruptions is associated with a poor prognosis and local control rate [94, 133, 139–141]. To minimize the risk of RT toxicity, the radiation field may be reduced, or multifield techniques are used to deliver the dose of RT more conformally to spare normal tissues.

Intensity-Modulated Radiation Therapy (IMRT)

IMRT involves the use of computer-aided optimization to deliver RT dose to the target in a highly conformal manner while minimizing dose to adjacent normal tissue or neighboring organ at risk (OAR) [28, 141–148]. The dosimetric advantage of IMRT over 3D CRT for OAR and healthy tissue sparing is established [28, 142, 144, 147, 149]. The outcome following treatment with IMRT does not differ from that with 3D CRT, but there is a marked decrease in the adverse effects and the need for treatment breaks and reduced total treatment time [28, 42, 126, 140, 143, 144, 147, 148, 150, 151]. With IMRT, there is a lower rate of acute and late gastrointestinal and genitourinary morbidity and decreased hematologic toxicity with bone marrow sparing IMRT [18, 141–144, 148, 152, 153]. Skin toxicity is reported in 0–38 % [28, 42, 126, 140, 143, 148].

Summary of CRT

Anal cancer is often a curable disease. Concurrent CRT is associated with good clinical response (80–94 %) and high 5-year OS (72–84 %), DFS (73 %), locoregional recurrence-free survival (70 %), and colostomy-free survival rates (70–80 %) [52, 55, 58, 102, 103, 106, 124, 154, 155]. In a cohort study of 19,195 patients treated for SCC between 1985 and 2000, the 5-year survival rates were 70 %, 59 %, 41 %, and 19 % for stage I, stage II, stage III, and stage IV disease, respectively [154]. The full benefit of CRT (UKCCCR trial, ACT I) is durable for at least 7 years, and most anal cancer-related deaths occur in the first few years (54 % in the first 2 years) [97]. The 5-year cumulative colostomy rate and actuarial 10-year OS and DSF rates are similar with MMC or cisplatin [156]. Metastatic disease is the cause of 40 % of cancer-specific deaths [55].

Pathologic factors that determine outcome include tumor size, local tumor extension, status of LN, and tumor grade [1, 102, 115, 124, 154, 157, 158]. Synchronous LN metastases are strictly related to tumor size and are found in 0 %, 8.5 %, 39 %, and 20–60 % with T1, T2, T3, and T4 tumors, respectively [53]. With tumors >5 cm and T4 lesions, LN metastasis is present 47 % and doubled with extension of tumor beyond the external sphincter 58 % [53]. Inguinal LN involvement is a major independent prognostic factor for LR, OS, and DFS [1, 97, 124, 154, 155]. Survival rates drop from 70 % with negative LN to 40–50 % with positive LN [1, 53]. The 5-year OS for T1–T2, T3, and T4 tumors is 80–90 %, 60 %, and <50 %, respectively. Prognosis is worsened by 50 % with nodal involvement and tumor size greater than 5 cm [1, 97, 102, 124, 154].

Clinical and treatment-related factors that influence the outcome include gender, race, socioeconomic status, age over 75 years, intolerance to treatment, fistulization, immunosuppression, and HIV positivity [159–161]. Worse outcome is noted in men than women, blacks than white, and Hispanic and all than Asian, age over 75 years, presence of immunosuppression and HIV positivity, intolerance to treatment, and presence of fistulization. Complete CR after CRT and performance status of the patient are independent predictors of OS [100, 142, 155, 157, 162]. Metabolic activity in the primary tumor at time of presentation and after treatment and metabolic response are potential biomarker for predicting response to treatment and prognosis of the cancer [68, 162, 163]. Treatment breaks and overall treatment time may influence local outcome [94, 102, 133, 140, 141, 164, 165].

Relapse

Patterns

The 5-year locoregional failure rates after definitive CRT vary from 10 to 33 % [1, 52, 55, 58, 97, 102, 115, 154] (Figs. 22.3a–c and 22.4). Relapse occurs within the first 3 years and rarely after 5 years, and 85 % of recurrences are detected within the first 2 years [1, 97]. Patient wih disease located laterally at presentation and later develop inguinal LN metastasis do so in the ipsilateral groin [53, 54]. Metachronous LN metastasis is found during follow-up in 5–25 % of patients within 6 months of treatment and is strictly related to tumor size [53]. About 17 % of patients treated with CRT develop metastatic disease and the liver is the most common site [5, 52]. Locoregional and/or distant recurrence occurs in up to 35 % of treated patients and is strongly associated with advanced T stage (T3 and T4) and nodal involvement [40].

Anal cancers regress slowly after CRT and patients are classified into complete responders and nonresponders with either residual/persistent disease or progressive disease (growth during treatment). Locoregional failure is equally divided between persistent, progressive, and true recurrent disease [1, 115]. The timing of when maximum response to CRT occurs is poorly defined. Hazard ratios indicate that assessment at 26 weeks is the most discriminating end point with the most significant effect on outcome and therefore the

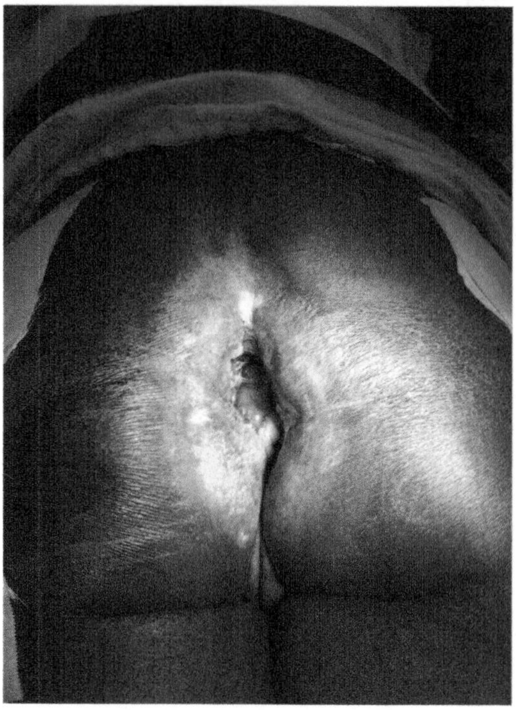

Fig. 22.4 Patient with a recurrent squamous cell carcinoma of the anal canal 2 years after Nigro protocol. This patient underwent an abdominosacral resection (Courtesy of Quyen D. Chu, MD, MBA, FACS)

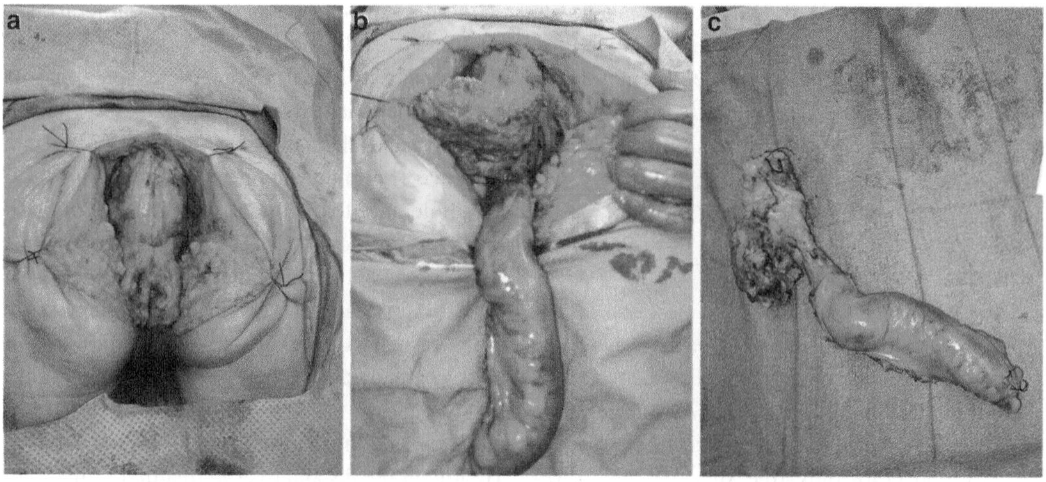

Fig. 22.3 (a–c) Abdominosacral resection of a patient with residual cancer following the Nigro protocol (Courtesy of Quyen D. Chu, MD, MBA, FACS)

optimum time for assessment [4]. Several studies suggest a waiting period of 8–10 weeks before final evaluation, but 6–12 weeks are commonly used. There is a debate regarding the best time to define lack of response and persistent disease. Most studies define residual disease as disease present within 6 months of CRT and recurrent disease when a tumor is discovered after 6 months. The ACT II trial showed that assessment of complete response at 11 weeks will discriminate those patients achieving and not achieving complete clinical response in terms of PFS and OS [104]. Some authors recommend biopsy only if a suspicious lesion is present [131].

Treatment of Relapse

With prophylactic RT, LN recurrence decreases to 2.5–3 % [58, 92, 115, 127, 166, 167]. If untreated, metachronous LN metastasis occurs in 7.4–7.8 % of patients [63, 100]. Inguinal LN dissection is indicated for persistent synchronous disease after radiotherapy and recurrent (metachronous) disease.

Despite effective CRT, 30–40 % of patients required salvage APR for tumor recurrence, incomplete pathological response, and progressive disease after treatment [79, 84, 86, 88–90, 158, 168]. In most studies, APR is performed for persistent disease after CRT [83, 131, 158, 169–171]. In a review of 13 studies, Renehan and O'Dwyer concluded that APR offers the only chance for cure [161]. Long-term survival varies from 25 to 60 %, reflecting the heterogeneity of the adjuvant therapy and individual characteristics of the patient and tumor [4, 124, 157, 161, 172, 173]. The most important prognostic factor after APR is margin status [169]. Other prognostic factors include T and LN status, size >5 cm, adjacent organ invasion, existence of metastases at time of surgery, male gender, and higher comorbidities [2, 86, 159, 171, 173]. Morbidity of salvage APR can be as high as 72 % due to urinary retention, impotence, poor healing, abscess, and perineal hernia formation [171]. Poor perineal wound healing is related to large defect created by the wide excision and prior RT. Wound breakdown occurred in 36–59 % of primary closure, 36 % of patients with omental flap, and 0 % with vertical rectus abdominis myocutaneous (VRAM) flap [171]. Salvage CRT (i.e., repeat Nigro protocol) for persistent disease has been evaluated, but the efficacy is not clear. Most commonly, 5-FU/cisplatin is used [58].

About 10–20 % of patients have extrapelvic metastatic disease at presentation, and 10–17 % of patients with initially local disease develop distant metastasis despite CRT. The liver is the most common site [5, 52, 55, 58, 102, 106, 107]. Few studies have addressed CT protocols for metastatic disease. Data indicate that treatment with 5-FU/cisplatin is associated with 50 % response rate and a median OS of 13–55 months [174–177]. In a retrospective analysis of patients treated with cetuximab and irinotecan, partial remission or stabilization of tumor was noted in patients with KRAS wild-type anal cancer compared to patients harboring KRAS mutations who had progressive disease [110]. An ongoing phase II (E3205) study is evaluating the efficacy of cetuximab+cisplatin, 5-FU, and RT [178].

Salient Points

- Anal SCC is considered a sexually transmitted disease and HPV is an important causative factor. Oncogenic HPV serotypes are strongly linked to premalignant and malignant anal and genital lesions.
- HIV-positive patients are more likely to be infected with HPV than HIV-negative patients regardless of sexual practices and have higher prevalence of AIN. They are at increased risk for the development of anal cancer. High-grade AIN progresses more frequently to cancer than HIV-negative patients.
- Studies by Nigro which demonstrated concurrent CRT (5-FU/MMC+low-dose radiation) resulted in high rates of local control, and subsequent randomized phase III trials have confirmed these findings. These studies have utilized 5-FU with MMC or cisplatin, but concurrent CRT with 5-FU and MMC remains the considered standard of care. However, MMC is associated with treatment-related deaths and life-threatening hematologic toxicity and

hemolytic-uremic syndrome. 5-FU/MMC is superior to 5-FU alone as it improves sphincter preservation and disease control despite greater associated toxicity.

- The addition of cisplatin-based neoadjuvant therapy prior to concurrent CRT is of no benefit in terms of colostomy-free survival (RTOG 98-11 and ACCORD-03).
- The administration of consolidation (adjuvant) 5-FU/cisplatin after concurrent CRT is also of no benefit in terms of CR, DFS, and OS (ACT II).
- Overall, HIV-positive individuals do not tolerate CRT (higher skin and hematologic toxicity) and carry a higher risk of local recurrence and risk of dying from the cancer after treatment, and OS correlates with CD 4+ count <200 cells/ml.
- IMRT reduces toxicity and maintains sphincter preservation without compromising local control.
- The role of alternative chemotherapeutic agents and biological therapy in the treatment of localized and metastatic anal canal is being tested.
- Abdominoperineal resection is the only hope for cure after failed concurrent CRT.

Questions and Answers

Questions

1. Tranformational epithelium
   A. Represents squamocolumnar zone spanning about 0–1.2 cm above the dentate line
   B. Is squamous metaplastic tissue that occurs above the dentate line and overlying columnar epithelium (6–10 cm)
   C. Is modified skin
   D. A and C
   E. None of the above
2. Low-grade AIN
   A. May regress
   B. May progress to high-grade AIN
   C. May progress directly to cancer
   D. A, B, and C
   E. A and B
3. HPV 16 and 18
   A. Have little oncogenic potential
   B. Are strongly linked to premalignant and malignant lesions of the anus but not the vulva and uterus
   C. Are present in small percentage of anal cancer cases
   D. Have oncogenic potential
   E. A, B, and C
4. In initial staging of anal cancer
   A. PET/CT scan is superior to CT scan in detecting groin LN metastasis.
   B. Sentinel LN biopsy is indicated when inguinal LNs are enlarged.
   C. Elective groin LN dissection is performed as a staging procedure routinely prior to combination CRT.
   D. CT scan is superior to PET scan in detecting metastasis to groin LN.
   E. None of the above.
5. Single-modality treatment with RT
   A. Has no role in the treatment of anal cancer
   B. Is as effective as concurrent CRT in the treatment of small anal cancers
   C. Is not indicated in the elderly patient
   D. A, B, and C
   E. A and C
6. Treatment with MMC
   A. May be eliminated from concurrent CRT because of toxicity
   B. Has no impact on local recurrence
   C. Has no impact on disease-free survival
   D. A, B and C
   E. None of the above
7. In HIV-positive patients on HAART treated with concurrent CRT
   A. Complete response rate, as in HIV-negative patients, is high.
   B. Patients have 5-year OS similar to HIV-negative patients.
   C. Patients have higher locoregional recurrence compared to HIV-negative patients.
   D. Unlike HIV-negative patients, majority die of anal cancer.
   E. All of the above.
8. The most important pathologic prognostic factors in anal SCC are:
   A. Tumor size and extent
   B. Location in relation to the dentate line
   C. Status of LN
   D. A, B, and C
   E. A and C

9. A 55-year old man presented with a large histologically proven SCC of the anal canal. Which of the following is the most appropriate treatment?
   A. Abdominoperineal resection (APR)
   B. Concurrent chemoradiation therapy with 5-FU and mitomycin C
   C. Chemotherapy alone
   D. Radiation therapy alone
   E. Neoadjuvant chemotherapy followed by an APR

Answers

1. B
2. E
3. D
4. A
5. B
6. E
7. E
8. E
9. B

References

1. Ryan DP, Compton CC, Mayer RJ. Carcinoma of the anal canal. N Engl J Med. 2000;342(11):792–800.
2. Jemal A, Murray T, Ward E, et al. Cancer statistics, 2005. CA Cancer J Clin. 2005;55(1):10–30.
3. Fuchshuber PR, Rodriguez-Bigas M, Weber T, Petrelli NJ. Anal canal and perianal epidermoid cancers. J Am Coll Surg. 1997;185(5):494–505.
4. Jemal A, Siegel R, Ward E, et al. Cancer statistics, 2006. CA Cancer J Clin. 2006;56(2):106–30.
5. Welton ML, Varma MG. Anal cancer. In: Wolff BG, Fleshman JW, Beck DE, Pemberton JH, Wexner SD editors. The ASCRS textbook of colon and rectal surgery. 1st ed. New York: Springer; 2007. p. 482–500.
6. Edge SB, Compton CC. The American Joint Committee on Cancer: the 7th edition of the AJCC cancer staging manual and the future of TNM. Ann Surg Oncol. 2010;17(6):1471–4.
7. Ries LAG, Harkin D, Krapcho M. SEER cancer statistics review, 1975–2003. Baltimore: National Cancer Institute; 2005. p. 1–103.
8. Patel P, Hanson DL, Sullivan PS, et al. Incidence of types of cancer among HIV-infected persons compared with the general population in the United States, 1992–2003. Ann Intern Med. 2008;148(10):728–36.
9. Frisch M, Glimelius B, van den Brule AJ, et al. Sexually transmitted infection as a cause of anal cancer. N Engl J Med. 1997;337(19):1350–8.
10. Johnson LG, Madeleine MM, Newcomer LM, Schwartz SM, Daling JR. Anal cancer incidence and survival: the surveillance, epidemiology, and end results experience, 1973–2000. Cancer. 2004; 101(2):281–8.
11. Siegel R, Ward E, Brawley O, Jemal A. Cancer statistics, 2011: the impact of eliminating socioeconomic and racial disparities on premature cancer deaths. CA Cancer J Clin. 2011;61(4):212–36.
12. Melbye M, Coté TR, Kessler L, Gail M, Biggar RJ. High incidence of anal cancer among AIDS patients. The AIDS/Cancer Working Group. Lancet. 1994; 343(8898):636–9.
13. Penn I. Cancers of the anogenital region in renal transplant recipients. Analysis of 65 cases. Cancer. 1986;58(3):611–6.
14. Daling JR, Weiss NS, Hislop TG, et al. Sexual practices, sexually transmitted diseases, and the incidence of anal cancer. N Engl J Med. 1987;317(16): 973–7.
15. Goedert JJ, Coté TR, Virgo P, et al. Spectrum of AIDS-associated malignant disorders. Lancet. 1998; 351(9119):1833–9.
16. Morson B. The pathology and results of treatment of squamous cell carcinoma of the anal canal and margin. Proc R Soc Med. 1960;53:416–20.
17. Renehan AG, O'Dwyer ST. Initial management through the anal cancer multidisciplinary team meeting. Colorectal Dis. 2011;13 Suppl 1:21–8.
18. Parikh J, Shaw A, Grant LA, et al. Anal carcinomas: the role of endoanal ultrasound and magnetic resonance imaging in staging, response evaluation and follow-up. Eur Radiol. 2011;21(4):776–85.
19. Czito BG, Willett CG. Current management of anal canal cancer. Curr Oncol Rep. 2009;11(3):186–92.
20. Tung W, Nivatvongs S. Perianal and anal canal neoplasms. In: Gordon PH, Nivatvongs S, editors. Principles and practice of surgery for the colon, rectum, and anus. 2nd ed. St. Louis: Quality Medical Publishing; 1999. p. 401–17.
21. Peters RK, Mack TM, Bernstein L. Parallels in the epidemiology of selected anogenital carcinomas. J Natl Cancer Inst. 1984;72(3):609–15.
22. Frisch M, Fenger C, van den Brule AJ, et al. Variants of squamous cell carcinoma of the anal canal and perianal skin and their relation to human papillomaviruses. Cancer Res. 1999;59(3):753–7.
23. Palefsky JM, Holly EA, Ralston ML, Da Costa M, Greenblatt RM. Prevalence and risk factors for anal human papillomavirus infection in human immunodeficiency virus (HIV)-positive and high-risk HIV-negative women. J Infect Dis. 2001; 183(3):383–91.
24. Daling JR, Madeleine MM, Johnson LG, et al. Human papillomavirus, smoking, and sexual practices in the etiology of anal cancer. Cancer. 2004; 101(2):270–80.
25. Marchesa P, Fazio VW, Oliart S, Goldblum JR, Lavery IC. Perianal Bowen's disease: a clinicopathologic study of 47 patients. Dis Colon Rectum. 1997;40(11):1286–93.

26. Marfing TE, Abel ME, Gallagher DM. Perianal Bowen's disease and associated malignancies. Results of a survey. Dis Colon Rectum. 1987; 30(10):782–5.
27. Watson AJ, Smith BB, Whitehead MR, Sykes PH, Frizelle FA. Malignant progression of anal intra-epithelial neoplasia. ANZ J Surg. 2006;76(8): 715–7.
28. Parkin DM. The global health burden of infection-associated cancers in the year 2002. Int J Cancer. 2006;118(12):3030–44.
29. Holly EA, Ralston ML, Darragh TM, Greenblatt RM, Jay N, Palefsky JM. Prevalence and risk factors for anal squamous intraepithelial lesions in women. J Natl Cancer Inst. 2001;93(11):843–9.
30. Duggan MA, Boras VF, Inoue M, McGregor SE, Robertson DI. Human papillomavirus DNA determination of anal condylomata, dysplasias, and squamous carcinomas with in situ hybridization. Am J Clin Pathol. 1989;92(1):16–21.
31. Hoots BE, Palefsky JM, Pimenta JM, Smith JS. Human papillomavirus type distribution in anal cancer and anal intraepithelial lesions. Int J Cancer. 2009;124(10):2375–83.
32. Rabkin CS, Biggar RJ, Melbye M, Curtis RE. Second primary cancers following anal and cervical carcinoma: evidence of shared etiologic factors. Am J Epidemiol. 1992;136(1):54–8.
33. Bjørge T, Engeland A, Luostarinen T, et al. Human papillomavirus infection as a risk factor for anal and perianal skin cancer in a prospective study. Br J Cancer. 2002;87(1):61–4.
34. Brotherton JM, Fridman M, May CL, Chappell G, Saville AM, Gertig DM. Early effect of the HPV vaccination programme on cervical abnormalities in Victoria, Australia: an ecological study. Lancet. 2011;377(9783):2085–92.
35. Ramamoorthy S, Liu YT, Luo L, Miyai K, Lu Q, Carethers JM. Detection of multiple human papillomavirus genotypes in anal carcinoma. Infect Agent Cancer. 2010;5:17.
36. Zbar AP, Fenger C, Efron J, Beer-Gabel M, Wexner SD. The pathology and molecular biology of anal intraepithelial neoplasia: comparisons with cervical and vulvar intraepithelial carcinoma. Int J Colorectal Dis. 2002;17(4):203–15.
37. de Sanjosé S, Palefsky J. Cervical and anal HPV infections in HIV positive women and men. Virus Res. 2002;89(2):201–11.
38. Piketty C, Darragh TM, Da Costa M, et al. High prevalence of anal human papillomavirus infection and anal cancer precursors among HIV-infected persons in the absence of anal intercourse. Ann Intern Med. 2003;138(6):453–9.
39. Winton E, Heriot AG, Ng M, et al. The impact of 18-fluorodeoxyglucose positron emission tomography on the staging, management and outcome of anal cancer. Br J Cancer. 2009;100(5):693–700.
40. Gervaz P, Calmy A, Durmishi Y, Allal AS, Morel P. Squamous cell carcinoma of the anus-an opportunistic cancer in HIV-positive male homosexuals. World J Gastroenterol. 2011;17(25):2987–91.
41. Hammad N, Heilbrun LK, Gupta S, et al. Squamous cell cancer of the anal canal in HIV-infected patients receiving highly active antiretroviral therapy: a single institution experience. Am J Clin Oncol. 2011;34(2):135–9.
42. Guiguet M, Boué F, Cadranel J, et al. Effect of immunodeficiency, HIV viral load, and antiretroviral therapy on the risk of individual malignancies (FHDH-ANRS CO4): a prospective cohort study. Lancet Oncol. 2009;10(12):1152–9.
43. Bower M, Powles T, Newsom-Davis T, et al. HIV-associated anal cancer: has highly active antiretroviral therapy reduced the incidence or improved the outcome? J Acquir Immune Defic Syndr. 2004;37(5):1563–5.
44. Chin-Hong PV, Vittinghoff E, Cranston RD, et al. Age-related prevalence of anal cancer precursors in homosexual men: the EXPLORE study. J Natl Cancer Inst. 2005;97(12):896–905.
45. Edgren G, Sparén P. Risk of anogenital cancer after diagnosis of cervical intraepithelial neoplasia: a prospective population-based study. Lancet Oncol. 2007;8(4):311–6.
46. Sillman FH, Sentovich S, Shaffer D. Ano-genital neoplasia in renal transplant patients. Ann Transplant. 1997;2(4):59–66.
47. Frisch M. On the etiology of anal squamous carcinoma. Dan Med Bull. 2002;49(3):194–209.
48. Daling JR, Sherman KJ, Hislop TG, et al. Cigarette smoking and the risk of anogenital cancer. Am J Epidemiol. 1992;135(2):180–9.
49. Tonolini M, Bianco R. MRI and CT of anal carcinoma: a pictorial review. Insights Imaging. 2013;4(1):53–62.
50. Carter PS, de Ruiter A, Whatrup C, et al. Human immunodeficiency virus infection and genital warts as risk factors for anal intraepithelial neoplasia in homosexual men. Br J Surg. 1995;82(4):473–4.
51. Pintor MP, Northover JM, Nicholls RJ. Squamous cell carcinoma of the anus at one hospital from 1948 to 1984. Br J Surg. 1989;76(8):806–10.
52. Bartelink H, Roelofsen F, Eschwege F, et al. Concomitant radiotherapy and chemotherapy is superior to radiotherapy alone in the treatment of locally advanced anal cancer: results of a phase III randomized trial of the European Organization for Research and Treatment of Cancer Radiotherapy and Gastrointestinal Cooperative Groups. J Clin Oncol. 1997;15(5):2040–9.
53. Gerard JP, Chapet O, Samiei F, et al. Management of inguinal lymph node metastases in patients with carcinoma of the anal canal: experience in a series of 270 patients treated in Lyon and review of the literature. Cancer. 2001;92(1):77–84.
54. Damin DC, Rosito MA, Schwartsmann G. Sentinel lymph node in carcinoma of the anal canal: a review. Eur J Surg Oncol. 2006;32(3):247–52.
55. UK Co-ordinating Committee on Cancer Research UKCCCR Anal Cancer Trial Working Party.

Epidermoid anal cancer: results from the UKCCCR randomised trial of radiotherapy alone versus radiotherapy, 5-fluorouracil, and mitomycin. UKCCCR Anal Cancer Trial Working Party. 1996;348(9034):1049–54.
56. Allal AS, Waelchli L, Bründler MA. Prognostic value of apoptosis-regulating protein expression in anal squamous cell carcinoma. Clin Cancer Res. 2003;9(17):6489–96.
57. Clark MA, Hartley A, Geh JI. Cancer of the anal canal. Lancet Oncol. 2004;5(3):149–57.
58. Flam M, John M, Pajak TF, et al. Role of mitomycin in combination with fluorouracil and radiotherapy, and of salvage chemoradiation in the definitive nonsurgical treatment of epidermoid carcinoma of the anal canal: results of a phase III randomized intergroup study. J Clin Oncol. 1996;14(9):2527–39.
59. Tarantino D, Bernstein MA. Endoanal ultrasound in the staging and management of squamous-cell carcinoma of the anal canal: potential implications of a new ultrasound staging system. Dis Colon Rectum. 2002;45(1):16–22.
60. Christensen AF, Nielsen MB, Engelholm SA, Roed H, Svendsen LB, Christensen H. Three-dimensional anal endosonography may improve staging of anal cancer compared with two-dimensional endosonography. Dis Colon Rectum. 2004;47(3):341–5.
61. Giovannini M, Bardou VJ, Barclay R, et al. Anal carcinoma: prognostic value of endorectal ultrasound (ERUS). Results of a prospective multicenter study. Endoscopy. 2001;33(3):231–6.
62. Martellucci J, Naldini G, Colosimo C, Cionini L, Rossi M. Accuracy of endoanal ultrasound in the follow-up assessment for squamous cell carcinoma of the anal canal treated with radiochemotherapy. Surg Endosc. 2009;23(5):1054–7.
63. Trautmann TG, Zuger JH. Positron Emission Tomography for pretreatment staging and posttreatment evaluation in cancer of the anal canal. Mol Imaging Biol. 2005;7(4):309–13.
64. Nguyen BT, Joon DL, Khoo V, et al. Assessing the impact of FDG-PET in the management of anal cancer. Radiother Oncol. 2008;87(3):376–82.
65. Mistrangelo M, Pelosi E, Bellò M, et al. Comparison of positron emission tomography scanning and sentinel node biopsy in the detection of inguinal node metastases in patients with anal cancer. Int J Radiat Oncol Biol Phys. 2010;77(1):73–8.
66. Borzomati D, Valeri S, Ripetti V, et al. Persisting perianal ulcer after radiotherapy for anal cancer: recurrence of disease or late radiation-related complication? Hepatogastroenterology. 2005;52(63):780–4.
67. Sato H, Koh PK, Bartolo DC. Management of anal canal cancer. Dis Colon Rectum. 2005;48(6):1301–15.
68. Day FL, Link E, Ngan S, et al. FDG-PET metabolic response predicts outcomes in anal cancer managed with chemoradiotherapy. Br J Cancer. 2011;105(4):498–504.
69. Cotter SE, Grigsby PW, Siegel BA, et al. FDG-PET/CT in the evaluation of anal carcinoma. Int J Radiat Oncol Biol Phys. 2006;65(3):720–5.
70. Anderson C, Koshy M, Staley C, et al. PET-CT fusion in radiation management of patients with anorectal tumors. Int J Radiat Oncol Biol Phys. 2007;69(1):155–62.
71. Bannas P, Weber C, Adam G, et al. Contrast-enhanced [(18)F]fluorodeoxyglucose-positron emission tomography/computed tomography for staging and radiotherapy planning in patients with anal cancer. Int J Radiat Oncol Biol Phys. 2011;81(2):445–51.
72. Meyer J, Willett C, Czito B. Current and emerging treatment strategies for anal cancer. Curr Oncol Rep. 2010;12(3):168–74.
73. Ortholan C, Resbeut M, Hannoun-Levi JM, et al. Anal canal cancer: management of inguinal nodes and benefit of prophylactic inguinal irradiation (CORS-03 Study). Int J Radiat Oncol Biol Phys. 2012;82(5):1988–95.
74. Wright JL, Patil SM, Temple LK, Minsky BD, Saltz LB, Goodman KA. Squamous cell carcinoma of the anal canal: patterns and predictors of failure and implications for intensity-modulated radiation treatment planning. Int J Radiat Oncol Biol Phys. 2010;78(4):1064–72.
75. De Nardi P, Carvello M, Staudacher C. New approach to anal cancer: individualized therapy based on sentinel lymph node biopsy. World J Gastroenterol. 2012;18(44):6349–56.
76. Gretschel S, Warnick P, Bembenek A, et al. Lymphatic mapping and sentinel lymph node biopsy in epidermoid carcinoma of the anal canal. Eur J Surg Oncol. 2008;34(8):890–4.
77. Péley G, Farkas E, Sinkovics I, et al. Inguinal sentinel lymph node biopsy for staging anal cancer. Scand J Surg. 2002;91(4):336–8.
78. Rabbitt P, Pathma-Nathan N, Collinson T, Hewett P, Rieger N. Sentinel lymph node biopsy for squamous cell carcinoma of the anal canal. ANZ J Surg. 2002;72(9):651–4.
79. de Jong JS, Beukema JC, van Dam GM, Slart R, Lemstrà C, Wiggers T. Limited value of staging squamous cell carcinoma of the anal margin and canal using the sentinel lymph node procedure: a prospective study with long-term follow-up. Ann Surg Oncol. 2010;17(10):2656–62.
80. Mistrangelo DM, Bellò M, Cassoni P, et al. Value of staging squamous cell carcinoma of the anal margin and canal using the sentinel lymph node procedure: an update of the series and a review of the literature. Br J Cancer. 2013;108(3):527–32.
81. Lampejo T, Kavanagh D, Clark J, et al. Prognostic biomarkers in squamous cell carcinoma of the anus: a systematic review. Br J Cancer. 2010;103(12):1858–69.
82. Boman BM, Moertel CG, O'Connell MJ, et al. Carcinoma of the anal canal. A clinical and pathologic study of 188 cases. Cancer. 1984;54(1):114–25.

83. Nigro ND, Vaitkevicius VK, Considine B. Combined therapy for cancer of the anal canal: a preliminary report. Dis Colon Rectum. 1974;17(3):354–6.
84. Staib L, Gottwald T, Lehnert T, et al. Sphincter-saving treatment in epidermoid anal cancer: cooperative analysis of 142 patients in five German university surgical centers. Int J Colorectal Dis. 2000;15(5–6):282–90.
85. Mariani P, Ghanneme A, De la Rochefordière A, Girodet J, Falcou MC, Salmon RJ. Abdominoperineal resection for anal cancer. Dis Colon Rectum. 2008;51(10):1495–501.
86. Lefèvre JH, Corte H, Tiret E, et al. Abdominoperineal resection for squamous cell anal carcinoma: survival and risk factors for recurrence. Ann Surg Oncol. 2012;19(13):4186–92.
87. Engstrom PF, Arnoletti JP, Benson AB, et al. NCCN clinical practice guidelines in oncology. Anal carcinoma. J Natl Compr Canc Netw. 2010;8(1):106–20.
88. Putta S, Andreyev HJ. Faecal incontinence: a late side-effect of pelvic radiotherapy. Clin Oncol (R Coll Radiol). 2005;17(6):469–77.
89. de Bree E, van Ruth S, Dewit LG, Zoetmulder FA. High risk of colostomy with primary radiotherapy for anal cancer. Ann Surg Oncol. 2007; 14(1):100–8.
90. Eeson G, Foo M, Harrow S, McGregor G, Hay J. Outcomes of salvage surgery for epidermoid carcinoma of the anus following failed combined modality treatment. Am J Surg. 2011;201(5):628–33.
91. Cummings B, Keane T, Thomas G, Harwood A, Rider W. Results and toxicity of the treatment of anal canal carcinoma by radiation therapy or radiation therapy and chemotherapy. Cancer. 1984; 54(10):2062–8.
92. Cummings BJ, Keane TJ, O'Sullivan B, Wong CS, Catton CN. Mitomycin in anal canal carcinoma. Oncology. 1993;50 Suppl 1:63–9.
93. Martenson JA, Gunderson LL. External radiation therapy without chemotherapy in the management of anal cancer. Cancer. 1993;71(5):1736–40.
94. Deniaud-Alexandre E, Touboul E, Tiret E, et al. Epidermoid carcinomas of the anal canal treated with definitive radiation therapy in a series of 305 patients. Cancer Radiother. 2003;7(4):237–53.
95. Lestrade L, De Bari B, Montbarbon X, Pommier P, Carrie C. Radiochemotherapy and brachytherapy could be the standard treatment for anal canal cancer in elderly patients? A retrospective single-centre analysis. Med Oncol. 2013;30(1):402.
96. Nigro ND, Vaitkevicius VK, Buroker T, Bradley GT, Considine B. Combined therapy for cancer of the anal canal. Dis Colon Rectum. 1981;24(2):73–5.
97. Northover J, Glynne-Jones R, Sebag-Montefiore D, et al. Chemoradiation for the treatment of epidermoid anal cancer: 13-year follow-up of the first randomised UKCCCR Anal Cancer Trial (ACT I). Br J Cancer. 2010;102(7):1123–8.
98. Martenson JA, Lipsitz SR, Wagner H, et al. Initial results of a phase II trial of high dose radiation therapy, 5-fluorouracil, and cisplatin for patients with anal cancer (E4292): an Eastern Cooperative Oncology Group study. Int J Radiat Oncol Biol Phys. 1996;35(4):745–9.
99. Rich TA, Ajani JA, Morrison WH, Ota D, Levin B. Chemoradiation therapy for anal cancer: radiation plus continuous infusion of 5-fluorouracil with or without cisplatin. Radiother Oncol. 1993; 27(3):209–15.
100. Gerard JP, Ayzac L, Hun D, et al. Treatment of anal canal carcinoma with high dose radiation therapy and concomitant fluorouracil-cisplatinum. Long-term results in 95 patients. Radiother Oncol. 1998; 46(3):249–56.
101. Peiffert D, Seitz JF, Rougier P, et al. Preliminary results of a phase II study of high-dose radiation therapy and neoadjuvant plus concomitant 5-fluorouracil with CDDP chemotherapy for patients with anal canal cancer: a French cooperative study. Ann Oncol. 1997;8(6):575–81.
102. Ajani JA, Winter KA, Gunderson LL, et al. Fluorouracil, mitomycin, and radiotherapy vs fluorouracil, cisplatin, and radiotherapy for carcinoma of the anal canal: a randomized controlled trial. JAMA. 2008;299(16):1914–21.
103. Gunderson LL, Winter KA, Ajani JA, et al. Long-term update of US GI intergroup RTOG 98-11 phase III trial for anal carcinoma: survival, relapse, and colostomy failure with concurrent chemoradiation involving fluorouracil/mitomycin versus fluorouracil/cisplatin. J Clin Oncol. 2012;30(35):4344–51.
104. Peiffert D, Giovannini M, Ducreux M, et al. High-dose radiation therapy and neoadjuvant plus concomitant chemotherapy with 5-fluorouracil and cisplatin in patients with locally advanced squamous-cell anal canal cancer: final results of a phase II study. Ann Oncol. 2001;12(3):397–404.
105. James R, Meadows H, Wan S. ACT II: the second UK phase III anal cancer trial. Clin Oncol (R Coll Radiol). 2005;17(5):364–6.
106. James R, Wan S, Glynn-Jones R, Sebago-Montefiore D, et al. On behalf of the II ACT study group: a randomized trial of chemoradiation using combination 5FU/mitomycin or 5FU/cisplatin, with or without maintenance cisplatin/5FU in squamous carcinoma of the anus (ACT II). J Clin Oncol. 2009;27(Suppl 797s):abstr LBA 4009.
107. Peiffert D, Tournier-Rangeard L, Gérard JP, et al. Induction chemotherapy and dose intensification of the radiation boost in locally advanced anal canal carcinoma: final analysis of the randomized UNICANCER ACCORD 03 trial. J Clin Oncol. 2012;30(16):1941–8.
108. Glynne-Jones R, Meadows H, Wan S, et al. EXTRA – a multicenter phase II study of chemoradiation using a 5 day per week oral regimen of capecitabine and intravenous mitomycin C in anal cancer. Int J Radiat Oncol Biol Phys. 2008;72(1):119–26.
109. Deenen MJ, Dewit L, Boot H, Beijnen JH, Schellens JH, Cats A. Simultaneous integrated boost-intensity

modulated radiation therapy with concomitant capecitabine and mitomycin C for locally advanced anal carcinoma: a phase 1 study. Int J Radiat Oncol Biol Phys. 2013;85(5):e201–7.

110. Lukan N, Ströbel P, Willer A, et al. Cetuximab-based treatment of metastatic anal cancer: correlation of response with KRAS mutational status. Oncology. 2009;77(5):293–9.
111. Barmettler H, Komminoth P, Schmid M, Duerr D. Efficacy of cetuximab in combination with FOLFIRI in a patient with KRAS wild-type metastatic anal cancer. Case Rep Oncol. 2012;5(2):428–33.
112. Zampino MG, Magni E, Sonzogni A, Renne G. K-ras status in squamous cell anal carcinoma (SCC): it's time for target-oriented treatment? Cancer Chemother Pharmacol. 2009;65(1):197–9.
113. Phan LK, Hoff PM. Evidence of clinical activity for cetuximab combined with irinotecan in a patient with refractory anal canal squamous-cell carcinoma: report of a case. Dis Colon Rectum. 2007; 50(3):395–8.
114. Olivatto LO, Vieira FM, Pereira BV, et al. Phase 1 study of cetuximab in combination with 5-fluorouracil, cisplatin, and radiotherapy in patients with locally advanced anal canal carcinoma. Cancer. 2013;119(16):2973–80.
115. Das P, Bhatia S, Eng C, et al. Predictors and patterns of recurrence after definitive chemoradiation for anal cancer. Int J Radiat Oncol Biol Phys. 2007;68(3): 794–800.
116. Peddada AV, Smith DE, Rao AR, Frost DB, Kagan AR. Chemotherapy and low-dose radiotherapy in the treatment of HIV-infected patients with carcinoma of the anal canal. Int J Radiat Oncol Biol Phys. 1997;37(5):1101–5.
117. Kim JH, Sarani B, Orkin BA, et al. HIV-positive patients with anal carcinoma have poorer treatment tolerance and outcome than HIV-negative patients. Dis Colon Rectum. 2001;44(10): 1496–502.
118. Chiao EY, Giordano TP, Richardson P, El-Serag HB. Human immunodeficiency virus-associated squamous cell cancer of the anus: epidemiology and outcomes in the highly active antiretroviral therapy era. J Clin Oncol. 2008;26(3):474–9.
119. Powles T, Robinson D, Stebbing J, et al. Highly active antiretroviral therapy and the incidence of non-AIDS-defining cancers in people with HIV infection. J Clin Oncol. 2009;27(6):884–90.
120. Oehler-Jänne C, Huguet F, Provencher S, et al. HIV-specific differences in outcome of squamous cell carcinoma of the anal canal: a multicentric cohort study of HIV-positive patients receiving highly active antiretroviral therapy. J Clin Oncol. 2008; 26(15):2550–7.
121. Edelman S, Johnstone PA. Combined modality therapy for HIV-infected patients with squamous cell carcinoma of the anus: outcomes and toxicities. Int J Radiat Oncol Biol Phys. 2006;66(1):206–11.
122. Wexler A, Berson AM, Goldstone SE, et al. Invasive anal squamous-cell carcinoma in the HIV-positive patient: outcome in the era of highly active antiretroviral therapy. Dis Colon Rectum. 2008;51(1): 73–81.
123. Berry JM, Palefsky JM, Welton ML. Anal cancer and its precursors in HIV-positive patients: perspectives and management. Surg Oncol Clin N Am. 2004;13(2):355–73.
124. Touboul E, Schlienger M, Buffat L, et al. Epidermoid carcinoma of the anal canal. Results of curative-intent radiation therapy in a series of 270 patients. Cancer. 1994;73(6):1569–79.
125. Chen YJ, Liu A, Tsai PT, et al. Organ sparing by conformal avoidance intensity-modulated radiation therapy for anal cancer: dosimetric evaluation of coverage of pelvis and inguinal/femoral nodes. Int J Radiat Oncol Biol Phys. 2005;63(1):274–81.
126. Dewas CV, Maingon P, Dalban C, et al. Does gap-free intensity modulated chemoradiation therapy provide a greater clinical benefit than 3D conformal chemoradiation in patients with anal cancer? Radiat Oncol. 2012;7:201.
127. Ferrigno R, Nakamura RA, Dos Santos Novaes PE, et al. Radiochemotherapy in the conservative treatment of anal canal carcinoma: retrospective analysis of results and radiation dose effectiveness. Int J Radiat Oncol Biol Phys. 2005;61(4):1136–42.
128. Huang K, Haas-Kogan D, Weinberg V, Krieg R. Higher radiation dose with a shorter treatment duration improves outcome for locally advanced carcinoma of anal canal. World J Gastroenterol. 2007;13(6):895–900.
129. Engineer R, Mallik S, Mahantshetty U, Shrivastava S. Impact of radiation dose on locoregional control and survival on squamous cell carcinoma of anal canal. Radiother Oncol. 2010;95(3):283–7.
130. Das P, Cantor SB, Parker CL, et al. Long-term quality of life after radiotherapy for the treatment of anal cancer. Cancer. 2010;116(4):822–9.
131. Fleshner PR, Chalasani S, Chang GJ, et al. Practice parameters for anal squamous neoplasms. Dis Colon Rectum. 2008;51(1):2–9.
132. Conroy T, Ducreux M, Lemanski C, et al. Treatment intensification by induction chemotherapy (ICT) and radiation dose escalation in locally advanced squamous cell anal canal carcinoma (LAAC): definitive analysis of the intergroup ACCORD 03 Trial. J Clin Oncol. 2009;27:4033.
133. Graf R, Wust P, Hildebrandt B, et al. Impact of overall treatment time on local control of anal cancer treated with radiochemotherapy. Oncology. 2003; 65(1):14–22.
134. Eng C. Anal cancer: current and future methodology. Cancer Invest. 2006;24(5):535–44.
135. Lim F, Glynne-Jones R. Chemotherapy/chemoradiation in anal cancer: a systematic review. Cancer Treat Rev. 2011;37(7):520–32.
136. Jung H, Beck-Bornholdt HP, Svoboda V, Alberti W, Herrmann T. Quantification of late complications

after radiation therapy. Radiother Oncol. 2001; 61(3):233–46.
137. Hung A, Crane C, Delclos M, et al. Cisplatin-based combined modality therapy for anal carcinoma: a wider therapeutic index. Cancer. 2003;97(5):1195–202.
138. Baxter NN, Habermann EB, Tepper JE, Durham SB, Virnig BA. Risk of pelvic fractures in older women following pelvic irradiation. JAMA. 2005;294(20):2587–93.
139. Konski A, Garcia M, John M, et al. Evaluation of planned treatment breaks during radiation therapy for anal cancer: update of RTOG 92-08. Int J Radiat Oncol Biol Phys. 2008;72(1):114–8.
140. Bazan JG, Hara W, Hsu A, et al. Intensity-modulated radiation therapy versus conventional radiation therapy for squamous cell carcinoma of the anal canal. Cancer. 2011;117(15):3342–51.
141. Weber DC, Kurtz JM, Allal AS. The impact of gap duration on local control in anal canal carcinoma treated by split-course radiotherapy and concomitant chemotherapy. Int J Radiat Oncol Biol Phys. 2001;50(3):675–80.
142. Chen YW, Yen SH, Chen SY, et al. Anus-preservation treatment for anal cancer: retrospective analysis at a single institution. J Surg Oncol. 2007;96(5):374–80.
143. Milano MT, Jani AB, Farrey KJ, Rash C, Heimann R, Chmura SJ. Intensity-modulated radiation therapy (IMRT) in the treatment of anal cancer: toxicity and clinical outcome. Int J Radiat Oncol Biol Phys. 2005;63(2):354–61.
144. Kachnic LA, Tsai HK, Coen JJ, et al. Dose-painted intensity-modulated radiation therapy for anal cancer: a multi-institutional report of acute toxicity and response to therapy. Int J Radiat Oncol Biol Phys. 2012;82(1):153–8.
145. Devisetty K, Mell LK, Salama JK, et al. A multi-institutional acute gastrointestinal toxicity analysis of anal cancer patients treated with concurrent intensity-modulated radiation therapy (IMRT) and chemotherapy. Radiother Oncol. 2009;93(2): 298–301.
146. Veldeman L, Madani I, Hulstaert F, De Meerleer G, Mareel M, De Neve W. Evidence behind use of intensity-modulated radiotherapy: a systematic review of comparative clinical studies. Lancet Oncol. 2008;9(4):367–75.
147. Vieillot S, Fenoglietto P, Lemanski C, et al. IMRT for locally advanced anal cancer: clinical experience of the Montpellier Cancer Center. Radiat Oncol. 2012;7:45.
148. Pepek JM, Willett CG, Wu QJ, Yoo S, Clough RW, Czito BG. Intensity-modulated radiation therapy for anal malignancies: a preliminary toxicity and disease outcomes analysis. Int J Radiat Oncol Biol Phys. 2010;78(5):1413–9.
149. Zanetta G, Rota S, Chiari S, Bonazzi C, Bratina G, Mangioni C. Behavior of borderline tumors with particular interest to persistence, recurrence, and progression to invasive carcinoma: a prospective study. J Clin Oncol. 2001;19(10):2658–64.
150. Kachnic LA, Winter K, Myerson RJ, et al. RTOG 0529: a phase 2 evaluation of dose-painted intensity modulated radiation therapy in combination with 5-fluorouracil and mitomycin-C for the reduction of acute morbidity in carcinoma of the anal canal. Int J Radiat Oncol Biol Phys. 2013;86(1):27–33.
151. Chuong MD, Freilich JM, Hoffe SE, et al. Intensity-modulated radiation therapy vs. 3D conformal radiation therapy for squamous cell carcinoma of the anal canal. Gastrointest Cancer Res. 2013; 6(2):39–45.
152. Mell LK, Schomas DA, Salama JK, et al. Association between bone marrow dosimetric parameters and acute hematologic toxicity in anal cancer patients treated with concurrent chemotherapy and intensity-modulated radiotherapy. Int J Radiat Oncol Biol Phys. 2008;70(5):1431–7.
153. Lujan AE, Mundt AJ, Yamada SD, Rotmensch J, Roeske JC. Intensity-modulated radiotherapy as a means of reducing dose to bone marrow in gynecologic patients receiving whole pelvic radiotherapy. Int J Radiat Oncol Biol Phys. 2003;57(2):516–21.
154. Bilimoria KY, Bentrem DJ, Rock CE, Stewart AK, Ko CY, Halverson A. Outcomes and prognostic factors for squamous-cell carcinoma of the anal canal: analysis of patients from the National Cancer Data Base. Dis Colon Rectum. 2009;52(4):624–31.
155. Kim HJ, Huh JW, Kim CH, et al. Long-term outcomes of chemoradiation for anal cancer patients. Yonsei Med J. 2013;54(1):108–15.
156. Olivatto LO, Cabral V, Rosa A, et al. Mitomycin-C- or cisplatin-based chemoradiotherapy for anal canal carcinoma: long-term results. Int J Radiat Oncol Biol Phys. 2011;79(2):490–5.
157. Roohipour R, Patil S, Goodman KA, et al. Squamous-cell carcinoma of the anal canal: predictors of treatment outcome. Dis Colon Rectum. 2008; 51(2):147–53.
158. Mullen JT, Rodriguez-Bigas MA, Chang GJ, et al. Results of surgical salvage after failed chemoradiation therapy for epidermoid carcinoma of the anal canal. Ann Surg Oncol. 2007;14(2):478–83.
159. Nilsson PJ, Svensson C, Goldman S, Glimelius B. Salvage abdominoperineal resection in anal epidermoid cancer. Br J Surg. 2002;89(11):1425–9.
160. Glynne-Jones R, Sebag-Montefiore D, Adams R, et al. Prognostic factors for recurrence and survival in anal cancer: generating hypotheses from the mature outcomes of the first United Kingdom Coordinating Committee on Cancer Research Anal Cancer Trial (ACT I). Cancer. 2013;119(4):748–55.
161. Renehan AG, Saunders MP, Schofield PF, O'Dwyer ST. Patterns of local disease failure and outcome after salvage surgery in patients with anal cancer. Br J Surg. 2005;92(5):605–14.
162. Schwarz JK, Siegel BA, Dehdashti F, Myerson RJ, Fleshman JW, Grigsby PW. Tumor response and survival predicted by post-therapy FDG-PET/CT in anal cancer. Int J Radiat Oncol Biol Phys. 2008; 71(1):180–6.

163. Bazan JG, Koong AC, Kapp DS, et al. Metabolic tumor volume predicts disease progression and survival in patients with squamous cell carcinoma of the anal canal. J Nucl Med. 2013;54(1):27–32.
164. Chakravarthy AB, Catalano PJ, Martenson JA, et al. Long-term follow-up of a Phase II trial of high-dose radiation with concurrent 5-fluorouracil and cisplatin in patients with anal cancer (ECOG E4292). Int J Radiat Oncol Biol Phys. 2011;81(4):e607–13.
165. Ben-Josef E, Moughan J, Ajani JA, et al. Impact of overall treatment time on survival and local control in patients with anal cancer: a pooled data analysis of Radiation Therapy Oncology Group trials 87-04 and 98-11. J Clin Oncol. 2010;28(34):5061–6.
166. Myerson RJ, Kong F, Birnbaum EH, et al. Radiation therapy for epidermoid carcinoma of the anal canal, clinical and treatment factors associated with outcome. Radiother Oncol. 2001;61(1):15–22.
167. Mitchell SE, Mendenhall WM, Zlotecki RA, Carroll RR. Squamous cell carcinoma of the anal canal. Int J Radiat Oncol Biol Phys. 2001;49(4):1007–13.
168. Saarilahti K, Arponen P, Vaalavirta L, Tenhunen M. The effect of intensity-modulated radiotherapy and high dose rate brachytherapy on acute and late radiotherapy-related adverse events following chemoradiotherapy of anal cancer. Radiother Oncol. 2008;87(3):383–90.
169. Sunesen KG, Buntzen S, Tei T, Lindegaard JC, Nørgaard M, Laurberg S. Perineal healing and survival after anal cancer salvage surgery: 10-year experience with primary perineal reconstruction using the vertical rectus abdominis myocutaneous (VRAM) flap. Ann Surg Oncol. 2009;16(1):68–77.
170. Ghouti L, Houvenaeghel G, Moutardier V, et al. Salvage abdominoperineal resection after failure of conservative treatment in anal epidermoid cancer. Dis Colon Rectum. 2005;48(1):16–22.
171. Schiller DE, Cummings BJ, Rai S, et al. Outcomes of salvage surgery for squamous cell carcinoma of the anal canal. Ann Surg Oncol. 2007;14(10):2780–9.
172. Papaconstantinou HT, Bullard KM, Rothenberger DA, Madoff RD. Salvage abdominoperineal resection after failed Nigro protocol: modest success, major morbidity. Colorectal Dis. 2006;8(2):124–9.
173. Akbari RP, Paty PB, Guillem JG, et al. Oncologic outcomes of salvage surgery for epidermoid carcinoma of the anus initially managed with combined modality therapy. Dis Colon Rectum. 2004;47(7):1136–44.
174. Jaiyesimi IA, Pazdur R. Cisplatin and 5-fluorouracil as salvage therapy for recurrent metastatic squamous cell carcinoma of the anal canal. Am J Clin Oncol. 1993;16(6):536–40.
175. Ajani JA, Carrasco CH, Jackson DE, Wallace S. Combination of cisplatin plus fluoropyrimidine chemotherapy effective against liver metastases from carcinoma of the anal canal. Am J Med. 1989;87(2):221–4.
176. Faivre C, Rougier P, Ducreux M, et al. 5-fluorouracile and cisplatinum combination chemotherapy for metastatic squamous-cell anal cancer. Bull Cancer. 1999;86(10):861–5.
177. Khater R, Frenay M, Bourry J, Milano G, Namer M. Cisplatin plus 5-fluorouracil in the treatment of metastatic anal squamous cell carcinoma: a report of two cases. Cancer Treat Rep. 1986;70(11):1345–6.
178. Garg M, Lee J, Kachnic L, Catalano P, et al. Phase II trials of cetuximab (CX) plus cisplatin (CDDP), 5-fluorouracil (5-FU) and radiation (RT) in immunocompetent (ECOG 3205) and HIV-positive (AMC045) patients with squamous cell carcinoma of the anal canal (SCAC): safety and preliminary efficacy results. J Clin Oncol. 2012;30(15):abstr 4030.
179. Compton C, Byrd D, Garcia-Aguilar J, et al. Anus. In: Compton C, Byrd D, Garcia-Aguilar J, Kurtzman S, Olawaiye A, Washington M, editors. AJCC cancer staging atlas. 2nd ed. New York: Springer; 2012. p. 203–13.

Part IV

Endocrine

Thyroid Cancer

23

Jocelyn F. Burke and Herbert Chen

Abbreviations

AJCC	American Joint Committee on Cancer
ATA	American Thyroid Association
AUS/FLUS	Atypia of undetermined significance/follicular lesion of undetermined significance
CEA	Carcinoembryonic antigen
CNS	Central nervous system
CT	Computed tomography
DTC	Differentiated thyroid cancer
EBRT	External beam radiation therapy
FDG-PET	Fluoro-deoxy-glucose positron emission tomography
FMTC	Familial medullary thyroid cancer
FN	Follicular neoplasms
FNA	Fine-needle aspiration
FTC	Follicular thyroid cancer
HCC	Hürthle cell carcinoma
HCN	Hürthle cell neoplasms
MEN	Multiple endocrine neoplasia
MRI	Magnetic resonance imaging
MTC	Medullary thyroid carcinoma
NCI	National Cancer Institute
PET	Positron emission tomography
PHPT	Primary hyperparathyroidism
PTC	Papillary thyroid carcinoma
PTH	Parathyroid hormone
RAI	Radioactive iodine
RET	Rearranged during transfection
rhTSH	Recombinant human TSH
SEER	Surveillance, epidemiology, and end results
Tg	Thyroglobulin
TSH	Thyroid-stimulating hormone
WBS	Whole-body RAI scans

J.F. Burke, M.D. • H. Chen, M.D. (✉)
Department of General Surgery, University of Wisconsin Hospital and Clinics, 600 Highland Ave, Madison 53792, WI, USA
e-mail: jburke@uwhealth.org; chen@surgery.wisc.edu

Learning Objectives

After reading this chapter, you should be able to:

- Describe the workup of a thyroid nodule.
- Choose the appropriate treatment based on fine-needle aspiration results.
- Appreciate the difference in cancer management based on thyroid cancer cell type.

Introduction

Thyroid nodules are a common finding in the global population, with 5 % of women and 1 % of men in industrialized nations having palpable thyroid nodules, and a further 19–67 % with nodules detectable by ultrasound imaging [1]. Thyroid nodules are of surgical concern in part due to the need to exclude thyroid cancer, which occurs in 5–15 % of nodules [1]. The overall incidence of thyroid cancer in the United States is increasing; between 1992 and 2006 it was 7.7 per 100,000 person-years, with a rate of 11.3 per 100,000

Q.D. Chu et al. (eds.), *Surgical Oncology: A Practical and Comprehensive Approach*,
DOI 10.1007/978-1-4939-1423-4_23, © Springer Science+Business Media New York 2015

woman-years and 4.1 per 100,000 man-years [2]. Papillary thyroid cancer is the most common, accounting for 84 % of new cases, followed by follicular (10 %), medullary (3–5 %), and anaplastic (1 %) thyroid cancer, with another 2 % of unspecified or miscellaneous thyroid cancer [2, 3]. This chapter will address the proper diagnostic, surgical, and surveillance techniques for thyroid cancers.

Initial Evaluation

While thyroid surgery requires expert precision and attention to detail, the preoperative workup is equally important. Any patient referred for a newly discovered thyroid nodule should undergo a diagnostic evaluation including a thorough history and physical exam, laboratory tests, imaging studies, and other procedures. To begin, a history of the nodule must be established. Any change in size and associated rate of growth should be noted, as this can indicate an aggressive lesion such as anaplastic cancer. Associated symptoms should also be evaluated, with attention to those that might indicate compression or invasion of surrounding anatomic structures. These include progressive dysphagia, cough, or dyspnea, which suggest compression of the esophagus and trachea, or dysphonia, which could indicate compression or invasion of the recurrent laryngeal nerve. Symptoms of hyper- or hypothyroid should be assessed, as these may indicate the presence of a functioning nodule or suppression of thyroid hormone production. A history of patient risk factors should then be acquired, including any head or neck irradiation, total body irradiation for bone marrow transplantation, exposure to ionizing radiation as a child, or family history of thyroid cancer or thyroid cancer syndromes (multiple endocrine neoplasia type 2 (MEN2), Cowden's syndrome, familial polyposis, Carney complex, Werner syndrome) in a first-degree relative [1, 4].

A physical exam focusing on the thyroid and associated cervical lymphadenopathy should then be performed. Evaluate the patient for signs of hyperthyroidism (tachycardia, tremor, restlessness, flushing, brisk deep tendon reflexes) and hypothyroidism (hair loss especially of the lateral eyebrows, pretibial edema, delayed deep tendon reflexes). Inspect the neck for jugular venous distention, tracheal deviation, and cervical lymphadenopathy. Palpate the thyroid gland for size, contour, and general mobility in reference to surrounding tissues. Note the size, mobility, firmness, and tenderness of any palpable nodules. With an especially large nodule or large substernal component to the thyroid gland, the patient should be evaluated for facial flushing, inspiratory stridor, and jugular venous distention together with both arms raised above their head – this triad is Pemberton's sign and can indicate superior vena cava obstruction.

After the history and physical exam, laboratory tests and imaging studies are necessary for diagnosis. A thyroid-stimulating hormone (TSH) level should be obtained in any patient with a thyroid nodule ≥1 cm in size [1]. If the serum TSH is low, a radionuclide thyroid scan should be obtained to determine if the nodule is hyperfunctioning ("hot"), isofunctioning ("warm"), or nonfunctioning ("cold"). Any hyperfunctioning nodule does not require biopsy, as the likelihood of a hot nodule containing a focus of malignancy is very low. Patients with hot nodules should undergo ultrasonography predominantly for the purpose of documenting the size and appearance of the nodule and should then go on for evaluation and treatment of their hyperthyroidism. On the contrary, if the serum TSH level is normal or high, the nodule requires further evaluation with ultrasonography and FNA (refer to Fig. 23.1). It is important to note that incrementally higher TSH levels, even on the high side of the normal range, are associated with an increased risk of malignancy [5, 6]. Additionally, if the patient has a strong family history of medullary thyroid cancer, a serum calcitonin and CEA level should be checked. In cases where the FNA is suspicious or suggestive of medullary thyroid cancer, serum calcitonin and CEA may be useful.

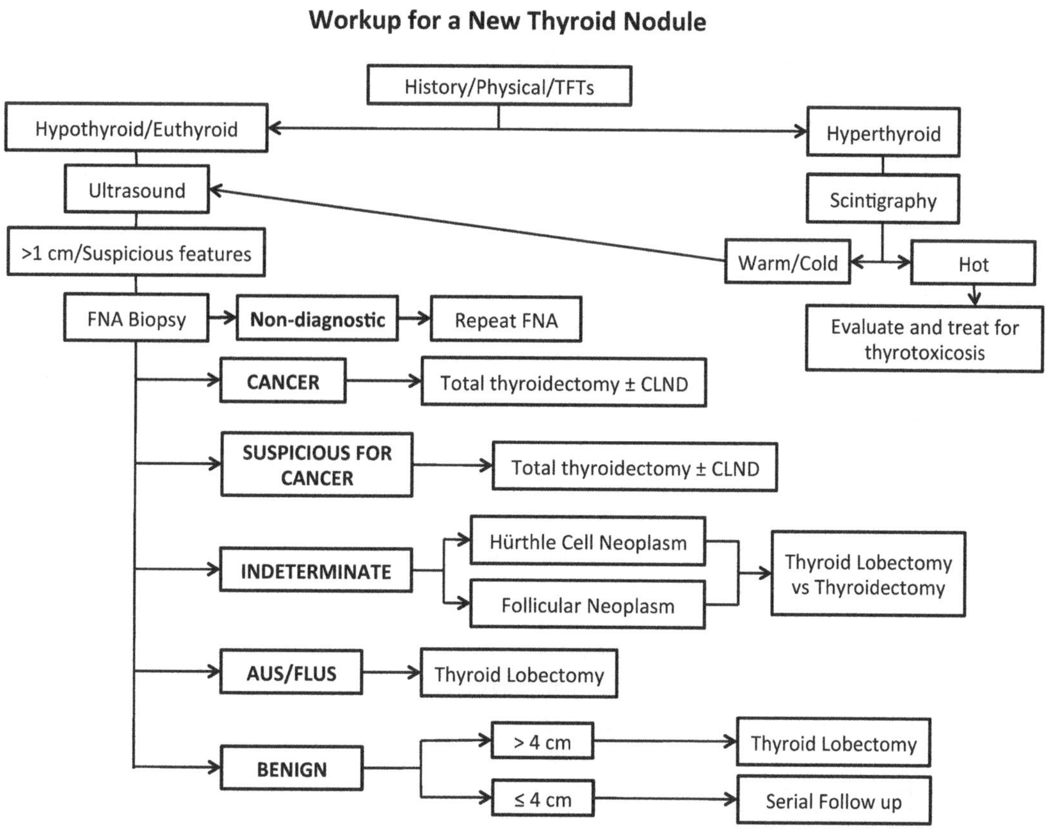

Fig. 23.1 The process recommended for evaluation of a new thyroid nodule. Surgical treatments are presented based on fine-needle aspiration (FNA) diagnosis and not by histological cell type. *TFTs* thyroid function tests, *CLND* central lymph node dissection

Diagnostic Imaging

Ultrasound

The American Thyroid Association (ATA) recommends ultrasound evaluation of all palpable thyroid nodules and all those discovered by incidental imaging [1]. This allows for the confirmation of the presence of a nodule, the identification of additional nodules, and the measurement and characterizations of any lesions. As above, only nodules that are ≥1 cm in greatest diameter should prompt continued evaluation, as these are more likely to harbor clinically significant cancers. Patients with normal or high TSH levels should be evaluated with particular attention to sonographic features that suggest malignancy. These suspicious features include poorly defined margins, predominantly solid composition, microcalcifications, hypoechogenicity, taller-than-wide shape, cervical lymphadenopathy, and hypervascularity by Doppler. While none of these findings are definitive, the combination of hypoechogenicity, microcalcifications, and irregular borders in a solitary nodule was associated with a 30-fold increased risk of malignancy in a retrospective study [7].

Computed Tomography/Magnetic Resonance Imaging

There are very few indications for CT or MRI imaging in the initial workup of a thyroid nodule. If a patient has had a previous thyroid operation, these imaging techniques can help better delineate the thyroid bed. In addition, if there are signs of tracheal deviation or superior vena cava obstruction, three-dimensional imaging can evaluate the extent of deviation or substernal/mediastinal component of the tumor. Any CT imaging must be done without intravenous iodinated contrast, as this blocks iodine uptake by the thyroid and thereby would delay any adjuvant therapy with radioactive iodine should it be necessary [8].

Fine-Needle Aspiration

Fine-needle aspiration (FNA) has become the gold standard for thyroid nodule evaluation. It is the most accurate and cost-effective method for evaluating thyroid nodules and should be performed on all nonfunctional nodules ≥1 cm in size, unless they are simple cysts with no solid components (refer to Fig. 23.1) [1]. In a patient with multiple nodules ≥1 cm (e.g., multinodular goiter), those nodules with suspicious sonographic findings should be preferentially biopsied with FNA. If none of the nodules have a suspicious appearance, the largest nodules should be evaluated with FNA. FNA of smaller nodules is also indicated in patients with a family history of thyroid cancer, a personal history of radiation exposure, or concerning ultrasound characteristics (see above). Additionally, if a thyroid nodule is detected incidentally on a positron emission tomography (PET) scan and is fluoro-deoxy-glucose (FDG) avid, it should be biopsied as these nodules have up to a 50 % risk of being malignant [9]. Ultrasound guidance is routinely used, but is especially essential in non-palpable nodules or those with >25–50 % cystic component to allow for more accurate targeting. Results from an FNA are reported in six general categories: benign, follicular lesion of undetermined significance, follicular neoplasm, suspicious for malignancy, malignant, and nondiagnostic. Each of these carries with it a certain risk of malignancy, as detailed in Table 23.1 [9]. See also Fig. 23.1 for guidance in management based on FNA results.

Table 23.1 Bethesda system for reporting thyroid cytopathology: implied risk and recommended management

Cytology classification	Risk of malignancy	Usual management
Nondiagnostic	N/A	Repeat FNA with US guidance
Benign	0–3 %	Clinical follow-up
Atypia or follicular lesion of undetermined significance	5–15 %	Repeat FNA
Follicular neoplasm	15–30 %	Thyroid lobectomy
Suspicious for malignancy	60–75 %	Total thyroidectomy or lobectomy
Malignant	97–100 %	Total thyroidectomy

Adapted from Layfield et al. [9]. With permission from John Wiley & Sons, Inc.
FNA fine-needle aspiration, *US* ultrasound

Nondiagnostic

Nondiagnostic or unsatisfactory samples are unable to be reliably interpreted due to limited cellularity or absence of follicular cells. This category also encompasses samples that suffer from poor fixation or preservation. Though this is not generally the final FNA diagnosis received, nondiagnostic results accounted for more than 9 % of all FNA results in a large series of patients that eventually went on to surgical removal at the Mayo Clinic [10]. This result in an FNA report should prompt a repeat US-guided FNA.

Benign

Generally, this category includes multinodular goiter, lymphocytic thyroiditis, and hyperplastic nonfunctional thyroid nodules. While benign aspiration cytology does not completely rule out malignancy, these nodules have a very low rate of pathological cancer diagnosis, with a risk of malignancy of 0–3 %. However, because the risk still exists, patients with a benign FNA result must continue active monitoring, with serial clinical and ultrasound examinations for 6–18 months after the first FNA. If the nodule is stable, then the periodic examinations can be extended to every 3–5 years [1]. Any changes in size or suspicious sonographic features should prompt a repeat FNA biopsy [9].

Any nodule ≥4 cm should undergo the same workup as smaller nodules, with serum laboratory tests, ultrasound evaluation, and FNA. However, surgical removal is recommended even if all of these tests indicate that the nodule is benign, for large nodules have a much higher rate of false-negative FNAs than smaller nodules do [11]. This holds true even if the nodule is functioning (or "hot") on thyroid scintigraphy.

Atypia of Undetermined Significance/ Follicular Lesion of Undetermined Significance (AUS/FLUS)

Cytopathology with atypia represents the most subjective category of results, with an associated malignancy risk of 5–15 %. These results include cells that do not represent benign lesions but do not have a degree of atypia sufficient to define them as follicular neoplasms. Recommendations vary as to how to manage patients with these FNA results. Since this category can include some biopsy results that have minimally sufficient cellularity for evaluation, a repeat FNA can be the most appropriate next step in these cases. The National Cancer Institute recommends obtaining an $iodine^{123}$ scan, especially if the patient's TSH level is low. If the nodule is "hot," the nodule can be followed clinically with a repeat FNA in 3–6 months [9]. If the nodule is "cold," the patient should undergo a thyroid lobectomy for further diagnostic evaluation and treatment [1, 9]. At our institution, the diagnosis of FLUS carries a malignancy rate that exceeds 15 %, and therefore virtually all patients with FLUS undergo surgery. Since FLUS can be a variable diagnosis, we recommend that each institution evaluates its own malignancy rate.

Follicular Neoplasm/Suspicious for Follicular Neoplasm

Biopsies categorized as follicular/Hurthle cell neoplasms include all non-papillary follicular patterned and Hürthle cell lesions and have a malignancy risk of 15–30 %. Since follicular neoplasms can only be truly differentiated from follicular carcinomas by evidence of capsular or vascular invasion on permanent histology, this distinction cannot be made with FNA alone. These patients must undergo a thyroid lobectomy for further diagnosis. We and others have previously demonstrated that the frozen section is not useful and extremely inaccurate in the evaluation of follicular neoplasms. It does not provide any diagnostic information 90 % of the time [12]. An initial thyroid lobectomy should be performed, and, if the surgical pathology indicates a diagnosis of follicular carcinoma, the patient can return for a completion thyroidectomy when clinically stable [1, 9]. If the patient has had a history of head/neck radiation, a family history of thyroid cancer, a bilateral nodular disease, and/or a preference for bilateral surgery, an initial total thyroidectomy can be considered.

Suspicious for Malignancy

Cytopathology in this category carries an intermediate to high risk of malignancy of 60–75 %. It is used to describe results that appear likely to be malignant but are lacking in sufficient evidence to confirm the diagnosis. These include results that are suspicious for papillary carcinoma (many in this group are eventually diagnosed with follicular variant of papillary carcinoma), suspicious for medullary carcinoma (with insufficient specimen available for confirmatory calcitonin immunostains), suspicious for lymphoma, suspicious for metastatic tumor, or suspicious for malignant neoplasm due to total necrosis of cells (e.g., anaplastic carcinoma). In cases where the FNA is suspicious for papillary thyroid cancer, thyroid lobectomy with intraoperative frozen section or total thyroidectomy is our preferred operation [13]. In the remaining suspicious cytologies, the patient may require diagnostic thyroid lobectomy. The appropriate operative approach depends on the histological diagnosis and is addressed in more detail below. Additionally, if a nodule is suspicious for medullary carcinoma, the patient should be evaluated for elevated serum calcitonin and CEA levels. Nodules suspicious for lymphoma may provide definitive diagnostic results if FNA is repeated with the resulting cells evaluated with flow cytometry for T- and B-lymphocyte markers.

Malignant

Nodules with FNA biopsies reported as malignant have a high risk of malignancy at 97–100 %. As described above, most but not all thyroid malignancies can be diagnosed by cytopathology, including papillary thyroid carcinoma, poorly differentiated thyroid carcinoma, anaplastic carcinoma, medullary carcinoma (with calcitonin immunostains and confirmatory serum tests), lymphoma (with the addition of flow cytometry), and metastatic tumors. While many prognostic scoring systems exist, they have predominantly been replaced by the TNM scoring system from the American Joint Committee on Cancer (AJCC) (Table 23.2) [14]. The ATA strongly recommends that any patient fit to undergo an operation receives at least a near-total or total thyroidectomy for a malignant FNA diagnosis in a carcinoma ≥1 cm, in contralateral disease, or if the patient has a personal history of head or neck radiation therapy or a family history of thyroid cancer [1]. Any additionally recommended procedures will be discussed in the detailed explanation of each histological diagnosis below.

Papillary Thyroid Cancer

Initial Evaluation and Treatment

Papillary thyroid carcinoma (PTC) is the most common thyroid cancer, accounting for 84 % of all thyroid cancers reported in the NCI's surveillance,

Table 23.2 American Joint Committee on Cancer (AJCC) TNM staging for thyroid carcinomas (7th edition)

Primary tumor (T)*			
All categories may be subdivided: (s) solitary tumor and (m) multifocal tumor (the largest determines the classification)			
TX	Primary tumor cannot be assessed		
T0	No evidence of primary tumor		
T1	Tumor ≤2 cm in greatest diameter limited to the thyroid		
T1a	Tumor ≤1 cm limited to the thyroid		
T1b	Tumor >1 cm ≤2 cm in greatest dimension, limited to the thyroid		
T2	Tumor >2 cm ≤4 cm in greatest dimension, limited to the thyroid		
T3	Tumor >4 cm in greatest dimension, limited to the thyroid or any tumor with minimal extrathyroid extension (e.g., extension to sternothyroid muscle or perithyroid soft tissues)		
T4	Moderately advanced disease		
	Tumor of any size extending beyond the thyroid capsule to invade the subcutaneous soft tissues, larynx, trachea, esophagus, or recurrent laryngeal nerve		
T4b	Very advanced disease		
	Tumor invades prevertebral fascia or encases the carotid artery or mediastinal vessels		
All anaplastic carcinomas are considered T4 tumors			
T4a	Intrathyroidal anaplastic carcinoma		
T4b	Anaplastic carcinoma with gross extrathyroid extension		
Regional lymph nodes (N) (comprises of central compartment, lateral cervical, and upper mediastinal lymph nodes)			
NX	Regional lymph nodes cannot be assessed		
N0	No regional lymph node metastasis		
N1	Regional lymph node metastasis		
N1a	Metastasis to Level VI (pretracheal, paratracheal and prelaryngeal/Delphian lymph nodes)		
N1b	Metastasis to unilateral, bilateral, or contralateral cervical (Levels I–V) or retropharyngeal or superior mediastinal lymph nodes (Level VII)		
Distant metastasis (M)			
M0	No distant metastasis		
M1	Distant metastasis		
Anatomic stage/prognostic groups			
	T	N	M
<45 years			
Papillary or follicular (differentiated)			
Stage I	Any T	Any N	M0
Stage II	Any T	Any N	M1

(continued)

Table 23.2 (continued)

Anatomic stage/prognostic groups			
	T	N	M
≥45 years			
Stage I	T1	N0	M0
Stage II	T2	N0	M0
Stage III	T3	N0	M0
	T1–T3	N1a	M0
Stage IVA	T4a	N0	M0
	T4a	N1a	M0
	T1–T3	N1b	M0
	T4a	N1b	M0
Stage IVB	T4b	Any N	M0
Stage IVC	Any T	Any N	M1
Medullary carcinoma (all age groups)			
Stage I	T1	N0	M0
Stage II	T2–T3	N0	M0
Stage III	T1–T3	N1a	M0
Stage IVA	T4a	N0	M0
	T4a	N1a	M0
	T1–T4a	N1b	M0
Stage IVB	T4b	Any N	M0
Stage IVC	Any T	Any N	M1
Anaplastic carcinoma (all are considered Stage IV)			
Stage IVA	T4a	Any N	M0
Stage IVB	T4b	Any N	M0
Stage IVC	Any T	Any N	M1

Adapted from Compton et al. [60]. With permission from Springer Verlag

epidemiology, and end results (SEER) database from 1992 to 2006 [2]. Fortunately, the prognosis is excellent, with an overall 20–25-year cancer-specific mortality rate of 5 % [15]. Interestingly, in the case of differentiated thyroid cancer, the staging system is additionally based on patient's age, with patients younger than 45 years old being classified only as Stage I or II (Table 23.2). Multiple subtypes of papillary cancer have been described, including the classical form, with areas that have mostly a papillary growth pattern as well as follicles; a follicular variant that has a predominantly follicular pattern; and the tall cell, columnar cell, diffuse sclerosing, and insular variants, which are all more aggressive than the other more common types [15]. The majority of patients are women, with female patients representing 60 % of new cases in the SEER program [2]. Specific risk factors for PTC include exposure to ionizing radiation and hereditary associations such as familial adenomatous polyposis, Cowden syndrome, and Carney complex. The goals of management for PTC include surgical removal of the primary tumor and any extrathyroidal disease including involved lymph nodes, radioablation of any remaining thyroid tissue, suppression of endogenous TSH, and continued long-term surveillance [16]. Since PTC spreads lymphatogenously, the preoperative workup should include a cervical ultrasound to evaluate the patient for lymphadenopathy. The rate of lymph node metastasis present at the time of diagnosis is 20–90 %, so any suspicious lymph nodes should be biopsied with FNA, as positive findings would increase the extent of the operation [17, 18]. If there is no evidence of lymphadenopathy, the initial operation in nodules ≥1 cm that are positive for papillary thyroid carcinoma should be a total thyroidectomy. The appropriate management of cervical lymph nodes in PTC is slightly more controversial. Some experts advocate a prophylactic dissection of the central neck (level VI, including the lower jugular node from the cricoid cartilage to the clavicle), citing the high percentage of nodal metastases at diagnosis and the inability to detect nodal micrometastases preoperatively with standard imaging. However, in the absence of any overt nodal disease, others recommend limiting the operation to a total thyroidectomy because extending the dissection can also increase complications, because prophylactic dissection has not been convincingly proven to reduce mortality or local recurrence and because, regardless of the significance of micrometastases, they can be treated with radioactive iodine ablation. The ATA recommends a central compartment (level VI) neck dissection for any patients with clinically significant FNA-positive central or lateral neck lymph nodes. For patients with no evidence of nodal disease, the recommendations are based only on consensus expert opinion and suggest that a prophylactic central compartment dissection can be performed in patients with more advanced primary tumors (T3 or T4, Table 23.2), but that total thyroidectomy is also a sufficient treatment, especially in T1 or T2 primary carcinomas [1]. We generally do not perform a prophylactic central neck dissection.

Postoperative Management

The second goal of PTC management is radioablation of any remnant tissue or unrecognized/unremoved micrometastases in selected patients. PTC cells are sensitive to iodine-131 (I^{131}), which is generally administered 4–12 weeks postoperatively. It should not be employed in patients who underwent less than a near-total thyroidectomy, as the remaining intact thyroid gland will absorb all or nearly all of the iodine, preventing it from treating the intended targets, micrometastases, and remnant tissue. Based on many previous studies of effective doses to achieve ablation while minimizing excess radiation, the ATA recommends 30–100 mCi doses in low-risk patients and allows for use of higher doses (100–200 mCi) in patients with known or suspected residual disease or with an aggressive variant cell type on tumor histology [1]. While the goal of radioactive iodine (RAI) ablation is specifically to ablate any small amount of remaining normal thyroid tissue, it can also be considered as adjuvant therapy to potentially treat any remaining thyroid cancer cells [19]. A scan approximately 2–10 days after administration of postoperative RAI ablation can also be useful in surveying patients for remaining disease, especially unrecognized disease in the neck that would have been masked by thyroid uptake in preoperative imaging. Two clear recommendations for RAI use exist: low-risk (stage I) patients under 45 years old should not undergo postoperative RAI ablation, and high-risk (stage III-IV) patients older than 45 years old or any with tumors >4 cm should receive postoperative RAI ablation [1, 20]. In the former group, use of RAI therapy does not show any overall or disease-free survival benefit [20, 21], while in the latter group, single-dose RAI adjuvant therapy has been shown to decrease disease recurrence and, in some cases, prolong survival [20, 22, 23]. Use of postoperative radioiodine therapy in all other groups is selective. The ATA recommends that patients older than 45 years with a T1–T2 carcinoma who also have N1 disease or other high risk factors should receive RAI adjuvant therapy. On the other hand, patients with multifocal cancer where none of the foci are >1 cm and no other high risk factors are present should not have RAI therapy [1].

Patients undergoing RAI ablation need to have high serum levels of circulating TSH (>30 mU/L) to stimulate uptake of iodine into cells. This can be achieved by withdrawal of levothyroxine over 4–6 weeks or by TSH stimulation with administration of recombinant human TSH (rhTSH). Baseline postoperative thyroglobulin (Tg) tests should also be performed at this time, when TSH will be at the highest level, around 72 h after administration of rhTSH [16] Thyroglobulin can only be synthesized by thyroid follicular cells, and it is thus used as a postoperative tumor marker for papillary or follicular thyroid cancer recurrence. While preoperative levels have no demonstrative predictive or prognostic utility, and thus should not be routinely measured, post-thyroidectomy levels should be consistently <2 ng/mL. Thyroid hormone suppression and rhTSH stimulation are provocative tests, and any Tg level >2 ng/mL under either of these conditions is indicative of recurrent (or persistent if in the first postoperative evaluation) disease [24].

The third goal for management of patients with PTC is suppression of endogenous TSH levels. TSH has a trophic effect on thyrocytes, and therefore suppressing circulating levels with supraphysiologic doses of levothyroxine has been demonstrated to reduce the risk of major clinical adverse events [25, 26]. The ATA consensus recommendations for degree of suppression are <0.1 mU/L for high- or intermediate-risk patients and 0.1–0.5 mU/L for low-risk patients.

Long-Term Surveillance

Surveillance in PTC consists of serial laboratory tests and imaging studies. The frequency of these tests is dictated in part by the TNM staging of the primary tumor and histological considerations such as resection margins and aggressive histological subtypes. The first evaluation should occur 6 months after RAI ablation. This consists of a physical exam, cervical ultrasound of the central and lateral compartments, and measurement of serum Tg, TSH, and antithyroglobulin (anti-Tg) antibodies. The anti-Tg antibodies should always be measured with Tg in surveillance as high levels of antibodies can falsely lower Tg levels. Rising serial anti-Tg antibody levels can be a surrogate marker for residual normal thyroid tissue or tumor. Tg levels can be measured with or without TSH stimulation, as long as the manner is consistent throughout. In low-risk patients, an undetectable Tg with undetectable anti-Tg antibody during TSH suppression and then confirmed with rhTSH stimulation is one of the criteria for disease-free status. Patients must also have undergone a total or near-total thyroidectomy and thyroid remnant ablation and have no clinical or imaging evidence of tumor on whole-body scans at follow-up examination.

Cervical ultrasounds evaluating the central and lateral compartment should be performed at 6 and 12 months post-RAI ablation and then annually for at least 3–5 years. If nodes are suspicious for disease involvement and are 5–8 mm in the smallest diameter, they should be biopsied by FNA with Tg measurement in the needle washout fluid. Lymph nodes suspicious for involvement smaller than 5–8 mm in largest diameter can be monitored without biopsy, but should be followed for growth and biopsied if changes occur.

Whole-body RAI scans (WBS) are used in surveillance of intermediate- or high-risk patients to detect any persistent or recurrence of iodine-avid disease. Any patient who had minimal to no uptake on the first WBS after RAI ablation treatment will have low sensitivity on any subsequent scans, so low-risk patients with undetectable Tg levels and negative cervical ultrasounds should not undergo a WBS as part of surveillance [1]. Intermediate- or high-risk patients should have a WBS with levothyroxine withdrawal or rhTSH stimulation 6–12 months after RAI ablation. However, since this test is for detection and not ablation, it should be done with lower radiation exposure levels, either by using ^{123}I or low-activity ^{131}I.

Management of Recurrent Disease

Recurrences in PTC are either locoregional or distant metastases. Locoregional disease detected by one of the above surveillance methods should be confirmed with FNA. The treatment of choice for locoregional recurrences is surgical resection. In general, the recommended approach to resection is either by formal compartmental resection of the involved side of the neck (level VI) or selective ipsilateral dissection of previously unexplored compartments with clinically significant involved nodes (>8 mm in diameter) (levels II–IV). With extensive disease, a modified neck dissection may be appropriate (levels II–V), with sparing of the spinal accessory nerve, internal jugular vein, and sternocleidomastoid muscle. These approaches are all preferred compared to selectively removing only nodes that appear positive, as micrometastases are generally more extensive than can be appreciated from imaging studies [1]. However, if the recurrent disease is in a previously dissected compartment, it may be appropriate to selectively remove only the involved nodes, as complete resection of the compartment may jeopardize surrounding vital structures [15].

Distant metastases most commonly occur in the lungs, bones, and central nervous system (CNS). Any iodine-avid disease should be treated with RAI ablation and therapy, with treatments completed every 6–12 months as long as the disease continues to take up the RAI. Macronodular disease in any location can be considered for surgical removal, especially for tumors that are not iodine avid. ^{18}FDG-PET scans should be considered if Tg levels are high (≥10 ng/mL), but a WBS does not show any uptake. This usually indicates that there is a present focus of recurrent disease that is not iodine avid but may be detectable with ^{18}FDG-PET. External beam radiation therapy (EBRT) or stereotactic radiosurgery may be considered for bone or CNS metastases, respectively, in the absence of iodine avidity when surgical resection would be unacceptably morbid [16]. This should be done in conjunction with corticosteroid administration to limit the risk of complications from acute tumor expansion.

Unfortunately, PTC is relatively insensitive to standard forms of cytotoxic chemotherapy, and it is thus not a recommended treatment option. In patients with recurrent disease that is resistant to all other forms of treatment, doxorubicin monotherapy is the only chemotherapy treatment that has been approved by the US Food and Drug Administration [1]. While this can show some cytotoxic tumor effect, it may also sensitize recurrent disease to EBRT, thus improving the efficacy of radiation treatment.

Follicular Thyroid Cancer

Initial Evaluation and Treatment

Follicular thyroid carcinoma (FTC) is the second most common type of thyroid cancer, accounting for 10 % of all new cases in the SEER program from 1992 to 2006 [2]. Hürthle cell carcinoma (HCC), while classified by the World Health Organization as a subtype of FTC, is actually a distinct clinical entity. It accounts for 4 % of all thyroid cancer cases, and, while it shares some similarities with FTC, they have different risk factors and considerations for treatment. The risk factors for developing FTC are similar to those for PTC, including radiation exposure and similar hereditary syndromes such as Cowden syndrome and Carney complex type 1. HCC has no associated genetic syndromes, but a connection between HCC and lymphoma has been proposed, though this requires more research to confirm. The imaging workup for FTC and HCC is as described above for PTC, though the common findings differ from those in PTC. On ultrasonography, follicular cancers tend to be iso- or hyperechoic (compared to the hypoechoic PTCs) and have a thick, irregular halo but lack microcalcifications [27].

FTC presents a diagnostic dilemma by FNA due to the inability to distinguish follicular adenomas from carcinomas by cytology alone because the distinction is based on invasion not apparent in an FNA. Additionally, efforts should be made to distinguish Hürthle cell neoplasms (HCN) from follicular neoplasms (FN). HCC has a higher risk of locally invasive (T4) disease at diagnosis (27 % vs. 9 %) and higher rate of recurrence (24 % vs. 8 %) than FTC [28]. HCC is also not generally iodine avid, so it cannot generally be treated by RAI ablation. Based on this information, patients with a diagnosis of FN/HCN on FNA should undergo a thyroid lobectomy and isthmusectomy at minimum, though high-risk patients, HCN patients with a nodule >4 cm or ≥70 years old, or patients with bilateral thyroid nodule(s) ≥1 cm should be considered for a total thyroidectomy as the initial operation [29–32]. Since follicular cancers spread hematogenously, the rate of synchronous lymph node metastases is very low (<10 %), though this risk may be slightly higher in HCC; routine prophylactic lymph node dissection is not recommended [1, 30]. If suspicious lymph nodes are detected in preoperative ultrasonography, these nodes should be biopsied with FNA to confirm involvement and removed during the initial operation, along with any nodes that appear grossly involved at the time of operation.

By pathology from the initial lobectomy, FTCs can be classified as minimally invasive or invasive variants. Minimally invasive FTC is encapsulated with a single focus of capsular invasion (differentiating it from a FN). Invasive FTC has sites of angioinvasion or extensive invasion beyond the capsule along with diffuse infiltration of the affected thyroid lobe [29]. Thyroid lobectomy is thus sufficient to treat a minimally invasive FTC, while a total thyroidectomy is necessary to treat invasive FTC. The management differs slightly in regard to lymph node dissection with a diagnosis of HCC from the initial lobectomy. Since HCC has higher rates of lymph node involvement and is often radioresistant, the ATA recommends considering central neck dissection (level VI) at the time of completion thyroidectomy.

Postoperative Management

Postoperative management follows the same principles for FTC and HCC as for PTC. Patients with minimally invasive FTC treated with a thyroid lobectomy need only have long-term surveillance, as described below. Patients treated with a total or completion thyroidectomy should undergo an evaluation for residual disease along with RAI ablation with ^{131}I, which should be done approximately 4–12 weeks postoperatively under conditions of either levothyroxine withdrawal or rhTSH stimulation, as described earlier. A WBS done 2–10 days after RAI administration can identify areas of residual iodine-avid thyroid tissue. Baseline postoperative Tg and anti-Tg antibody should be drawn at this time also, to obtain it under levothyroxine withdrawal or rhTSH stimulation. Although the majority of HCCs will not be iodine avid, this should not preclude undergoing a RAI ablation. Even if this does not treat any residual microcarcinomatous disease, it will ablate any remaining thyroid tissue, making Tg surveillance testing and future WBS more sensitive. Additionally, both FTC and HCC have TSH receptors, and so chronic TSH suppression should be initiated postoperatively in both, following the same process and to the same suppression levels as described for PTC.

Long-Term Surveillance

Patients with FTC or HCC should follow the same surveillance pattern as PTC, with physical examination, cervical ultrasound, and serum levels of Tg and anti-Tg antibodies at 6 and 12 months postoperatively and then annually for at least 3–5 years. In surveillance, any patient whose Tg becomes detectable after previously being undetectable should have a cervical ultrasound to attempt to locate the source. If this is negative, a diagnostic RAI scan should be performed. If both of these imaging studies fail to localize a site of recurrence, an ^{18}FDG-PET scan is indicated to find the radioiodine-resistant focus of recurrence.

Management of Recurrent Disease

Management of recurrent FTC and HCC is similar to recurrent PTC. Microscopic (i.e., negative on cervical ultrasound) local recurrences of iodine-avid tissue should be treated with high-dose (~150 mCi) ^{131}I. Any macroscopic local recurrences should be resected following the same principle described for PTC management, with comprehensive compartment lymphadenectomy except in the case of a recurrence in a previously dissected compartment. With central neck recurrences, a central neck dissection (level VI) should be performed, and with lateral nodal disease, a modified radical neck dissection of levels II–V is indicated, sparing the internal jugular vein, the spinal accessory nerve, and the sternocleidomastoid muscle. Unresectable locoregional metastases can be treated with external beam radiation therapy (EBRT), which may show slightly more efficacy in HCC than FTC.

Distant metastases are more common in HCC than FTC and occur in different locations: HCC more commonly occurs in the lungs, while FTC more commonly occurs in bones. These metastases should be managed the same as for PTC, with RAI ablation for micronodular disease and attempted resection for macronodular disease. In cases where resection of the metastases would be too morbid or disfiguring, and in cases of metastasis-related bone pain, EBRT can be employed. Special attention must be paid to avoid cerebral edema if EBRT is used for brain metastases by ensuring concurrent steroid administration. If the metastases can be resected, this has been shown to improve patient survival in FTC, HCC, or PTC [33, 34]. Unfortunately, for cases of disease recurrence that are unresectable and are not sensitive to either RAI or EBRT treatment, few options remain. As in PTC, doxorubicin has been approved for chemotherapeutic use, but response rates are uniformly poor.

Medullary Thyroid Cancer

Initial Evaluation and Treatment

Medullary thyroid carcinoma (MTC) arises from the parafollicular C cells rather than the follicular epithelial thyroid cells. The C cells are neuroendocrine in origin and responsible for producing calcitonin, which participates in calcium regulation. These accounted for 3–5 % of all newly diagnosed thyroid cancers in the SEER program from 1992 to 2006 [2]. In cases of MTC, the cells continue to produce calcitonin, which then serves as a highly sensitive tumor marker that plays a role in diagnosis and postoperative management. While the majority of MTC cases occur sporadically, approximately 25 % of patients have a hereditary form that occurs as a result of a germline mutation in the rearranged during transfection (RET) proto-oncogene.

RET is located on chromosome 10q11.2 and codes for the receptor tyrosine kinase RET, which is involved in cell growth and survival. Somatic mutations of *RET* are present in the majority of sporadic MTC cases, and germline mutations cause the MEN2 syndromes. These syndromes are inherited in an autosomal dominant fashion and carry a near 100 % lifetime risk of developing MTC, as well as the risk of developing other tumors based on the subtype of the syndrome. The described subtypes of MEN2 are MEN2a, MEN2b, and familial medullary thyroid cancer (FMTC).

MEN2a is the most common subtype, accounting for approximately 80 % of the MEN2 cases [35]. It is characterized by development of MTC in virtually 100 % of patients, of pheochromocytomas (either unilateral or bilateral) in 50 % of patients, and of hyperparathyroidism in 20–35 % of patients [36]. MEN2b is the second most common subtype, making up most of the remaining 20 % of MEN2 patients. It is characterized by development of MTC in 100 % of patients, pheochromocytomas in 50 %, and characteristic physical findings. These include a thin, marfanoid body habitus; increased joint laxity; and mucosal ganglioneuromas of the gastrointestinal tract, lips, tongue, and eyelids. MEN2b is more aggressive than MEN2a, and MTC develops at a younger age in this patient cohort – this subtype therefore needs to be identified as early in infancy as possible. FMTC is now recognized by the ATA as a clinical variant of MEN2a in which MTC is the only manifestation [37]. Because this is an uncommon diagnosis, and because improper diagnosis could lead to missing a pheochromocytoma preoperatively, the qualifications for diagnosis are relatively rigid. Patients must have four or more family members over two generations with MTC and a documented absence of pheochromocytoma and hyperparathyroidism and long-term follow up. Workup and management varies based on the type of MTC and the manner of initial detection, and so each will be addressed separately.

Evaluation and Management of Sporadic MTC

Generally, patients with sporadic MTC (or those who are the index case in a family for MEN2a or FTMC) present with thyroid nodules in the third and fourth decades of life. A patient's history should be obtained regarding symptoms of a neck mass and recurrent laryngeal nerve invasion, such as dysphagia and voice changes; symptoms of distant metastasis such as bone pain; symptoms of hypercalcitoninemia such as flushing and diarrhea; and symptoms of tumors associated with MEN2 syndromes, such as kidney stones, pancreatitis, and osteoporosis from hyperparathyroidism and anxiety, tremor, and panic attacks from pheochromocytoma. While over 80 % of patients with a palpable MTC nodule will have locoregional disease at the time of diagnosis, only 15 % of patients with sporadic MTC will present with symptoms of this locally advanced disease, such as hoarseness, dysphagia, and dyspnea, and 10 % of patients will have symptoms of hypercalcitoninemia, such as flushing and diarrhea [38].

Patients with an FNA biopsy suspicious or diagnostic for MTC should go through further workup and treatment that differs from the previously described well-differentiated cancers. First, a serum calcitonin level must be obtained – a level ≥100 pg/mL confirms the diagnosis of MTC. Serum calcium, parathyroid hormone (PTH), carcinoembryonic antigen (CEA), and free metanephrine and normetanephrine levels should be checked at the same time. Elevated calcium and/or PTH levels could indicate hyperparathyroidism, consistent with the MEN2a syndrome, and elevated CEA levels can help to diagnose some MTC cases in which the tumor does not initially oversecrete calcitonin. High levels of CEA have also been associated with a worse prognosis in MTC [35]. Evaluation of the plasma free metanephrine levels can help rule out the presence of a pheochromocytoma.

Patients with elevated plasma-free metanephrines or normetanephrines should be evaluated for the presence of a pheochromocytoma with an adrenal CT or MRI. Patients with concern for concomitant hyperparathyroidism should be evaluated by ultrasound and technetium-99m sestamibi scan. Additionally, the ATA recommends offering all patients with a new diagnosis of MTC testing for germline *RET* mutations, as any of these patients may represent the index case of MEN2 in a family [37]. Patients should then undergo an extended neck ultrasound to evaluate for additional nodules and lymphadenopathy in the superior mediastinum, central, and bilateral lateral neck compartments. As in PTC and FTC, metastasis to suspicious locoregional lymph nodes can be confirmed with FNA prior to thyroidectomy. Finally, any patient with a serum calcitonin level ≥400 pg/mL is likely to have radiographically detectable distant metastases and so should be evaluated with a chest CT, neck CT, and three-phase contrast-enhanced multidetector liver CT or contrast-enhanced MRI [37, 39].

Any patients with biochemical and imaging workup suggestive of a pheochromocytoma should receive treatment for that prior to removal of their MTC with α-adrenergic followed by β-adrenergic blockers in the setting of adequate hydration and then surgical removal via laparoscopic adrenalectomy. The extent of surgical resection in the neck is then determined by the presence or absence of local invasion or calcitonin levels suggestive of the presence of distant metastases. Patients with no evidence of advanced local invasion by the tumor, no clinically involved cervical lymph nodes, and no evidence of distant metastases, and a serum calcitonin level <400 pg/mL should undergo a total thyroidectomy with central compartment (level VI) neck dissection [37, 39]. Patients thought by imaging to have limited local metastatic disease (≤T3 and ≤N1b) to lymph nodes in the central and lateral neck compartments who have either no evidence of distant metastases or limited (<1 cm) distant metastases should undergo a total thyroidectomy with central (level VI) and lateral neck (levels IIA, III, IV, and V) dissection [37]. If there is evidence of bilateral primary tumors or extensive ipsilateral lymphadenopathy, a contralateral lateral neck dissection should be considered. In patients with evidence of distant metastatic disease >1 cm, less aggressive neck surgery can be considered to manage local symptoms while preserving speech, swallowing, and parathyroid function [37].

Evaluation and Management of Hereditary Disease

MTC occurring in patients with one of the MEN2 variants occurs much earlier than in sporadic MTC patients, usually before the third decade of life. The overall risk of developing MTC is nearly 100 % in carriers of *RET* mutations. For this reason, any child in a family with known MEN2 syndromes should be evaluated as early as possible for the presence of germline *RET* mutations and be considered for a prophylactic thyroidectomy if mutations are present. Much study has been devoted to the timing of prophylactic thyroidectomy in this population, and this has led to an understanding of the variation in aggressiveness of MTC based on the *RET* codon that is mutated.

The patterns of these *RET* mutations vary with each MEN2 syndrome. In MEN2a, 85 % of cases involve a mutation in codon 634 within exon 11; with codons 609, 611, 618, and 620 in exon 10; and codon 804 in exon 14 accounting for the majority of the remaining cases. In MEN2b, 95 % of patients have a single point mutation at a codon in exon 16 that changes a methionine into a threonine, which is thought to cause autophosphorylation and activation of the RET receptor. The other codon mutations associated with MEN2b are 922, also on exon 16, and 883 on exon 15. The investigations into the aggressiveness of MTC development based on codon mutation has led to classification of the most common mutations and recommendations for timing and extent of prophylactic thyroidectomy based on *RET* sequencing. In the most recent consensus guidelines regarding MTC, the ATA went one step further to evaluate all previously described mutations and rank them according to risk of aggressive MTC (A–D, with D being the highest risk) [37].

Table 23.3 Codon-directed timing of surgery by MTC-associated *RET* mutations

Risk level for MTC	*RET* codon mutation	Recommended age for prophylactic thyroidectomy
Level 1 (high)	609, 630, 768, 790, 791, 804, 891	Between ages 5 and 10
Level 2 (higher)	611, 618, 620, 634	Before age 5
Level 3 (highest)	883, 918, 922	Before 6 months (preferably in the first month)

MTC medullary thyroid cancer, *RET* *re*arranged during *t*ransfection gene

These correlate closely with the risk levels assigned to a smaller group of identified codons at the Seventh International Workshop (Table 23.3) and should be consulted if an *RET* mutation is identified that is not listed here. Based on the mutations listed in Table 23.3, level 3 mutations (those associated with MEN2b, codons 883, 918, and 922) correlate strongly with development of MTC in the first years of life [40]. Prophylactic thyroidectomy is therefore recommended in this group within the first 6 months of life and preferably within the first month [37, 41, 42]. Level 2 mutations (codons 634, 611, 618, and 620) are associated with an intermediate risk to develop early MTC and should undergo prophylactic thyroidectomy within the first 5 years of life. Level 1 mutations (codons 609, 630, 768, 790, 791, 804, and 891), while highly likely to develop MTC early in life, have the lowest risk of those categorized here. Thyroidectomy by the end of the first decade of life is recommended in this group; however, due to the variability in age of onset of MTC, many recommend completing thyroidectomy by age 5 in all patients who will tolerate the operation at that time. With strict serial calcitonin and ultrasound monitoring, the operation can be delayed up to age 10 in those for whom it would be preferential to wait.

Since these operations are generally performed prophylactically, most patients are asymptomatic at the time of evaluation. However, cervical ultrasound should be performed in every patient prior to operation to evaluate for the presence of thyroid nodules and lymphadenopathy. Similarly, baseline calcitonin and CEA levels should be drawn, though caution should be used in interpreting these levels in patients <3 years old because sufficient data are lacking regarding normal values in young children. That said, any MEN2b patient >1 year old or MEN2a patient >5 years old must undergo preoperative calcitonin testing because the possibility of metastatic MTC is much higher at these ages, and knowledge of metastatic disease changes the surgical approach [37]. If any patient has thyroid nodules ≥5 mm in diameter, lymphadenopathy, or a calcitonin level ≥40 pg/mL, they should be managed according to the guidelines for sporadic disease presented above [35]. In patients being considered for prophylactic thyroidectomy, the ATA recommends evaluation for the presence of the MEN2-associated neoplasms, parathyroid adenomas, and pheochromocytomas only in patients who exhibit signs or symptoms of either. The risk of either occurring in asymptomatic patients younger than 8 years old with no adrenal mass detected by physical exam or parathyroid adenoma/hyperplasia detected by cervical ultrasound is so low that the ATA recommends against screening these children preoperatively [37].

All surgery for children should be performed in a tertiary care setting by highly experienced surgeons whenever possible due to the concern for higher risks of complications in children, especially those <1 year old. However, a study of a single-institution endocrine surgery center demonstrates that, when operations are performed by experienced surgeons in a tertiary hospital accustomed to caring for pediatric endocrine patients, the complication rate was similar to adults [43]. Patients with MEN2b operated on before 1 year of age should undergo only a total thyroidectomy; when there is evidence of lymph node involvement at the time of surgery, dissection should be extended to the level VI compartment. Imaging positive compartments in the lateral neck should also be dissected out in their entirety. Additionally, any MEN2b patient undergoing their operation after 1 year of age should have a prophylactic central neck dissection (level VI) due to high risk of lymph node micrometastases in these patients. Patients with MEN2a of FTMC with level 2 risk codon mutations should undergo a prophylactic thyroidectomy alone by 5 years of age, as long as all nodules are <5 mm, serum calcitonin is <40 pg/mL, and all lymph nodes are clinically negative. Again, if lymphadenopathy becomes apparent at the time of surgery, a central neck dissection (level VI) should be performed, as well as a complete dissection of any compartment in the lateral neck that demonstrates positive nodes at the time of surgery [37]. One of the most common complications of central neck dissection in children is devascularization of parathyroid glands. At the time of operation, parathyroid glands can be autotransplanted to retain function. If a patient has minimal risk of developing primary hyperparathyroidism (PHPT) in the future (e.g., MEN2b and FMTC patients), devascularized parathyroid glands can be autotransplanted into the sternocleidomastoid muscle(s). However, if a patient has a high risk of developing PHPT (e.g., MEN2a patients), any autotransplanted parathyroid glands should be implanted in the forearm so as to not confuse future imaging examinations of the neck [37].

Postoperative Management

Contrary to postoperative management in PTC or FTC, MTC cells do not concentrate iodine nor do they respond to TSH stimulation. Therefore, there is no role for RAI ablation or for TSH suppression in the postoperative period. Levothyroxine should be dosed to replace thyroid function, with a target serum TSH level between 0.5 and 2.5 mIU/L [37].

Instead of using thyroglobulin as a thyroid hormone tumor marker, calcitonin and CEA levels are used for postoperative surveillance. The initial basal postoperative levels should be obtained 2–3 months postoperatively, which is when the levels reach their nadir. If the basal levels are undetectable, the risk of persistent or residual recurrent disease is low, and these patients can enter long-term follow-up. Patients that have a detectable initial postoperative basal calcitonin have a more complicated postoperative course. If the calcitonin is detectable but <150 pg/mL, the patient should have a neck ultrasound to detect any apparent lymphadenopathy. Any suspicious lymph nodes should be biopsied with FNA. The washout fluid from the FNA can also be tested for calcitonin, which may increase the sensitivity and specificity of the test for MTC recurrence [44]. Additional imaging can be obtained to serve as a baseline comparison as the likelihood of detecting residual disease or distant metastases with a low serum level of calcitonin is very small. This imaging could include the same imaging outlined for detection of metastases in the setting of high preoperative serum calcitonin levels, i.e., neck CT, chest CT, triple-phase contrast-enhanced multidetector liver CT, or contrast-enhanced MRI, bone MRI, and a bone scan. While this is optional for patients with a low detectable calcitonin level and can be decided on through discussion between the patient and the managing surgeon, patients with a basal postoperative serum calcitonin ≥150 pg/mL should undergo all of the outlined imaging tests. If these imaging tests fail to localize locoregional or metastatic disease, a central and ipsilateral compartment dissection can be considered, but should be weighed against the risk of damage to surrounding vital structures. Further discussion is addressed in "Management of recurrent disease" below.

Long-Term Surveillance

The manner and frequency of long-term surveillance is dependent in part on basal postoperative calcitonin levels. In patients who have an undetectable calcitonin level post-thyroidectomy, basal calcitonin levels and physical exams should be performed every 6–12 months initially, then annually for 3–5 years if the levels remain undetectable. If a patient's calcitonin level increases at any time during surveillance, they should be evaluated following the same steps described for postoperative management. Patients with MEN2a and MEN2b should also have annual biochemical screening along with history and physical exam for pheochromocytoma and hyperparathyroidism (MEN2a only). These serial screening exams can begin at age 8 in patients with MEN2b or codon 630 or 634 mutations and at age 20 in carriers of all other MEN2a *RET* mutations [37].

Multiple studies have demonstrated that serum calcitonin levels do not always return to normal levels postoperatively, even without any evidence of persistent disease. In patients who continue to have low level detectable calcitonin levels (<150 pg/mL) and no evidence of metastatic disease on multiple imaging studies (described above), close serial surveillance can be continued. Calcitonin and CEA levels should be obtained every 6 months to allow for determination of their doubling times. These patients should then be followed with basal calcitonin and CEA levels and physical exam at intervals that are 1/4th the shortest doubling time or annually, whichever is more frequent. If any nodes become clinically positive, or if either the CEA or calcitonin rises 20–100 % above postoperative levels, a cervical ultrasound and metastatic workup are indicated. Those patients with basal calcitonin levels ≥150 pg/mL in the postoperative period are considered to have persistent disease and are managed as such.

Management of Recurrent Disease

Compared to those with well-differentiated thyroid cancers, patients with MTC more frequently develop multifocal metastases early in their disease course. Since the goal to be free of disease at this point is, for most, unachievable, the aims for these patients involve palliative and strategically prophylactic care. These include locoregional control, palliation of symptoms of hormone excess, palliation of symptoms caused by distant metastases, and prevention of potential damage that could be caused by existent metastases [37]. As a neuroendocrine tumor, metastatic MTC can produce hormones that cause debilitating syndromes, including diarrhea, hypercalcemia, and Cushing syndrome. When metastases are positively localized, treatment decisions involve weighing the morbidity and toxicity involved in available treatments with the usually indolent course of tumor growth and current quality of life (including the presence of hormonal syndromes). Patients with long calcitonin and CEA doubling times (>2 years) who have no symptoms from the recurrent disease can continue to be managed with surveillance. Those with at least one doubling time, <2 years should be considered for further treatment. Treatment for recurrent and metastatic disease involves three modalities: surgery, EBRT, and systemic therapy.

Surgery for recurrent locoregional disease in the neck should be considered in patients that had an inadequate initial operation (e.g., hemithyroidectomy, no lymphadenectomy with clinically positive disease) or have no other apparent distant metastatic disease. Threat to vital structures in the neck, intractable pain, and unremitting symptoms from hormonal syndromes caused by recurrent disease are also indications for neck reoperation [45]. Distant metastases can be treated by surgery in some cases. Any bone metastasis that is causing spinal cord compression or threatening fracture in a weight-bearing bone should be evaluated for surgical removal. Any lung or mediastinal lesions that compress or threaten to compress the airway can be considered for surgery, as can isolated or limited brain metastases and single or limited large liver metastases that are causing diarrhea syndromes or pain.

External beam radiation therapy has been shown to be effective in selective patients with recurrent neck disease. When microscopic residual disease, extrathyroidal invasion, or lymph node involvement is present postoperatively, postoperative EBRT could improve disease-free survival, though no overall survival benefit has been demonstrated [46, 47]. Metastases to the brain, bone, lung, and mediastinum that are not amenable to surgical removable can be treated with EBRT. In addition, EBRT can be used to palliate bone pain that arises with bony metastases. Liver metastases are usually disseminated throughout the organ and are thus harder to treat with radiation.

Systemic chemotherapy for MTC is the focus of much ongoing clinical study. Standard cytotoxic chemotherapies have limited effect, with the best responses being partial remission in 10–20 % of patients who use the most successful agents: dacarbazine, fluorouracil, and doxorubicin. Recently, the US Food and Drug Administration has approved the tyrosine kinase inhibitors vandetanib and cabozantinib for treatment of disseminated MTC. Phase III clinical trials with vandetanib indicate that progression-free survival and biochemical control can be increased in both sporadic and hereditary MTC with daily oral dosing of the drug, though its applications may be limited by its toxicities [48]. Clinical trials of other targeted therapies are ongoing, and the ATA recommends enrolling suitable patients in these when systemic treatment is sought.

Anaplastic Thyroid Cancer

Initial Evaluation

The most aggressive of the thyroid cancers, anaplastic thyroid cancer (ATC) is also the most rare, accounting for 39 % of all thyroid cancer deaths while representing only 1 % of all new cases of thyroid cancer from 1992 to 2006 [2, 49]. ATC more often occurs in older patients and generally presents with a rapidly enlarging thyroid mass. Patients often have symptoms of local compression and invasion in the neck, such as dysphagia, dyspnea, and dysphonia. ATC is thought by some to arise from dedifferentiated papillary or follicular thyroid cancers, as these often appear in conjunction in pathological specimens [50, 51]. Additionally, poorly differentiated thyroid cancer, which is a potential differential diagnosis for ATC, may represent an intermediate form of cancer between well-differentiated thyroid cancer and ATC.

When ATC is suspected based on the clinical presentation and physical exam, prompt diagnosis and treatment is necessary. FNA biopsy is recommended, though there is a higher chance that the FNA will be nondiagnostic, with only necrotic or inflamed tissue identified due to necrotic centers in the carcinoma. While in these cases FNA can be repeated, an open core biopsy is recommended [52]. A sufficient biopsy should reveal one or a mixture of the following cell types: spindle cell, pleomorphic giant cells, or squamoid pattern. When the diagnosis of ATC is confirmed, further investigation is required to determine extent of tumor, functional status of other glands, and general health status of the patient.

Laboratory studies obtained at diagnosis should include: complete blood count (for anemia, platelet count, leukocytosis, or neutropenia from tumor-associated immunosuppression), chemistry panel (for impaired parathyroid gland function due to tumor invasion), liver function tests (in part to evaluate for liver metastases), free thyroxine and thyrotropin (for potential hypothyroidism with advanced tumor or hyperthyroidism with thyrotoxicosis from a functional tumor), coagulation studies, and blood type and cross-match (in preparation for the difficulty of the resection that will be required). Imaging to determine the extent of disease should be obtained, but not at the sacrifice of delaying therapeutic intervention. Neck ultrasound can evaluate the quality and extent of the primary thyroid mass and of nodal involvement. Contrast-enhanced CT or MRI of the neck and chest can further demonstrate tumor extent as well as identify obstruction or invasion of the vasculature, trachea, and esophagus. ^{18}FDG-PET whole-body scans are the most useful in evaluating metastatic sites, but a contrast-enhanced CT or MRI through the head, neck, chest, abdomen, and pelvis can be done if ^{18}FDG-PET imaging cannot be obtained quickly. Since differentiated thyroid cancer (DTC) and ATC tend to coexist in patients, ^{18}FDG-PET scans can help distinguish between ATC and DTC metastases. ATC is more hypermetabolic than DTC; thus, these sites will appear brighter on ^{18}FDG-PET, and PET/CT fusion scans can help more precisely localize these tumors. Evaluation of vocal cord function with laryngoscopy is also necessary in all patients, as many present with hoarseness and unilateral vocal cord paralysis. Laryngoscopy can also help identify direct invasion of the airway, giving information regarding resectability and possible need for postoperative tracheostomy [52].

Initial Management

Once diagnosis and extent of disease is confirmed, the tumor should be staged and initial management planned. Due to its aggressive behavior and poor prognosis (median survival is 5–6 months, and 1 year survival rate is 23 % [49, 50]), the AJCC classifies all ATC as Stage IV disease (Table 23.2). In the case of ATC, T4a tumors are any that are intrathyroidal (and thus surgically resectable), while T4b tumors have extrathyroidal extension [53]. Stage IVA tumors are T4a with any N and M0; stage IVB tumors are T4b, any N, and M0; and any distant metastasis confers stage IVC status. Many patient series suggest that younger age (<45–70 years) and smaller primary tumor size (<5–7 cm) carry a more promising prognosis [49, 54, 55].

Most experts recognize ATC as a systemic disease requiring multiple modalities for treatment. After diagnosis and staging, a treatment plan should be devised with a team including, ideally, endocrine surgery, radiation oncology, medical oncology, radiology, nutrition, palliative care, social work, psychology/psychiatry, and clergy if desired. For the majority of patients, ATC is a fatal disease, and end-of-life care should be discussed with patients. Families should be involved in care planning and be aware of the extent of morbidities and likelihood of success in all treatment modalities undertaken.

Locoregional Disease

The initial management of Stage IVA or IVB tumors depends on their resectability. If a tumor is resectable for curative intent, meaning disease is confined to the neck, does not involve unresectable structures, and a satisfactory resection could be achieved down to a grossly negative margin without unacceptable morbidity (R1 resection), surgery should be attempted as it is associated with prolonged disease-free survival [52, 56, 57]. ATC is confined to the thyroid at diagnosis in only 10 % of patients, and in these patients, a total thyroidectomy without further extent of resection should be performed [52]. In those with lymph node spread, resection of compartments with grossly positive nodes should be performed, with no evidence of any benefit in prophylactic central or lateral neck dissection [50, 52, 58]. Resections of the larynx, pharynx, or esophagus are discouraged, unless this would allow for an R1 resection with minimal morbidity. Partial surgical removals or tumor debulking should only be considered for symptomatic control or to preserve threatened vital structures.

For patients who desire aggressive rather than palliative treatment, definitive radiation therapy treatment should be offered as it may be beneficial in controlling locoregional disease and improving progression-free survival in those who had a successful R0 (no evidence of disease)/R1 resection [55, 57, 59]. Locoregional control with aggressive radiation therapy can also improve overall survival in patients with metastatic disease, if only by a few months [59]. However, the morbidity involved in high-dose radiation therapy must be appreciated as it may go against any palliative goals for treatment. Radiation therapy can be started as soon as the patient is sufficiently recovered from the operation, usually within 2–3 weeks postoperatively [52].

The use of chemotherapy in ATC may offer some benefit when combined with radiation therapy in multimodal treatment. Cytotoxic compounds that are known to radiosensitize tumor cells are the most recommended and can be used in combination, including taxanes (paclitaxel or docetaxel), anthracyclines (doxorubicin), and platins (cisplatin or carboplatin) [52]. While these may improve success rates of combined chemoradiation treatment, they will also increase the treatment-specific morbidity to a patient and so must be used only in patients who continue to have a good performance status postoperatively. No specific recommendations exist for when to begin treatment postoperatively, but it can be given concurrently with radiation therapy and may be started when the patient is sufficiently recovered from surgery, as early as 1 week postoperatively.

Metastatic Disease

Stage IVC ATC is almost uniformly fatal with no prospects for a curative outcome. It is therefore important for the treatment team and the patient to define the desired goals of treatment in these cases and for end-of-life planning to occur. The chemotherapies described above (taxanes, anthracyclines, and platins) may have some effect in disease stabilization or even regression and can be considered for patients desiring an aggressive treatment approach. Ongoing clinical trials of new, targeted therapies should also be sought for these patients, as many are ongoing and have shown some initial promise.

Follow-Up and Surveillance

For the small group of patients that achieve a complete therapeutic surgical resection with adjuvant chemoradiation therapy, close follow-up is recommended. The ATA suggests this consist of CT or MRI imaging of the brain, neck, chest, abdomen, and pelvis every 1–3 months for the first 6–12 months posttreatment, then every 4–6 months for another year. This frequency can be reduced after 2 years with no evidence of disease or in patients who do not want aggressive treatment for any recurrence. A PET scan can be used at 3–6 months postoperatively for its higher sensitivity for detection of metastases.

The treatment for metastases in patients who respond to chemoradiation with disease stabilization is controversial. ATC most commonly metastasizes to the lung, bone, and brain. In general, surgical removal or directed radiotherapy of brain or bone metastases can be considered in patients with good functional status. Patients with neurological symptoms from brain metastases should have early initiation of glucocorticoids prior to surgery; otherwise, in asymptomatic patient, glucocorticoid treatment is not recommended [52]. Metastases in weight-bearing bones should be evaluated by orthopedic surgery prior to treatment to allow for fixation if necessary. Lung metastases in ATC are usually numerous and thus not amenable to either surgical or radiation treatment. Patients with recurrent disease after an extended tumor-free period (>1 year) should be evaluated and managed in the same manner as for their initial disease.

Neither RAI ablation nor TSH suppression therapy plays a role in the postoperative management of ATC as this cancer does not concentrate iodine nor respond to growth stimulation from TSH. Similarly, ATC rarely produces Tg, so monitoring serum Tg levels is not warranted.

Summary

Newly discovered thyroid nodules requiring evaluation are a common presentation, and the incidence of thyroid cancer continues to increase in the US population. While the majority of thyroid nodules are benign, each must be evaluated appropriately for the presence of thyroid cancer. Fine-needle aspiration (FNA) is the most valuable diagnostic tool in this evaluation. Papillary and follicular thyroid cancers represent the most common diagnoses in malignant thyroid masses, and they have an excellent prognosis if treated appropriately. For these malignancies, the pattern of treatment involves evaluation and diagnosis with FNA, surgical removal of the primary tumor with cervical lymphadenectomy if indicated, radioactive iodine ablation, TSH suppression, and long-term surveillance. Medullary thyroid cancer presents a variation from this pattern of treatment due to its genetic inheritance in 25 % of cases, which makes prophylactic treatment an option for some. As a neuroendocrine tumor, patients with medullary thyroid cancer also develop hormonal syndromes that sometimes determine the extent of treatment. Finally, anaplastic thyroid cancer is rarely curable, though research is ongoing to discover targeted systemic therapies to better address this disease. All patients can benefit from multidisciplinary team involvement in their care, with an endocrinologist, endocrine surgeon, medical oncologist, or radiation oncologist directing care when appropriate.

Salient Points

- Thyroid nodules are a common finding, and the surgeon's role is to determine which contain malignancy and treat them appropriately.
- Papillary cancer is the most common thyroid cancer, followed by follicular cancer, Hürthle cell cancer, medullary cancer, and anaplastic cancer.
- The most important diagnostic test in the workup of new thyroid nodules is fine-needle aspiration.
- An important part of treatment is taking the correct steps after FNA results:

- Benign → Monitor with serial ultrasound and physical exams.
- Nondiagnostic → Repeat the FNA.
- AUS/FLUS → Should be determined by each institution based on malignancy rate. Further evaluation with scintigraphy scan and lobectomy of any cold nodules versus initial lobectomy.
- Suspicious for malignancy → Thyroid lobectomy; total thyroidectomy if multifocal disease or in some cases of suspicious for papillary cancer.
- Malignant → Total thyroidectomy ± lymph node dissection based on histological diagnosis.

- If a thyroid nodule is ≥4 cm, the risk of a false-negative FNA is much higher; even if these nodules are benign by FNA, they should be removed with a thyroid lobectomy.

Questions

1. A 45-year-old woman presents to her primary care office with a newly discovered neck mass and progressive difficulty swallowing solid foods. The most appropriate next steps of a workup are:
   A. History and physical exam, TSH, ^{131}iodine scintigraphy, ultrasound, MRI, FNA
   B. History and physical exam, TSH, ultrasound, CT, FNA
   C. History and physical exam, TSH, ultrasound, FNA
   D. History and physical exam, TSH, ultrasound, MRI, FNA
2. Cervical lymph node dissection is important to control the extent of local disease in all of the thyroid cancer types except:
   A. Papillary
   B. Follicular
   C. Medullary
   D. Anaplastic
3. Radioactive iodine ablation is the most appropriate next step after total thyroidectomy when treating each of the following cancers except:
   A. Papillary
   B. Follicular
   C. Hürthle cell
   D. Medullary
4. The most appropriate operation for an incidental diagnosis of anaplastic thyroid cancer confined to the thyroid in a lobectomy for follicular cancer is:
   A. Completion thyroidectomy
   B. Completion thyroidectomy with central neck dissection
   C. Completion thyroidectomy with modified radical neck dissection
   D. Completion thyroidectomy with modified radical neck dissection and radioactive iodine ablation
5. A 47-year-old woman presents for evaluation of a new asymptomatic neck mass. A cervical ultrasound shows a hypoechoic mass measuring 3×4.3×2.5 cm with no evidence of lymphadenopathy. An FNA shows benign follicular thyroid cells and colloid. What is the most appropriate next step?
   A. Serial exams and ultrasounds to monitor
   B. Thyroid lobectomy
   C. Total thyroidectomy
   D. Repeat FNA
6. A 52-year-old man with a history of radiation exposure presents with a new asymptomatic neck mass. Cervical ultrasound demonstrates a 2×2×1 cm hyperechoic nodule in the right thyroid lobe and a subcentimeter hyperechoic nodule in the left lobe. FNA results are consistent with follicular lesion of unknown significance. What is the most appropriate next step?
   A. Serial exams and ultrasounds to monitor
   B. Thyroid lobectomy
   C. Total thyroidectomy
   D. Repeat FNA
7. A 36-year-old woman presents with a new thyroid nodule diagnosed as medullary cancer by FNA. Ultrasound demonstrates a 3×2.4×1.5 mass in the left thyroid lobe, a second subcentimeter nodule in the left lobe, and two lymph nodes 1 cm in length in the central compartment. The most appropriate operation is:
   A. Thyroid lobectomy (left)
   B. Total thyroidectomy
   C. Total thyroidectomy with central neck dissection
   D. Total thyroidectomy with modified radical neck dissection

8. A 27-year-old male undergoes a total thyroidectomy for medullary thyroid cancer. His mother also had an operation for thyroid cancer. The *RET* gene from his carcinoma is sequenced, and it shows a codon 634 mutation. His 18-month-old daughter also has a codon 634 *RET* mutation. Which of the following is the most appropriate course of treatment?
   A. Immediate thyroidectomy
   B. Thyroidectomy at 3 years old
   C. Thyroidectomy at 6 years old
   D. Thyroidectomy at 10 years old

Answers

1. C
2. B
3. D
4. A
5. B
6. C
7. C
8. B

References

1. Cooper DS, Doherty GM, Haugen BR, et al. Revised American Thyroid Association management guidelines for patients with thyroid nodules and differentiated thyroid cancer. Thyroid. 2009;19(11):1167–214.
2. Aschebrook-Kilfoy B, Ward MH, Sabra MM, Devesa SS. Thyroid cancer incidence patterns in the United States by histologic type, 1992–2006. Thyroid. 2011;21(2):125–34.
3. Mazeh H, Chen H. Advances in surgical therapy for thyroid cancer. Nat Rev Endocrinol. 2011;7(10):581–8.
4. Melck AL, Carty SE. Evaluation of a new thyroid nodule. In: Sippel RS, Chen H, editors. The handbook of endocrine surgery. Singapore: World Scientific Publishing; 2012. p. 39–48.
5. Boelaert K, Horacek J, Holder RL, Watkinson JC, Sheppard MC, Franklyn JA. Serum thyrotropin concentration as a novel predictor of malignancy in thyroid nodules investigated by fine-needle aspiration. J Clin Endocrinol Metab. 2006;91(11):4295–301.
6. Haymart MR, Repplinger DJ, Leverson GE, et al. Higher serum thyroid stimulating hormone level in thyroid nodule patients is associated with greater risks of differentiated thyroid cancer and advanced tumor stage. J Clin Endocrinol Metab. 2008;93(3):809–14.
7. Jabiev AA, Ikeda MH, Reis IM, Solorzano CC, Lew JI. Surgeon-performed ultrasound can predict differentiated thyroid cancer in patients with solitary thyroid nodules. Ann Surg Oncol. 2009;16(11):3140–5.
8. Bomeli SR, LeBeau SO, Ferris RL. Evaluation of a thyroid nodule. Otolaryngol Clin North Am. 2010;43(2):229–38, vii.
9. Layfield LJ, Cibas ES, Baloch Z. Thyroid fine needle aspiration cytology: a review of the National Cancer Institute state of the science symposium. Cytopathology. 2010;21(2):75–85.
10. Seningen JL, Nassar A, Henry MR. Correlation of thyroid nodule fine-needle aspiration cytology with corresponding histology at Mayo Clinic, 2001–2007: an institutional experience of 1,945 cases. Diagn Cytopathol. 2012;40 Suppl 1:E27–32.
11. Pinchot SN, Al-Wagih H, Schaefer S, Sippel R, Chen H. Accuracy of fine-needle aspiration biopsy for predicting neoplasm or carcinoma in thyroid nodules 4 cm or larger. Arch Surg. 2009;144(7):649–55.
12. Chen H, Nicol TL, Udelsman R. Follicular lesions of the thyroid. Does frozen section evaluation alter operative management? Ann Surg. 1995;222(1):101–6.
13. Haymart MR, Greenblatt DY, Elson DF, Chen H. The role of intraoperative frozen section if suspicious for papillary thyroid cancer. Thyroid. 2008;18(4):419–23.
14. Randolph G, Duh QY, Heller KS, et al. The prognostic significance of nodal metastases from papillary thyroid carcinoma can be stratified based on the size and number of metastatic lymph nodes, as well as the presence of extranodal extension ATA Surgical Affairs Committee's Taskforce on Thyroid Cancer Nodal Surgery. Thyroid. 2012;11:1144–52.
15. Elaraj DM, Sturgeon C. Papillary thyroid carcinoma. In: Morita SY, Dackiw APB, Zeiger MA, editors. Endocrine surgery. New York: McGraw-Hill; 2010. p. 47–64.
16. Elaraj DM, Sturgeon C. Management of papillary thyroid cancer. In: Sippel RS, Chen H, editors. The handbook of endocrine surgery. Singapore: World Scientific Publishing; 2012. p. 49–61.
17. Grebe SK, Hay ID. Thyroid cancer nodal metastases: biologic significance and therapeutic considerations. Surg Oncol Clin N Am. 1996;5(1):43–63.
18. Kouvaraki MA, Shapiro SE, Fornage BD, et al. Role of preoperative ultrasonography in the surgical management of patients with thyroid cancer. Surgery. 2003;134(6):946–54, discussion 54–5.
19. Pinchot SN, Sippel RS, Chen H. Multi-targeted approach in the treatment of thyroid cancer. Ther Clin Risk Manag. 2008;4(5):935–47.
20. Patel SS, Goldfarb M. Well-differentiated thyroid carcinoma: the role of post-operative radioactive iodine administration. J Surg Oncol. 2013;107(6):665–72.
21. Kim HJ, Kim NK, Choi JH, et al. Radioactive iodine ablation does not prevent recurrences in patients with papillary thyroid microcarcinoma. Clin Endocrinol (Oxf). 2013;78(4):614–20.
22. Jonklaas J, Sarlis NJ, Litofsky D, et al. Outcomes of patients with differentiated thyroid carcinoma following initial therapy. Thyroid. 2006;16(12):1229–42.

23. Podnos YD, Smith DD, Wagman LD, Ellenhorn JD. Survival in patients with papillary thyroid cancer is not affected by the use of radioactive isotope. J Surg Oncol. 2007;96(1):3–7.
24. Poehls JL, Sippel RS. Thyroid evaluation – laboratory testing. In: Sippel RS, Chen H, editors. The handbook of endocrine surgery. Singapore: World Scientific Publishing; 2012. p. 3–13.
25. Mazzaferri EL. Long-term outcome of patients with differentiated thyroid carcinoma: effect of therapy. Endocr Pract. 2000;6(6):469–76.
26. McGriff NJ, Csako G, Gourgiotis L, Lori CG, Pucino F, Sarlis NJ. Effects of thyroid hormone suppression therapy on adverse clinical outcomes in thyroid cancer. Ann Med. 2002;34(7–8):554–64.
27. Jeh SK, Jung SL, Kim BS, Lee YS. Evaluating the degree of conformity of papillary carcinoma and follicular carcinoma to the reported ultrasonographic findings of malignant thyroid tumor. Korean J Radiol. 2007;8(3):192–7.
28. Kushchayeva Y, Duh QY, Kebebew E, D'Avanzo A, Clark OH. Comparison of clinical characteristics at diagnosis and during follow-up in 118 patients with Hurthle cell or follicular thyroid cancer. Am J Surg. 2008;195(4):457–62.
29. McHenry CR, Wilhelm SM. Management of follicular and Hürthle cell cancer. In: Sippel RS, Chen H, editors. The handbook of endocrine surgery. Singapore: World Scientific Publishing; 2012. p. 79–88.
30. Yip L, Carty SE. Follicular thyroid carcinoma and oncocytic (Hürthle cell) carcinoma. In: Morita SY, Dackiw APB, Zeiger MA, editors. Endocrine surgery. New York: McGraw-Hill; 2010. p. 65–88.
31. Chen H, Nicol TL, Zeiger MA, et al. Hürthle cell neoplasms of the thyroid: are there factors predictive of malignancy? Ann Surg. 1998;227(4):542–6.
32. Zhang YW, Greenblatt DY, Repplinger D, et al. Older age and larger tumor size predict malignancy in hürthle cell neoplasms of the thyroid. Ann Surg Oncol. 2008;15(10):2842–6.
33. Zettinig G, Fueger BJ, Passler C, et al. Long-term follow-up of patients with bone metastases from differentiated thyroid carcinoma – surgery or conventional therapy? Clin Endocrinol (Oxf). 2002;56(3):377–82.
34. McWilliams RR, Giannini C, Hay ID, Atkinson JL, Stafford SL, Buckner JC. Management of brain metastases from thyroid carcinoma: a study of 16 pathologically confirmed cases over 25 years. Cancer. 2003;98(2):356–62.
35. Pinchot SN, Sippel RS. Management of medullary thyroid cancer. In: Sippel RS, Chen H, editors. The handbook of endocrine surgery. Singapore: World Scientific Publishing; 2012. p. 63–78.
36. Chen H, Sippel RS, O'Dorisio MS, et al. The North American Neuroendocrine Tumor Society consensus guideline for the diagnosis and management of neuroendocrine tumors: pheochromocytoma, paraganglioma, and medullary thyroid cancer. Pancreas. 2010; 39(6):775–83.
37. Kloos RT, Eng C, Evans DB, et al. Medullary thyroid cancer: management guidelines of the American Thyroid Association. Thyroid. 2009;19(6):565–612.
38. Kebebew E, Ituarte PH, Siperstein AE, Duh QY, Clark OH. Medullary thyroid carcinoma: clinical characteristics, treatment, prognostic factors, and a comparison of staging systems. Cancer. 2000;88(5): 1139–48.
39. Machens A, Schneyer U, Holzhausen HJ, Dralle H. Prospects of remission in medullary thyroid carcinoma according to basal calcitonin level. J Clin Endocrinol Metab. 2005;90(4):2029–34.
40. Sippel RS, Kunnimalaiyaan M, Chen H. Current management of medullary thyroid cancer. Oncologist. 2008;13(5):539–47.
41. Truong M, Cook MR, Pinchot SN, Kunnimalaiyaan M, Chen H. Resveratrol induces Notch2-mediated apoptosis and suppression of neuroendocrine markers in medullary thyroid cancer. Ann Surg Oncol. 2011; 18(5):1506–11.
42. Callender GG, Hu MI, Evans DB, Perrier ND. Medullary thyroid carcinoma. In: Morita SY, Dackiw APB, Zeiger MA, editors. Endocrine surgery. New York: McGraw-Hill; 2010. p. 89–109.
43. Burke JF, Sippel RS, Chen H. Evolution of pediatric thyroid surgery at a tertiary medical center. J Surg Res. 2012;177(2):268–74.
44. Boi F, Maurelli I, Pinna G, et al. Calcitonin measurement in wash-out fluid from fine needle aspiration of neck masses in patients with primary and metastatic medullary thyroid carcinoma. J Clin Endocrinol Metab. 2007;92(6):2115–8.
45. Chen H, Roberts JR, Ball DW, et al. Effective long-term palliation of symptomatic, incurable metastatic medullary thyroid cancer by operative resection. Ann Surg. 1998;227(6):887–95.
46. Brierley J, Sherman E. The role of external beam radiation and targeted therapy in thyroid cancer. Semin Radiat Oncol. 2012;22(3):254–62.
47. Brierley J, Tsang R, Simpson WJ, Gospodarowicz M, Sutcliffe S, Panzarella T. Medullary thyroid cancer: analyses of survival and prognostic factors and the role of radiation therapy in local control. Thyroid. 1996;6(4):305–10.
48. Campbell MJ, Seib CD, Gosnell J. Vandetanib and the management of advanced medullary thyroid cancer. Curr Opin Oncol. 2013;25(1):39–43.
49. Hundahl SA, Fleming ID, Fremgen AM, Menck HR. A National Cancer Data Base report on 53,856 cases of thyroid carcinoma treated in the U.S., 1985–1995 [see comments]. Cancer. 1998;83(12): 2638–48.
50. Ruan DT, Clark OH. Anaplastic thyroid carcinoma, metastases to the thyroid gland, and thyroid lymphoma. In: Morita SY, Dackiw APB, Zeiger MA, editors. Endocrine surgery. New York: McGraw-Hill; 2010. p. 110–24.
51. Nishiyama RH. Overview of surgical pathology of the thyroid gland. World J Surg. 2000;24(8):898–906.

52. Smallridge RC, Ain KB, Asa SL, et al. American Thyroid Association guidelines for management of patients with anaplastic thyroid cancer. Thyroid. 2012;22(11):1104–39.
53. Neff RL, Farrar WB, Kloos RT, Burman KD. Anaplastic thyroid cancer. Endocrinol Metab Clin North Am. 2008;37(2):525–38, xi.
54. Kim TY, Kim KW, Jung TS, et al. Prognostic factors for Korean patients with anaplastic thyroid carcinoma. Head Neck. 2007;29(8):765–72.
55. Pierie JP, Muzikansky A, Gaz RD, Faquin WC, Ott MJ. The effect of surgery and radiotherapy on outcome of anaplastic thyroid carcinoma. Ann Surg Oncol. 2002;9(1):57–64.
56. McIver B, Hay ID, Giuffrida DF, et al. Anaplastic thyroid carcinoma: a 50-year experience at a single institution. Surgery. 2001;130(6):1028–34.
57. Passler C, Scheuba C, Prager G, et al. Anaplastic (undifferentiated) thyroid carcinoma (ATC). A retrospective analysis. Langenbecks Arch Surg. 1999;384(3):284–93.
58. Guerrero MA, Kebebew E. Management of aggressive variants and anaplastic thyroid cancers. In: Sippel RS, Chen H, editors. The handbook of endocrine surgery. Singapore: World Scientific Publishing; 2012. p. 89–100.
59. Levendag PC, De Porre PM, van Putten WL. Anaplastic carcinoma of the thyroid gland treated by radiation therapy. Int J Radiat Oncol Biol Phys. 1993;26(1):125–8.
60. Compton C, Byrd D, Garcia-Aguilar J. Thyroid. In: Compton C, Byrd D, Garcia-Aguilar J, Kurtzman S, Olawaiye A, Washington M, editors. AJCC cancer staging atlas. 2nd ed. New York: Springer Science+Business Media; 2012. p. 113–20.

24 Pancreatic Neuroendocrine Tumors (PNETs)

Rouzbeh Daylami, Dhruvil Shah, and Richard J. Bold

Learning Objectives

After reading this chapter, you should be able to:

- Recognize the signs and symptoms of PNET
- Understand the preoperative biochemical and radiologic evaluation
- Discern the biologic factors involved in treatment decision making
- Decide appropriate surgical options for localized PNET

Background

Pancreatic neuroendocrine tumors (PNETs) are a heterogenous group of tumors characterized histopathologically by expression of somatostatin receptor, chromogranin A (CgA) and synaptophysin/neuron-specific enolase. Based on SEER database data, the pancreas represents the primary site of disease development for 7 % of all neuroendocrine neoplasms in the USA from 1973 to 2007 [1]. Patients who present with metastatic disease to the liver from PNET have a worse survival than those with midgut neuroendocrine carcinomas [2]. PNETs occur in approximately 1 in 100,000 individuals each year and are typically diagnosed in the fifth and sixth decade of life. Of all pancreatic neoplasms, PNETs account for only 1–2 % of all tumors [3, 4].

The division of PNETs into functional and nonfunctional classes is mostly of academic and historical interest to the surgeon for a number of reasons. Firstly, the functional status of the PNET rarely changes the surgical management of the primary tumor. Furthermore, clinical outcomes appear to be driven more by tumor biology and burden of disease (grade and stage). Finally, the definition of "functional tumors" has not been standardized across the literature as some symptoms of PNETs may be attributed to local effects or systemic symptoms that may be seen in progressive malignancy.

Functional tumors, however, are significantly associated with familial syndromes, for which therapy and outcome may be significantly different than sporadic PNETs. More helpful classifications of PNETs into well differentiated *vs.* poorly differentiated, local *vs.* metastatic, and resectable *vs.* unresectable will be the focus of this chapter.

R. Daylami, M.D.
Department of Surgery, Kaiser Permanente, 6600 Bruceville Rd, 95823 Sacramento, CA, USA
e-mail: rouzbeh.daylami@kp.org

D. Shah, M.D.
Department of Surgery, UC Davis Cancer Center, 2315 Stockton Blvd, 95817 Sacramento, CA, USA
e-mail: dhruvil.shah@ucdmc.ucdavis.edu

R.J. Bold, M.D. (✉)
Division of Surgical Oncology, UC Davis Cancer Center, 4501 X Street, Suite 3010, Sacramento, CA, USA 95817
e-mail: richard.bold@ucdmc.ucdavis.edu

Q.D. Chu et al. (eds.), *Surgical Oncology: A Practical and Comprehensive Approach*,
DOI 10.1007/978-1-4939-1423-4_24,

Evaluation of Suspected PNET

Patients with PNETs will typically present in one of three primary fashions: (1) suspected functional PNET due to constellation of symptoms, (2) due to mass effect on local/adjacent organs, or (3) incidentally identified based on radiologic imaging obtained for other reasons. Nonfunctional PNETs are seen more frequently and account for 60 % of these tumors [5]. Occasionally, patients will be screened for PNETs due to family members who are part of a kindred of familial syndromes associated with PNETs.

Unique biochemical and clinical manifestation of functional PNETs warrant discussion related to diagnosis (Table 24.1). It must be noted that patients with these functional tumors should be investigated for the possibility of having MEN 1 syndrome (see below). The clinical manifestation of insulin-secreting PNETs (insulinoma) has been termed Whipple's triad and includes symptoms of hypoglycemia, fasting glucose <40 mg/dL, and relief of symptoms following administration of glucose. The biochemical diagnosis can be made in the absence of plasma sulfonylurea by a serum glucose <45 mg/dL, an insulin level >6 uU/ml, and a C-peptide >300 pm/L. Diabetic drugs, notably insulin and sulfonylureas, are the most common cause of hypoglycemia, which needs to be excluded in the work-up for insulinoma. Most insulinomas are located intrapancreatic and distributed evenly throughout the pancreas.

The clinical manifestation of gastrin-secreting PNETs (gastrinoma, or Zollinger-Ellison syndrome) is related to the hypersecretion of gastric acid and includes severe peptic ulcer disease/gastroesophageal reflux disease (GERD), epigastric pain, and diarrhea. The biochemical diagnosis is highly suspected with a fasting gastrin of tenfold above normal (e.g., >1,000 pg/mL). Secretin stimulation test can help secure the diagnosis of gastrinoma; a gastrin level ≥200 pg/ml following secretin stimulation is diagnostic. Nearly 90 % of gastrinomas can be found in the "gastrinoma triangle" or the "Passaro Triangle" [6], a triangle that is formed by the confluence of the cystic duct and common bile duct superiorly, the second and third portion of the duodenum inferiorly, and the neck and body of the pancreas medially (Fig. 24.1).

PNETs that hypersecrete vasoactive intestinal peptide (VIPoma, Verner-Morrison syndrome, WDHA) cause the clinical constellation of symptoms of diarrhea, dehydration, and hypokalemia. Plasma hormone levels of VIP are typically >500 pg/mL (normal is typically <190 pg/ mL).

The clinical manifestation of PNETs that hypersecrete glucagons (glucagonoma) include glucose intolerance/diabetes mellitus, weight loss, and a unique dermatitis (necrolytic migratory erythema) [7]. The supporting biochemical study of a glucagonoma is that plasma levels of glucagons are generally >500 pg/mL.

Lastly, the PNETs that are associated with increased secretion of somatostatin do not consistently produce clinical manifestations, but symptoms may include diabetes mellitus, cholelithiasis, and weight loss. In addition, PNETs may secrete a variety of other hormones (e.g., pancreatic polypeptide, serotonin, calcitonin, growth-hormone-releasing factor) that may or may not be associated with the clinical manifestations.

Familial Syndromes Associated with PNETs

Three familial syndromes are associated with the development of PNETS: (1) multiple endocrine neoplasia type I (MEN1), (2) von Hippel-Lindau disease (VHL), and (3) von Recklinghausen disease (VRH, also termed neurofibromatosis type 1 or NF1). MEN1 is an autosomal dominant syndrome associated with mutation of the MEN1 gene which encodes the menin protein that regulates transcription of a variety of genes involved in cell growth and cell cycle progression. In addition to PNETs, MEN1 is associated with pituitary adenomas (typically prolactin secreting) and

Table 24.1 Summary of functional PNETs

	Clinical presentation	Diagnosis	Malignant potential	Location in the pancreas	Localization studies
Insulinoma	Symptoms of hypoglycemia Whipple's triad Hypoglycemia Fasting glucose <40 mg/dl Symptomatic relief with glucose	Glucose <45 mg/dl (no sulfonylurea) Insulin >6 u/ml C-peptide >300 pm/l	10 %	1/3 in head 1/3 in body 1/3 in tail Most are intrapancreatic	CT, MRI, US, ^{111}In-pentetreotide imaging ^{18}F-DOPA PET, IOUS Selective angiography with calcium stimulation and hepatic venous sampling
Gastrinoma	ZES PUD GERD Diarrhea 50 % present with metastases	Fasting gastrin >1,000 pg/ml Secretin stimulation test: gastrin level ≥200 pg/ml	50–60 %	Gastrinoma triangle	Upper endoscopy, EUS CT, MRI, SRS Selective angiography with secretin stimulation and hepatic venous sampling IOUS, transillumination of duodenum, duodenotomy
VIPomas (Verner-Morrison syndrome, WDHA)	WDHA: Watery diarrhea Dehydration Hypokalemia Achlorhydria Most present with metastases	Plasma level of VIP >500 pg/ml (normal <190 pg/ml)	60–80 %	Body and tail 95 % solitary	CT, MRI, SRS, EUS
Glucagonoma	Diabetes Weight loss Low albumin Necrolytic migratory erythema 50 % present with metastases	Plasma level of glucagon > 500pg/ml	75–85 %	Body and tail	CT, MRI, SRS, EUS Angiography
Somatostatinoma	Cholelithiasis Steatorrhea Diabetes Weight loss Most present with metastases	Plasma level of somatostatin, generally 1,000-fold higher than reference range	65 %	Ampullary, periampullary region	CT, MRI, SRS, EUS

Courtesy of Quyen D. Chu, MD, MBA, FACS
ZES Zollinger-Ellison syndrome, *EUS* endoscopic ultrasound; *IOUS* intraoperative ultrasound

hyperparathyroidism (typically four-gland hyperplasia). The PNET most commonly associated with MEN1 is a gastrinoma, though to a lesser degree, insulinomas and glucagonomas are seen; although rare, VIPomas and somatostatinomas can also be associated with MEN 1 syndrome. The hallmark of PNETs associated with MEN1 is the multicentric nature of the tumors distributed throughout the pancreatic gland. A more in-depth discussion of MEN 1 is found in Chap. 25, Multiple Endocrine Neoplasia (MEN) Syndromes.

VHL is an autosomal dominant syndrome associated with mutation of the VHL gene, which encodes for a protein regulating transcription of proteins involved in angiogenesis. VHL is

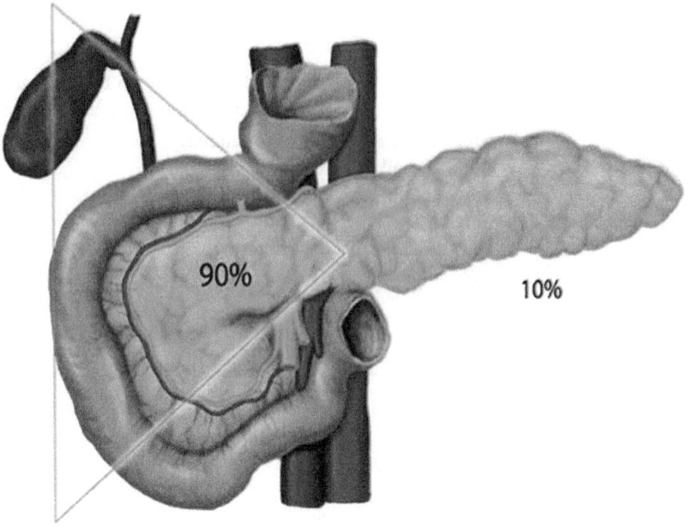

Fig. 24.1 *Gastrinoma Triangle (Passaro Triangle)*: A triangle that is formed by the confluence of the cystic duct and common bile duct superiorly, the second and third portion of the duodenum inferiorly, and the neck and body of the pancreas medially (Reprinted from Hernandez-Jover et al. [6]. With permission from Springer Verlag)

characterized by hemangioblastomas of the eye or cerebral nervous system, renal cell carcinomas, and pheochromocytomas. The PNETs associated with VHL are typically nonfunctional and present in less than 20 % of VHL patients.

VRH is due to mutations in the NF-1 gene which encodes the neurofibromin protein; through binding to microtubules, neurofibromin affects the cellular cytoskeleton. VRH is a relatively common familial syndrome with cutaneous manifestations of café-au-lait spots, neurofibromas, and a variety of cognitive developmental disorders. PNETs are relatively uncommon for VRH patients, though the prototypic tumor is duodenal somatostatinoma.

Classification/Staging

The World Health Organization (WHO) 2010 classification of PNETs divides tumors into well differentiated and poorly differentiated based on histopathologic grading (mitotic rate and proliferative index as measured by Ki-67 staining). This grading system is useful in determining overall prognosis (Table 24.2). Both the European Neuroendocrine Tumor Society and the American Joint Commission on Cancer have proposed a TNM staging system to predict overall prognosis. These systems incorporate presence of the tumor size (T stage), metastasis to regional lymph nodes (N stage), and absence or presence of distant metastasis (M stage) [8] (Table 24.3).

Table 24.2 Pancreatic neuroendocrine tumors: WHO classification

WHO[a] classification	Grade	Ki-67 Proliferation rate	Mitotic count per 10 HPF
1	G1	≤2 %	<2
2	G2	3–20 %	2–20
3	G3	>20 %	>20

[a]*WHO* World Health Organization

The liver represents the most common site of distant metastatic disease. Additional adverse prognostic factors (beyond the WHO histologic classification system) include younger age, male gender, and perhaps extent of extrapancreatic disease.

Radiologic Evaluation of Resectable vs. Unresectable Disease

In a patient with suspected PNET, the most important question to answer is whether the disease is resectable as curative resection remains the cornerstone of treatment in nonmetastatic PNETs. Management of PNETs should be based upon a multidisciplinary approach with the surgeon determining resectability. This decision incorporates

Table 24.3 TNM System of staging for pancreatic neuroendocrine tumors

Primary tumor size (cm)	
TX	Primary tumor cannot be assessed
T0	No evidence of primary tumor
Tis	Carcinoma in situ
T1	≤2, limited to pancreas
T2	>2, limited to pancreas
T3	Beyond pancreas, but without involvement of the celiac axis or the superior mesenteric artery
T4	Tumor involves the celiac axis or the superior mesenteric artery (unresectable primary tumor)
Regional lymph nodes	
NX	Regional lymph nodes cannot be assessed
N0	No regional lymph node metastasis
N1	Regional lymph node metastasis
Distant metastases	
M0	No distant metastasis
M1	Distant metastasis
Staging	
Stage 0	TisN0 M0
Stage IA	T1N0 M0
Stage IB	T2N0 M0
Stage IIA	T3N0 M0
Stage IIB	T1-3 N1
Stage III	T4, Any N, M0
Stage IV	Any T, any N, M1

Reprinted from [25]. With permission from Springer Verlag

Symptoms (functioning tumors)	Surgical management
– Resection of solitary disease confined to the pancreas – Systemic somatostatin for metastatic disease – Liver directed therapy (e.g. RFA, embolization)	– Enucleation vs. anatomic resection – Observation for small, benign, non-functional tumors

RFA: Radiofrequency ablation

Fig. 24.2 *Approaches to PNET therapy*. Tabular list of options for therapy to address both symptoms arising from hormonal hypersecretion or surgical management directed at tumor resection

the ability to achieve a complete resection of disease which is termed an R0 resection. Patients who present with symptomatic hypersecreting tumors may be palliated if an optimal cytoreductive (>85 %) resection can be achieved. It should be stressed that an optimal cytoreduction procedure should not be considered in an asymptomatic patient. A generalized approach to managing PNETs is shown in Fig. 24.2.

The resectability of the tumor depends on the location and extent of the primary disease as well as whether there is any radiologic evidence of metastatic lesions. There are a number of radiographic tools that can be employed to help the surgeon including ultrasound, computed tomography (CT), magnetic resonance imaging (MRI), selective angiography, somatostatin receptor scintigraphy (SRS), positron emission tomography (PET), and single-photon emission computed tomography (SPECT). SRS is useful for localizing all of PNETs except for insulinomas; SRS may miss up to 40 % of insulinomas because these tumors lack sufficient amount of subtype 2 somatostatin receptors [9].

Due to its wide availability and high sensitivity (approaching 90 %), contrast-enhanced triple-phase multidetector CT of the abdomen is the most common and useful imaging modality [10] (see Fig. 24.3). CT has decreased sensitivity for identifying lesions <0.5 cm and if clinical suspicion persists based either on patient symptoms or biochemical evaluation, endoscopic ultrasound (EUS) shows great sensitivity for the identification of PNETs less than 0.5 cm in size, particularly in the head of the pancreas. For radiologically occult functional PNETs, additional selective angiography with provocative testing (secretin for gastrinomas and calcium gluconate for insulinomas) and venous sampling may be helpful for localization of small tumors, but high-resolution radiographic imaging and intraoperative ultrasound have decreased the use of this technique.

Determining distant metastasis is best accomplished with some form of somatostatin receptor imaging. The most widely available and studied imaging modality for this purpose has been SRS using ^{111}In-DTPA-octreotide which has a sensitivity and specificity of 90 and 80 %, respectively, except in the case of insulinoma in which the sensitivity drops to <70 % [11]. Somatostatin receptors are decreased in high-grade tumors and absent on carcinoid tumors; therefore ^{18}FDG-PET may be a better modality for identifying metastatic disease or monitoring for disease progression [12].

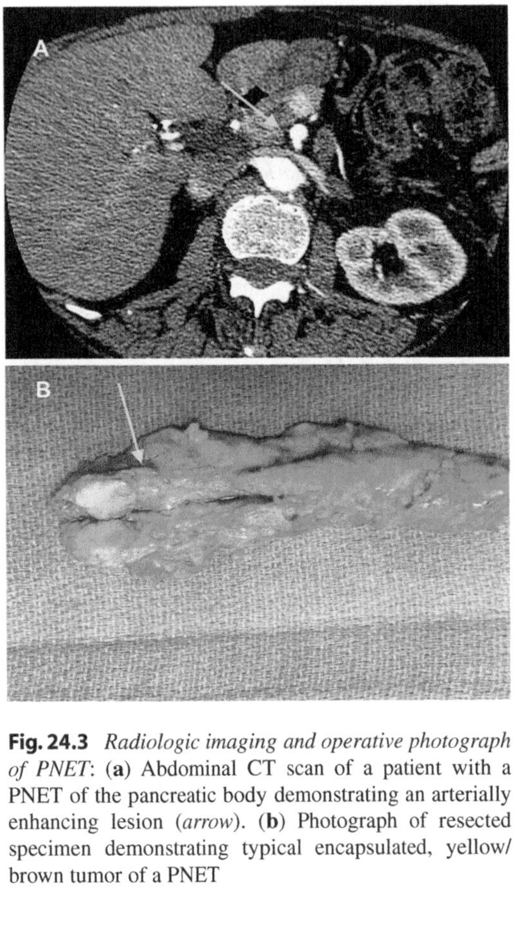

Fig. 24.3 *Radiologic imaging and operative photograph of PNET*: (**a**) Abdominal CT scan of a patient with a PNET of the pancreatic body demonstrating an arterially enhancing lesion (*arrow*). (**b**) Photograph of resected specimen demonstrating typical encapsulated, yellow/brown tumor of a PNET

Management of Local Disease

Surgical options can be broadly divided into parenchyma-preserving resections (i.e., enucleation) or anatomic resections (i.e., distal pancreatectomy, central pancreatectomy, or pancreaticoduodenectomy). Figures 24.4 and 24.5 show general guidelines in deciding whether to enucleate or resect anatomically. Several factors must be taken into account when deciding whether a patient is good candidate for

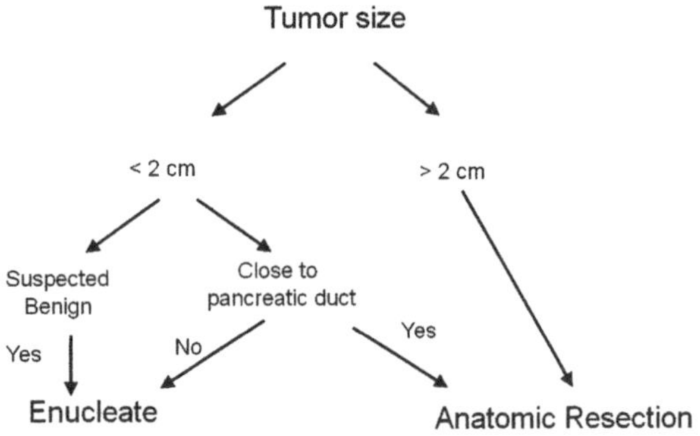

Fig. 24.5 *Decision tree for guidance of enucleation versus anatomic resection*. Characteristics of the tumor size and relationship to the pancreatic duct can be used to guide the decision to enucleate or resect a PNET

- Observation - <5mm, asymptomatic can be observed
- 5mm to 2cm –Gray Zone
  - ENETS guideline :"no data exist with respect to a positive effect of surgery on overall survival in small (<2 cm), possibly benign or intermediate-risk pancreatic endocrine tumors."
  - Histologic sampling to guide risk of malignancy:
    - More likely to be benign
      - <2cm
      - <2 mitoses per 10HPF
      - Ki-67 index <2%
  - > 3cm: Resection

Fig. 24.4 *Therapeutic options for nonfunctioning tumors*. Guidelines for surgical intervention of nonfunctioning PNETs based on size of the primary tumor. In the intermediate "gray zone" of 5 mm–2.0 cm, histologic sampling may be used to guide the decision of observation versus resection based on factors more likely to be associated with benign tumors enucleation. For practical purposes, enucleation is performed on tumors on the ventral surface of the pancreas and on tumors that are small enough that enucleation does not significantly disrupt the parenchyma. The relationship of the tumor to the main pancreatic duct is also critical in order to diminish the risk of pancreatic duct leak post resection. The relationship between the PNET and the main pancreatic duct is best done with intraoperative ultrasound. Furthermore, tumors that are high grade, have a high likelihood of being malignant (e.g., gastrinoma or glucagonoma), or have clear radiologic evidence of direct invasion into adjacent structures or regional lymph nodes, should not be considered for enucleation. For tumors in the body and tail of the pancreas, a laparoscopic approach to a distal pancreatectomy can be performed safely [13]. The oncologic outcomes for laparoscopic pancreatectomy when compared to open pancreatectomy have not been clearly reported, though it is reasonable to assume equivalent outcomes based on the equivalence of laparoscopic techniques for other abdominal malignancies. Furthermore, laparoscopic pancreatectomy is associated with decreased hospital length of stays, higher rates of spleen preservation, and a pancreatic duct leak in most series of 10–20 % [14]. Tumors in the head of the pancreas which are amenable to resection should be considered for pancreaticoduodenectomy in patients who will tolerate it. There may be a role for observation in patients with small (<1 cm), benign, nonfunctional, incidentally identified PNETs [15].

Advanced and Metastatic Disease

Over 60 % of patients with PNET present with unresectable or metastatic disease, and the median survival time for those with distant disease is approximately 24 months [16]. Until recently, the primary therapeutic modalities for hepatic metastasis from PNETs were resection, ablation, or embolization. These approaches provide both survival benefit and symptomatic relief for patients with functioning PNETs. In selected patients with resectable liver metastasis who undergo hepatectomy, 5-year survival of 60–80 % has been reported. There is a paucity of data regarding the role of surgical management of PNET metastasis outside of the liver. Hepatic artery embolization (with or without chemotherapy) and ablative modalities (such as radiofrequency ablation or microwave ablation) have also been used for patients not amenable to hepatic resection. Somatostatin injections are also useful in controlling the symptoms of patients with metastatic functional PNETs and may confer a modest survival benefit. Streptozocin, either alone or in combination with doxorubicin, is the only agent that was approved for the treatment of advanced PNETs [17]. Unfortunately, its efficacy has been questioned [18].

Advances have been made in the targeted molecular therapy of advanced, unresectable, and metastatic PNET. Vascular endothelial growth factor (VEGF) [19] and platelet-derived growth factor receptors (PDGFRs) α and β [20] are known to be involved in the pathogenesis of PNET. Sunitinib (Pfizer), a tyrosine kinase inhibitor that inhibits VEGFR and PDGFR signaling, was shown in a phase III clinical trial to be better than placebo at improving overall survival (OS) as well as progression-free survival (PFS) in patients with well-differentiated tumors who were deemed unresectable due to having locally advanced or metastatic disease [21]. The median PFS for patients receiving sunitinib was twice longer than those who received placebo (11.4 vs. 5.5 months; $p<0.001$). At the cutoff date, there were nine deaths (10 %) in the sunitinib group versus 21 deaths (25 %) in the placebo group ($P=0.02$) [21].

Mammalian target of rapamycin (mTOR) stimulates cell growth, proliferation, and angiogenesis and is also believed to play a role in the pathogenesis of PNET [22]. The mTOR inhibitor, everolimus (Afinitor, Novartis Pharmaceuticals), was recently found in a phase III clinical trial to increase PFS in patients with unresectable low- to medium-grade PNETs who had radiographic progression of their disease [23] (Table 24.4).

Despite these encouraging results, the role of these targeted agents prior to or following curative resection has yet to be determined. Furthermore, whether combination of sunitinib

Table 24.4 Phase III Trials of Targeted Therapy for Advanced PNETs

Authors/year	# patients	Study groups	Outcomes
Raymond/2011 [21]	171	Sunitinib versus placebo	Median PFS:
			Sunitinib: 11.4 mos
			Placebo: 5.5 mos
			($P<0.001$)
			Deaths:
			Sunitinib: 10 %
			Placebo: 25 %
			($P=0.02$)
Yao/2011 [23] RADIANT-3	410	Everolimus versus placebo	Median PFS:
			Everolimus: 11 mos
			Placebo: 4.6 mos
			($P<0.001$)
			OS: $P=0.59$

Courtesy of Quyen D. Chu, MD, MBA, FACS
RADIANT-3 RAD001 in Advanced Neuroendocrine Tumors, Third Trial Study Group
PFS Progression Free Survival; OS: Overall Survival

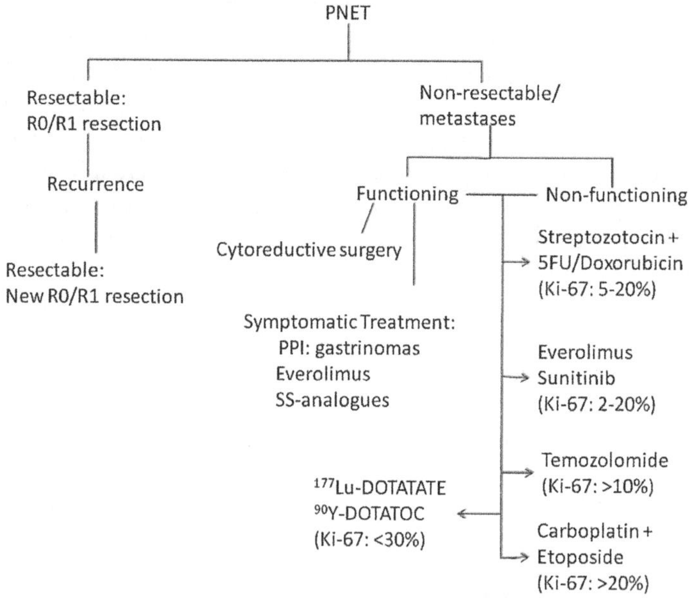

Fig. 24.6 *Algorithmic multidisciplinary approach to PNETs*: DOTA (1,4,7,10-tetraazacyclododecane-1,4,7,10-tetra-acetic acid); ^{177}Lu (^{177}Lutetium); DOTATOC ([DOTA^0,Tyr^3]octreotide); DOTATATE ([DOTA^0,Tyr^3] octreotate) (Modified from Öberg et al. [24]. With permission from Oxford University Press)

and everolimus will result in better outcome than either alone is not known. Figure 24.6 demonstrates an algorithmic multidisciplinary approach to PNETs [24].

The 5-year overall survival rate for all patients with PNET is approximately 60 %, localized disease ~100 %, regional disease ~40 %, and distant disease ~25 %. However, the 5-year survival rate for metastatic disease can reach as high as 60 % in dedicated centers [24]

Salient Points

- Tumor size, histologic grade, proliferative index, and function can be used to guide risk of malignancy.
- PNETs infrequently are part of familial syndromes, though management may be different than sporadic tumors due to the multicentric nature of the lesions.

- Primary resection options include enucleation for small, benign tumors not closely approximated to the main pancreatic duct.
- Primary methods for localization of functional tumors include contrast-enhanced CT scan and ultrasound performed either endoscopically or intraoperatively.
- Targeted therapies (e.g., sunitinib and everolimus) are now approved for the treatment of locally advanced, unresectable, and metastatic disease, although surgical resection should still be considered for patients with resectable hepatic metastasis.

Questions

1. A 45-year-old woman with persistent secretory diarrhea is found to have a 3-cm pancreatic mass. Endoscopic ultrasound biopsy shows a neuroendocrine cell tumor. Of the following hormones that could be produced by this tumor, the one that is most likely to account for this patient's diarrhea is:
   A. Neurotensin
   B. Serotonin
   C. VIP
   D. Gastrin
   E. Pancreatic polypeptide
2. The clinical manifestations of which of the following neoplasms are LEAST likely to be alleviated by administration of somatostatin analogue.
   A. PPoma
   B. Glucagonoma
   C. Carcinoid tumor
   D. VIPoma
   E. Gastrinoma
3. Which of the following statements about insulinomas is TRUE?
   A. They are associated with a low insulin/glucose ratio.
   B. Intraoperative ultrasonography is not helpful in localizing these tumors.
   C. Anatomic resection is the preferred operation.
   D. They are usually solitary in sporadic cases.
   E. Tumors are found primarily in the head of the pancreas.
4. Which of the following is not a prognostic variable of PNETs?
   A. Histologic grade
   B. Proliferative index
   C. Tumor location within the pancreas
   D. Tumor size
   E. Lymph node status
5. Gastrinomas associated with MEN1 are characterized by all of the following EXCEPT?
   A. They are poorly imaged by endoscopic ultrasound.
   B. They are usually located in the head of the pancreas.
   C. Most commonly they are malignant.
   D. Gastrinomas are the most common PNETs of MEN1.
   E. Gastrin levels are usually > 200 pg/mL.
6. A 55-year-old otherwise healthy man is found to have an enhancing 3.5 cm lesion in the tail of his pancreas on a CT scan obtained for kidney stones. He has no symptoms. The best method of treatment would be:
   A. Observation with repeat CT scan in 6 months
   B. Laparoscopic distal pancreatectomy
   C. Pancreaticoduodenectomy
   D. Radiofrequency ablation
   E. Sunitinib therapy

Answers

1. C
2. E
3. D
4. C
5. A
6. B

References

1. Lawrence B, Gustafsson BI, Chan A, Svejda B, Kidd M, Modlin IM. The epidemiology of gastroenteropancreatic neuroendocrine tumors. Endocrinol Metab Clin North Am. 2011;40(1):1–18, vii.
2. Johanson V, Tisell LE, Olbe L, Wängberg B, Nilsson O, Ahlman H. Comparison of survival between malignant neuroendocrine tumours of midgut and pancreatic origin. Br J Cancer. 1999;80(8):1259–61.
3. Muniraj T, Vignesh S, Shetty S, Thiruvengadam S, Aslanian HR. Pancreatic neuroendocrine tumors. Dis Mon. 2013;59(1):5–19.

4. Ito T, Igarashi H, Jensen RT. Pancreatic neuroendocrine tumors: clinical features, diagnosis and medical treatment: advances. Best Pract Res Clin Gastroenterol. 2012;26(6):737–53.
5. Sharma J, Duque M, Saif MW. Emerging therapies and latest development in the treatment of unresectable pancreatic neuroendocrine tumors: an update for clinicians. Therap Adv Gastroenterol. 2013;6(6):474–90.
6. Hernandez-Jover D, Pernas JC, Gonzalez-Ceballos S, Lupu I, Monill JM, Pérez C. Pancreatoduodenal junction: review of anatomy and pathologic conditions. J Gastrointest Surg. 2011;15(7):1269–81.
7. Chu Q, Al-Kasspooles M, Smith J, et al. Is glucagonoma of the pancreas a curable disease? Int J Gastrointest Cancer. 2001;29(3):155–62.
8. Edge SB, Compton CC. The American Joint Committee on Cancer: the 7th edition of the AJCC cancer staging manual and the future of TNM. Ann Surg Oncol. 2010;17(6):1471–4.
9. Mirallié E, Pattou F, Malvaux P, et al. Value of endoscopic ultrasonography and somatostatin receptor scintigraphy in the preoperative localization of insulinomas and gastrinomas. Experience of 54 cases. Gastroenterol Clin Biol. 2002;26(4):360–6.
10. Zhou C, Zhang J, Zheng Y, Zhu Z. Pancreatic neuroendocrine tumors: a comprehensive review. Int J Cancer. 2012;131(5):1013–22.
11. Rufini V, Calcagni ML, Baum RP. Imaging of neuroendocrine tumors. Semin Nucl Med. 2006;36(3): 228–47.
12. Strosberg JR, Coppola D, Klimstra DS, et al. The NANETS consensus guidelines for the diagnosis and management of poorly differentiated (high-grade) extrapulmonary neuroendocrine carcinomas. Pancreas. 2010;39(6):799–800.
13. Tseng WH, Canter RJ, Bold RJ. Perioperative outcomes for open distal pancreatectomy: current benchmarks for comparison. J Gastrointest Surg. 2011;15(11):2053–8.
14. Kooby DA, Hawkins WG, Schmidt CM, et al. A multicenter analysis of distal pancreatectomy for adenocarcinoma: is laparoscopic resection appropriate? J Am Coll Surg. 2010;210(5):779–85. 786–777.
15. Lee LC, Grant CS, Salomao DR, et al. Small, nonfunctioning, asymptomatic pancreatic neuroendocrine tumors (PNETs): role for nonoperative management. Surgery. 2012;152(6):965–74.
16. Yao JC, Hassan M, Phan A, et al. One hundred years after "carcinoid": epidemiology of and prognostic factors for neuroendocrine tumors in 35,825 cases in the United States. J Clin Oncol. 2008;26(18):3063–72.
17. Moertel CG, Lefkopoulo M, Lipsitz S, Hahn RG, Klaassen D. Streptozocin-doxorubicin, streptozocin-fluorouracil or chlorozotocin in the treatment of advanced islet-cell carcinoma. N Engl J Med. 1992;326(8):519–23.
18. Cheng PN, Saltz LB. Failure to confirm major objective antitumor activity for streptozocin and doxorubicin in the treatment of patients with advanced islet cell carcinoma. Cancer. 1999;86(6):944–8.
19. Casanovas O, Hicklin DJ, Bergers G, Hanahan D. Drug resistance by evasion of antiangiogenic targeting of VEGF signaling in late-stage pancreatic islet tumors. Cancer Cell. 2005;8(4):299–309.
20. Fjällskog ML, Hessman O, Eriksson B, Janson ET. Upregulated expression of PDGF receptor beta in endocrine pancreatic tumors and metastases compared to normal endocrine pancreas. Acta Oncol. 2007;46(6):741–6.
21. Raymond E, Dahan L, Raoul JL, et al. Sunitinib malate for the treatment of pancreatic neuroendocrine tumors. N Engl J Med. 2011;364(6):501–13.
22. von Wichert G, Jehle PM, Hoeflich A, et al. Insulin-like growth factor-I is an autocrine regulator of chromogranin A secretion and growth in human neuroendocrine tumor cells. Cancer Res. 2000;60(16):4573–81.
23. Yao JC, Shah MH, Ito T, et al. Everolimus for advanced pancreatic neuroendocrine tumors. N Engl J Med. 2011;364(6):514–23.
24. Öberg K, Knigge U, Kwekkeboom D, Perren A, Group EGW. Neuroendocrine gastro-entero-pancreatic tumors: ESMO Clinical Practice Guidelines for diagnosis, treatment and follow-up. Ann Oncol. 2012;23 Suppl 7:vii 124–30.
25. Compton C, Byrd D, Garcia-Aguilar J. Exocrine and Endocrine Pancreas. In: Compton C, Byrd D, Garcia-Aguilar J, Kurtzman S, Olawaiye A, Washington M, (eds). AJCC Cancer Staging Atlas. 2nd ed. New York, NY: Springer; 2012:297–308.

25 Multiple Endocrine Neoplasia (MEN) Syndromes

Jeffrey J. Brewer

Learning Objectives

By the end of this chapter, the reader should be able to understand:

- The endocrine disorders and associated findings of MEN 1 and MEN 2A and B
- The genetic causes of MEN 1 and MEN 2
- The indications for screening and genetic testing in those with MEN-associated tumors
- The treatment—both surgical and medical—of MEN-related endocrinopathies

Background

MEN syndromes are rare autosomal dominant conditions that affect hormone-secreting organs such as the pituitary, parathyroid, thyroid, adrenal, pancreas, paraganglia, and/or non-endocrine organs. These tumors can be benign or malignant. MEN syndromes are generally characterized by hyperactivity of the endocrine glands with overproduction of hormones. It is an inheritable condition and stems from germline mutations. In MEN 1, the mutated tumor suppressor gene MEN1 is inactivated, while in MEN 2, the mutated rearranged-during-transfection (RET) proto-oncogene is activated.

J.J. Brewer, M.D. (✉)
Department of Surgery, University at Buffalo, 462 Grider Street, Buffalo 14215, NY, USA
e-mail: jbrewer@ecmc.edu

Multiple Endocrine Neoplasia Type 1

Epidemiology

MEN 1 syndrome, also known as "Wermer syndrome," affects the pituitary, pancreas, and parathyroid (the 3 "Ps"). It is a relatively rare condition and appears in one in 30,000 with a prevalence of 2–3 per 100,000. The disorder affects both genders equally with a broad distribution of age at diagnosis. There does not appear to be any preferential ethnic, geographic, or socioeconomic patterns of distribution. No known risk factors have been established other than family history, although approximately 10 % of patients have a sporadic de novo mutation without having any evidence of a family history.

MEN 1 is also associated with other tumors such as carcinoid, lipoma, meningioma, leiomyoma, and adrenal tumors. Because of the number of different possible combinations of tumor types that can occur, the clinical diagnosis of MEN 1 can become difficult at times. In general, patients who have tumors affecting two of the three endocrine organs (pituitary, neuroendocrine tumors of the pancreas, hyperparathyroidism) are diagnosed as having MEN 1. Any first-degree relative of a patient with MEN 1 with a single-associated endocrinopathy is diagnosed as having familial MEN 1.

Q.D. Chu et al. (eds.), *Surgical Oncology: A Practical and Comprehensive Approach*,
DOI 10.1007/978-1-4939-1423-4_25, © Springer Science+Business Media New York 2015

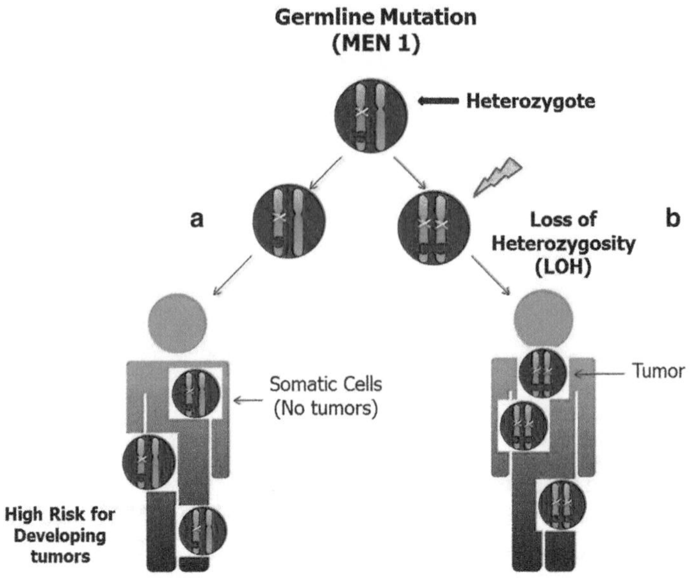

Fig. 25.1 Patients who inherited the menin mutation have an inactivated allele and a functioning allele (heterozygous). Because the functioning allele is a functioning tumor suppressor gene, these patients do not have cancer, although they are at an increased risk of developing it. When the second functioning allele is inactivated by epigenetic silencing, errors in chromosomal segregation, deletions, etc. (loss of heterozygosity), this predisposes the patient to developing tumors (Courtesy of Quyen D. Chu, MD, MBA, FACS)

Genetics

MEN 1 syndrome is the result of a germline mutation of the MEN1 gene on chromosome 11q13 which codes for the 610-amino acid protein menin. While the normal function of menin remains elusive, it is felt to be a tumor suppressor protein. In general, a tumor suppressor gene encodes protein(s) that acts as the "brakes" for the cell cycle. Mutation of a tumor suppressor gene is said to have a loss-of-function mutation. The inherited defect leads to one nonfunctioning gene and one functional gene. However, somatic deletion of the functional allele during the individual's lifetime subsequently leads to a loss of heterozygosity, a situation that leads to a complete loss of tumor suppressor function, or loss of the "brakes." This loss of the "brakes" is believed to lead to uncontrolled cellular growth, resulting in the clinical manifestation of MEN 1 (Fig. 25.1). Of note, at the level of the individual cells, mutations of tumor suppressor genes are said to be recessive, even though the pattern of inheritance is autosomal dominant.

More than 1,300 different germline mutations have been identified thus far and most of these mutations are either frameshift or nonsense mutations. Germline mutations in the menin gene are found in over 75 % of patients with familial forms of MEN 1. About 30 % of sporadic type MEN 1 patients demonstrate the mutation, suggesting that other proteins may play a role in the development of the syndrome.

Loss of function of the menin gene has also been found in other sporadic endocrine tumors such as parathyroid adenomas, bronchial carcinoids, and gastrinomas; this observation further supports the importance of menin in normal endocrine organ tumor surveillance.

Clinical Presentation of MEN 1

The most common initial presenting symptom is often related to the sequelae of primary hyperparathyroidism. Because symptoms of primary hyperparathyroidism (PHPT) in patients with MEN 1 syndrome are similar to patients with sporadic PHPT, the diagnosis of MEN 1 is often overlooked and delayed for several years. Such patients may present with mild hypercalcemia, renal stones, peptic ulcer disease, and depression (Table 25.1). Nearly all patients with MEN 1 will eventually develop PHPT; there is an 80–100 % penetrance by the age of 50 [1].

Table 25.1 Conditions and symptoms seen in patients with hyperparathyroidism

Nephrolithiasis	Depression
Osteopenia	Fatigue
Pancreatitis	Nausea and vomiting
Gout	Dyspepsia
Peptic ulcer disease	Polyuria
Weight loss	Muscle aches
Lethargy	Pruritus

In contrast to sporadic PHPT, which tends to manifest as single gland adenoma in upward of 85 % of cases, the PHPT seen in MEN 1 patients is typically multigland hyperplasia. The average age of onset in MEN 1 is in the third decade compared to the sixth decade for sporadic lesions [2]. Despite the prevalence of hyperparathyroidism in MEN 1 patients, parathyroid carcinoma remains rare.

The second most common manifestation of MEN 1 is the pancreatic neuroendocrine tumor (PNET) origin. These tumors can develop in up to 60 % of patients over the age of 40 [3, 4]. The morbidity associated with these tumors depends on the tumor type. Gastrinomas account for over 50 % of PNET lesions in MEN 1. Associated with persistent gastric acid hypersecretion and a predisposition to refractory ulcer disease, these are usually small and multicentric at the time of diagnosis and are found almost exclusively in the duodenum. Nearly half of gastrinomas are malignant at the time of diagnosis and often have lymph node or hepatic metastases.

Insulinomas are the second most common tumor of PNET origin (10–20 %) with a morbidity that is related to profound hypoglycemia. Besides gastrinomas and insulinomas, nonfunctioning neuroendocrine tumors have been recently reported to occur in up to 55 % of patients when screened with endoscopic ultrasound. Although they are referred to as nonfunctioning, these neuroendocrine tumors can secrete low levels of polyamines without having any associated symptoms. Glucagonomas, vasoactive intestinal peptide tumors (VIPomas), and somatostatinomas have all been reported, though in much less frequency. In glucagonomas, necrolytic migratory erythema (NME) is the pathognomonic dermatologic lesion [5].

Treatment of PNET tumors generally involves medical control of symptoms, while operative intervention is somewhat controversial, except for insulinomas. The prognosis of malignant PNETs tends to be more favorable in MEN 1 patients than that seen in sporadic cases; for MEN 1 patients, the mean survival is approximately 15 years after diagnosis compared to 5 years for patients with sporadic tumors. However, these results may be due to biases related to earlier diagnosis.

Pituitary tumors are seen in up to 50 % of patients diagnosed with MEN 1 [6]. The vast majority are microadenomas, which are defined as being smaller than 10 mm. The mean age at diagnosis is late 30s to early 40s. Prolactinoma is the most common functional tumor followed by growth hormone secreters and nonfunctional tumors, although somatotropinomas and corticotropinomas have also been reported. Pituitary tumors associated with MEN 1 tend to progress to macroadenomas and become more resistant to medical therapy over time.

Less common manifestations of MEN 1 include carcinoids of the upper aerodigestive tract (5–10 %), which includes the bronchus, thymus, and stomach [7]. Benign skin and subcutaneous lesions including angiofibromas and lipomas are commonly seen in up to 80 % of patients with MEN 1 [8].

Diagnosis and Screening

Genetic testing for the MEN1 gene mutation and further workup should be initiated in those patients that demonstrate any two of the three common endocrine tumors (hyperparathyroidism, pituitary tumor, PNET tumors). Patients with a family history of MEN 1 who have an associated endocrine tumor should also undergo genetic testing. Genetic testing of the offspring of MEN patient should begin at an early age. Some investigators recommend screening of individuals who have early hyperparathyroidism (under age 30), gastrinoma at any age, or multifocal pancreatic neuroendocrine tumors (PNET).

Table 25.2 Screening recommendations for MEN 1

Hyperparathyroidism	Intact PTH and serum calcium—yearly starting at age 8
Pituitary tumor	Serum prolactin and insulin-like growth factor—yearly starting at age 5
	Brain MRI based on abnormal result
Gastrinoma	Fasting serum gastrin yearly starting at age 20
	Abdominal CT based on result
Insulinoma	Fasting insulin and glucose starting at age 5
	Abdominal CT based on result

In those who harbor the MEN 1 mutation, it is recommended that they should undergo yearly screening for all of the common MEN 1-related tumors starting at the age of 5 years (Table 25.2). Any biochemical abnormalities should prompt further radiologic investigation such as a magnetic resonance imaging (MRI) of the brain for suspected pituitary tumors or computed tomography (CT)/ultrasound for PNET-related tumors. Unfortunately, genetic mutations are detected in only 75 % of patients with MEN I and early detection has yet to demonstrate an improvement in morbidity or mortality in MEN 1 patients.

Treatment

As the involved endocrine organs vary greatly from patient to patient, so does the therapy for MEN 1-affected individuals. True surgical cures are very difficult to achieve, and any intervention is typically guided toward alleviation of medically resistant symptoms and prevention of progression toward malignancy and metastatic disease. The following are recommendations for treating the most common MEN 1-related disorders.

Management of Hyperparathyroidism in MEN 1

As mentioned, nearly all patients with MEN 1 will develop hyperparathyroidism, often as the primary presenting symptom of the disorder. Confirmatory diagnosis is typically laboratory based with elevated levels of parathyroid hormone in the presence of hypercalcemia.

Much controversy surrounds the timing of intervention as well as the type of resection. Earlier intervention at the time of diagnosis limits the deleterious effects of long-standing hypercalcemia such as osteopenia, nephrolithiasis, ulcer disease, etc. but at the cost of a higher likelihood of recurrence and need for reintervention. Most patients will recur over time, often requiring further resection of any remaining parathyroid tissue. The risk of recurrence increases over time with recurrence rates being well over 50 % at 10 years in patients who had undergone subtotal or total parathyroidectomy with reimplantation surgery [9]. Given the high rate of recurrence over time, the goal of parathyroidectomy should be to achieve the longest durable remission time from hyperparathyroidism in the safest fashion for the patient.

No consensus exists with regard to whether a subtotal 3½ gland excision should be performed or a total parathyroidectomy with reimplantation. The general benefit of a subtotal resection is the low risk of developing profound hypocalcemia. However, the disadvantage with this approach is the greater risk of developing earlier recurrence and the need for reoperation in the neck. Total parathyroidectomy and reimplantation in the forearm carries a higher incidence of recalcitrant hypocalcemia but with the benefit of a less taxing operation at the forearm to remove implanted parathyroid tissue for recurrent disease.

Prior to planning any operative resection of the parathyroids, a thorough examination and evaluation of the thyroid gland should be undertaken because of the high rate of having synchronous thyroid tumors. This includes obtaining biochemical and ultrasound analysis. There is evidence that performing a cervical thymectomy at the initial resection decreases recurrence rates as well as reduces the risk of developing thymic carcinoids, a situation that can be seen in up to 10 % of MEN 1 patients [1].

Management of Pancreatic Neuroendocrine Tumors (PNET) in MEN 1

Over 60 % of patients with MEN 1 will have a PNET over their lifetime. The treatment of these tumors is predicated on whether the lesion is a functional or nonfunctional tumor, the most common being gastrinoma followed by insulinoma as previously discussed.

As gastrinoma accounts for the majority of these lesions, therapy traditionally has been medical symptom control with the use of H2 blockers and proton pump inhibitors. It is important to remember that surgical intervention should be delayed until after hypercalcemia has been addressed as calcium plays a role in acid hypersecretion. Correction of the hypercalcemic state often leads to a reduction of serum gastrin levels. As gastrinomas are often multifocal, surgical cures are rare and often require a subtotal pancreatectomy, duodenal exploration, as well as regional lymph node dissection [10]. Surgical interventions should be reserved for malignant gastrinomas or those with disease refractory to medical management.

In contrast to gastrinoma, insulinoma often requires surgical resection and is rarely malignant though symptomatic control is often more difficult. These lesions can typically be treated effectively with surgical enucleation (either with open or laparoscopic technique) and are found almost exclusively within the pancreatic parenchyma.

As with sporadic PNETs, there is a role for surgical debulking of tumor mass in all types of PNETs, and the goal is to achieve symptom control rather than surgical cure. In those patients in whom surgery is not possible, medical therapy including diazoxide, sunitinib, somatostatin, or other therapies can be employed for palliation.

Management of Pituitary Neoplasms in MEN 1

Therapy of associated pituitary neoplasm is typically directed toward controlling symptoms such as headaches and vision changes due to the mass effect of the tumor. Pituitary tumors associated with MEN 1 can also exert hormonal effects, the most common tumor being prolactinoma, followed by growth-hormone- secreting tumors and adrenocorticotropic-hormone (ACTH)-secreting tumors. The first-line therapy of prolactinoma is medical management, employing dopamine agonists such as bromocriptine or cabergoline. For growth-hormone-secreting tumors and ACTH-secreting tumors, as well as prolactinomas that are refractory to medical therapy, a transsphenoidal hypophysectomy offers a safe and effective alternative to medical management. Somatostatin analogs and/or radiation are sometimes employed with some success as primary medical therapy or for recurrences of these tumors.

Multiple Endocrine Neoplasia Type 2

Multiple endocrine neoplasia type 2 (MEN 2) includes two subtypes—A and B—as well as a third entity, familial medullary thyroid carcinoma (FMTC), all linked by mutations of the RET proto-oncogene and a tendency for the development of medullary thyroid cancers (MTC) (Table 25.3). MTC was first described in 1959 by Hazard et al. [11]. Two years later, Sipple described a patient in which MTC and pheochromocytoma were found implying a common linkage [12]. It was not until 1968 that a report of a family with MTC, pheochromocytoma, and hyperparathyroidism was reported [13].

Table 25.3 Manifestation of clinical features by MEN 2 subtypes

Subtype	Hyperparathyroidism	Pheochromocytoma	MTC
MEN 2A	20–30 %	50 %	95 %
MEN 2B	Rare	50 %	100 %
FMTC	0 %	0 %	100 %

MTC Medullary thyroid carcinoma, *FMTC* Familial medullary thyroid carcinoma

This syndrome was later termed "Sipple syndrome" now known as MEN 2A.

MTC is a rare form of sporadic thyroid cancer arising from the parafollicular C cells and accounts for approximately 5 % of all thyroid malignancies. MTC tends to be more aggressive than the more common thyroid malignancies—papillary, follicular—with a predilection for lymphatic spread. Calcitonin is the product of the parafollicular C cells, and elevated serum levels can be seen in advanced disease. It can also be used as a surveillance modality after a thyroidectomy. A more thorough discussion of MTC can be found in Chap. 23, Thyroid Cancer.

Unlike MEN 1 which can have high variability in the timing as well as the types of tumors seen in the disorder, MEN 2 tends to be more predictable and early diagnosis by genetic testing has resulted in a significant reduction in the morbidity and mortality associated with the disease.

Genetics

Mutations of the RET proto-oncogene on chromosome 10 leading to MEN 2 were first discovered in 1993 [14]. The mutations were found to encode for a transmembrane tyrosine kinase receptor involved in the processes of cell migration, division, and proliferation. RET is normally expressed in neural crest-derived tissues and is key to the normal embryological development of these derived organs. Under-expression of RET has been associated with neonatal Hirschsprung's disease with aganglionogenesis leading to colonic dysfunction. Upregulation and activation leads to MEN 2 and FMTC.

The mutation is transmitted in an autosomal dominant fashion with 50 % of offspring expected to develop the disease. Unlike tumor suppressor genes, which act as brakes for the cell cycle, oncogenes are more analogous to the gas pedal of a car. Consequently, only one-altered copy of a proto-oncogene is required to affect the individual. Mutation of the proto-oncogene is a gain-of-function mutation.

The most common mutations associated with MEN 2A involve a missense mutation substituting cysteine for another amino acid. The majority of these occurs on the extracellular portion of the receptor with mutation of exon 11 at codon 634 being by far the most common and is found in up to 85 % of MEN 2A patients. MEN 2B is most often associated with mutations encoding for the intracellular domain of RET which allow for direct intracellular activation and downstream amplification. Over 95 % of MEN 2B patients have a point mutation at codon 918 at exon 16 substituting threonine for methionine [15]. FMTC has been linked to a number of various sporadic mutations often in non-cysteine-rich regions.

Unlike MEN 1 in which similar mutations may have widely variable expression, the mutations found in MEN 2 tend to follow predictable patterns in regard to the development of tumors and the severity of disease. This has led to the quantification of the risks associated with each specific mutation and allows for the generation of specific guidelines regarding surveillance and treatment of affected patients. The American Thyroid Association (ATA) Guidelines Task Force stratifies aggressiveness of MTC into four categories (low, medium, high, highest) based on specific RET mutations [16].

MEN 2A

MEN 2A is by far the most common form of MEN type 2, occurring in one in 30,000–40,000 individuals. Affected patients may develop MTC, hyperparathyroidism, and pheochromocytoma. Nearly all individuals with MEN 2A will develop MTC, with most developing it by their teenage years and often with metastatic disease at the time of diagnosis.

MTC is not amenable to radioactive iodine ablation as these tumors do not readily take up iodine, thus making it difficult to treat recurrent disease. While MEN 2A, MEN 2B, and FMTC only account for 20 % of all MTCs, the tumor observed in these conditions tends to be more aggressive, be multifocal, and arise at a far younger age than the sporadic form of the disease. MTC is often the only related endocrine malignancy manifested in these patients.

Therefore, early intervention with prophylactic total thyroidectomy has greatly increased survival rates. The penetrance of the disease often dictates the timing of thyroidectomy, and in some patients, the procedure was performed as early as the first year of life.

Pheochromocytomas arise from the catecholamine-producing chromaffin cells of the adrenal medulla and are most commonly discovered within or near the adrenal glands. Pheochromocytomas are seen in up to 50 % of patients with MEN 2A, typically between the second and fourth decades of life; it is rarely the first sign of the syndrome. In contrast to the sporadic forms of pheochromocytomas, pheochromocytomas in MEN 2A individuals are often bilateral, multifocal, and extra-adrenal, and the most common symptoms are hypertension and headache.

Primary hyperparathyroidism (PHPT) can develop in nearly 25 % of MEN 2A patients, but in contrast to MEN 1, it is rarely the presenting symptom and often occurs later in life (i.e., fourth and fifth decades). Many of these patients will have single-gland adenomas and minimal elevations in serum calcium levels, further highlighting its differences from MEN 1. The age at which pheochromocytomas and PHPT occur often directly correlates with the specific RET mutation. Those with more aggressive mutations tend to present at an earlier age. Cutaneous lichen amyloidosis, a benign pruritic skin lesion generally found on the upper back of MEN 2A individuals, occurs in 10 % of patients with MEN 2A.

MEN 2B

The syndrome, like MEN 2A, involves nearly 100 % development of MTC and 50 % occurrence of pheochromocytomas. MEN 2B is rarer than MEN 2A, occurring in approximately 1/1,000,000. The average onset of MTC is 10 years younger than those with MEN 2A, and the MTC associated with MEN 2B tends to be very aggressive with reports of malignancy found at birth. Such aggressiveness accounts for the reduced lifespan of this patient population. However, unlike MEN 2A, hyperparathyroidism does not occur and patients can present with marfanoid body habitus. Additionally, affected individuals can also present with telltale mucosal neuromas, which are demonstrated in nearly 100 % of patients. These neuromas can lead to the development of prominent lumpy lips as well as thickened eyelid, which can cause eversion of the upper canthus. Ganglioneuromatosis of the GI (gastrointestinal) and urinary tracts are also a prominent feature of MEN 2B. The overall prognosis tends to be much worse when compared to MEN 2A.

Familial Medullary Thyroid Carcinoma (FMTC)

Familial medullary thyroid carcinoma (FMTC) is considered by many to be the mildest form of MEN 2. While by definition, all affected individuals will develop MTC, there is no predilection to the development of other endocrine tumors. The behavior of the tumors and age of onset mirrors that of MEN 2A. The diagnosis of FMTC is made when MTC is found in four members of a family over two generations and without evidence of pheochromocytoma or parathyroid dysfunction. The diagnosis has been made with increasing frequency given the widespread use of genetic testing for the RET mutation. Some authors believe FMTC to be a variant of MEN 2A with a delay in the discovery of the other associated tumors.

Diagnosis and Screening

Unfortunately, the initial manifestation of all forms of MEN 2 is typically MTC, which often occurs at a young age. Survival is related to the extent of the disease at diagnosis. Patients often have cervical lymph node metastases at the time of diagnosis and may complain only of a neck mass or more frequently diarrhea. Diarrhea is often seen in patients with elevated calcitonin levels and is a marker of advanced disease. Prior to genetic testing, serial calcitonin levels were drawn in those who were deemed to be at high risk. This type of testing has largely been abandoned due to a delay in patients receiving a thyroidectomy and the advent of genetic testing.

Screening for MEN 2 by genetic testing should be offered to any patient who is diagnosed with MTC or primary C-cell hyperplasia. While only 20 % of patients with MTC will have MEN 2, there is a benefit in screening all who have MTC so as to identify affected MEN 2 patients for both screening of their offspring and further surveillance of their related endocrinopathies (hyperparathyroidism, pheochromocytoma).

Children of known MEN 2 patients should undergo RET genetic screening within the first 6 months of life for those with high-risk mutations or no later than the third year of life. Ultrasound of the thyroid gland and serum calcitonin levels are also part of the early screening program of offspring. Prophylactic thyroidectomy is largely guided by the identified mutation [16]. For patients in the low-risk to high-risk group, prophylactic thyroidectomy is recommended by age 5. However, for those in the highest-risk group, prophylactic thyroidectomy is recommended as early as possible, before age 1 [16].

Evaluation for the presence of a pheochromocytoma should be undertaken in any patient found to have a RET-associated MTC as well as any RET carrier who is planning on becoming pregnant. Evaluation can be limited to obtaining serum and urinary levels of metanephrines, epinephrine, norepinephrine, and urinary catecholamines. Elevation in any of these biomarkers should prompt imaging with CT, MRI, or metaiodobenzylguanidine (MIBG) scan. If a pheochromocytoma is found, it should be addressed prior to thyroidectomy due to the risk of a hypertensive crisis during surgery. Those diagnosed with MEN 2 should undergo annual screening for pheochromocytoma with serum and urinary studies starting at age 20 for MEN 2A and age 8 for MEN 2B.

In those patients found to have mutations in the most common codons linked to MEN 2A—codons 630 and 634—screening with blood sample assays for the presence of hyperparathyroidism should begin at age 8. Albumin-corrected calcium level or ionized calcium and intact parathyroid hormone level is sufficient to make the determination of hyperparathyroidism. MEN 2A patients with other mutations as well as those diagnosed with FMTC should begin screening at age 20 on an annual basis.

Treatment and Prophylactic Thyroidectomy Guidelines

MTC is the most common tumor seen in all of the RET-associated MEN 2 disorders and has the greatest impact on overall survival. Historically, a thyroidectomy was withheld until patients demonstrated a rise in calcitonin serum level above the normal level or was found to have an abnormal response to stimulation with pentagastrin or calcium infusion. Unfortunately, delaying a thyroidectomy until after the tumor had expressed excess level of calcitonin led to poor outcomes because these tumors tend to have regional lymph node spread or distant metastases, leading to the need for greater, more morbid dissections and shortened survival from metastatic disease. With the institution of early genetic testing at early childhood, a prophylactic thyroidectomy often at a very young age has lengthened lives and spared patients from more morbid resections.

Calcitonin has since become an important serum marker for detecting recurrence of disease after resection. In those patients found to have MTC at presentation, the recommended resection is a total thyroidectomy with a central lymph node dissection of zones VI and VII (Figs. 25.2 and 25.3). Further lymphatic resection is mandated by the presence of palpable-involved nodes in the surrounding nodal basins. The timing of prophylactic total thyroidectomy prior to malignant transformation is based on the specific inherited mutation. Those in the highest-risk groups are recommended to undergo resection within the first year of life, while others are typically advised to undergo removal by the age of 5. Only those with the lowest-risk mutations are recommended to delay resection beyond the age of 5 years with stringent follow-up and continued yearly testing. In those undergoing a prophylactic thyroidectomy without evidence of tumor, there is no need for a nodal dissection.

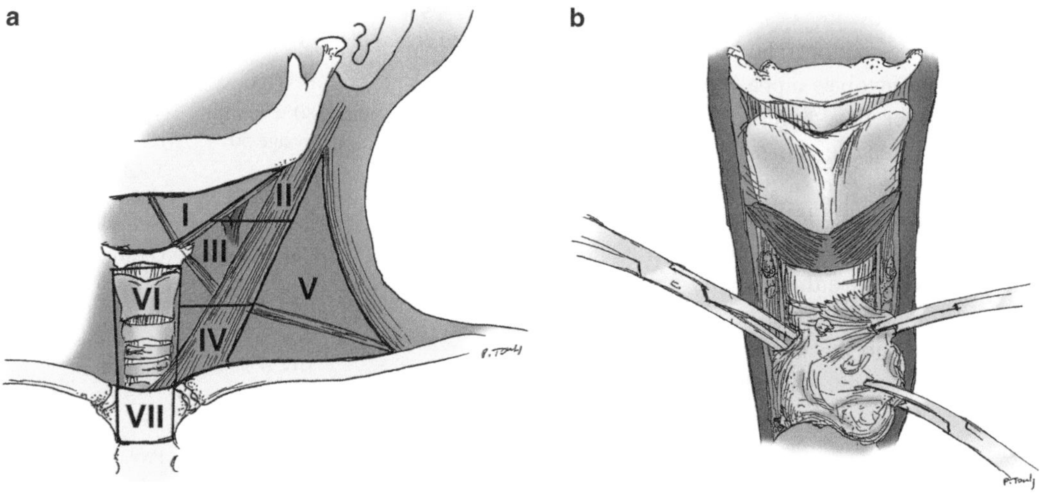

Fig. 25.2 (**a**) Neck level for neck dissection. Note that central neck dissection includes levels 6 and 7. (**b**) The anatomic boundaries of central neck dissection include the hyoid bone superiorly, the bilateral carotid arteries laterally, and the innominate vein inferiorly (Illustrator-Paul Tomljanovich, MD; modified by Lory Tubbs; Courtesy of Quyen D. Chu, MD, MBA, FACS)

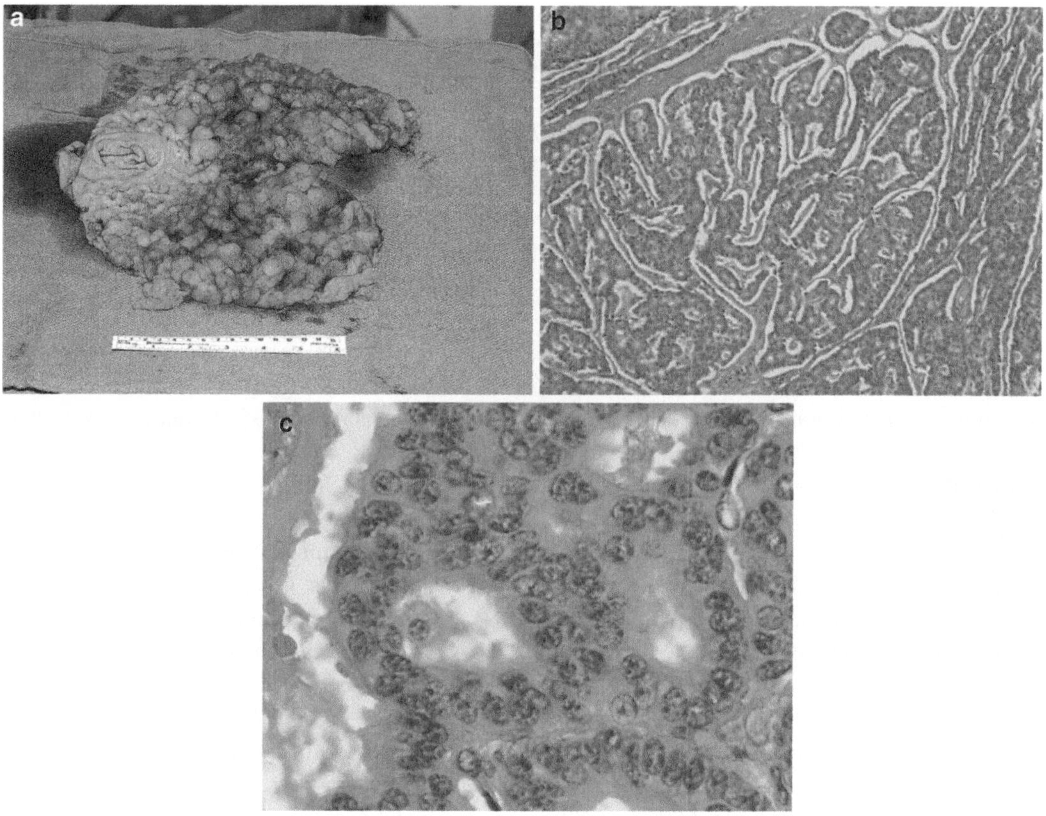

Fig. 25.3 A patient with MEN 1 and diffuse symptomatic gastrinomas. (**a**) Gross picture of lesions in the stomach. (**b**) 40X: The tumor shows characteristic organoid pattern with anastomosing of nests and trabeculae that are composed of uniform endocrine cells. (**c**) 200X: The tumor cells have a moderate amount of cytoplasm and uniform nuclei. The nuclei are characterized with "salt-and-pepper" pattern (Courtesy of Quyen D. Chu, MD, MBA, FACS)

Pheochromocytomas, when discovered, often require resection. The initial treatment of these tumors involves alpha blockade and may require further beta blockade to prevent and control hypertensive crises. Patients should be well hydrated as part of the preoperative management. Like sporadic pheochromocytomas, a surgical resection is ultimately required, which can be done with either a laparoscopic or an open technique. Of note, the left adrenal vein drains directly to the left renal vein or the left inferior phrenic vein, while the right adrenal vein tends to be short and drains directly into the vena cava.

As many of these patients have, or will develop, bilateral disease, every effort should be made to perform cortical-sparing or partial adrenal-sparing resections to avoid the development of Addison's disorders. There have been several reports of deaths following bilateral adrenalectomy due to insufficient use of exogenous steroids, especially in times of stress and also due to lack of proper patient education.

Hyperparathyroidism discovered in the setting of MEN 2A is most commonly seen in relation to mutations of codon 634. When discovered, the disease tends to be found in older patients and behave in a milder fashion than those seen in MEN 1. Treatment typically mirrors that seen in sporadic four-gland hyperplasia, which typically requires a subtotal parathyroidectomy. Such an operation provides long-term remission since recurrence is uncommon.

Salient Points

- MEN 1 and MEN 2: autosomal dominant conditions
- MEN 1 = mutated MEN1 gene, a tumor suppressor gene. The menin is the gene product. Affected individuals need to have both mutated alleles
- MEN 2 = mutated *RET* proto-oncogene. Affected individuals only need to have one mutated allele
- MEN 1 (Wermer syndrome) = 3 "P"s: parathyroid, pancreas, and pituitary (Table 25.4)

Table 25.4 Degree of penetrance and treatment of affected organs in MEN 1 syndrome

Organ	Penetrance	Treatment
Hyperparathyroidism	80 % has this by age 50	31/2 gland resection Total parathyroidectomy with reimplantation
Pancreas (PNET)	Gastrinoma: 50 %	Gastrinoma: medical management
	Insulinoma: 10–20 %	Insulinoma: enucleation
	Nonfunctioning tumor	
Pituitary	50 % Prolactinoma: most common	Prolactinoma: medical management

  - Necrolytic migratory erythema: pathognomonic for glucagonoma
- MEN 2 (Sipple syndrome): Test for *RET* oncogene: All have medullary thyroid cancer (MTC)
  - MEN 2A:
    Most common MEN 2
    MTC, pheochromocytoma, and hyperparathyroidism
  - MEN 2B
    MTC, pheochromocytoma, marfanoid body habitus, and neuromas
  - FMTC
    Four members of a family over two generations
    No pheochromocytoma or parathyroid dysfunction
- Medullary thyroid cancer:
  - Parafollicular C cells: secretes calcitonin (marker of recurrence following surgery)
  - Treatment: total thyroidectomy and central neck dissection (level 6 and 7)
  - Timing of prophylactic thyroidectomy depends on specific inherited mutation
  - American Thyroid Association (ATA) Guidelines assist with determining timing of prophylactic thyroidectomy

Questions

1. The most common pancreatic neuroendocrine tumors associated with multiple endocrine neoplasia type 1 (MEN 1) are:
   A. Somatostatinoma
   B. Insulinoma
   C. Gastrinoma
   D. Glucagonoma
2. The most common pancreatic neuroendocrine tumors associated with MEN 1 which require operative resection are:
   A. Somatostatinoma
   B. Insulinoma
   C. Gastrinoma
   D. Glucagonoma
3. Genetic testing for MEN 1:
   A. Is indicated for all patients with hyperparathyroidism
   B. Is positive demonstrating a mutation in >95 % of patients with MEN 1
   C. Should be offered to any patient with an insulinoma
   D. Has not improved overall survival or morbidity in MEN 1 patients
4. *RET* proto-oncogene is associated with all of the following except:
   A. Medullary thyroid cancer
   B. Hirschsprung's disease
   C. Hyperparathyroidism
   D. Pheochromocytoma
5. Appropriate evaluation of offspring of patient with MEN 2 includes:
   A. Immediate thyroidectomy
   B. Genetic testing followed by thyroidectomy before age 1 if highest risk
   C. Genetic testing if calcitonin level found to be elevated
   D. Yearly ultrasound and calcitonin testing on highest-risk mutations
6. In regard to genetic testing in MEN 2, all of the following are true except:
   A. Mutations are found in over 95 % of patient with the disease.
   B. Mutations discovered at codon 918 should prompt immediate thyroidectomy.
   C. Genetic testing should be offered in all newly diagnosed medullary thyroid cancer cases.
   D. Genetic testing has not improved overall survival.
7. Necrolytic migratory erythema (NME) is pathognomonic for:
   A. Glucagonoma
   B. Insulinoma
   C. VIPoma
   D. Somatostatinoma
8. Which of the following statement is true of pancreatic neuroendocrine tumor (PNET)?
   A. There is no role for debulking large, symptomatic tumor.
   B. Enucleation of insulinoma is the preferable treatment, if possible.
   C. PNET is seen in both MEN 1 and MEN 2.
   D. Surgical resection of gastrinoma is the primary treatment.

Answers

1. C
2. B
3. D
4. C
5. B
6. D
7. A
8. B

References

1. Pieterman CR, van Hulsteijn LT, den Heijer M, et al. Primary hyperparathyroidism in MEN1 patients: a cohort study with longterm follow-up on preferred surgical procedure and the relation with genotype. Ann Surg. 2012;255(6):1171–8.
2. Eller-Vainicher C, Chiodini I, Battista C, et al. Sporadic and MEN1-related primary hyperparathyroidism: differences in clinical expression and severity. J Bone Miner Res. 2009;24(8):1404–10.
3. Tonelli F, Giudici F, Fratini G, Brandi ML. Pancreatic endocrine tumors in multiple endocrine neoplasia type 1 syndrome: review of literature. Endocr Pract. 2011;17 Suppl 3:33–40.
4. Thakker RV. Multiple endocrine neoplasia type 1 (MEN1). Best Pract Res Clin Endocrinol Metab. 2010;24(3):355–70.
5. Chu Q, Al-Kasspooles M, Smith J, et al. Is glucagonoma of the pancreas a curable disease? Int J Gastrointest Cancer. 2001;29(3):155–62.
6. Trump D, Farren B, Wooding C, et al. Clinical studies of multiple endocrine neoplasia type 1 (MEN1). QJM. 1996;89(9):653–69.
7. Machens A, Schaaf L, Karges W, et al. Age-related penetrance of endocrine tumours in multiple endocrine neoplasia type 1 (MEN1): a multicentre study of 258 gene carriers. Clin Endocrinol (Oxf). 2007;67(4):613–22.

8. Darling TN, Skarulis MC, Steinberg SM, Marx SJ, Spiegel AM, Turner M. Multiple facial angiofibromas and collagenomas in patients with multiple endocrine neoplasia type 1. Arch Dermatol. 1997;133(7):853–7.
9. Carling T, Udelsman R. Parathyroid surgery in familial hyperparathyroid disorders. J Intern Med. 2005;257(1):27–37.
10. Dickson PV, Rich TA, Xing Y, et al. Achieving eugastrinemia in MEN1 patients: both duodenal inspection and formal lymph node dissection are important. Surgery. 2011;150(6):1143–52.
11. Hazard JB, Hawk WA, Crile G. Medullary (solid) carcinoma of the thyroid; a clinicopathologic entity. J Clin Endocrinol Metab. 1959;19(1):152–61.
12. Sipple JH. The association of pheochromocytoma with carcinoma of the thyroid gland. Am J Med. 1961;31:163–6.
13. Steiner AL, Goodman AD, Powers SR. Study of a kindred with pheochromocytoma, medullary thyroid carcinoma, hyperparathyroidism and Cushing's disease: multiple endocrine neoplasia, type 2. Medicine (Baltimore). 1968;47(5):371–409.
14. Mulligan LM, Kwok JB, Healey CS, et al. Germ-line mutations of the RET proto-oncogene in multiple endocrine neoplasia type 2A. Nature. 1993;363(6428): 458–60.
15. Eng C, Clayton D, Schuffenecker I, et al. The relationship between specific RET proto-oncogene mutations and disease phenotype in multiple endocrine neoplasia type 2. International RET mutation consortium analysis. JAMA. 1996;276(19):1575–9.
16. Kloos RT, Eng C, Evans DB, et al. Medullary thyroid cancer: management guidelines of the American Thyroid Association. Thyroid. 2009;19(6):565–612.

Carcinoid Tumors

26

Christopher N. Scipione and Mark S. Cohen

Learning Objectives

After reading this chapter, you should be able to:

- Describe the epidemiology, clinical presentation, and staging of carcinoid tumors.
- Understand the importance of classification, histology, and genetic markers in the diagnosis, prognosis, and treatment of carcinoid tumors.
- Describe diagnostic work-up and options for imaging of carcinoid tumors for disease evaluation and staging.
- Describe the factors which predict recurrence or poorer outcomes.
- Understand the surgical treatment for gastric, small intestine, and colorectal carcinoid tumors.
- Understand the role for medical management including hormonal therapy with somatostatin analogs as well as the role for adjuvant therapies.
- Describe postsurgical follow-up for patients with carcinoid tumors.

C.N. Scipione, M.D. • M.S. Cohen, M.D. (✉)
Department of General Surgery, University of Michigan Hospital and Health Systems, 1500 East Medical Center Drive, 2920 Taubman Center, 48109-5331 Ann Arbor, MI, USA
e-mail: scipione@umich.edu; cohenmar@umich.edu

Introduction

Carcinoid tumors have an incidence of 2 per 100,000 people in the United States [1]. They are most commonly diagnosed in the fifth or sixth decade of life and have a slight female preponderance [1, 2]. The most commonly identified locations of carcinoid tumors are the vermiform appendix and the distal ileum. These locations each account for approximately 20–30 % of carcinoid tumors [1, 3]. Carcinoid tumors of the vermiform appendix occur in approximately 0.17 % of autopsy specimens and 0.5–1.6 % of pathology specimens for following appendectomy for presumed appendicitis [4, 5]. Carcinoids are the most common primary neoplasm of the appendix, accounting for 32–57 % of appendiceal tumors [6–8]. Appendiceal carcinoid is also the most common neoplasm of the gastrointestinal tract in childhood and adolescence [9]. The stomach, bronchopulmonary tree, and the rectum are also the frequently involved sites.

Histopathology and Pathophysiology

The carcinoid tumor was first reported in the ileum by Ranson in 1890; however, Lubarsh first described it pathologically in 1888 and Oberdorfer coined these tumors as "karzinoide" in 1907 due to the fact that they are more indolent

Q.D. Chu et al. (eds.), *Surgical Oncology: A Practical and Comprehensive Approach*,
DOI 10.1007/978-1-4939-1423-4_26, © Springer Science+Business Media New York 2015

than adenocarcinomas of the bowel [10–12]. In 1928, carcinoid was defined as a neuroendocrine tumor (NET) whose cells demonstrate the amine precursor uptake and decarboxylation (APUD) system [13]. Serotonin was isolated in carcinoid tumors in 1953, and in 1955, the carcinoid syndrome was noted to have elevated levels of urinary 5-hydroxyindoleacetic acid (5-HIAA) [14]. Carcinoid tumors, in fact, produce a number of biologically active substances including growth hormone, tachykinins, chromogranin A, neuron-specific enolase, neurotensin, adrenocorticotropic hormone, bombesin, substance P, gastrin, insulin, pancreatic polypeptide, 5-hydroxytryptophan, 5-HIAA, platelet-derived growth factor, and transforming growth factors [15]. A variety of clinical symptoms may develop when these substances escape the enteral-hepatic circulation as in the case of metastatic disease or the carcinoid syndrome. Patients may describe flushing, bronchospasm with wheezing, hypotension, abdominal cramping, diarrhea, pellagra, and right-sided heart failure from plaque-like deposits on the valvular cusps. It is thought that the left side of the heart is protected by the lungs' inactivation of the biologically active substances.

Malignant appendiceal NETs are classified into four main histological subtypes according to 2010 World Health Organization recommendations: well-differentiated NET which is also known as malignant carcinoid tumor (MCT), poorly differentiated (high-grade) neuroendocrine carcinoma, goblet cell carcinoid (GCC), and composite goblet cell carcinoid-adenocarcinoma (CGCCA) [16, 17]. GCC is the most common type of NET (60 %), followed by MCT (32 %) and CGCCA (7 %). The CGCCA subtype confers a poorer prognosis when compared with the GCC and MCT subtypes (5 year overall survival: 56 % vs. 78 % and 86 %, respectively) [18].

Carcinoid tumors may be found anywhere in the gastrointestinal (GI) tract as well in the pancreas and bronchopulmonary system. In the GI tract, these tumors are further differentiated by their location with "midgut" carcinoids (those involving the ileum and appendix) being the most common, followed by "hindgut" carcinoids in the rectum, and lastly "foregut" carcinoids in the stomach and duodenum [19]. Very rarely these tumors will also present in the esophagus, jejunum, and colon.

As an aside, classification is based on the three blood supplies to the GI tract. In general, the celiac artery supplies the "foregut" (stomach, duodenum proximal to the opening of the bile duct, liver, pancreas, and biliary apparatus), the superior mesenteric artery (SMA) supplies the "midgut" (the rest of the duodenum, small bowel, and proximal transverse colon), and the inferior mesenteric artery (IMA) supplies the "hindgut" (the rest of the distal transverse colon and sigmoid colon) [20].

Diagnosis and Staging

Carcinoid tumors can be difficult to diagnose preoperatively as most of these tumors are clinically silent, without overproduction of hormones or biologically active substances. Many of these tumors are found incidentally in the setting of emergency surgery for appendicitis or due to clinical symptoms associated with metastatic spread to the liver and development of the carcinoid syndrome [21].

MCTs of the appendix have a female predominance of 70 % and tend to present at a younger age than carcinoids at other sites, with a median age at time of diagnosis of around 40 years of age. The GCC subtype presents at the median age of around 50 with a more equal distribution between genders [16–18].

Carcinoid tumors associated with acute appendicitis are usually noted incidentally as up to 62–78 % of these specimens reside in the distal third of the appendix and are not the cause of luminal obstruction leading to inflammation [7, 19]. Lesions less than 1 cm in size (which account for more than 70 % of specimens) do not require tumor staging unless there is a high suspicion for malignancy based on histology [4]. Patients with tumors greater than 1 cm may benefit from additional staging and work-up, and for patients with tumors greater than 2 cm, further investigation is mandatory.

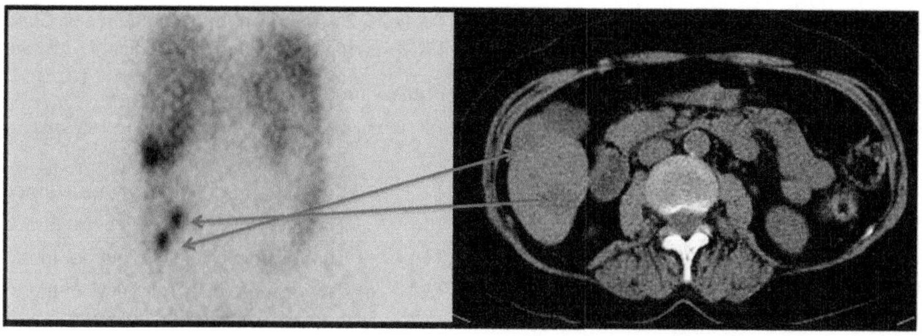

Fig. 26.1 Octreoscan (*left*) with a soft tissue mass in the distal ileum demonstrating increased radiotracer uptake, likely representing the primary carcinoid. There are also two hepatic lesions (*arrows*) in the inferior aspect of the right hepatic lobe concerning for multifocal metastatic disease (with corresponding CT scan showing the two liver metastases) (Courtesy of Dr. Tobias Else, University of Michigan, Ann Arbor, MI)

Tumor evaluation involves biochemical as well as endoscopic and imaging studies including computed tomography (CT), magnetic resonance imaging (MRI), positron emission tomography (PET), radiolabeled metaiodobenzylguanidine (^{123}I-MIBG), and octreotide scintigraphy labeled with Indium^{111} (octreoscan). Standard PET imaging with 18-fluorodeoxyglucose has been shown to image carcinoid tumors with high proliferative activity; however, it is not as sensitive as octreoscan [22]. MIBG is concentrated in carcinoid tumors and ^{123}I-MIBG imaging carries a sensitivity of 55–70 % with a specificity of 95 % [23]. Octreoscan, however, is the study of choice with an overall sensitivity for carcinoid tumors in the range of 80–90 % [24]. Figure 26.1 is a representative example of an octreoscan showing a small bowel carcinoid with concurrent liver metastases. Recent studies have shown that PET imaging with ^{68}Ga-DOTA-somatostatin analogs may be useful in diagnosing NET and provide higher special resolution and radiopharmaceutical distribution characteristics when compared to octreotide scintigraphy [25–27].

Biochemical analysis includes plasma chromogranin A and urine 5-HIAA levels. Elevated chromogranin A levels are currently the most important blood marker for the disease, and a level greater than 5,000 μg/l correlates with a poor outcome [28, 29]. Chromogranin A levels, however, may also be elevated in pancreatic neuroendocrine tumors [30]. Collection of 24 h urine 5-HIAA levels is a useful marker for carcinoid tumors with a specificity of 88 % [31]. Patients should avoid eating nuts, bananas, plantains, pineapple, plums, kiwis, or tomatoes prior to collection as these foods may significantly increase urine 5-HIAA levels.

There is a lack of consensus for a unified staging system. Consequently, a number of different systems from the American Joint Committee on Cancer (AJCC), Union for International Cancer Control (UICC), World Health Organization (WHO), and European Neuroendocrine Tumor Society (ENETS) exist to stage NETs. In many cases, GI carcinoids are often staged using similar system with minor variations that is used for other cancers of the same organ. For example, stomach carcinoids are similarly staged as stomach adenocarcinoma with some variations such as the inclusion of tumor size for stomach carcinoids (Table 26.1).

Regardless, a number of these staging systems do take into account prognostic information such as tumor size, location of tumor origin, extent of invasion into organ of origin, evidence of regional/distant disease, and tumor grade (mitotic rate and/or Ki67 proliferation index).

The current AJCC proposed staging system for appendiceal carcinoid tumors has yet to be validated prospectively with survival statistics. T1 tumors are ≤2 cm in diameter; T2 tumors are between 2 and 4 cm, or involving the cecum; T3 tumors are >4 cm or extending into the ileum; and T4 tumors directly invade other structures. Stage I disease consists of T1 tumors, Stage II

Table 26.1 American Joint Committee on Cancer (AJCC) TNM staging for gastric carcinoid (7th edition)

Primary tumor (T)	
TX	Primary tumor cannot be assessed
T0	No evidence of primary tumor
Tis	Carcinoma in situ/dysplasia (tumor size less than 0.5 mm), confined to mucosa
T1	Tumor invades lamina propria or submucosa and 1 cm or less in size
T2	Tumor invades muscularis propria or more than 1 cm in size
T3	Tumor penetrates subserosa
T4	Tumor invades visceral peritoneum (serosal) or other organs or adjacent structures (Fig. 17.9)
	For any T, add (m) for multiple tumors

Regional lymph nodes (N)	
NX	Regional lymph nodes cannot be assessed
N0	No regional lymph node metastasis
N1	Regional lymph node metastasis (Fig. 17.10)

Distant metastases (M)	
M0	No distant metastases
M1	Distant metastasis

Anatomic stage/prognostic groups			
Stage 0	Tis	N0	M0
Stage I	T1	N0	M0
Stage IIA	T2	N0	M0
Stage IIB	T3	N0	M0
Stage IIIA	T4	N0	M0
Stage IIIB	Any T	N1	M0
Stage IV	Any T	Any N	M1

Adapted from Compton C, Byrd D, Garcia-Aguilar J, et al. Neuroendocrine Tumors. In: Compton C, Byrd D, Garcia-Aguilar J, Kurtzman S, Olawaiye A, Washington M (eds). AJCC Cancer Staging Atlas. 2nd ed. New York, NY: Springer Science; 2012: 221–240. With permission from Springer Verlag

disease includes T2 and T3 tumors, Stage III disease includes T4 tumors or positive regional lymph nodes, and Stage IV disease involves distant metastatic disease [32] (Table 26.2). Most cases of appendiceal carcinoid present as localized disease (60 % of cases). However, regional spread (28 %) and metastatic disease (12 %) can be present at the time of diagnosis [33].

The ENETS/UICC staging for small bowel such as jejunoileal primaries is similar to colorectal

Table 26.2 American Joint Committee on Cancer (AJCC) TNM staging for appendiceal carcinoid (7th edition)

Primary tumor (T)	
TX	Primary tumor cannot be assessed
T0	No evidence of primary tumor
T1	Tumor 2 cm or less in greatest dimension
T1a	Tumor 1 cm or less in greatest dimension
T1b	Tumor more than 1 cm but not more than 2 cm
T2	Tumor more than 2 cm but not more than 4 cm or with extension to the cecum
T3	Tumor more than 4 cm or with extension to the ileum
T4	Tumor directly invades other adjacent organs or structures, e.g., abdominal wall and skeletal muscle*

Note: Tumor that is adherent to other organs or structures, grossly, is classified cT4. However, if no tumor is present in the adhesion, microscopically, the classification should be classified pT1-3 depending on the anatomical depth of wall invasion

*Penetration of the mesoapppendix does not seem to be as important a prognostic factor as the size of the primary tumor and is not separately categorized

Regional lymph nodes (N)	
NX	Regional lymph nodes cannot be assessed
N0	No regional lymph node metastasis
N1	Regional lymph node metastasis

Distant metastasis (M)	
M0	No distant metastasis
M1	Distant metastasis

pTNM Pathologic Classification. The pT, pN, and pM categories correspond to the T, N, and M categories except that pM0 does not exist as a category

pN0. Histological examination of a regional lymphadenectomy specimen will ordinarily include 12 or more lymph nodes. If the lymph nodes are negative, but the number ordinarily examined is not met, classify as pN0

Anatomic stage/prognostic groups			
Stage I	T1	N0	M0
Stage II	T2, T3	N0	M0
Stage III	T4	N0	M0
	Any T	N1	M0
Stage IV	Any T	Any N	M1

Adapted from Compton C, Byrd D, Garcia-Aguilar J, et al. Appendix. In: Compton C, Byrd D, Garcia-Aguilar J, Kurtzman S, Olawaiye A, Washington M (eds). AJCC Cancer Staging Atlas. 2nd ed. New York, NY: Springer Science; 2012: 169–184. With permission from Springer Verlag cancer with T1 tumors confined to the submucosa and ≤1 cm, T2 tumors invade the submucosa or >1 cm, T3 tumors invade the subserosa, and T4 tumors invade adjacent structures. Stage I, IIA, IIb, and IIIA correspond to T1–T4 tumors, respectively. Stage IIIb represents metastatic disease to regional lymph nodes and Stage IV denotes distant metastatic disease [34, 35] (Table 26.3).

TNM staging system for carcinoid tumors of the colon and rectum is as follow: T1 are lesions that have not invaded the muscularis propria and ≤2 cm in size, T2 are lesions that have invaded the muscularis propria or >2 cm in size with invasion of lamina propria or submucosa, T3 are those that invade through the muscularis propria into the subserosa or into non-peritonealized pericolic or perirectal tissues, and T4 are those that invade peritoneum or other organs. Stage 1 is T1N0M0; stage 2 is T2N0M0 or T3N0M0; stage 3 is T4N0 or evidence of nodal disease, regardless of T-stage; and stage 4 is evidence of distant metastasis (Table 26.4). Lung carcinoid tumor is staged the same as non-small cell lung cancer (NSCLC).

Carcinoid tumors can also be classified into one of the three stages: localized disease, regional spread and distant disease. In a localized carcinoid tumor, disease is confined within the wall of the primary organ, such as the stomach, colon, or intestine. Tumors with regional spread include spread through the wall of the primary organ to nearby tissues, such as fat, muscle, or lymph nodes. Finally for distant spread, the carcinoid tumor has spread to tissues or organs far away from the primary organ, such as the liver, bones, or lungs.

Table 26.3 American Joint Committee on Cancer (AJCC) TNM staging for duodenum/ampulla/jejunum/ileum carcinoid (7th edition)

Primary tumor (T)	
TX	Primary tumor cannot be assessed
T0	No evidence of primary tumor
T1	Tumor invades lamina propria or submucosa and size 1 cm or less* (small intestinal tumors); tumor 1 cm or less (ampullary tumors)
T2	Tumor invades muscularis propria or size >1 cm (small intestinal tumors); tumor >1 cm (ampullary tumors)
T3	Tumor invades through the muscularis propria into subserosal tissue without penetration of overlying serosa (jejunal or ileal tumors) or invades pancreas or retroperitoneum (ampullary or duodenal tumors) or into non-peritonealized tissues
T4	Tumor invades visceral peritoneum (serosa) or invades other organs
	For any T, add (m) for multiple tumors

**Note*: Tumor limited to ampulla of Vater for ampullary gangliocytic paraganglioma

Regional lymph nodes (N)	
NX	Regional lymph nodes cannot be assessed
N0	No regional lymph node metastasis
N1	Regional lymph node metastasis

Distant metastases (M)	
M0	No distant metastases
M1	Distant metastasis

Anatomic stage/prognostic groups			
Stage 0	Tis	N0	M0
Stage I	T1	N0	M0
Stage IIA	T2	N0	M0
Stage IIB	T3	N0	M0
Stage IIIA	T4	N0	M0
Stage IIIB	Any T	N1	M0
Stage IV	Any T	Any N	M1

Adapted from Compton C, Byrd D, Garcia-Aguilar J, et al. Neuroendocrine Tumors. In: Compton C, Byrd D, Garcia-Aguilar J, Kurtzman S, Olawaiye A, Washington M (eds). AJCC Cancer Staging Atlas. 2nd ed. New York, NY: Springer Science; 2012: 221–240. With permission from Springer Verlag

Genetic and Prognostic Factors

The genetic alterations leading to carcinoid tumorigenesis is an ongoing scientific investigation. Pancreatic NETs are associated with numerous genetic syndromes such as MEN-1, von Hippel-Lindau, neurofibromatosis type 1, and tuberous sclerosis [36]. More in-depth discussion of this topic is found in Chap. 24, Pancreatic Neuroendocrine Tumors (PNETs). Genomic aberrations in gastrointestinal carcinoids seem to be fewer than those seen in pancreatic NETs, which suggests a different molecular pathogenesis. Loss of heterozygosity mutations of chromosome 18 are the most common genetic abnormality [37].

Table 26.4 American Joint Committee on Cancer (AJCC) TNM staging for colorectal carcinoid (7th edition)

Primary tumor (T)	
TX	Primary tumor cannot be assessed
T0	No evidence of primary tumor
T1	Tumor invades lamina propria or submucosa and size 2 cm or less
T1a	Tumor size less than 1 cm in greatest dimension
T1b	Tumor size 1–2 cm in greatest dimension
T2	Tumor invades muscularis propria or size more than 2 cm with invasion of lamina propria or submucosa
T3	Tumor invades through the muscularis propria into the subserosal or into non-peritonealized pericolic or perirectal tissues
T4	Tumor invades peritoneum or other organs. For any T, add (m) for multiple tumors

Regional lymph nodes (N)	
NX	Regional lymph nodes cannot be assessed
N0	No regional lymph node metastasis
N1	Regional lymph node metastasis

Distant metastases (M)	
M0	No distant metastases
M1	Distant metastasis

Anatomic stage/prognostic groups			
Stage 0	Tis	N0	M0
Stage I	T1	N0	M0
Stage IIA	T2	N0	M0
Stage IIB	T3	N0	M0
Stage IIIA	T4	N0	M0
Stage IIIB	Any T	N1	M0
Stage IV	Any T	Any N	M1

Adapted from Compton C, Byrd D, Garcia-Aguilar J, et al. Neuroendocrine Tumors. In: Compton C, Byrd D, Garcia-Aguilar J, Kurtzman S, Olawaiye A, Washington M (eds). AJCC Cancer Staging Atlas. 2nd ed. New York, NY: Springer Science; 2012: 221–240. With permission from Springer Verlag

The most frequently reported mutated gene in gastrointestinal carcinoid tumors is beta-catenin, which plays an important role in the Wnt signaling pathway. Cyclin D1 and cMyc overexpression have also been reported in these tumors, while a set of genes (NAP1L1, MAGE-2D, and MTA1) has been correlated with malignant behavior of small intestinal carcinoids [38].

For appendiceal carcinoids, tumor characteristics that predict aggressive behavior include tumor size greater than 2 cm, mesoappendiceal involvement, and histologic subtype [39]. Mesoappendiceal invasion has been shown to correlate with malignant potential and nodal spread in tumors less than 2 cm in size [40].

Table 26.5 World Health Organization Grading System for Neuroendocrine Tumors

Grade	Mitotic count per 10 HPF	Ki-67 index (percent)
G1	<2	≤2
G2	2–20	3–20
G3	>20	>2

HPF high power field

The World Health Organization (WHO) has proposed a tumor grading system for neuroendocrine tumors based on mitotic rate and the Ki67 proliferation index where G1 is Ki67 ≤ 2 % or mitotic count <2/10 high powered fields (HPF), G2 is Ki67 3–20 % and mitotic count 2–20/10 HPF, and G3 if Ki67 > 20 % and mitotic count >20/10 HPF [41] (Table 26.5). Multi-institutional studies have demonstrated increasing age at diagnosis, plasma chromogranin A levels, high tumor volume, and Ki67 level to be associated with a poorer prognosis [42].

For bronchial carcinoids, atypical histology predicts a poorer outcome as these tumors have higher mitotic rates as well as nodal metastases with an overall 5-year survival of 60 %. In gastric carcinoids, type 3 tends to be larger and more likely to have metastatic spread than types 1 and 2; it carries a 50 % 5-year survival rate. Type 4 gastric carcinoids tend to be unresectable at the time of presentation and carry the poorest outcome. Colorectal carcinoid tumors tend to be diagnosed later than small bowel carcinoid tumor and are associated with a worse prognosis (5-year survival 40–50 %).

Medical Management of Advanced Disease and the Carcinoid Syndrome

Patients with metastatic disease to the liver are more likely to develop carcinoid syndrome, a clinical situation that is a result of the overproduction of biologically active substances and hormones produced by carcinoid tumors and secreted directed into the systemic circulation. Although nonmetastatic carcinoids can secrete bioactive products, these products are inactivated by the liver as they enter the portal circulation. Thus, nonmetastatic carcinoids do not generally produce carcinoid syndrome, except for ovarian and bronchial carcinoids, which can secrete bioactive hormones directly into the systemic circulation.

Symptoms associated with the carcinoid syndrome include flushing, bronchospasm, hypotension, abdominal cramping, diarrhea, or even right-sided heart failure. It occurs in only 5 % of patients with carcinoid tumors. In the past, supportive care was the mainstay of treatment. Bronchodilators were prescribed for bronchospasm and wheezing. Antidiarrheals such as loperamide were used for diarrhea, although severe cases were sometimes given cyproheptadine which decreased diarrhea in up to 50 % of patients [43]. Heart failure was treated with diuretics and if severe, valve replacement.

Modern management of carcinoid syndrome and advanced carcinoid tumors involves surgical resection and debulking of identified disease combined with medical management of unresectable disease utilizing a multidisciplinary approach. Somatostatin analogs (SA) have been the mainstay of medical therapy for advanced carcinoid tumors. These substances inhibit the symptoms of carcinoid syndrome quite effectively in many patients. Octreotide is administered by subcutaneous injection every 6–12 h and has a half-life of approximately 90 min [44]. Numerous retrospective studies exist suggesting that a partial response to SAs are demonstrated in less than 10 % of patients and stable disease is seen in 40–87 % of patients without evidence of prior disease progression [45–50]. In addition to standard octreotide injections, long-acting depot injections are available and provide an excellent option for patients requiring long-term maintenance therapy.

The placebo-controlled, double-blind, prospective randomized study on the effect of octreotide LAR in the control of tumor growth in patients with metastatic neuroendocrine midgut tumors (PROMID) study group presented a compelling randomized control trial with evidence of enhanced disease-free survival in patients receiving octreotide long-acting repeatable (LAR) injections compared to placebo. The median time to tumor progression was 14.3 months in the octreotide LAR group compared to 6 months in the placebo group [51]. The benefit was most pronounced in those patients who underwent primary resection and those with a lower hepatic tumor burden.

Interferon-alpha (IFN-α) has also been explored as a second-line therapy for patients with carcinoid symptoms refractory to SA monotherapy. Prospective, randomized data exists demonstrating a statistically insignificant increase in survival with combination therapy versus SA therapy alone (5-year survival 57 % vs. 37 %) [52]. There did appear to be a significantly reduced risk of tumor progression with combination therapy. Several other studies of IFN-α have similarly failed to demonstrate significant progression-free and long-term survival advantage to combination treatment over SA monotherapy and increased side effects in the groups receiving IFN-α [53–55].

Chemotherapy has been evaluated in multiple phase II clinical trials evaluating single agent regimens as well as combination regimens utilizing agents such as 5-fluorouracil, streptozocin, cyclophosphamide, doxorubicin, and cisplatin. Results have overall been poor, with no trial demonstrating a sustained partial response rate greater than 15 % [56–58]. Trials have been reported using hepatic arterial vascular occlusion therapy in selected patients with metastatic disease to the liver [59–67]. Tumor responses were observed in up to 60 % of patients with a reduction in biochemical symptoms in 12–75 % of patients [65, 67].

Novel agents utilizing targeted radiotherapy such as [^{111}In-DTPA-D-Phe] octreotide, yttrium-labeled compounds [^{90}Y-DOTATOC], and lutetium-labeled SA analogs [^{177}Lu-DOTA0, Tyr3] octreotate have shown promise for the treatment of metastatic or inoperable carcinoid tumors. Indium-labeled compounds have shown response rates between 13 and 20 %, symptomatic improvement in 60 % of patients, and biochemical responses in as high as 80 % of subjects [68–71]. Yttrium-labeled compounds have shown a similar tumor regression in 14 % of patients with stable disease in an additional 41 % of patients [72, 73]. The newest SA radiolabeled analog, lutetium, has shown the most promising results with one study reporting a 48 % tumor regression 3 months after therapy [74, 75].

Recently, bevacizumab (vascular endothelial growth factor inhibitor) has been explored as a target for carcinoid therapy. Patients with metastatic or unresectable carcinoid tumor on octreotide therapy were randomized to receive bevacizumab or pegylated IFN-α. Progression-free survival was significantly higher in the bevacizumab group (95 %) when compared to the pegylated IFN-α group (68 %) at 18 weeks [76].

Phase 3 trials in patients with advanced pancreatic neuroendocrine tumors have shown that the mammalian target of rapamycin (mTOR) inhibitor, everolimus, significantly increased median progression-free survival versus placebo when used in addition to octreotide LAR (16 months vs. 11 months) [77]. Although everolimus has shown potential benefit in progressive pancreatic neuroendocrine tumors, it has not yet been used in the treatment of carcinoid tumors.

Principles of Surgical Resection by Site

Bronchopulmonary Carcinoids

Bronchopulmonary carcinoid tumors account for approximately 2 % of lung neoplasms. As high as 25 % of well-differentiated NETs are located in the bronchopulmonary tree [78]. Carcinoid syndrome occurs in less than 2 % of patients who present with pulmonary carcinoid compared to 10 % of patients presenting with a gastrointestinal tract primary [79]. The overall prognosis of pulmonary carcinoid depends heavily on the underlying histological appearance, typical versus atypical carcinoid. Atypical carcinoid tumors have increased mitotic activity, nuclear pleomorphism, and tumor necrosis while typical carcinoid tumors have more organized architecture and rarely show mitotic figures [80].

Typical carcinoid tumors behave more indolently than atypical carcinoid tumors, but lymph node metastasis does occur in 10–15 % of cases with distant metastatic disease occurring in 3–5 % of cases [81, 82]. The 5-year survival rate exceeds 90 % following resection. In contrast, atypical carcinoids have nodal metastases 50 % of the time, distant metastases 20 % of the time, and a 5-year survival of 60 % [83].

The standard surgical treatment for bronchial carcinoids involving complete surgical resection with regional lymphadenectomy [84]. Lobectomy is most often required, but lung-sparing operations such as a sleeve resection or wedge resection can occasionally be adequate. Endoscopic resection is typically inadequate and is associated with high recurrence rates [79]. In cases where resection is not possible, palliation can often be achieved with external beam radiation where a course of 45–50 Gy can achieve partial responses in many cases but long-term responses are not expected. Additionally spinal or bone metastases often will respond to XRT while liver metastases do not.

Gastric Carcinoids

Gastric carcinoid tumors compromise 20 % of gastroentero-pancretic NETs and 1 % of gastric neoplasms [85]. These tumors are divided into four distinct types based on clinical presentation and histological features (Table 26.6). Type 1 gastric carcinoid tumors are typically small and behave in a benign fashion [86]. These tumors are the most common type of gastric carcinoid tumors (75 %) and are associated with chronic atrophic gastritis and hypergastrinemia. Most type 1 tumors are <2 cm and are amenable to endoscopic resection if endoscopic ultrasound does not demonstrate regional lymph node involvement or wall invasion [87, 88]. Yearly endoscopic surveillance is recommended because these lesions are highly recurrent. Surgical excision is recommended for larger type 1 tumors >3 cm due to their higher malignant potential and those tumors that are demonstrated to be invasive. For patients with multiple type 1 gastric carcinoids, somatostatin analogs have been shown to halt regression and prevent recurrence [89, 90]. Death as a result of type 1 lesions is uncommon.

Table 26.6 Characteristics of subtypes of gastric carcinoids

	Type	Gastrin level	Treatment	Prognosis
Type 1	Most common (70–80 %) Tend to be small and multiple Associated with chronic atrophic gastritis and hypergastrinemia	High in response to gastric achlorhydria	Endoscopic resection for tumors ≤2 cm Gastrectomy for tumors >3 cm or suspicious for invasion Somatostatin analog	Good
Type 2	Occurs in 5 % of gastric carcinoids Associated with MEN and ZES Tend to be small and multiple	High due to gastrinoma from MEN or ZES	Resection Somatostatin analog	Good
Type 3	Occurs in 20 % of gastric carcinoids Sporadic type Tend to be solitary lesion Aggressive	Normal	Treat like gastric adenocarcinoma (gastrectomy and lymph node dissection)	50 % 5-year survival for nonmetastatic 15 % 5 year survival for metastatic

Courtesy of Quyen D. Chu, MD, MBA, FACS
MEN multiple endocrine neoplasia, *ZES* Zollinger-Ellison syndrome

Type 2 gastric carcinoid lesions are associated with multiple endocrine neoplasia type 1 and Zollinger-Ellison syndrome. These tumors tend to be somewhat larger than type 1 tumors, but also usually behave in a benign fashion. Often patients will present with multiple tumors [90]. Surgical treatment is aimed at correcting the hypergastrinemia by resection of the gastrinoma as long as the lesions do not demonstrate invasion. Somatostatin analogs are used to halt tumor growth for this type of gastric carcinoid as well [91]. Death due to type 2 gastric carcinoid tumors is rare, but these tumors do require yearly surveillance similar to type 1 tumors.

Type 3 gastric carcinoid tumors arise sporadically in the setting of a normal gastrin level and gastric pH, unlike type 1 and type 2 carcinoid tumors. These tumors tend to behave similar to gastric adenocarcinoma and are usually 3–5 cm at the time of their discovery [92]. Most of these tumors show infiltration into the gastric wall. Treatment for type 3 lesions involves surgical resection which may require subtotal or total gastrectomy and lymphadenectomy [93]. Five-year survival for type 3 gastric carcinoid tumors is 50 % overall and 15 % in those that present with metastatic disease [94]. Type 4 gastric carcinoids are poorly differentiated neuroendocrine cancers that will often present with disseminated disease at the time of diagnosis. Curative surgical therapy is usually not possible, but surgical debulking with chemotherapy can be considered in selected patients.

Jejunoileal Carcinoids

Carcinoid tumors of the small intestine tend to progress slowly with an extended disease course. These tumors often will present with symptoms of obstruction or ischemia and are typically located within the distal ileum. Five-year survival rates are 50–60 %; however, the prognosis is better in patients who present with localized disease (5-year survival of 80–90 %) than those who present with lymph node metastasis or distant spread (5-year survival 70 % and 55 %, respectively) [94]. The histological grading of the tumor is also important in the overall prognosis. Tumors with low Ki-67 and well-differentiated tumors show an overall survival advantage [55]. Although surgical resection can relieve symptoms, patients must have lifelong surveillance due to the high risk of recurrence.

Prior to operative intervention, tumor localization and staging is critical because patients may present with multiple tumors and localization can be challenging intraoperatively. Endoscopic identification can be achieved through standard colonoscopy with intubation of the terminal ileum.

Double-balloon enteroscopy and video-capsule endoscopy may also be effective in directly visualizing the tumor [95–98]. Octreotide scintigraphy is an important tool for initial staging and ruling out liver metastases. Gallium-68-PET scan may be even more sensitive than octreoscan and useful for detecting smaller tumors.

Curative resection of primary tumors of the jejunum or ileum typically yields excellent results with near 100 % survival in stage I and II patients. Principles of surgical resection involve resection of the primary tumor and the lymphatic drainage within the mesentery [99–106]. If the tumor involves the terminal ileum, performing a right hemicolectomy is a consideration if the tumor is felt to involve the lymphatic drainage of the right colon. Bulky lymphatic metastases should be cleared from the mesentery while preserving the vasculature to limit the extent of small bowel resection. Cholecystectomy may be performed at the initial operation because of a propensity for gallstone formation in patients with NETs receiving SAs; however, no prospective benefit has been detected [107].

Appendiceal Carcinoids

Most appendiceal carcinoids are found incidentally at the time of appendectomy. It is important to make the diagnosis correctly prior to resection, as other more aggressive appendiceal neoplasms such as colonic adenocarcinoma may require more extensive anatomic resection. Frozen section analysis intraoperatively may help in ascertaining the tumor histology. For carcinoid tumors, however, the greatest determinant of operative strategy is the size of the tumor. The literature has continued to support the following guidelines for operative resection of carcinoids. Small tumors less than 1 cm in diameter are almost always benign and may be treated with simple appendectomy, although there has been one case report in the literature of a small 0.6 cm appendiceal carcinoid having metastatic spread to the liver at the time of diagnosis [108]. This tumor was noted to be at the base of the appendix with invasion of the mesoappendix, a finding associated with more aggressive tumor behavior.

For tumors larger than 2 cm, a radical resection involving a right hemicolectomy and regional lymphadenectomy is recommended as up to 30 % of these tumors will have lymph node metastases at the time of presentation [21]. However, since a majority of these larger tumors will not have metastatic spread, some authors would recommend simple appendectomy for elderly patients or patients at high operative risk [109]. Other authors report that all appendiceal carcinoids in children under the age of 15 may be treated by simple appendectomy regardless of tumor size, depth of invasion, or presence of perineural involvement as proven by 24 year follow-up without recurrence [110].

In addition to tumor size, mesoappendiceal involvement, angioinvasion, high mitotic index and Ki67 index, and GCC/CGCCA, poorly differentiated histological subtypes should be treated more aggressively with right hemicolectomy when feasible [39, 102].

Surgeons should also be aware that 18–33 % of carcinoids are associated with synchronous or metachronous colorectal malignancies [7, 111]. In cases of synchronous colon lesions, appropriate anatomic resection for colorectal cancer is warranted in addition to appendectomy or right hemicolectomy for the carcinoid tumor. For patients presenting with unresectable disease, mesenteric metastases, and symptoms of small bowel obstruction or ischemia, cytoreductive surgery is beneficial at providing palliation of symptoms [112].

Colorectal Carcinoids

Colonic carcinoid tumors comprise only 7 % of all NETs in the United States. In contrast, rectal carcinoids comprise approximately 15 % [33, 111, 113]. Due to their relative lack of symptoms, colorectal carcinoid tumors tend to be diagnosed later than small bowel carcinoid tumor and are associate with a worse prognosis (5-year survival 40–50 %) [85, 114]. Colonic carcinoids tend to have a poorer prognosis than rectal carcinoids. Part of the reasons for this may be that colonic carcinoids are more likely to occur on the right colon, which can be clinically silent until it

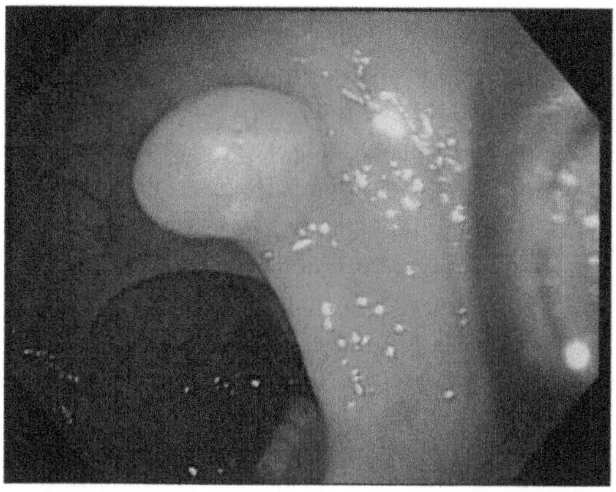

Fig. 26.2 Endoscopic picture of a rectal carcinoid (Courtesy of Dr. Scott Regenbogen, University of Michigan, Ann Arbor, MI)

becomes advanced. Consequently, patients with colon NETs will present with distant metastatic disease; about 66 % have nodal or distant disease at the time of diagnosis [115]. As with colorectal adenocarcinoma, colonoscopy and CT scanning are useful in the diagnostic work-up. Pelvic MRI is the imaging modality of choice for T2–T4 or node positive tumors of the rectum to determine local extension. Endoscopic ultrasound can provide important information on the tumor depth of invasion and local lymph node metastasis for rectal carcinoid tumors [116].

Colonic carcinoid tumors are generally treated in a similar fashion to colonic adenocarcinoma. Small lesions <2 cm may be excised endoscopically; however, most lesions are advanced at the time of diagnosis. Lesions >2 cm, G3 tumor grade, or those that are incompletely resected endoscopically should undergo surgical resection in a similar fashion to colonic adenocarcinoma.

Rectal carcinoid tumors that are <1 cm have a low risk of metastatic spread and can be excised endoscopically or via a transanal technique [117, 118] (Fig. 26.2). The 5-year survival rate for resected stage 1 tumors was 97 % [119]. Tumors between 1 and 2 cm can display more aggressive behavior and 10–15 % will have metastatic disease. Tumors that are between 1 and 2 cm with a low grade and no invasion of the muscularis propria can be removed by local excision, but those displaying higher grade or with invasion of the muscularis propria should undergo surgical resection following similar surgical principles to the treatment of rectal adenocarcinoma (anterior resection versus abdominal-perineal resection) [120, 121]. Tumors >2 cm generally present with metastatic disease 60–80 % of the time [122]. These larger tumors should be removed by low anterior resection or abdominal-perineal resection if they are believed to be curable or to palliate symptoms of rectal obstruction. For tumors >2 cm with diffuse metastatic disease and no evidence of obstruction, surgical resection may not provide survival benefit and medical management or ablative therapies should be considered with a multidisciplinary approach.

Metastatic Disease to the Liver

Liver resection of metastatic neuroendocrine tumors, including carcinoid, resulted in an overall 4 year survival of 73 % [123]. General requirements for resection of liver metastasis with a curative intent include anatomically resectable disease, G1–G2 tumor grade, absence of other unresectable lymph node or intra-abdominal metastases, and no evidence of peritoneal carcinomatosis. Resection of metastatic liver disease with G3 tumor grade is generally not advisable given the overall poor prognosis. For patients with hepatic metastasis that are not completely resectable, evidence exists that palliative tumor cytoreduction prolongs survival when compared to hepatic embolization (mean survival 32 month vs. 24 months, $p<0.001$) [124]. Combination approaches with anatomical liver resection ± embolization or ablation procedures have shown increased 3-year survival compared to medical therapy or embolization procedures alone [125]. Patients with diffuse liver metastases should not be treated via surgical approach.

Initial results of liver transplantation for carcinoid tumors in 15 patients with carcinoid tumors were promising with reports of a 5-year survival of 69 % [126]. A review of the UNOS database regarding the outcomes of liver transplantation for 150 patients with metastatic neuroendocrine tumors revealed 1-, 3-, and 5-year survival rates for patients with NETs undergoing isolated liver transplantation were 81, 65, and 49 % [127].

This is comparable to the results of liver transplantation for non-carcinoid tumors such as hepatocellular carcinoma.

Surgical Management of Other Distant Metastases

Overall survival in patients with distant metastatic disease is highly influenced by tumor grade. Patients with G1 or G2 tumor grade have a median survival of 33 months, whereas those with G3 tumor grade have a median survival of 5 months [33]. Trials do exist that suggest early tumor debulking with regional lymph node dissection may be associated with improved survival outcomes [91, 128]. However, the data supporting tumor-debulking surgery is retrospective in nature and may be influenced by some patient-selection bias. Nevertheless, tumor debulking does appear to palliate symptoms related to endocrine hypersecretion or obstruction caused by the tumor and may durably improve quality of life in patients who are failing medical management [129–131]. The extent of debulking necessary to produce symptomatic benefit is unknown.

Long-Term Follow-Up and Outcomes

As appendiceal carcinoid tumors are often slow growing and most (70 %) are less than 1 cm in size at time of resection, prognosis is relatively good [4]. Overall 5- and 10-year survival for patients with appendiceal carcinoid are 86 % and 80 %, respectively [7, 102]. Five-year survival rates for appendiceal carcinoid tumors are superior when compared to other primary sites such as gastric (49 %), pancreatic (34 %), bronchopulmonary (77 %), small bowel (80 %), colon (42 %), and rectum (72 %) [17, 132]. Mortality is observed almost exclusively in patients with metastatic spread and tumors greater than 1 cm in size [133]. Metastases with appendiceal carcinoid occur primarily to regional lymph nodes rather than the liver [134]. A long-term follow-up study spanning five decades of tumors demonstrated a 5-year survival of 92 % for patients with local disease only, 81 % for patients with regional disease, and 31 % for patients with distant metastases [111].

Follow-up for patients with advanced disease or tumors greater than 2 cm after resection includes imaging every 6–12 months with octreoscan as well as biochemical follow-up with plasma chromogranin A and urine 5-HIAA levels. Development of symptoms suggestive of carcinoid syndrome is also an indication for radiographic and biochemical reevaluation.

Salient Points

- The most common locations of carcinoids are in the appendix and distal ileum
- Diagnosis of appendiceal carcinoids can be difficult and most are found incidentally at the time of appendectomy (approximately 1 % of appendectomy specimens). Tumor size, histology, and molecular markers are important in determining malignant potential.
- Prognosis depends on tumor size, location of tumor, extent of invasion into organ of origin, evidence of regional/distant disease, and tumor grade (mitotic rate and/or Ki67 proliferation index).
- Diagnostic work-up of patients with suspected advanced carcinoid tumors includes plasma chromogranin A, urine 5-HIAA levels, and octreoscan imaging.
- A right hemicolectomy is recommended for appendiceal tumors: 2 cm or greater in size; involvement of the base of the appendix with positive margins or cecal spread; mesoappendiceal extension or angioinvasion; high-grade malignant tumors demonstrating a high mitotic index and Ki67 levels; and histological subtypes with more aggressive behavior such as goblet cell carcinoid.
- Principles of surgical resection for other primary sites of carcinoid tumors typically involve complete surgical resection of the mass with regional lymphadenectomy.
- Jejunoileal carcinoids: Multiple tumors may be present. Therefore, preoperative tumor localization using endoscopic and imaging modality (i.e., octreotide scintigraphy, CT scan) may be required.

- Hindgut carcinoids (i.e., colorectal), in general, have the worse prognosis of all the types of carcinoids.
- Small rectal carcinoids (<1 cm) are treatable if they can be completely excised endoscopically. Larger rectal carcinoids (>2 cm) require formal surgical excision (anterior resection versus abdominal-perineal resection).
- The carcinoid syndrome refers to a constellation of symptoms that are due to metastatic disease to the liver. Because these overproduced biologically active substances bypassed the portal circulation, patients can experience flushing, diarrhea, bronchospasm, wheezing, and/or right heart failure. Treatment is best achieved with the somatostatin analogs and surgical treatment of resectable disease.
- Prognosis for malignant appendiceal carcinoid is better than jejunoileal or colonic primaries with an 80 % 10-year overall survival rate. 5-year survival is greater than 90 % in patients with local disease, 80 % for patients with regional lymph node metastases, and 30 % or less for the few patients who develop distant spread to the liver and other organs.
- Somatostatin analogs have been used with success in patients with advanced disease. While chemotherapy has not shown great promise, metabolically directed radiotherapy, hepatic artery embolization, hepatic resection, liver transplantation, and bevacizumab may have a role in selected patients.
- The PROMID randomized trial demonstrated a median time to tumor progression of 14.3 months in the octreotide long-acting repeatable (LAR) injections group versus 6 months in the placebo group.

Questions

1. The most important blood marker for carcinoid tumors is:
   A. Somatostatin
   B. 5-HIAA
   C. Chromogranin A
   D. Carcinoembryonic antigen (CEA)
2. Regarding gastric carcinoids, which of the following is false:
   A. Type 1 gastric carcinoid tumors are typically small and behave in a benign fashion.
   B. Type 2 gastric carcinoid lesions are not associated with multiple endocrine neoplasia type 1 or Zollinger-Ellison syndrome.
   C. Five-year survival for type 3 gastric carcinoid tumors is 50 % overall.
   D. Type 4 gastric carcinoids often present with disseminated disease at the time of diagnosis.
3. Which of the following is correct regarding appendiceal carcinoid tumors and their management:
   A. Tumors >2 cm involving the base of the appendix or mesoappendix should be removed by formal right hemicolectomy including resection of locoregional lymph nodes.
   B. Tumors 1–2 cm in size can always be treated with simple appendectomy.
   C. Appendiceal carcinoids rarely are associated with acute appendicitis.
   D. It is never adequate to do a simple appendectomy for these tumors as they are malignant in nature.
4. The most frequently reported mutation in gastrointestinal carcinoid tumors is:
   A. MAGE-2D
   B. c-Myc
   C. Beta-catenin
   D. Cyclin D1
5. Regarding the epidemiology of carcinoid tumors, all of the following are correct *EXCEPT*:
   A. The incidence in the United States is around 1 in 50,000 people.
   B. There is a slight female preponderance for the disease.
   C. The average age of diagnosis is in the fifth or sixth decade of life.
   D. Gastric carcinoids represent the most common location for the disease.

6. Adjuvant chemotherapeutics evaluated recently for metastatic carcinoid include all of the following except:
   A. Docetaxel
   B. Everolimus
   C. Pegylated IFN-α
   D. Bevacizumab
7. The imaging modality most often used to identify carcinoid tumors is :
   A. FDG-PET
   B. Octreoscan
   C. DOTATEC-PET
   D. MRI
   E. Ultrasound
8. Rectal carcinoids <1 cm in size should best be treated with:
   A. Low anterior resection with primary anastomosis
   B. Abdominal-perineal resection with colostomy
   C. Transanal excision
   D. Close clinical observation
9. Five-year overall survival is highest for which of the following types of carcinoid tumors:
   A. Gastric
   B. Rectal
   C. Pancreatic
   D. Appendiceal
10. Which of the following statement regarding jejunoileal carcinoid is correct?
   A. They have the worse prognosis among the carcinoids of the GI tract.
   B. They tend to present with multiple synchronous lesions.
   C. Histological grading has no prognostic role.
   D. Five-year survival rate is 30 % for those with localized disease.

Answers

1. C
2. B
3. A
4. C
5. D
6. A
7. B
8. C
9. D
10. B

References

1. Modlin IM, Sandor A. An analysis of 8305 cases of carcinoid tumors. Cancer. 1997;79(4):813–29.
2. Woods HF, Bax ND, Ainsworth I. Abdominal carcinoid tumours in Sheffield. Digestion. 1990;45 Suppl 1:17–22.
3. Lu Cortez L, Clemente C, Puig V, Mirada A. Carcinoid tumor. An analysis of 131 cases. Rev Clin Esp. 1994;194(4):291–3.
4. Moertel CG, Dockerty MB, Judd ES. Carcinoid tumors of the vermiform appendix. Cancer. 1968;21(2):270–8.
5. Chandrasegaram MD, Rothwell LA, An EI, Miller RJ. Pathologies of the appendix: a 10-year review of 4670 appendicectomy specimens. ANZ J Surg. 2012;82(11):844–7.
6. Connor SJ, Hanna GB, Frizelle FA. Appendiceal tumors: retrospective clinicopathologic analysis of appendiceal tumors from 7,970 appendectomies. Dis Colon Rectum. 1998;41(1):75–80.
7. Sandor A, Modlin IM. A retrospective analysis of 1570 appendiceal carcinoids. Am J Gastroenterol. 1998;93(3):422–8.
8. Deans GT, Spence RA. Neoplastic lesions of the appendix. Br J Surg. 1995;82(3):299–306.
9. Moertel CL, Weiland LH, Telander RL. Carcinoid tumor of the appendix in the first two decades of life. J Pediatr Surg. 1990;25(10):1073–5.
10. Lubarsch O. Uber den pimaeren krebs des ileum nebst Bemerkungen ueber das gleichzeitige Vorkommen von krebs und Tuberculos. Virchows Arch. 1888;11:280–317.
11. Ransom W. Case of primary carcinoma of ileum. Lancet. 1890;136:1020–3.
12. Oberndorfer S. Karzinoide Rumoren des Dunndarms. Frankf. 1907;1:425–9.
13. Masson P. Carcinoids (argentaffin-cell tumors) and nerve hyperplasia of the appendicular mucosa. Am J Pathol. 1928;4(3):181–212.
14. Page IH, Corcoran AC, Udenfriend S, Szoedsma A, Weissbach H. Argentaffinoma as endocrine tumour. Lancet. 1955;268(6856):198–9.
15. Schnirer II, Yao JC, Ajani JA. Carcinoid – a comprehensive review. Acta Oncol. 2003;42(7):672–92.
16. Komminoth P, Arnold R, Capella C. Neuroendocrine neoplasms of the appendix. 4th ed. Lyon: IARC2010; 2010. p. 217–24.
17. Hsu C, Rashid A, Xing Y, et al. Varying malignant potential of appendiceal neuroendocrine tumors: importance of histologic subtype. J Surg Oncol. 2013;107(2):136–43.
18. McGory ML, Maggard MA, Kang H, O'Connell JB, Ko CY. Malignancies of the appendix: beyond case series reports. Dis Colon Rectum. 2005; 48(12):2264–71.
19. Chejfec G, Falkmer S, Askensten U, Grimelius L, Gould VE. Neuroendocrine tumors of the gastrointestinal tract. Pathol Res Pract. 1988;183(2): 143–54.

20. Moore K, Dalley AF, Agur AM. The developing human. Clinically oriented embryology. 7th ed. W.B. Saunders Company; 2013. 1982. p. 226–46. Saint Louis, Missouri.
21. Stinner B, Kisker O, Zielke A, Rothmund M. Surgical management for carcinoid tumors of small bowel, appendix, colon, and rectum. World J Surg. 1996;20(2):183–8.
22. Adams S, Baum R, Rink T, Schumm-Dräger PM, Usadel KH, Hör G. Limited value of fluorine-18 fluorodeoxyglucose positron emission tomography for the imaging of neuroendocrine tumours. Eur J Nucl Med. 1998;25(1):79–83.
23. Hanson MW, Feldman JM, Blinder RA, Moore JO, Coleman RE. Carcinoid tumors: iodine-131 MIBG scintigraphy. Radiology. 1989;172(3):699–703.
24. Krenning EP, Kooij PP, Bakker WH, et al. Radiotherapy with a radiolabeled somatostatin analogue, [111In-DTPA-D-Phe1]-octreotide. A case history. Ann N Y Acad Sci. 1994;733:496–506.
25. Srirajaskanthan R, Kayani I, Quigley AM, Soh J, Caplin ME, Bomanji J. The role of 68Ga-DOTATATE PET in patients with neuroendocrine tumors and negative or equivocal findings on 111In-DTPA-octreotide scintigraphy. J Nucl Med. 2010;51(6):875–82.
26. Gabriel M, Decristoforo C, Kendler D, et al. 68Ga-DOTA-Tyr3-octreotide PET in neuroendocrine tumors: comparison with somatostatin receptor scintigraphy and CT. J Nucl Med. 2007;48(4):508–18.
27. Krausz Y, Freedman N, Rubinstein R, et al. 68Ga-DOTA-NOC PET/CT imaging of neuroendocrine tumors: comparison with ^{111}In-DTPA-octreotide (OctreoScan®). Mol Imaging Biol. 2011;13(3):583–93.
28. Stivanello M, Berruti A, Torta M, et al. Circulating chromogranin A in the assessment of patients with neuroendocrine tumours. A single institution experience. Ann Oncol. 2001;12 Suppl 2:S73–7.
29. Janson ET, Holmberg L, Stridsberg M, et al. Carcinoid tumors: analysis of prognostic factors and survival in 301 patients from a referral center. Ann Oncol. 1997;8(7):685–90.
30. Eriksson B. Tumor markers for pancreatic endocrine tumors, including chromogranins, HCG-alpha and HCG-beta. Basel: Karger; 1995. p. 121.
31. Tormey WP, FitzGerald RJ. The clinical and laboratory correlates of an increased urinary 5-hydroxyindoleacetic acid. Postgrad Med J. 1995;71(839):542–5.
32. Edge SB, Compton CC. The American Joint Committee on Cancer: the 7th edition of the AJCC cancer staging manual and the future of TNM. Ann Surg Oncol. 2010;17(6):1471–4.
33. Yao JC, Hassan M, Phan A, et al. One hundred years after "carcinoid": epidemiology of and prognostic factors for neuroendocrine tumors in 35,825 cases in the United States. J Clin Oncol. 2008;26(18):3063–72.
34. Sobin LH, Gospodarowicz M, Wittekind C, editors. TNM classification of malignant tumours. 7th ed. Chichester: Wiley/Blackwell; 2009. p. 94–100.
35. Rindi G, Klöppel G, Couvelard A, et al. TNM staging of midgut and hindgut (neuro) endocrine tumors: a consensus proposal including a grading system. Virchows Arch. 2007;451(4):757–62.
36. Toumpanakis CG, Caplin ME. Molecular genetics of gastroenteropancreatic neuroendocrine tumors. Am J Gastroenterol. 2008;103(3):729–32.
37. Löllgen RM, Hessman O, Szabo E, Westin G, Akerström G. Chromosome 18 deletions are common events in classical midgut carcinoid tumors. Int J Cancer. 2001;92(6):812–5.
38. Oberg K. Genetics and molecular pathology of neuroendocrine gastrointestinal and pancreatic tumors (gastroenteropancreatic neuroendocrine tumors). Curr Opin Endocrinol Diabetes Obes. 2009; 16(1):72–8.
39. Goede AC, Caplin ME, Winslet MC. Carcinoid tumour of the appendix. Br J Surg. 2003;90(11): 1317–22.
40. Syracuse DC, Perzin KH, Price JB, Wiedel PD, Mesa-Tejada R. Carcinoid tumors of the appendix. Mesoappendiceal extension and nodal metastases. Ann Surg. 1979;190(1):58–63.
41. Rindi G, Arnold R, Bosman FT, et al. Nomenclature and classification of neuroendocrine neoplasms of the digestive system. In: Bosman TF, Carneiro F, Hruban RH, Theise ND, editors. WHO classification of tumours of the digestive system. 4th ed. Lyon: International Agency for Research on cancer (IARC); 2010. p. 13.
42. Ahmed A, Turner G, King B, et al. Midgut neuroendocrine tumours with liver metastases: results of the UKINETS study. Endocr Relat Cancer. 2009;16(3):885–94.
43. Moertel CG. Karnofsky memorial lecture. An odyssey in the land of small tumors. J Clin Oncol. 1987;5(10):1502–22.
44. Kvols LK, Moertel CG, O'Connell MJ, Schutt AJ, Rubin J, Hahn RG. Treatment of the malignant carcinoid syndrome. Evaluation of a long-acting somatostatin analogue. N Engl J Med. 1986;315(11):663–6.
45. Eriksson B, Renstrup J, Imam H, Oberg K. High-dose treatment with lanreotide of patients with advanced neuroendocrine gastrointestinal tumors: clinical and biological effects. Ann Oncol. 1997;8(10):1041–4.
46. Tomassetti P, Migliori M, Gullo L. Slow-release lanreotide treatment in endocrine gastrointestinal tumors. Am J Gastroenterol. 1998;93(9):1468–71.
47. Wymenga AN, Eriksson B, Salmela PI, et al. Efficacy and safety of prolonged-release lanreotide in patients with gastrointestinal neuroendocrine tumors and hormone-related symptoms. J Clin Oncol. 1999;17(4):1111.

48. Ricci S, Antonuzzo A, Galli L, et al. Long-acting depot lanreotide in the treatment of patients with advanced neuroendocrine tumors. Am J Clin Oncol. 2000;23(4):412–5.
49. Tomassetti P, Migliori M, Corinaldesi R, Gullo L. Treatment of gastroenteropancreatic neuroendocrine tumours with octreotide LAR. Aliment Pharmacol Ther. 2000;14(5):557–60.
50. Toumpanakis C, Garland J, Marelli L, et al. Long-term results of patients with malignant carcinoid syndrome receiving octreotide LAR. Aliment Pharmacol Ther. 2009;30(7):733–40.
51. Rinke A, Müller HH, Schade-Brittinger C, et al. Placebo-controlled, double-blind, prospective, randomized study on the effect of octreotide LAR in the control of tumor growth in patients with metastatic neuroendocrine midgut tumors: a report from the PROMID Study Group. J Clin Oncol. 2009; 27(28):4656–63.
52. Kölby L, Persson G, Franzén S, Ahrén B. Randomized clinical trial of the effect of interferon alpha on survival in patients with disseminated midgut carcinoid tumours. Br J Surg. 2003; 90(6):687–93.
53. Faiss S, Pape UF, Böhmig M, et al. Prospective, randomized, multicenter trial on the antiproliferative effect of lanreotide, interferon alfa, and their combination for therapy of metastatic neuroendocrine gastroenteropancreatic tumors – the International Lanreotide and Interferon Alfa Study Group. J Clin Oncol. 2003;21(14):2689–96.
54. Frank M, Klose KJ, Wied M, Ishaque N, Schade-Brittinger C, Arnold R. Combination therapy with octreotide and alpha-interferon: effect on tumor growth in metastatic endocrine gastroenteropancreatic tumors. Am J Gastroenterol. 1999;94(5):1381–7.
55. Arnold R, Rinke A, Klose KJ, et al. Octreotide versus octreotide plus interferon-alpha in endocrine gastroenteropancreatic tumors: a randomized trial. Clin Gastroenterol Hepatol. 2005;3(8):761–71.
56. Oberg K, Norheim I, Alm G. Treatment of malignant carcinoid tumors: a randomized controlled study of streptozocin plus 5-FU and human leukocyte interferon. Eur J Cancer Clin Oncol. 1989;25(10):1475–9.
57. Moertel CG. Treatment of the carcinoid tumor and the malignant carcinoid syndrome. J Clin Oncol. 1983;1(11):727–40.
58. Moertel CG, Hanley JA. Combination chemotherapy trials in metastatic carcinoid tumor and the malignant carcinoid syndrome. Cancer Clin Trials. 1979;2(4):327–34.
59. Eriksson BK, Larsson EG, Skogseid BM, Löfberg AM, Lörelius LE, Oberg KE. Liver embolizations of patients with malignant neuroendocrine gastrointestinal tumors. Cancer. 1998;83(11):2293–301.
60. Nobin A, Månsson B, Lunderquist A. Evaluation of temporary liver dearterialization and embolization in patients with metastatic carcinoid tumour. Acta Oncol. 1989;28(3):419–24.
61. Carrasco CH, Charnsangavej C, Ajani J, Samaan NA, Richli W, Wallace S. The carcinoid syndrome: palliation by hepatic artery embolization. AJR Am J Roentgenol. 1986;147(1):149–54.
62. Diaco DS, Hajarizadeh H, Mueller CR, Fletcher WS, Pommier RF, Woltering EA. Treatment of metastatic carcinoid tumors using multimodality therapy of octreotide acetate, intra-arterial chemotherapy, and hepatic arterial chemoembolization. Am J Surg. 1995;169(5):523–8.
63. Therasse E, Breittmayer F, Roche A, et al. Transcatheter chemoembolization of progressive carcinoid liver metastasis. Radiology. 1993;189(2): 541–7.
64. Kimmig BN. Radiotherapy for gastroenteropancreatic neuroendocrine tumors. Ann N Y Acad Sci. 1994;733:488–95.
65. Drougas JG, Anthony LB, Blair TK, et al. Hepatic artery chemoembolization for management of patients with advanced metastatic carcinoid tumors. Am J Surg. 1998;175(5):408–12.
66. Ruszniewski P, Rougier P, Roche A, et al. Hepatic arterial chemoembolization in patients with liver metastases of endocrine tumors. A prospective phase II study in 24 patients. Cancer. 1993;71(8): 2624–30.
67. Kim YH, Ajani JA, Carrasco CH, et al. Selective hepatic arterial chemoembolization for liver metastases in patients with carcinoid tumor or islet cell carcinoma. Cancer Invest. 1999;17(7):474–8.
68. McCarthy KE, Woltering EA, Espenan GD, Cronin M, Maloney TJ, Anthony LB. In situ radiotherapy with 111In-pentetreotide: initial observations and future directions. Cancer J Sci Am. 1998; 4(2):94–102.
69. De Jong M, Breeman WA, Bernard HF, et al. Therapy of neuroendocrine tumors with radiolabeled somatostatin-analogues. Q J Nucl Med. 1999;43(4): 356–66.
70. Anthony LB, Woltering EA, Espenan GD, Cronin MD, Maloney TJ, McCarthy KE. Indium-111-pentetreotide prolongs survival in gastroenteropancreatic malignancies. Semin Nucl Med. 2002;32(2):123–32.
71. Buscombe JR, Caplin ME, Hilson AJ. Long-term efficacy of high-activity 111in-pentetreotide therapy in patients with disseminated neuroendocrine tumors. J Nucl Med. 2003;44(1):1–6.
72. Otte A, Herrmann R, Heppeler A, et al. Yttrium-90 DOTATOC: first clinical results. Eur J Nucl Med. 1999;26(11):1439–47.
73. Virgolini I, Britton K, Buscombe J, Moncayo R, Paganelli G, Riva P. In- and Y-DOTA-lanreotide: results and implications of the MAURITIUS trial. Semin Nucl Med. 2002;32(2):148–55.
74. Teunissen JJ, Kwekkeboom DJ, Krenning EP. Quality of life in patients with gastroenteropancreatic tumors treated with [^{177}Lu-DOTA0, Tyr^{3}]octreotate. J Clin Oncol. 2004;22(13): 2724–9.

75. Kwekkeboom DJ, Mueller-Brand J, Paganelli G, et al. Overview of results of peptide receptor radionuclide therapy with 3 radiolabeled somatostatin analogs. J Nucl Med. 2005;46 Suppl 1:62S–6.
76. Yao JC, Phan A, Hoff PM, et al. Targeting vascular endothelial growth factor in advanced carcinoid tumor: a random assignment phase II study of depot octreotide with bevacizumab and pegylated interferon alpha-2b. J Clin Oncol. 2008;26(8): 1316–23.
77. Pavel ME, Hainsworth JD, Baudin E, et al. Everolimus plus octreotide long-acting repeatable for the treatment of advanced neuroendocrine tumours associated with carcinoid syndrome (RADIANT-2): a randomised, placebo-controlled, phase 3 study. Lancet. 2011;378(9808):2005–12.
78. Gustafsson BI, Kidd M, Modlin IM. Neuroendocrine tumors of the diffuse neuroendocrine system. Curr Opin Oncol. 2008;20(1):1–12.
79. McCaughan BC, Martini N, Bains MS. Bronchial carcinoids. Review of 124 cases. J Thorac Cardiovasc Surg. 1985;89(1):8–17.
80. Vuitch F, Sekido Y, Fong K, Mackay B, Minna JD, Gazdar AF. Neuroendocrine tumors of the lung. Pathology and molecular biology. Chest Surg Clin N Am. 1997;7(1):21–47.
81. Fink G, Krelbaum T, Yellin A, et al. Pulmonary carcinoid: presentation, diagnosis, and outcome in 142 cases in Israel and review of 640 cases from the literature. Chest. 2001;119(6):1647–51.
82. Scott WJ. Surgical treatment of other bronchial tumors. Chest Surg Clin N Am. 2003;13(1):111–28.
83. Beasley MB, Thunnissen FB, Brambilla E, et al. Pulmonary atypical carcinoid: predictors of survival in 106 cases. Hum Pathol. 2000;31(10):1255–65.
84. Cardillo G, Sera F, Di Martino M, et al. Bronchial carcinoid tumors: nodal status and long-term survival after resection. Ann Thorac Surg. 2004;77(5): 1781–5.
85. Niederle MB, Hackl M, Kaserer K, Niederle B. Gastroenteropancreatic neuroendocrine tumours: the current incidence and staging based on the WHO and European Neuroendocrine Tumour Society classification: an analysis based on prospectively collected parameters. Endocr Relat Cancer. 2010;17(4):909–18.
86. Ichikawa J, Tanabe S, Koizumi W, et al. Endoscopic mucosal resection in the management of gastric carcinoid tumors. Endoscopy. 2003;35(3):203–6.
87. Borch K, Ahrén B, Ahlman H, Falkmer S, Granérus G, Grimelius L. Gastric carcinoids: biologic behavior and prognosis after differentiated treatment in relation to type. Ann Surg. 2005;242(1):64–73.
88. Delle Fave G, Capurso G, Milione M, Panzuto F. Endocrine tumours of the stomach. Best Pract Res Clin Gastroenterol. 2005;19(5):659–73.
89. Campana D, Nori F, Pezzilli R, et al. Gastric endocrine tumors type I: treatment with long-acting somatostatin analogs. Endocr Relat Cancer. 2008; 15(1):337–42.
90. Klöppel G, Scherübl H. Neuroendocrine tumors of the stomach. Risk stratification and therapy. Pathologe. 2010;31(3):182–7.
91. Akerström G, Hellman P. Surgery on neuroendocrine tumours. Best Pract Res Clin Endocrinol Metab. 2007;21(1):87–109.
92. Ruszniewski P, Delle Fave G, Cadiot G, et al. Well-differentiated gastric tumors/carcinomas. Neuroendocrinology. 2006;84(3):158–64.
93. Rindi G, Bordi C, Rappel S, La Rosa S, Stolte M, Solcia E. Gastric carcinoids and neuroendocrine carcinomas: pathogenesis, pathology, and behavior. World J Surg. 1996;20(2):168–72.
94. Eriksson B, Klöppel G, Krenning E, et al. Consensus guidelines for the management of patients with digestive neuroendocrine tumors – well-differentiated jejunal-ileal tumor/carcinoma. Neuroendocrinology. 2008;87(1):8–19.
95. van Tuyl SA, van Noorden JT, Timmer R, Stolk MF, Kuipers EJ, Taal BG. Detection of small-bowel neuroendocrine tumors by video capsule endoscopy. Gastrointest Endosc. 2006;64(1):66–72.
96. Johanssen S, Boivin M, Lochs H, Voderholzer W. The yield of wireless capsule endoscopy in the detection of neuroendocrine tumors in comparison with CT enteroclysis. Gastrointest Endosc. 2006;63(4):660–5.
97. Bailey AA, Debinski HS, Appleyard MN, et al. Diagnosis and outcome of small bowel tumors found by capsule endoscopy: a three-center Australian experience. Am J Gastroenterol. 2006;101(10):2237–43.
98. Bellutti M, Fry LC, Schmitt J, et al. Detection of neuroendocrine tumors of the small bowel by double balloon enteroscopy. Dig Dis Sci. 2009;54(5):1050–8.
99. Akerström G, Makridis C, Johansson H. Abdominal surgery in patients with midgut carcinoid tumors. Acta Oncol. 1991;30(4):547–53.
100. Rothmund M, Kisker O. Surgical treatment of carcinoid tumors of the small bowel, appendix, colon and rectum. Digestion. 1994;55 Suppl 3:86–91.
101. Ahlman H, Wängberg B, Jansson S, et al. Interventional treatment of gastrointestinal neuroendocrine tumours. Digestion. 2000;62 Suppl 1:59–68.
102. Makridis C, Oberg K, Juhlin C, et al. Surgical treatment of mid-gut carcinoid tumors. World J Surg. 1990;14(3):377–83; discussion 384–375.
103. Norton JA. Surgical management of carcinoid tumors: role of debulking and surgery for patients with advanced disease. Digestion. 1994;55 Suppl 3:98–103.
104. Goede AC, Winslet MC. Surgery for carcinoid tumours of the lower gastrointestinal tract. Colorectal Dis. 2003;5(2):123–8.
105. Sutton R, Doran HE, Williams EM, et al. Surgery for midgut carcinoid. Endocr Relat Cancer. 2003; 10(4):469–81.
106. Han SL, Cheng J, Zhou HZ, Guo SC, Jia ZR, Wang PF. Surgically treated primary malignant tumor of small bowel: a clinical analysis. World J Gastroenterol. 2010;16(12):1527–32.

107. Norlén O, Hessman O, Stålberg P, Akerström G, Hellman P. Prophylactic cholecystectomy in midgut carcinoid patients. World J Surg. 2010; 34(6):1361–7.
108. MacGillivray DC, Heaton RB, Rushin JM, Cruess DF. Distant metastasis from a carcinoid tumor of the appendix less than one centimeter in size. Surgery. 1992;111(4):466–71.
109. Moertel CG, Weiland LH, Nagorney DM, Dockerty MB. Carcinoid tumor of the appendix: treatment and prognosis. N Engl J Med. 1987;317(27):1699–701.
110. Ryden SE, Drake RM, Franciosi RA. Carcinoid tumors of the appendix in children. Cancer. 1975;36(4):1538–42.
111. Modlin IM, Lye KD, Kidd M. A 5-decade analysis of 13,715 carcinoid tumors. Cancer. 2003;97(4):9 34–59.
112. Omohwo C, Nieroda CA, Studeman KD, et al. Complete cytoreduction offers longterm survival in patients with peritoneal carcinomatosis from appendiceal tumors of unfavorable histology. J Am Coll Surg. 2009;209(3):308–12.
113. Jetmore AB, Ray JE, Gathright JB, McMullen KM, Hicks TC, Timmcke AE. Rectal carcinoids: the most frequent carcinoid tumor. Dis Colon Rectum. 1992;35(8):717–25.
114. Garcia-Carbonero R, Capdevila J, Crespo-Herrero G, et al. Incidence, patterns of care and prognostic factors for outcome of gastroenteropancreatic neuroendocrine tumors (GEP-NETs): results from the National Cancer Registry of Spain (RGETNE). Ann Oncol. 2010;21(9):1794–803.
115. Ballantyne GH, Savoca PE, Flannery JT, Ahlman MH, Modlin IM. Incidence and mortality of carcinoids of the colon. Data from the Connecticut Tumor Registry. Cancer. 1992;69(10):2400–5.
116. Matsumoto T, Iida M, Suekane H, Tominaga M, Yao T, Fujishima M. Endoscopic ultrasonography in rectal carcinoid tumors: contribution to selection of therapy. Gastrointest Endosc. 1991;37(5): 539–42.
117. Kwaan MR, Goldberg JE, Bleday R. Rectal carcinoid tumors: review of results after endoscopic and surgical therapy. Arch Surg. 2008;143(5):471–5.
118. Onozato Y, Kakizaki S, Iizuka H, Sohara N, Mori M, Itoh H. Endoscopic treatment of rectal carcinoid tumors. Dis Colon Rectum. 2010;53(2):169–76.
119. Landry CS, Brock G, Scoggins CR, McMasters KM, Martin RC. A proposed staging system for rectal carcinoid tumors based on an analysis of 4701 patients. Surgery. 2008;144(3):460–6.
120. Shields CJ, Tiret E, Winter DC, Group IRCS. Carcinoid tumors of the rectum: a multi-institutional international collaboration. Ann Surg. 2010;252(5):750–5.
121. Sauven P, Ridge JA, Quan SH, Sigurdson ER. Anorectal carcinoid tumors. Is aggressive surgery warranted? Ann Surg. 1990;211(1):67–71.
122. Pavel M, Baudin E, Couvelard A, et al. ENETS Consensus Guidelines for the management of patients with liver and other distant metastases from neuroendocrine neoplasms of foregut, midgut, hindgut, and unknown primary. Neuroendocrinology. 2012;95(2):157–76.
123. Que FG, Nagorney DM, Batts KP, Linz LJ, Kvols LK. Hepatic resection for metastatic neuroendocrine carcinomas. Am J Surg. 1995;169(1):36–42; discussion 42–33.
124. Osborne DA, Zervos EE, Strosberg J, et al. Improved outcome with cytoreduction versus embolization for symptomatic hepatic metastases of carcinoid and neuroendocrine tumors. Ann Surg Oncol. 2006; 13(4):572–81.
125. Musunuru S, Chen H, Rajpal S, et al. Metastatic neuroendocrine hepatic tumors: resection improves survival. Arch Surg. 2006;141(10):1000–4; discussion 1005.
126. Le Treut YP, Delpero JR, Dousset B, et al. Results of liver transplantation in the treatment of metastatic neuroendocrine tumors. A 31-case French multicentric report. Ann Surg. 1997;225(4):355–64.
127. Gedaly R, Daily MF, Davenport D, et al. Liver transplantation for the treatment of liver metastases from neuroendocrine tumors: an analysis of the UNOS database. Arch Surg. 2011;146(8):953–8.
128. Durante C, Boukheris H, Dromain C, et al. Prognostic factors influencing survival from metastatic (stage IV) gastroenteropancreatic well-differentiated endocrine carcinoma. Endocr Relat Cancer. 2009;16(2):585–97.
129. Chen H, Hardacre JM, Uzar A, Cameron JL, Choti MA. Isolated liver metastases from neuroendocrine tumors: does resection prolong survival? J Am Coll Surg. 1998;187(1):88–92; discussion 92–83.
130. Sarmiento JM, Que FG. Hepatic surgery for metastases from neuroendocrine tumors. Surg Oncol Clin N Am. 2003;12(1):231–42.
131. Elias D, Lasser P, Ducreux M, et al. Liver resection (and associated extrahepatic resections) for metastatic well-differentiated endocrine tumors: a 15-year single center prospective study. Surgery. 2003;133(4):375–82.
132. Srirajaskanthan R, Ahmed A, Prachialias A, et al. ENETS TNM staging predicts prognosis in small bowel neuroendocrine tumours. ISRN Oncol. 2013;2013:420795.
133. Godwin JD. Carcinoid tumors. An analysis of 2,837 cases. Cancer. 1975;36(2):560–9.
134. MacGillivray DC, Synder DA, Drucker W, ReMine SG. Carcinoid tumors: the relationship between clinical presentation and the extent of disease. Surgery. 1991;110(1):68–72.

Part V

Sarcoma

27 Soft Tissue Sarcoma

Rachel D. Aufforth, Justin John Baker, and Hong Jin Kim

Learning Objectives

After reading this chapter you should be able to:

- List the common locations of soft tissue sarcomas.
- Understand the presenting symptoms of extremity and retroperitoneal sarcomas (RPS).
- Implement the standard workup for extremity and RPS.
- Understand the advantages and limitations of different biopsy techniques.
- List the five prognostic markers of soft tissue sarcomas.
- Understand the AJCC staging system for sarcomas.
- Understand the goals and role of surgical resection in extremity and RPS.
- Understand the indications for radiation therapy and chemotherapy in both extremity and RPS.
- Understand the management of recurrent disease in both extremity and retroperitoneal sarcomas.
- Understand the anatomic location of gastrointestinal stromal tumors (GIST).
- List the common genetic mutation associated with GISTs.
- Understand the treatment goal of GISTs.
- List the indications for and duration of imatinib treatment for primary GISTs.

Soft tissue sarcomas represent a diverse group of tumors that arise from mesenchymal cells. These tumors develop from a wide variety of different cell types, with over 50 different histologic varieties [1]. These tumors can develop anywhere in the body but most commonly occur on the extremities and in the retroperitoneum [2]. They are rare tumors representing less than 1 % of all solid tumors in adults [2].

Epidemiology

In 2012, the American Cancer Society estimated 11,280 new cases of sarcoma in the United States. 6,110 of these cases were in men and the remaining 5,170 occurred in women. It is estimated that there were 3,900 deaths in 2012 from soft tissue sarcomas [3]. In 2008, for a patient under the age of 20, soft tissue sarcomas were the fourth leading cause of cancer death for males and the fifth

R.D. Aufforth, M.D.
Division of Surgical Oncology and Endocrine Surgery, University of North Carolina, 170 Manning Drive, Chapel Hill 27599, NC, USA
e-mail: Aufforth@med.unc.edu

J.J. Baker, M.D.
Department of Surgery, Maine Medical Center/Tufts University School of Medicine, 22 Bramhall St., Portland 04102, ME, USA
e-mail: bakerj2@mmc.org

H.J. Kim, M.D. (✉)
Division of Surgical Oncology and Endocrine Surgery, University of North Carolina at Chapel Hill, Lineberger Comprehensive Cancer Center, P1150 Physicians Office Building, CB 7213, 170 Manning Drive, Chapel Hill 27599-7213, NC, USA
e-mail: kimhj@med.unc.edu

Q.D. Chu et al. (eds.), *Surgical Oncology: A Practical and Comprehensive Approach*,
DOI 10.1007/978-1-4939-1423-4_27, © Springer Science+Business Media New York 2015

for females [3]. Even though sarcoma is a leading cause of cancer death in young persons, the vast majority of sarcoma deaths are in those over the age of 45 [4]. The overall incidence of sarcoma increases with age [2]. The incidence of soft tissue sarcomas has been relatively consistent over the last 30 years [5]. The incidence is 3.7 and 2.6 per 100,000 in males and females, respectively [2]. There is some variation in incidence by race, with Caucasians, Blacks, and Hispanics having the highest incidence and Asians and Native Americans the lowest [2]. According to the data from the MD Anderson Cancer Center from 1996 to 2005, the common anatomic locations for sarcoma include: extremity (45 %), retroperitoneal (27 %), visceral (13 %), thoracic (9 %), and head and neck (6 %) [6].

Risk Factors

The development of some sarcomas can be partially attributed to specific risk factors such as: radiation, environmental toxins, immunodeficiency, and lymphedema. Although radiation-induced sarcoma is a rare event accounting for only 0.5–5 % of all sarcomas, it has been linked to the development of osteogenic sarcoma, malignant fibrous histiocytoma (MFH), angiosarcoma, lymphangiosarcoma, spindle cell neoplasms, fibrosarcoma, liposarcoma, leiomyosarcoma, chondrosarcoma, and desmoid tumors [2, 7]. In breast cancer patients receiving radiation, the incidence of developing a radiation-induced sarcoma is 0.13 % at 10 years [8]. In addition to radiation, other environmental exposures may increase the development of sarcomas [2, 4]. Specifically, chemical exposures have been linked to certain sarcomas. The most notable chemicals include vinyl chloride, thorotrast, and arsenic; all have been associated with an increased risk of hepatic angiosarcoma [9].

A compromised immune system and chronic lymphedema have both been associated with an increased risk of sarcoma development. Human herpesvirus 8 (HHV8) in the setting of severe immunodeficiency such as AIDS has a strong predilection for the development of Kaposi's sarcoma [4]. Patients with solid organ transplants who are on chronic immunosuppressive medications have a twofold-increased incidence of sarcoma [10]. There also appears to be an association between Epstein-Barr virus and the development of leiomyosarcoma in certain immunosuppressed patients [11]. Untreated chronic lymphedema exposes patients to an increased risk of developing lymphangiosarcoma or Stewart-Treves syndrome [12, 13].

In addition to environmental and immunologic risk factors, there are a number of familial syndromes associated with an increased risk of sarcoma. Familial gastrointestinal stromal tumor (GIST) syndrome causes an activating mutation in *c-kit* and *PDGFRA* genes that lead to multiple GISTs [14]. Li-Fraumeni syndrome is a germline mutation in the tumor suppressor gene *p53*. This mutation is responsible for an increased risk of sarcoma as well as other epithelial-based cancers [15]. Neurofibromatosis is associated with a germline mutation in NF-1, a tumor suppressor gene, and imparts an increased risk of malignant peripheral nerve sheath tumors [16]. Inactivating germline mutations in Rb1, a tumor suppressor gene, results in retinoblastoma during childhood and carries an increased risk of other cancers throughout the patient's lifetime [17]. Werner syndrome, Bloom syndrome, and Rothmund-Thomson syndrome are three rare autosomal recessive syndromes associated with sarcomas that have germline mutations in genes responsible for DNA recombination, replication, and repair [2].

Histology

The histology of sarcoma is varied and is dependent upon the specific histologic type of sarcoma identified. Typically these tumors arise from embryonic mesodermal cells but they may also arise from ectoderm. The embryonic mesoderm eventually develops into vessels, muscle, bone, cartilage, synovium, and connective tissue [18]. These differentiated cell lines give rise to the vast array of sarcomas and are responsible for the varied location of development in the body. The exact number of patients with each particular subtype of sarcoma is unknown. In a study conducted at MD Anderson Cancer Center, the three most common histologic subtypes were malignant fibrous histiocytoma (28 %), liposarcoma (15 %), and leiomyosarcoma (12 %) [2]. This is slightly different than a large review of the SEER database, which showed 23.9 % of sarcomas to be leiomyosarcomas, 17.1 % MFH, 11.5 % liposarcoma, 10.5 % dermatofibrosarcoma, 4.6 % rhabdomyosarcoma, and 12.8 % sarcoma NOS [19].

The histologic determination of specific sarcomas is initially based on the morphology of cells using standard staining techniques [18]. Special immunostains are used to help differentiate specific tissue types. Certain sarcomas have specific chromosomal alterations, allowing the use of molecular genetics to identify and determine specific histologic subtypes [20]. These techniques are not perfect, and there is still much to discover in regard to the histologic determination of sarcomas.

Genetic and Molecular Alterations

Molecular alterations of soft tissue sarcomas are identified and described through multiple techniques like DNA sequencing and gene expression profiling. Recent studies have shown recurring molecular alterations among soft tissue sarcomas. Barretina et al. demonstrated that *TP53, NF1*, and *PIK3CA* are frequently mutated genes in different subtypes of liposarcomas [21]. Alterations in *N-myc* and *c-erbB2* oncogenes have been linked with Ewing's sarcoma. Deletions in the *PTEN* tumor suppressor gene and alterations in the *RB1* gene and *p53* are also common among soft tissue sarcomas [22]. The genomic mutations associated with soft tissue sarcomas can either be classified as (1) simple genetic alterations or (2) complex unbalanced karyotypes. Most molecular alterations arise de novo; however, some sarcomas acquire and accumulate genetic mutations as the cell progresses through different stages leading to complex karyotypes [23]. One-third of all sarcomas will have simple genetic alterations or translocations. Translocations end in gene fusion proteins that ultimately upregulate genes for tumor growth or serve as tumor formation drivers [24]. Ewing's sarcoma is associated with a translocation involving the *ews* gene on chromosome 22 and *fli1* gene on chromosome 11. The resulting *EWS-FLI1* fusion protein is associated with 85 % of Ewing's sarcomas [25]. The majority of soft tissue sarcomas however have nonspecific genetic alterations ending in complex karyotypes [26]. The progression of atypical lipoma or well-differentiated liposarcoma to dedifferentiated liposarcoma, neurofibroma to malignant peripheral nerve sheath tumor, or enchondroma to chondrosarcoma are all examples of well-behaved tumors acquiring genetic mutations and becoming more aggressive tumors with complex karyotypes [27–29]. Liposarcomas acquire increasing aberrant chromosomal copy numbers as tumors progress from well-differentiated to dedifferentiated liposarcomas [30]. Gene expression profiling has revealed amplification of 12q13-q15 in all liposarcomas with differing levels of *CDK4*, *HMGA2*, and *MDM2* oncogenes [30].

Understanding the molecular alterations responsible for sarcomagenesis is critical for assisting with diagnosis and identification of potential prognostic biomarkers. Currently, molecular testing using conventional cytogenetic analysis, fluorescence in situ hybridization (FISH), and polymerase chain reaction (PCR) are being used to assist in the diagnosis of soft tissue sarcomas [31, 32]. In addition to diagnosis, the identification of certain fusion proteins has resulted in prognostic biomarkers for some sarcomas. The identification of *PAX7-FOX01* fusion gene in patients with metastatic alveolar rhabdomyosarcoma is associated with a better prognosis than the *PAX3-FOX01* fusion gene [33]. In synovial sarcomas, the prognostic role of fusion genes is unclear. As the understanding of molecular alterations for specific soft tissue sarcomas becomes more evident, the opportunity for developing new, more effective treatments with targeted therapies will arise.

Grading and Staging Sarcomas

Staging of soft tissue sarcomas is done in accordance to the guidelines outlined in the 7th edition of the American Joint Committee on Cancer (AJCC) staging system [34] (Tables 27.1 and 27.2). This system includes grade with the traditional T, N, and M stage. The T stage is based on the size of tumor with T1 assigned to all tumors 5 cm or less and T2 for tumors greater than 5 cm. The T stage is further subdivided into *a* and *b* based on superficial or deep tumors. Superficial tumors are defined as tumors located entirely above the superficial fascia. Note that all retroperitoneal sarcomas are considered deep sarcomas. The AJCC grading system incorporates the Fédération Nationales des Centres de Lutte Contre le Cancer (FNCLCC) grading system, which assigns a score for each of the following three parameters: differentiation, mitotic rate, and extent of necrosis [35, 36]. Final histologic grade (G) is assigned based on a summation of each of the three parameters (Table 27.2) [37].

Grading of soft tissue sarcomas has important prognostic implications. Histologic grade is the strongest predictor of patient outcome. Other prognostic factors for sarcomas include primary tumor site, resection margin status, size of tumor, and primary versus recurrent disease [38, 39]. Linehan and colleagues found that tumor location significantly impacted 5-year survival among patients with completely resected liposarcomas [39]. The overall 5-year survival rate for retroperitoneal sarcomas is significantly lower compared to high-risk extremity sarcomas, 25–55 % versus 60–75 % [38]. Along with grade and tumor location, margin status also impacts survival rates. A study at Memorial Sloan Kettering Cancer Center found an 83 % disease-specific survival for margin-negative patients, compared

Table 27.1 American Joint Committee on Cancer (AJCC) TNM staging for soft tissue sarcoma (7th edition)

Primary tumor (T)	
TX	Primary tumor cannot be assessed
T0	No evidence of primary tumor
T1	Tumor ≤5 cm in greatest dimension*
T1a	Superficial tumor
T1b	Deep tumor
T2	Tumor >5 cm in greatest dimension*
T2a	Superficial tumor
T2b	Deep tumor

*Note: Superficial tumor is located exclusively above the superficial fascia without invasion of the fascia; deep tumor is located either exclusively beneath the superficial fascia, superficial to the fascia with invasion of or through the fascia, or both superficial yet beneath the fascia

Regional lymph nodes (N)	
NX	Regional lymph nodes cannot be assessed
N0	No regional lymph node metastasis
N1*	Regional lymph node metastasis

*Note: Presence of positive nodes (N1) in M0 tumors is considered stage III

Distant metastasis (M)	
M0	No distant metastasis
M1	Distant metastasis

Anatomic stage/prognostic groups				
Group	T	N	M	Grade
Stage IA	T1a, T1b	N0	M0	G1, GX
Stage IB	T2a, T2b	N0	M0	G1, GX
Stage IIA	T1a, T1b	N0	M0	G2, G3
Stage IIB	T2a, T2b	N0	M0	G2
Stage III	T2a, T2b	N0	M0	G3
	Any T	N1	M0	Any G
Stage IV	Any T	Any N	M1	Any G

*Grade (G) is determined by using the Fédération Nationale des Centres de Lutte Contre le Cancer (FNCLCC) grading system (see Table 27.2)

Adapted from Compton et al. [109]. With permission from Springer Verlag

Table 27.2 Fédération Nationale des Centres de Lutte Contre le Cancer (FNCLCC) histologic grade criteria

Tumor differentiation	Mitotic count	Necrosis
1: Well	1: $n<10$ per 10HPF	0: No necrosis
2: Moderate	2: 10–19 per 10HPF	1: <50 %
3: Poor	3: $n\geq20$ per 10HPF	2: ≥50 %

Modified from Trojani et al. [110], with permission from John Wiley & Sons, Inc.
The sum of the scores from each column determines the final grade:
G1: Score 2, 3
G2: Score 4, 5
G3: Score 6–8
HPF high power fields

to 75 % for margin-positive patients [40]. Margin status at the time of resection significantly impacts the rate of recurrence, which has been shown to predict future recurrences and affect survival [41]. Local recurrence rates for retroperitoneal sarcomas range from 40 to 65 % [42].

Evaluation of Extremity Sarcomas

According to the National Comprehensive Cancer Network (NCCN) guidelines, all patients with a new mass concerning sarcoma should undergo management by a multidisciplinary team [42]. The specific sarcoma workup should include a history and physical imaging of the tumor, a carefully planned biopsy, and a staging workup for distant disease [42] (Fig. 27.1).

Workup of a patient with an extremity soft tissue mass always begins with a thorough history. Important information to gather includes: time course, circumstances preceding the mass, and a thorough family history to rule out familial cancer syndromes. Patients with extremity sarcomas often present with a newly found painless mass [43]. One of the more common presentations is a recent history of trauma to the area where the mass is identified. Trauma does not necessarily cause sarcoma development, but it allows for a heightened awareness to a particular area leading to examination and imaging of that area [2]. Patients may also present with pain and neurologic symptoms at the site of the mass. After a detailed history is obtained, a full physical examination should be performed with particular focus on the mass. The mass will be more noticeable depending on whether it is deep or superficial and the body habitus of the patient. Sarcomas located below the fascia usually attain a large size prior to diagnosis. For example, a deep thigh mass is often significantly larger at the time of diagnosis compared to a more superficial mass on the forearm [44]. The size, exact anatomic location, overlying skin changes, neurological defects or muscle weakness, and vascular compromise are all important aspects of the physical exam (Fig. 27.2).

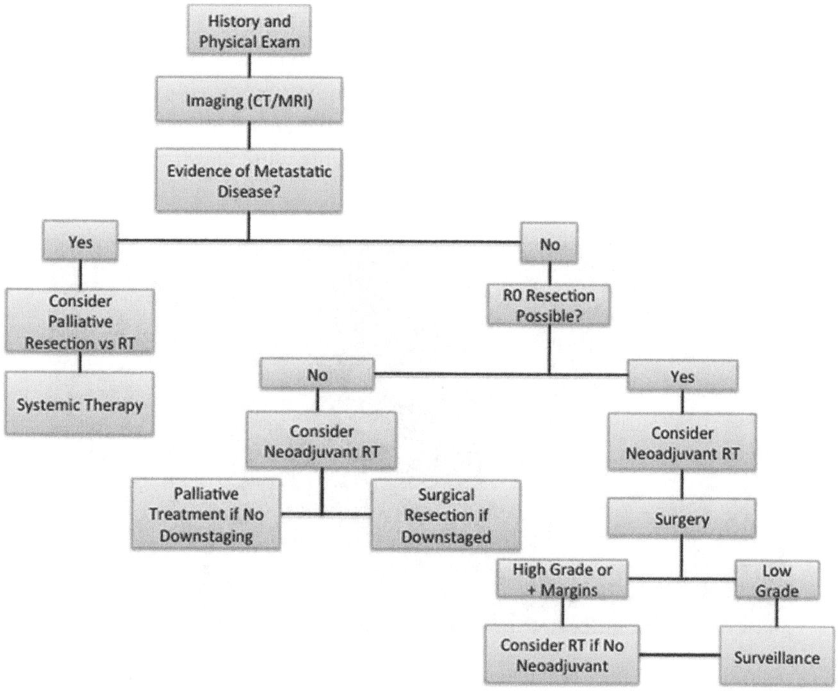

Fig. 27.1 Treatment algorithm for soft tissue sarcomas (*RT* radiation therapy, *R0* no gross or microscopic disease)

The next phase in an extremity sarcoma workup is to image the mass. Imaging allows for treatment planning prior to surgical resection by determining its size, location, association with surrounding structures, and potentially even histologic information. Imaging modalities include conventional radiography, ultrasound, computed tomography (CT) scan, and magnetic resonance imaging (MRI) (Fig. 27.3); each of these modalities has their relative merit and downsides. Conventional radiography provides good resolution of the bone trabecular, therefore providing information regarding bony involvement of the mass [45]. Ultrasound is helpful in determining if the mass is cystic or solid. It also helps guide tissue biopsy. CT provides cross-sectional imaging with the benefits of rapid image acquisition, decreased cost compared to MRI, and excellent bony and solid organ detail [45]. It can also be utilized when MRI is contraindicated. The addition of intravenous contrast allows for further determination of the vascularity of the tumor, the tumor size and location, and its anatomic association with large arteries and veins [46]. CT should also be used in the initial staging workup and in follow-up for the detection of metastatic disease in the lungs and liver, particularly for high-grade tumors. The issues with CT imaging include exposure to radiation, risk of allergic reactions to the contrast dye, and risk of contrast-induced nephropathy. MRI is the imaging modality of choice for soft tissue sarcomas of the extremity. This modality gives precise anatomical definition, revealing the relationship of the tumor to the investing fascia, size of the tumor, potential histologic characteristics, and proximity to neurovascular structures [47]. MRI can also be used to determine the enhancement pattern and amount of necrosis that can be followed during treatment [48]. The benefits of MRI include the lack of radiation exposure; problems include long acquisition time, increased expense, the contraindication in patients with metal implants, and anxiety in patients with claustrophobia [45].

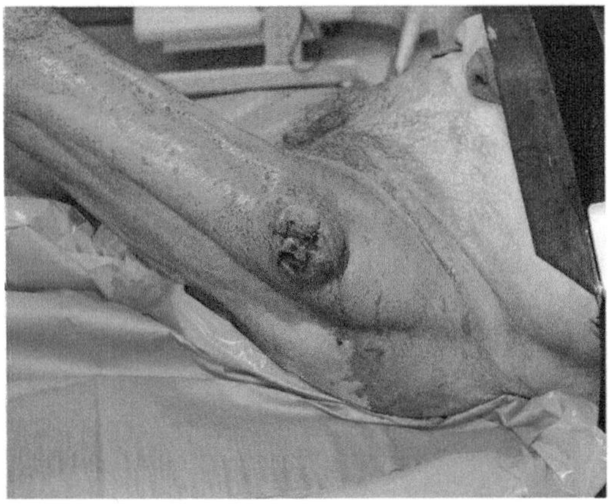

Fig. 27.2 Extremity sarcoma located on the lateral aspect of the patient's thigh (Courtesy of Quyen D. Chu, MD, MBA, FACS)

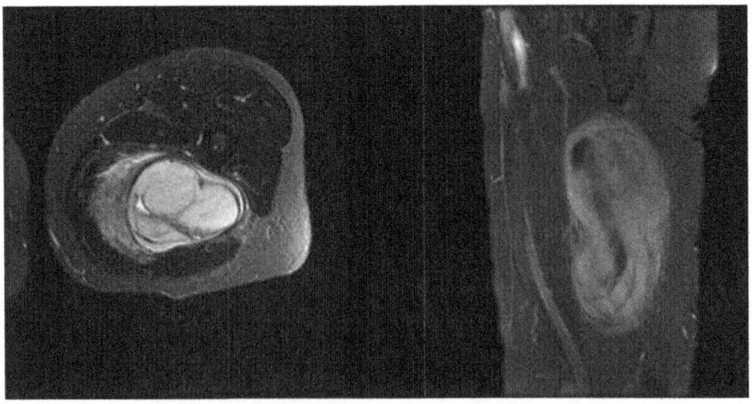

Fig. 27.3 MRI of a patient with a malignant fibrous histiocytoma (MFH) of the medial thigh. The patient underwent preoperative chemotherapy followed by a complete resection with a negative margin greater than 1 cm. Final pathology demonstrated no residual tumor (Courtesy of Quyen D. Chu, MD, MBA, FACS)

Once imaging has been completed, tissue biopsy may be indicated for tissue diagnosis. There are two ways to obtain tissue for a pathological diagnosis: needle biopsy and surgical biopsy. Needle biopsy can be divided into fine needle aspiration (FNA) and core needle biopsy. Both of these techniques can be done with and without radiological guidance. In the setting of extremity sarcoma, ultrasound is typically the radiologic guidance of choice. FNA is performed using a small gauge needle, passing it through the lesion multiple times on negative pressure. The downside of FNA is that it does not provide tissue architecture and supplies only a limited number of cells for evaluation and specialized pathologic investigations. Core needle biopsy is performed using a specialized biopsy needle that removes a core of tissue. This technique preserves the architecture of the tissue and typically provides enough cells for specialized immunostains while remaining minimally invasive. For these reasons, core needle biopsy has become the biopsy technique of choice [49]. When performing needle biopsy, the needle should enter through the proposed incision for resection on the skin so that the needle tract can be excised with the specimen. This eliminates the chance of local recurrence at the biopsy site [50]. Some have advocated tattooing the needle biopsy site to ensure removal at final resection.

The other choice for obtaining tissue is through an excisional or incisional surgical biopsy. Excisional surgical biopsy is an inadequate method for performing a biopsy on a mass concerning for sarcoma because a margin is not taken. In the setting of sarcoma, a second operation would need to be performed to obtain appropriate surgical margins. Incisional surgical biopsy is a reasonable approach when access to core needle biopsy is unavailable. To minimize recurrence at the biopsy site, a small incision along the direction of the proposed resection is performed.

Management of Primary Extremity Sarcoma

The mainstay of management of extremity sarcoma is surgical resection with negative margins [43]. This type of local control was historically obtained through amputation of the affected limb causing severe functional and psychological ramifications to the patient. Regardless, amputation was allowed for good local control and was the treatment of choice for decades [51]. In 1982, a prospective randomized clinical trial from the National Cancer Institute was published comparing limb-sparing surgery with radiation versus amputation for extremity sarcoma. The results showed no difference in 5-year overall survival rates between the two groups, and there was a nonsignificant increase in local recurrence rates in the limb-sparing surgery with radiation group [52]. These data support the use of limb-sparing surgery for the treatment of extremity sarcoma. Despite these results, amputation may still be the preferred choice of treatment depending on the involvement of major neurovascular structures and potential functional outcome after treatment.

The ultimate goal of resection includes complete removal of the tumor including the biopsy site and tract, while preserving a functional limb. An important aspect of limb-sparing resection is to ensure that negative margins are obtained. A number of studies have shown that gross and even microscopic margins lead to an increased risk of local recurrence [44, 53]. Although the prognostic significance of a positive margin is clear, the question remains what should a surgeon do if faced with a positive margin after resection. A retrospective review from MD Anderson Cancer Center of patients with positive margins after surgery showed that those who underwent re-resection to negative microscopic margins had a better local control than those who did not, despite the use of postoperative radiation therapy [54]. Therefore, it is recommended that a re-resection be preformed, if anatomically possible, to obtain negative margins. When performing these oncologic resections, it is important to make incisions longitudinally along the limb so that the mass may be resected with the best chance of primary closure. If the patient did not have preoperative radiation, it is important to keep the drains near the surgical field so they can be incorporated within the radiation field. If a large surgical defect is expected after resection, reconstruction planning is an important aspect of the perioperative surgical care.

For the most part, there is no role for lymph node sampling/dissection because the risk of regional metastasis is ≤5 %. However, it should be considered for patients with synovial sarcoma, epithelioid sarcomas, clear cell sarcomas, vascular sarcomas, and rhabdomyosarcomas since lymph node metastasis can occur in up to 24 % of patients [55].

Radiation therapy is used to improve local control when combined with limb-sparing surgery. A study from the National Cancer Institute highlighted the role of radiation therapy in a study randomizing patients undergoing limb-sparing surgery for sarcoma to receive postoperative radiation or no postoperative radiation. In patients with either high-grade sarcomas or low-grade sarcomas, there was a statistically significant improvement in local control if postoperative radiation was received. In this study, there was no difference in the overall survival between the two groups [56]. This study highlights the importance of radiation in the local control of sarcoma for patients undergoing limb-sparing surgery. External beam radiation has been the delivery method of choice; however, some groups have studied brachytherapy and intraoperative radiation therapy with and without external beam radiation, with good local control rates [57].

After surgical resection, the radiation field for external beam radiation can be quite extensive. There are also theoretical and logistical benefits associated with neoadjuvant radiation therapy [58]. Radiation doses in the preoperative setting tend to be lower, and the radiation field tends to be smaller if performed preoperatively. There is a decrease in long-term radiation effects, such as fibrosis and limb/joint dysfunction, if the radiation is given preoperatively [59]. In a prospective randomized study of preoperative radiation versus postoperative radiation in extremity sarcomas, there was no difference in local control rates between the two groups. There was also no difference in the margin status after the resection between the two groups. There was, however, an increase in the wound complication rate: 17 % for the postoperative radiation group compared to 35 % for the preoperative radiation group. Preoperative radiation also resulted in an increased rate of secondary wound closures (grafts and flaps). However, preoperative radiation was associated with decrease toxic skin effects from radiation, as compared to postoperative radiation [60]. The utility of radiation in a subset of patients with small or low-grade tumors remains controversial and deserves further investigation. According to the NCCN guidelines for stage I tumors with resection margins >1 cm, it is acceptable to omit radiation [5, 42].

Despite the good local control obtained from surgery and radiation therapy, there are a significant number of patients with high-grade sarcomas that will develop metastatic disease. The role of adjuvant chemotherapy with the goal of decreasing metastatic rates in primary sarcoma is uncertain. Most chemotherapy regimens have included Adriamycin, with well-defined toxicities. A meta-analysis of randomized trials showed an improvement in time-to-local and distant recurrence for those who received chemotherapy, but no improvement in overall survival [61]. The European Organization for Research and Treatment of Cancer concluded a multicenter randomized trial (EORTC 62931), in which patients with resected soft tissue sarcomas were randomized to receive a chemotherapy regimen or no chemotherapy. The trial showed no difference in overall survival (66 % vs. 67 %) or relapse-free survival between the two groups [62]. Given the unclear benefits of adjuvant chemotherapy, patients at high risk for metastatic disease should consider a discussion of the risks and benefits to chemotherapy with a medical oncologist.

The neoadjuvant approach to chemotherapy in sarcoma has been studied and may be even more controversial than the adjuvant approach. A single institution review of neoadjuvant chemotherapy alone in high-grade extremity sarcomas failed to show improvement in local control or overall survival [63]. Radiation has been added to the chemotherapy regimens in an attempt to improve both local control and decrease distant metastasis. A single institution review of this approach has shown that it has good long-term survival and tolerable toxicities, but there has yet to be a randomized study comparing the different approaches [64]. Another group is looking at the role of regional hyperthermia at the time of neoadjuvant chemotherapy for extremity sarcomas. In a prospective randomized multicenter trial comparing neoadjuvant chemotherapy to neoadjuvant chemotherapy with hyperthermia, they found that patients who had hyperthermia had improved local recurrence and disease-free survival [65]. Despite this interesting work, there is little data comparing an adjuvant approach for chemotherapy to a neoadjuvant approach so patients who are interested in this approach should consider clinical trials.

It is important to address the management of patients who present with synchronous metastatic disease, a clinical scenario that occurs in 12–23 % of patients with sarcomas [66, 67]. Kane et al. reported the outcome of 48 patients from a single institution who presented with synchronous metastases and treated with aggressive surgical resection of both the primary and metastatic sites [68]. Pulmonary metastases were most commonly encountered ($n=30$), followed by nodal ($n=11$) and liver ($n=4$) disease. Seventeen patients underwent resection of their metastatic site. Although the median survival for patients undergoing metastasectomy was slightly longer than that of patients with unresectable disease, the difference was not statistically significant. The authors concluded that resection of soft tissue sarcoma and synchronous metastases should be approached with caution and reserved for patients requiring symptomatic palliation [68].

Follow-Up and Surveillance

Once treatment has been completed, patients enter the surveillance phase. The goal of surveillance is to identify local regional recurrence or metastatic disease while it is still treatable. The clinical follow-up and surveillance of extremity sarcoma patients include a combination of history, physical examination, and imaging. Most recurrences occur within the first five years of initial treatment; therefore the surveillance schedule is more intense in the early phase and decreases after five years. It is recommended that a history and physical examination focusing on the local regional area of resection should be done every 3 months for the first 3 years, every 6 months for years 4–5, and annually after 5 years. There are no specific lab tests that are needed secondary to the lack of tumor markers available for this disease. MRI of the primary site should be obtained to look for local regional recurrence every 6 months for the first 3 years, annually from years 4–5, and only if suspected after year 5. If the patient has contraindication to MRI, then CT should be performed of the primary site. CT imaging of the chest in patients with high-grade sarcomas to rule out lung metastases is also important, with images recommended every 6 months for the first 3 years, and annually during years 4–5. Patients should also perform self-examinations on a regular basis at home and alert their treatment team if there are any changes. The above recommendations comply with the NCCN guidelines for surveillance of sarcoma patients [42].

Management of Recurrent and Metastatic Extremity Sarcoma

Extremity sarcomas may recur locally or at distant sites. A number of groups have reviewed prognostic factors that increase the likelihood of a local recurrence. There is a consensus that a positive margin and a recurrent sarcoma are both independent prognostic factors for local recurrence [69, 70]. The unfortunate event of locally recurrent extremity sarcoma provides significant challenges to the treatment team. If the recurrence was detected on physical examination, imaging is important to delineate relationship to surrounding anatomic structures and vasculature. A metastatic workup should also be done with CT scan of the chest to rule out synchronous metastasis. It is also important to obtain all prior clinical documentation (treatments, pathology) for treatment planning [71]. In patients with isolated local recurrence and no prior history of radiation treatments, it would be appropriate to consider preoperative radiation followed by surgical resection or surgical resection with adjuvant radiotherapy. If the patient has already received radiation, the options after re-excision include limited additional external beam radiotherapy, brachytherapy, or intraoperative radiation therapy. Isolated limb perfusion can be considered at centers conducting clinical trials. Surgically aggressive limb-sparing therapy can lead to very good local control rates. In a single institution retrospective review, 87 % of patients obtained durable local control with or without re-irradiation [72].

In addition to local recurrence, patients may also develop distant metastases. 20–40 % of patients with extremity sarcoma will have or develop pulmonary metastases. In a review from Memorial Sloan Kettering Cancer Center, the only prognostic factor that determined good outcome in patients with sarcoma metastatic to the lung was complete resection [73]. In a more recent retrospective review of 48 patients with metastatic sarcoma to the lung that had undergone pulmonary resection, the 5-year overall survival rate was found to be 52 % [74]. These data highlight that careful selection of patients combined with an aggressive approach in resection of pulmonary metastases can result in favorable outcomes.

If resection is not possible, the efficacy of chemotherapy regimens is currently limited. The standard doxorubicin-based regimens have modest clinical efficacy and significant treatment-associated toxicities [75]. However, newer regimens show promise in early phase testing. In a phase II trial of gemcitabine and docetaxel compared to gemcitabine alone, there was an increase in both progression-free survival and overall survival. Unfortunately, the combined regimen was also quite toxic [76]. Trabectedin, a marine-derived antineoplastic compound, has also shown promise in treating metastatic liposarcoma and leiomyosarcoma [77].

Evaluation of Retroperitoneal Sarcomas

Patients with retroperitoneal sarcomas (RPS) commonly present with symptoms of abdominal fullness or obstruction involving the gastrointestinal or renal systems. Pain, neurologic symptoms, and weight loss are other common presenting symptoms. Symptoms are initially vague in nature, precluding many patients from seeking early medical attention. The relatively non-confining space of the retroperitoneum can conceal a mass for an extended period of time, allowing tumors to become quite large prior to the development of clinical symptoms.

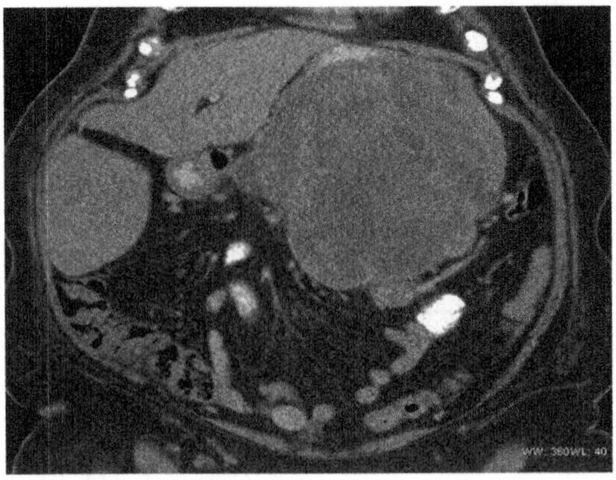

Fig. 27.4 Retroperitoneal sarcoma: large mass suspicious for a retroperitoneal sarcoma (Courtesy of Quyen D. Chu, MD, MBA, FACS)

Patients who present with suspicious symptoms of an abdominal mass should undergo imaging with a CT of the abdomen and pelvis (Fig. 27.4). A CT chest is performed to complete the staging workup and evaluate for metastatic disease. A well-described fatty tumor of the retroperitoneum without hyperdense areas is considered a well-differentiated lipomatous tumor or well-differentiated liposarcoma. Both diagnoses require surgical resection and biopsy is not usually indicated. A lipomatous tumor of the retroperitoneum with higher dense areas is diagnostic for retroperitoneal liposarcoma. The higher dense areas may represent areas of dedifferentiation or simply areas of different liposarcoma histologic subtypes. Image-guided biopsy is indicated if therapy other than surgery is considered as first-line treatment [78]. Retroperitoneal masses with little or no fatty component have a large differential diagnosis that includes germ cell tumors, lymphoma, abscess, renal and adrenal tumors, neurogenic tumors, undifferentiated carcinoma of primary or metastatic origin, and sarcoma. Because of the extensive differential diagnosis, most authors advocate for an image-guided tissue biopsy in these tumors. Any soft tissue mass in an adult that is larger than 5 cm, growing or persistent beyond 4–6 weeks, that is not characteristic of a liposarcoma should be biopsied [6]. FNA and core biopsy can both be used for diagnosing soft tissue sarcomas. Core biopsy is 95 % accurate in diagnosing sarcomas, whereas the accuracy of FNA biopsy is largely dependent on the experience of the cytopathologist interpreting the results [41]. One advantage of core biopsy over FNA is that cores provide tumor architecture, and this allows for identification of histologic subtype and grading. The benefit of assessing tumor grade has made core biopsy the first choice for biopsy techniques. Biopsies should be approached from the retroperitoneum and should avoid the peritoneal cavity to decrease contamination with tumor cells. Additional imaging such as high-resolution CT or MRI may be indicated to help plan surgical approach and better delineate involvement of the muscles, nerves, vessels, bone, and vertebral foramen. If resection includes removal of a kidney, a preoperative nuclear renal function scan is indicated to assess the function of the remaining kidney. The only lab work indicated is the usual preoperative labs of electrolytes, coagulation studies, hemoglobin, and platelet count. Currently there are no serum tumor markers available for soft tissue sarcomas.

Management of Primary Retroperitoneal Sarcomas

A multidisciplinary approach involving surgical oncology, medical oncology, and radiation oncology is crucial to the management of these tumors. Treatment requires thoughtful planning and timing of different modalities to offer the best functional and oncologic outcomes for patients.

As in extremity sarcomas, surgical resection with negative margins is the standard of care and primary treatment for localized retroperitoneal sarcomas (RPS). En bloc resection of involved surrounding organs may be necessary to obtain clear margins. Resection of the colon, mesocolon, and muscle as part of the en bloc resection is well tolerated with limited consequences. The resection of a kidney, spleen, or distal pancreas as part of the en bloc resection has minimal short-term morbidities, and the removal of such organs is usually tolerated (Fig. 27.5). When the en bloc resection involves the head of the pancreas, duodenum, major vessels and nerves, or the liver, complication rates can be significant, and resection of such organs is usually not performed unless there is macroscopic involvement [78]. Complete negative margin resections of retroperitoneal sarcomas have been reported between 50 and 67 % [79]. Obtaining negative microscopic margins is difficult due to the extremely large mass of tumors, the extent of surface area involved, and the anatomic constraints of tumor location in the retroperitoneum. Although achieving negative margins is difficult, it has been illustrated that the patient who obtain negative margins has better outcomes [38]. Complete surgical resection improves median survival in patients with primary retroperitoneal sarcomas [80]. The 5-year survival rate for patients with complete surgical resection and R0 margins is 103 months compared to 18 months for incomplete surgical resection and positive margins [42, 81]. Surgery remains the mainstay of treatment for patients with locally resectable disease.

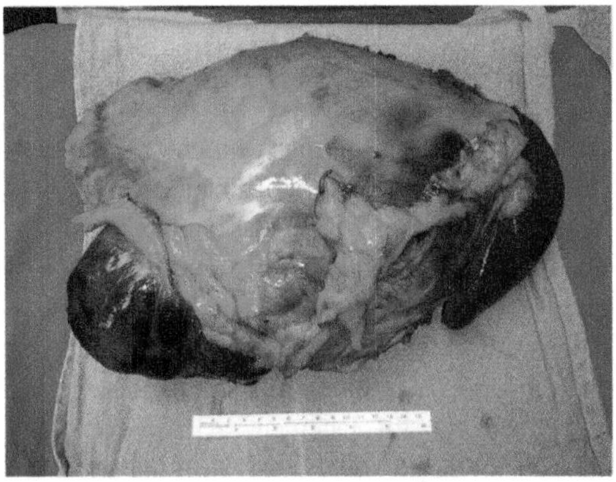

Fig. 27.5 Gross specimen of a retroperitoneal sarcoma. Patient underwent a total gastrectomy, distal pancreatectomy, and splenectomy for a large retroperitoneal leiomyosarcoma (Courtesy of Quyen D. Chu, MD, MBA, FACS)

The exact role of radiation therapy in retroperitoneal sarcoma is difficult to define. Radiation has a well-established role in extremity sarcomas;

however, the adjacent radiosensitive structures in the retroperitoneum limit the use of this modality in retroperitoneal sarcomas. Single institutional studies have shown an improvement in local control rates with the addition of radiation therapy to surgery for retroperitoneal sarcomas [82, 83]. The advantages, disadvantages, and feasibility of preoperative, intraoperative, and postoperative radiation therapies are based on observational and retrospective studies [6]. Preoperative radiation allows for displacement of adjacent structures by the large tumor mass, limiting exposure of other critical structures (i.e., small bowel) to radiation thus decreasing the rate of toxicity. Preoperative radiation also clearly establishes boundaries of the intended treatment fields. Postoperative radiation on the other hand allows for better assessment of tumor histology and grade, which enables selection of patients most likely to benefit from radiation therapy. However, when the large tumor is removed, a void is created and filled with other critical structures. These structures are exposed to the radiation, resulting in increased gastrointestinal toxicity with postoperative radiation therapy. The lack of level 1 evidence and the varied radiation treatment plans in published series make discernment of the timing of radiation in retroperitoneal sarcomas difficult to determine. Preoperative radiation therapy with complete surgical resection has been associated with improved recurrence-free survival, disease-specific survival, and overall survival. The 5-year local recurrence-free survival of 60 %, disease-specific survival of 46 %, and overall survival of 61 % were demonstrated in two prospective trials of patients with intermediate and high-grade retroperitoneal sarcomas who had preoperative radiation therapy and aggressive surgical resection with R0 or R1 status [84]. Postoperative radiation has been associated with improved relapse-free survival but has not impacted overall survival [85, 86]. The addition of intraoperative radiation therapy to aggressive surgical resection and preoperative external beam radiation improves local recurrence-free rates to 83 % from 61 % and overall survival rates to 74 % from 30 % when compared to surgical resection alone [87, 88]. At our institution, preoperative radiation with or without intraoperative radiation has become the standard approach to RPS. Published data from our institution has shown one- and two-year local control rates of 64 and 50 % and OS of 90 % at 1 year and 74 % at 2 years with minimal toxicity from preoperative radiation [58].

Current recommendations state that for all patients with surgically resected disease and R1 margins who did not receive preoperative radiation should undergo postoperative radiation [42]. Radiation should also be considered in patients with an R0 resection and high-grade tumors [42]. Patients who received preoperative radiation and underwent surgical resection with R1 margins may receive an additional radiation boost to the tumor bed [42].

The role of chemotherapy for localized soft tissue sarcomas of the retroperitoneum is limited. Most commonly, chemotherapy for localized disease is used as a radiation sensitizer or as neoadjuvant cytoreductive therapy to improve achievement of an R0 resection. A recent meta-analysis by Pervaiz et al. found a marginal benefit to adjuvant chemotherapy with respect to local recurrence, distant recurrence, overall recurrence, and overall survival [89]. Their work demonstrated an odds ratio (OR) for local recurrence of 0.73 (95 % CI 0.56–0.94; $p=0.02$) and an OR for overall survival of 0.56 (95 % CI 036–0.85; $p=0.01$) in favor of adjuvant chemotherapy. The greatest benefit was achieved with a combination-based chemotherapy of doxorubicin and ifosfamide [89].

Follow-Up and Surveillance

Local recurrence is a major morbidity and a leading cause of mortality in patients with retroperitoneal sarcomas. Because 40–60 % of patients with retroperitoneal sarcomas will develop a recurrence, close follow-up is vital to improving patient outcomes [42].

According to the NCCN guidelines, patients who undergo surgical resection and have an R0 margin status should have a history and physical exam and CT of the abdomen and pelvis every

3–6 months for 2–3 years and then annually. Patients who undergo surgical resection and have an R1 margin status or have a high-grade tumor with an R0 margin status should have a history and physical exam and CT of the abdomen and pelvis every 3–6 months for 2–3 years, then every 6 months for 2 years, then annually.

Management of Recurrent and Metastatic Retroperitoneal Sarcomas

Recurrence is common with retroperitoneal sarcomas. 40–60 % of resected retroperitoneal sarcomas will develop recurrence. Each local recurrence makes complete surgical resection more difficult and less likely.

Recurrent retroperitoneal sarcomas are evaluated with a biopsy and staged with CT imaging of the chest, abdomen, and pelvis (Figs. 27.7 and 27.8). Once metastatic disease is ruled out and the recurrence is determined to be local, the patient should undergo complete surgical resection with a curative intent, if feasible (Figs. 27.6, 27.7, 27.8, 27.9 and 27.10). The success for complete resection is favorable with the first recurrence but significantly decreases with each additional recurrence. Lewis et al. showed that 57 % of patients with a first local recurrence were able to undergo complete surgical resection where only 22 % of second and 10 % of third recurrences were completely resected [81].

The role of surgery in metastatic disease is dependent on multiple factors. Data suggest that patients with isolated pulmonary metastases may have an improved disease-free survival with pulmonary metastasectomy [90]. Patients with abdominal sarcomatosis, which is more common with retroperitoneal sarcomas, may also benefit from metastasectomy. The liver is a common site of metastatic disease for patients with retroperitoneal sarcomas. Rehders et al. showed 5- and

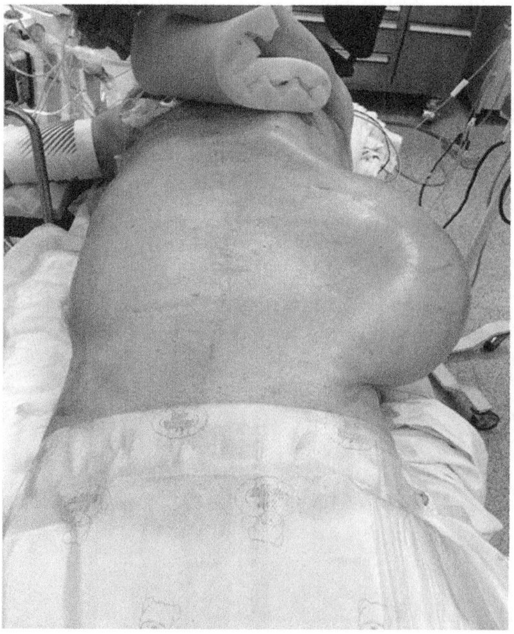

Fig. 27.6 A patient with a recurrent liposarcoma (Courtesy of Quyen D. Chu, MD, MBA, FACS)

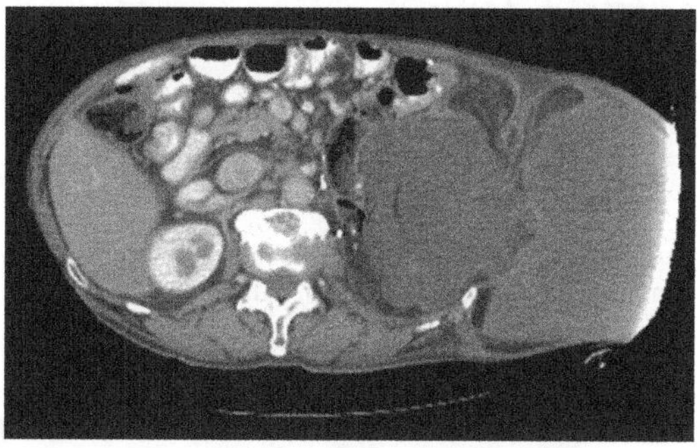

Fig. 27.7 A patient with a recurrent liposarcoma (Courtesy of Quyen D. Chu, MD, MBA, FACS)

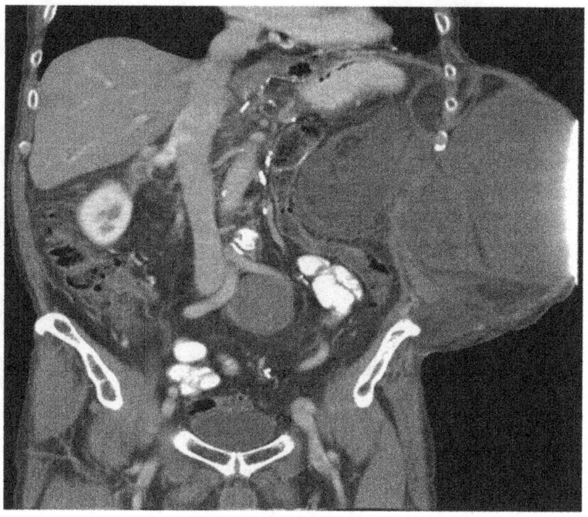

Fig. 27.8 A patient with a recurrent liposarcoma (Courtesy of Quyen D. Chu, MD, MBA, FACS)

10-year survival rates of 49 % and 33 % respectively with median survival of 44 months after hepatic metastasectomy [91]. An important consideration for metastasectomy is the number and location of metastases and the behavior of the tumors. Complete surgical resection of metastatic disease is a significant prognostic factor for improved survival [73]. Patients with slow-growing, low-grade metastases that are stable over a significant period of time and have a lengthy disease-free interval between the primary sarcoma and development of metastases are likely to achieve the most benefit from surgical resection [90, 91]. The majority of patients with advanced retroperitoneal sarcomas are often too advanced to benefit from metastasectomy. However, many of these patients will develop significant symptoms that require surgery for palliation. Yeh et al. showed that 71 % of patients had relief of symptoms at 30 days after palliative surgery [92]. The durability of symptom relief is limited, and at 100 days from palliative surgery, only 54 % of patients had relief of symptoms [92]. Surgical intervention for advanced disease requires highly selected patients to ensure the best chance of improved disease-free survival or palliation of symptoms.

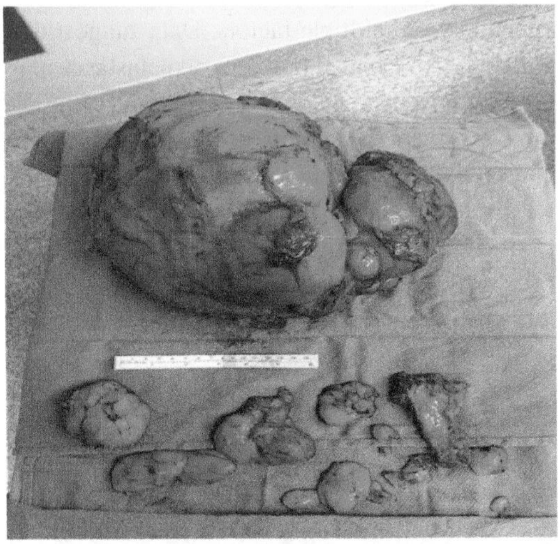

Fig. 27.9 A patient with a recurrent liposarcoma (Courtesy of Quyen D. Chu, MD, MBA, FACS)

Patients with recurrent or advanced disease should also receive radiation therapy and chemotherapy if not included in prior treatments. Despite the limited benefit of chemotherapy in localized retroperitoneal sarcomas, there is a role for chemotherapy in advanced sarcomas. Doxorubicin is considered first-line treatment for

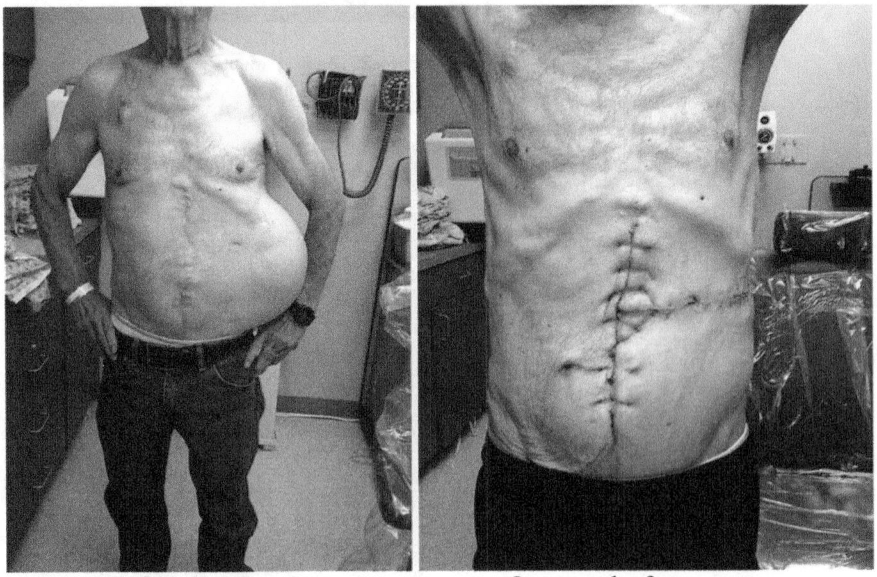

Before Surgery One month after surgery

Fig. 27.10 A patient with a recurrent liposarcoma (Courtesy of Quyen D. Chu, MD, MBA, FACS)

stage IV disease. The addition of ifosfamide to doxorubicin improves the response rate but does not impact overall survival compared to single-agent doxorubicin [5, 93]. Other cytotoxic medications that can be used as single agents or in combination with doxorubicin include gemcitabine, epirubicin, or paclitaxel. The drugs most commonly used for palliation of symptoms are doxorubicin and ifosfamide [5].

The administration of chemotherapy and/or radiation therapy preoperatively or postoperatively in the setting of metastasectomy is unknown, and discussion at a multidisciplinary tumor board is highly recommended.

Gastrointestinal Stromal Tumors (GIST)

For completeness, GISTs will be briefly discussed. A more in-depth discussion can be found in Chap. 28 on GIST. GISTs are the most common mesenchymal tumors. They can arise anywhere along the gastrointestinal tract, but the stomach and the small intestine are the most common sites [94]. These tumors are extraluminal in location, involving the muscularis propria of the intestinal wall. 95 % of tumors are associated with an activating tyrosine kinase receptor protein mutation: *KIT* or *CD117* [95]. 5 % of GIST tumors do not contain this mutation and are considered *KIT*-negative GISTs. A small percentage of the *KIT*-negative tumors will have a mutation in the platelet-derived growth factor receptor-alpha gene [96].

Most GISTs do not elicit symptoms and are found incidentally during physical examinations or endoscopic procedures. If symptoms are present, they are usually related to mass effect of the tumor and result in nausea, emesis, early satiety, pain, and/or abdominal distention. A significant number of GIST tumors are discovered on cross-sectional imaging for abdominal pain. Once the diagnosis of GIST has been suggested by imaging, endoscopic ultrasound may be performed to help delineate the full depth of the tumor. Preoperative biopsy is only indicated if (1) the diagnosis is in question, (2) a diagnosis of lymphoma is to be excluded, or (3) neoadjuvant therapy is being considered.

Surgical resection is the mainstay of treatment. Microscopically negative margin is the goal of surgery. A 1 cm gross surgical margin should be taken to ensure an R0 resection. 85 % of patients with primary GIST will be candidates for complete surgical resection, and 70–90 % of cases will have negative margins [97–99]. The recurrence rate for primary GIST after complete surgical resection ranges from 26 to 44 % [97, 98, 100].

Patients with high-risk pathologic findings (size >5 cm, mitotic rate >5 per 50 high-powered field) benefit from postoperative imatinib therapy. Imatinib is a selective inhibitor of the *KIT* protein-tyrosine kinase. Multiple studies have shown an improvement in recurrence-free survival when imatinib therapy is given postoperatively to completely resected GIST tumors. A double-blinded randomized trial done by the American College of Surgeons Oncology Group (ACOSOG Z9001) showed a prolonged recurrence-free survival of 98 % *versus* 83 % for patients given 400 mg/day of imatinib therapy for one year after surgical resection compared to patients receiving placebo [101]. Another recently published trial by the Scandinavian Sarcoma Group XVIII found that 36 months of postoperative imatinib therapy improved recurrence-free survival and overall survival when compared to 12 months for patients at high risk of recurrence [102]. Currently the NCCN guidelines recommend 36 months of imatinib therapy for primary resected GIST at high risk of recurrence [42].

The treatment of choice for unresectable primary gastrointestinal stromal tumors and recurrent or metastatic gastrointestinal stromal tumors is imatinib therapy. Phase II and III trials have shown good response rates and improved progression-free survival (PFS) among unresectable or metastatic GIST patients taking imatinib therapy [103–106]. The B2222 trial confirmed durable disease control with imatinib in patients with advanced GIST. The estimated 9-year overall survival from this trial was 35 %. Thirty-eight percent of patients responded to treatments and

49 % of patients had stabilization of their disease [107]. Current recommendations include 400 mg/day of imatinib therapy with dose escalation upon tumor progression [42]. For patients with nonmetastatic unresectable primary GIST, preoperative imatinib therapy has been associated with a 60 % partial response rate and eventual surgical resection in 36 % of patients [108]. The NCCN guidelines recommend preoperative imatinib therapy in locally advanced GIST with the hope of downstaging for surgical resection [42]. Preoperative treatment should continue as long as cross-sectional imaging shows continued response to therapy.

Follow-Up and Surveillance

According to the current NCCN guidelines, patients with resected localized GIST should undergo a complete history and physical exam every 3–6 months with cross-sectional imaging of the abdomen and pelvis every 3–6 months for 5 years, then annually after 5 years [42].

Salient Points

- Soft tissue sarcomas can be located throughout the body. The extremity and retroperitoneum are the two most common sites of soft tissue sarcomas.
- The majority of soft tissue sarcomas have complex unbalanced karyotypes resulting from a variety of genetic mutations.
- Most common subtypes are malignant fibrous histiocytoma, liposarcoma, and leiomyosarcoma.
- Tumor grade, tumor size, tumor location, margin status, and primary tumor versus recurrent tumor have all been shown to carry prognostic implications for soft tissue sarcomas.
- Grade is the strongest predictor of patient outcome.
- Workup and evaluation of sarcomas involve a complete history and physical exam, cross-sectional imaging studies, evaluation of distant disease, and discussion at a multidisciplinary tumor board for a definitive treatment plan.
- CT of the chest should be considered for high-grade and large extremity sarcomas.
- Fine-needle aspiration or core needle biopsy can be performed to obtain a diagnosis for extremity masses.
- For extremity lesions larger than 5 cm, an incisional biopsy is recommended.
- The goal of surgery for extremity sarcomas is functional limb-sparing surgery.
- Re-resection to achieve a negative margin is recommended for extremity sarcoma.
- Incision should be placed longitudinally along the limb for extremity sarcoma.
- There is no role for lymph node sampling except for synovial sarcoma, epithelioid sarcomas, clear cell sarcomas, vascular sarcomas, and rhabdomyosarcoma.
- Postoperative radiation improves local control but not overall survival for extremity sarcoma.
- Postoperative radiation can be omitted for stage 1 tumor with a resection margin >1 cm.
- There is no difference in local control rates or overall survival rates between preoperative radiation versus postoperative radiation, although there is an increased in wound complication rate in the preoperative group.
- The goal of surgery for RPS is en bloc resection of tumor and involved adjacent organs.
- Radiation therapy plays an important role in local tumor control for both extremity and retroperitoneal sarcomas.
- The role of chemotherapy is not well understood in the setting of adjuvant therapy. However, for metastatic disease, combination therapy with doxorubicin and ifosfamide plays an important role in palliative treatment.
- 40–60 % of soft tissue sarcomas will recur. Treatment of local recurrences involves complete surgical resection when appropriate.
- 95 % of GISTs have a *KIT* mutation.
- Standard treatment of GIST involves complete surgical resection and 3 years of adjuvant imatinib for high-risk tumors.

Study Questions

1. The most common location of soft tissue sarcoma is:
   A. Retroperitoneum
   B. Extremity

   C. Head and neck
   D. Visceral
2. The three most common histologic subtypes of soft tissue sarcomas are:
   A. Liposarcoma, angiosarcoma, and leiomyosarcoma
   B. Synovial sarcoma, leiomyosarcoma, and rhabdomyosarcoma
   C. Liposarcoma, leiomyosarcoma, and malignant peripheral nerve sheath tumors
   D. Liposarcoma, leiomyosarcoma, and malignant fibrous histiocytoma
3. Prognostic markers for soft tissue sarcomas include:
   A. Tumor size, tumor grade, gender, and mutational status
   B. Tumor size, tumor location, resection margin, and tumor grade
   C. Tumor location, tumor grade, mutational status, and recurrent versus primary tumor
   D. Tumor grade, tumor size, tumor location, and gender
4. A 33-year-old male was recently diagnosed with a well-differentiated liposarcoma of the posterior lower left leg. MRI revealed a 7 cm lobulated mass superficial to the fascia. Treatment options include:
   A. Surgery followed by adjuvant doxorubicin
   B. Radiation alone
   C. Amputation of the left leg
   D. Limb-sparing surgical resection of the left lower leg mass
5. A 67-year-old female with a history of a well-differentiated retroperitoneal liposarcoma resected 3 years ago presents for routine follow-up. On CT of the abdomen/pelvis, two new lesions are identified. One is located in the right psoas perirenal area (primary surgical bed) without invasion or involvement of surrounding organs. The second lesion is located in the right pelvis with concern for involvement of the right ureter. The next step in treatment is:
   A. Cytotoxic chemotherapy with doxorubicin and ifosfamide
   B. CT of the chest to r/o pulmonary metastases
   C. Surgical resection of the primary bed tumor alone
   D. En bloc surgical resection of both tumors and surrounding involved organs
6. The mutation associated with GIST is:
   A. p53
   B. Rb1
   C. APC
   D. KIT
7. Treatment for localized high-risk GIST includes:
   A. Surgical resection alone
   B. Surgical resection with radiation therapy
   C. Surgical resection with adjuvant imatinib for 1 year
   D. Surgical resection with adjuvant imatinib for 3 years
8. The characteristics of high-risk GIST include:
   A. Size >10 cm, mitoses >5/50 hpf
   B. Size >5 cm, mitoses >5/50 hpf
   C. Size >5 cm, mitoses >10/50 hpf
   D. Size >10, mitoses >10/50 hpf
9. The drug treatment of choice for metastatic GIST is:
   A. Imatinib
   B. Vemurafenib
   C. Doxorubicin
   D. Gemcitabine

Sarcoma Chapter Question Answers

1. B
2. D
3. B
4. D
5. B
6. D
7. D
8. B
9. A

References

1. Association of Directors of Anatomic and Surgical Pathology. Recommendations for the reporting of soft tissue sarcomas. Hum Pathol. 1999;30(1):3–7. PubMed PMID: 9923919. Epub 1999/01/29. eng.
2. Lahat G, Lazar A, Lev D. Sarcoma epidemiology and etiology: potential environmental and genetic factors. Surg Clin North Am. 2008;88(3):451–81, v. PubMed PMID: 18514694. Epub 2008/06/03. eng.
3. Siegel R, Naishadham D, Jemal A. Cancer statistics, 2012. CA Cancer J Clin. 2012;62(1):10–29. PubMed PMID: 22237781. Epub 2012/01/13. eng.
4. Burningham Z, Hashibe M, Spector L, Schiffman JD. The epidemiology of sarcoma. Clin Sarcoma Res. 2012;2(1):14. PubMed PMID: 23036164.

Pubmed Central PMCID: 3564705. Epub 2012/10/06. eng.
5. General Information about Adult Soft Tissue Sarcoma: National Cancer Institute; [updated 8/8/2012]. Available from: www.cancer.gov.
6. Pisters P, O'Sullivan B, Maki RG. Soft tissue sarcomas. In: Hong WK, Bast R, Hait WN, Kufe DW, Pollock RE, Weichselbaum RR, Holland JF, Frei III E, editors. Holland Frei Cancer Medicine 8. Shelton: People's Medical Publishing House; 2010.
7. Brady MS, Gaynor JJ, Brennan MF. Radiation-associated sarcoma of bone and soft tissue. Arch Surg. 1992;127(12):1379–85. PubMed PMID: 1365680. Epub 1992/12/01. eng.
8. Karlsson P, Holmberg E, Samuelsson A, Johansson KA, Wallgren A. Soft tissue sarcoma after treatment for breast cancer – a Swedish population-based study. Eur J Cancer. 1998;34(13):2068–75. PubMed PMID: 10070313. Epub 1999/03/10. eng.
9. Falk H, Herbert J, Crowley S, Ishak KG, Thomas LB, Popper H, et al. Epidemiology of hepatic angiosarcoma in the United States: 1964–1974. Environ Health Perspect. 1981;41:107–13. PubMed PMID: 7199426. Pubmed Central PMCID: 1568861. Epub 1981/10/01. eng.
10. Penn I. Sarcomas in organ allograft recipients. Transplantation. 1995;60(12):1485–91. PubMed PMID: 8545879. Epub 1995/12/27. eng.
11. Deyrup AT, Lee VK, Hill CE, Cheuk W, Toh HC, Kesavan S, et al. Epstein-Barr virus-associated smooth muscle tumors are distinctive mesenchymal tumors reflecting multiple infection events: a clinicopathologic and molecular analysis of 29 tumors from 19 patients. Am J Surg Pathol. 2006;30(1):75–82. PubMed PMID: 16330945. Epub 2005/12/07. eng.
12. Stewart FW, Treves N. Lymphangiosarcoma in postmastectomy lymphedema; a report of six cases in elephantiasis chirurgica. Cancer. 1948;1(1):64–81. PubMed PMID: 18867440. Epub 1948/05/01. eng.
13. Woodward AH, Ivins JC, Soule EH. Lymphangiosarcoma arising in chronic lymphedematous extremities. Cancer. 1972;30(2):562–72. PubMed PMID: 5051679. Epub 1972/08/01. eng.
14. Rubin BP, Heinrich MC, Corless CL. Gastrointestinal stromal tumor. Lancet. 2007;369(9574):1731–41. PubMed PMID: 17512858. Epub 2007/05/22. eng.
15. Li FP, Fraumeni Jr JF, Mulvihill JJ, Blattner WA, Dreyfus MG, Tucker MA, et al. A cancer family syndrome in twenty-four kindreds. Cancer Res. 1988;48(18):5358–62. PubMed PMID: 3409256. Epub 1988/09/15. eng.
16. Pollack IF, Mulvihill JJ. Neurofibromatosis 1 and 2. Brain Pathol. 1997;7(2):823–36. PubMed PMID: 9161732. Epub 1997/04/01. eng.
17. Moll AC, Imhof SM, Bouter LM, Kuik DJ, Den Otter W, Bezemer PD, et al. Second primary tumors in patients with hereditary retinoblastoma: a register-based follow-up study, 1945–1994. Int J Cancer. 1996;67(4):515–9. PubMed PMID: 8759610. Epub 1996/08/07. eng.
18. Wu JM, Montgomery E. Classification and pathology. Surg Clin North Am. 2008;88(3):483–520, v–vi. PubMed PMID: 18514695. Epub 2008/06/03. eng.
19. Toro JR, Travis LB, Wu HJ, Zhu K, Fletcher CD, Devesa SS. Incidence patterns of soft tissue sarcomas, regardless of primary site, in the surveillance, epidemiology and end results program, 1978–2001: an analysis of 26,758 cases. Int J Cancer. 2006;119(12):2922–30. PubMed PMID: 17013893. Epub 2006/10/03. eng.
20. Thway K. Pathology of soft tissue sarcomas. Clin Oncol. 2009;21(9):695–705. PubMed PMID: 19734027. Epub 2009/09/08. eng.
21. Barretina J, Taylor BS, Banerji S, Ramos AH, Lagos-Quintana M, Decarolis PL, et al. Subtype-specific genomic alterations define new targets for soft-tissue sarcoma therapy. Nat Genet. 2010;42(8):715–21. PubMed PMID: 20601955. Pubmed Central PMCID: 2911503. Epub 2010/07/06. eng.
22. Gibault L, Perot G, Chibon F, Bonnin S, Lagarde P, Terrier P, et al. New insights in sarcoma oncogenesis: a comprehensive analysis of a large series of 160 soft tissue sarcomas with complex genomics. J Pathol. 2011;223(1):64–71. PubMed PMID: 21125665. Epub 2010/12/03. eng.
23. Taylor BS, Barretina J, Maki RG, Antonescu CR, Singer S, Ladanyi M. Advances in sarcoma genomics and new therapeutic targets. Nat Rev Cancer. 2011;11(8):541–57. PubMed PMID: 21753790. Pubmed Central PMCID: 3361898. Epub 2011/07/15. eng.
24. Teicher BA. Searching for molecular targets in sarcoma. Biochem Pharmacol. 2012;84(1):1–10. PubMed PMID: 22387046. Epub 2012/03/06. eng.
25. Bernstein M, Kovar H, Paulussen M, Randall RL, Schuck A, Teot LA, et al. Ewing's sarcoma family of tumors: current management. Oncologist. 2006;11(5):503–19. PubMed PMID: 16720851. Epub 2006/05/25. eng.
26. Bovee JV, Hogendoorn PC. Molecular pathology of sarcomas: concepts and clinical implications. Virchows Arch. 2010;456(2):193–9. PubMed PMID: 19787372. Pubmed Central PMCID: 2828555. Epub 2009/09/30. eng.
27. Horvai AE, DeVries S, Roy R, O'Donnell RJ, Waldman F. Similarity in genetic alterations between paired well-differentiated and dedifferentiated components of dedifferentiated liposarcoma. Mod Pathol. 2009;22(11):1477–88. PubMed PMID: 19734852. Epub 2009/09/08. eng.
28. Gregorian C, Nakashima J, Dry SM, Nghiemphu PL, Smith KB, Ao Y, et al. PTEN dosage is essential for neurofibroma development and malignant transformation. Proc Natl Acad Sci U S A. 2009;106(46):19479–84. PubMed PMID: 19846776. Pubmed Central PMCID: 2765459. Epub 2009/10/23. eng.
29. van Beerendonk HM, Rozeman LB, Taminiau AH, Sciot R, Bovee JV, Cleton-Jansen AM, et al.

Molecular analysis of the INK4A/INK4A-ARF gene locus in conventional (central) chondrosarcomas and enchondromas: indication of an important gene for tumour progression. J Pathol. 2004;202(3):359–66. PubMed PMID: 14991902. Epub 2004/03/03. eng.
30. Singer S, Socci ND, Ambrosini G, Sambol E, Decarolis P, Wu Y, et al. Gene expression profiling of liposarcoma identifies distinct biological types/subtypes and potential therapeutic targets in well-differentiated and dedifferentiated liposarcoma. Cancer Res. 2007;67(14):6626–36. PubMed PMID: 17638873. Epub 2007/07/20. eng.
31. Pfeifer JD, Hill DA, O'Sullivan MJ, Dehner LP. Diagnostic gold standard for soft tissue tumours: morphology or molecular genetics? Histopathology. 2000;37(6):485–500. PubMed PMID: 11122430. Epub 2000/12/21. eng.
32. Hill DA, O'Sullivan MJ, Zhu X, Vollmer RT, Humphrey PA, Dehner LP, et al. Practical application of molecular genetic testing as an aid to the surgical pathologic diagnosis of sarcomas: a prospective study. Am J Surg Pathol. 2002;26(8):965–77. PubMed PMID: 12170083. Epub 2002/08/10. eng.
33. Sorensen PH, Lynch JC, Qualman SJ, Tirabosco R, Lim JF, Maurer HM, et al. PAX3-FKHR and PAX7-FKHR gene fusions are prognostic indicators in alveolar rhabdomyosarcoma: a report from the children's oncology group. J Clin Oncol. 2002;20(11):2672–9. PubMed PMID: 12039929. Epub 2002/06/01. eng.
34. Edge SB, Compton CC. The American Joint Committee on Cancer: the 7th edition of the AJCC cancer staging manual. New York: Springer; 2010.
35. Costa J, Wesley RA, Glatstein E, Rosenberg SA. The grading of soft tissue sarcomas. Results of a clinicohistopathologic correlation in a series of 163 cases. Cancer. 1984;53(3):530–41. PubMed PMID: 6692258. Epub 1984/02/01. eng.
36. Guillou L, Coindre JM, Bonichon F, Nguyen BB, Terrier P, Collin F, et al. Comparative study of the National Cancer Institute and French Federation of Cancer Centers Sarcoma Group grading systems in a population of 410 adult patients with soft tissue sarcoma. J Clin Oncol. 1997;15(1):350–62. PubMed PMID: 8996162. Epub 1997/01/01. eng.
37. Myhre-Jensen O, Kaae S, Madsen EH, Sneppen O. Histopathological grading in soft-tissue tumours. Relation to survival in 261 surgically treated patients. Acta Pathol Microbiol Immunol Scand A. 1983;91(2):145–50. PubMed PMID: 6846018. Epub 1983/03/01. eng.
38. Kotilingam D, Lev DC, Lazar AJ, Pollock RE. Staging soft tissue sarcoma: evolution and change. CA Cancer J Clin. 2006;56(5):282–91, quiz 314–5. PubMed PMID: 17005597. Epub 2006/09/29. eng.
39. Linehan DC, Lewis JJ, Leung D, Brennan MF. Influence of biologic factors and anatomic site in completely resected liposarcoma. J Clin Oncol. 2000;18(8):1637–43. PubMed PMID: 10764423. Epub 2000/04/14. eng.
40. Stojadinovic A, Leung DH, Hoos A, Jaques DP, Lewis JJ, Brennan MF. Analysis of the prognostic significance of microscopic margins in 2,084 localized primary adult soft tissue sarcomas. Ann Surg. 2002;235(3):424–34. PubMed PMID: 11882765. Pubmed Central PMCID: 1422449. Epub 2002/03/08. eng.
41. Jones NB, Iwenofu H, Scharschmidt T, Kraybill W. Prognostic factors and staging for soft tissue sarcomas: an update. Surg Oncol Clin N Am. 2012;21(2):187–200. PubMed PMID: 22365514. Epub 2012/03/01. eng.
42. NCCN Guidelines Soft tissue Sarcoma [updated 2/2012]. Available from: www.nccn.org.
43. Hueman MT, Thornton K, Herman JM, Ahuja N. Management of extremity soft tissue sarcomas. Surg Clin North Am. 2008;88(3):539–57, vi. PubMed PMID: 18514697. Epub 2008/06/03. eng.
44. McKee MD, Liu DF, Brooks JJ, Gibbs JF, Driscoll DL, Kraybill WG. The prognostic significance of margin width for extremity and trunk sarcoma. J Surg Oncol. 2004;85(2):68–76. PubMed PMID: 14755506. Epub 2004/02/03. eng.
45. Fadul D, Fayad LM. Advanced modalities for the imaging of sarcoma. Surg Clin North Am. 2008;88(3):521–37, vi. PubMed PMID: 18514696. Epub 2008/06/03. eng.
46. Lois JF, Fischer HJ, Deutsch LS, Stambuk EC, Gomes AS. Angiography in soft tissue sarcomas. Cardiovasc Intervent Radiol. 1984;7(6):309–16. PubMed PMID: 6099221. Epub 1984/01/01. eng.
47. Miller SL, Hoffer FA. Malignant and benign bone tumors. Radiol Clin North Am. 2001;39(4):673–99. PubMed PMID: 11549165. Epub 2001/09/11. eng.
48. Fayad LM, Jacobs MA, Wang X, Carrino JA, Bluemke DA. Musculoskeletal tumors: how to use anatomic, functional, and metabolic MR techniques. Radiology. 2012;265(2):340–56. PubMed PMID: 23093707. Pubmed Central PMCID: 3480818. Epub 2012/10/25. eng.
49. Heslin MJ, Lewis JJ, Woodruff JM, Brennan MF. Core needle biopsy for diagnosis of extremity soft tissue sarcoma. Ann Surg Oncol. 1997;4(5):425–31. PubMed PMID: 9259971. Epub 1997/07/01. eng.
50. Schwartz HS, Spengler DM. Needle tract recurrences after closed biopsy for sarcoma: three cases and review of the literature. Ann Surg Oncol. 1997;4(3):228–36. PubMed PMID: 9142384. Epub 1997/04/01. eng.
51. Hardin CA. Radical amputation for sarcoma of the extremities including postoperative resection of pulmonary metastasis. Ann Surg. 1968;167(3):359–66. PubMed PMID: 5638521. Pubmed Central PMCID: 1387065. Epub 1968/03/01. eng.
52. Rosenberg SA, Tepper J, Glatstein E, Costa J, Baker A, Brennan M, et al. The treatment of soft-tissue sarcomas of the extremities: prospective randomized evaluations of (1) limb-sparing surgery plus radiation therapy compared with amputation and (2) the

role of adjuvant chemotherapy. Ann Surg. 1982;196(3):305–15. PubMed PMID: 7114936. Pubmed Central PMCID: 1352604. Epub 1982/09/01. eng.
53. Heslin MJ, Woodruff J, Brennan MF. Prognostic significance of a positive microscopic margin in high-risk extremity soft tissue sarcoma: implications for management. J Clin Oncol. 1996;14(2):473–8. PubMed PMID: 8636760. Epub 1996/02/01. eng.
54. Zagars GK, Ballo MT, Pisters PW, Pollock RE, Patel SR, Benjamin RS. Surgical margins and resection in the management of patients with soft tissue sarcoma using conservative surgery and radiation therapy. Cancer. 2003;97(10):2544–53. PubMed PMID: 12733154. Epub 2003/05/07. eng.
55. Fong Y, Coit DG, Woodruff JM, Brennan MF. Lymph node metastasis from soft tissue sarcoma in adults. Analysis of data from a prospective database of 1772 sarcoma patients. Ann Surg. 1993;217(1):72–7. PubMed PMID: 8424704. Pubmed Central PMCID: 1242736.
56. Yang JC, Chang AE, Baker AR, Sindelar WF, Danforth DN, Topalian SL, et al. Randomized prospective study of the benefit of adjuvant radiation therapy in the treatment of soft tissue sarcomas of the extremity. J Clin Oncol. 1998;16(1):197–203. PubMed PMID: 9440743. Epub 1998/01/24. eng.
57. Pisters PW, Harrison LB, Leung DH, Woodruff JM, Casper ES, Brennan MF. Long-term results of a prospective randomized trial of adjuvant brachytherapy in soft tissue sarcoma. J Clin Oncol. 1996;14(3):859–68. PubMed PMID: 8622034. Epub 1996/03/01. eng.
58. Caudle AS, Tepper JE, Calvo BF, Meyers MO, Goyal LK, Cance WG, et al. Complications associated with neoadjuvant radiotherapy in the multidisciplinary treatment of retroperitoneal sarcomas. Ann Surg Oncol. 2007;14(2):577–82. PubMed PMID: 17119868. Epub 2006/11/23. eng.
59. Davis AM, O'Sullivan B, Turcotte R, Bell R, Catton C, Chabot P, et al. Late radiation morbidity following randomization to preoperative versus postoperative radiotherapy in extremity soft tissue sarcoma. Radiother Oncol. 2005;75(1):48–53. PubMed PMID: 15948265. Epub 2005/06/11. eng.
60. O'Sullivan B, Davis AM, Turcotte R, Bell R, Catton C, Chabot P, et al. Preoperative versus postoperative radiotherapy in soft-tissue sarcoma of the limbs: a randomised trial. Lancet. 2002;359(9325):2235–41. PubMed PMID: 12103287. Epub 2002/07/10. eng.
61. Adjuvant chemotherapy for localised resectable soft-tissue sarcoma of adults: meta-analysis of individual data. Sarcoma Meta-analysis Collaboration. Lancet 1997;350(9092):1647–54. PubMed PMID: 9400508. Epub 1997/12/24. eng.
62. Woll PJ, van Glabbeke M, Hohenberger P, et al. Adjuvant chemotherapy (CT) with doxorubicin and ifosfamide in resected soft tissue sarcoma (STS): interim analysis of a randomised phase III trial. J Clin Oncol. 2007;25 Suppl 18:A-10008.
63. Pisters PW, Patel SR, Varma DG, Cheng SC, Chen NP, Nguyen HT, et al. Preoperative chemotherapy for stage IIIB extremity soft tissue sarcoma: long-term results from a single institution. J Clin Oncol. 1997;15(12):3481–7. PubMed PMID: 9396401. Epub 1997/12/13. eng.
64. Look Hong NJ, Hornicek FJ, Harmon DC, Choy E, Chen YL, Yoon SS, et al. Neoadjuvant chemoradiotherapy for patients with high-risk extremity and truncal sarcomas: a 10-year single institution retrospective study. Eur J Cancer. 2013;49(4):875–83. PubMed PMID: 23092789. Epub 2012/10/25. eng.
65. Issels RD, Lindner LH, Verweij J, Wust P, Reichardt P, Schem BC, et al. Neo-adjuvant chemotherapy alone or with regional hyperthermia for localised high-risk soft-tissue sarcoma: a randomised phase 3 multicentre study. Lancet Oncol. 2010;11(6):561–70. PubMed PMID: 20434400. Pubmed Central PMCID: 3517819. Epub 2010/05/04. eng.
66. Suit HD. Patterns of failure after treatment of sarcoma of soft tissue by radical surgery or by conservative surgery and radiation. Cancer Treat Symp. 1983;2:241–6.
67. Lawrence Jr W, Donegan WL, Natarajan N, Mettlin C, Beart R, Winchester D. Adult soft tissue sarcomas. A pattern of care survey of the American College of Surgeons. Ann Surg. 1987;205(4):349–59. PubMed PMID: 3566372. Pubmed Central PMCID: 1492738.
68. Kane JM, Finley JW, Driscoll D, Kraybill WG, Gibbs JF. The treatment and outcome of patients with soft tissue sarcomas and synchronous metastases. Sarcoma. 2002;6(2):69–73. PubMed PMID: 18521331. Pubmed Central PMCID: 2395477.
69. Singer S, Corson JM, Gonin R, Labow B, Eberlein TJ. Prognostic factors predictive of survival and local recurrence for extremity soft tissue sarcoma. Ann Surg. 1994;219(2):165–73. PubMed PMID: 8129487. Pubmed Central PMCID: 1243118. Epub 1994/02/01. eng.
70. Zagars GK, Ballo MT, Pisters PW, Pollock RE, Patel SR, Benjamin RS, et al. Prognostic factors for patients with localized soft-tissue sarcoma treated with conservation surgery and radiation therapy: an analysis of 1225 patients. Cancer. 2003;97(10):2530–43. PubMed PMID: 12733153. Epub 2003/05/07. eng.
71. Hohenberger P, Schwarzbach MH. Management of locally recurrent soft tissue sarcoma after prior surgery and radiation therapy. Recent Results Cancer Res. 2009;179:271–83. PubMed PMID: 19230546. Epub 2009/02/24. eng.
72. Fontanesi J, Mott MP, Lucas DR, Miller PR, Kraut MJ. The role of irradiation in the management of locally recurrent non-metastatic soft tissue sarcoma of extremity/truncal locations. Sarcoma. 2004;8(2–3):57–61. PubMed PMID: 18521396. Pubmed Central PMCID: 2395609. Epub 2008/06/04. eng.
73. Billingsley KG, Burt ME, Jara E, Ginsberg RJ, Woodruff JM, Leung DH, et al. Pulmonary metastases

from soft tissue sarcoma: analysis of patterns of diseases and postmetastasis survival. Ann Surg. 1999;229(5):602–10, discussion 10–2. PubMed PMID: 10235518. Pubmed Central PMCID: 1420804. Epub 1999/05/11. eng.
74. Predina JD, Puc MM, Bergey MR, Sonnad SS, Kucharczuk JC, Staddon A, et al. Improved survival after pulmonary metastasectomy for soft tissue sarcoma. J Thorac Oncol. 2011;6(5):913–9. PubMed PMID: 21750417. Epub 2011/07/14. eng.
75. Bramwell VH, Anderson D, Charette ML. Doxorubicin-based chemotherapy for the palliative treatment of adult patients with locally advanced or metastatic soft tissue sarcoma. Cochrane Database Syst Rev. 2003;3, CD003293. PubMed PMID: 12917960. Epub 2003/08/15. eng.
76. Maki RG, Wathen JK, Patel SR, Priebat DA, Okuno SH, Samuels B, et al. Randomized phase II study of gemcitabine and docetaxel compared with gemcitabine alone in patients with metastatic soft tissue sarcomas: results of sarcoma alliance for research through collaboration study 002 [corrected]. J Clin Oncol. 2007;25(19):2755–63. PubMed PMID: 17602081. Epub 2007/07/03. eng.
77. Demetri GD, Chawla SP, von Mehren M, Ritch P, Baker LH, Blay JY, et al. Efficacy and safety of trabectedin in patients with advanced or metastatic liposarcoma or leiomyosarcoma after failure of prior anthracyclines and ifosfamide: results of a randomized phase II study of two different schedules. J Clin Oncol. 2009;27(25):4188–96. PubMed PMID: 19652065. Epub 2009/08/05. eng.
78. Bonvalot S, Raut CP, Pollock RE, Rutkowski P, Strauss DC, Hayes AJ, et al. Technical considerations in surgery for retroperitoneal sarcomas: position paper from E-Surge, a master class in sarcoma surgery, and EORTC-STBSG. Ann Surg Oncol. 2012;19(9):2981–91. PubMed PMID: 22476756. Epub 2012/04/06. eng.
79. Anaya DA, Lev DC, Pollock RE. The role of surgical margin status in retroperitoneal sarcoma. J Surg Oncol. 2008;98(8):607–10. PubMed PMID: 19072853. Epub 2008/12/17. eng.
80. Mendenhall WM, Zlotecki RA, Hochwald SN, Hemming AW, Grobmyer SR, Cance WG. Retroperitoneal soft tissue sarcoma. Cancer. 2005;104(4):669–75. PubMed PMID: 16003776. Epub 2005/07/09. eng.
81. Lewis JJ, Leung D, Woodruff JM, Brennan MF. Retroperitoneal soft-tissue sarcoma: analysis of 500 patients treated and followed at a single institution. Ann Surg. 1998;228(3):355–65. PubMed PMID: 9742918. Pubmed Central PMCID: 1191491. Epub 1998/09/22. eng.
82. Stoeckle E, Coindre JM, Bonvalot S, Kantor G, Terrier P, Bonichon F, et al. Prognostic factors in retroperitoneal sarcoma: a multivariate analysis of a series of 165 patients of the French Cancer Center Federation Sarcoma Group. Cancer. 2001;92(2):359–68. PubMed PMID: 11466691. Epub 2001/07/24. eng.
83. Zlotecki RA, Katz TS, Morris CG, Lind DS, Hochwald SN. Adjuvant radiation therapy for resectable retroperitoneal soft tissue sarcoma: the University of Florida experience. Am J Clin Oncol. 2005;28(3):310–6. PubMed PMID: 15923806. Epub 2005/06/01. eng.
84. Pawlik TM, Pisters PW, Mikula L, Feig BW, Hunt KK, Cormier JN, et al. Long-term results of two prospective trials of preoperative external beam radiotherapy for localized intermediate- or high-grade retroperitoneal soft tissue sarcoma. Ann Surg Oncol. 2006;13(4):508–17. PubMed PMID: 16491338. Epub 2006/02/24. eng.
85. Heslin MJ, Lewis JJ, Nadler E, Newman E, Woodruff JM, Casper ES, et al. Prognostic factors associated with long-term survival for retroperitoneal sarcoma: implications for management. J Clin Oncol. 1997;15(8):2832–9. PubMed PMID: 9256126. Epub 1997/08/01. eng.
86. Catton CN, O'Sullivan B, Kotwall C, Cummings B, Hao Y, Fornasier V. Outcome and prognosis in retroperitoneal soft tissue sarcoma. Int J Radiat Oncol Biol Phys. 1994;29(5):1005–10. PubMed PMID: 8083069. Epub 1994/07/30. eng.
87. Alektiar KM, Hu K, Anderson L, Brennan MF, Harrison LB. High-dose-rate intraoperative radiation therapy (HDR-IORT) for retroperitoneal sarcomas. Int J Radiat Oncol Biol Phys. 2000;47(1):157–63. PubMed PMID: 10758318. Epub 2000/04/12. eng.
88. Gieschen HL, Spiro IJ, Suit HD, Ott MJ, Rattner DW, Ancukiewicz M, et al. Long-term results of intraoperative electron beam radiotherapy for primary and recurrent retroperitoneal soft tissue sarcoma. Int J Radiat Oncol Biol Phys. 2001;50(1):127–31. PubMed PMID: 11316555. Epub 2001/04/24. eng.
89. Pervaiz N, Colterjohn N, Farrokhyar F, Tozer R, Figueredo A, Ghert M. A systematic meta-analysis of randomized controlled trials of adjuvant chemotherapy for localized resectable soft-tissue sarcoma. Cancer. 2008;113(3):573–81. PubMed PMID: 18521899. Epub 2008/06/04. eng.
90. van Geel AN, Pastorino U, Jauch KW, Judson IR, van Coevorden F, Buesa JM, et al. Surgical treatment of lung metastases: the European Organization for Research and Treatment of Cancer-Soft Tissue and Bone Sarcoma Group study of 255 patients. Cancer. 1996;77(4):675–82. PubMed PMID: 8616759. Epub 1996/02/15. eng.
91. Rehders A, Peiper M, Stoecklein NH, Alexander A, Boelke E, Knoefel WT, et al. Hepatic metastasectomy for soft-tissue sarcomas: is it justified? World J Surg. 2009;33(1):111–7. PubMed PMID: 18949511. Epub 2008/10/25. eng.
92. Yeh JJ, Singer S, Brennan MF, Jaques DP. Effectiveness of palliative procedures for intra-abdominal sarcomas. Ann Surg Oncol.

2005;12(12):1084–9. PubMed PMID: 16244805. Epub 2005/10/26. eng.
93. Verma S, Younus J, Stys-Norman D, Haynes AE, Blackstein M. Meta-analysis of ifosfamide-based combination chemotherapy in advanced soft tissue sarcoma. Cancer Treat Rev. 2008;34(4):339–47. PubMed PMID: 18313854. Epub 2008/03/04. eng.
94. Miettinen M, Lasota J. Gastrointestinal stromal tumors: review on morphology, molecular pathology, prognosis, and differential diagnosis. Arch Pathol Lab Med. 2006;130(10):1466–78. PubMed PMID: 17090188. Epub 2006/11/09. eng.
95. Hirota S, Isozaki K, Moriyama Y, Hashimoto K, Nishida T, Ishiguro S, et al. Gain-of-function mutations of c-kit in human gastrointestinal stromal tumors. Science. 1998;279(5350):577–80. PubMed PMID: 9438854. Epub 1998/02/07. eng.
96. Heinrich MC, Corless CL, Duensing A, McGreevey L, Chen CJ, Joseph N, et al. PDGFRA activating mutations in gastrointestinal stromal tumors. Science. 2003;299(5607):708–10. PubMed PMID: 12522257. Epub 2003/01/11. eng.
97. DeMatteo RP, Lewis JJ, Leung D, Mudan SS, Woodruff JM, Brennan MF. Two hundred gastrointestinal stromal tumors: recurrence patterns and prognostic factors for survival. Ann Surg. 2000;231(1):51–8. PubMed PMID: 10636102. Pubmed Central PMCID: 1420965. Epub 2000/01/15. eng.
98. Kim TW, Lee H, Kang YK, Choe MS, Ryu MH, Chang HM, et al. Prognostic significance of c-kit mutation in localized gastrointestinal stromal tumors. Clin Cancer Res. 2004;10(9):3076–81. PubMed PMID: 15131046. Epub 2004/05/08. eng.
99. Bumming P, Ahlman H, Andersson J, Meis-Kindblom JM, Kindblom LG, Nilsson B. Population-based study of the diagnosis and treatment of gastrointestinal stromal tumours. Br J Surg. 2006;93(7):836–43. PubMed PMID: 16705644. Epub 2006/05/18. eng.
100. Wu TJ, Lee LY, Yeh CN, Wu PY, Chao TC, Hwang TL, et al. Surgical treatment and prognostic analysis for gastrointestinal stromal tumors (GISTs) of the small intestine: before the era of imatinib mesylate. BMC Gastroenterol. 2006;6:29. PubMed PMID: 17062131. Pubmed Central PMCID: 1633731. Epub 2006/10/26. eng.
101. Dematteo RP, Ballman KV, Antonescu CR, Maki RG, Pisters PW, Demetri GD, et al. Adjuvant imatinib mesylate after resection of localised, primary gastrointestinal stromal tumour: a randomised, double-blind, placebo-controlled trial. Lancet. 2009;373(9669):1097–104. PubMed PMID: 19303137. Pubmed Central PMCID: 2915459. Epub 2009/03/24. eng.
102. Joensuu H, Eriksson M, Sundby Hall K, Hartmann JT, Pink D, Schutte J, et al. One vs three years of adjuvant imatinib for operable gastrointestinal stromal tumor: a randomized trial. JAMA. 2012;307(12):1265–72. PubMed PMID: 22453568. Epub 2012/03/29. eng.
103. Demetri GD, von Mehren M, Blanke CD, Van den Abbeele AD, Eisenberg B, Roberts PJ, et al. Efficacy and safety of imatinib mesylate in advanced gastrointestinal stromal tumors. N Engl J Med. 2002;347(7):472–80. PubMed PMID: 12181401. Epub 2002/08/16. eng.
104. Blanke CD, Demetri GD, von Mehren M, Heinrich MC, Eisenberg B, Fletcher JA, et al. Long-term results from a randomized phase II trial of standard- versus higher-dose imatinib mesylate for patients with unresectable or metastatic gastrointestinal stromal tumors expressing KIT. J Clin Oncol. 2008;26(4):620–5. PubMed PMID: 18235121. Epub 2008/02/01. eng.
105. Blanke CD, Rankin C, Demetri GD, Ryan CW, von Mehren M, Benjamin RS, et al. Phase III randomized, intergroup trial assessing imatinib mesylate at two dose levels in patients with unresectable or metastatic gastrointestinal stromal tumors expressing the kit receptor tyrosine kinase: S0033. J Clin Oncol. 2008;26(4):626–32. PubMed PMID: 18235122. Epub 2008/02/01. eng.
106. Verweij J, Casali PG, Zalcberg J, LeCesne A, Reichardt P, Blay JY, et al. Progression-free survival in gastrointestinal stromal tumours with high-dose imatinib: randomised trial. Lancet. 2004;364(9440):1127–34. PubMed PMID: 15451219. Epub 2004/09/29. eng.
107. von Mehren M, Heinrich M, Joensuu H, et al. Follow-up results after 9 years (yrs) of the ongoing, phase II B2222 trial of imatinib mesylate (IM) in patients (pts) with metastatic or unresectable KIT+ gastrointestinal stromal tumors (GIST) [abstract]. J Clin Oncol. 2011;29(Suppl 15):Abstract 10016.
108. Blesius A, Cassier PA, Bertucci F, Fayette J, Ray-Coquard I, Bui B, et al. Neoadjuvant imatinib in patients with locally advanced non metastatic GIST in the prospective BFR14 trial. BMC Cancer. 2011;11:72. PubMed PMID: 21324142. Pubmed Central PMCID: 3052196. Epub 2011/02/18. eng.
109. Compton C, Byrd D, Garcia-Aguilar J, et al. Soft Tissue Sarcoma. In: Compton C, Byrd D, Garcia-Aguilar J, Kurtzman S, Olawaiye A, Washington M, editors. AJCC cancer staging atlas. 2nd ed. New York: Springer; 2012. p. 349–54.
110. Trojani M, et al. Soft tissue sarcomas of adults: study of pathological prognostic variables and definition of histopathological grading system. Int J Cancer. 1984;33:37–42.

28 Gastrointestinal Stromal Tumor (GIST)

Lesly A. Dossett and Nipun B. Merchant

Abbreviations

ACOSOG	American College of Surgeons Oncology Group
ACRIN	American College of Radiology Imaging Network
AGITG	Australasian Gastro-Intestinal Trials Group
AJCC	American Joint Commission on Cancer
CALGB	Cancer and Leukemia Group B
CT	Computed tomography
DOG1	Discovered on GIST 1
ECOG	Eastern Cooperative Group
EORTC	European Organization for Research and Treatment of Cancer
ESMO	European Sarcoma Network Working Group
EUS	Endoscopic ultrasound
FNA	Fine-needle aspiration
GIST	Gastrointestinal stromal tumor
HPF	High-powered field
ISG	Italian Sarcoma Group
MRI	Magnetic resonance imaging
NCCN	National Comprehensive Cancer Network
OS	Overall survival
PDGFRA	Platelet-derived growth factor receptor alpha
PET	Positron emission tomography
RFS	Recurrence-free survival
SCF	Stem cell factor
SSG	Scandinavian Sarcoma Group
SWOG	Southwest Oncology Group
TKI	Tyrosine kinase inhibitor
TNM	Tumor/node/metastasis
UICC	International Union Against Cancer

L.A. Dossett, M.D., M.P.H.
Department of Surgery, Naval Hospital Jacksonville, 2080 Child Street, Jacksonville 32214, FL, USA
e-mail: ladossett@gmail.com

N.B. Merchant, M.D., F.A.C.S. (✉)
Department of Surgical Oncology and Endocrine Surgery, Vanderbilt University Medical Center, 2220 Pierce Ave 597 PRB, Nashville 37232, TN, USA
e-mail: nipun.merchant@vanderbilt.edu

Learning Objectives

After reading this chapter, you should be able to:

- Describe the epidemiology, clinical presentation, and staging of GISTs.
- Understand the importance of mutations in tyrosine kinase receptors KIT and platelet-derived growth factor receptor alpha (PDGFRA) in the diagnosis, prognosis, and treatment of GISTs.
- Describe the factors which predict recurrence.
- Select options for local and systemic/recurrent control of the disease.
- Understand the criteria for adjuvant and neo-adjuvant therapy.

Q.D. Chu et al. (eds.), *Surgical Oncology: A Practical and Comprehensive Approach*,
DOI 10.1007/978-1-4939-1423-4_28, © Springer Science+Business Media New York 2015

- Describe the controversies surrounding optimal dose and duration of therapy for imatinib.
- Describe treatment options for imatinib-resistant GISTs.

Background

Gastrointestinal stromal tumors (GISTs) are the most common sarcoma of the gastrointestinal (GI) tract, accounting for 1–3 % of all GI malignancies in the United States (US). The estimated incidence of GISTs is 3,000 to 5,000 new cases per year, with other studies suggesting that asymptomatic, incidentally detected sub-centimeter gastric GISTs may occur more frequently. GISTs are slightly more common in males (53 %) and are most commonly diagnosed between the ages of 55 and 65 years of age. GISTs are rare in children and occur almost exclusively in the stomach in this population [1].

GISTs arise from the interstitial cells of Cajal, an intestinal pacemaker cell located in and around the myenteric plexus. GISTs may be present throughout the GI tract, but they are most frequently located in the stomach (65–70 %) or small intestine (25–45 %), followed by the colon and rectum (5–15 %) and esophagus (<5 %) (Figs. 28.1, 28.2, and 28.3 and 28.4). Primary omental or mesenteric GISTs have been reported but are exceptionally rare [2, 3].

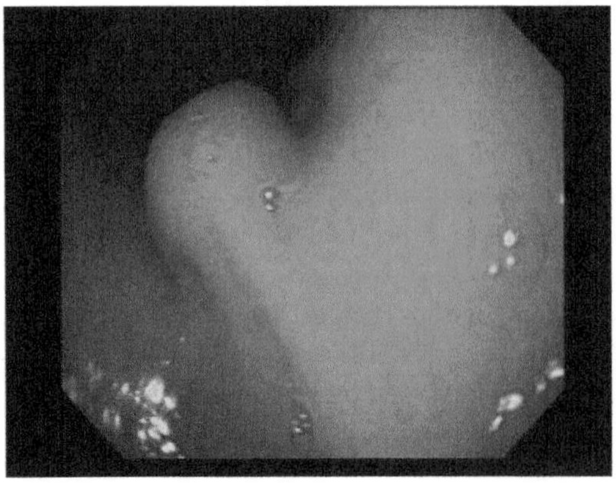

Fig. 28.1 Upper endoscopy of a stomach GIST (Courtesy of David Schwartz, MD, Vanderbilt University Medical Center)

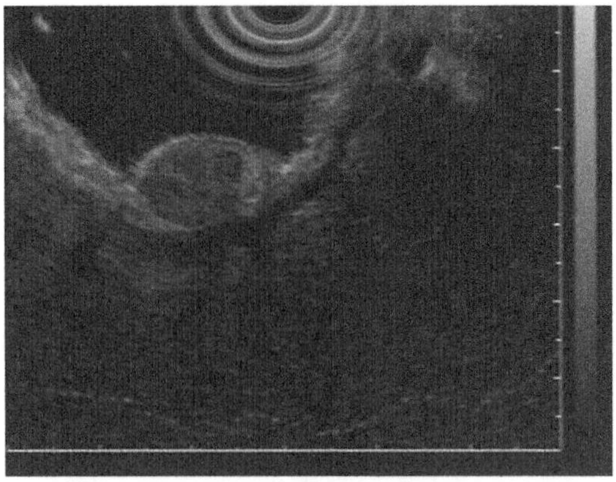

Fig. 28.2 Endoscopic ultrasound (EUS) of a stomach GIST (Courtesy of David Schwartz, MD, Vanderbilt University Medical Center)

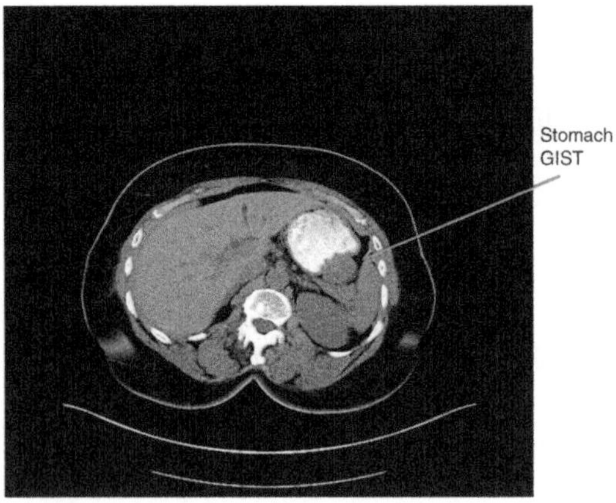

Fig. 28.3 CT of a stomach GIST (Courtesy of Quyen D. Chu, MD, MBA, FACS)

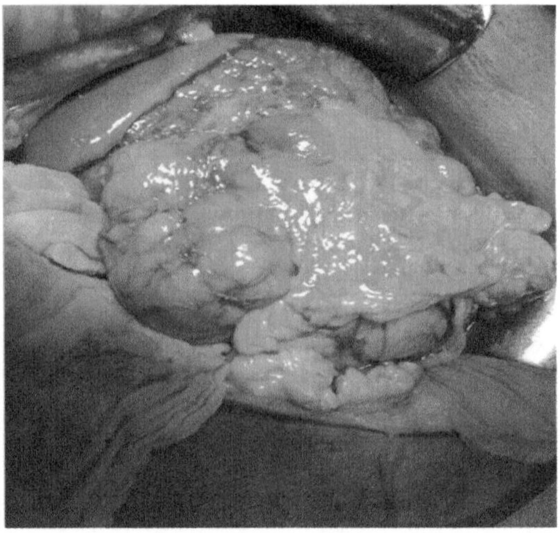

Fig. 28.4 Patient with a large stomach GIST (Courtesy of Quyen D. Chu, MD, MBA, FACS)

CD-117 antigen by almost all (80–95 %) GISTs represented a major breakthrough in the classification, approach, and treatment of these tumors over the last 30 years [4]. Other spindle cell neoplasms arising in the GI tract such as lipomas, true leiomyomas, and leiomyosarcomas are typically CD-117 negative. The CD-117 molecule is part of the KIT receptor tyrosine kinase that is a product of the KIT proto-oncogene. This gene encodes a transmembrane receptor for a growth factor named stem cell factor (SCF). Binding of SCF to KIT induces KIT dimerization and activation. Constitutive activation of KIT signaling leads to uncontrolled cell proliferation and inhibition of apoptosis. The KIT product is expressed on the interstitial cells of Cajal, mast cells, and melanocytes, but a mesenchymal spindle cell tumor in the GI tract that stains diffusely positive for CD117 is characteristic of a GIST.

KIT mutations generally occur in one of four of the 21 exons of the gene. The most common mutation is of exon 11 which encodes for the intracellular component of the transmembrane portion, but mutations of exon 9 (the extracellular component of the transmembrane portion) are also common (7 %). Mutations of exon 13 and exon 17 are rare. Mutations make KIT function independent of activation, leading to a high rate of mitosis and genomic instability [5].

A small percentage of GISTs (5–7 %) have a mutation in the platelet-derived growth factor receptor-alpha (PDGFRA) instead of the more common KIT mutation [6]. PDGFRA is a receptor tyrosine kinase which shares extensive similarities with KIT, but the mutations are distinct in that they do not respond to the same growth factors. Almost all GISTs will harbor either the KIT or PDGFRA mutation, but not both since each is an alternative path to uncontrolled proliferation. As many as 60 % of PDGFRA mutations occur in exon 18 (specific mutation noted as D842V). Emerging data suggest that mutation type has important implications for prognosis, recurrence, response to therapy, and the development of tyrosine kinase inhibitor resistance.

Diagnosis and Staging

GISTs originate from the interstitial cell of Cajal or its precursor, within the submucosa or muscularis propria, but may extend toward the serosa (extraluminal or exophytic type) or lumen (endoluminal type). Clinical symptoms typically vary depending on the tumor size, growth type, and location. Most patients presenting with symptoms have tumors that exceed 5 cm in maximum dimension, and some tumors are as large as 30–40 cm at presentation. The most frequent symptoms include early satiety, gastrointestinal or intraperitoneal hemorrhage, and abdominal mass or pain. Intestinal obstruction and intestinal perforation can also occur. Associated symptoms may include nausea, vomiting, anorexia, and weight loss. Other patients with GISTs are asymptomatic and are incidentally diagnosed by abdominal imaging or endoscopy. No laboratory test can confirm or exclude the diagnosis of a GIST [7].

Radiologic exams are often essential in determining the size, location, extent of local invasion, and operative strategy for the treatment of GISTs. Imaging is also critical in restaging, monitoring the response to therapy, and performing follow-up surveillance for recurrence. Contrast-enhanced computed topography (CT) is preferred for initial screening and staging because of its superior ability to provide a comprehensive evaluation of the abdomen (Fig. 28.3). Magnetic resonance imaging (MRI) may be preferred for the evaluation of GISTs in certain anatomic sites such as the rectum or liver. Tumors that are greater than 5 cm, lobulated, enhance heterogeneously, and have mesenteric fat infiltration, ulceration, or an exophytic growth pattern are more likely to demonstrate metastatic or recurrent behavior. Conversely, smaller GISTs, those with an endoluminal growth pattern, and those with a homogeneous pattern of enhancement tend to demonstrate less aggressive behavior.

While positron emission tomography (PET) imaging of GISTs is rarely required for the evaluation of localized disease, PET is capable of detecting sub-centimeter lesions and may therefore be useful for detecting an unknown primary site or monitoring the response to systemic therapy. PET can also help differentiate active tumor from necrotic or inactive scar tissue, malignant from benign tissue, and recurrence from nondescript postsurgical changes.

On upper gastrointestinal endoscopy, a smooth, mucosa-lined protrusion of the bowel wall may be present, with or without signs of ulceration (Fig. 28.1). Standard endoscopic biopsies usually do not obtain sufficient tissue for a definite diagnosis. Endoscopic ultrasound (EUS)-guided fine-needle aspiration (FNA) or forceps biopsies have a higher yield and may also be useful for excluding the diagnosis of other submucosal lesions (Fig. 28.2). Definitive tissue diagnosis is not required for a resectable lesion in which there is a high suspicion for a GIST, but biopsy should be performed to confirm the diagnosis when metastatic disease is present or suspected. A biopsy is also required for patients with a locally advanced GIST who are being considered for neoadjuvant therapy. EUS-FNA of the primary site is preferred over percutaneous biopsy due to the risk of tumor hemorrhage and dissemination.

The gross pattern of GISTs is diverse but most are well-circumscribed nodular masses. However, they can also be multinodular and exhibit foci of cystic degeneration, hemorrhage, and necrosis. Microscopically, most GISTs can be divided into histologic subgroups including both spindle cell type, epithelioid type, and mixed variants. Intestinal variants are histologically more homogenous group of tumors. Differentiation between GISTs and other spindle cell tumors is typically based upon morphology, immunohistochemistry staining, and molecular analysis. Approximately 85–90 % of GISTs has gain-of-function mutations of KIT and PDGFRA genes and characteristically stain positive for either KIT (CD117), CD34, or DOG1. The level of expression can vary from diffuse and strong to focal and weakly positive. CD34, however, is not a sensitive or specific marker, staining only 50–80 % of gastric and small intestinal GIST. The morphologic identification of KIT negative remains a diagnostic challenge, but a newly discovered antigen known as DOG1 (discovered on GIST-1) can help to identify certain KIT-negative GISTs. DOG1 is a calcium-dependent, receptor-activated chloride channel protein, and it is expressed in GISTs independent of mutation type. In view of the cross-reactivity and expression of these antibodies in a variety of other spindle cell mesenchymal tumors considered in the differential diagnosis of GIST, a panel of antibodies is recommended and include CD117, DOG1, CD34, S10, desmin, smooth muscle actin, and keratin as indicated.

Several factors have been identified as contributing to clinical outcomes in patients with GISTs. The most reliable prognostic factors for GISTs are tumor size, location of the primary tumor, and the mitotic index [8]. Gastric tumors have a more favorable prognosis than the intestinal ones with similar characteristics [9]. Risk of metastatic disease or recurrence is higher for tumors greater than 5 cm and those demonstrating high cellularity, prominent nuclear pleomorphism, necrosis, greater than 5 mitoses per 50 high-power field (HPF), and invasion into adjacent structures. Historically, some GISTs were classified as "benign" based on a size less than 2 cm and favorable histologic features, but with long-term follow-up, it is becoming increasingly clear that virtually all GISTs have the potential for malignant behavior and recurrence.

The American Joint Commission on Cancer (AJCC) and International Union Against Cancer (UICC) first included a TNM (tumor/node/metastasis) classification and staging system for GISTs in the 2010 7th edition of the cancer staging manual (Table 28.1) [10]. The T-categories are based on tumor size and then combined with mitotic rate and tumor site to define a clinical stage. Given the rarity of nodal metastasis with GISTs, any patient without examined regional nodes is considered to be N0. The presence of either nodal or distant disease is classified as stage IV. There remains some controversy as to whether or not the TNM system applies well to GISTs since factors known to predict outcomes such as mutation type and tumor rupture are not included.

Table 28.1 American Joint Committee on Cancer (AJCC) TNM staging for gastrointestinal stromal tumor (7th edition)

Primary tumor (T)	
TX	Primary tumor cannot be assessed
T0	No evidence of primary tumor
T1	Tumor ≤2 cm
T2	Tumor >2 cm but <5 cm
T3	Tumor >5 cm but <10 cm
T4	Tumor >10 cm in greatest diameter

Regional lymph nodes (N)	
N0	No regional lymph node metastasis*
N1	Regional lymph node metastasis

*Note: If regional node status is unknown, use N0, not NX

Distant metastasis (M)	
M0	No distant metastasis
M1	Distant metastasis

Anatomic stage/prognostic groups				
Group	T	N	M	Mitotic rate
*Gastric GIST**				
Stage IA	T1 or T2	N0	M0	Low
Stage IB	T3	N0	M0	Low
Stage II	T1, T2	N0	M0	High
	T4	N0	M0	Low
Stage IIIA	T3	N0	M0	High
Stage IIIB	T4	N0	M0	High
Stage IV	Any T	N1	M0	Any rate
	Any T	Any N	M1	Any rate
*Small intestinal GIST***				
Stage I	T1 or T2	N0	M0	Low
Stage II	T3	N0	M0	Low
Stage IIIA	T1	N0	M0	High
	T4	N0	M0	Low
Stage IIIB	T2–T4	N0	M0	High
Stage IV	Any T	N1	M0	Any rate
	Any T	Any N	M1	Any rate

*Note: Also to be used for omentum

**Note: Also to be used for esophagus, colorectal, mesentery, and peritoneum

Any patient with N or M disease is classified as stage IV, irrespective of T stage

Histopathologic grade
Low mitotic rate: ≤5 per 50 HPF
High mitotic rate: >5 per 50 HPF

Adapted from Compton et al. [33]. With permission from Springer Verlag

Operative Therapy for Localized GISTs

Operative resection remains the treatment of choice for a localized GIST (Table 28.2). Complete surgical resection of the gross tumor and pseudocapsule including en bloc resection of any involved adjacent organs is recommended if possible. GISTs are fragile and should be handled with care to avoid tumor rupture. Both nonradical resection with a positive margin (R1) and tumor rupture are associated with adverse outcomes. Because lymph node involvement is exceedingly rare, extensive lymphadenectomy does not provide a survival advantage and is not recommended. Repeat resection is generally not indicated for microscopically positive margins on final pathology, although every effort should be made to obtain negative microscopic margins at the initial operation.

Most gastric GISTs can be resected using a wedge resection with a 1–2 cm margin. For tumors along the greater curvature of the stomach, the omentum is removed from the stomach

Table 28.2 Treatment summary for localized, recurrent, and metastatic GIST

Clinical scenario	Management
Local disease	Complete en bloc resection with tumor-free margins
	Consider neoadjuvant therapy for patients with marginally resectable disease or those who would require total gastrectomy, pancreaticoduodenectomy, or an abdominoperineal resection or if the tumor is particularly large
	Consider adjuvant therapy with imatinib for higher-risk tumors (>5 cm, >5 mitoses/50 HPF)
	No role for conventional radiation or chemotherapy
Recurrent or metastatic disease	Treat with imatinib until treatment failure
	Consider dose escalation or other tyrosine kinase inhibitors for imatinib-refractory or resistance GISTs
	Surgical resection of residual tumors of responding patients or symptomatic tumors may be considered

near the tumor. For lesser curvature lesions, a pyloromyotomy should be performed if the vagal nerves supplying the pylorus are disrupted. Many GISTs may be resected using a laparoscopic approach. Extraluminal tumors (serosal based) are easily localized laparoscopically, while endoluminal tumors may require concurrent upper endoscopy. In laparoscopic resections, the specimen should be removed from the abdomen in an endoscopic retrieval bag to avoid spillage or seeding of port sites. Sphincter-sparing surgery should be considered for rectal GISTs. In selected cases, neoadjuvant imatinib therapy may enable sphincter-sparing surgery and improve outcomes in patients with low rectal GISTs. Even when complete resection is achieved, many tumors can recur, often involving the liver and peritoneum.

Systemic Therapy

Systemic chemotherapy and radiation have minimal activity against GISTs and are not routinely recommended. Since tyrosine kinase activation occurs in the majority of cases, tyrosine kinase inhibition (TKI) has emerged as the primary therapeutic modality for metastatic or recurrent GISTs (Table 28.3).

Table 28.3 Summary of selected clinical trials on GISTs

Study [Ref]	Findings
US-CDN (phase 3) [14]	No difference in PFS or OS between 400 mg qd and 800 mg qd dosing schedule
EU-AUS (phase 3) [15]	Initial report: PFS advantage with 800 mg qd over 400 mg qd
	Follow-up report: No advantage with 800 mg qd dose
MetaGIST [18]	Combined data from UC-CDN and EU-AUS
	No OS with 800 mg qd schedule
	Improved PFS for patients with KIT exon 9 mutation
ACOSOG Z9001 (phase 3) [25]	Adjuvant imatinib prolonged RFS but not OS
SSG XVIII (phase 3) [26, 27]	3-year adjuvant imatinib prolonged both RFS and OS over 1 year
RTOG 0132/ACRIN 6665 (phase 2) [30]	Demonstrates role of neoadjuvant imatinib
Demetri [31]	Sunitinib improved PFS and OS for patients with advanced GIST who were resistant to or intolerant of imatinib

US-CDN Joint trial by the Southwest Oncology Group, Cancer and Leukemia Group B, National Cancer Institute of Canada, and the Eastern Cooperative Oncology Group EU-AUS Joint trial by European Organisation for Research and Treatment of Cancer, Italian Sarcoma Group, Australasian Gastro-Intestinal Trials Group *ACOSOG* American College of Surgeons Oncology Group, *SSG XVIIII* Scandinavian Sarcoma Group, *RTOG* Radiation Therapy Oncology Group, *ACRIN* American College of Radiology Imaging Network, *PFS* progression-free survival, *OS* overall survival, *Qd* daily

Imatinib Mesylate

Imatinib mesylate (Gleevec®, Novartis Pharmaceuticals) is an oral agent that is a selective molecular inhibitor of the KIT tyrosine kinase. In 2000, imatinib was found to be effective against metastatic GISTs in a single patient [11], and its efficacy was confirmed in multiple subsequent phase II and phase III clinical trials [12–15].

Due to the uncertainty about the optimal dose of imatinib for patients with unresectable or metastatic disease, a series of clinical trials evaluated different regimens for which dosing regimen varies from 400 mg/day to 400 mg twice a day [12, 13, 16]. Blanke et al., reporting for the US/Finnish B2222 trial, randomized 147 patients with unresectable or metastatic gastrointestinal stromal tumors to either 400 mg/day or 600 mg/day of imatinib. The response rates, median progression-free survival (PFS), and median overall survival (OS) were nearly identical for both arms [13]. The overall response rate was 68 %, the median duration of response was 29 months, and the median time to progression was 24 months overall, 20 months in the 400 mg/day group and 26 months in the 600 mg/day group [13].

Two phase III trials were launched to further delineate the optimal effective dose of imatinib—one was conducted jointly in the United States by the Southwest Oncology Group (SWOG), Cancer and Leukemia Group B (CALGB), National Cancer Institute of Canada, and the Eastern

Cooperative Oncology Group (ECOG) (trial S0033, referred to as US-CDN) [14], and the other was conducted jointly in Europe and Australia by the European Organisation for Research and Treatment of Cancer (EORTC), the Italian Sarcoma Group (ISG), and the Australasian Gastro-Intestinal Trials Group (AGITG) (trial 62005, referred to as EU-AUS) [15]. The US-CDN trial randomized 746 patients to receive either 400 mg (standard dose) or 800 mg (high dose) of imatinib daily, and in a median follow-up of 4.5 years, there was no difference in dose response, PFS, or OS [14]. The EU-AUS trial, however, found that although OS was identical in both arms, there was a small but significant PFS advantage for the high-dose arm [15]. However, a further follow-up report of the study found the difference in PFS became statistically insignificant [17].

While these results confirmed the safety and efficacy of imatinib at 400 mg daily as the standard initial dose, high-dose imatinib might benefit a select group of patients, specifically those with the KIT exon 9 mutation. A meta-analysis of 1,640 patients from the combined data of the two large phase III randomized trials demonstrated that although there was no OS advantage with the high-dose regimen, there was a small improvement in PFS for those with the KIT exon 9 mutation [18]. The National Comprehensive Cancer Network (NCCN) recommends dose escalation up to 800 mg daily for patients with documented mutations in KIT exon 9 [19].

Four clinical trials have found that mutation type can serve as an important predictor of response to therapy [20–23]. Patients with KIT exon 11 mutations respond better to imatinib than those with KIT exon 9 mutations [21, 22]. Using archival pathology specimens from patients enrolled in the B2222 trial, Heinrich et al. found that patients with the exon 11 mutation had a partial response rate of 84 % compared to only 48 % for those with exon 9 mutations [22]. Results from the EORTC phase III trial (EORTC-62005) [21] and the North American phase III study SWOG (Southwest Oncology Group) [23] also confirmed that the KIT exon 11 genotype is associated with a favorable outcome as compared to the exon 9 genotype. Despite these encouraging results, however, there is no data to support that mutational analysis improves OS.

Rapid disease progression is seen within months after imatinib is discontinued, and therefore, imatinib interruption is not recommended. Continuous therapy until disease progression (or lifelong if disease does not progress) is currently the standard of care for patients with metastatic GIST. In select patients, metastasectomy may improve survival if a complete (R0) resection can be achieved, or resection may be mandatory if tumors become infected or cause bleeding or intestinal obstruction.

Adjuvant Therapy

While surgery is the optimal therapy for localized GISTs, it does not routinely produce a durable cure. Complete resection is possible in approximately 85 % of patients, but a majority of these patients will recur or develop distant disease. The 5-year survival rate approximates 50 %, and the median time to recurrence following resection is 2 years. Given the success of imatinib in the advanced setting and the high recurrence rates after complete resection of GIST, there is a substantial rationale for testing imatinib in the adjuvant setting.

The American College of Surgeons Oncology Group (ACOSOG) conducted a phase II trial (ACOSOG Z9000) to evaluate the safety and efficacy of adjuvant imatinib (400 mg daily) for 1 year following a complete resection [24]. This study demonstrated prolonged RFS and OS compared to historical controls in patients who were considered as having a high risk of recurrence. The results of ACOSOG Z9000 were confirmed in a subsequent phase III trial (ACOSOG Z9001) [25]. In this trial, 713 patients with completely resected primary GISTs of at least 3 cm or greater were randomly assigned to receive either 1 year of adjuvant imatinib (400 mg daily) or placebo. Those that received adjuvant imatinib had an improved RFS over the placebo group (98 % vs.

83 %; $p<0.0001$). Accrual was stopped early based on an interim analysis that demonstrated superiority of imatinib over placebo. However, there was no difference in OS, but this may have been due to the short duration of follow-up, the limited number of relapses, and the high degree of efficacy of imatinib in patients who were allowed to cross over to active treatment, thus obscuring potential difference in overall survival.

Because recurrence following cessation of imatinib after 1 year of treatment is common, the Scandinavian Sarcoma Group (SSG) XVIII randomized 400 patients with high-risk GISTs to either 1 year or 3 years of adjuvant imatinib [26, 27]. At a median follow-up of 54 months, the 3-year treatment arm had a significantly longer RFS and OS than the 1-year group. Although prolonged treatment was associated with more treatment-related adverse events, these were generally mild (grade 1 or 2).

A question remains as to whether or not an even longer duration of therapy would be beneficial. Answer to this question depends on data maturation of two key trials: (1) EORTC 62024, a phase III trial randomizing 750 patients to either imatinib 400 mg daily for 2 years versus observation with a primary endpoint of overall survival [28], and (2) Post-resection Evaluation of Recurrence-free Survival for gastroIntestinal Stromal Tumors (PERSIST-5), a phase II trial treating 85 postsurgical patients with imatinib 400 mg daily for 5 years with a primary outcome of time to progression [29].

Selecting high-risk patients for adjuvant imatinib therapy has not been well established. The SSGXVIII trial defined the high-risk group as tumor size >10 cm, mitotic rate >10/50 HPF, tumor size >5 cm and >5 mitoses/HPF, or a ruptured GIST [27]. NCCN currently recommends at least 36 months of imatinib therapy for patients with tumors larger than 5 cm in size with a high mitotic rate (>5 mitoses/50 HPF) or a risk of recurrence that is greater than 50% [19]. Alternatively, 1 year of imatinib is considered by many medical oncologists to be appropriate for intermediate-risk GIST (≤5 cm, ≥mitoses/50 HPF or >10 cm, ≤5 mitoses/50 HPF).

Neoadjuvant Imatinib

For patients with extensive involvement of adjacent organs and borderline resectability, preoperative imatinib therapy may be considered. The Radiation Therapy Oncology Group/American College of Radiology Imaging Network (RTOG 0132/ACRIN 6665) trial was the first to evaluate the efficacy of neoadjuvant imatinib [30]. In this phase II trial, 63 patients with resectable primary GIST of 5 cm or larger or resectable metastatic/recurrent disease were treated preoperatively with imatinib 600 mg daily for 8–12 weeks. Following resection, all patients received at least 24 months of postoperative imatinib. Partial response rates of 5–7 % and stable disease rates of 83–91 % were observed with preoperative imatinib. The estimated 2-year PFS rate was 83 % for those patients with primary disease and 77 % for those with recurrent or metastatic disease [30]. While this trial confirmed the safety of neoadjuvant imatinib, the short duration of therapy may have blunted any substantial response rates since in patients with metastatic disease, maximal radiographic response to imatinib generally occurs after 3–9 months.

There currently is no consensus as to the indications for neoadjuvant imatinib, with most limiting treatment to those with high-risk tumors or tumors in anatomic locations which would result in a potentially morbid resection. The NCCN recommends initial treatment with imatinib for patients with marginally resectable GISTs and in those with tumors in anatomic locations where resection presents significant morbidity (esophagus, esophagogastric junction, duodenum, and distal rectum) [19]. The most commonly recommended treatment regimen is 3–12 months of 400 mg daily of imatinib, with the duration of time dependent on ongoing radiographic response. If genotyping is performed, patients with KIT exon 9 mutations should be treated with 800 mg of imatinib, and those with mutations typically resistant to imatinib (PDGFRA exon 18 D842V) should proceed directly to resection [19].

Resistance to Imatinib

Unfortunately, most patients who initially respond to imatinib ultimately acquire resistance to the drug and demonstrate disease progression. Median time to progression is typically 2–3 years. Acquired resistance to imatinib is a frequent event in patients with metastatic GISTs. Primary resistance is defined as evidence of clinical progression in the first 6 months of imatinib therapy. Primary resistance is most commonly seen in patients with KIT exon 9, PDGFRA exon 18, or those with wild-type GISTs. Secondary resistance typically presents with progression at 18–24 months and is often due to a secondary mutation in KIT. Secondary resistance occurs primarily in patients with exon 11 mutations. Once clinical progression occurs, dose escalation from 400 mg daily to 800 mg daily or switching to sunitinib may be considered.

Sunitinib Malate

Sunitinib malate (Sutent®, Pfizer Inc.) targets multiple tyrosine kinases, and an increasing number of reports indicate efficacy in imatinib-refractory or intolerant patients. In a randomized phase III placebo-controlled trial, sunitinib was associated with an improved time to tumor progression (27.3 vs. 6.4 weeks) and greater estimated OS [31]. In a subsequent open-label, multicenter, randomized placebo-controlled phase II study, patients with advanced GIST and imatinib failure were randomized to either sunitinib or placebo. Patients receiving sunitinib had a better outcome; the overall clinical benefit rate was 53 %, with median PFS and OS of 34 and 107 weeks, respectively [32].

Emerging data also suggests that the clinical activity of sunitinib in imatinib-resistant patients is significantly influenced by mutation type. Sunitinib induced higher response rates in patients with primary KIT 9 exon mutations as compared to exon 11 mutations (58 % vs. 34 %). PFS and OS were also longer for patients with the exon 9 mutation, while patients with the PDGFRA mutation had no clinical benefit. Combination therapy either concurrently or sequentially with agents of different tyrosine kinase inhibitor classes may have a synergistic effect. Some patients, particularly those with certain types of PDGFRA mutations, exhibit primary resistance to both imatinib and sunitinib. Patients with this phenotype should seek enrollment in a clinical trial.

Posttreatment Follow-Up

There is no consensus on optimal posttreatment follow-up for patients with GISTs. Recurrences are common, and they typically occur in the liver or peritoneum. The NCCN recommends a history and physical examination and CT scan every 3–6 months for 5 years, then annually [10]. The European Sarcoma Network Working Group (ESMO) emphasizes risk assessment in selecting the frequency and makeup of follow-up regimens (19). For high-risk tumors, routine follow-up with CT every 3–6 months for 3 years during adjuvant therapy is recommended, followed by imaging every 3–6 months for 5 years, then annually for five additional 5 years. For low-risk tumors, the usefulness of routine follow-up is not known.

Salient Points

- GISTs arise from the interstitial cells of Cajal, an intestinal pacemaker cell.
- 80–95 % of GISTs have KIT mutation; 5–7 % have platelet-derived growth factor receptor alpha (PDGFRA) mutation.
- Discovered on GIST-1 (DOG1) helps identify KIT-negative and PDGFRA-negative GISTs.
- Gastric GISTs generally have more favorable prognosis than intestinal GISTs.
- The most reliable prognostic factors for GISTs are tumor size, location of the primary tumor, and the mitotic index.
- Definitive tissue diagnosis is not required for resectable lesions.
- Surgical resection remains the treatment of choice for localized GISTs.
- Systemic chemotherapy and radiation are not routinely recommended.
- Lymphadenectomy is not recommended.

- Surgery alone does not routinely produce a durable cure, providing rationale for adjuvant imatinib therapy.
- Consider adjuvant imatinib therapy for tumor >5 cm with >5 mitoses/50 HPF, tumor >10 cm, mitotic rate >10/50 HPF, tumor >5 cm and >5 mitoses/HPF, or a ruptured GIST.
- Imatinib mesylate (GLEEVEC™) is a selective molecular inhibitor of the KIT tyrosine kinase which is an effective treatment for GISTs. Mutation type is emerging as an important predictor of the response to targeted therapy.
- Two phase III trials demonstrated no survival advantages with 800 mg regimen over 400 mg.
- Patients with a KIT exon 9 mutation have a prolonged progression-free survival with the higher-dose regimen.
- Patients with a KIT exon 11 mutation respond better to Gleevec than those with a KIT exon 9 mutation. However, patients with a KIT exon 9 mutation respond better to sunitinib than those with a KIT exon 11 mutation.
- Most patients who initially respond to Gleevec ultimately acquire resistance and demonstrate disease progression.
- Sunitinib malate targets multiple tyrosine kinases and is effective in imatinib-refractory or intolerant patients.
- There is no consensus as to the indications for neoadjuvant imatinib; it has been used in high-risk tumors or tumors located in regions in which surgical resection can result in serious morbidity.

Questions

1. Which of the following statement is false?
   A. Pediatric GISTs are rare, but when they do occur, they are typically in the small intestine.
   B. The estimated incidence of GISTs in the United States is 3,000–5,000 new cases, though this estimate may not account for small incidentally diagnosed tumors.
   C. GISTs are most commonly located in the stomach and small intestine, but colon, rectal, and esophageal tumors also occur.
   D. GISTs are the most common sarcoma of the GI tract, accounting for 1–3 % of all GI malignancies.
   E. GISTs are sensitive to chemotherapy and radiation therapy.
2. Which of the following is NOT helpful in diagnosing GISTs?
   A. c-KIT
   B. k-ras
   C. PDGFRA
   D. DOG1
   E. CD34
3. A 55-year-old man is noted to have a 2.5 cm submucosal greater curve mass on an upper endoscopy performed for gastroesopagheal reflux. He is asymptomatic and CT scan reveals the mass and no further disease. The next step in management is:
   A. Distal gastrectomy, vagotomy, and omentectomy
   B. Wedge resection
   C. Imatinib therapy
   D. Systemic chemotherapy
   E. Observation
4. Which of the following features is NOT a prognosticator in GISTs?
   A. Tumor size
   B. Mitotic rate
   C. 2 cm resection margin
   D. Staining for PDGFR-alpha
   E. Location of primary tumor
5. A 65-year-old woman presents with upper abdominal pain and early satiety. A large 7 cm GIST is noted on CT scan which appears to invade the spleen, transverse colon, and celiac axis. The next step in management is:
   A. En bloc resection including splenectomy and transverse colectomy
   B. Imatinib therapy followed by resection after maximal response
   C. Radiation therapy and chemotherapy
   D. Referral to palliative care
   E. Treatment with sunitinib
6. Which of the following features are NOT associated with a worse prognosis on CT imaging?
   A. Exophytic growth phase
   B. Heterogeneity of contrast and evidence of tumor necrosis
   C. Size less than 2 cm

   D. Invasion into adjacent organs
   E. Size greater than 10 cm
7. Which of the following statements is TRUE?
   A. Sunitinib is used as initial therapy for large GISTs.
   B. There is no consensus as to the indications for neoadjuvant imatinib.
   C. Most patients will not develop resistance to imatinib.
   D. Lymphadenectomy should be routinely performed.
   E. Intestinal GISTs have more favorable prognosis than gastric GISTs.
8. Options for imatinib-refractory or resistance GIST include which of the following:
   A. Systemic doxorubicin-based chemotherapy
   B. External beam radiation
   C. Second-line tyrosine kinase inhibitor (sunitinib)
   D. Palliative care
   E. Combined chemoradiation therapy
9. Which of the following statements is INCORRECT?
   A. Adjuvant imatinib given at 800 mg daily is better than 400 mg daily.
   B. Patients with mutations in KIT exon 9 should be considered for imatinib at 800 mg qd.
   C. Patients with KIT exon 11 mutations are more responsive to imatinib than those with KIT exon 9 mutations
   D. Despite having a better response with a particular mutation, mutational analysis has not been shown to improve overall survival.
   E. Neoadjuvant imatinib should be considered for patients with marginally resectable GISTs.
10. Which of the following is considered NOT to be high risk?
   A. Tumor >10 cm
   B. Ruptured GIST
   C. Tumor >5 cm with >5 mitoses/50 HPF
   D. Tumor size 2 cm
   E. Mitotic rate >10/50 HPF

Answers

1. A
2. B
3. B
4. D
5. B
6. C
7. B
8. C
9. A
10. D

References

1. Nilsson B, Bumming P, Meis-Kindblom JM, Oden A, Dortok A, Gustavsson B. Gastrointestinal stromal tumors: the incidence, prevalence, clinical course and prognostication in the preimatinib mesylate era – a population based study in western Sweden. Cancer. 2005;15(4):821–9.
2. Joensuu H. Gastrointestinal stromal tumor (GIST). Ann Oncol. 2006;17 Suppl 10:x280–6.
3. Pidhorecky I, Cheney RT, Kraybill WG, et al. Gastrointestinal stromal tumors: current diagnosis, biologic behavior, and management. Ann Surg Oncol. 2000;135:1070.
4. Hirota S, Isozaki K, Moriyama Y, et al. Gain-of-function mutations of c-kit in human gastrointestinal stromal tumors. Science. 1998;279:577–80.
5. Joensuu H, DeMatteo RP. The management of gastro-intestinal stromal tumors: a model for targeted and multidisciplinary therapy of malignancy. Annu Rev Med. 2012;63:247–58.
6. Heinrich MC, Corless CL, Duensing A, et al. PDGFRA activating mutations in gastrointestinal stromal tumors. Science. 2003;299:708–10.
7. Joensuu H, Fletcher C, Dimitrijevic S, Silberman S, Roberts P, Demetri G. Management of malignant gas-trointestinal stromal tumours. Lancet Oncol. 2002;3: 655–64.
8. Joensuu H. Risk stratification of patients diagnosed with gastrointestinal stromal tumor after surgery: an analysis of pooled population-based cohorts. Lancet Oncol. 2012;13:265.
9. Miettinen M, Lasota J. Gastrointestinal stromal tumors: pathology and prognosis at different sites. Semin Diagn Pathol. 2006;23:70–83.
10. American Joint Committee on Cancer. Gastrointestinal stromal tumor. In: Edge SB, Byrd DR, Compton CC, et al., editors. American Joint Committee on cancer staging manual. 7th ed. New York: Springer; 2010. p. 175.
11. Joensuu H, Roberts PJ, Sarlomo-Rikala M, Andersson LC, Tervahartiala P, Tuveson D, et al. Brief report: effect

of the tyrosine kinase inhibitor STI571 in a patient with a metastatic gastrointestinal stromal tumor. N Engl J Med. 2001;344:1052–6.
12. Verweji J, Van OA, Blay JY, Judson I, Rodenhuis S, van der Graaf W. Imatinib mesylate (STI-571 Glevec, Gleevec) is an active agent for gastrointestinal stromal tumours, but does not yield responses in other soft-tissue sarcomas and bone sarcoma group phase II study. Eur J Cancer. 2003;39:2006–11.
13. Blanke CD, Demetri GD, von Mehren M, Heinrick MC, Eisenberg G, Flethcher JA. Long-term results from a randomized phase II trial of standard- versus higher-dose imatinib mesylate for patients with unresectable or metastatic gastrointestinal stromal tumors expressing KIT. J Clin Oncol. 2008;26:620–5.
14. Blanke C, Rankin C, Demetri G, Ryan C, von Mehren M, Benjamin R, et al. Phase III randomized, intergroup trial assessing imatinib mesylate at two dose levels in patients with unresectable or metastatic gastrointestinal stromal tumors expressing the kit receptor tyrosine kinase: S0033. J Clin Oncol. 2008;26:626–32.
15. Verweij J, Casali P, Zalcberg J, LeCesne A, Reichardt P, Jean-Yves B, et al. Progression-free survival in gastrointestinal stromal tumours with high-dose imatinib: randomized trial. Lancet. 2004;364:1127–34.
16. Demetri G, von Mehren M, Blanke C, et al. Efficacy and safety of imatinib mesylate in advanced gastrointestinal stromal tumors. N Engl J Med. 2002;347:472–80.
17. Casali P, Verweij J, Kotasek D, LeCesne A, Reichardt P, Blay J, et al. Imatinib mesylate in advanced gastrointestinal stromal tumors (GIST): survival analysis of the intergroup EORTC/ISG/AGITG randomized trial in 946 patients. Eur J Cancer Suppl. 2005;3:201–2 (abstract 711).
18. Gastrointestinal Stromal Tumor Meta-Analysis Group (MetaGIST). Comparison of two doses of imatinib for the treatment of unresectable or metastatic gastrointestinal stromal tumors: a meta-analysis of 1,640 patients. J Clin Oncol. 2010;28:1247–53.
19. National Comprehensive Cancer Network. NCCN clinical practice guidelines in Oncology: soft tissue sarcoma. Version 3. http://www.nccn.org/professionals/physician_gls/pdf/sarcoma.pdf (2012). Last accessed 7 Sept 2013.
20. Debiec-Rychter M, Dumez H, Judson I, et al. Use of c-KIT/PDGFRA mutational analysis to predict the clinical response to imatinib in patients with advanced gastrointestinal stromal tumours entered on phase I and II studies of the EORTC Soft Tissue and Bone Sarcoma Group. Eur J Cancer. 2004;40:689–95.
21. Debiec-Rychter M, Sciot R, LeCesne A, Schlemmer M, Hohenberger P, van Oosterom A, et al. KIT mutations and dose selection for imatinib in patients with advanced gastrointestinal stromal tumours. Eur J Cancer. 2006;42:1093–103.
22. Heinrich M, Corless C, Demetri G, Blanke C, von Mehren M, Joensuu H, et al. Kinase mutations and imatinib response in patients with metastatic gastrointestinal stromal tumor. J Clin Oncol. 2003;21:4342–9.
23. Heinrich M, Shoemaker J, Corless C, et al. Correlation of target kinase genotype with clinical activity of imatinib mesylate (IM) in patients with metastatic GI stromal tumors (GISTs) expressing KIT (KIT+). J Clin Oncol. 2005;23 Suppl 16:(3s). Abstract 7.
24. DeMatteo RP, Owzar K, Antonescu CR, et al. Efficacy of adjuvant imatinib mesylate following complete resection of localized. primary gastrointestinal stromal tumor (GIST) at high risk of recurrence: the US Intergroup phase II trial ACOSOG Z9000 (abstract). Data presented at the 2008 ASCO Gastrointestinal Cancers Symposium; 2008;Jan 25–27; Orlando
25. DeMatteo RP, Ballman KV, Antonescu CR, et al. Adjuvant imatinib mesylate after resection of localized, primary gastrointestinal stromal tumour: a randomized, double-blind, placebo-controlled trial. Lancet. 2009;373:1097.
26. Joensuu H, Eriksson M, Hatrmann J, et al. Twelve versus 36 months of adjuvant imatinib (IM) as treatment of operable GIST with a high risk of recurrence: final results of a randomized trial (SSGXVIII/AIO). J Clin Oncol. 2011;29 Suppl: Abstr LBA1.
27. Joensuu H, Eriksson M, Sundby Hall K, et al. One vs three years of adjuvant imatinib for operable gastrointestinal stromal tumor: a randomized trial. JAMA. 2012;307:1265.
28. Casali P, Le Cesne A, Velasco A, et al. Imatinib failure-free survival (IFS) in patients with localized gastrointestinal stromal tumors (GIST) treated with adjuvant imatinib (IM): the EORTC/AGITG/FSG/GEIS/ISG randomized controlled phase III trial (abstract). J Clin Oncol. 2013 (Supple: abstr 10500).
29. PERSIST-5. Five year adjuvant imatinib mesylate (Gleevec®) in Gastrointestinal Stromal Tumor (GIST). NCT Identifier: NCT00867113. http://clinicaltrials.gov/show/NCT00867113. Last accessed 7(Sept 2013.
30. Wang D, Zhang Q, Blanke C, Demetri G, Heinrich M, Watson J, et al. Phase II trial of neoadjuvant/adjuvant imatinib mesylate for advanced primary and metastatic/recurrent operable gastrointestinal stromal tumors: long-term follow-up results of Radiation Therapy Oncology Group 0132. Ann Surg Oncol. 2012;19:1074–80.
31. Demetri G, van Oosterom A, Garrett C, Blackstein M, Shah M, Verweij J, McArthur G, et al. Efficacy and safety of sunitinib in patients with advanced gastrointestinal stromal tumour after failure of imatinib: a randomised controlled trial. Lancet. 2006;368:1329–38.
32. Demetri GD, Heinrich MC, Fletcher AJ, Fletcher CD, Van den Abbeele AD, et al. Molecular target modulation, imaging and clinical evaluation of gastrointestinal stromal tumor patients treated with sunitinib malate after imatinib failure. Clin Cancer Res. 2009;15(18):5902–9.
33. Compton C, Byrd D, Garcia-Aguilar J, et al. Gastrointestinal stromal tumor. In: Compton C, Byrd D, Garcia-Aguilar J, Kurtzman S, Olawaiye A, Washington M, editors. AJCC cancer staging atlas. 2nd ed. New York: Springer Science; 2012. p. 215–9.

Part VI

Gynecology

29 Ovarian and Adnexal Masses

Elena Pereira, Liane Deligdisch, and Linus T. Chuang

Learning Objectives

After reading this chapter, you should be able to:

- Describe the epidemiology and clinical presentation of different adnexal masses.
- Understand the approach to adnexal masses for patients in each age group: premenarchal patients, patients of childbearing age, and postmenopausal patients.
- Describe the World Health Organization classification system for histologic subtypes of ovarian neoplasms.
- Understand the prognostic factors associated with the malignant subtypes of adnexal malignancies.
- Identify when fertility-sparing surgery is appropriate.
- Appropriately utilize well-described tumor markers.
- Describe the staging procedures for malignant adnexal masses and understand the FIGO staging system.
- Identify patients requiring adjuvant therapy.

E. Pereira, M.D.
Department of Obstetrics, Gynecology and Reproductive Science, Icahn School of Medicine at Mount Sinai, New York, NY, USA
e-mail: elena.pereira@mountsinai.org

L. Deligdisch, M.D.
Department of Pathology, Obstetrics-Gynecology and Reproductive Science, Icahn School of Medicine at Mount Sinai, New York, NY, USA
e-mail: liane.deligdisch@mssm.edu

L.T. Chuang, M.D., M.P.H., F.A.C.O.G. (✉)
Division of Gynecologic Oncology, Department of Obstetrics, Gynecology and Reproductive Science, Icahn School of Medicine at Mount Sinai,
1176 Fifth Avenue, Box 1173,
10029 New York, NY, USA
e-mail: linus.chuang@mssm.edu

Introduction

The differential diagnosis of an adnexal mass can be complex and can include a multitude of processes in both the ovaries and fallopian tubes (Table 29.1). The likelihood that an ovarian mass is malignant is largely dependent on the age of the individual patient. Therefore, intraoperative management of an adnexal mass will be guided by the age of the patient and whether preservation of fertility is desired. In young women and women of childbearing age, approximately 90 % of adnexal masses are benign; this is in contrast to women of postmenopausal age in whom up to 25 % of adnexal masses are malignant [1]. Another important group, premenarchal patients, must also be considered carefully as adnexal masses in this group are rare, but are more likely to be malignant. While age is the most important risk factor for malignancy, other important risk factors include family history, nulliparity, early menarche, and late menopause. The approach to each patient should depend on whether or not there is suspicion of malignancy with consideration

Q.D. Chu et al. (eds.), *Surgical Oncology: A Practical and Comprehensive Approach*,
DOI 10.1007/978-1-4939-1423-4_29, © Springer Science+Business Media New York 2015

Table 29.1 Differential diagnosis of adnexal masses

Ovarian
Simple cyst
Corpus luteum
Follicular cyst
Benign serous
Benign mucinous
Complex
Endometrioma
Dermoid
Malignant ovarian tumor
Malignant metastatic tumor
Malignant tumors
Epithelial
Germ cell
Sex cord
Extraovarian
Ectopic pregnancy
Tubo-ovarian abscess
Hydrosalpinx
Pedunculated fibroid

toward preservation of fertility in young women and women of childbearing age.

Adnexal masses encountered incidentally at time of abdominal surgery can present as a challenge to the surgeons. Proper management of these masses often depends on patient's age and findings from preoperative workup. Ideally preoperative workup should include a transvaginal ultrasound and evaluation of tumor markers. Simple-appearing cystic masses with normal tumor markers are less suspicious for malignancy, whereas complex cystic masses with solid components and elevated tumor markers may raise concern for an adnexal malignancy. However, an understanding of possible types of adnexal masses, both benign and malignant, may assist the general surgeon in appropriately managing adnexal masses incidentally found at time of surgery.

Generally when a suspicious mass is encountered, if a gynecologic oncologist is available, it is always advisable to call for an intraoperative consultation in the case of gynecologic malignancy. When either a gynecologist or gynecologic oncologist is not available or frozen section is unable to yield definitive histologic diagnosis, conservative approach of removing the abnormal adnexal mass while preserving the contralateral adnexa should always be considered.

Additional surgical procedures including hysterectomy, contralateral salpingo-oophorectomy can be performed if needed in a subsequent setting. The conservative approach will allow the pathologist to properly analyze the entire specimen and the gynecologic oncologist to have the opportunity to counsel the patient and her family regarding any further additional surgical procedures and adjuvant therapies that may be required prior to definitive surgery.

In the following section, different types of ovarian neoplasm will be discussed. Salient features will be presented to assist the surgeons and gynecologists in understanding the ovarian tumor that is encountered during the surgery. Specific surgical approaches as they pertain to adnexal masses in women of different age groups will then be discussed in order to aid in intraoperative decision-making.

Histologic Types of Ovarian Neoplasms

The ovaries are made up of three types of cells: epithelial cells, germ cells, and stromal cells. Generally, adnexal neoplasms are grouped into five larger categories based on histologic type according to the World Health Organization classification system. The most commonly encountered are: epithelial, germ cell, sex cord-stromal tumors, metastatic tumors, and a miscellaneous group. There exist both benign and malignant entities in the three larger subtypes. Epithelial ovarian tumors are the most commonly encountered, which account for approximately 75 % of all ovarian tumors and 90–95 % of ovarian malignancies. Germ cell tumors are the second most common, accounting for about 15–20 % of ovarian neoplasms. Approximately 5–10 % of all ovarian neoplasms are categorized as sex cord-stromal tumors [2–4] (Table 29.2). Lastly, it must always be considered that an ovarian tumor may represent metastatic disease from another primary, most commonly from the breast, colon, stomach, and other gynecologic organs such as the endometrium or the cervix.

Epithelial Tumors

Epithelial-type tumors are the most commonly encountered of the ovarian tumors, and the majority of these tumors are benign [2, 4]. Epithelial-type tumors are classified as either benign, malignant, or tumors of low malignant potential. Epithelial-type tumors can be further divided according to the type of cells into which they differentiate: serous, mucinous, endometrioid, clear cell, and Brenner tumors. Malignant tumors of epithelial origin are then further subdivided according to their degree of differentiation (well, moderately, and poorly differentiated neoplasm), which is reflected in their clinical behavior. Tumors of low malignant potential, also referred to as borderline tumors, represent a group of tumors that demonstrate a pattern of proliferation greater than those found in benign tumors, but lacking destructive invasion of the stromal components of the ovary. Borderline tumors have a substantially more favorable prognosis compared to their malignant counterpart, with an overall 10-year survival of 83–93 % [4, 5].

Table 29.2 Ovarian tumors and incidence

Histologic types	Incidence of ovarian tumors
Epithelial ovarian tumors	75 %
Germ cell tumors	15–20 %
Sex cord-stromal tumors	5–10 %

The pattern of spread among the epithelial tumors is unique in that it involves exfoliation of surface ovarian tumor into the peritoneal cavity, resulting in peritoneal surface spread. Important risk factors have been identified for malignant epithelial tumors. Among these the strongest correlation has been found with BRCA mutations. Approximately 5–10 % of ovarian cancers are associated with mutations in BRCA1 and BRCA2 tumor suppressor genes. The average lifetime risk for ovarian cancer in patients with BRCA1 mutations is approximately 30–40 % and a smaller risk for patients with BRCA2 mutations (10–18 %) [6]. Management of patients with BRCA1 and BRCA2 are further discussed in Chap. 6, BRCA1 and BRCA2 in Breast Cancer and Ovarian Cancer. Other important risk factors include age, nulliparity, obesity, and family history. Oral contraceptive use has been found to be protective [2, 4, 7, 8].

Serous epithelial tumors are the most common of all ovarian tumors (Figs. 29.1, 29.2, and 29.3). These tumors are subcategorized into benign, malignant, and tumors of low malignant potential. The mean age at presentation of malignant serous tumors is in the sixth decade of life, and this tumor type is uncommon in women less than 35 years of age. Serous carcinomas are further

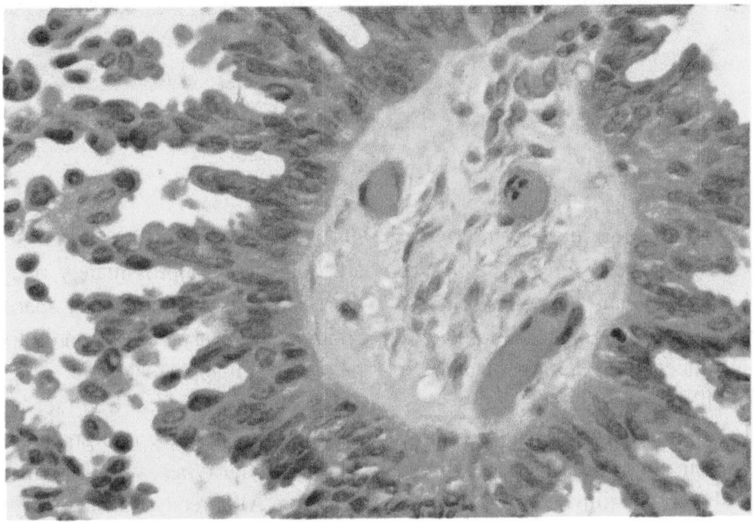

Fig. 29.1 Microscopic view of serous cystadenoma of low malignant potential (micropapillary type)

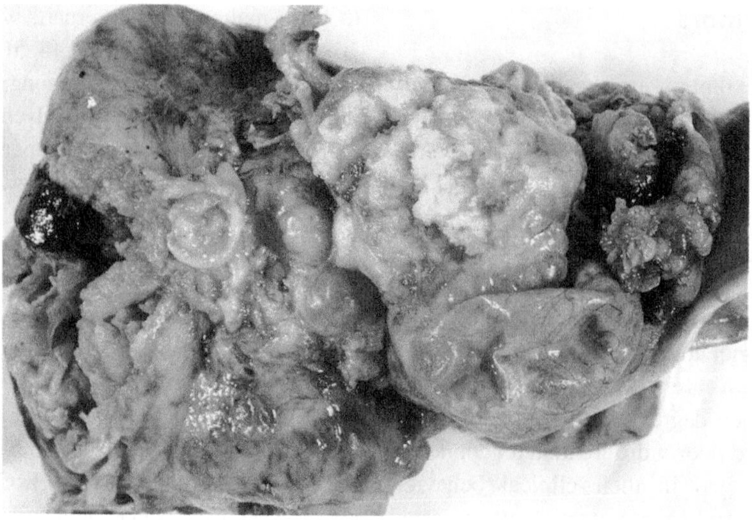

Fig. 29.2 Gross specimen of serous cystadenocarcinoma

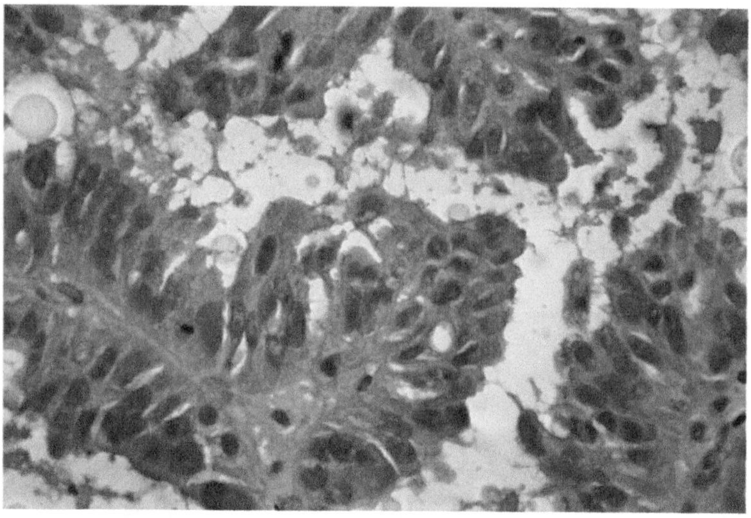

Fig. 29.3 Microscopic picture of serous cystadenocarcinoma

divided into low-grade and high-grade types. Low-grade histologic types tend to be slower growing with better survival outcomes, whereas high-grade serous carcinomas are associated with rapid growth, advanced presentation of disease, and poor survival [2, 9].

Benign and low malignant potential serous tumors tend to present slightly earlier in life, more commonly in and before the fifth decade of life [2]. Well-staged borderline tumors that are confined to the ovary have an excellent prognosis. These tumors are bilateral in approximately one-third of cases; therefore, in cases of fertility-sparing surgery, the contralateral ovary must be carefully inspected and preserved if it appears normal.

Mucinous tumors like serous tumors are divided into benign, malignant, and low malignant potential types, with benign being the most common. All three types classically present as very large ovarian tumors with a mean size of 18 cm.

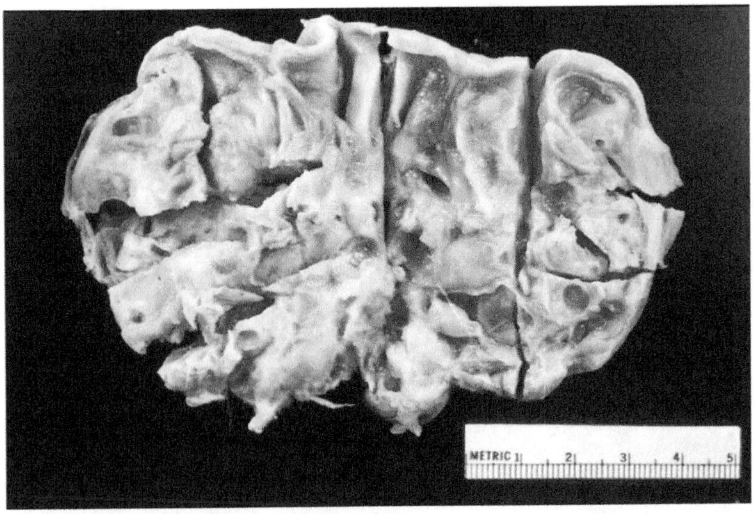

Fig. 29.4 Gross specimen of a mature cystic teratoma

These tumors are less common than their serous counterpart representing only 10 % of epithelial-type ovarian tumors. The age distribution of these tumors is similar to that of the serous types with malignancy occurring more commonly beyond the fifth decade of life. It must be kept in mind when encountering this tumor type that these masses may represent metastasis, most commonly from the gastrointestinal tract. These tumors are usually bilateral in nature. This can make diagnosis challenging, as the ovarian tumor may be the first visible sign of disease. Careful inspection of the gastrointestinal tract should be carried out when mucinous tumor is encountered incidentally and routine appendectomy is recommended for patient with malignant ovarian mucinous tumor.

Endometrioid tumors make up a smaller portion of epithelial-type ovarian tumors. Like other epithelial tumors, they are also classified as benign, malignant, and borderline. The age distribution is similar to other epithelial-type tumors. The malignant tumors can present synchronously with endometrioid-type endometrial cancers of the uterus in up to 30 % of cases.

Clear cell tumors are uncommon and are classically thought to be more aggressive than the other epithelial tumors; however, data regarding this is inconsistent. Clear cell tumors can present as tumors of low malignant potential; however, it is very difficult to differentiate these from the malignant subtype. Clear cell tumors are most often associated with endometriosis.

Ovarian Germ Cell Tumors

These tumors account for 15–20 % of all ovarian tumors but represent less than 5 % of all ovarian malignancies. The benign mature cystic teratoma, also referred to as a dermoid cyst, makes up the largest component of tumors in this category and is the most common ovarian neoplasm overall (Figs. 29.4 and 29.5).

Dermoids often contain components from all three embryonic germ layers, but most commonly of the ectoderm layer containing elements such as hair and sebum. These tumors often have a high-fat content, and their buoyancy places these tumors at higher risk for ovarian torsion. It is important in cases of dermoid cysts that thorough inspection of the other ovary is performed, as 20 % of these cysts are bilateral. As these tumors are usually benign, conservative approach such as ovarian cystectomy should be attempted if possible. Tumors of this category also represent

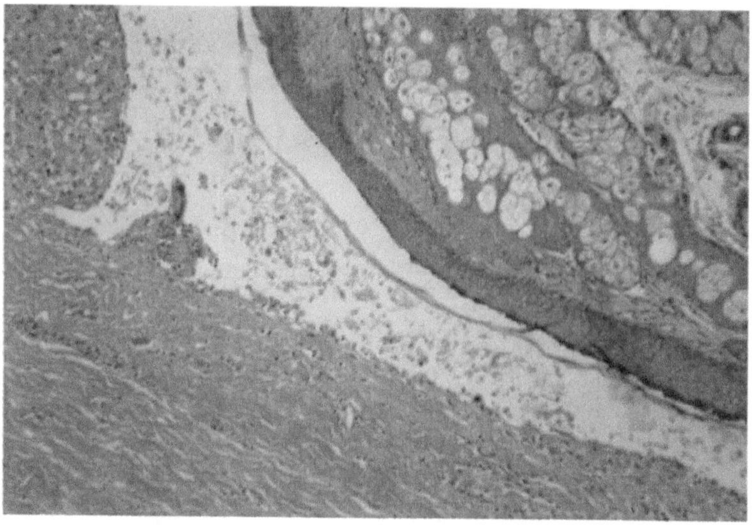

Fig. 29.5 Microscopic picture of a mature cystic teratoma

the most common ovarian malignancies affecting women younger than 20 years of age, and in fact, approximately 70 % of these tumors occur in this age group. Malignant tumors in this category include dysgerminomas, endodermal sinus tumors (yolk sac tumors), immature teratomas, mixed germ cell tumors, and embryonal tumors.

Dysgerminomas are the most common of the malignant type, and although they can be seen in patients with normal karyotypes, they are also classically seen in patients with gonadal dysgenesis, such as patients with testicular feminization. The risk of bilaterality is approximately 10 %, and the contralateral ovary should be inspected carefully. The risk of dysgerminomas peaks at age 20 but can range from age 6 to 40 depending on the histologic type. These tumors tend to be predominantly solid, large fleshy masses [10, 11].

Yolk sac tumors are the next most common of the germ cell tumors and tend to grow quite rapidly (Figs. 29.6 and 29.7). These tumors are typically unilateral; however, metastasis to the contralateral ovary may occur. In adults, yolk sac tumors account for approximately 15 % of all germ cell tumors. Yolk sac tumors are relatively more common in children. These tumors tend to be more cystic than dysgerminomas and may exhibit more substantial areas of necrosis. Yolk sac tumors are aggressive and these patients require adjuvant chemotherapy [10, 11].

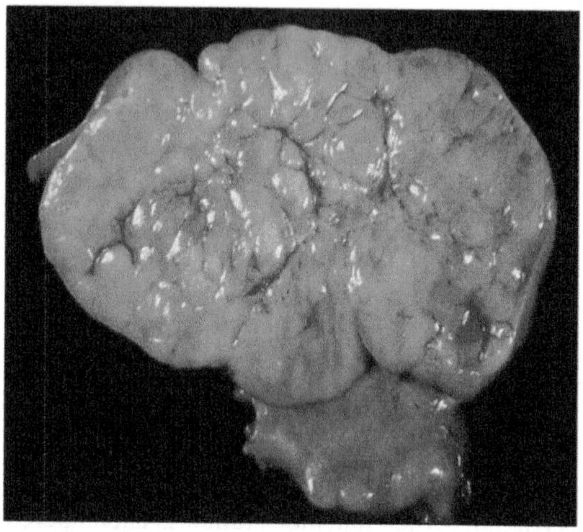

Fig. 29.6 Gross specimen of yolk sac tumor

Immature teratomas are the third most common malignant tumor in this category (Figs. 29.8 and 29.9). It contains variable amounts of immature tissue from all three germ cell layers. Again, most patients are diagnosed as stage I disease, and survival is most closely associated with grade of the tumor. Survival of women with grade 1 disease is 100 %, grade 2 disease is 70 %, and grade 3 disease is 33 %. Adjuvant therapies are usually recommended for patients with stage I grade 3 tumors or advanced stage diseases [11].

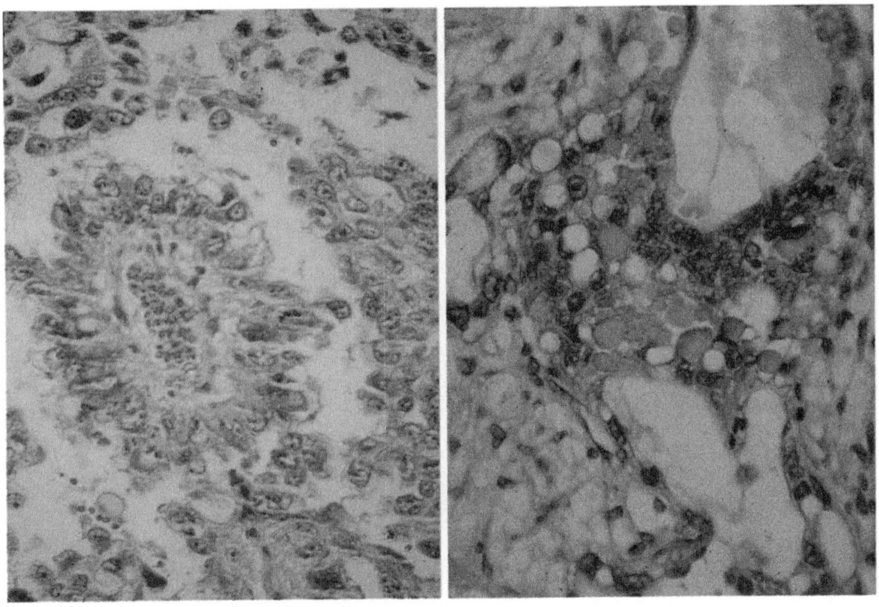

Fig. 29.7 Microscopic picture of yolk sac tumors

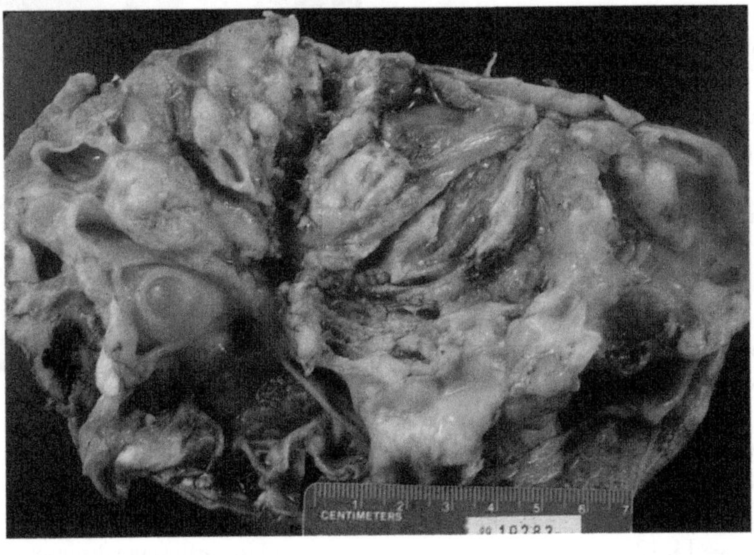

Fig. 29.8 Gross specimen of immature tumor

Ovarian Sex Cord-Stromal Tumors

Sex cord-stromal tumors are significantly less common and comprise only 5–10 % of all ovarian tumors. These tumors are derived from the sex cord and stromal components of the ovary. Because of this derivation tumors of this type can contain a variety of cell types including granulosa cells, theca cells, lutein cells, Sertoli cells, Leydig cells, and fibroblasts. Fibromas and thecomas make up the benign category, which rarely demonstrate malignant counterparts. Fibromas account for the most common tumor among the sex cord-stromal tumors. Often with sex cord-stromal tumors, the histologic components of the tumor are a combination of more than one of these types of cell.

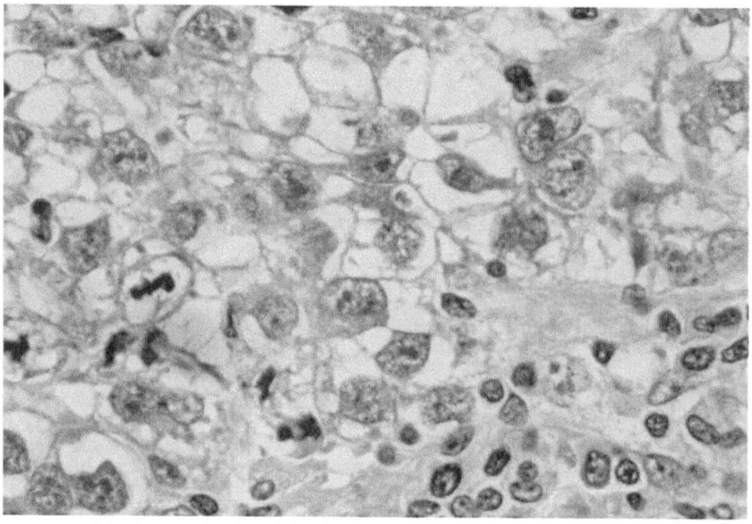

Fig. 29.9 Microscopic picture of immature tumor

Granulosa cell tumors are the next most common tumors in this category (Figs. 29.10 and 29.11). They are an estrogen-producing malignant type of ovarian tumor. Granulosa cells comprise 70 % of the tumors in this category and are divided in adult type and juvenile type, which differ morphologically and in the age distribution of patients affected. The adult-type histology is the more common of the two accounting for approximately 95 % of cases. Both types often present with signs of unopposed estrogen (abnormal vaginal bleeding, precocious puberty, etc.); however, the juvenile-type granulosa cell tumor is known to be far more aggressive with one small study demonstrating only a 23 % survival in stages II–IV disease. The average size of tumor at presentation is 12 cm, and these tumors should be suspected in patients from this age group who present with large unilateral adnexal masses [4, 12, 13].

Sertoli-Leydig cell tumors are rarer than granulosa cell tumors, making up less than 1 % of all ovarian tumors. In some cases, they can be associated with virilization as they may secrete testosterone but like granulosa cell tumors often present with symptoms of an abdominal mass and menstrual disorders. These tumors are also quite large at presentation with an average 16 cm tumor size noted at time of detection. Also like granulosa cell tumors, these tumors tend to be diagnosed in early stage disease with only 2–3 % demonstrating extraovarian spread at time of diagnosis [4].

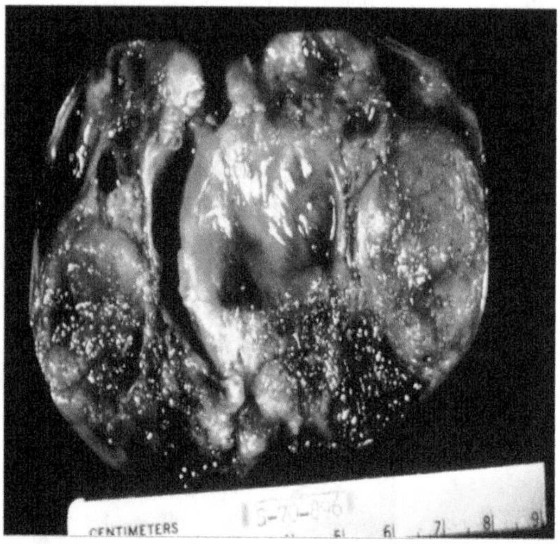

Fig. 29.10 Gross specimen of granulosa-theca cell tumor

Fallopian Tube and Peritoneal Surface Tumors

Benign cysts of the fallopian tube are referred to as paratubal cysts. They are often simple and of no consequence. Therefore, surgical intervention

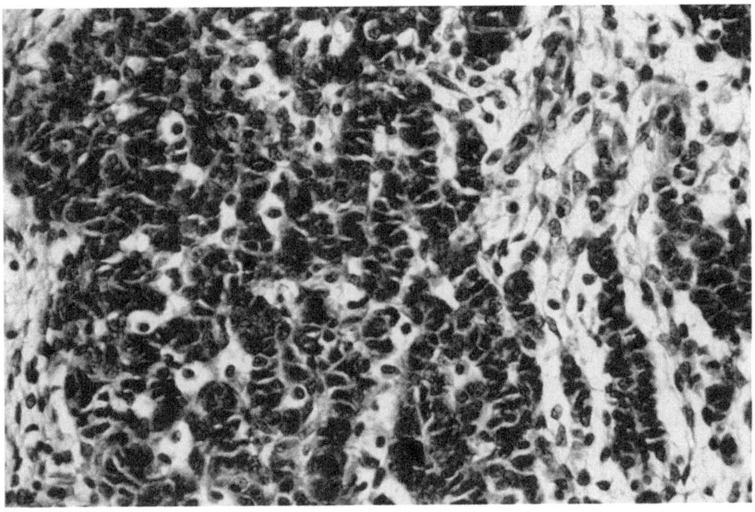

Fig. 29.11 Microscopic picture of juvenile granulosa cell tumor

is not necessary for this incidental finding. Malignant tumors of the fallopian tube and primary peritoneal surface tumors behave very similarly to epithelial ovarian malignancies. In fact, recent studies have suggested that high-grade serous carcinoma may actually originate from the fimbriated end of the fallopian tubes. Given the proximity of the fallopian tube to the ovary, and the typically advanced nature of these malignancies, it is often difficult to distinguish between primary fallopian tube and primary ovarian tumors. In contrast, although primary peritoneal tumors behave similarly to epithelial ovarian malignancies, at time of diagnosis, the ovaries are either only minimally involved or not involved at all. Carcinomatosis can be present in all three entities [14].

Evaluation of the Surgical Specimen

Diagnosis is typically made via frozen section, which is both highly specific and sensitive in the evaluation of adnexal masses. The sensitivity and specificity are highest for malignant and benign tumors (88–97 %), with less accuracy being seen in the diagnosis of borderline tumors (33–62 %). Once a diagnosis of adnexal malignancy is made by frozen section, an appropriate staging procedure should be initiated. *However, in cases of uncertainty, a conservative approach should be taken. The patient can always return at a later time to complete the staging procedure once a final pathologic diagnosis is achieved* [15–17].

Table 29.3 Tumor markers by histologic subtype

Histology	Tumor marker
Epithelial type	CA-125
Germ cell tumors	Alpha-fetoprotein (AFP)
Yolk sac tumor Choriocarcinoma	Lactate Dehydrogenase b-hCG
Granulosa cell tumor	Inhibin B and A Estradiol

Tumor Markers

Although tumor markers are not considered useful for routine screening in ovarian tumors, they may assist with preoperative diagnosis by increasing suspicion of particular tumor types. Tumor markers are also useful after initial diagnosis for evaluation of therapeutic response and can be an indicator of recurrent disease (Table 29.3).

Surgical Approach to Young Patients and Women of Childbearing Age

When approaching malignancy in the younger patient, fertility-sparing surgery, when appropriate, is at the focus of management. Malignant tumors in this age group tend to present at an early stage and can often be staged conservatively, sparing the uterus and the contralateral ovary. If both ovaries are involved, sparing of the uterus may be considered. If possible, consultation with a reproductive endocrinologist should be utilized as they may provide guidance regarding egg or embryo cryopreservation for future fertility. Prevalence of different histology types is important to keep in mind, as many of these tumors are less aggressive than their epithelial counterparts and present at early stage disease. In one review of patients with germ cell tumors, survival for stage I disease was 98.2 % and that for patients with advanced disease stages was 94.4 % [18]. The favorable survival of these tumors is due in part to the diagnosis at early stage disease and largely because these tumors respond well to current chemotherapeutic regimens. In cases of more advanced disease, metastatic disease should be appropriately resected (cytoreduced), which may be possible even with consideration to fertility sparing. *In short, all visible disease should be cytoreduced while sparing the uterus and contralateral ovary if possible*. Again, in cases of uncertainty, a conservative approach should be taken. The patient can always return at a later time to complete the staging procedure once a final pathologic diagnosis is achieved [15–17]. Although these patients respond well to current chemotherapy regimens, those who have complete cytoreduction of disease at time of surgery fare better [19].

Ovarian masses in premenarchal girls are rare; however, when encountering a mass in this population, it is important to keep in mind that up to 20 % of ovarian masses in children are malignant [1]. Therefore, all adnexal masses in this age group should be approached carefully. Ideally if tumor markers can be sent prior to surgery, they may help guide management.

Appropriate tumor markers to send include AFP, LDH, 4. bHCG, inhibin B, and CA-125. It must be emphasized that the surgical approach in young women must be balanced between adequate removal of all tumor and fertility preservation. Conservative management should always be considered with this age group, keeping in mind the option of returning for surgical staging once a full discussion has been made with the patient and her family.

In contrast to epithelial malignant tumors, which exhibit surface spread, germ cell tumors tend to exhibit early lymphatic spread. This becomes important in surgical planning. Evaluation must begin with careful inspection of the affected ovary and the contralateral ovary. Biopsy of the contralateral ovary may be considered in cases of dysgerminoma; however, unnecessary biopsy should be avoided as it may cause damage to the remaining ovary. Additionally in cases of gonadal dysgenesis, removal of the other ovary should also be considered. The staging procedure should begin with collection of ascites, if present, and pelvic washings to be sent for evaluation. If disease appears to be limited to the ovary, then biopsies of the omentum and peritoneal surfaces are recommended. Suspicious pelvic and para-aortic nodes should be removed. If there are no palpable nodes, then random sampling is recommended. In rare cases of advanced disease, complete removal of all visible disease is recommended [20]. These procedures should be performed by a gynecologic oncologist or a surgeon who is trained to perform lymphadenectomy.

Surgical Approach to Women Beyond Childbearing and Postmenopausal Patients

The approach to women beyond childbearing age is different than that in younger patients. For one, the histologic malignant tumor types in this age group tend to be more aggressive and present at later stages of disease. Secondly, as preservation of fertility no longer is of concern, full staging surgery, including hysterectomy, is typically recommended. The predominant malignant tumor type in this age group is the epithelial tumor. Common presenting symptoms are fairly nonspecific and include bloating, pelvic pain, decreased appetite, and early satiety. Multiple retrospective reviews have demonstrated that complete cytoreduction is directly correlated with improved overall survival [21–23]. However, 5-year survival is poor and epithelial ovarian tumors

Table 29.4 International Federation of Gynecology and Obstetrics (FIGO) classification of ovarian cancer staging

FIGO stage	Description
I	*Tumor limited to ovaries (1 or both)*
1A	Tumor limited to 1 ovary, capsule intact, no tumor on ovarian surface, no malignant cells in pelvic ascites or washings
1B	Tumor limited to both ovaries, capsules intact, no tumor on ovarian surface, no malignant cells in pelvic ascites or washings
1C	Tumor limited to one or both ovaries with any of the following: capsule ruptured, tumor on ovarian surface, malignant cells in ascites or in pelvic washings
II	*Tumor involves one or both ovaries with pelvic extension*
IIA	Extension and/or implants on the uterus and/or tubes, no malignant cells in ascites or peritoneal washings
IIB	Extension to other pelvic tissues, no malignant cells in ascites or peritoneal washings
IIC	Pelvic extension as described in IIA and IIB with malignant cells in ascites or pelvic washings
III	*Tumor involves one or both ovaries with microscopically confirmed peritoneal metastasis outside the pelvis*
IIIA	Microscopic peritoneal metastasis beyond the pelvis
IIIB	Macroscopic peritoneal metastasis beyond the pelvis, ≤2 cm in greatest dimension
IIIC	Macroscopic peritoneal metastasis beyond the pelvis, >2 cm in greatest dimension, or regional lymph node metastasis
IV	*Distant metastasis, includes liver parenchyma and supradiaphragmatic spread*

continue to be one of the great challenges of gynecologic oncology in spite of improved chemotherapeutic regimens and surgical technique.

The approach to surgical staging is dependent on the histologic type of ovarian tumor. In this age group, epithelial-type malignancies are most common and often multiple surfaces within the peritoneum are involved. Surgical staging primarily involves obtaining pelvic and abdominal cytologic washings, careful exploration of the upper and lower abdomen, recommend removal of the bilateral fallopian tubes and ovaries, removal of the uterus, pelvic and para-aortic lymph node sampling, omentectomy, and removal of all visible disease. Various procedures including bowel resection, splenectomy, and upper abdominal resections may be required to achieve an optimal cytoreduction. Adequate staging is important for both prognosis and for determination of appropriate adjuvant therapy (Table 29.4). Staging may be done via laparotomy or laparoscopy. In skilled hands, laparoscopic approaches appear to confer similar survival advantage; however, the rate of rupture is noted to be higher in laparoscopic surgery [17, 24].

The approach to borderline disease may be more conservative as many studies demonstrate that although conservative surgery may be associated with higher incidence of recurrence, in most cases, secondary cytoreduction is possible and recurrence in those cases has not been found to affect overall survival. However, the surgical approach for each patient should be individualized, and in cases where fertility is not a consideration, many gynecologic oncologists would recommend removal of the bilateral fallopian tubes and ovaries [17, 25–27].

Adjuvant Chemotherapy

Appropriate adjuvant chemotherapy is guided both by the histology of the tumor and by the grade of the tumor. Patients can be referred to a gynecologic oncologist for the continuation of their care and for adjuvant therapy planning. For several decades, chemotherapy has been the standard treatment for all but early stage and well-differentiated tumors. Combination platinum and paclitaxel-based chemotherapy has become the first-line treatment for advanced epithelial ovarian tumors with an overall response rate of approximately 75 %, and adjuvant therapy is recommended for patients with stage IC disease or greater. Recently the inclusion of intraperitoneal chemotherapy has been reported to result in improved survival in patients with optimally cytoreduced advanced ovarian cancers [28]. It has also been demonstrated that patients with epithelial high-grade stage 1A/1B tumors benefit from adjuvant chemotherapy [29–31]. Patients with stage IA dysgerminoma and immature teratoma tumors can be followed closely and do not require adjuvant therapy. Chemotherapy is recommended for all patients with yolk sac tumors and for dysgerminoma and immature teratoma patients with stage IB disease or greater. The current recommended regimen is a platinum-based combination therapy: bleomycin, etoposide, and cisplatin [32]. These chemotherapy regimens can all be quite toxic, and full understanding of adverse effects is important.

Other Considerations

Other benign entities to consider in the differential diagnosis of adnexal masses are tubo-ovarian abscess, ectopic pregnancy, and ovarian torsion. Classically, tubo-ovarian abscesses present with gradual onset pain and can be associated with fevers, nausea, emesis, and purulent vaginal discharge. In fact, the presentation of a tubo-ovarian abscess and appendicitis can be very similar. Ruptured tubo-ovarian abscesses are considered a life-threatening emergency and require prompt surgical intervention. Surgery should be combined with antimicrobial therapy in such cases. The goal of surgery should be to remove as much of the abscess cavity and infectious material as possible. In patients who have completed childbearing, a hysterectomy and bilateral salpingo-oophorectomy may be appropriate [32, 33]. Patients who are clinically stable with no evidence of sepsis or large abscess may be treated with antibiotics alone [33].

Ovarian torsion refers to the partial or complete rotation of the ovary about its ligamentous support. Classically, the pain associated with ovarian torsion is sudden onset, severe, intermittent, and unilateral. Although torsion more commonly occurs in the case of adnexal masses, ovarian torsion can also occur in normal ovaries. Patients with ovarian torsion may also present with nausea and vomiting. Prompt diagnosis is important as the surgeon's ability to salvage the ovary decreases as the ovary becomes necrotic. Detorsion of the ovary should be attempted and the ovary should be observed for return of normal color. In cases where the color does not return or the ovary appears necrotic, a salpingo-oophorectomy should be performed.

If an ectopic pregnancy is suspected, a blood pregnancy level (bHCG) should be sent. Patients with ectopic pregnancy often present with abdominal pain, amenorrhea, or abnormal vaginal bleeding. Surgically, hemoperitoneum may be noted in the case of a ruptured ectopic pregnancy. Surgical management involves a salpingectomy, with care taken not to disrupt the blood supply to the ovary.

Salient Points

- The management of adnexal masses must be guided with respect to the age of the patient and whether fertility is desired.
- The likelihood of malignancy is less likely in women of childbearing age and more likely in premenarcheal and postmenopausal women.
- Generally if a suspicious lesion is encountered, a frozen section should be performed.
- When either a gynecologist or gynecologic oncologist is not available or frozen section is unable to yield definitive histologic diagnosis, conservative approach of removing the abnormal adnexal mass while preserving the contralateral adnexa should always be considered for women of childbearing age. Additional surgical procedures including hysterectomy and contralateral salpingo-oophorectomy can be performed if needed in a subsequent setting.
- Full surgical staging of ovarian malignancy should include pelvic and abdominal washings, exploration of the upper and lower abdomen, removal of bilateral tubes and ovaries, removal of the uterus, pelvic and para-aortic lymph node sampling, removal of omentum, and *removal of all visible disease*.
- *Epithelial neoplasms* are the most commonly encountered of the ovarian tumors, and the

majority of these tumors are benign. Subtypes are serous, mucinous, endometrioid, clear cell, and Brenner tumors.

- *Ovarian germ cell tumors* account for 15–20 % of all ovarian tumors but represent less than 5 % of all ovarian malignancies. Most tumors in this category are benign dermoid cysts; however, malignant subtypes are the most common ovarian malignancies affecting women younger than 20 years. The most common malignant subtypes are dysgerminoma, yolk sac tumor, and immature teratomas.
- Ovarian sex cord-stromal tumors comprise only 5–10 % of all ovarian tumors. Benign fibromas are the most common tumors in this category. The most common malignant subtypes are granulosa cell and Sertoli-Leydig cell.

Surgical Approach to Young Women and Women of Childbearing Age

- Fertility preservation, when appropriate, is at the focus of management in these patients.
- Tumors in this age group tend to be lower grade and can often be staged conservatively.
- *All visible disease should be removed while sparing the contralateral ovary and uterus if possible.*
- It must be emphasized that the surgical approach in young women must be balanced between adequate removal of all tumor and fertility preservation.

Surgical Approach to Women Beyond Childbearing and Postmenopausal Patients

- Malignant tumor types in this age group tend to be more aggressive histologic types and present at later stages of disease.
- As preservation of fertility no longer is of concern, *full staging surgery* is typically recommended.
- Adequate staging is important for both prognosis and for determination of appropriate adjuvant therapy.

Questions

1. A 28-year-old nulliparous woman was incidentally found at the time of cholecystectomy to have serous adenocarcinoma of the right ovary. Inspection of the uterus and left adnexa, omentum, and the abdominal and pelvic cavities did not reveal any other abnormal findings. All of following procedures should be considered except?
   A. No additional surgical intervention at this time
   B. Pelvic washings for cytology and right salpingo-oophorectomy
   C. Pelvic washings for cytology, right salpingo-oophorectomy, peritoneal biopsy, and pelvic and para-aortic lymphadenectomy
   D. Pelvic washings for cytology, hysterectomy, bilateral salpingo-oophorectomy, peritoneal biopsy, and pelvic and para-aortic lymphadenectomy
   E. Call for gynecologic oncology consultation
2. The average lifetime risk for ovarian cancer in patients with BRCA1 mutations is approximately:
   A. 15 %
   B. 30 %
   C. 45 %
   D. 60 %
3. Which of the following tumor category represents the most common ovarian malignancies affecting women younger than 20 years of age.
   A. Epithelial
   B. Sex cord-stromal
   C. Germ cell
4. Which of the following sex cord tumor is an estrogen-producing ovarian tumor.
   A. Granulosa cell tumors
   B. Yolk sac tumors
   C. Dysgerminomas
   D. Sertoli-Leydig cell tumors
5. Match the tumor marker with the correct tumor category. Tumor markers may be used more than once.
   A. Papillary serous adenocarcinoma
   B. Germ cell tumor
   C. Granulosa cell tumor
   D. Yolk sac tumor
      1. CA-125
      2. Alpha-fetoprotein
      3. Inhibin A and B
      4. bHCG

6. True or false. Patients with stage IA dysgerminoma and immature teratoma tumors can be followed closely and do not require adjuvant therapy.
7. True or false. In young women and women of childbearing age, approximately 90 % of adnexal masses are benign.
8. A 32-year-old, sexually active patient presents with gradual onset pain, fevers, nausea, and emesis. Appendicitis is suspected and she is taken to the operating room. Her appendix is found to be normal. Which of the following adnexal masses is most likely to present with the above symptoms?
   A. Papillary serous adenocarcinoma
   B. Ectopic pregnancy
   C. Tubo-ovarian abscess
   D. Dermoid cyst

Answers

1. D
2. B
3. C
4. A
5. A-1, B-2, C-3, D-4
6. True
7. True
8. C

References

1. Hassan E, Creatsas G, Deligeorolgou E, Michalas S. Ovarian tumors during childhood and adolescence. A clinicopathological study. Eur J Gynaecol Oncol. 1999;20(2):124–6.
2. Kumar V, Abbas A, Aster J, editors. Robbins basic pathology. 9th ed. Philadelphia: Saunders/Elsevier; 2013. p. 695–700.
3. Lee-Jones L. Ovarian tumours: an overview. Atlas Genet Cytogenet Oncol Haematol. 2004;8(2):115–9.
4. Scully RE. Classification of human ovarian tumors. Environ Health Perspect. 1987;73:15–25.
5. Nikrui N. Survey of clinical behavior of patients with borderline epithelial tumors of the ovary. Gynecol Oncol. 1981;12(1):107–19.
6. Chen S, Parmigiani G. Meta-analysis of BRCA1 and BRCA2 penetrance. J Clin Oncol. 2007;25(11): 1329–33.
7. Barakat R, Markman M, Randall M, editors. Principles and practice of gynecologic oncology. 6th ed. Philadelphia: Wolters Kluwer Health/Lippincott Williams & Wilkins; 2013. p. 757–836.
8. Engeland A, Tretli S, Bjørge T. Height, body mass index, and ovarian cancer: a follow-up of 1.1 million Norwegian women. J Natl Cancer Inst. 2003;95(16): 1244–8.
9. Heintz AP, Odicino F, Maisonneuve P, et al. Carcinoma of the ovary. Int J Gynaecol Obstet. 2003;83 Suppl 1:135–66.
10. Roth L. Variants of yolk sac tumor. Pathol Case Rev. 2005;10:186–92.
11. Kurman RJ, Norris HJ. Malignant germ cell tumors of the ovary. Hum Pathol. 1977;8(5):551–64.
12. Malmström H, Högberg T, Risberg B, Simonsen E. Granulosa cell tumors of the ovary: prognostic factors and outcome. Gynecol Oncol. 1994;52(1):50–5.
13. Evans AT, Gaffey TA, Malkasian GD, Annegers JF. Clinicopathologic review of 118 granulosa and 82 theca cell tumors. Obstet Gynecol. 1980;55(2): 231–8.
14. Kindelberger DW, Lee Y, Miron A, et al. Intraepithelial carcinoma of the fimbria and pelvic serous carcinoma: evidence for a causal relationship. Am J Surg Pathol. 2007;31(2):161–9.
15. Brun JL, Cortez A, Rouzier R, et al. Factors influencing the use and accuracy of frozen section diagnosis of epithelial ovarian tumors. Am J Obstet Gynecol. 2008;199(3):244.e1–e7.
16. Boriboonhirunsarn D, Sermboon A. Accuracy of frozen section in the diagnosis of malignant ovarian tumor. J Obstet Gynaecol Res. 2004;30(5):394–9.
17. Covens AL, Dodge JE, Lacchetti C, et al. Surgical management of a suspicious adnexal mass: a systematic review. Gynecol Oncol. 2012;126(1):149–56.
18. Low JJ, Perrin LC, Crandon AJ, Hacker NF. Conservative surgery to preserve ovarian function in patients with malignant ovarian germ cell tumors. A review of 74 cases. Cancer. 2000;89(2):391–8.
19. Brookfield KF, Cheung MC, Koniaris LG, Sola JE, Fischer AC. A population-based analysis of 1037 malignant ovarian tumors in the pediatric population. J Surg Res. 2009;156(1):45–9.
20. Zalel Y, Piura B, Elchalal U, Czernobilsky B, Antebi S, Dgani R. Diagnosis and management of malignant germ cell ovarian tumors in young females. Int J Gynaecol Obstet. 1996;55(1):1–10.
21. Hoskins WJ. Epithelial ovarian carcinoma: principles of primary surgery. Gynecol Oncol. 1994;55(3 Pt 2):S91–6.
22. Curtin JP, Malik R, Venkatraman ES, Barakat RR, Hoskins WJ. Stage IV ovarian cancer: impact of surgical debulking. Gynecol Oncol. 1997;64(1):9–12.
23. Chi DS, Liao JB, Leon LF, et al. Identification of prognostic factors in advanced epithelial ovarian carcinoma. Gynecol Oncol. 2001;82(3):532–7.
24. Ghezzi F, Cromi A, Siesto G, Serati M, Zaffaroni E, Bolis P. Laparoscopy staging of early ovarian cancer: our experience and review of the literature. Int J Gynecol Cancer. 2009;19 Suppl 2:S7–13.
25. Donnez J, Munschke A, Berliere M, et al. Safety of conservative management and fertility outcome in women with borderline tumors of the ovary. Fertil Steril. 2003;79(5):1216–21.

26. Zanetta G, Rota S, Chiari S, Bonazzi C, Bratina G, Mangioni C. Behavior of borderline tumors with particular interest to persistence, recurrence, and progression to invasive carcinoma: a prospective study. J Clin Oncol. 2001;19(10):2658–64.
27. Camatte S, Morice P, Pautier P, Atallah D, Duvillard P, Castaigne D. Fertility results after conservative treatment of advanced stage serous borderline tumour of the ovary. BJOG. 2002;109(4):376–80.
28. Armstrong DK, Bundy B, Wenzel L, et al. Intraperitoneal cisplatin and paclitaxel in ovarian cancer. N Engl J Med. 2006;354(1):34–43.
29. McGuire WP, Markman M. Primary ovarian cancer chemotherapy: current standards of care. Br J Cancer. 2003;89 Suppl 3:S3–8.
30. Seamon LG, Richardson DL, Copeland LJ. Evolution of the Gynecologic Oncology Group protocols in the treatment of epithelial ovarian cancer. Clin Obstet Gynecol. 2012;55(1):131–55.
31. Williams S, Blessing JA, Liao SY, Ball H, Hanjani P. Adjuvant therapy of ovarian germ cell tumors with cisplatin, etoposide, and bleomycin: a trial of the Gynecologic Oncology Group. J Clin Oncol. 1994;12(4):701–6.
32. Ginsburg DS, Stern JL, Hamod KA, Genadry R, Spence MR. Tubo-ovarian abscess: a retrospective review. Am J Obstet Gynecol. 1980;138(7 Pt 2):1055–8.
33. Lareau SM, Beigi RH. Pelvic inflammatory disease and tubo-ovarian abscess. Infect Dis Clin North Am. 2008;22(4):693–708. vii.

Index

Q.D. Chu et al. (eds.), *Surgical Oncology: A Practical and Comprehensive Approach*,
DOI 10.1007/978-1-4939-1423-4, © Springer Science+Business Media New York 2015

H

M

N